If you need to (take a break/rest
(right/left) hand.
Si usted necesita (tomar un des
por favor levante su mano (dere

How many times a day do you
¿Cuántas veces al día usted se

Do you floss your teeth every day?
¿Usted limpia sus dientes con hilo dental todos los días?

(Open/close) your mouth.
(Abra/Cierre) su boca.

(Rest/tilt/lift) your head.
(Descanse/Incline/Levante) su cabeza.

Tilt your chin down.
Incline su cabeza hacia abajo.

Rinse your mouth. Swish the water around in your mouth.
Enjuague su boca. Agite el agua en su boca.

When did you last have radiographs taken?
¿Cuándo fue la última vez que le tomaron radiografías?

We will (anesthetize/numb) the tooth before starting.
(Anestesiaremos/Adormeceremos) el diente antes de comenzar.

We have determined that you have periodontal disease, and we need to treat it now.
Hemos determinado que usted tiene enfermedad periodontal y necesitaremos tratarla ahora.

You have an abscess of this tooth.
Usted tiene un absceso de este diente.

You have an infection in this tooth.
Usted tiene una infección en este diente.

You need to have a root canal.
Usted necesita tener un canal radicular.

Would you like to improve your (smile/bite)?
¿Le gustaría mejorar su (sonrisa/mordedura)?

Would you like to (whiten/bleach) your teeth?
¿Le gustaría blanquear sus dientes?

(You/Your child) will need to have (braces/teeth straightened).
(Usted/Su niño(a)) necesitará tener (frenillos/los dientes enderezados).

Do you like your denture's appearance?
¿Le gusta la apariencia de su dentadura?

A crown is a (protective covering/cap) that will fit over your tooth.
Una corona es un revestimiento protector que encajará sobre su diente.

From *Spanish Terminology for the Dental Team*, Mosby, St. Louis, 2004.

Mosby's DENTAL DICTIONARY

Second Edition

With **305** *illustrations*

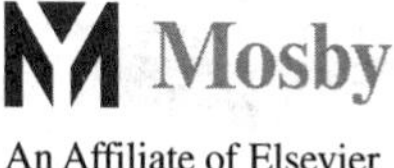

An Affiliate of Elsevier

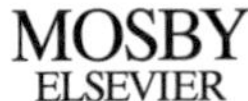

11830 Westline Industrial Drive
St. Louis, Missouri 63146

MOSBY'S DENTAL DICTIONARY, SECOND EDITION

ISBN: 978-0-323-04963-4

NOTICE

Knowledge and best practice in this field are constantly changing. As new research and experience broaden our knowledge, changes in practice, treatment and drug therapy may become necessary or appropriate. Readers are advised to check the most current information provided (i) on procedures featured or (ii) by the manufacturer of each product to be administered, to verify the recommended dose or formula, the method and duration of administration, and contraindications. It is the responsibility of the practitioner, relying on their own experience and knowledge of the patient, to make diagnoses, to determine dosages and the best treatment for each individual patient, and to take all appropriate safety precautions. To the fullest extent of the law, neither the Publisher nor the Editor assumes any liability for any injury and/or damage to persons or property arising out of or related to any use of the material contained in this book.

The Publisher

Library of Congress Control Number 2007933380

Vice President and Publisher: Linda Duncan
Senior Editor: John Dolan
Developmental Editor: Courtney Sprehe
Publishing Services Manager: Melissa Lastarria
Cover Design Direction: Paula Catalano
Text Designer: Paula Catalano

Printed in the United States of America

Last digit is the print number: 9 8 7 6 5 4 3 2

Editorial Consultants

Charles A. Babbush, DDS, MScD
Director, The Dental Implant Center;
Clinical Professor, Oral and Maxillofacial Surgery
Case Western Reserve University School of Dentistry;
Director, Dental Implant Research
Case Western Reserve University School of Dentistry
Cleveland, Ohio

Margaret J. Fehrenbach, RDH, MS
Oral Biologist and Dental Hygienist
Adjunct Faculty, Marquette University, Milwaukee, Wisconsin;
Educational Consultant and Private Practice
Seattle, Washington

Mary Emmons, CDH, Med
Co-Director of Dental Hygiene Program
School of Dental Hygiene, Parkland College
Champaign, Illinois

David W. Nunez, DDS, MS
Oral and Maxillofacial Pathologist
Chief of Dental Services
Vance Air Force Base
Enid, Oklahoma

Key staff members of Publication Services, Inc., worked cooperatively to expand the concentration subject areas in the realm of dental hygiene and dental assisting:
Project Manager: Ted Young
Editor: Scott Stocking
Associate Editor: Carol McGillivray
Pronunciation Editor: Jerome Colburn
Database Design: Richard Bronson
Audio CD Producers: Dominic Menichetti and Phil Wall
Elocutionists: Greg Whitlock and Dorothy Evans

Preface

Today's dental professionals face the challenge of competition, specialization, and a more educated patient pool, placing ever-increasing demands on the entire dental team. Innovations, research, new technology, and new products drive the changes in the field, and whether you are a recent graduate or an experienced professional the new edition of *Mosby's Dental Dictionary* is an essential tool to help you meet the responsibilities and expectations of the field.

The second edition of *Mosby's Dental Dictionary* is a contemporary, comprehensive glossary of more than 10,000 terms useful for the entire dental team. Definitions are included for words used in immunology, microbiology, radiography, special needs, dentistry, pediatric dentistry, anesthesiology, and common medicines, as well as terminology from the legal and insurance fields. Audio pronunciations of complex terms ensure accuracy. Synonyms are included where applicable to help users comprehend related terms.

Dental professionals need to continue to educate themselves and their patients. If you work as a dental professional you know that the dental team is moving beyond initial care and cleaning, requiring expertise in a broader range of subject matters. *Mosby's Dental Dictionary* will provide you with a comprehensive, chair-side resource that you will use on a daily basis.

NEW TO THIS EDITION

In the new edition of *Mosby's Dental Dictionary* you will find:

- Thoroughly revised and updated content that has been carefully scrutinized to eliminate any obsolete terms, update current definitions, and add additional terms.
- More than 800 new terms. These terms cover all areas of dentistry, but special attention has been given to oral surgery, anatomy, and pathology.
- A thoroughly revised art program that includes more implant and pathology photos.
- Updated appendices that include new information on:
    - CDT-2007/2008—the coding system from American Dental Association (ADA)
    - Chemical Agents for Surface Disinfection
    - The ADA's Guidelines for Prescribing Dental Radiographs
    - Implant Prosthetics

FORMAT

Mosby's Dental Dictionary has been designed to be a convenient chair-side or computer-side reference. The colored thumb bleeds aid in locating definitions quickly while its pocket-size and durable cover make it the perfect portable resource. More than 300 photographs and line drawings help bring the terms to life before your eyes, including a number of unique conditions, new to this edition, that can be encountered throughout your dental career. Extensive appendices provide quick, easy-to-use resources for vital information.

ABOUT THE CD-ROM

Included in the back is an accompanying mini CD-ROM. This easy-to-use CD format contains the entire dictionary text in a searchable format, as well as an audio feature that allows users to hear the correct pronunciation of the most complex terms (approximately 50% of all terms, 20% more than the first edition!). Words that include a bold pronunciation indicate which terms can be heard on the mini CD-ROM. Also included are thumbnails of all illustrations, which can be enlarged for optimal viewing.

This mini CD-ROM will work only when placed into tray-loaded CD-ROM drives. If your computer is set to autorun, just load the CD-ROM into the drive. The CD-ROM will do the rest!

ACKNOWLEDGMENT

The editorial staff of Elsevier wishes to express our gratitude to the Editorial Consultants who took time away from their teaching, research, and private practice to move this project forward in such a positive and compelling direction. The insights and candor of Charles A. Babbush, Margaret J. Fehrenbach, Mary Emmons, and David W. Nunez are much appreciated in the development of this project.

The Publishers

Contents

Pronunciation Guide

VOWEL SOUNDS

Print	Key words
a	h**a**t
ä	f**a**ther
ā	pl**ay**, f**a**te, f**ei**gn
e	fl**e**sh
ē	sh**e**, sw**ee**t
er	**air**, f**err**y
i	s**i**t
ī	**eye,** k**i**nd, m**i**ne
ir	**ear**, w**eir**d
o	pr**o**per
ō	n**o**se, c**oa**l
ô	s**aw**, f**aw**n
oi	c**oi**n, (German) f**eu**er
$\overline{oo}$	m**oo**n, m**o**ve
ŏŏ	p**u**t, b**oo**k
ou	**ou**t
u	c**u**p, l**o**ve
Y	(German) gr**ü**n, F**ü**hrer; (French) t**u**
ur	f**ur**, f**ir**st
ə	**a**go, car**ee**r
œ	(German) sch**ö**n, G**oe**the
N	This symbol does not represent a sound but indicates that the preceding vowel is nasal, as in (French) b**on**.

CONSONANTS

Print	Key words
b	**b**ook
ch	**ch**ew, wa**tch**
d	**d**ay, **d**ea**d**
f	**f**ast, **ph**one, enou**gh**
g	**g**ood
h	**h**appy
j	**j**ump, **g**em
k	**c**oo**k**, **qu**ick
l	**l**ate
m	**m**a**mm**al
n	**n**oo**n**
ng	si**ng**, dri**n**k
ng-g	fi**ng**er
p	**p**ul**p**
r	**r**eady, **r**ely

s	**s**a**ss**y
sh	**sh**ine, **s**ure, lo**ti**on
t	**t**o
th	**th**in (voiceless)
th	**th**an, wi**th** (voiced)
v	**v**al**v**e
w	**w**ork
y	**y**es
z	**z**eal, ha**s**
zh	a**z**ure, vi**si**on
(h)w	**wh**en, **wh**ile
kh	(Scottish) lo**ch**, (German) Ba**ch**
kh	(German) i**ch**
nyə	o**ni**on, (Spanish) se**ñ**or, (French) Boulo**gne**

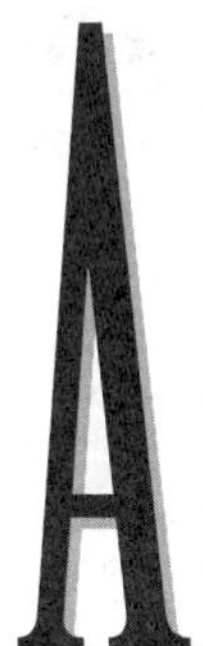

a nativitate (ä′ nətiv′itāt, -tä′tā), *adj* the state of existing at birth or from infancy; denotes a congenital disability.

A point, *n* See point, A.

A-P discrepancy, *n* See anterior-posterior discrepancy.

A:G ratio, *n* See ratio, A:G.

aa, *adv* an abbreviation for the Greek term ana, used in prescription writing, meaning "of each."

A-alpha fibers, *n.pl* See fibers, nerve.

ab (antecedent), *prep* beforehand; a notice given previously or a condition existing earlier.

abacterial (ā′baktir′ē-əl), *adj* nonbacterial; free from bacteria.

abandonment (of a patient), *n* the withdrawing of a patient from treatment without giving reasonable notice or providing a competent replacement.

abatement (əbāt′ment), *n* a decrease in severity of pain or symptoms.

Abbé-Estlander operation (ab′ē-est′landur), *n* See operation, Abbé-Estlander.

abdomen, *n* the portion of the body between the thorax and the pelvis.

abdominal thrust, *n* See Heimlich maneuver.

abduct (abdukt′), *v* to draw away from the median line or from a neighboring part or limb.

abduction (abduk′shən), *n* the process of abducting; opposite of adduction.

aberrant (aber′ənt), *adj* deviating from the usual or normal course, location, or action.

A-beta fibers, See fibers, nerve.

abfraction (abfrak′shən), *n* a mechanism that explains the loss of dentin tissue and tooth enamel caused by flexure and ultimate material fatigue of susceptible teeth at locations away from the point of loading. The breakdown is dependent on the magnitude, duration, frequency, and location of the forces.

abfraction area (abfrak′shən), *n* the part of the tooth, most commonly the cervical area, that is affected by the loss of dentin and enamel due to flexure and material fatigue.

ablation (ablā′shən), *n* an amputation or excision of any part of the body, or a removal of a growth or harmful substance.

abnormal, *adj* departing from the norm, however defined; departing from the mean of a distribution (statistics); departing from the usual, from a state of integration or adjustment.

abnormal tooth mobility, *n* excessive movement of a tooth within its socket as a result of changes in the supporting tissues caused by injury or disease.

abrade (əbrād), *v* to wear away by friction.

abrasion (əbrā′zhən), *n* **1.** the abnormal wearing away of a substance or tissue by a mechanical process. *n* **2.** the pathologic wearing away of tooth structure by an external mechanical source, most commonly incorrect toothbrushing methods.

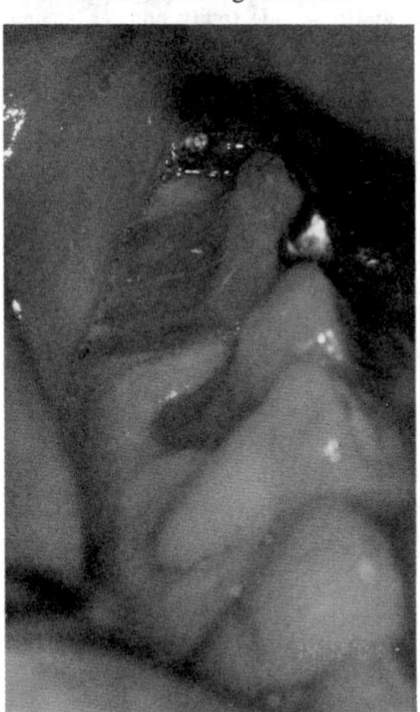

Abrasion. (Courtesy Dr. Charles Babbush)

abrasion, dentifrice, *n* the wearing away of the cementum and dentin of an exposed root by an abrasive-containing dentifrice.

abrasion resistance, *n* See resistance, abrasion.

A

abrasive (əbrā′siv), *n* a substance used for grinding or polishing that will wear away a material or tissue.
abrasive disk, n See disk, abrasive.
abrasive, finishing, n the application of abrasive materials in order to eliminate surface imperfections.
abrasive point, rotary, n See point, abrasive, rotary.
abrasive polishing agent, n a paste containing sharp-edged particles that are moved over the surface of a material with varying pressure and speed. The movement abrades the surface with microscopic scratches, which creates a polished finish. See also dentifrice and polishing.
abrasive strip, n See strip, abrasive.
abrasive system, n the materials used for polishing and cleansing. Common materials include calcium carbonate (calcite, chalk, whiting), diamond particles (for porcelain), some aluminum derivatives (not for enamel), rouge (jeweler's rouge; applied to gold and precious metal alloys), and tin oxide (putty powder, stannic oxide).

abscess (ab′ses), *n* a localized accumulation of suppuration in a confined space formed by tissue disintegration.

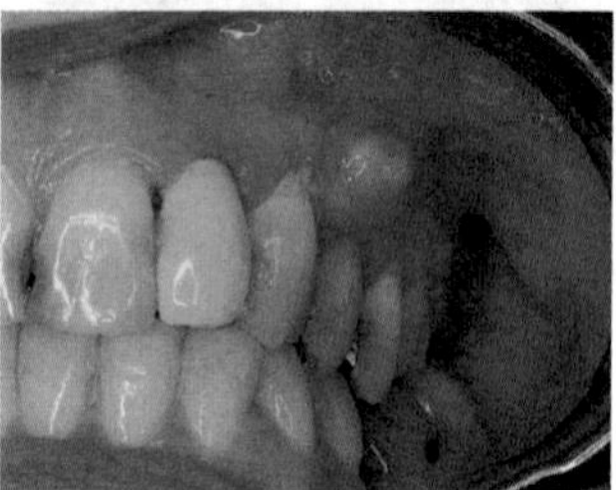

Abscess. (Regezi/Sciubba/Jordan, 2008)

abscess, alveolar, n See periapical abscess.
abscess, apical, n See periapical abscess.
abscess, dentoalveolar, n See periapical abscess.
abscess, gingival, n a superficial periodontal abscess occurring within the free gingival sulcus surrounding the tooth, frequently caused by the impaction of food.
abscess, lateral, n See periodontal abscess.
abscess, periapical **(per′ēā′pikəl),** *n* an abscess involving the apical region of the root, alveolus, and surrounding bone as a result of pulpal disease.
abscess, pericoronal, n See pericoronitis.
abscess, periodontal, n an abscess involving the attachment tissues and alveolar bone as a result of periodontal disease.
abscess, periradicular **(per′ērədik′-yələr),** *n* an abscess involving the periradicular region of the root, alveolus, and surrounding bone as a result of pulpal disease.
abscess, pulpal, n an abscess occurring within pulpal tissue.
abscess, staphylococcal **(staf′-əlōkok′əl),** *n* an abscess caused by the bacteria *S. aureus,* an infectious agent that can be transmitted via saliva and other discharges of the body. The incubation period is 4 to 10 days; the duration of the abscess varies and is indefinite. The bacteria are communicable throughout the drainage period of the lesions and while the carrier state continues.

absorb (əbzôrb′), *v* **1.** to suck up or be removed. *v* **2.** to incorporate or assimilate a liquid or gas into tissue or cells.

absorbable gelatin sponge, *n brand name:* Gelfoam; *drug class:* hemostatic; *action:* absorbs blood and provides area for clot formation; *uses:* hemostasis during and following surgery.

absorbefacient (abzôr′bifā′shənt), *adj/n* causing absorption, or an agent that promotes absorption.

absorbent (abzôrb′ənt), *adj* a substance that causes absorption of diseased tissue; taking up by suction.

absorptiometry, dual energy radiograph, *n* the standard technique that uses two radiographic beams to diagnose osteoporosis and to assess the efficacy of treatment.

absorption (abzôrp′shən), *n* **1.** the passage of a substance into the interior of another by solution or penetration. *n* **2.** the taking up of fluids or other substances by the skin, mucous surfaces, absorbent vessels, or dental materials so that they are removed. *n* **3.** the process by which radiation imparts some or all of its energy to any material through which it passes.

absorption coefficient, *n* the ratio of the linear rate of change of intensity of roentgen rays in a given homogeneous material to the intensity at a given point within the same mass.

absorption, drug, *n* in dentistry, the factors that determine the speed and duration of response to a local anesthetic. The faster the absorption, the higher the chance of systemic toxicity and the lower the duration of effectiveness. The rate is altered by route of administration, use of vasoconstrictors, and patient factors.

abstinence (ab′stənəns), *n* self-restraint, especially from harmful substances or morally questionable behaviors. See also withdrawal.

abstraction (abstrak′shən), *n* teeth or other maxillary and mandibular structures that are inferior to (below) their normal position; away from the occlusal plane.

abuse, *n* the improper use of program benefits, resources, and/or services by either dental professionals, institutions, or patients.

abuse, child, *n* See child abuse.

abuse, drug, *n* the misuse of legal or illegal substances with the intent to alter the user's feelings, behavior, or perception.

abuse, elder, *n* the behavior or treatment toward an elderly person, by another person in a position of care, that has the purpose or effect of harming the elderly person's well-being. Such harm may include economic, physical, sexual, or mental abuse.

abuse, nitrous oxide, *n* the deliberate inhalation of nitrous oxide to produce mood-altering effects. A type of substance abuse.

abuse, polysubstance, *n* the physical dependence on at least three substances that have been classified as habit forming, but without any one of the substances having greater importance or influence than the others. The concept does not include caffeine or nicotine.

abuse, sexual, *n* sexual acts performed with children or with nonconsenting adults in a criminal manner.

abuse, substance, *n* the misuse of legal or illegal substances with the intent to alter some aspect of the user's experience. May include medications, illicit drugs, legal substances with potential mood-altering effects (such as alcohol or tobacco), or substances whose primary use may not be for human consumption (such as inhalants).

abutment (əbut′mənt), *n* a tooth, root, or implant used for support and retention of a fixed or removable prosthesis. See also pontic.

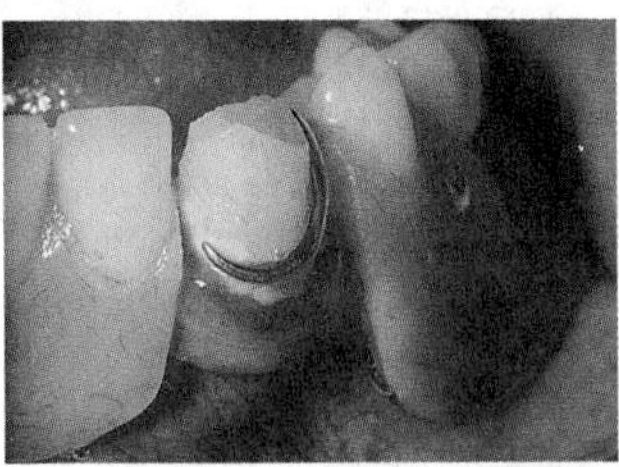

Abutment. (Daniel/Harfst/Wilder, 2008)

abutment, angulated **(ang′gyəlātid),** *n* an abutment whose body is not parallel to the long axis of the implant. It is utilized when the implant is at a different inclination in relation to the proposed prosthesis.

abutment, custom, *n* a custom-made post attached to the superior part of the metal dental implant that protrudes through the gingival tissues and onto which the restoration is fitted; either machined or cast, and used in situations where prefabricated abutments cannot be used.

abutment, healing, *n* a cylinder or screw used during the second stage of dental restoration. This serves two purposes: to allow gingival tissues to heal prior to the placement of the permanent abutment, and to maintain proper spacing in the oral cavity before the final restoration (prosthesis) is placed.

abutment, intermediate, *n* an abutment located between the abutments that form the ends of the prosthesis.

abutment, multiple, *n* abutments splinted together as a unit to support and retain a fixed prosthesis.

abutment, prefabricated, *n* a machine-manufactured post attached to the superior part of a dental implant that protrudes through the gingival tissues and onto which a restoration is fitted.

A

abutment, preparable, *n* a dental implant abutment that can be prepared and changed from the manufacturer's original design.

abutment, screw, *n* a screw that secures an abutment to an implant. It is usually torqued to a final seating position.

abutment, UCLA, *n* a cast component used to create a custom abutment for a prosthesis. Also known as a *castable abutment.*

a.c., *adv* the abbreviation for ante cibum, a Latin phrase meaning "before eating."

Academy of General Dentistry (AGD), *n.pr* a nonprofit, international organization dedicated to serving the needs and representing the general interests of dental professionals.

acanthesthesia (əkan′thesthē′zēə, -zhə), *n* a form of paresthesia experienced as numbness, tingling, or "pins and needles."

acanthion (əkan′thēon), *n* the tip of the anterior nasal spine.

acantholysis (ak′anthol′isis), *n* the loosening, separation, or disassociation of individual prickle cells within the epithelium from their neighbor, often seen in conditions such as pemphigus vulgaris and keratosis follicularis.

acanthosis (ak′ənthō′sis), *n* an increase in the number of cells in the prickle cell layer of stratified squamous epithelium, with thickening of the entire epithelial cell layer and a broadening and fusing of rete pegs.

acapnia (akap′nēə), *n* a condition characterized by diminished carbon dioxide in the blood.

acarbia (akär′bēə), *n* a condition in which the blood bicarbonate level is decreased.

acarbose, *n brand name:* Precose, Prandase; *drug class:* oligosaccharide, glucosidase enzyme inhibitor; *action:* inhibits α-glucosidase enzyme in the GI tract to slow the breakdown of carbohydrates to glucose; *uses:* a single drug or in combination with others when diet control is ineffective in controlling blood glucose levels such as with type 2 diabetes mellitus.

acatalasemia (a′katələsē′mēə), *n* a congenital lack of the enzyme catalase in blood and other tissues that leads to a progressive necrosis of the oral tissues (Takahara's disease).

accelerator (aksel′ərātur), *n* **1.** a substance that increases rapidity of action or function. *n* **2.** a catalyst or other substance that hastens a chemical reaction (e.g., NaCl added to water and plaster to hasten the set). *n* **3.** a film-developing solution of potassium hydroxide or sodium carbonate used to enlarge the emulsion and to establish an alkaline medium.

accelerator, platelet thrombin, *n* See factor, platelet 2.

accelerator, prothrombin conversion, I **(prōthrom′bin kənvur′zhən),** *n* (factor V, labile factor, plasma accelerator globulin, proaccelerin, serum accelerator globulin), a substance that is considered by some to be a factor in serum and plasma that catalyzes the conversion of inactive prothrombin to an active form.

accelerator, prothrombin conversion, II, *n* (extrinsic thromboplastin, factor VII, serum prothrombin conversion accelerator [SPCA], stable factor), a substance that is considered by some to be one of the factors in the blood that accelerates the conversion of active prothrombin to thrombin by thromboplastin. Vitamin K deficiency reduces the activity of this factor.

accelerator, serum, *n* See factor V.

accelerin (aksel′ərin), *n* See factor V.

acceptability, *n* an overall assessment of the dental care available to a person or group; includes accessibility, cost, quality, results, convenience, and attitudes of dental professionals and patients.

acceptance, *n* the act of a person to whom something is offered or tendered by another, whereby he receives that which is offered with the intention of retaining it. A contract is not valid without the acceptance of an offer by the party to whom the offer is made, either expressly or by conduct.

acceptance, absolute, *n* an express and positive agreement to pay a bill according to its text.

acceptance, conditional, *n* an agreement to pay a bill on the fulfillment of a condition.

acceptance, implied, *n* an acceptance interpreted by law from the acts or conduct of the patient.

access (ak′ses), *n* **1.** the means of approach. *n* **2.** a surgical preparation of hard or soft tissue to allow entrance to a treatment site and adequate space for visualization and instrumentation of the field.

access, cavity, *n* a coronal opening required for effective cleaning, shaping, and filling of the pulp space.

access, computer, *n* **1.** the process of transferring information into or out of a storage location. *n* **2.** the time required to begin and complete the read and write functions of a specified piece of data.

access flap, *n* a periodontal surgical technique that provides visualization of the root in conjunction with curettage and root planing. Types of access flaps include supracrestal, subcrestal-full thickness, and partial thickness flaps. See also flaps, periodontal.

access, form, *n* the surgical removal of tooth structure sufficient for visualization and instrumentation of a restorative preparation.

accessibility standards (akses′-abil′itē), *n.pl* the requirements designed by the Americans with Disabilities Act (ADA), by which public places must provide disabled individuals with barrier-free access to buildings, forms of communication, and modes of transportation such as dental offices and clinics.

accessory, *adj* providing complementary or supplementary assistance.

accessory canal (akses′ərē), *n* See canal, accessory root.

accident, *n* **1.** an unusual, unforeseen event. *n* **2.** an unusual or unexpected result attending the performance of a usual or necessary act or event. *n* **3.** occurring without intent or happening by chance. The term does not have a precise legal definition but is generally used to indicate that an occurrence was not the result of negligence.

accident, cerebrovascular (CVA) **(ser′əbrōvas′kyələr),** (stroke) *n* apoplexy resulting from hemorrhage into the brain or occlusion of the cerebral vessels from an embolism or thrombosis. It can result in paralysis (mainly one side), speech difficulties, and difficulty in maintaining personal hygiene, including oral care.

accident, unavoidable, *n* an accident not occasioned, either remotely or directly, by the want of such care or skill as the law holds every person bound to exercise; occurring without fault or negligence.

accident prevention, *n* a set of precautionary measures taken to avoid possible bodily harm. Devices that can be especially important in preventing damage to the orofacial area are seat belts and bicycle helmets; the use of these should be encouraged in all patients.

accidental exposure management, *n* a set of regulations followed in case of inadvertent exposure to hazardous materials.

account, *n* a basic storage unit in an accounting system. Individual accounts accept debit and credit entries that reflect the different types of transactions made by the practice.

account book, *n* a book in which the financial transactions of a business or profession are entered. Such books may be admitted as evidence.

account, open, *n* a straightforward arrangement between the dental provider and the patient for the handling of financial payments due the dental provider and owed by the patient.

account, payable, *n* a dollar amount owed to creditors for items or services purchased from them.

accountability, *n* an obligation to periodically disclose appropriate information in adequate detail and consistent form to all contractually involved parties.

accreditation, *n* a process of formal recognition of a school or institution attesting to the required ability and performance in an area of education, training, or practice. In dentistry, this process is controlled by the Commission on Dental Accreditation (CODA).

accretions (əkrē′shənz), *n.pl* an older term for accumulations of foreign material such as plaque, materia alba, calculus, and other debris on teeth. Now called deposits.

accrual, *n* continually recurring short-term liabilities. Examples are accrued wages, taxes, and interest.

A

accrued needs, *n.pl* the amount of treatment needed by an individual or a group at any given time. In dental plans, usually refers to conditions present at the time of enrollment. Synonym: accumulated needs.

acebutolol HCl (as′əbyōō′təlôl), *n brand names:* Monitan, Sectral; *drug class:* antihypertensive, selective β_1 blocker; *action:* produces fall in blood pressure without reflex tachycardia or significant reduction in heart rate; *uses:* mild-to-moderate hypertension and ventricular dysrhythmias.

acellular, *adj* not composed of or having cells.

acenesthesia (əsen′esthē′zēə, -zhə), *n* the loss, or lack, of the normal perception of one's own body; absence of the feelings of a physical existence, a symptom that is common with many psychiatric disorders.

acentric relation (āsen′trik), *n* See relation, jaw, eccentric.

acesulfame-K, *n* a synthetic non-nutritive sweetener.

acetabulum (as′ətab′yələm), *n* a cup-shaped attachment site located laterally on the hip bone for the head of the femur.

acetaminophen (əsē′təmin′əfin), *n brand names:* Tylenol, Anacin-3; *drug class:* nonnarcotic analgesic; *action:* thought to block initiation of pain impulses by inhibition of prostaglandin synthesis; *uses:* mild-to-moderate pain, fever; also used in combination with narcotic analgesics. See also Percocet.

acetate (as′ətāt), *n* **1.** a salt of acetic acid. *n* **2.** a short form for cellulose acetate, the film base for radiographs.

acetazolamide/acetazolamide sodium (əsē′təzō′ləmīd sō′dēəm), *n brand names:* Dazamide, Acetazolam, Apo-Acetazolamide; *drug class:* diuretic; carbonic anhydrase inhibitor; *action:* inhibits carbonic anhydrase activity in proximal renal tubular cells to decrease reabsorption of water, sodium, potassium, bicarbonate; *uses:* open-angle glaucoma, epilepsy, drug-induced edema.

acetic acid, *n* a clear, colorless, pungent liquid that is miscible with water, alcohol, glycerin, and ether and that constitutes 3% to 5% of vinegar.

acetohexamide, *n brand names:* Dimelor, Dymelor; *drug class:* sulfonylurea; antidiabetic; *action:* causes functioning β cells in the pancreas to release insulin, leading to a drop in blood glucose level; *uses:* stable type 2 diabetes mellitus.

acetone (as′ətōn), *n* Dimethylketone; **1.** an organic solvent. **2.** in the body, a chemical that is formed when the body uses fat instead of glucose for energy. The formation of acetone means that cells lack insulin or cannot effectively use available insulin to burn glucose for energy. It passes through the body into the urine as ketone bodies. **3.** the simplest ketone. It is normally present in urine in small amounts but can increase in those who have diabetes mellitus. Results in having "fruity" acetone breath.

acetone abuse, *n* a deliberate inhalation of acetone to produce mood-altering effects. See also huffing.

acetone breath, *n* a characteristic "fruity" or acetone breath odor that occurs with a life-threatening condition of diabetic ketoacidosis. See diabetic ketoacidosis and acetone.

acetyl groups, *n.pl* the carbon- and hydrogen-containing groups required for synthesis of lipids.

acetylcholine (as′ətilkō′lēn, əsē′til), *n* **1.** an acetate ester of choline that serves as a neurohumoral agent in the transmission of an impulse in autonomic ganglia, parasympathetic postganglionic fibers, and somatic motor fibers. *n* **2.** an ester of choline actively involved as a chemical mediator at the neuromuscular junction, at autonomic ganglia, and between parasympathetic nerve endings and visceral effectors.

acetylcysteine (əsē′tlsis′tēn), *n brand name:* Mucosil; *drug class:* mucolytic; *action:* decreases viscosity of pulmonary secretions by breaking disulfide links of mucoproteins; *uses:* acetaminophen toxicity, bronchitis, pneumonia, cystic fibrosis, emphysema, atelectasis tuberculosis, and complications of thoracic surgery.

achlorhydria (ā′klôrhī′drēə), *n* the absence of free hydrochloric acid in the stomach, even with histamine stimulation.

achondroplasia (ākon′drōplā′zēə, -zhə), *n* a hereditary disturbance of endochondral bone formation transmitted as a mendelian dominant factor and resulting in dwarfism. Malocclusion and prognathism may occur.

achromatopsia (əkrōmətōp′sēə), *n* the condition of total color blindness.

Achromycin V, *n.pr* a brand name for the antibiotic tetracycline hydrochloride.

achylia (ākē′lēə), *n* the absence or lack of hydrochloric acid and the enzyme pepsinogen in the stomach.

acid (as′id), *n* a chemical substance that, in an aqueous solution, undergoes dissociation with the formation of hydrogen ions; pH levels range from 0 to 6.9. See also pH and acidic. Opposite: base.

acid, acetic, *n* the acid of vinegar, sometimes used as a solvent for the removal of calculus from a removable dental prosthesis. See also solvent.

acid, ascorbic, *n* See vitamin C.

acid, carbolic, *n* See phenol.

acid, cevitamic, *n* See vitamin C.

acid conditioning, *n* the use of acid (such as phosphoric acid) to prepare the tooth surface for bonding of dental adhesives or enamel sealants.

acid etchant, *n* an application of phosphoric acid used to prepare enamel surfaces to aid enamel sealant placement.

acid etching, *n* the process of treating the tooth enamel, generally with phosphoric acid, by removal of approximately 40 mm of enamel rod to provide retention for enamel sealant, restorative material, or orthodontic bracket.

acid, folic, *n* See vitamin B complex.

acid, hydroxypropionic **(hī′drōok′-sēprōpēon′ik),** *n* See acid, lactic.

acid, lactic (hydroxypropionic acid), *n* a monobasic acid, $C_3H_6O_3$, formed as an end product in the intermediary metabolism of carbohydrates. The accumulation of lactic acid in the tissues is in part responsible for the lowering of pH levels during inflammatory states; that is, the drop in pH level is believed to increase bone loss level.

acid, nicotinic, *n* **1.** a vitamin of the B complex group and its vitamer, niacinamide, specific for the treatment of pellagra. Niacinamide functions as a constituent of coenzyme I (DPN) and coenzyme II (TPN). Nicotinic acid is found in lean meats, liver, yeast, milk, and leafy green vegetables. *n* **2.** an acid (C_5H_4N [COOH]) that forms part of the B complex group of vitamins. It acts as a cofactor in intermediary carbohydrate metabolism. It is a constituent of certain coenzymes that function in oxidative-reductive metabolic systems. With niacinamide, it is a pellagra-preventive factor. Also called *niacin, P.-P. factor, pyridine 3-carboxylic acid, vitamin P.-P.*

acid, orthophosphoric **(ôr′thōfos-fôr′ik),** *n* See acid, phosphoric.

acid, pantothenic **(pan′tōthen′ik),** *n* a vitamin of the B complex group, the importance of which has not been established. It is a constituent of coenzyme A.

acid phosphatase, *n* an enzyme found in the kidneys, serum, semen, and prostate gland. It is elevated in serum blood levels in individuals with prostate cancer and in individuals who have recently experienced trauma.

acid, phosphoric (**H_3PO_4**, orthophosphoric acid), *n* the principal ingredient of silicate and zinc phosphate cement liquids.

acid, pteroylglutamic, *n* See vitamin B complex.

acid salt, *n* a salt containing one or more replaceable hydrogen ions.

acid, strong, *n* an acid that is completely ionized in aqueous solution.

acid-base balance, *n* the balance of acid to base necessary to keep the blood pH level normal (between 7.35 and 7.43).

acidemia (as′idē′mēə), *n* a decreased pH level of the blood, irrespective of changes in the blood bicarbonate.

acidemia, isovaleric, *n* a genetic disorder of amino acid metabolism in which isovaleric acid accumulates in the blood and urine at abnormally high levels; may respond to a low-protein diet and the administration of synthetic amino acids. See also homocystinuria.

acidic, *adj* having the properties of an acid; acid-forming properties.

acidifier (əsid′ifī′ur), *n* a chemical ingredient (acetic acid) that maintains the required acidity of the fixer and stop-bath solutions in the photographic development process.

acidogenic, *adj* generating acid or acidity. See also acid and acidic.

acidophilic (as′idōfil′ik), *adj* **1.** readily stained with acid dyes. *adj* **2.** growing well in an acid medium.

acidosis (as′idō′sis), *n* a pathologic disturbance of the acid-base balance of the body characterized by an excess of acid or inadequate base. Causes include acid ingestion, increased acid production such as that seen in diabetes mellitus or starvation, or loss of base through the kidneys or intestine.

acidosis, compensated, *n* a condition of acidosis in which the body pH level is maintained within the normal range through compensatory mechanisms involving the kidneys or lungs.

acidosis, respiratory, *n* an acidemia resulting from retention of an excess of CO_2 caused by hypoventilation.

acidosis, uncompensated, *n* an acidosis in which compensatory mechanisms are unable to maintain the body pH level within the normal range.

acidulated phosphate fluoride, *n* a topical agent with a low pH that is used in the prevention of dental caries.

Acinetobacter **(əsin′ətōbak′tər),** *n* a genus of nonmotile, aerobic bacteria of the family *Neisseriaceae* that often occurs in clinical specimens.

acinus (*pl.* acini) (as′inəs), *n* **1.** a saclike cavity present in a gland or the lungs. **2.** a group of secretory cells of the salivary gland.

acinus, serous **(as′inəs sēr′əs),** *n* a group of serous cells producing serous secretory product such as in the salivary glands.

Ackerman-Proffit orthogonal analysis, *n.pr* a taxonomy of malocclusion based on set theory or Boolean algebra, which is organized using combinations and permutations of malocclusions within the three planes of space. See also Appendix F.

acne, *n* an inflammatory, papulopustular skin eruption occurring most often in or near the sebaceous glands on the face, neck, shoulders, and upper back.

acne rosacea, *n* a condition of the facial skin typically indicated by blushing, swelling, and the appearance of broken blood vessels in a "spider web" pattern that may lead to severe scarring of the skin surface. Etiology is not fully understood.

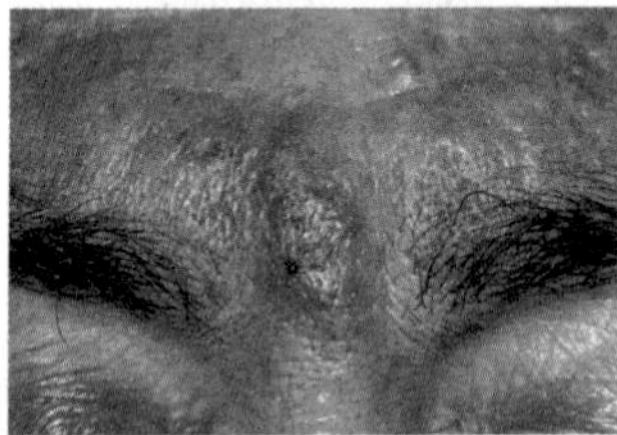

Acne rosacea. (Regezi/Sciubba/Jordan, 2008)

acne vulgaris, *n* a common form of acne seen predominantly in adolescents and young adults. Probably an effect of the rise of androgenic hormones.

acoustic turbulence, *n* agitation observed in fluids by mechanical vibrations of an ultrasonic tip; used to disrupt bacterial cell walls.

acquired centric relation (sen′trik), *n* See relation, centric, and relation, jaw, eccentric.

acquired immunodeficiency syndrome (AIDS), *n* a disease caused by a retrovirus known as human immunodeficiency virus type 1 (HIV-1). A related but distinct retrovirus (HIV-2) has recently appeared in a limited number of patients in the United States. Patients are considered to have AIDS when one or more indicator diseases, as defined by the Centers for Disease Control and Prevention (CDC), are present. See also human immunodeficiency virus (HIV). The CDC has classified stages of the disease as follows:

Group I: acute HIV infection, *n* a group who within one month of exposure develops the first clinical evidence of HIV infection, which may appear as an acute retroviral syndrome. This is a mononucleosis-like syndrome with symptoms including fever, rash, diarrhea, lymphadenopathy, myalgia, arthralgia, and fatigue. Development of antibodies usually follows.

Group II: asymptomatic HIV infection, *n* a group in which most persons develop antibodies to the HIV within 6 to 12 weeks after exposure. Although individuals may remain asymptomatic for months or years, they can transmit the virus.

Group III: persistent generalized lymphadenopathy (PGL), *n* a group who develops persistent generalized lymphadenopathy that lasts longer than 3 months. See also lymphadenopathy, persistent generalized.

Group IV: HIV-associated diseases, *n* a group who is clinically variable and has signs and symptoms of HIV infection other than or in addition to lymphadenopathy. Based on clinical findings, patients in Group IV may be assigned to one or more of the following subgroups: (A) constitutional disease, also known as wasting syndrome. This subgroup is characterized by fever that lasts more than one month, involuntary weight loss of greater than 10% for baseline, or diarrhea persisting for more than one month, (B) neurological disease, (C) secondary infectious disease, (D) secondary cancers, and (E) other conditions resulting from HIV infections.

acridine (orange) (ak′ridēn), *n* a dibenzopyridine compound used in the synthesis of dyes and drugs. In dentistry, has been used to research dental deposits.

acroanesthesia (ak′rōan′esthē′zēə, -zhə), *n* anesthesia of the extremities.

acrocephalia (ak′rōsefal′ēə), *n* a deformity of the head characterized by a superior and anterior bulge of the frontal bones and a flat occiput. Synonym: oxycephalia.

acrodermatitis (ak′rōder′mətī′-tis), *n* an eruption of the skin of the hands and feet caused by a parasitic mite, which is a member of the order Acarina.

acrodynia (ak′rōdī′nēə), *n* (erythredema polyneuropathy, Feer's syndrome, pink disease, Swift's syndrome, Selter's disease), a disease that occurs in infants and young children in which manifestations occur with the eruption of the primary teeth. Symptoms include raw-beef hands and feet, superficial sensory loss, photophobia, tachycardia, muscular hypotonia, changes in temperament, stomatitis, periodontitis, and premature loss of teeth. The etiology has been related to mercury and deficiency of vitamin B6 and essential fatty acids. See also erythredema polyneuropathy.

acroesthesia (ak′rōesthē′zēə, -zhə), *n* **1.** increased sensitivity. *n* **2.** pain in the extremities.

acromegaly (akrəmeg′əlē), *n* (Marie's disease), a condition caused by hyperfunction of the pituitary gland in adults. Characterized by enlargement of the skeletal extremities, including the feet, hands, mandible, and nose.

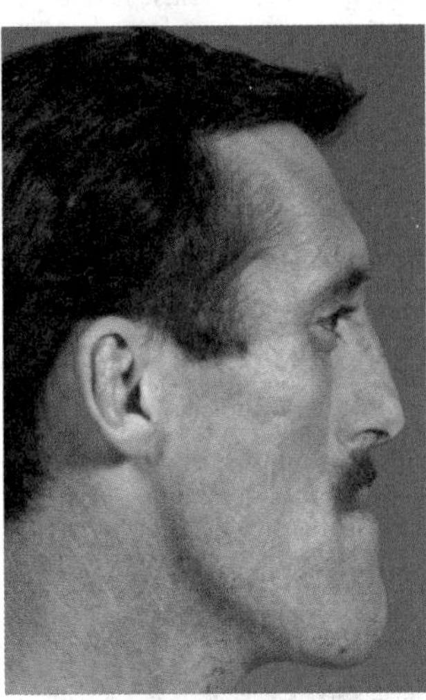

Acromegaly. (Proffit/White/Sarver, 2007)

acrosclerosis (ak′rōsklerō′sis), *n* a special form of scleroderma that affects the extremities, head, and face and is associated with Raynaud's phenomenon. There may be significant thickening of the periodontal ligament.

acrylic (/əkril′ik), *adj* formed from acrylic acid; e.g., acrylic resin, acrylic resin denture, and acrylic resin tooth. See also denture, acrylic resin; and tooth, acrylic resin.

acrylic resin, *n* See resin, acrylic.

ACTH (adrenocorticotropic hormone) (ədrē′nōkor′tikōtrō′pik hor′mōn), *n* a hormone produced by basophilic cells of the anterior lobe of the pituitary gland that exerts a reciprocal regulating influence on the production of corticosteroids by the adrenal cortex.

actinic cheilitis (aktin′ik), *n* See cheilitis, actinic.

***Actinobacillus,* (ak′tənōbəsil′is)** *n* a genus of nonmobile, gram-negative aerobic and facultatively anaerobic bacteria of the family Brucellaceae.

***Actinomyces* (ak′tənōmī′sēz),** *n.pl* filamentous microorganisms that have been implicated in the formation of dental calculus and serve as a mode of attachment of dental calculus to the tooth surface. These microorganisms have also been found in pathologic lesions of the alveolar processes (actinomycosis).

***A. israelii* (ak′tənōmī′sēz izrā′lē),** *n.pl* a normally occurring oral bacteria that aggressively causes infection (actinomycosis) when oral health is compromised.

***A. naeslundii* (ak′tənōmī′sēz nāz-lun′dē),** *n* a specific strain of bacteria resident in open sores in the oral cavity.

A. viscosus, *n* a species of *Actinomyces* occurring in high numbers in the dental plaque, cemental caries, and tonsillar crypts.

actinomycosis (ak′tinōmīkō′sis), *n* (lumpy jaw), an infection of humans and some animal species caused by species of *Actinomyces,* which are gram-positive, filamentous, microaerophilic microorganisms.

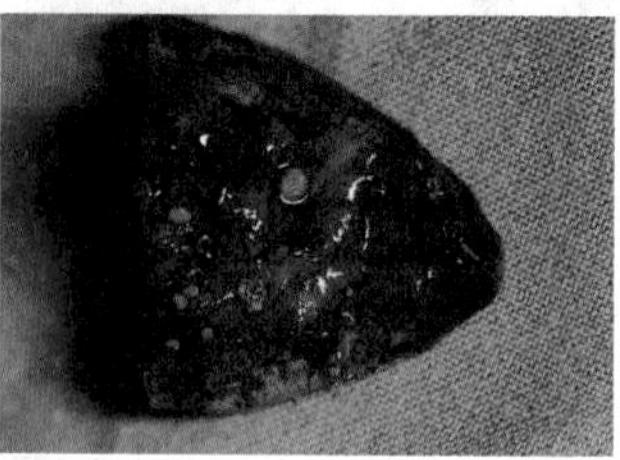

Actinomycosis. (Regezi/Sciubba/Pogrel, 2000)

action, *n* the coordinated movement of a group of muscles, relative to the resting position of the body.

action potential, *n* **1.** an electric impulse consisting of a self-propagating series of polarizations and depolarizations, transmitted across the cell membranes of a nerve fiber during the transmission of a nerve impulse and across the cell membranes of a muscle cell during contraction. *n* **2.** the electrical potential developed in a muscle or nerve during activity.

activate (ak′tivāt), *v* in orthodontics, to adjust an appliance so that it will exert effective force on the teeth and jaws.

activated resin, *n* See resin, autopolymer.

activator (ak′tivātur), *n* **1.** an alkali, sodium carbonate, which is a component of photographic developing solution that softens and swells the gelatin of the film emulsion and provides the necessary alkaline medium for the developing agents to react with the sensitized silver halide crystals. *n* **2.** in orthodontics, a removable orthodontic appliance intended to function as a passive transmitter and sometimes stimulator of the forces of the perioral muscles. One in the myofunctional category of appliances also known by such names as *Andresen, Bimler, Monobloc,* and *Frankel.*

active, *adj* in orthodontics, pertaining to the condition of an orthodontic appliance that has been adjusted to apply effective force to the teeth or jaws.

active reciprocation, *n* See reciprocation, active.

acts, practice, *n.pl* the statutory requirements of a state for the education, training, examination, credentialing, supervision, and accountability of dental professionals.

acuity (əkyōōitē), *n* sharpness; clearness; keenness.

acuity, auditory, *n* the sensitivity of the auditory apparatus; sharpness of hearing. The ability to hear a given tone with respect to the degree of intensity required to produce a sensation that is just perceptible.

acuity, visual, *n* sharpness, acuteness, clearness of vision. Visual acuity may be defective because of optical or neurologic dysfunction.

A

acupuncture, *n* a method of producing analgesia or altering the function of a system of the body by inserting fine, wire-thin needles into the skin at specific sites along a series of lines or channels called meridians. The needles may be twirled, energized electrically, or warmed.

acute, *adj* pertaining to a traumatic, pathologic, or physiologic phenomenon or process having a short and relatively severe course. Antonym: chronic.

acute phase reactions, *n.pl* the abnormalities in the blood associated with acute and chronic inflammatory and necrotic processes and detected by a variety of tests, including erythrocyte sedimentation rate, C-reactive protein, serum hexosamine, serum mucoprotein, and serum nonglucosamine polysaccharides.

acyanotic (āsī′yənot′ik), *adj* refers to the absence of cyanosis, or deficient oxygenation of blood. Typically used in reference to types of congenital heart defects that do not prevent blood from being properly oxygenated by the lungs.

acyclovir (āsī′klōvir), *n brand name:* Zovirax; *drug class:* antiviral. *Uses:* a 5% ointment; may be used systemically. Drug of choice in simple mucocutaneous herpes simplex, in immunocompromised patients with initial herpes genitalis. Active against herpes viruses such as herpes zoster and varicella (chickenpox).

ADA Seal of Acceptance, *n.pr* the insignia of the American Dental Association's Council on Scientific Affairs, given to products used in all aspects of oral health and maintenance. Designed to help the public and dental professionals make informed decisions about safe and effective dental products.

adamantinoma (adəman′tinō′mə), *n* See ameloblastoma.

adamantoblastoma (adəman′tōblastō′mə), *n* See ameloblastoma.

Adams' clasp, *n* a retention clasp to stabilize removable appliances by engaging the mesiobuccal and distobuccal surfaces of buccal teeth.

adaptation, *n* **1.** an alteration that an organ or organism undergoes to adjust to its environment. **2.** a close approximation of a tissue flap, an appliance, or a restorative material to natural tissue. **3.** an accurate adjustment of a band or a shell to a tooth. **4.** a condition in reflex activity marked by a decline in the frequency of impulses when sensory stimuli are repeated several times.

adaptation, instrument, *n* the process of manually adjusting and positioning the functional end, edge, or surface of a dental instrument for safe and effective use according to its purpose and relative to the shape of the tooth.

adapter, band, *n* an instrument used as an aid in fitting an orthodontic band to a tooth.

adaptive functioning, *n* the relative ability of a person to effectively interact with society on all levels and care for one's self; affected by one's willingness to practice skills and pursue opportunities for improvement on all levels. Often used to describe levels of mental retardation.

addict (ad′ikt), *n* an individual who has developed physiologic or psychologic dependence on a chemical such as alcohol or other drugs.

addiction (ədik′shən), *n* the state of being addicted. Although there is no universally accepted definition, addiction is generally considered a condition involving two factors: (1) a compulsive behavior pattern, and (2) an altered physiologic state that requires continued use of the drug to prevent withdrawal symptoms.

addictive (ədik′tiv), *adj* pertaining to a drug whose repeated use may produce addiction.

Addison's disease, *n.pr* See disease, Addison's.

Addison-Biermer anemia (ad′isən-bir′mur), *n.pr* See anemia, pernicious.

additive, *n* an ingredient added to a food, drug, or other preparation to produce a desired result, such as color or consistency, unrelated to the primary purpose of the preparation.

adduct (ədukt′), *v* to draw toward the center or midline.

adduction (əduk′shən), *n* the process of bringing two objects toward each other; the opposite of abduction.

A-delta fibers, *n.pl* See fiber, nerve.

A

adenine (ad′ənēn), *n* a component of the nucleic acids, DNA and RNA, and a constituent of cyclic AMP and the adenosine portion of AMP, ADP, and ATP.

adenitis (ad′ənī′tis), *n* an inflammation of glandular tissue, often accompanied by pain.

adenocarcinoma (ad′ənōkarsinō′mə), *n* a large group of malignant epithelial cell tumors of the glands. Specific tumors are diagnosed and named by the cell type of the tissue affected.

adenocarcinoma, acinic cell, n a cancer of the salivary glands, primarily the parotid gland.

adenocarcinoma, polymorphous low-grade (PLGA) **(pol′ēmor′fəs),** *n* a cancer of the salivary glands, primarily in the minor salivary glands.

adenoidectomy, *n* the removal of the lymphoid tissue in the nasopharynx, usually in conjunction with the surgical removal of the palatine tonsils.

adenoids (ad′ənoidz′), *adj* See tonsil, pharyngeal.

adenoid facies, n an older term used to describe patients who exhibit a long, narrow face, short upper lip, oral cavity breathing, and a hyperactive swallowing pattern. Newer term is *long face syndrome.*

adenoma (ad′ənō′mə), *n* a benign epithelial neoplasm or tumor with a basic glandular (acinar) structure, suggesting derivation from glandular tissue.

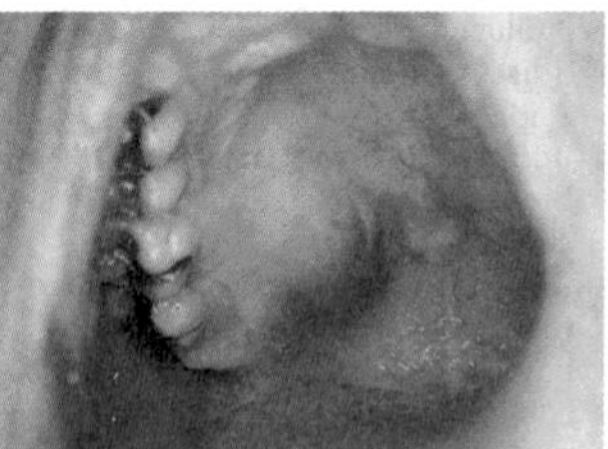

Adenoma. (Regezi/Sciubba/Jordan, 2008)

adenoma, acidophilic, n See oncocytoma.

adenoma, oxyphilic, n See oncocytoma.

adenomatosis oris (ad′ənōmətō′sis), *n* an enlargement of the mucous glands of the lip without secretion or inflammation.

adenopathy (ad′ənop′əthē), *n* an enlargement or increase in size of glandular organs or tissues usually resulting from disease processes.

adenosine (əden′əsēn′), *n* a compound derived from nucleic acid, composed of adenine and a sugar, D-ribose. Major molecular component of nucleotides and the nucleic acids.

adenosine monophosphate (AMP), n an ester, composed of adenine, D-ribose, and phosphoric acid, that affects energy release in work done by a muscle.

adenosine triphosphate (ATP), n a compound consisting of the nucleotide adenosine attached through its ribose group to three phosphoric acid molecules. Stores energy in muscles, which is released when it is hydrolized to adenosine diphosphate.

***Adenoviridae* (ad′ənōvēr′idē),** *n* a family of unenveloped, 20-sided DNA viruses found in mammals (Mastadenovirus) and birds (Aviadenovirus). The human variety can cause a number of diseases, from conjunctivitis to urinary tract infection.

adequacy, velopharyngeal, *n* a functional closure of the velum to the postpharyngeal wall that restricts air and sound from entering the nasopharyngeal and nasal cavities.

adequate intake (AI), *n* the consumption and absorption of sufficient food, vitamins, and essential minerals necessary to maintain health. See also dietary reference intakes; estimated average requirement; recommended dietary allowances; and upper intake levels, tolerable.

ADH, *n* See hormone, antidiuretic.

adhesion (adh′zhən), *n* **1.** the attraction of unlike molecules for one another. **2.** the molecular attraction existing between surfaces in close contact. **3.** the condition in which a material sticks to itself or another material. **4.** the abnormal joining of tissues, generally by fibrous connective tissue, to each other after repair of an injury.

adhesion, bacterial, n a microbial

surface antigen that frequently exists in the form of filamentous projections and binds to specific receptors on epithelial cell membranes.

adhesion, sublabial, n the abnormal union of the sublabial mucosa of the upper lip to the alveolar process; usually present in a unilateral or bilateral cleft of the lip.

adhesive, *n* an intermediate material that causes two materials to stick together; a luting agent.

adhesives, bonding, for desensitization, n sealant materials applied to the open ends of dentinal tubules that block the stimuli linked to tooth sensitivity.

adhesive foil, n See foil, adhesive.

adipose tissue (ad′əpōs′), *n* a connective tissue composed of a collection of fat cells.

adjudicate (əjōō′dikāt′), *v* the final step in dental peer review at which the dental peer review committee renders a formal, nonlegal decision on a case.

adjunct (aj′ungkt), *n* a drug or other substance that serves a supplemental purpose in therapy.

adjust (əjust′), *v* to make correspondent, comfortable, or to fit.

adjustment (əjust′ment), *n* a modification of a restoration or of a denture after insertion in the oral cavity.

adjustment, occlusal, n a grinding of the occluding surfaces of teeth to develop harmonious relationships between each other, their supporting structures, muscles of mastication, and temporomandibular joints.

adjuvant (aj′əvənt), *n* an auxiliary active ingredient that supports the action of the basic drug. See also basis.

administration, *n* the giving of, dispensing of, or application of medicines, drugs, or remedies to relieve or cure an illness.

administration, buccal, n the delivery of a medication by application to the buccal mucosa.

administration, inhalation, n the delivery of a medication by breathing it.

administration, intranasal, n See administration, inhalation.

administration, oral, n the delivery of a medication by oral cavity.

administration, rectal, n the delivery of a medication through the rectum.

administration, sublingual, n the delivery of a medication by placing it under the ventral surface of the tongue for dissolution and absorption through the mucous membrane.

administration, topical, n the delivery of a medication by application to the skin or mucous membrane.

administrative costs, *n.pl* the overhead expenses incurred in the operation of a dental benefits program, excluding costs of dental services provided.

administrative services only (ASO), *n* an arrangement in which a third party, for a fee, processes claims and handles paperwork for a self-funded group. This frequently includes almost all insurance company services, including actuarial services, underwriting, and benefit description, and excluding assumption of risk.

administrator, *n* a person who manages or directs a dental benefits program on behalf of the program's sponsor. See also third-party administrator and dental benefits organization.

admission, *n* the voluntary concession or admission that a fact or allegation is true.

admission, hospital, n **1.** a full stay. The formal acceptance by a hospital or other inpatient health care facility of a patient who is to be provided with room, board, and continuous nursing service in an area of the hospital or facility where patients generally reside at least overnight. *n* **2.** a surgicenter with short stays. Day bed only with nursing; patient does not stay overnight. *n* **3.** an outpatient admission. Pertains to a patient who enters the hospital but requires no bed; the patient enters for treatment and leaves after treatment.

adnexa (adnek′sə), *n* the conjoined anatomic parts, or tissues adjacent to or contained within a nearby space.

adolescence, *n* the period of development between the onset of puberty and adulthood. This period is generally marked by the appearance of secondary sex characteristics, usually from 11 to 13 years of age, and spans the teen years.

adolescent growth spurt, *n* a pe-

riod of rapid increase in height, weight, and muscle mass, which for boys takes place at age 12 to 16 and for girls at age 11 to 14. See also adolescence.

adrenal cortex (ədrē′nəl kor′teks), *n* the greater portion of the adrenal gland fused with the gland's medulla and producing mineralocorticoids, androgens, and glucocorticoids, hormones essential to homeostasis. The outer cortex is normally a deep yellow; the inner part is dark red or brown.

adrenal corticoid (ədrē′nəl kor′təkoid′), *n* See corticoid, adrenal.

adrenal crisis, *n* See crisis, adrenal.

adrenal steroids, *n.pl* See corticoid, adrenal.

adrenalectomy (ədrē′nəlek′təmē), *n* the surgical removal of one or both of the adrenal glands or the resection of a portion of one or both of the adrenal glands.

Adrenalin (ədren′əlin), *n* the brand name for epinephrine. See also epinephrine.

adrenaline (ədren′əlin), *n* the British term for epinephrine.

adrenergic (ad′rinur′jik), *adj* **1.** transmitted by norepinephrine or activated by norepinephrine or the other sympathomimetic agents. *n* **2.** a term applied to nerve fibers that liberate epinephrine or norepinephrine at a synapse when a nerve impulse passes. *n* **3.** a drug that mimics the action of adrenergic nerves.

adrenergic agonists, *n.pl* drugs that mimic the actions of norepinephrine, a neurotransmitter, resulting in stimulation of the sympathetic nervous system.

adrenergic blocking agent, *n* See agent, adrenergic blocking.

adrenergic fibers, *n.pl* See fibers, adrenergic.

adrenergic receptors, *n.pl* See receptors, adrenergic.

adrenic (ədrē′nik), *adj* pertaining to the adrenal gland.

adrenocortical insufficiency (ədrē′nōkôr′tikəl), *n* an acute or chronic adrenocortical hypofunction, as in Waterhouse-Friderichsen syndrome or Addison's disease. See hypoadrenocorticalism.

adrenocorticotropin (ədrē′nōkôr′tikōtrō′pin), *n* See ACTH.

adrenolytic (ədrē′nōlit′ik), *adj* capable of impeding the action of epinephrine, levarterenol (norepinephrine), or both (sympatholytic).

adrenolytic agent, *n* See agent, adrenergic blocking.

adrenotropic (ədrē′nōtrōp′ik), *adj* having a special affinity for the adrenal gland.

adsorb, *v* to attract molecules of a substance to the surface of another solid substance.

adsorbent (adsor′bənt), *adj* a substance that adsorbs, such as activated charcoal and clay.

adsorption, *n* a natural process whereby molecules of a gas or liquid adhere to the surface of a solid.

adult, *n* **1.** a person who has the fully developed characteristics of a mature person. *n* **2.** a person who has reached full legal age.

adumbration (ad′əmbrā′shən), *n* a geometric lack of sharpness of the radiograph shadow. See also penumbra, geometric.

advances, *n.pl* monies paid before the scheduled time of payment.

adverse drug effect, *n* a harmful, unintended reaction to a drug administered at normal dosage.

adverse reaction, *n* a harmful, unintended effect of a medication, diagnostic test, or therapeutic intervention.

adverse reactions, *n.pl* unfavorable reactions resulting from administration of a local anesthetic; responsible factors include the drug used, concentration, and route of administration.

adverse selection, *n* a statistical condition within a group when there is a greater demand for dental services and/or more services necessary than the average expected for that group.

advertising, *n* a paid form of nonpersonal presentation and promotion of ideas, goods, or services by an identified sponsor.

aeration (erā′shən), *n* the passage of air or gases into liquid (e.g., the passage of oxygen from pulmonary alveoli into the blood).

aerobiosis (er′ōbīō′sis), *n* life occurring in the presence of oxygen.

A

aerodontalgia (er′ōdontal′jə), *n* pulpal pain with decreased barometric pressure.

***Aeromonas* (er′ōmō′nas),** *n* a genus of bacteria usually found in water.

aerosol (er′əsôl), *n* **1.** the suspension of materials in a gas or vapor (e.g., saliva vaporized in air-water spray from a high-speed handpiece). **2.** a substance dispensed as a constituent of a gas or vapor suspension.

aesthetic factors, *n.pl* See esthetic dentistry.

affect (af′ekt), *n* **1.** the feeling of pleasantness or unpleasantness produced by a stimulus. *n* **2.** the emotional complex influencing a mental state. *n* **3.** the feeling experienced in connection with an emotion.

affective domain, *n* the area of learning involved in appreciation, interests, and attitudes.

afferent (af′ərənt), *adj* conveying from a periphery to a center.

afferent impulse, *n* an impulse that arises in the periphery and is carried into the central nervous system. An afferent nerve conducts the impulse from the site of origin to the central nervous system.

afferent nerves, *n.pl* See nerves, afferent, in pulp. See also afferent impulse.

afferent nervous system, *n.* the sensory nerves, a subdivision of the peripheral nervous system. Afferent nerves receive sensory input.

affiliation (əfil′ēā′shən), *n* the incorporation or formation of a partnership by dental professionals for the purpose of practicing the profession of dentistry.

afflux (af′luks), *n* the rush of blood to a body part.

affricative (əfrik′ətiv), *n* a fricative speech sound initiated by a plosive.

aflatoxins (af′lətok′sins), *n.pl* a group of carcinogenic and toxic factors produced by *Aspergillus flavus* food molds.

afterperception, the perception of a sensation after the stimulus producing it has ceased. (not current)

agar, hydrocolloid (ä′gär), *n* a reversible hydrocolloid made from agar-agar.

age, *n* the period of time a person has existed or an object has existed.

age, biological, *n* the age determined by physiology rather than chronology. Factors include changes in the physical structure of the body as well as changes in the performance of motor skills and sensory awareness.

age, chronologic, *n* age determined by the passage of time since birth.

age determination, *n* (by teeth), an estimate of age from the stage of tooth development and/or pattern of wear.

age distribution, *n* a grouping of the persons within a population on the basis of birth date.

age factors, *n.pl* variables affected by time since birth.

age hardening, *n* See hardening, age.

age of onset, *n* the chronologic age of the patient at which the disease, affliction, or disability appeared.

age, psychological, *n* a subjectively experienced age based on a person's behavior, or "how old they feel."

age, skeletal, *n* the age based on skeletal measurements relative to chronological skeletal development.

aged, *n* a state of having grown older or more mature than others of the population. See also geriatrics.

agenesis (ājen′əsis), *n* the defective development or congenital absence of parts.

agent(s), *n* **1.** a person or product that causes action. *n* **2.** a person authorized to act for, or in place of, another.

agent, adrenergic blocking, *n* a drug that blocks the action of the neurohormones norepinephrine and/or epinephrine or of adrenergic drugs at sympathetic neuroeffectors.

agent, adrenolytic blocking **(ədrē′nəlit′ik),** *n* an uncertain term sometimes used in reference to adrenergic blocking agents.

agent, anesthetic, *n* a drug that produces local or general loss of sensation.

agent, antianxiety, *n* any medication prescribed to relieve anxiety disorder symptoms, primarily stress and insomnia. The most common forms are benzodiazepine derivatives.

agent, antiarrhythmic **(an′tiərith′mik),** *n.pl* a substance used to prevent or relieve an irregular rhythm of heartbeat. Also mistakenly called *antidysrhythmic.*

A

agent, antigingivitis, *n* compound that inhibits, controls, or kills organisms associated with the formation of gingivitis.

agent, antihypertensive, *n* a medication used to lower elevated blood pressure (e.g., diuretics, beta-blockers, and vasodilators).

agent, antiinflammatory, *n* a drug that reduces inflammation.

agent, antimanic, *n* a substance used to treat various nervous system and psychiatric disorders; possible effects on fetal development include sluggishness, oxygen deficiency, and physical malformations.

agent, antiparasitic, *n* an antimicrobe that specifically targets pathogenic microorganisms.

agent, blocking, *n* an agent that occupies or usurps the receptor site normally occupied by a drug or a biochemical intermediary (e.g., acetylcholine or epinephrine).

agent, bonding, *n* a substance used to bond fillings and tooth restorations to the tooth surface.

agent, chemotherapeutic **(kē′mō-therəpyōō′tik),** *n* a chemical of natural or synthetic origin used for its specific action against disease, usually against infection.

agent, cholinergic blocking **(kō′-ləner′jik),** *n* **1.** a drug that inhibits the action of acetylcholine or cholinergic drugs at the postganglionic cholinergic neuroeffectors. *n* **2.** an anticholinergic agent.

agent, cleaning, *n.pl* an abrasive substance contained in toothpastes, gels, and powders that polishes teeth and aids in the removal of stains and plaque biofilm. See also abrasion, dentifrice.

agent, coloring, *n.pl* any substance contained in toothpastes, gels, and powders purely to make the product more appealing.

agent, coupling, *n* a substance or material that binds to both resin and reinforcement material and helps join them to make a composite.

agent, ganglionic blocking **(gang′-lēon′ik),** *n* a drug that prevents passage of nerve impulses at the synapses between preganglionic and postganglionic neurons.

agent, myoneural blocking, *n* a drug that prevents transmission of nerve impulses at the junction of the nerve and the muscle.

agent, oxidizing, *n* an agent that provides oxygen in reaction with another substance or, in the broader and more definitive chemical sense, a chemical capable of accepting electrons and thereby decreasing the negative charge on an atom of the substance being oxidized.

agent, polishing, *n* an abrasive that produces a smooth, lustrous finish.

agent, postganglionic sympathetic blocking, *n.pl* a medication used to treat hypertension by blocking the release of the naturally occurring hormone norepinephrine.

agent, reducing, *n* a category of chemicals used in film processing that brings out the gray tones of an image by creating black metallic silver from silver halide crystals.

agent, wetting, *n* any agent that will reduce the surface tension of water. Generally used in investing wax patterns.

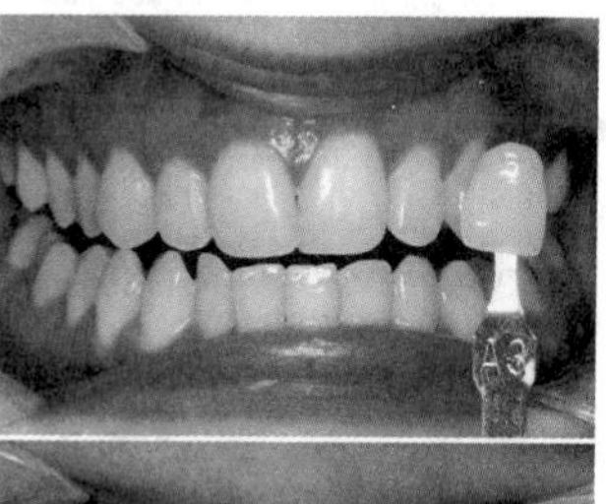

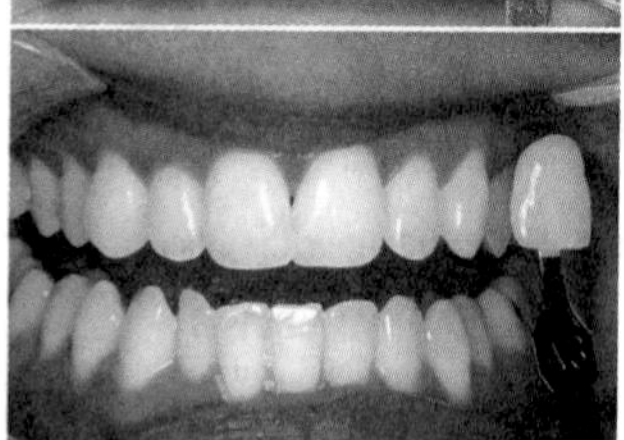

Whitening agent, before and after.
(Bird/Robinson, 2005)

agent, whitening, *n* a bleaching substance applied to teeth to lighten their appearance.

agents, antiadrenergic, centrally acting **(an′tēad′rəner′jik),** *n.pl* antihypertensive drugs used to lower blood pressure, specifically those that operate by stimulating α-receptors in the central nervous system and arterioles.

agents, antianginal, *n* one of several types of medication used to treat heart disease; alleviates pain associated with angina by lowering blood pressure during systole. See also vasodilator.

agents, oxygenating, *n.pl* the substances, such as hydrogen peroxide, that, when used as mouthrinses, release oxygen into gingival tissues and reduce inflammation. The process has not proved to reduce the bacteria causing the inflammation. Long-term use may cause tissue damage.

agents, sympathetic, *n.pl* the medications that stimulate the sympathetic nervous system by imitating the actions of naturally occurring norepinephrine and epinephrine. They may be used to treat cardiac arrest, nasal congestion, asthma, glaucoma, and attention deficit hyperactivity disorder and may cause anxiety, loss of appetite, and arrythmias. Also called *adrenergic agents.*

age-related macular degeneration (AMD), *n* the loss of central (as opposed to peripheral) vision due to diminished functioning of the macula of the retina. In those age 60 years and older, it is the most common cause of blindness.

ageusia (əgōō'sēə), *n* a loss or impairment of the sense of taste.

agglutination (əglōō'tinā'shən), *n* the aggregation or clumping together of cells as a result of their interaction with specific antibodies called agglutinins, commonly used in blood typing and in identifying or estimating the strength of immunoglobulins or immune sera.

agglutinin (əglōō'tinin), *n* **1.** a specific kind of antibody whose interaction with antigens is manifested as agglutination. **2.** an antibody that agglutinates red blood cells or renders them agglutinable.

aging, *n* in human development, the process of growing old. Physically, aging is marked by the reduction in the ability of cells to function normally or to produce new body cells at an optimal rate.

aging schedule, *n* a report showing how long accounts receivable have been outstanding. It gives the percentage of receivables not past due and the percentage past due by 1 month, 2 months, or other periods.

agitation, *n* **1.** the shaking of a substance, either for mixing ingredients or to remove debris or buildup from an object within the substance, such as a removable oral prosthetic. **2.** the intentional, usually mild, disturbance of the skin, mucosa, or other surface (e.g., with a wooden interdental cleaner or probe instrument) to determine if infection or disease is present. If agitated surfaces bruise or bleed easily, or are otherwise disrupted (e.g., develop a lesion), the presence of a pathologic condition should be suspected. **3.** a psychosomatic condition represented by uncontrollable or excessive body movements. The psychologic aspect may often indicate the presence of unresolved stress.

aglossia (aglôs'ēə), *n* a developmental anomaly in which a portion or all of the tongue is absent.

agnathia (agnath'ēə), *n* an absence of the mandible.

agnosia (agnō'zēə, -zhə), *n* a loss of ability to recognize common objects (that is, a loss of ability to understand the significance of sensory stimuli [e.g., tactile, auditory, or visual] resulting from brain damage).

agonist (ag'ənist), *n* **1.** an organ, gland, muscle, or nerve center that is so connected physiologically with another that the two function simultaneously in forwarding a given process, such as when two muscles pull on the same skeletal member and receive a nervous excitation at the same time. Opposite: antagonist. **2.** a drug or other substance having a specific cellular affinity that produces a predictable response.

agony, *n* severe pain or extreme suffering.

agoraphobia (ag'ərəfō'bēə), *n* an anxiety disorder characterized by a fear of being in an open, crowded, or public place where escape may be difficult or help may not be available if needed.

agranulocytosis (āgran'yŏŏlōsītō'sis), *n* a decrease in the number of granulocytes in peripheral blood resulting from bone marrow depression by drugs and chemicals or replacement by a neoplasm. Oral lesions are ulceronecrotic, involving the gingivae, tongue, buccal mucosa, or lips. Regional lymphadenopathy and lymphadenitis are prevalent.

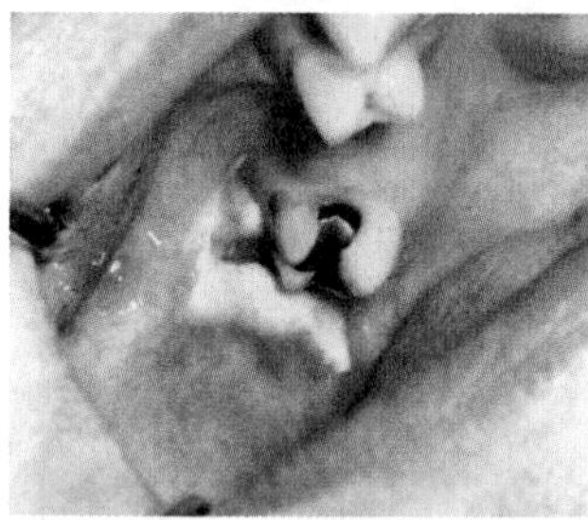

Agranulocytosis. (Sapp/Eversole/Wysocki, 2004)

agreement, *n* the coming together in accord of two minds on a given proposition.

AH-26, *n* an epoxy resin root canal sealer.

AHF, *n* the abbreviation for antihemophilic factor. See also factor VIII.

aid, *n* assistance; support.

aid in physiotherapy, *n* an agent used by the patient to cleanse the teeth and oral tissues and provide pseudofunctional stimulation of the gingival tissues to maintain periodontal health.

aid, speech therapy, *n* a restoration, appliance, or electronic device used to improve speech.

aid, visual, *n* a model, drawing, or photograph used to help the patient understand proposed treatment.

AIDS, *n* the abbreviation for acquired immunodeficiency syndrome. See also human immunodeficiency virus (HIV).

AIDS-related complex (ARC), *n* See acquired immunodeficiency syndrome.

air, *n* the invisible, odorless, gaseous mixture that makes up the earth's atmosphere.

air, ambient, *n* the encircling or enveloping environment; surrounding air.

air chamber, *n* See chamber, relief.

air, complemental, *n* See volume, inspiratory reserve.

air, functional residual, *n* See capacity, functional residual.

air, minimal, *n* the volume of air in the air sacs themselves (part of the residual air).

air reserve, *n* See volume, expiratory reserve.

air, residual, *n* See volume, residual.

air, supplemental, *n* See volume, expiratory reserve.

air syringe, *n* See syringe, air.

air, tidal, *n* See volume, tidal.

air turbine handpiece, *n* See handpiece, air turbine.

air application in calculus identification, *n* See calculus, identification of, by air application.

air bubbles on radiographic film, *n* See film fault, white spots.

air embolism, *n* an obstruction of a blood vessel caused by the entrance of air into the bloodstream. See also embolism.

air tip, *n* a part of a compressed air-water syringe, with an angled end that facilitates dental examination procedures.

air-powder polishing, *n* a technique for plaque and stain removal in which sodium bicarbonate particles and water are propeled against the teeth in a regulated flow using air and water pressure. Also called *airabrasive* or *airbrasive.*

airborne, *adj* carried through the air. In health care settings, viruses or bacteria may become airborne, e.g., when someone sneezes or coughs.

airborne contaminants, *n.pl* materials in the atmosphere that can affect the health of persons in the same or a nearby environment. Also referred to as *air pollution.*

airway, *n* **1.** a clear passageway for air into and out of the lungs. **2.** a device for securing unobstructed respiration during general anesthesia or in states of unconsciousness.

airway, chin lift, *n* a method of opening the trachea of an individual by manually changing the position of his or her head in order to perform rescue breathing.

airway obstruction, *n* an abnormal condition of the respiratory pathway characterized by a mechanical impediment to the delivery or to the absorption of oxygen in the lungs, as in choking, bronchospasm, obstructive lung disease, or laryngospasm.

airway obstruction, chest thrust, *n* an alternate method of removing an obstacle lodged in the airway by compressing the sternum; used when pregnancy or a patient's body size render the Heimlich maneuver impossible or inappropriate. See Heimlich maneuver.

airway obstruction, infant chest thrust, *n* a method of removing an obstacle lodged in the airway of an infant by placing the child facedown along the forearm and striking the child's back with the opposite hand. See Heimlich maneuver.

airway resistance, *n* the ratio of pressure difference between the oral cavity, nose, or other airway opening and the alveoli to the simultaneously measured resulting volumetric gas flow rate.

akinesia (ā′kənē′zhə), *n* a loss of controllable motion and feelings of exhaustion. It is a common consequence of Parkinson's disease, causing dopamine loss in the direct pathway of movement.

Al-Anon, *n.pr* group connected to Alcoholics Anonymous specifically organized for individuals connected to the recovering alcoholic.

ala (ā′lə), *n* winglike cutaneous-covered cartilaginous structure on the lateral aspect of the external naris of the nose.

alanine (al′ənēn), *n* a nonessential amino acid found in many proteins in the body. It is metabolized in the liver to produce pyruvate and glutamate.

ALARA concept, *n* an acronym for "As Low As Reasonably Achievable"; it pertains to radiation exposure encountered when taking radiographs. This idea requires that every possible precaution is taken to limit radiation levels when exposing the patient or clinician to radiation.

alarm reaction, *n* See reaction, alarm and syndrome, general adaptation.

Alateen, *n.pr* group connected to Alcoholics Anonymous specifically organized for teenage children of recovering alcoholics.

Albers-Schönberg disease (al′berz-shœn′berg), *n.pr* See osteopetrosis.

Albright's syndrome, *n.pr* See syndrome, McCune-Albright.

albumin (albyōō′min), *n* the primary protein of plasma (4.5% g) that aids in maintaining capillary osmotic pressure.

albuminuria (albyōō′minyōō′rēə), *n* (hyperproteinuria, proteinuria, proteuria), the presence of clinically detectable amounts of protein in the urine. Usually less than 100 mg/24 hr may be found normally by special methods. The usual protein is albumin, although globulins, Bence Jones protein, and fibrinogen may be present and may exceed the amount of albumin. The condition may be caused by prerenal or renal disease or by inflammation of the urinary tract.

albuterol, *n brand names:* Proventil, Proventil Repetabs, Nova-Salmol, Ventodisk, Ventolin, Ventolin Rotacaps; *drug class:* adrenergic β_2-agonist; *action:* causes bronchodilation; *uses:* prevents exercise-induced asthma, bronchospasm.

Alcaligenes (al′kəlij′ənēz), *n.pl* (literally, "alkali-generating") aerobic, gram-negative eubacteria, commonly found in invertebrate intestinal tracts and normally occurring on the skin.

alcohol (al′kəhôl), *n* a transparent, colorless liquid that is mobile and volatile. Alcohols are organic compounds formed from hydrocarbons by the substitution of hydroxyl radicals for the same number of hydrogen atoms.

alcohol, absolute, *n* an alcohol containing no more than 1% H_2O.

alcohol abuse, *n* the frequent intake of large amounts of alcohol, typically distinguished by decreased health and physical and social functioning impairment. See also alcoholism.

alcohol blood level, *n* See blood alcohol concentration.

alcohol dependence, *n* a mental and physical need to consume alcohol in order to prevent the pains of withdrawal and obtain certain results; causes a limited capacity to control actions during consumption of alcohol. See also alcohol abuse.

alcohol hallucinosis **(həlōō'sənō'sis),** *n* a complication of the last stage of withdrawal from alcohol, occurring within 48 hours of sudden decrease or halt of increased consumption after a lengthy period of dependence. It is indicated by severely impairing visual and auditory hallucinations similar to schizophrenia symptoms that may persist for weeks or months.

alcohol withdrawal delirium, *n* a complication of the last stage of withdrawal from alcohol, occurring within 1 week of sudden decrease or halt of increased consumption after a lengthy period of dependence; indicated by dramatic auditory, visual, and tactile hallucinations, confusion, delusions, disorientation, tremors, nervous actions, sweating, and rapid heartbeat. Also called *DTs* or *delirium tremens.*

alcoholic group therapy, *n* an association of men and women devoted to helping each other treat alcohol dependence. Participants and facilitators may use psychotherapy, behavior therapy, and the recruitment of family members and friends to achieve objectives.

alcoholic, recovering, *n* a person who is attempting to refrain from the compulsive consumption of alcohol and thereby escape the physiologic, psychologic, and social impairments associated with it.

Alcoholics Anonymous (AA), *n.pr* a group program in which the members help themselves and each other defeat alcoholism.

alcoholism, *n* the continued extreme dependence on excessive amounts of alcohol, accompanied by a cumulative pattern of deviant behaviors. The most frequent consequences are chronic gastritis, central nervous system depression, and cirrhosis of the liver, each of which can compromise the delivery of dental care. Oral cancer and increased levels of periodontal disease are also risks.

aldehyde (al'dəhīd'), *n* a large category of organic compounds derived from a corresponding alcohol by the removal of two hydrogen atoms, as in the conversion of ethyl alcohol to acetaldehyde.

aldesleukin (al'dəslōō'kin), *n* (interleukin-2, IL-2), *brand name:* Proleukin; *drug class:* antineoplastic; *action:* enhancement of lymphocyte mitogenesis and stimulation of IL-2-dependent cell lines; *uses:* metastatic renal cell carcinoma in adults.

aldosterone (aldos'tərōn), *n* an adrenal corticosteroid hormone that acts primarily to accelerate the exchange of potassium for sodium in the renal tubules and other cells. It is a potent mineralocorticoid but also has some regulatory effect on carbohydrate metabolism.

aldosteronism, primary (aldos'tərō'nizəm), *n* a hyperadrenal syndrome caused by abnormal elaboration of aldosterone and characterized by excessive loss of potassium and resultant muscle weakness. The symptoms suggest tetany. The condition is often associated with an adenoma or cortical hyperplasia of the adrenal glands.

alendronate sodium (əlen'drənāt' sō'dēəm), *n brand name:* Fosamax; *drug class:* amino biphosphonate; *action:* acts as a specific inhibitor of bone resorption; *uses:* osteoporosis in postmenopausal women, Paget's disease of bone.

alganesthesia (algan'esthē'zhə), *n* the absence of a normal sense of pain.

algesia (aljē'zēə), *n* sensitivity to pain; hyperesthesia; a sense of pain.

algesic (aljē'sik), *adj* painful.

algesimetry (aljəsim'etrē), *n* the measurement of response to painful stimuli.

algetic (aljet'ik), *adj* painful.

alginate (al'jināt), *n* a salt of alginic acid (e.g., sodium alginate), which, when mixed with water in accurate proportions, forms an irreversible hydrocolloid gel used for making impressions or molds of the dentition. See also hydrocolloid, irreversible.

algorithm, *n* an explicit protocol with well-defined rules to be followed in solving a complex problem.

align (əlīn), *v* to move the teeth into their proper positions to conform to the line of occlusion.

alignment, tooth (əlīn'ment), *n* the arrangement of the teeth in relation-

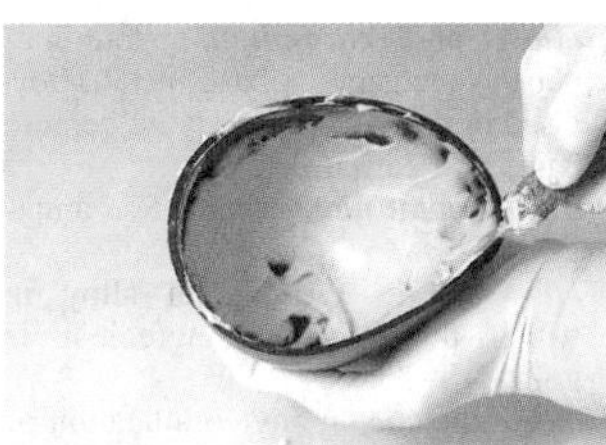

Alginate. (Bird/Robinson, 2005)

ship to their supporting bone (alveolar process), adjacent teeth, and opposing dentition.

alkali (al′kəlī), *n* a strong water-soluble base. A chemical substance that, in aqueous solution, undergoes dissociation, resulting in the formation of hydroxyl (OH) ions.

alkaline (al′kəlin), *adj* having the reductions of an alkali. A pH level of 7.1 to 14 designates an alkaline solution. See also basic.

alkaline diet, n See diet, alkaline.

alkaline phosphatase, n an enzyme present in bone, the kidneys, the intestines, plasma, and teeth. It may be elevated in the serum in some diseases associated with disturbances in bone, liver, or other tissues.

alkaline reserve, n See reserve, alkaline.

alkaloid (al′kəloid), *n* the many nitrogen-containing organic bases derived from plants. They are bitter and physiologically active. A number are useful therapeutic agents.

alkaloid, synthetic, n a synthetically prepared compound having the chemical characteristics of the alkaloids.

alkalosis (alkəlō′sis), *n* a disturbance of acid-base balance and water balance, characterized by an excess of alkali or a deficiency of acids.

alkalosis, compensated, n a condition in which the blood bicarbonate is usually higher than normal but compensatory mechanisms have kept the pH level within normal range. See also alkalosis, uncompensated.

alkalosis, hypochloremic, n a metabolic abnormality caused by an increase in blood bicarbonate after significant chloride loss.

alkalosis, respiratory, n alkalemia produced by hypoventilation. Plasma bicarbonate is therefore decreased in respiratory alkalosis but raised in metabolic alkalosis.

alkalosis, uncompensated, n alkalemia usually accompanied by an increased blood bicarbonate.

allele (əlēl′), *n* (allelomorph), one or more genes occupying the same location in a chromosome but differing because of a mutational change of one.

allergen (al′urjen), *n* a substance capable of producing an allergic response or antigen. Common allergens are pollens, dust, drugs, and foods. See also antigen.

allergy (al′urjē), *n* a hypersensitive reaction to an allergen; an antigen-antibody reaction is manifested in several forms—anaphylaxis, asthma, hay fever, urticaria, angioedema, dermatitis, and stomatitis.

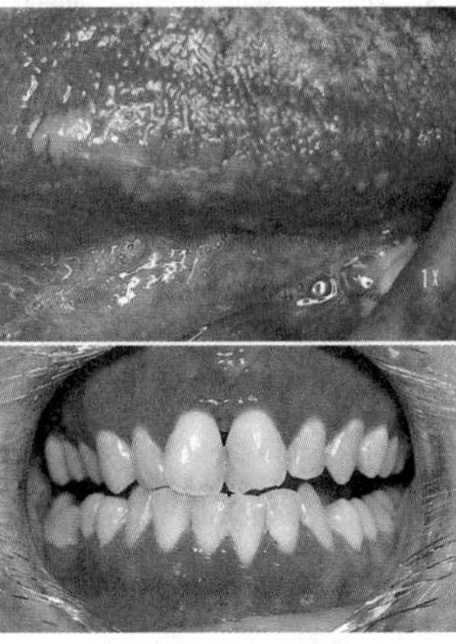

Manifestations of allergies. (Regezi/Sciubba/Pogrel, 2000)

allergy, cross-reactive, n a condition in which a patient allergic to one medication will experience an allergic reaction to all other medications and their derivatives (i.e., cross-sensitivity between penicillin derivatives, cephalosporins and carbapenems). See also resistance, cross.

allergy, "spontaneous" clinical, n See atopy.

allied health personnel, *n.pl* the health care professionals, other than physicians, dental professionals, clinical psychologists, pharmacists, and nurses, with education, training, and

A

experience to serve as members of the health care delivery team.

allochiria (al'ōkī'rēə, al'ōkir'ēə), *n* the tactile sensation experienced at the side opposite its origin.

allogenic, *adj* from individuals of the same species. Tissue transplanted from one person to another is said to be allogenic.

allografts (al'əgraf'ts), *n.pl* the transplantation of tissue between genetically nonidentical individuals of the same species. Also known as *homoplastic grafts* or *homografts.*

alloplast (al'lōplast), *n* inorganic material used as a bone substitute or an implant.

alloplastic (al'ōplas'tik), *adj* nonbiologic material such as metal, ceramic, and plastic.

alloplasty (al'ōplas'tē), *n* a plastic surgery procedure in which material not from the human body is used.

allopurinol (al'əpyōō'rinol), *n* *brand names:* Lopurin, Zyloprim; *drug class:* antigout drug; *action:* inhibits the enzyme xanthine oxidase, reducing uric acid synthesis; *uses:* chronic gout, hyperuricemia associated with malignancies.

allowable benefits, *n.pl* necessary, reasonable, and customary items of service or treatments covered in whole or in part under an insurance plan.

allowable charge, *n* the maximum dollar amount on which benefit payment is based for each dental procedure.

allowable expenses, *n.pl* the dollar amounts allowable for each dental procedure covered by a dental insurance policy.

alloxan (əlok'san), *n* a substance, mesoxalyl urea, capable of producing experimental diabetes by destroying the islet cells of the pancreas.

alloy (al'oi), *n* **1.** a solution composed of two metals dissolved in each other when in the liquid state. *n* **2.** the product of the fusion of two or more metals.

alloy, amalgam **(əmal'gəm),** *n* the alloy or product of the fusion of several metals, usually supplied as filings, that is mixed with mercury to produce dental amalgam. Colloquial term is silver fillings.

alloy, cobalt-chromium, n (chrome-cobalt amalgam), a base metal alloy. Used in dentistry for metallic denture bases and partial dentures.

alloy, dental amalgam, n See amalgam.

alloy, dental gold, n an alloy in which the principal ingredient is gold.

alloy, eutectic, n any combination of metals the melting point of which is lower than that of any of the individual metals of which it consists. An alloy in which the components are mutually soluble in the solid state. A eutectic alloy has a nonhomogeneous grain structure and is therefore likely to be brittle and subject to tarnishing and corrosion.

alloy, nickel-chromium, n a stainless steel.

alopecia (al'əpē'shə), *n* the loss of hair. Baldness. Various types with varying causes.

alpha-adrenergic blockers (al'fə-ad'rəner'jik), *n.pl* drugs prescribed for hypertension that impede α-receptors, which in turn halts sympathetic autonomic nervous system action. See also agent, adrenergic blocking.

alpha-amylase (al'fə-am'əlās'), *n* a starch-splitting enzyme used in the treatment of inflammatory conditions and edema of soft tissues associated with traumatic injury.

alpha-estradiol (al'fə-estrədī'ôl), *n* an estrogenic steroid, prepared by dehydrogenation of estrone, which is one of the factors responsible for the maintenance of the epithelial integrity of the oral tissues. A deficiency results in epithelial desquamation.

alpha-glucosidase inhibitors (al'fə-glōōkō'sidās'), *n.pl* an orally administered agent used in the treatment of type 2 diabetes mellitus. Examples include acarbose, which slows the digestion and absorption of glucose into the bloodstream.

alpha-hemihydrate (al'fə-hem'ēhī'drāt), *n* a physical form of the hemihydrate of calcium sulfate $(CaSO_4)$-H_2O; dental artificial stone.

alpha-interferon, *n* See interferon, alpha.

alpha-selective blockers, *n.pl* antihypertensive drugs that lower blood pressure by blocking α-receptors in the arterioles and venules.

alpha-tocopherol, *n* See vitamin E.

alphabet, international phonetic, *n* a set of internationally agreed upon alphabetical symbols, one for each sound; supplements the existing alphabet to fill out needed representation of sounds.

alphanumeric, *adj* pertaining to a character set that contains letters and numerals and usually other special characters.

alprazolam (alprāz′əlam′), *n brand names:* Xanax, Apo-Alpraz, Novo-Alprazol, Nu-Alpraz; *drug class:* benzodiazepine (Controlled Substance Schedule IV); *action:* produces CNS depression; *uses:* anxiety, panic disorders, anxiety with depressive symptoms.

alprostadil (alpros′tədil′), *n brand name:* Caverject; *drug class:* naturally occurring prostaglandin; *action:* induces erection by relaxation of trabecular smooth muscle and by dilation of cavernosal arteries; *uses:* treatment of erectile dysfunction caused by neurogenic, vasculogenic, psychogenetic, or mixed etiology.

alternate benefit, *n* a provision in a dental plan contract that allows the third-party payer to determine the benefit based on an alternative procedure that is generally less expensive than the one provided or proposed.

alternate treatment, *n* the contract provisions that authorize the insurance carrier to determine the amount of benefits payable, giving consideration to alternate procedures, services, or courses of treatment that may be performed to accomplish the desired result. The attending dental provider and the patient have the option of which procedure to use, although payment for the procedure may be based on the alternate treatment principle.

alternative benefit plan, *n* a plan other than a traditional (fee-for-service, freedom of choice) indemnity or service corporation plan for reimbursing a participating dental provider for providing treatment to an enrolled patient population.

alternative delivery system, *n* an arrangement for the provision of dental services in other than the traditional way (e.g., licensed dental provider providing treatment in a fee-for-service dental office).

alternative treatment plan, *n* a compromise plan of treatment deviating from the ideal plan in scope and financial investment.

altitude, *n* pertaining to any location on earth with reference to a fixed surface point, which is usually sea level. The higher the altitude, the lower the oxygen concentration and the greater the ultraviolet radiation, both of which can cause health problems.

altretamine (altret′əmēn′), *n brand name:* Hexalen; *drug class:* antineoplastic; *action:* products of metabolism interact with tissue macromolecules, including DNA, which may be responsible for cytotoxicity; *uses:* palliative treatment of recurrent, persistent ovarian cancer.

alumina (əlōōminə), *n* aluminum oxide, an abrasive sometimes used as a polishing agent.

aluminum, *n* a widely used metallic element and the third most abundant of all the elements. Aluminum is a principal component of many compounds used in antacids, antiseptics, astringents, and styptics. Aluminum hydroxychloride is the most commonly used agent in antiperspirants.

aluminum carbonate gel, *n brand name:* Basajel; *drug class:* antacid; *action:* neutralizes gastric acidity, binds phosphates in GI tract; *uses:* antacid, prevention of phosphate stones, phosphate binder in chronic renal failure.

aluminum filters/disks, *n.pl* the extremely thin (0.05 cm) pieces of aluminum that are placed over the aperture of the radiographic tube to eliminate x rays over a certain wavelength.

aluminum hydroxide, *n brand names:* AlternaGEL, Alu-Cap, Alu-Tab, Amphojel, Dialume; *drug class:* antacid; *action:* neutralizes gastric acidity, binds phosphates in GI tract; *uses:* antacid, hyperphosphatemia in chronic renal failure.

aluminum oxide, *n* a metallic oxide that includes alpha single crystal (an inert, biocompatible strong ceramic material used in the fabrication of some endosseous implants) and polycrystal (a constituent of dental porce-

A

lain that increases viscosity and strength).

Aluwax (al′yəwaks), *n* a commercially prepared wax wafer containing aluminum that is used to register jaw relationship.

alveolalgia (al′vēōlal′jēə), *n* See socket, dry.

alveolar (alvē′ōlär), *adj* pertaining to an alveolus.

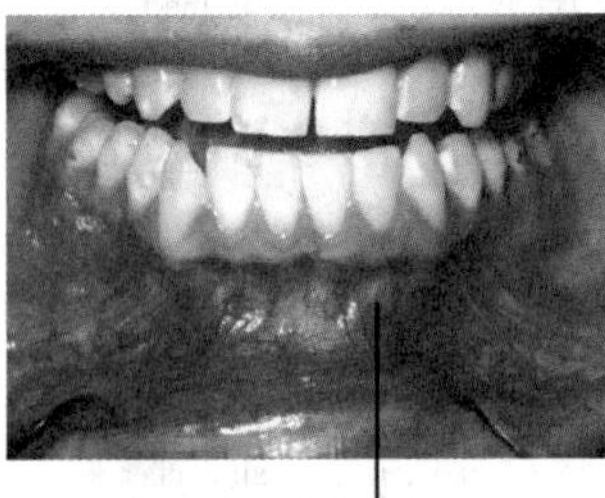

Alveolar mucosa. (Liebgott, 2001)

alveolar bone loss, *n* See bone loss, periodontal.

alveolar crest, *n* See crest, alveolar.

alveolar process, *n* See process, alveolar.

alveolar ridge, *n* See ridge, alveolar.

alveolar ridge augmentation, *n* a surgical procedure to improve the shape and size of the alveolar ridge(s) in preparation to receive and retain a dental prosthesis.

alveolectomy (al′vēəlek′təmē), *n* the excision of a portion of the alveolar process to aid in the removal of teeth, modification of the contour after the removal of teeth, and preparation of the oral cavity for dentures.

alveolitis, *n* the inflammation of a tooth socket.

alveoloplasty (alvē′əlōplas′tē), *n* the surgical shaping and smoothing of the margins of the tooth socket after extraction of the tooth, generally in preparation for the placement of a prosthesis.

alveolus (alvē′əlus), *n* **1.** an air sac of the lungs formed by terminal dilations of the bronchioles. *n* **2.** the socket in the bone in which a tooth is attached by means of the periodontal ligament.

Alzheimer's disease, *n.pr* a presenile dementia characterized by confusion, memory failure, disorientation, restlessness, agnosia, hallucinosis, speech disturbances, and the inability to carry out purposeful movement. The disease usually begins in later middle life with slight defects in memory and behavior that become progressively more severe. Also known as primary progressive aphasia.

amalgam (əmal′gəm), *n* (dental amalgam alloy), an alloy, one of the constituents of which is mercury.

amalgam, bonded, *n* **1.** a composite of tooth-colored acrylic resin and finely ground glass-like particles that is bonded or adhered to the tooth during dental restoration. The advantage is that less of the tooth structure needs to be removed during the restoration, resulting in a smaller filling compared with traditional amalgams. **2.** a composite filling.

amalgam carrier, *n* See carrier, amalgam.

amalgam carver, *n* See carver, amalgam.

amalgam condenser, *n* See condenser, amalgam.

amalgam, copper, *n* an alloy composed principally of copper and mercury. See also amalgam.

amalgam, dental, *n* an amalgam used for dental restorations and dyes.

amalgam matrix, *n* See matrix, amalgam.

amalgam pigmentation, *n* See amalgam tattoo.

amalgam plugger, *n* See condenser, amalgam.

amalgam, silver, *n* a dental amalgam, the main constituent of which is silver. The ADA composition specifications are as follows: silver, 65% minimum; tin, 25% minimum; copper, 6% maximum; zinc, 2% maximum.

amalgam squeeze cloth, *n* a piece of linen used to hold plastic amalgam from which excess mercury is to be squeezed. Used with hand trituration.

amalgam tattoo, *n* a solitary discrete gray, blue, or black discoloration of tissue usually located in the gingiva, alveolar ridge, or buccal mucosa caused by small amounts of dental amalgam that became embedded under the surface. The asymptomatic lesion is static and requires no treatment. If doubt exists about the lesion or if the lesion is unsightly, excisional biopsy is recommended.

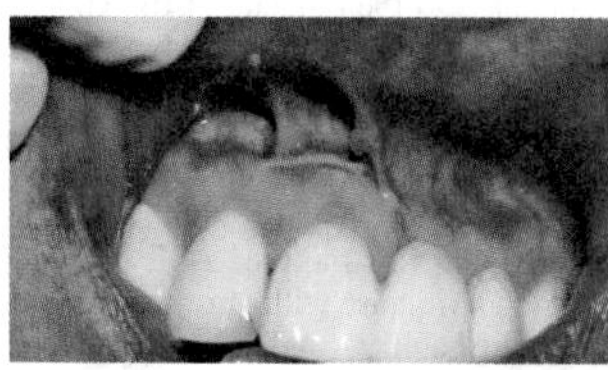

Amalgam tattoo. (Sapp/Eversole/Wysocki, 2004)

amalgam well, *n* a small, bowl-shaped container that holds mixed amalgam prior to its being loaded into the amalgam carrier.

amalgamation (əmal′gəmā′shən), *n* the formation of an alloy by mixing mercury with another metal or other metals. See also trituration.

amalgamation amalgamator **(əmal′gəmātur),** *n* a mechanical device used to triturate the ingredients of dental amalgam into a plastic mass. See trituration.

amantadine (əman′tidēn), *n* an antiviral that prevents uncoating and replication of the influenza A virus; most effectively used in the early stages of exposure.

ambulatory care, *n* the health services provided on an outpatient basis to those who can visit a health care facility and return home the same day.

ambulatory surgery, *n* the surgical care provided to persons who do not require overnight nursing care.

amcinonide, *n brand name:* Cyclocort; *drug class:* topical fluorinated corticosteroid, group II high potency; *action:* antipruritic, antiinflammatory; *uses:* psoriasis, eczema, contact dermatitis, pruritus.

amelia (əmel′ēə, əmē′lēə), *n* a congenital abnormality characterized by the absence of one or more limbs.

ameloblast (am′əlōblast′), *n* an epithelial cell associated with the enamel organ that, during tooth development, secretes enamel matrix.

ameloblast atrophy, *n* a wasting of or decrease in the epithelial cells, which form tooth enamel; may occur as the result of a deficiency in vitamin A. See also atrophy, periodontal.

ameloblastic fibroma, *n* See fibroma, ameloblastic.

ameloblastic fibro-odontoma (am′əlōblas′tik fī′brō-ō′dontō′mə), *n* an aggressive, generally benign tumor of the oral tissues, most commonly occurring in the posterior mandible. It is generally associated with developing teeth and thus is usually found in children or adolescents.

ameloblastic sarcoma (am′əlōblas′tik sarkō′mə), *n* See sarcoma, ameloblastic.

ameloblastoma (am′əlōblastō′mə), *n* an epithelial neoplasm with a basic structure resembling the enamel organ and suggesting derivation from ameloblastic cells. It is usually benign but aggressive. Also called *adamantinoblastoma* or *adamantinoma.*

ameloblastoma, acanthomatous, *n* a type that differs from the simple form in that the central cells within the cell nests are squamous and may be keratinized rather than stellate. The peripheries of the cell nests are composed of ameloblastic cells. See also ameloblastoma.

amelogenesis, *n* the process during which the enamel matrix is formed by ameloblasts. See also ameloblast.

amelogenesis imperfecta **(am′əlōjen′əsis),** *n* a broad category of developmental disturbances in the structural formation of enamel. The disease is divided into four main types (type 1, Hypoplastic; type 2, Hypomaturation; type 3, Hypocalcified; type 4, mixed) and 15 subtypes, which range from mild to severe.

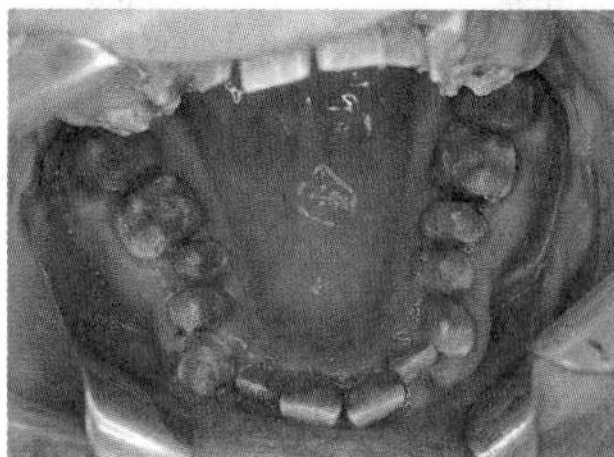

Amelogenesis imperfecta. (Regezi/Sciubba/Pogrel, 2000)

amenorrhea (əmen′ōrē′ə), *n* the absence or abnormal cessation of the menstrual cycle.

American Academy of Periodontology (AAP), *n.pr* a nonprofit professional association of dental professionals specializing in the prevention, diagnosis, and treatment of diseases affecting the periodontium and in the placement and maintenance of dental implants.

American Cancer Society (ACS), *n.pr* a national advocacy and fund-raising organization, headquartered in Atlanta, Georgia, that is dedicated to raising public awareness about cancer and to providing support for cancer patients and their families.

American Dental Association (ADA), *n.pr* a nonprofit professional association whose membership is dental professionals in the United States. Its purpose is to assist its members in providing the highest professional and ethical care to the citizens of the United States and to serve as an advocate for the advancement of the profession.

American Dental Hygienists Association (ADHA), *n.pr* a nonprofit professional association of dental hygienists in the United States created to assist its members in providing the highest professional and ethical care to the citizens of the United States and to serve as an advocate for the advancement of the profession.

American Foundation for the Blind, *n.pr* an advocacy group for individuals with visual disabilities.

American Heart Association (AHA), *n.pr* a national voluntary health agency that has the goal of increasing public and medical awareness of cardiovascular diseases and stroke, and thereby reducing the number of associated deaths and disabilities.

American Hospital Association (AHA), *n.pr* a nonprofit national organization of individuals, institutions, and organizations engaged in direct patient care. The association works to promote the improvement of health care services.

American manual alphabet, *n.pr* a representation of alphabet letters using a variety of finger positions.

American Medical Association (AMA), *n.pr* a nonprofit professional association of physicians in the United States, including all medical specialties. Its purpose is to assist its members in providing the highest professional and ethical medical care to the citizens of the United States and to serve as an advocate for the advancement of the profession.

American Sign Language (ASL), *n.pr* a mode of communication using gestures and visuals with a unique grammatical structure. ASL is used by individuals with limited or no hearing ability and by those who communicate regularly with such individuals.

Americans with Disabilities Act (ADA), *n.pr* a federal law that defines a private dental office as a place of public accommodation, thereby requiring that dental offices serve persons with disabilities.

amide (am'īd), *n* **1.** an ammonia-derived organic compound formed through the displacement of a hydrogen atom by an acyl radical. **2.** An ammonia-derived inorganic compound formed through the replacement of an acid's hydroxyl group (OH) with that of an amino group such as $-NH_2$. **3.** type of local anesthetic agent. See also anesthetic, amide.

amiloride HCl (əmil'ərīd'), *n brand name:* Midamor; *drug class:* potassium-sparing diuretic; *action:* acts primarily on the distal renal tubule, increasing the retention of potassium; *uses:* edema in chronic heart failure in combination with other diuretics, for hypertension, with INH solution for cystic fibrosis.

amines (əmēnz'), *n.pl* organic compounds that contain nitrogen.

amino acid, *n* an organic acid in which one of the CH hydrogen atoms has been replaced by NH_2. Amino acids are the building blocks of proteins.

amino acid, essential, *n* the group of amino acids that cannot be synthesized by the organism but are required by the organism. They must be supplied by the diet. Isoleucine, leucine, lysine, methionine, phenylalanine, threonine, tryptophan, and valine are essential for adults; these eight plus arginine and histidine are considered essential for infants and children.

amino acid, glucogenic **(gloo͞okō-jen′ik),** *n* the group of amino acids that produce enzymes that may be converted to glucose if necessary.

amino acid, ketogenic **(kē′tōjen′ik),** *n* an amino acid that produces ketone bodies following chemical alteration of its carbon skeleton.

amino acid, nonessential, *n* the group of amino acids that can be synthesized by the organism and are not required in the diet.

amino acid pool, *n* an accumulation of amino acids in the liver and blood that adjusts to meet the body's need for protein and amino acids.

aminocaproic acid (əmē′nōkə-prō′ik), *n brand name:* Amicar; *drug class:* hemostatic; *action:* inhibits fibrinolysis by inhibiting plasminogen activator substances; *uses:* hemorrhage from hyperfibrinolysis; adjunctive therapy in hemophilia; unapproved, hemorrhage following dental surgery in hemophilia.

aminoglutethimide (əmē′nōgloo͞-teth′əmīd), *n brand name:* Cytadren; *drug class:* antineoplastic, adrenal steroid inhibitor; *action:* acts by inhibiting the enzymatic conversion of cholesterol to pregnenolone, thereby blocking synthesis of all adrenal steroids; *uses:* suppression of adrenal function in Cushing's syndrome, metastatic breast cancer, and adrenal cancer.

aminoglycosides (əmē′nōglī′kə-sīdz′), *n.pl* the bacteriocidal antibiotics obtained from *Streptomyces* that inhibit protein synthesis in bacterial ribosomes and are effective against aerobic gram-negative bacilli.

aminophylline (theophylline ethylenediamine), *n brand names:* Phyllocontin; *drug class:* xanthine; *action:* relaxes smooth muscle of the respiratory system; *uses:* bronchial asthma, bronchospasm, Cheyne-Stokes respirations.

amiodarone HCl (əmē′ōdərōn′), *n brand name:* Cordarone; *drug class:* antidysrhythmic (drug class III); *action:* prolongs action potential duration and effective refractory period; *uses:* documented life-threatening ventricular tachycardia.

amitriptyline HCl (am′itrip′təlēn), *n brand names:* Apo-Amitriptyline, Elavil, Emitrip, Endep, Enovil, Levate, Novotriptyn; *drug class:* tricyclic antidepressant; *action:* inhibits both norepinephrine and serotonin (5-HT); *uses:* major depression.

amlodipine besylate (amlō′dipēn bes′əlāt), *n brand name:* Norvasc; *drug class:* calcium channel blocker; *action:* inhibits calcium ion influx across cell membrane during cardiac depolarization; produces relaxation of coronary vascular smooth muscle and dilates coronary arteries; decreases SA/AV node conduction; *uses:* hypertension as a single agent or in combination with other antihypertensives, chronic stable angina pectoris, vasospastic angina.

ammeter (am′ētur), *n* a contraction of amperemeter. An apparatus that measures the amperage of an electric current.

ammonia, *n* a colorless aromatic gas consisting of nitrogen and hydrogen, produced by the decomposition of nitrogenous organic matter. Some of its many uses are as an aromatic stimulant, a detergent, and an emulsifier.

ammonia thiosulfate **(əmō′nyə thī-ōsul′fāt),** *n* an ingredient of the photographic fixing solution that acts as a solvent for silver halides.

ammoniacal silver nitrate, *n* See silver nitrate, ammoniacal.

ammonium chloride, *n* the chlorine salt of the ammonium ion. It is a popular deliquescent agent (i.e., it attracts and absorbs water from the atmosphere).

amnesia (amnē′zēə, -zhə), *n* the lack or loss of memory.

amnesiac (amnē′zēak), *n* a person affected by amnesia.

amnesic (amnē′zik), *n/adj* affected with, or characterized by, amnesia.

amnestic (amnes′tik), *adj* amnesic; causing amnesia.

amniotic fluid (am′nēot′ik), *n* a serum within the amniotic sac in which the embryo is immersed and cushioned.

amniotic sac, *n* a thin membrane that completely surrounds the embryo and contains a protective fluid in which the embryo is immersed. Also called the *amnion.*

amobarbital/amobarbital sodium (am′ōbär′bital), *n brand name:* Amytal; *drug class:* barbiturate

A

sedative-hypnotic (Controlled Substance Schedule II); *action:* nonselective depression of CNS ranging from sedation to hypnosis to anesthesia to coma, depending on dose administered; *uses:* sedation, preanesthetic sedation, insommia, anticonvulsant, adjunct in psychiatry, hypnotic.

amoeba (əmē′bə), *n* a Rhizopod protozoa that uses extensions of its cytoplasm, called pseudopodia, to move. Some varieties of amoebae are implicated in human infection. Also spelled *ameba(s).*

amorphous (āmôr′fus, əmôr′fus), *adj* having no specific space lattice, the molecules being distributed at random.

amortization, *n* a generic term that includes various specific practices, such as depreciation, depletion, write-off of intangibles, prepaid expenses, and deferred charges.

amoxapine (əmok′səpēn), *n brand name:* Asendin; *drug class:* tricyclic antidepressant; *action:* inhibits both norepinephrine and serotonin (5-HT) uptake in brain; *uses:* depression.

amoxicillin trihydrate (əmok′-səsil′in trīhī′drāt), *n brand names:* Amoxil, Apo-Amoxi, Novamoxin, Nu-Amoxi and others; *drug class:* aminopenicillin; *action:* interferes with cell wall replication of susceptible organisms; *uses:* sinus infections, pneumonia, otitis media, skin, urinary tract infections. This is a drug of choice for antibiotic premedication for patients at risk for bacterial endocarditis unless there is an allergy to penicillin-related antibiotics.

amoxicillin/clavulanate potassium, *n brand names:* Augmentin, Clavulin; *drug class:* aminopenicillin with a β-lactamase inhibitor; *action:* interferes with cell wall replication of susceptible organisms; *uses:* sinus infections, pneumonia, otitis media, skin, urinary tract infections; effective for strains of *E. coli, H. influenzae, S. pneumoniae,* and β-lactamase-producing organisms.

ampere (am′pir), *n* (Amp), a unit of measurement of the quantity of electric current, equal to a flow of 1 coulomb per second or 6.25 time 10^{18} electrons per second. The current produced by 1 volt acting through a resistance of 1 ohm.

amphetamines (amfet′əmēnz′), *n.pl* a group of nervous system stimulants that are subject to abuse because of their ability to reduce appetite and produce wakefulness and euphoria. Abuse of amphetamines may lead to compulsive behavior, paranoia, hallucinations, and suicidal tendencies.

amphotericin B, topical (am′fəter′əsin), *n brand name:* Fungizone; *drug class:* polyene antifungal; *action:* increases cell membrane permeability in susceptible organisms by binding to sterols; *uses:* cutaneous, mucocutaneous infections caused by *Candida.*

ampicillin (am′pisil′in), *n* an acid-stable semisynthetic penicillin antibiotic with a broader spectrum of effectiveness than penicillin G.

amputation neuroma, *n* See neuroma, traumatic.

amputation, root, *n* the removal of a root of a multirooted tooth.

amylase (am′ilās), *n* an enzymatic protein essential for changing starches into sugars.

amyloid (am′əloid′), *n* a starchlike protein-carbohydrate complex that is deposited abnormally in some tissues during certain chronic disease states, such as amyloidosis, rheumatoid arthritis, and tuberculosis.

amyloidosis (am′iloidō′sis), *n* a condition in which amyloid, a glycoprotein, is deposited intercellularly in tissues and organs. Four types of amyloidosis are recognized, two of which, primary amyloidosis and amyloid tumor, frequently produce nodules in the tongue and gingiva.

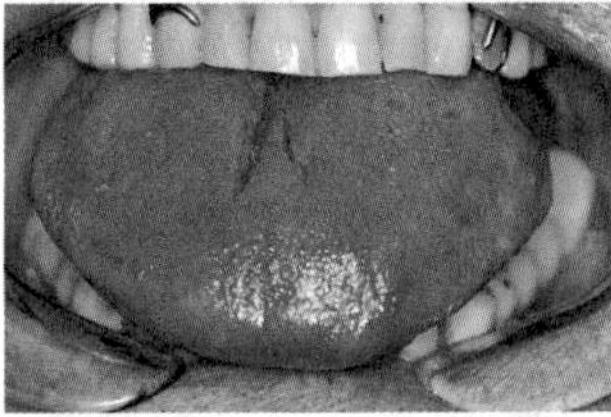

Amyloidosis. (Regezi/Sciubba/Jordan, 2008)

amyloidosis, primary, *n* a type occurring without a known predisposing cause. Amyloid deposits are found in the tongue, lips, skeletal muscles, and other mesodermal structures. The disease may be manifested by polyneuropathy, purpura, hepatosplenomegaly, heart failure, and the nephrotic syndrome.

amyloidosis, secondary, *n* a type occurring secondary to chronic diseases such as tuberculosis, leprosy, rheumatoid arthritis, multiple myeloma, and prolonged bacterial infections. Amyloid deposits are found in parenchymal organs. The disease is usually manifested by proteinuria and hepatosplenomegaly.

amyotonia (ā′mīōtō′nēə), *n* an abnormal flaccidity or flabbiness of a muscle or group of muscles.

amyotrophic lateral sclerosis (ALS) (ā′mīətrō′fik lat′ərəl sklərō′sis), *n* a degenerative disease of the motor neurons, characterized by atrophy of the muscles of the hands, forearms, and legs, and spreading to involve most of the body. Colloquial term is Lou Gehrig's disease.

anabolic steroids, *n.pl* a group of compounds derived from testosterone or prepared synthetically to promote general growth. Anabolic steroids are used in the treatment of aplastic anemia, anemias associated with renal failure, myeloid metaplasia, and leukemia. Anabolic steroids are subject to abuse to promote muscle mass in athletes.

anabolism (ənab′əlizəm), *n* the constructive process by which substances are converted from simple to complex forms by living cells; constructive metabolism.

anaerobe (an′ərōb), *n* a microorganism that can exist and grow only in the partial or complete absence of molecular oxygen.

anaerobe, facultative **(fak′ultātiv),** *n* an organism that can grow in the absence or presence of oxygen.

analeptic (an′əlep′tik), *n* **1.** an agent that acts to overcome depression of the central nervous system. *n* **2.** a strong central nervous system stimulant that is used to restore consciousness, especially from a drug-induced coma.

analgesia (an′əljē′zēə), *n* an insensibility to pain without loss of consciousness; a state in which painful stimuli are not perceived or interpreted as pain; usually induced by a drug, although trauma or a disease process may produce a general or regional analgesia.

analgesia, diagnostic, *n* the administration of a local anesthetic to determine the location, source, or cause of pain.

analgesia, endotracheal **(en′dətrā′kēəl),** *n* an inhalation technique in which the anesthetic agent and respiratory gases are passed through a tube inserted in the trachea via either the nose or oral cavity.

analgesia, infiltration, *n* the arrest of the sensory responses of nerve endings at the surgical site by injections of an anesthetic at that site.

analgesia, insufflation, *n* the delivery of anesthetic gases or vapors directly to the airway of a patient while he or she is breathing room air. Insufflation is usually an open drop method.

analgesia, intranasal, *n* the delivery of an analgesic agent to the membrane of the nose by either topical application or insufflation.

analgesia, nonnarcotic, *n* drugs that relieve pain by action at the site of the pain. Generally, nonnarcotic analgesics do not produce tolerance or dependence.

analgesia, patient-controlled, *n* mechanisms by which the patient can administer and/or control the application of an analgesic agent to an area. One such mechanism is the use of transcutaneous electric nerve stimulation (TENS) to control facial pain. The TENS unit is a variable controlled device designed to deliver a controlled electrical stimulus to the skin surface overlying a painful muscle.

analgesia, regional, *n* the reversible loss of pain sensation over an area by blocking the afferent conduction of its innervation with a local anesthetic agent.

analgesic (anəljē′zik), *adj* (analgetic), **1.** the property of a drug that enables it to raise the pain threshold (e.g., nitrous oxide). *n* **2.** an analgesic may be classified in one of two groups: an analgesic that blocks the sensory neural pathways of pain (e.g., xylocaine) or an analgesic that acts directly on the thalamus to raise the pain threshold.

analgetic (anəljet′ik), *adj* See analgesic.

analgia (anal′jēə), *n* an absence of pain.

analysis (ənal′isis), *n* a separation into component parts.

analysis, anthropometric **(an′thrəpəmet′rik),** *n* a study of the human body that uses such tools as body mass index, basal metabolic rate, bioelectrical impedance, and dual energy radiograph absorptiometry, along with measurements of skinfold thickness and arm muscle circumference, to assess the structure, form, and composition of the body for purposes of comparison.

analysis, bite mark, *n* a technique in forensic dentistry for comparing a bite mark to a dental cast for purposes of identifying the person who made the mark.

analysis, cephalometric **(sef′əlōmet′rik),** *n* the evaluation of the growth pattern or morphologic conoval of teeth, modification of the contour after the removal of teeth, and preparation of the oral cavity for dentures.

analysis, dietary, *n* a comparison of an individual's typical food choices with those recommended in the Food Guide Pyramid; deviations are noted, and recommendations are given.

analysis, occlusal, *n* a study of the relations of the occlusal surfaces of the opposing teeth and their functional harmony.

analyzing rod, *n* See rod, analyzing.

anamnesis (an′amnē′sis), *n* a history of disease or injury based on the patient's memory or recall at the time of dental and/or medical interview and examination.

anaphylactic (an′əfilak′tik), *adj* pertaining to decreasing, rather than increasing, immunity.

anaphylactic hypersensitivity, *n* (Arthus' reaction), a local tissue response that is the result of an Ag-AB reaction caused by repeated intradermal injections with one antigen, resulting in inflammation and necrosis.

anaphylactoid (an′əfilak′toid), *adj* resembling anaphylaxis; pertaining to a reaction, the symptoms of which resemble those of the anaphylactic response produced by the injection of serum and other nonspecific proteins.

anaphylactoid reaction, *n* See reaction, anaphylactoid.

anaphylaxis (an′əfilak′sis), *n* a violent allergic reaction characterized by sudden collapse, shock, or respiratory and circulatory failure after injection of an allergen.

anaplasia (an′əplā′zhə), *n* a regressive change in cells toward a more primitive or embryonic cell type. It is a prominent characteristic of malignancy in tumors.

anasarca (an′əsär′kə), *n* (dropsy), generalized edema.

anastomosis (pl. anastomoses) (ənas′təmō′sis), *n* the joining together of two blood vessels or other tubular structures to furnish a direct or indirect communication between the two structures.

anastomosis graft, *n* the connection of two autogenous tubular structures as a part of reconstructive surgery.

anatomic (anətom′ik), *adj* pertaining to the anatomy of a structure.

anatomic dead space, *n* the actual capacity of the respiratory passages that extend from the nostrils to and including the terminal bronchioles.

anatomic form, *n* See form, anatomic.

anatomic height of contour, *n* See contour, height of.

anatomic impression, *n* See impression, anatomic.

anatomic landmark, *n* See landmark, anatomic.

anatomic teeth, *n.pl* See tooth, anatomic.

anatomical root, *n* See root.

anatomical crown, *n* See crown, anatomical.

anatomy (ənat′ōmē), *n* the science of the form, structure, and parts of animal organisms.

anatomy, dental, *n* the science of the structure of the teeth and the relationship of their parts. The study involves macroscopic and microscopic components.

anatomy, radiographic, *n* the images on a radiographic film of the combined anatomic structures through which the roentgen rays (radiographs) have passed.

ANB angle, *n* a cephalometric measurement of the anterior-posterior relationship of the maxilla with the mandible.

anchorage, *n* **1.** the supporting base for orthodontic forces applied to stimulate tooth movement. *n* **2.** the area of application of the reciprocal forces generated when corrective forces are applied to teeth. Anchorage units may be one tooth or more or may include a portion of the neck or cranium.

anchorage bends, *n.pl* bends placed in an orthodontic wire to enhance the resistance to the anterior displacement of teeth during orthodontic treatment; primarily used in the Tweed and Begg techniques.

anchorage, cervical, *n* an extraoral anchorage based at the back of the neck.

anchorage, cranial, *n* an extraoral anchorage based at the back of the skull.

anchorage, extraoral, *n* in orthodontics, an orthodontic anchorage based outside the oral cavity. Dental attachments are typically linked to a wire bow or hooks extending between the lips and attached elastically to a cap, a strap around the neck, or another extraoral device.

anchorage, facial, *n* an extraoral anchorage based on the face, usually the chin or forehead.

anchorage, intermaxillary, *n* an anchorage based in the opposite jaw.

anchorage, intramaxillary, *n* an anchorage based on teeth within the same jaw.

anchorage, intraoral, *n* an anchorage based within the oral cavity (intermaxillary, intramaxillary, or myofunctional).

anchorage, occipital, *n* a cranial anchorage based in the occipital area.

anchorage, reciprocal, *n* all anchorage is reciprocal; sometimes used to describe a force system in which the resistance units are similar.

anchorage, simple, *n* the use of a tooth as a resistance unit without tipping control.

anchorage, stationary, *n* a genus of Nematoda commonly known as *hookworm.*

Andresen appliance, *n.pr* See appliance, Andresen.

androgen (an′drōjen), *n* a substance that possesses masculinizing qualities, such as testosterone.

anemia (ənē′mēə), *n* a term indicating that the concentration of hemoglobin or the number of red blood cells is below the accepted normal value with respect to age and gender. In true anemia the total concentration of hemoglobin, or the total number of erythrocytes, is below normal regardless of concentration values. Symptoms, which may not be evident, include weakness, pallor, anorexia, and those related to the cause of the anemia.

anemia, Addison-Biermer, *n.pr* See anemia, pernicious.

anemia, aplastic, *n* a type characterized by a decrease in all marrow elements, including platelets, red blood cells, and granulocytes.

anemia, Biermer's, *n.pr* See anemia, pernicious.

anemia, Cooley's, *n.pr* See thalassemia major.

anemia, displacement, *n* See anemia, myelophthisic.

anemia, erythroblastic, *n* See thalassemia major.

anemia, hemolytic, *n* a type characterized by an increased rate of destruction of red blood cells, reticulocytosis, hyperbilirubinemia, and/or increased urinary and fecal urobilinogen, and, generally, splenic enlargement. Hereditary ones include congenital hemolytic jaundice, sickle cell anemia, oval cell anemia, and thalassemia. Included are paroxysmal nocturnal hemoglobinuria and those caused by immune mechanisms (erythroblastosis fetalis), transfusions of incompatible blood, infections, drugs, and poisons. Autoimmune ones are acquired hemolytic anemias associated with antibody-like substances that may not be true autoantibodies or even antibodies; they may be primary (idiopathic), or they may be secondary to lymphoma, lymphatic leukemia, disseminated lupus erythematosus, or sensitization to drugs and pollens.

anemia, hemorrhagic **(hem′əraj′ik),** *n* a type due to deficiency in red blood cells and/or hemoglobin resulting from excessive bleeding.

anemia, hyperchromic, *n* a type in which the erythrocytes are larger than normal so that the content but not the concentration of hemoglobin is increased.

anemia, hypochromic, *n* a type caused by impaired hemoglobin synthesis resulting from a deficiency of iron or pyridoxine and from chronic lead poisoning.

anemia, iron deficiency, *n* a type resulting from a deficiency of iron, characterized by hypochromic microcytic erythrocytes and a normoblastic reaction of the bone marrow. Iron deficiency may result from an increased demand during growth or repeated pregnancies; chronic or recurrent hemorrhage such as from menstrual abnormalities, hemorrhoids, or peptic ulcer; a low intake of iron; or impaired absorption, as often occurs with chronic diarrhea.

anemia, macrocytic normochromic **(mak′rəsit′ik nor′məkrō′mik),** *n* a type related to a failure of nucleoprotein synthesis caused by a deficiency of vitamin B_{12}, folic acid, or related substances.

anemia, Mediterranean, *n* See thalassemia major.

anemia, megaloblastic, *n* a type characterized by hyperplastic bone marrow changes and maturation arrest resulting from a dietary deficiency, impaired absorption, impaired storage and modification, or impaired use of one or more hematopoietic factors. Included are pernicious anemia, nutritional macrocytic anemias associated with gastrointestinal disturbances, anemias associated with impaired liver function (e.g., macrocytic anemia of pregnancy), hypothyroidism, leukemia, and achrestic anemia.

anemia, microcytic hypochromic, *n* a type in which the mean corpuscular volume (MCV), mean corpuscular hemoglobin (MCH) content, and mean corpuscular hemoglobin concentration (MCHC) are all low (e.g., iron deficiency anemia, hereditary leptocytosis, hemoglobin C anemia, and anemias resulting from pyridoxine deficiency and chronic lead poisoning).

anemia, myelophthisic **(mī′əloffthizik),** *n* (displacement anemia), a type resulting from displacement or crowding out of erythropoietic cells of the bone marrow by foreign tissue, as in leukemia, metastatic carcinoma, lymphoblastoma, multiple myeloma, osteoradionecrosis, and xanthomatosis.

anemia, normocytic normochromic **(nor′məsit′ik nor′məkrō′mik),** *n* a type associated with disturbances of red cell formation and related to endocrine deficiencies, chronic inflammation, and carcinomatosis.

anemia, nutritional macrocytic, *n* macrocytic normochromic type occurring as a result of a deficiency of substances necessary for deoxyribonucleic acid synthesis; e.g., vitamin B_{12} and folic acid deficiency may result from a lack of intrinsic factors, sprue, or regional enteritis or with chronic alcoholism, as a result of a diet deficient in meats and vegetables, and in diseases causing intestinal malabsorption.

anemia, oval cell, *n* See elliptocytosis.

anemia, pernicious **(per′nishəs),** *n* (Addison-Biermer anemia), a macrocytic normochromic (megaloblastic) type associated with achlorhydria and lack of a gastric intrinsic factor necessary for the binding and absorption of vitamin B_{12}, which is an erythrocyte maturing factor. In addition to hematologic findings, atrophic glossitis and gastrointestinal and nervous disorders occur.

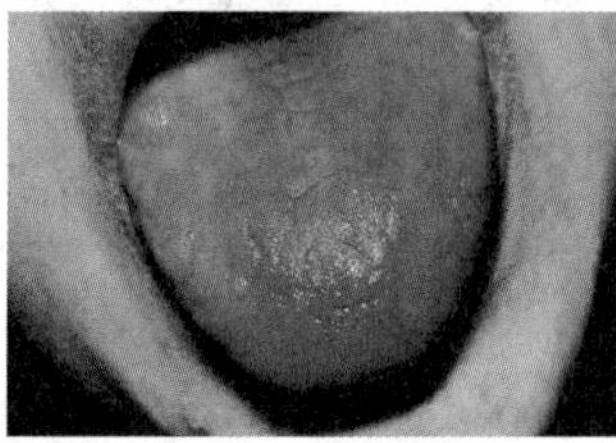

Pernicious anemia. (Sapp/Eversole/Wysocki, 2004)

anemia, physiologic, *n* a type characterized by lowered blood values resulting from an increase in plasma volume that occurs most markedly during the sixth and seventh months of pregnancy.

anemia, sickle cell, *n* (drepanocythemia, sicklemia), a hereditary hemolytic type in which the presence of an abnormal hemoglobin (hemoglobin S) results in distorted, sickle-shaped erythrocytes. Manifestations include episodic crises of muscle, joint, and abdominal pain; neurologic symptoms; and leg ulcers. Sickle cell anemia occurs almost exclusively in African Americans. See also trait, sickle cell.

anemia, spherocytic **(sfē′rōsit′ik),** *n* See jaundice, congenital hemolytic.

anergy (an′urjē), *n* in terms of hypersensitivity, an inability to react to specific antigens (i.e., lack of reaction to intradermally injected antigens in measles, Hodgkin's sarcoma, and overwhelming tuberculosis).

anesthesia (an′esthē′zēə, an′esthē′zhə), *n* the loss of feeling or sensation, especially loss of tactile sensibility, with or without loss of consciousness, resulting from the use of certain drugs or gases that serve as inhibitory neurotransmitters.

anesthesia, basal, *n* a state of narcosis, induced before the administration of a general anesthetic, that permits the production of states of surgical anesthesia with greatly reduced amounts of general anesthetic agents.

anesthesia, block, *n* a local anesthesia induced by injecting the local anesthetic drug close to the nerve trunk, at some distance from the operative field. See also anesthesia, infiltration, and block.

anesthesia, conduction, *n* a local anesthesia induced by injecting the local anesthetic agent close to the nerve trunk, at some distance from the operative field.

anesthesia, general, *n* an irregular, reversible depression of the cells of the higher centers of the central nervous system that makes the patient unconscious and insensible to pain.

anesthesia, glove, *n* an anesthesia with a distribution corresponding to the part of the skin covered by a glove.

anesthesia, infiltration, *n* a local anesthesia induced by injecting the anesthetic agent directly into or around the tissues to be anesthetized; used for operative procedures on the maxillary premolar, anterior teeth, and mandibular incisors. Also called *field block.* See also anesthesia, block.

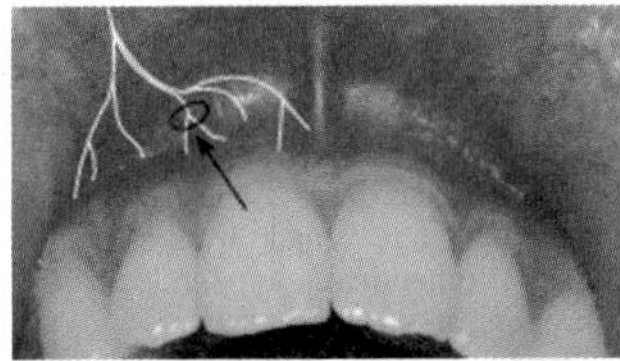

Infiltration anesthesia. (Malamed, 2004)

anesthesia, intraosseous, *n* the local anesthesia produced by the injection of a local anesthetic agent into the cancellous portion of a bone.

anesthesia, intrapulpal, *n* the injection of a local anesthetic agent directly into pulpal tissue under pressure.

anesthesia, local, *n* (regional anesthesia), the loss of pain sensation over a specific area of the anatomy without loss of consciousness.

anesthesia, regional, *n* a term used for local anesthesia. See also anesthesia, local.

anesthesia, topical, *n* a form of local anesthetic agent with which the surface free nerve endings in accessible structures are rendered incapable of stimulation by applying a suitable solution directly to the surface of the area. Used on the surface soft tissue before a local anesthetic injection to anesthetize surface soft tissues for minor operative procedures.

anesthesiologist (an′əsthē′zēol′əjist), *n* a physician specializing in the administration of anesthetics.

anesthesiology (an′isthē′zēol′ōjē), *n* the branch of medicine concerned with the relief of pain and the administration of medication to relieve pain during surgery or other invasive procedures.

anesthetic (an′esthet′ik), *n* a drug that produces loss of feeling or sensation generally or locally.

anesthetic, aerosol spray topical, *n* application of an aerosol spray directly on the surface of a mucous membrane, resulting in loss of nerve conduction.

anesthetic agent, *n* See agent, anesthetic.

anesthetic, allergy to, *n* hypersensitivity to a local agent, which is fairly common with esters but rarely occurs

A

with amides. Allergy to bisulfites in vasoconstrictors also needs to be considered, as well as agents containing sulfites.

anesthetic, amide (am'īd), *n* a local anesthetic agent made from a specific class of chemical compounds that are broken down by the liver and are generally considered more effective and longer-lasting than esters. This type of anesthetic rarely causes allergic reactions.

anesthetic, antioxidants in, *n* a preservative substance added by the manufacturer to a local anesthetic cartridge containing a vasoconstrictor. Metabisulfite and sodium bisulfite are the most commonly used antioxidants.

anesthetic, cartridge, *n* a capsulelike vessel containing the local anesthetic solution that is inserted into the syringe in preparation for an injection. Older term is carpule.

anesthetic, ester, *n* a short-acting local anesthetic agent made from a specific class of chemical compounds that are broken down by blood enzymes. They are less effective than amide anesthetics and more likely to cause allergic reactions. No longer used as an injection in the United States but still used as a topical agent. See also benzocaine.

anesthetic, hydrophilic group **(hī'drōfil'ik),** *n* a portion of a local anesthetic agent's chemical structure, with strong water-attracting properties that enable the diffusion of the agent through the water portions of the tissues to the final destination in the nerves. Typically described in opposition to the lipophilic portion of a local anesthetic agent.

anesthetic, intermediate chain linkage, *n* the connecting linkage between the lipophilic and hydrophilic portions of a local anesthetic agent's chemical structure. Local anesthetic agent's classification is performed on the basis of whether the intermediate chain is made up of an ester or an amide. See also ester and amide.

anesthetic, lipophilic group **(lip'əfil'ik),** *n* a portion of a local anesthetic agent's chemical structure, with its fat-attracting properties that enable the agent to pass through the lipid-membrane of the tissues in order to reach the nerve destination. Typically described in opposition to the hydrophilic portion of the local anesthetic agent.

anesthetic, local, *n* a drug that, when injected into the tissues and absorbed into a nerve, will temporarily interrupt its property of conduction. See also anesthetic, ester and anesthetics, amide.

anesthetic, topical, *n* a drug applied to the surface of the skin or mucosal tissues that produces local insensibility to pain. See also benzocaine.

anesthetist (ənes'thətist), *n* a person who administers anesthetics.

anesthetize (ənes'thətīz), *v* to place under anesthesia.

aneurysm (an'yōōrizəm), *n* a localized dilation of an artery in which one or more layers of the vessel walls are distended.

aneurysm, arteriovenous, *n* See shunt, arteriovenous.

angiitis, visceral (an'jēī'tis), *n* See disease, collagen.

angina (anjīnə), *n* a spasmodic, choking pain. The term is sometimes applied to the disease producing the pain (e.g., Ludwig's angina).

angina, agranulocytic **(ā'gran'yəlōsit'ik),** *n* See agranulocytosis.

angina, Ludwig's, *n.pr* a cellulitis involving the submandibular space and characterized clinically by a firm swelling of the floor of the oral cavity, with elevation of the tongue.

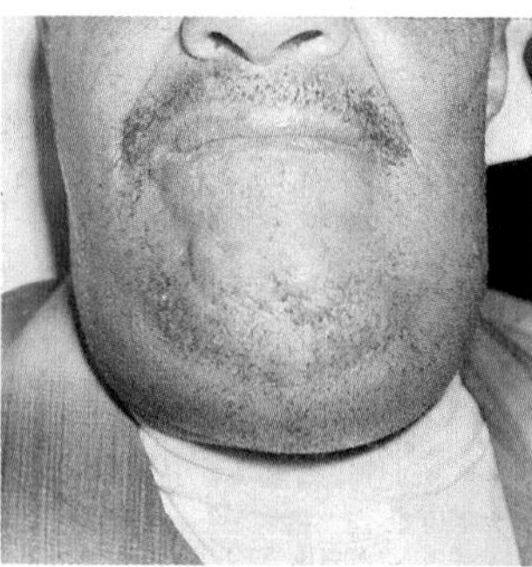

Ludwig's angina. (Courtesy Dr. Charles Babbush)

angina, monocytic, *n* a "sore throat" associated with infectious mononucleosis.

angina pectoris, *n* a symptom of cardiovascular diseases; characterized by a severe, viselike pain behind the sternum that sometimes radiates to the arms, neck, or mandible. It also includes a sense of constriction or pressure of the chest. Angina pectoris is caused by exertion or excitement and is relieved by rest.

angina, Vincent's, *n* an older term for involvement of the pharynx by the spread of necrotizing ulceromembranous gingivitis. See also gingivitis, necrotizing ulcerative.

angioedema (angioneurotic edema, Quincke's disease) (an'jēō-ədē'mə), *n* the spontaneous swelling of the lips, cheeks, eyelids, tongue, soft palate, pharynx, and glottis, frequently associated with allergy to food or drugs and lasting from several hours to several days. Involvement of the glottis results in obstruction of the airway.

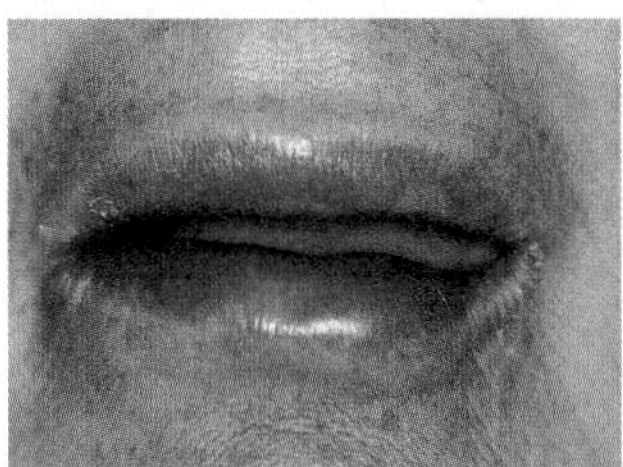

Angioedema. (Regezi/Sciubba/Pogrel, 2000)

angiography (an'jēog'rəfē), *n* the radiographic visualization of the internal anatomy of the heart and blood vessels after the intravascular introduction of radiopaque contrast medium.

angioma (an'jēō'mə), *n* a benign tumor of vascular nature. See also hemangioma and lymphangioma.

angiomatosis, Sturge-Weber (an'jēōmətō'sis sturj'-web'ər), *n.pr* an encephalofacial angiomatosis characterized by cutaneous facial cerebral angiomatosis, ipsilateral gyriform calcifications of the brain, mental retardation, seizures, contralateral hemiplegia, and ocular involvement. The facial lesions (port-wine stain) may present along with intraoral angiomas on the buccal mucosa and gingival tissues.

angioneurotic edema (an'jē-ōnyōōrot'ik), *n* See edema, angioneurotic.

angioplasty (an'jēəplas'tē), *n* a medical procedure used to treat angina or blockage of the coronary arteries. The procedure involves the insertion of a balloon-tipped catheter into the body through a small incision, usually in the groin. The catheter is guided to the blockage using radiographs and injected dye. Once the blockage is reached, the balloon on the catheter is gently inflated to open the blood vessel. Also called *percutaneous transluminal coronary angioplasty (PTCA).*

angle, *n* the degree of divergence of two or more lines or planes that meet each other; the space between such lines. Measured in degrees of an arc.

angle, bayonet former, *n* a hoe-shaped, paired cutting instrument; biangled with the blade parallel with the axis of the shaft. The cutting edge is not perpendicular to the axis of the blade. Used to accentuate angles in an "invisible" class 3 cavity.

angle, Bennett, *n* the angle formed by the sagittal plane and the path of the advancing condyle during lateral mandibular movement, as viewed in the horizontal plane.

angle board, *n* a device used to facilitate the establishment of reproducible angular relationships between a patient's head, the radiographic beam, and the radiograph film.

angle, cavosurface **(kā'vōsur'fəs),** *n* the angle in a prepared cavity, formed by the junction of the wall of the cavity with the surface of the tooth.

angle, contact, *n* the angle at which a liquid or vapor meets a solid surface; e.g., the angle at which a droplet of water rests on an oily surface.

angle, cranial base, *n* the angle formed by a line representing the floor of the anterior cranial fossa intersecting a line representing the axis of the clivus of the base of the skull.

angle, cusp, *n* **1.** the angle made by the slopes of a cusp with the plane that passes through the tip of the cusp and is perpendicular to a line bisecting the cusp; measured mesiodistally

A

or buccolingually. Half of the included angle between the buccolingual or mesiodistal cusp inclines. *n* **2.** the angle made by the slopes of a cusp with a perpendicular line bisecting the cusp; measured mesiodistally or buccolingually.

angle, facial, *n* an anthropometric expression of the degree of protrusion of the lower face, assessed by measuring the inclination of the facial plane relative to a horizontal reference plane.

angle, former, *n* a paired, hoe-shaped cutting instrument that has the cutting edge at an angle other than a right angle in relation to the axis of the blade.

angle, Frankfort-mandibular incisor (FMIA) **(frank′fərt-mandib′yələr insī′zər),** *n* a measure of the mandibular incisor to the Frankfort horizontal plane.

angle, incisal **(insī′zal),** *n* the degree of slope between the axis-orbital plane and the palatal discluding skidway of the maxillary incisor.

angle, incisal guidance, *n* the angle formed with the occlusal plane by drawing a line in the sagittal plane between the incisal edges of the maxillary and mandibular central incisors when the teeth are in centric occlusion.

angle, incisal guide, *n* the inclination of the incisal guide on the articulator.

angle, lateral incisal guide, *n* the inclination of the incisal guide in the frontal plane.

angle, line, *n* an angle formed by the junction of the two walls along a line; designated by combining the names of the walls forming the angle.

angle, occlusal rest, *n* the angle formed by the occlusal rest with the upright minor connector.

angle of mandible, *n* an angle at the intersection of the posterior and inferior borders of the ramus.

angle, point, *n* an angle formed by the junction of three walls at a common point; designated by combining the names of the walls forming the angle.

angle, prophylaxis **(prōfəlak′sis),** *n* the term for an angled instrument that holds a rubber cup or bristle brush used to polish teeth. It may be either contra- or right-angled. May also be called a *prophy angle.*

angle, protrusive incisional guide, *n* the inclination of the incisal guide in the sagittal plane.

angle, rest, *n* See angle, occlusal rest.

angle, symphyseal **(sim′fisē′əl),** *n* the angle of the chin, which may be protruding straight or receding, according to type.

Angle's classification of malocclusion (modified), *n.pr* a classification of the different forms of malocclusion. See also malocclusion.

Class I, *n* the normal anteroposterior relationship of the mandible to the maxillae. The mesiobuccal cusp of the permanent maxillary first molar occludes in the buccal groove of the permanent mandibular first molar.

Type I, *n.pr* dentition in linguoversion.

Type II, *n.pr* with narrow arches; labioversion of the maxillary anterior teeth and linguoversion of the mandibular anterior teeth.

Type III, *n.pr* with linguoversion of the maxillary anterior teeth; crowded; lack of development in the proximal region.

Class II, *n.pr* the posterior relationship of the mandible to the maxillae. The mesiobuccal cusp of the permanent maxillary first molar occludes mesial to the buccal groove of the permanent mandibular first molar.

Division 1, *n.pr* with labioversion of the maxillary teeth.

Subdivision, *n.pr* signifies a unilateral condition.

Division 2, *n.pr* with linguoversion of the maxillary central incisor teeth.

Subdivision, *n.pr* signifies a unilateral condition.

Class III, *n.pr* the anterior relationship of the mandible to the maxillae, may have a subdivision. The mesiobuccal cusp of the permanent maxillary first molar occludes distal to the buccal groove of the permanent mandibular first molar.

Type I, *n.pr* with good alignment generally but arch relationship abnormal.

Type II, *n.pr* with good alignment of the maxillary anterior teeth but linguoversion of the mandibular anterior teeth.

Type III, n.pr an underdeveloped maxillary arch; linguoversion of maxillary anterior teeth; good mandibular alignment.

angled shank, *n* an adaptation to the design of a handheld instrument in order to allow easier access to posterior teeth or to individual tooth surfaces which might otherwise be difficult to reach. See also instrument, hand.

angstrom (Å) unit (ang′strəm), *n* See unit, angstrom.

angular cheilitis (kīlī′təs), *n* a disease that most often occurs among the elderly but is caused by parasitic fungi, along with bacterial involvement, or a deficiency in vitamin B rather than age; angular cheilitis appears as skin lesions on the lips, particularly as breaks in the tissue at the corners of the oral cavity (commissures). Often occurs in conjunction with reduced mobility and strength in the oral cavity. See perlèche.

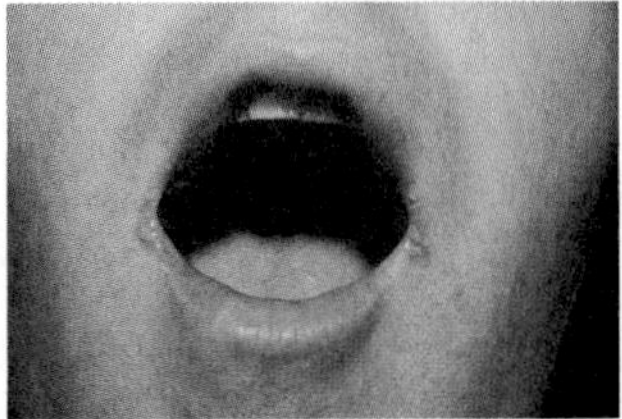

Angular cheilitis. (Courtesy Dr. Donald Schermer)

angular cheilosis, *n* See cheilosis, angular.

angular thickening, *n* a widening of the periodontal space between the periodontal ligament and the root of a tooth that indicates the presence of periodontal disease, possibly that of trauma or infection. This shows up on radiographs as a thick radiolucent line next to the root.

angulation (instrumental) (ang′gyōōlā′shən), *n* the angle formed between the blade of an instrument and a tooth or tissue to provide increased access and more effective treatment.

angulation, bisecting error, n See bisecting-the-angle error.

angulation, bisecting-angle technique, n the proper angle to take a periapical survey radiograph using the bisecting angle technique. Horizontally angled so that the ray passes through the interproximal space as close to the center of the area being radiographed as possible, and vertically angled so that the ray travels perpendicular to the bisection of the angle formed by the film and the long axes of the targeted teeth.

angulation for air-powder polishing, n the correct angle at which the polisher's handpiece must be positioned in order to reduce the backflow of aerosol spray during treatment. The position varies according to tooth position and surface.

angulation, horizontal, n the angle measured within the occlusal plane at which the central ray of the radiographic beam is projected relative to a reference point in the vertical or sagittal plane.

angulation, mandibular midline projection, n the proper angle to take a mandibular midline radiograph. The position-indicating device should be pointed at the end of the chin at a –55° angle to the film for a view of the incisal region. To view the floor of the oral cavity, the position-indicating device should be perpendicular to the film, directly below the chin.

angulation, maxillary midline projection, n the proper angle to take a maxillary midline radiograph. The position-indicating device should be aimed at a +65° angle at the bridge of the nose.

angulation of central ray/beam, n the horizontal and vertical angles at which the central ray is aimed. Too much horizontal angulation causes superimposed images, while too much vertical angulation causes foreshortening. Also, too little vertical angulation causes elongation of the image.

angulation, paralleling technique, n the technique that gives the proper angle for taking a periapical radiograph using the paralleling technique. The central ray should be directed through the interproximal area roughly at the center of the film while the vertical angle should be at a precise right angle to the film. This is sometimes preferable because, un-

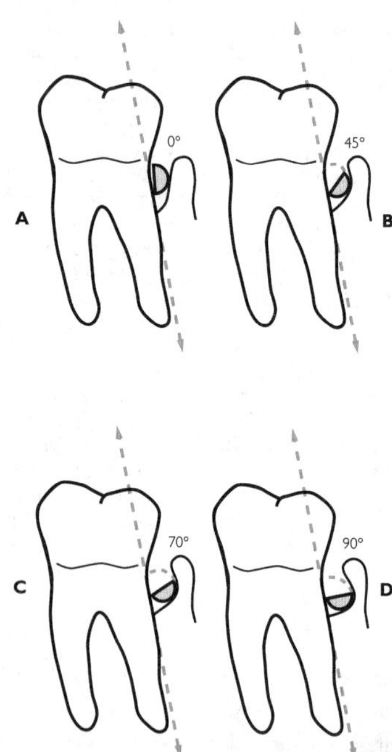

Instrumental angulation. A, Ideal initial placement. **B,** Too close to effectively remove calculus. **C,** Ideal for debridement. **D,** Too open. (Daniel/Harfst/Wilder, 2008)

like the bisecting angle technique, no radiographs are directed at the thyroid.

angulation, vertical, *n* the angle measured within the vertical plane at which the central ray of the radiographic beam is projected relative to a reference in the horizontal or occlusal plane.

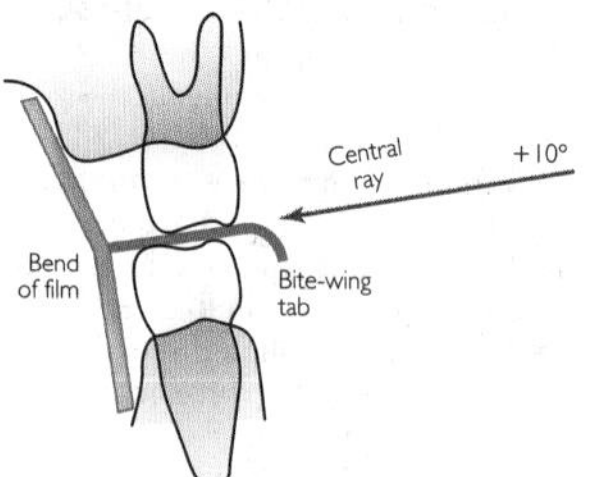

Vertical angulation. (Iannucci/Jansen Howerton, 2006)

angulation (radiographic) (ang′-gyōōlā′shən), *n* the direction of the primary beam of radiation in relation to object and film.

anhidrosis (an′hīdrō′sis), *n* a severe deficiency in the production of sweat; may be associated with hypodontia or anodontia in ectodermal dysplasia.

anhidrotic ectodermal dysplasia (an′hīdrot′ik ek′tōder′məl displā′zhə), *n* See hypohidrotic ectodermal dysplasia.

anhydrous (anhī′drus), *adj* without water.

anion (an′īən), *n* a negatively charged ion.

anionic detergent (an′īon′ik), *n* See detergent, anionic.

anirodia (an′irō′dēə), *n* the absence of the iris. Usually a congenital condition.

anisocytosis (anī′sōsītō′sis), *n* a wide variation in cell size, especially of red blood cells.

anisognathous (an'īsog'nathəs), *adj* having maxillary and mandibular dental arches or jaws that are of different sizes.

anisotropy (an'āsôt'rəpē), *n* the condition of not having properties or characteristics that are the same in all directions.

ankyloglossia (ang'kilōglôs'ēə), *n* an abnormally short lingual frenum that limits movement of the tongue. Method of treatment may involve myofunctional therapy instead of surgical release. Older term: tongue-tie. See also lingual frenum.

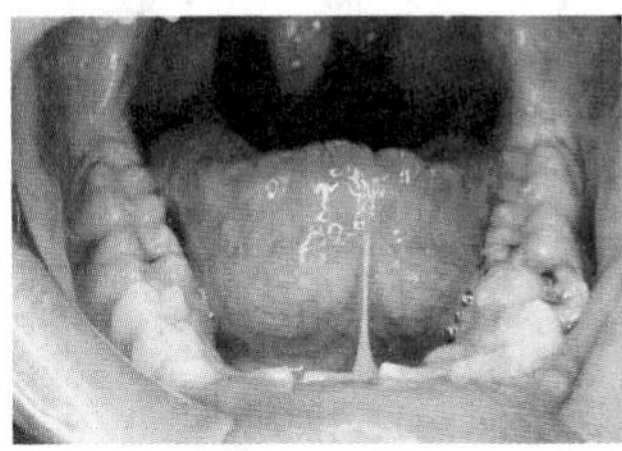

Ankyloglossia. (Ibsen/Phelan, 2004. Courtesy Dr. George Blozis)

ankylosis (ang'kilō'sis), *n* an abnormal fixation and immobility of a joint.

ankylosis, bony, *n* a joining of bone with tooth or bone with bone that causes total loss of movement. See also tooth, ankylosed.

ankylosis, false, *n* an inability to open the oral cavity because of trismus rather than disease of the joint.

ankylosis, fibrous, *n* the fixation of a joint by fibrous tissue.

ankylosis of tooth, *n* See tooth, ankylosed.

anlage (on'lägə), *n* the first cells in the embryo that form any distinct part or organ.

anneal (anēl'), *n* (homogenizing heat treatment, softening heat treatment), the softening of a metal by controlled heating and cooling.

anneal foil, *n* a process of subjecting noncohesive foil to heat to volatilize a protective gaseous coating on its surface, thus leaving the surface clean, making it cohesive.

anneal glass, *n* a process of regulated heating and subsequent cooling to remove strain hardening or work hardening of glass.

anneal metal, *n* a process of regulated heating and subsequent cooling to remove strain hardening or work hardening of metal.

announcement, *n* a communication, usually printed, that states office policies or practice limitations to the public and profession.

annual reports, *n.pl* the statistical, fiscal, and descriptive yearly reports used to inform a constituency of the status of the institution or organization.

annual statement, *n* the report of an insurer or carrier showing assets and liabilities, receipts and disbursements, and other information for a specified 12-month period (fiscal or calendar year).

anochromasia (an'ōkrōmā'zēə, -zhə), *n* a variation in the staining quality of cells, particularly of degenerating red blood cells.

anociassociation (ənō'sēəsōsēā'-shən), *n* the blocking of neuroses, fear, pain, and harmful influences or associations to prevent shock.

anode (an'ōd), *n* the electrically positive terminal of a roentgen ray (radiographic) tube; a tungsten block embedded in a copper stem and set at an angle of 20° or 45° to the cathode. The anode emits roentgen rays (radiographs) from the point of impact of the electronic stream from the cathode.

anode, rotating, *n* an anode that rotates during radiograph production to present a constantly different focal spot to the electron stream and to permit use of small focal spots or higher tube voltages without overheating the tube.

anodontia (an'ōdon'tēə), *n* (aplasia of dentition), the complete failure of teeth to form; the total absence of teeth.

anodontia, partial, *n* an obsolete term referring to hypodontia or oligodontia.

anodontia, total, *n* an obsolete term referring to anodontia.

anodyne (an'ōdīn), *n* an agent or drug that relieves pain; milder than analgesia.

anomaly (ənom'əlē), *n* an aberration or deviation from normal anatomic growth, development, or function.

A

anomaly, dental, n an abnormality in which a tooth or teeth have deviated from normal in form, function, or position.

anomaly, developmental **(divel′əpmen′təl),** *n* **1.** an abnormality originating in fetal development. **2.** deficiencies or imperfections occurring in the teeth as a consequence of irregular tooth growth.

anomaly, dysgnathic **(disnath′ik),** *n* an older term for an abnormality that extends beyond the teeth and includes the maxillae, the mandible, or both.

anomaly, eugnathic **(yōōnath′ik),** *n* an older term for an abnormality limited to the teeth and their immediate alveolar supports.

anomaly, gestant **(jes′tənt),** *n* See odontoma.

anomaly, maxillofacial, n a distortion of normal development of the face and jaws; a dysgnathic anomaly.

anomaly, oral, n an abnormal structure of the oral cavity other than of the teeth.

anomaly, orofacial, n a term indicating an oral or facial abnormality.

anomaly, root, n a general term for describing any deviation from normal found in a tooth root.

anophaxia (anōfax′ēə), *n* a tendency for one eye to turn upward.

anophthalmos (an′opthal′məs), *n* a congenital absence of all tissues of the eyes.

anorexia (anōrek′sēə), *n* the partial or complete loss of appetite for food.

anorexia nervosa, n a psychoneurotic disorder characterized by a prolonged refusal to eat, resulting in emaciation, amenorrhea in women, emotional disturbance concerning body image, and an abnormal fear of becoming fat. See also disorder, body dysmorphic.

anoxemia (an′oksē′mēə), *n* a deficient aeration of the blood; a total lack of oxygen content in the blood.

anoxia (anok′sēə), *n* a condition of total lack of oxygen; a term frequently misused as a synonym of hypoxia.

anoxic hypoxia, *n* See hypoxia, anoxic.

antagonist, *n* **1.** a drug that counteracts, blocks, or abolishes the action of another drug. *n* **2.** a muscle that acts in opposition to the action of another muscle (e.g., flexor vs. extensor). *n* **3.** a tooth in one jaw that occludes with a tooth in the other jaw.

antagonist, narcotic, n a narcotic drug that acts specifically to reverse depression of the central nervous system.

antagonists, insulin, n.pl the circulating hormonal and nonhormonal substances that stimulate glyconeogenesis (e.g., 11-oxysteroids and S hormones).

ante cibum (an′tē sī′bum), *adv* See a.c.

antegonial notch (an′təgō′nēəl), *n* the notch or concavity usually present at the junction between the ramus and body of the mandible, near the anterior margin of the masseter muscle attachment.

anterior, *adj* **1.** situated in front of. *adj* **2.** a term used to denote the incisor and canine teeth or the forward region of the oral cavity. *adj* **3.** the forward position.

anterior cervical triangle, n See triangle, anterior cervical.

anterior cranial base, n the anterior cranial fossa, sometimes identified by related landmarks such as the sella turcica and nasion.

anterior determinants of occlusion, n.pl See occlusion, anterior determinants of cusp.

anterior discrepancy, n a difference (as in tooth size or another characteristic) between the members of a pair of corresponding teeth in the anterior sextant.

anterior guide, n See guide, anterior.

anterior nasal spine, n See spine, anterior nasal.

anterior palatal bar, n See connector, anterior palatal major.

anterior tooth arrangement, n See arrangement, tooth, anterior.

anterior-posterior discrepancy (antē′rēər-postē′rēər), *n* an anterior-posterior morphologic imbalance between the maxilla and mandible and consequently between structures attached to either.

anterior-posterior spread, *n* a calculation of the greatest amount of cantilever allowed for a dental implant within its bilateral distal ranges. It is measured by determining the distance from the center of the most posterior to the center of the most anterior implants and multiplying by 1.5.

anterocclusion (an′terōklōō′zhən), *n* a malocclusion of the teeth, in which the mandibular teeth are in a position anterior to their normal position relative to the teeth in the maxillary arch.

anteroposterior plane of space, *n* See sagittal plane.

anteversion, *n* the tipping or tilting of teeth or other maxillary and mandibular structures too far forward (anterior) from the normal or generally accepted standard.

anthelmintic (an′thelmin′tik), *n* a drug that acts against parasitic worms, especially intestinal worms.

anthrax (an′thraks), *n* an infectious disease in herbivorous animals caused by a spore-forming *Bacillus* organism. Primary lesions in human beings may be on the lips or cheeks.

anthrocyclanins (an′thrōsī′-klənin z), *n.pl* a group of floral pigments existing as glycosides that may be used as hematoxylin substitutes.

anthropology, *n* the science of human beings ranging from physical characteristics to cultural, social, and environmental aspects.

anthropology, cultural, *n* the study of the interpersonal and community mores of a society or isolate.

anthropology, physical, *n* the study of the physical attributes of a society or isolate.

anthropometry (an′thrəpom′-ətrē), *n* the measurement of the body and its parts.

anti-HAV, *n* a passively acquired antibody to the hepatitis A virus that provides protective immunity against recurrences of the infection. It may be detected in the blood of infected individuals within 14 days after they show the first symptoms of hepatitis A.

anti-HBc, IgM, *n* an antibody to the core antigen of the hepatitis B virus. Its presence in the blood indicates a previous infection with the hepatitis B virus.

anti-HBe, *n* an antibody to the e antigen of the hepatitis B virus. Its detection in the blood indicates the presence of a low-titer hepatitis B infection and decreased ability of the infected person to pass the virus on to another person.

anti-HBs, *n* an antibody to the surface antigen of the hepatitis B virus; indicative of either active immunity to the hepatitis B virus as a result of prior infection or passive immunity from the presence of hepatitis B immunoglobulin in the blood. It may also be an immune response triggered as the result of having received vaccination against the hepatitis B virus.

anti-HCV, *n* an antibody to the hepatitis C virus. Its presence in the blood is indicative of an active or chronic hepatitis C infection.

anti-HDV, *n* an antibody to the hepatitis D virus. Its presence in the blood is indicative of a hepatitis D infection that may be either active, chronic, or under control.

anti-HSV antibodies, *n.pl* an immunoglobulin contained in the fluid of the gingival sulcus that may or may not provide immunity to recurrent attacks of the herpes simplex virus.

antibiotic (an′tibīot′ik), *n* an organic substance produced by one of several microorganisms, especially certain molds, that is capable, in low concentration, of destroying or inhibiting the growth of certain other microorganisms.

antibiotic, oral reactions to, *n* the manifestations on the oral mucous membrane of reactions to antibiotics; characterized by glossitis, angular cheilosis, and/or a hairy tongue. Reactions may result from an imbalance of oral flora produced by the antibiotics or from hypersensitivity to the antibiotics.

antibiotic prophylaxis **(prōfəlak′-sis),** *n* the use of an antibiotic to protect a patient from an anticipated bacterial invasion associated with a medical or dental invasive procedure, particularly patients with a compromised cardiovascular system and risk of bacterial endocarditis.

antibiotic, subgingival placement, *n* the administration of antimicrobials in the subgingival region to control bacterial infections and manage periodontal disease.

antibiotic therapy, *n* See therapy, antibiotic.

Antibiotic: mode of action

Mode of action	*Representative antibiotics*
Inhibition of bacterial cell wall synthesis	Penicillins
Alteration of membrane permeability	Cephalosporins
Inhibition of microbial DNA translation and transcription	Bacitracins
	Polymyxin B
Inhibition of essential metabolite synthesis	Amphotericin B
	Nystatin
	Erythromycin
	Tetracyclines
	Streptomycin
	Lincomycin
	Kanamycin
	Chloramphenicol
	Paraminosalicylic acid
	Sulfonamides

antibody (an′tibodē), *n* **1.** a specific substance that is produced by an animal as a reaction to the presence of an antigen and that reacts specifically with an antigen in some observable way. *n* **2.** an immunoglobulin (preferred term), essential to the immune system, produced by lymphoid tissue in response to bacteria, viruses, or other antigenic substances. Each type is identified by its action, agglutinins, bacteriolysins, opsonins, and precipitins. See also immunoglobulins.

antibody, antinuclear, *n* an antibody having an affinity for the cell nuclei.

antibody formation, *n* the response of the lymphatic system to the presence of foreign substances in the body such as bacteria, viruses, food substances, pollens, and other antigens.

antibody, monoclonal **(mon′ōklon′əl),** *n* an antibody produced by a clone or genetically homogeneous population of hybrid cells.

antibody, specificity, *n* the lymphatic system produces antibodies specific to each antigen. Viruses have the capacity to alter an antigen's genetic makeup, thereby creating a mutant antigen that requires new antibodies to combat it.

antibody-mediated hypersensitivity, *n* **1.** an anaphylactic (Type I) reaction, also known as "immediate"; allergen-induced IgE antibodies remember the target antigen and proliferate against it, producing mediators such as histamines. *n* **2.** a cytotoxic (Type II) reaction; antigens and antibodies come together on the surface of a cell, causing lysis of the cell or other cell membrane damage. *n* **3.** an immune complex (Type III) reaction; a complex of antigens and antibodies that is attracted to tissue.

anticariogenic (an′tīker′ēōjen′ik), *adj* describing foods, chemicals, or other agents that tend to contribute favorably to dental health by remineralizing teeth and discouraging the acid that causes dental caries.

anticariogenic agents (an′tīker′ēōjen′ik), *n.pl* substances that inhibit or arrest dental caries formation. See also fluorides, sealants.

anticholinergic (an′tīkō′linur′jik), *n* (parasympatholytic, cholinolytic), a drug that acts to inhibit the effects of the neurohormone acetylcholine or to inhibit its cholinergic neuroeffects. A cholinergic blocking agent.

anticholinesterase (an′tīkō′lines′tərās), *n* a drug or chemical that inhibits or inactivates the enzyme cholinesterase, resulting in the actions produced by the accumulation of acetylcholine at cholinergic sites.

anticoagulant (an′tīkōag′yələnt), *n* a drug that delays or prevents coagulation of blood.

anticonvulsive (an′tīkonvul′siv), *adj* relieving or preventing convulsion.

antidepressants, *n.pl* agents used to counteract or treat depression.

antidepressants, tricyclic (TCA), *n.pl* a classification of antidepressant drugs used to treat a variety of psychiatric conditions, including mental depression, social phobia, and mood, panic, or obsessive-compulsive disorders, as well as other conditions.

antidiabetes mellitus agents (an′tēdī′əbē′tēz məlī′təs), *n.pl* drugs used to combat diabetes mellitus, particularly insulin; also drugs that combat the common side effects of diabetes mellitus, hypoglycemia, and hyperglycemia. See also diabetes.

antidiarrheals (an′tēdī′ərē′əlz), *n.pl* drugs that combat diarrhea by decreasing gastrointestinal motility; may cause sedation of the central nervous system and xerostomia.

antidote (an′tidōt), *n* a substance that acts to antagonize the toxic effects of a drug, especially in overdose, or of a poison. See also poison.

antidysrhythmics (an′tīdisrith′miks), *n.pl* a misnomer for antiarrhythmia. See antiarrhythmia.

antiemetic (an′tēəmet′ik, an′tīəmet′ik), *n* drug used to prevent, stop, or relieve nausea and emesis (vomiting).

antiepileptic drugs, *n.pl* agents that inhibit or control seizures associated with epilepsy or other conditions.

antifibrinolytics (an′tēfī′brənolit′iks), *n* a type of substance that prevents the breakdown of fibrin in blood clots. Used to prevent excessive bleeding.

antiflux, *n* a material that prevents and confines the flow of solder (e.g., graphite).

antifungal agents, *n.pl* agents that inhibit, control, or kill fungi. The most common yeastlike fungus occurring in or near the oral cavity is *C. albicans.*

antigen (an′tijen), *n* a substance, usually a protein, that elicits the formation of antibodies that react with it when introduced parenterally into an individual or species to which it is foreign. See also immunogens.

antigen, human leukocyte (HLA), *n* the group of genes contained within the major histocompatibility complex (MHC), these antigen-bearing proteins are encoded by multiple genetic loci on human chromosome 6 and are found on the outer regions of the cellular structure.

antigenic drift (an′tējen′ik), *n* the ability of viruses to alter their genetic makeup, thereby creating mutant antigens and bypassing the antibody barrier of the host.

antihemophilic factor (an′tīhē′mōfil′ik), *n* See factor VII.

antihistamine (an′tīhis′təmin), *n* a drug that counteracts the release of histamine such as occurs in allergic reactions; also has topical anesthetic and sedative effects, as well as a drying effect on the nasal mucosa.

antihistaminic (an′tīhistəmin′ik), *adj* referring to a drug that acts to prevent or antagonize the pharmacologic effects of histamine released in the tissues.

antihypertensive drugs, *n.pl* agents that lower or reduce high blood pressure.

antihypnotic (an′tīhipnot′ik), *adj* preventing or hindering sleep. (not current)

antiinflammatory agents, *n.pl* compounds that counteract or reduce inflammation.

antileptic (an′tilep′tik), *adj* assisting, supporting, revulsive.

antimicrobial, systemic, *n* an antimicrobial agent, usually in the form of an antibiotic, that is generally administered orally and absorbed into the bloodstream through the intestine. They move from the circulatory system to the tissues where they reach the periodontal pocket through the gingival sulcus fluid.

antimony, *n* a bluish crystalline metallic element occurring in nature both free and as salts. Antimony compounds are used in the treatment of filariasis, leishmaniasis, and other parasitic diseases. Antimony is also used as an emetic.

antineoplastic agent, *n* a drug that prevents the development, maturation, or spread of neoplastic cells.

antiodontalgic, *adj* pertaining to a toothache remedy.

antioxidants, *n.pl* agents that reduce or prevent oxidation, such as occurs in the deterioration of fats, oils, and nonprecious metals.

antiphlogistic (an′tīflōjis′tik), *adj* an older term for antiinflammatory or antipyretic.

antiplaque agents, *n.pl* compounds that inhibit, control, or kill organisms associated with plaque formation.

A

antipruritic (an′tīprōōrit′ik), *adj* relieving or preventing itching.

antipsychotics (an′tēsīkot′iks), *n.pl* medications used to decrease hallucinations, delusions, and other symptoms associated with schizophrenia and other psychotic disorders; enables functioning in daily life for individuals.

antipyretic (an′tīpīret′ik), *n* a drug that reduces fever primarily through action on the hypothalamus, thereby resulting in increased heat dissipation through augmented peripheral blood flow and sweating.

antipyrine (an′tēpī′rēn), *n* an analgesic and antipyretic used in conjunction with salicylates.

antisepsis (an′tīsep′sis), *n* the prevention of infection of a body surface, usually skin or oral mucosa, through the application of an antimicrobial agent.

antiseptic (an′tisep′tik), *n* an antimicrobial agent for application to a body surface, usually skin or oral mucosa, in an attempt to prevent or minimize infection at the area of application.

antisialic (an′tīsīal′ik), *adj* checking or that which checks salivary secretions.

antisialogogue (an′tīsīal′əgog), *n* a drug that reduces, slows, or prevents the flow of saliva.

antispasmodic (an′tīspazmod′ik), *n* (antispastic), a drug that relieves muscle spasms.

antispastic, *adj* See antispasmodic.

antistreptolysin O (an′tīstreptol′əsin), *n* an antibody against streptolysin O, a hemolysin produced by group A streptococci. A high titer is supporting evidence of rheumatic fever.

antithermic, *adj* reducing temperature. See also antipyretic.

antitoxin (an′tētok′sin), *n* a subgroup of antisera usually prepared from the serum of horses immunized against a particular toxin-producing organism, such as botulism antitoxin and diphtheria antitoxin given prophylactically to prevent those infections.

antitragus (an′titrā′gus), *n* the structure located opposite the tragus, a cartilaginous prominence in front of the external opening of the ear.

antitussive (an′tītus′iv), *n* a drug that relieves or prevents cough.

antrodynia (an′trōdī′nēə), *n* an older term for pain in the maxillary antrum.

antrostomy (antros′təmē), *n* a surgical opening into an antrum, either through the medial wall into the nose or through the lateral wall into the oral cavity.

antrum (an′trum), *n* a general term for cavity or chamber that may have specific meaning in referencing certain organs or sites in the body. For example, referring to paranasal sinuses, the maxillary sinus can be referred to as a maxillary antrum.

antrum, maxillary, *n* See sinus, maxillary.

antrum of Highmore, *n.pl* See sinus, maxillary.

ANUG, *n* the abbreviation for acute necrotizing ulcerative gingivitis. An obsolete term. See gingivitis, necrotizing ulcerative.

anxiety, *n* a condition of heightened and often disruptive tension accompanied by an ill-defined and distressing aura of impending harm or injury. It can disrupt physiologic functions through its effect on the autonomic nervous system. The patient may assume a tense posture, show excessive vigilance, move the hands and feet restlessly, and speak with a strained, uneven voice. The pupils may be widely dilated, giving the appearance of unrestrained fright, and the hands and face may perspire excessively. In extremely acute forms the patient may have generalized visceral reactions of respiratory, cardiac, vascular, and gastrointestinal dysfunction. The dental professional must recognize the existence of it, seek its etiology and relation to dental treatment, and determine ways that the patient's defenses against it can be used to facilitate rather than inhibit treatment.

anxiety control, *n* the combination of measures that are used to eliminate patient apprehension and control pain during the performance of a dental procedure. The determination of the appropriate measures to be taken depends on the patient's overall periodontal health and tolerance for pain, as well as the specific treatment to be delivered.

anxiety neurosis, *n* an extreme manifestation of anxiety characterized by acute anxiety attacks (sympathetic overreactivity) and phobias, causing avoidance of the anxiety-provoking situations.

anxiolytic medication (angk′sē-ōlit′ik), *n* a drug used to decrease emotional stress or anxiety. Also called *antianxiety agent.*

aorta (āor′tə), *n* the main arterial trunk of the systemic circulation. Consists of four parts: the ascending aorta, the arch of the aorta, the thoracic portion of the descending aorta, and the abdominal portion of the descending aorta. Gives rise to the common carotid and subclavian arteries on the left side and to the brachiocephalic artery on the right side.

aortic aneurysm, *n* a localized dilation or ballooning of the wall of the aorta caused by atherosclerosis, hypertension, or a combination.

aortic valve, *n* a valve in the heart between the left ventricle and the aorta; also known as the tricuspid valve.

apathism (ap′əthizm), *n* the state of being slow in responding to stimuli.

apatite (ap′ətīt), *n* the inorganic mineral substance of teeth and bone. See also carbonate hydroxyapatite.

APC, *n* See aspirin, phenacetin, caffeine.

Apert syndrome, *n.pr* See syndrome, Apert.

apertognathia (əpur′tōnath′ēə), *n* an occlusion characterized by a vertical separation between the maxillary and mandibular anterior teeth. Commonly called an *open bite.*

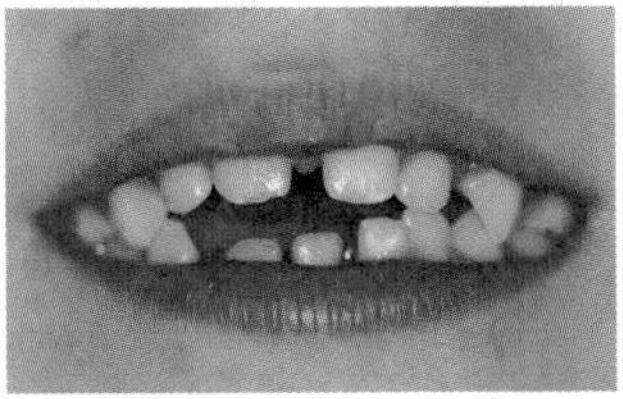

Apertognathia. (Courtesy Dr. David Nunez)

aperture, *n* an opening such as in bone.

apex, *n* **1.** the pointed end of a conical structure. **2.** the end of the root.

apex blunderbuss, *n* an open or everted apex of a tooth, resembling the divergent form of the barrel of a blunderbuss rifle.

apexification (āpek′sifikā′shə), *n* the process of induced root development or apical closure of the root by hard tissue deposition.

apexigraph (āpek′sigraf), *n* a device for determining the position of the apex of a tooth root.

APF, *n* the abbreviation for **acidulated phosphate fluoride.**

aphagia (əfā′jēə), *n* the inability to swallow.

aphasia (əfa′zhə), *n* a loss of power of expression through speech, writing, or signs of comprehension of spoken or written language resulting from disease or injury of the brain centers.

aphtha (af′thə), *n* (aphthous stomatitis), **1.** a small ulcer on the mucous membrane. **-hae** *n.pl* **2.** vesicles that undergo subsequent ulceration and are surrounded by a raised erythematous area.

aphtha, Bednar's **(bed′närz),** *n.pr* (pterygoid ulcer), an ulcer on the soft palate near the greater palatine foramen; seen in newborns.

aphtha, Mikulicz' **(mik′ulich),** *n.pr* a recurrent ulceration of the oral mucosa, resembling herpes. See also periadenitis mucosa necrotica recurrens.

aphtha, recurrent, *n* See stomatitis, herpetic and ulcer, aphthous, recurrent.

aphtha, recurrent scarring, *n* See periadenitis mucosa necrotica recurrens.

aphthosis (afthō′sis), *n* a clinical manifestation of apthae.

aphthous (af′thus), *adj* characterized by aphthae or aphthosis.

aphthous fever, *n* a fever associated with aphthosis.

aphthous pharyngitis **(af′thus far′-injī′tis),** *n* aphthosis of the pharynx.

aphthous stomatitis, *n* See aphtha and stomatitis, aphthous.

apical (ap′ikəl), *adj* pertaining to the end portion of the root.

apical curettage, *n* the surgical removal of diseased tissue surrounding a root apex.

A

apical fiber, *n* See fiber, apical.
apical foramen, *n* See foramen, apical.
apical third, *adj* the inferior third of a tooth's root or root canal.

apicectomy, See apicoectomy.

apicoectomy (ap′ikōek′təmē), *n* (apicectomy, apiectomy, root amputation, root resection), the surgical removal of the apex or apical portion of a root.

***Apicomplexa* protozoa** (ap′ikomplek′sə), *n* a parasitic group that sometimes needs multiple hosts to survive. Some varieties are implicated in diarrhea and malaria.

aplasia (əplā′zhə), *n* a lack of origin or development (e.g., aplasia of dentition associated with ectodermal dysplasia).
aplasia of dentition, *n* See anodontia.

apnea (apnē′ə, ap′nēə), *n* a temporary cessation of respiratory movements.

apneumatic (apnōōmat′ik), *adj* free from air; used to describe something accomplished with the exclusion of air, such as an apneumatic operation. (not current)

apoplexy (ap′ōplek′sē), *n* a sudden loss or decrease of neurologic function often caused by cerebrovascular accident (CVA).

apoptosis (ap′ətō′sis), *n* cell reduction by fragmentation into membrane-bound particles that are phagocytosed by other cells.

apostematosa, cheilitis glandularis (kīlī′təs glan′jəlar′is), *n* See cheilitis glandularis apostematosa.

apothecaries' system (əpoth′əkar′ēz), *n* See system, apothecaries'.

apoxesis (ap′əksē′sis), *n* See curettage, apical.

apparatus (ap′ərat′us), *n* **1.** an arrangement of a number of parts that act together to perform some special function. **2.** a device.
apparatus, attachment, *n* an older term for the tissues that invest and support the teeth for function and include gingivae, cementum of the tooth, periodontal ligament, and alveolar bone. Now commonly called *periodontium.*
apparatus, masticating, *n* an older term for the structures involved in chewing (i.e., the teeth, mandibular musculature, mandible and its temporomandibular joints, accessory mandibular and facial musculature, and tongue), which are controlled by an exquisitely functioning neuromuscular mechanism. See also system, stomatognathic.

appellant (əpel′ənt), *n* the party who, dissatisfied with the disposition of a case on the trial level, appeals to a higher court.

appendicitis, *n* an inflammation of the vermiform appendix, usually acute, which, if undiagnosed and not surgically removed, leads rapidly to perforation and peritonitis.

appendix, *n* **1.** an accessory part of a main structure or text; **2.** the term generally refers to the *vermiform appendix,* which is located at the junction of the small and large intestines.

appetite suppressant, *n* an agent that diminishes the desire for eating.

appliance (əplī′əns), *n* a device used to provide function or therapeutic effect. See also restoration.
appliance, Andresen removable orthodontic, *n.pr* an appliance intended to function as a passive transmitter and sometimes stimulator of the forces of the perioral muscles. One of the activator types of orthodontic appliances that induces or directs oral forces to contribute to improved tooth position and jaw relationship.
appliance, Begg fixed orthodontic, *n.pr* an appliance based on a modified ribbon-arch attachment.
appliance, Bimler removable orthodontic, *n.pr* an activator-type appliance.
appliance, chin cup extraoral orthodontic, *n* an extraoral traction appliance used to restrain the forward positioning of the mandible and/or the forward growth of the mandible.
appliance, Crozat removable orthodontic, *n.pr* a wrought wire appliance originally introduced by George Crozat.
appliance, edgewise fixed orthodontic, *n* an orthodontic appliance characterized by attachment brackets with a rectangular slot for engagement of a round or rectangular arch wire.
appliance, extraoral orthodontic, *n* a device that uses a portion of the face, neck, or back of the head as a

base from which to deliver traction force to the teeth or jaws.

appliance, fixed orthodontic, *n* an appliance that is cemented to the teeth or attached by an adhesive material.

appliance, fracture, *n* (biphase pin fixation, external pin fixation, Stader splint), any one of the various devices for extraoral reduction and fixation of fractures in which pins, clamps, or screws are placed in the fractured segments, the fractured parts are aligned, and then the pins, clamps, or screws are joined with metal bars or rigid plastic connectors (e.g., the Stader splint or Roger-Anderson pin-fixation appliance).

appliance, Frankel removable orthodontic, *n.pr* an activator-type appliance.

appliance, Hawley retaining orthodontic, *n.pr* See retainer.

appliance, hay rake fixed orthodontic, *n* a device used to limit abnormal swallowing excursions of the tongue. In this manner, harmful effects of tongue thrusting are mitigated until the patient learns a new swallowing pattern.

appliance, intraoral orthodontic **(in′trəor′əl ôr′thədän′tik),** *n* a device placed inside the oral cavity to correct or alleviate a malocclusion.

appliance, Kloehn cervical extraoral orthodontic **(kloen ser′vikəl ek′strəôr′əl ôr′thədän′tik),** *n.pr* the classical cervical extraoral traction appliance. Uses a relatively light and flexible (0.045 inch; 1.15 mm) inner arch rigidly attached to a long outer bow.

appliance, labiolingual fixed orthodontic **(lā′bēōling′gwəl fikts ôr′thədän′tik),** *n* an appliance using the maxillary and mandibular first permanent molars as anchorage, with labial arches 0.036 to 0.040 inch (0.090 to 0.10 cm) in diameter introduced into horizontal buccal tubes attached to the anchor bands and lingual arches of the same diameter fitted into vertical or horizontal tubes fastened to the lingual side of the anchor bands.

appliance, obturator **(ob′tərātər),** *n* a dental prosthesis used to close an opening such as cleft palate.

appliance, orthodontic, *n* a device used for influencing tooth position. Orthodontic appliances may be classified as fixed or removable, active or retaining, and intraoral or extraoral.

appliance, pin and tube fixed orthodontic, *n* a labial arch with vertical posts that insert into tubes attached to bands on the teeth.

appliance, prosthetic **(prosthet′ik),** *n* an older term referring to a complete or partial denture for children when groups of teeth are lost or are congenitally missing. Used to maintain space or masticatory function or for aesthetic reasons.

appliance, removable orthodontic, *n* an appliance designed so that it can be removed and replaced by the patient.

appliance, retaining orthodontic, *n* an orthodontic device used to hold the teeth in place, following orthodontic tooth movement, until the occlusion is stabilized.

appliance, straight-wire fixed orthodontic, *n* a variation of the edgewise appliance in which an effort is made to obviate the need for many arch-wire adjustments by reorientation of the arch-wire slots.

appliance, therapeutic, *n* a vehicle used to transport and retain some agent for therapeutic purposes (e.g., a radium carrier).

appliance, twin-wire fixed orthodontic, *n* an orthodontic appliance typically using a pair of 0.010-inch (0.25-mm) wires to form the midsection of the arch wire.

appliance, universal fixed orthodontic, *n* an orthodontic appliance developed by S.R. Atkinson, combining some of the principles of edgewise and ribbon-arch appliances with very light arch wires.

application program, *n* a standard and frequently used computer program tailored to medical and dental needs. It may be supplied to the user by the manufacturer, purchased from a software house, or written by the user.

applicator, *n* a device for applying medication; usually a slender rod of glass or wood, used with a pledget of cotton on the end.

appointment, *n* a mutually agreed-on time reserved for the patient to receive treatment.

A

appointment book, *n* a ledger or table of workdays divided into segments of time to enable the dental staff to reserve specified lengths of time for patient treatment. Now appointments are usually on the computer, but the computer program is still referred to using this term.

appointment card, *n* a small card given to the patient as a reminder of the time reserved for the appointment. Even if sent via e-mail, it is still referred to as this.

apposition (ap′əzish′ən), *n* **1.** the condition of being placed or fitted together; juxtaposition; coaptation. *n* **2.** a layered formation of a firm or hard tissue such as cartilage, bone, enamel, dentin, and cementum.

appropriate, *adj* **1.** the determination that the service provided is suited for the condition. *adj* **2.** being suitable for a particular person, group, community, condition, occasion, and/or place. *adj* **3.** proper.

approved services, *n.pl* **1.** all services provided in a dental plan. In some plans, authorization must be obtained before approved service is provided; other plans make exception for treatment of emergency needs; still others require no prior authorization for any treatment approved under the program. *n.pl* **2.** dental services that meet quality standards maintained in a dental plan.

approximal (əprôk′səməl), *adj* (approximating), contiguous; adjacent; next to each other.

approximating, *adj* See approximal.

apraclonidine (ap′rəklon′idēn), *n* *brand name:* Iopidine; *drug class:* selective α_2-adrenergic agonist; *action:* reduces intraocular pressure; *uses:* control or prevention of increases in intraocular pressure related to laser surgery of eye.

apraxia (əprak′sēə), *n* a loss of ability to execute a purposeful, goal-oriented, or skilled act resulting from selective damage to certain high-level brain centers, either sensory, motor, or both.

apron, *n* a piece of clothing worn in front of the body for protection.

apron band, *n* a labioincisal or gingival extension of an orthodontic band that aids in retention of the band and in proper positioning of the bracket.

apron, lead, *n* an apron made of materials containing metallic lead or lead compounds used to reduce radiation hazards.

apron, lingual, *n* See connector, linguoplate major.

apron, rubber dam, *n* a small strip of rubber dam, perforated to fit over an implant abutment that is used to inhibit introduction of cement into the periimplant space.

aprotinin (āprō′tənin), *n* a protease and kallikrein inhibitor useful in the treatment of pancreatitis.

aqueous (ā′kwēus), *adj* containing or relating to water.

arachidonic acid (ar′əkədon′ik), *n* an essential fatty acid that is a component of lecithin and a basic material for the biosynthesis of some prostaglandins.

Arachnia propionica, **(ərak′nēə prō′pēon′ikə)** *n* an opportunistic, naturally occurring organism in the body, especially in body cavities and on the skin. It is sometimes implicated in actinomycosis, especially in open wounds.

arboviruses (ar′bōvī′rəsəz), *n.pl* an acronym for hemophagic **ar**thropod-**bo**rne viruses, passed on to the host by a bite; implicated in viral encephalitis. The term is not accepted as an official taxonomic nomenclature.

ARC, *n* the abbreviation for **AIDS-related complex.** See also acquired immunodeficiency syndrome.

arc, reflex, *n* a system of nerves used in a reflex or involuntary act, consisting primarily of an afferent nerve with sensory receptor, a nerve center, and an efferent nerve that stimulates the effector muscle or gland.

arch (pl. es), *n* a structure with a curved outline, such as bone.

arch bar, *n* See bar, arch.

arch, basal, *n* See base, apical.

arch, branchial, *n* the small pouches that emerge during embryonic development on each side of the pharynx. Also known as the *pharyngeal arches.*

arch, dental, *n* the composite structure of the dentition and alveolar ridge or the remains thereof after the loss of some or all of the natural teeth.

arch, dental, contraction, *n* See contraction.

arch, dentulous dental **(den′-chələs),** *n* a dental arch containing natural teeth.

arch, edentulous dental **(ē′den′-chələs),** *n* a dental arch from which all natural teeth are missing. Also called the *residual alveolar ridge.*

arch expansion, *n* See expansion.

arch form, See form, arch.

arch, high labial, *n* a labial arch wire adapted so that it lies gingival to the anterior tooth crowns; it has auxiliary springs extending downward in contact with the teeth to be moved.

arch, inferior dental, *n* See arch, lower.

arch length, *n* the length of a dental arch, usually measured through the points of contact between adjoining teeth.

arch length, available, *n* the space available for all teeth.

arch length, deficiency, *n* the difference between required and available arch length.

arch length, required, *n* the sum of the mesiodistal widths of all teeth.

arch, lower, *n* the arch-like curve of the cutting edges and surfaces of the teeth on the mandible. Also known as the *inferior dental arch.*

arch, ovoid, *n* an arch that curves continuously from the molars on one side to the molars on the opposite side so that two such arches placed back to back describe an oval.

arch, palatine, *n* (glossopalatine arch), the pillars of the fauces; the two arches of mucous membrane enclosing the muscles at the sides of the passage from the oral cavity to the pharynx.

arch, partially edentulous dental, *n* a dental arch from which one or more but not all teeth are missing.

arch, passive lingual, *n* an orthodontic appliance effective in maintaining space and preserving arch length when bilateral primary molars are prematurely lost.

arch, pharyngeal, *n* See arch, branchial.

arch, removable lingual, *n* an arch wire designed to fit the lingual surface of the teeth. It has two posts soldered on each end that fit snugly into the vertical tubes of the molar anchor bands.

arch, stationary lingual, *n* an arch wire designed to fit the lingual surface of the teeth and soldered to the anchor bands.

arch, tapering, *n* a dental arch that converges from molars to central incisors to such an extent that lines passing through the central grooves of the molars and premolars intersect within 1 inch (2.5 cm) anterior to the central incisors.

arch, trapezoidal **(trap′əzoid′əl),** *n* an arch that has the same convergence as a tapering arch but to a lesser degree. The anterior teeth are somewhat square to abruptly rounded from canine tip to canine tip. The canines act as corners of the arch.

arch, U-shaped, *n* a dental arch in which there is little difference in diameter (width) between the first premolars and the last molars; the curve from canine to canine is abrupt, so a dental arch in the shape of a capital U is formed.

arch width, *n* the width of a dental arch. The width, which varies in all diameters between the right and left opposites, is determined by direct measurement between the canines, between the first molars, and between the second premolars. These intercanine, interpremolar, and intermolar distances can be cited as arch width.

arch wire, *n* a wire applied to two or more teeth through fixed attachments to cause or guide orthodontic tooth movement.

arch wire, full, *n* a wire extending from the molar region of one side of an arch to the other.

arch wire, sectional, *n* a wire extending to only a few teeth, usually on one side or in the anterior segment.

architecture, *n* in medicine and dentistry, usually refers to the framework of a structure or system.

architecture, gingival, *n* See gingival architecture.

archive (ar′kīv), *n* the storage of older, rarely required data or patient information in a cheaper and/or more compact form.

arcus senilis (är′kəs senil′is), *n* an opaque, grayish-white ring at the periphery of the cornea occurring in older adults.

area, *n* region.

area, apical, n See base, apical.

area, basal seat, n (denture-bearing area, denture-supporting area, stress-bearing area, stress-supporting area), the portion of the oral structures available to support a denture.

area, contact, n See point, contact.

area, denture-bearing, n See area, basal seat.

area, denture-supporting, n See area, basal seat.

area, impression, n the surface of the oral structures recorded in an impression.

area, pear-shaped, n See pad, retromolar.

area, post dam, n See area, posterior palatal seal.

area, posterior palatal seal, n the soft tissues along the junction of the hard and soft palates on which compression, within the physiologic limits of the tissues, can be applied by a denture to aid in its retention.

area, postpalatal seal **(post′pal′ətəl),** *n* See area, posterior palatal seal.

area, pressure, n an area of excessive displacement of soft tissue by a prosthesis.

area, recipient, n the portion of the body on which a skin, bone, tooth, or other graft is placed.

area, relief, n the portion of the surface of the oral cavity under prosthesis on which pressures are reduced or eliminated.

area, rest (rest seat), n the prepared surface of a tooth or fixed restoration into which the rest fits, giving support to a removable partial denture.

area, rugae **(rōō′jē),** *n* (rugae zone), that portion of the hard palate in which rugae are found.

area, saddle, n See area, basal seat.

area, stress-bearing, n See area, basal seat.

area, stress-supporting, n See area, basal seat.

area, supporting, n the areas of the maxillary and mandibular edentulous ridges best suited to carry the forces of mastication when the dentures are in use. See also area, basal seat.

area, work, n the entire space in which the dental hygienist moves and works while treating a patient. This includes the instrument tray and dental chair, unit, and light.

Arenaviridae **(ərē′nəvī′ridē),** *n* a grouping of enveloped, helix-shaped RNA viruses implicated in a relatively benign form of meningitis (lymphoctyic choriomeningitis; severe encephalitic forms do occur rarely) that affects young adults.

arginine, *n* an essential amino acid for infants and children. See also amino acid.

Argyll Robertson pupil (ärgil′), *n.pr* See pupil, Argyll Robertson.

argyria, local (ärjir′ēə), *n* a localized blue pigmentation of the oral mucosa from the deposition of silver amalgam in the submucosal connective tissue.

argyrosis (ärjirō′sis), *n* a pathologic bluish-black pigmentation in a tissue resulting from the deposition of an insoluble albuminate of silver.

ariboflavinosis (ərī′bōflāvinō′sis), *n* a nutritional disease resulting from a deficiency of riboflavin (vitamin B_2); characterized by angular cheilosis, seborrheic dermatitis, a magenta tongue, and ocular disturbance.

Arkansas stone (är′kənsô), *n* See stone, Arkansas.

arm, *n* an extension or projection of a removable partial denture framework.

arm, neutral position of, n a body position to be assumed while treating a patient that prevents cumulative trauma to the arm; incorporates proper placement of the wrist, elbow, and shoulder.

arm, reciprocal, n a clasp arm used on a removable partial denture to oppose any force arising from an opposing clasp arm on the same tooth. See also arm, retention.

arm, retention, n an extension or projection that is part of a removable partial denture and is used to aid in the retention and stabilization of the restoration. See also retainer divet.

arm, truss, n See connector, minor.

arm, upright, n See connector, minor.

armamentarium (är′məmenter′ē-əm), *n* the equipment and materials of the clinician.

arrangement, *n* the pattern into which a group of things is organized.

arrangement, financial, n an agreement between the dental provider and patient on the method of handling the patient's account.

arrangement, tooth, n the placement of teeth on a denture or temporary base with definite objectives in mind.

arrhythmia (ərith′mēə), *n* a variation from the normal rhythm of the heart.

arteriole (ärtir′ēōl), *n* a smaller arterial branch off an artery and connecting to a capillary.

arteriosclerosis (ärtir′ēōsklerō′sis), *n* a term applied to a group of diseases that affect the elasticity of the blood vessels. It may refer to atherosclerosis, hyperplastic arteriosclerosis, or Mönckeberg's sclerosis. These degenerative processes generally affect only the tunica media and tunica intima. The effect is narrowing of the lumen of a blood vessel, causing rupture of the blood vessel or ischemia of an area of tissue that the vessel supplies.

arteriosclerotic heart disease (ärtir′ēōsklerot′ik), *n* See disease, heart, arteriosclerotic.

arteriovenous shunt (ärtir′ēōvē′nus), *n* See shunt, arteriovenous.

arteritis (ärtərī′tis), *n* an inflammatory condition of the inner layers or the outer coat of one or more arteries. It may occur as a separate clinical entity or accompanying another disorder, such as rheumatoid arthritis, rheumatic fever, or systemic lupus erythematosus.

arteritis, temporal, n an inflammation of the temporal artery that produces a nodular, tortuous swelling of the temporal artery accompanied by a burning, throbbing pain, initially in the teeth, temporomandibular joint, and eye, but ultimately localized over the artery. This disorder occurs primarily in persons over 55 years of age.

artery, *n* a blood vessel through which the blood passes away from the heart to the various structures. There are three layers: the inner coat (tunica intima), composed of an inner endothelial lining, connective tissue, and an outer layer of elastic tissue (inner elastic membrane); the middle coat (tunica media), composed mainly of muscle tissue; and the outer coat (tunica adventitia), composed mainly of connective tissue. The structure of the three layers varies with the location, size, and purpose of the blood vessel.

artery arthograms, n.pl radiographs of a joint usually with the introduction of a contrast compound into the joint capsule. In dentistry, an arthogram usually involves the temporomandibular joint.

artery, large, n an elastic artery with an abundant supply of elastic tissue and a great reduction of smooth muscle. The tunica intima is thick, and the endothelial cells are round or polygonal. The tunica media is the thickest of the three layers. It contains few smooth muscle fibers, and its outer border has a special concentration of elastic fibers—the external elastic membrane. The tunica adventitia is relatively thin and ill defined and is continuous with the loose connective tissue surrounding the vessel.

artery, lingual, n the artery that branches off the external carotid artery and carries blood to the tissues superior to the hyoid bone, the tongue, and the inferior part of the oral cavity.

artery, medium-sized, n most of the arteries in the body (e.g., facial, maxillary, radial, ulnar, and popliteal). Thick muscular bands are found in the tunica media. Thin elastic fibers course circularly in the tunica media and run longitudinally in the tunica adventitia. The tunica adventitia is as thick as the tunica media, and its outer layer gradually blends with the connective tissue that supports the artery and surrounding structures.

artery, mental, n the mental branch of the inferior alveolar artery, running from the mandibular canal to the apical foramen of the teeth.

artery, posterior superior alveolar, n the artery that originates from the maxillary artery; its branches supply the maxillary molars.

arthralgia (ärthral′jēə), *n* pain in a joint or joints.

A

arthritis (ärthrī′tis), *n* any of a number of types of inflammation of a joint or joints.

arthritis, allergic, n an arthralgia, swelling, and stiffness of joints associated with food and drug allergies and serum sickness.

arthritis, atrophic, n See arthritis, rheumatoid.

arthritis, bacterial, n See arthritis, infective.

arthritis, hypertrophic **(hī′pertrō′-fik),** *n* See osteoarthritis.

arthritis, infective, n (bacterial arthritis), a primary and secondary bacterial infection of the joints (e.g., by staphylococcal, gonococcal, streptococcal, or pneumococcal organisms).

arthritis, rheumatic **(rōōmat′ik),** *n* an acute polyarticular and migratory arthritis of unknown cause but assumed to be related to group A streptococcal infection of the upper respiratory tract.

arthritis, rheumatoid **(rōō′mətoid),** *n* a chronic destructive inflammation of the joints due to an autoimmunity with unknown etiology, with associated systemic manifestations such as weakness, weight loss, anemia, leukopenia, splenomegaly, lymphadenopathy, and the formation of subcutaneous nodules. Chronic synovitis and regressive changes in the articular cartilage occur with pain, swelling, deformity, limitation of motion, and occasionally ankylosis of the joints. Small joints are principally affected, with onset in the third or fourth decade of life.

arthritis, senile, n an arthritis occurring in persons of advanced age.

arthritis, specific infectious, n an arthritis caused by direct invasion and subsequent infection of joint structures by microorganisms from the bloodstream. Nearly all pathogenic bacteria have been isolated as etiologic agents.

arthritis, traumatic, n an acute or chronic inflammation of a joint as a result of acute or chronic injury.

Arthrobacter, *n* a genus of a strictly aerobic gram-positive bacteria found in soil and present in dental caries.

arthroplasty (är′thrəplas′tē), *n* the surgical correction of a joint abnormality.

arthroplasty, gap, n See gap arthroplasty.

arthroplasty, interposition, n See interposition arthroplasty.

arthroscope (ar′thrōskōp′), *n* an instrument used to view the inside of a joint.

arthrostomy (ärthros′təmē), *n* the surgical formation of an opening into a joint.

articaine (ar′tikān′), *n* an immediate-acting local anesthetic drug of the amide group that is used to anesthetize the treatment site during a dental procedure.

articular cartilage, *n* See cartilage, articular.

articular eminence (artik′yələr em′ənəns), *n* a raised area located on the articulated surface of the temporal bone, in conjunction with the condyle of the mandible it allows for the opening and closing of the jaw.

articulare (artik′yəlār′), *n* the point of intersection of the dorsal contour of the mandibular condyle and the temporal bone.

articulate (ärtik′yōōlāt), *v* **1.** to arrange or place in connected sequence. See also arrangement, tooth. *v* **2.** to connect by articulating strips, paper, or cloth coated with ink-containing or dye-containing wax, used for marking or locating occlusal contacts.

articulating paper, *n* a paper treated with brightly colored material, such as dye or wax, that marks the points of contact made by the teeth when a patient bites or grinds on it.

articulation (ärtik′yōōlā′shən), *n* **1.** a joint where the bones are joined together. See also joint. *n* **2.** the relationship of cusps of teeth during jaw movement.

articulation, anatomic, n a rigid or movable junction of a bony part.

articulation, articulator, n the use of a device that incorporates artificial temporomandibular joints that permit the orientation of casts in a manner duplicating or simulating various positions or movements of the mandible.

articulation, balanced, n the simultaneous contacting of the maxillary and mandibular teeth as they glide over each other when the mandible is moved from centric relation to the various eccentric relations. See also occlusion, balanced.

articulation, mandibular, *n* See articulation, temporomandibular.

***articulation, temporomandibular* (tem′pərōmandib′yələr),** *n* (temporomandibular joint, mandibular joint), **1.** the joint formed by the two condyles of the mandible. *n* **2.** the bilateral articulation between the glenoid or mandibular fossae of the temporal bones and condyles (condyloid processes) of the mandible.

articulation, temporomandibular, capsule, *n* the ligamentous covering of the temporomandibular joint.

articulation, temporomandibular, collagen disease, *n* a rheumatoid arthritis in which the joint may be so involved because of bone changes that the mandibular condyle is fused to the articular fossa in the base of the cranium.

articulation, temporomandibular, hormonal disturbances, *n.pl* hormonal disorders that frequently affect growth patterns of the skeleton, involving the temporomandibular joint (e.g., acromegaly).

articulation, temporomandibular, neuromuscular disorders, *n.pl* neuromuscular disorders involving the temporomandibular joint in which the patient is unable to maintain appropriate patterns of mandibular closure consistent with good dental occlusion. The natural teeth degenerate rapidly and are frequently lost prematurely; when dentures are substituted, they cause the residual tissues to deteriorate rapidly. In addition to the chronic masticatory disability, the deglutitive mechanism functions poorly because of incoordinated lip and tongue action.

articulation, temporomandibular, pain-dysfunction syndrome, *n* See temporomandibular joint disorder.

articulator, adjustable (ärtik′yōōlātur), *n* an articulator that may be adjusted to permit movement of the casts into various recorded eccentric relationships.

articulator, crescent, *n* a device used in creating dental prostheses and evaluating casts. It represents the temporomandibular joints and simulates jaw movement.

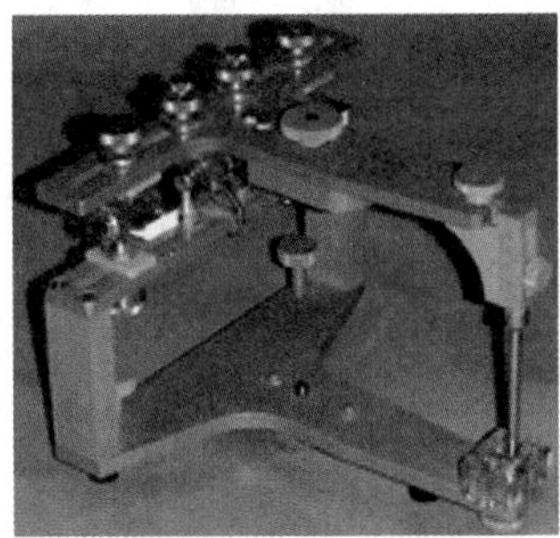

Adjustable articulator. (Rosenstiel/Land/Fujimoto, 2006)

artifact (är′təfakt), *n* a blemish or image in the radiograph that is not present in the roentgen image of the object.

artificial intelligence (A-I), *n* a system that makes it possible for a machine to perform functions similar to human intelligence. Computer technology produces many systems and functions that mimic and surpass some human capabilities, such as the ability to play chess.

artificial organs, *n.pl* the devices used to support life because of the failure or limited capacity of the human organ. The most effective is the artificial kidney, which consists of a set of tubes that pass the blood through a dialysate solution where wastes are removed by osmosis and diffusion. See also hemodialysis.

artificial respiration, *n* See respiration, artificial.

artificial stone, *n* See stone, artificial.

arytenoepiglottic (er′ətē′nō-ep′iglot′ik), *adj* pertaining to the arytenoid cartilage and the epiglottis.

ASA classification, *n* See health, ASA classification.

asbestos (asbes′təs), *n* a group of fibrous impure magnesium silicate minerals. Inhalation of the fibers can lead to pulmonary fibrosis.

***Ascaris* (as′kəris),** *n* a genus of large parasitic intestinal roundworms such as *A. lumbricoides.*

Aschheim-Zondek (AZ) test (ash′hīm tson′dek), *n* See test, pregnancy.

ascites (əsīˈtēz), *n* an abnormal accumulation of serous fluid, containing large amounts of protein and electrolytes, in the peritoneal cavity. Ascites is a complication of cirrhosis, congestive heart failure, nephrosis, malignant neoplastic disease, and various fungal and parasitic diseases.

ascorbic acid (vitamin C), *n* generic; many brand names; *drug class:* vitamin C, water-soluble vitamin; *action:* needed for wound healing, collagen synthesis, antioxidant, carbohydrate metabolism; *uses:* vitamin C deficiency, scurvy, delayed wound and bone healing, chronic disease, urine acidification, before gastrectomy.

asepsis (əsepˈsis), *n* the condition of being without infection; of being free of viable pathogenic microorganisms.

asepsis, chain of, *n* a series of tasks, each step of which is performed in a bacteria-free environment, which serves to maintain the sterility of the entire process.

aseptic (əsepˈtik), *adj* not producing microorganisms or free from microorganisms.

asialia (əsēāˈlēə), *n* See asialorrhea.

asialorrhea (əsīˈəlōrēˈə), *n* (asialia), a decrease in or lack of salivary flow. See also hyposalivation.

asparagine, *n* a nonessential amino acid found in many proteins in the body.

aspartame (asˈpərtām), *n brand name:* NutriSweet, a low-calorie sweetening agent about 200 times as sweet as sucrose.

aspect, buccal (bukˈəl), *n* the facial surface or cheek side of posterior teeth.

aspergillosis (aspˈərjəlōsis), *n* an infection caused by a fungus of the genus *Aspergillus.* Most commonly affects the ear but is capable of causing inflammatory, granulomatous lesions on or in any organ.

Aspergillus, *n* a genus of fungi that is a common contaminant in the laboratory and a cause of nosocomial infection. See also aspergillosis.

asphyxia (asfikˈsēə), *n* a condition of suffocation resulting from restriction of oxygen intake and interference with the elimination of carbon dioxide.

aspirate (asˈpirāt), *v* **1.** to draw or breathe in. *v* **2.** to remove materials by vacuum. *n* **3.** a phonetic unit whose identifying characteristic is the sound generated by the passage of air through a relatively open channel; the sound of *h;* a sound followed by or combined with the sound of *h.*

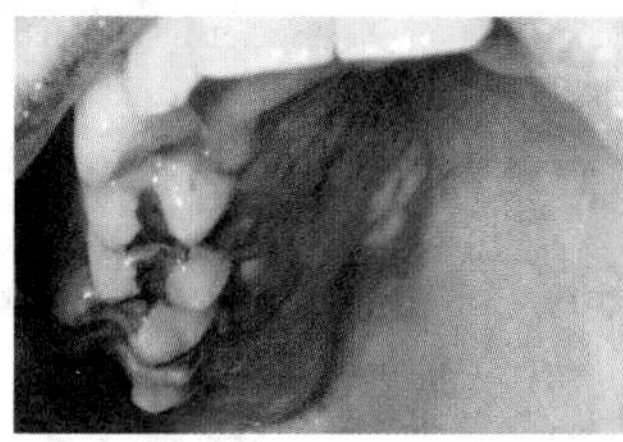

Aspergillosis. (Neville/Damm/Allen/Bouquot, 2002)

aspirated materials, managing, *n* steps taken to keep a patient from ingesting tools or materials during treatment, (e.g., a rubber dam). See also risk management.

aspiration (asˈpirāˈshən), *n* **1.** the act of breathing or drawing in. *n* **2.** the removal of fluids, gases, or solids from a cavity by means of a vacuum pump.

aspiration biopsy, *n* See aspiration, fine needle (FNA).

aspiration, fine needle (FNA), *n* the procedure of obtaining a biopsy specimen by aspiration through a needle; used for diagnosing bone or deep soft tissue lesions. Also known as a *needle biopsy.*

aspiration pneumonia, *n* pneumonia produced by aspiration of foreign material into the lungs.

aspirator (asˈpərātur), *n* a device used for removal of fluids, gases, or solids from a cavity by vacuum.

aspirin, *n brand names:* ASA, Aspirin, Ecotrin; *drug class:* nonnarcotic analgesic salicylate; *action:* inhibits prostaglandin synthesis, possesses analgesic, antiinflammatory, antipyretic properties; *uses:* mild to moderate pain or fever. It was the first discovered member of the class of drugs known as nonsteroidal antiinflammatory drugs (NSAIDs), not all of which are salicylates, although they all have similar effects and a similar action mechanism. Its primary undesirable side effects, especially in stronger doses, are gastrointestinal distress (including ulcers and stomach bleeding) and tinnitus. Another side effect, due to its anticoagulant properties, is increased bleeding.

aspirin burn, n See burn, aspirin.

aspirin, phenacetin, caffeine (APC, PAC) **(fənas′itin),** *n* a pharmaceutical preparation used as an analgesic.

assault, *n* an intentional, unlawful offer of bodily injury to another by force or unlawfully directing force toward another person to create a reasonable fear of imminent danger, coupled with the apparent ability to do the harm threatened if not prevented. A completed assault is a battery. In a medical setting, the unconsented touching of the body would be an assault and battery.

assessment, *n* the qualified opinion of a healthcare provider, informed by patient feedback and examination results, with regard to a specific health issue, whether critical, pending, or routine.

assessment, extraoral, n a preliminary examination of the head, neck, and face, usually made in conjunction with an intraoral examination, to recognize anomalies that might impact the patient's health; may require observation, listening, touch, and smell.

assessment, risk, n process of evaluating a potential hazard, likelihood of suffering, or any adverse effects.

assessment stroke, n the light movement of an instrument against a tooth to detect calculus, caries, overhangs, or other surface irregularities; the movement of a probe to determine pocket depth. Also called *exploratory stroke.*

assets, *n.pl* everything a business owns or that is owned. Cash, investments, money due, materials, and inventories are current assets. Buildings and equipment are fixed assets.

assignment of benefits, *n* a procedure whereby a beneficiary or patient authorizes the administrator of the program to forward payment for a covered procedure directly to the treating dental professional.

assistant, *n* an agent or employee.

assistant, dental, n an auxiliary to the dental operator. See also certified dental assistant.

assistant's stool, n an adjustable chair with additional base support and footrest used to maintain the comfort of the individual assisting the clinician during an examination.

association, *n* a connection, union, joining, or combination of things.

astemizole (əstem′izōl), *n brand name:* Hismanal; *drug class:* antihistamine, H_1-histamine antagonist; *action:* decreases allergic response by blocking pharmacologic effects of histamine; *uses:* rhinitis, allergy symptoms.

asthenia (asthē′nēə), *n* the loss of vitality or strength; a condition of debility; weakness.

asthenic (asthēn′ik), *adj* describing an individual with a long, slender appearance who is thin and flat-chested and has long limbs and a short trunk; comparable to the ectomorph in Sheldon's classification.

asthma (az′mə), *n* a condition characterized by paroxysmal wheezing and difficulty in breathing resulting from bronchospasms. Frequently has an allergic basis and occasionally an emotional origin. See also status asthmaticus.

asthma, cardiac, n a condition characterized by shortness of breath (paroxysmal dyspnea), sonorous rales, and expiratory wheezes that resemble bronchial asthma; related to cardiac failure.

astigmatism (əstig′mətizəm), *n* a defective curvature of the refractive surfaces of the eye, resulting in a condition in which a ray of light is not focused sharply on the retina but is spread over a more or less diffuse area.

astringent (əstrin′jənt), *n* styptic; an agent that checks the secretions of mucous membranes and contracts and hardens tissues, limiting the secretions of glands.

astrocytes (as′trōsī′ts), *n* a large, star-shaped cell found in certain tissues of the nervous system. A mass of astrocytes is called astroglia. See also astrocytoma.

astrocytoma (as′trōsītō′mə), *n* a primary tumor of the brain composed of astrocytes and characterized by slow growth, cyst formation, invasion of surrounding structures, and often, the development of a highly malignant glioblastoma within the primary tumor mass.

asymmetric (āsimet′rik), *adj* unevenly arranged; out of balance; not the same on both sides; not a mirror image on both sides.

asymmetry, *n* an inharmonious relationship between the maxillary and mandibular teeth during closure or functional jaw movements or facial features.

asymptomatic, *n* the absence of any evidence or symptoms of illness or condition.

asymptomatic carrier, *n* an individual who serves as host for an infectious agent but who does not show any apparent signs of the illness; may serve as a source of infection for others.

asynergy (āsin′urjē), *n* a lack of muscular coordination in special functions (e.g., hand-to-oral cavity movements for feeding).

asystole (āsis′təlē), *n* the faulty contraction of the ventricles of the heart, resulting in incomplete or imperfect systole.

ataractic (at′ərak′tik), *n* (ataraxic, tranquilizer), a poorly defined group of drugs designed to produce ataraxia. The former concept, that the use of ataractics involved no mental or motor impairment, is subject to question.

ataraxia (at′ərak′sēə), *n* a state of complete serenity without impairment of mental or physical functions.

ataxia (ātak′sēə), *n* a muscular incoordination characterized by irregular muscle activity.

ataxia, locomotor, *n* See tabes dorsalis.

atelectasis (at′ilek′təsis), *n* the complete or partial collapse of a lung.

atenolol (əten′əlôl), *n brand name:* Nova-Atenol, Tenormin; *drug class:* antihypertensive, selective β_1 blocker; *action:* produces fall in blood pressure without reflex tachycardia or significant reduction in heart rate; *uses:* acute myocardial infarction, mild to moderate hypertension, prophylaxis of angina pectoris.

atheroma (ath′ərō′mə), *n* a fatty, fibrous deposit developing on the artery lining. Also called *atheromatous plaque.*

atherosclerosis (ath′ərōsklərō′sis), *n* a degenerative disease principally affecting the aorta and its major branches, the coronary artery, and the larger cerebral arteries. The arterial changes include narrowing of the lumen of the vessels; weakening of the arterioles, leading to rupture; an increased tendency toward development of atheromatous plaques; and thrombi. Atherosclerosis is a common cause of myocardial infarctions and cerebrovascular accident.

athetosis (ath′ətō′sis), *n* a neuromuscular impairment in which extensive twisting and swaying spasms of the skeletal musculature interfere with voluntary control of movement; the spasms are especially conspicuous and disconcerting during emotional stress and on initiation of conscious voluntary acts.

athiaminosis (əthī′əminō′sis), *n* a deficiency of thiamine. See also beriberi.

athletic (athlet′ik), *adj* pertaining to a bodily constitution characterized by a strong, muscular, robust appearance.

athletic injuries, *n.pl* injuries sustained by persons while engaged in sports, more frequently while engaged in contact sports such as football.

atlantooccipital joint (atlan′toksip′itl), *n* condyloid joint formed by the articulation of the atlas of the vertebral column with the occipital bone of the skull.

atlas, *n* the first cervical vertebra articulating superiorly with the occipital bone and inferiorly with the axis (second cervical vertebra).

atmosphere (atm), *n* the natural body of air, composed of approximately 20% oxygen, 78% nitrogen, and 2% carbon dioxide and other gases.

atom (at′əm), *n* the smallest part of an element capable of entering into a chemical reaction.

atomic (ətom′ik), *adj* pertaining to the atom.

atomic energy, *n* See energy, atomic.

atomic mass number, *n* (symbol: A), the total number of nucleons (protons and neutrons) of which an atom is composed.

atomic number (Z), *n* **1.** the number of electrons outside the nucleus of a neutral atom. *n* **2.** the number of protons in the nucleus.

atomic structure theory, *n* the theory that matter is composed of a vast number of particles, or atoms, bound together by a force of attraction of electrical charges.

atomic weight, *n* the weight of one atom of an element as compared with the weight of an atom of hydrogen.

atomizer (at′əmīzur), *n* a device for changing a jet of liquid into a spray.

atonia, in cerebral palsy (ātō′nēə), *n* an inability to stand or lift the head and diminished capacity to speak or swallow due to weak muscular tone.

atonic, *adj* lacking rigidity or regular tone.

atopy (ā′tōpē), *n* (atopic hypersensitivity, "spontaneous" clinical allergy), a group of "allergic" disorders showing a marked familial distribution; although the susceptibility appears to be inherited, contact with the antigen must occur before hypersensitivity can develop. Disorders include asthma or hay fever resulting from pollens and gastrointestinal tract and skin reactions resulting from food.

atovaquone (ətō′vəkōn′), *n brand name:* Mepron; *drug class:* antipneumocystic; *action:* unknown, may inhibit synthesis of ATP and nucleic acids; *uses:* treatment of *Pneumocystis jiroveci (carinii)* pneumonia in patients who are intolerant of trimethoprim-sulfamethoxazole.

atresia (ətrē′zēə), *n* the congenital absence or occlusion of a normal opening of one or more ducts in an organ.

atresia, aural, *n* the absence of closure of the auditory canal.

atrial fibrillation, *n* a heart condition characterized by rapid random contractions of the atria at the rate of 130 to 150 ventricular beats per minute.

atrophy (at′rōfē), *n/v* a progressive, acquired decrease in the size of a normally developed cell, tissue, or organ. Atrophy may result from a decrease in cell size, number of cells, or both.

atrophy, adipose **(ad′əpōz),** *n* an atrophy resulting from a reduction in fatty tissue.

atrophy, alveolar, *n* a depletion of the size of the alveolar process of the jaws from disuse, overuse, or pathologic disturbance of the bone.

atrophy, bone, *n* **1.** the bone resorption internally (in density) and externally (in form) (e.g., of residual ridges). *n* **2.** a loss of bone substance or volume. Atrophy of bone ordinarily occurs without a corresponding change in the volume or external dimensions of bone, but the mass of bone tissue may be reduced by as much as 75%. The internal architecture of the bone gradually becomes attenuated and finally disappears. Atrophied bone is brittle and has a more spongy consistency than normal bone. In cross-section the cortex is thin, and the periosteal surface is smooth and unchanged, but the intramedullary substance is composed of a yellow, fatty, cancellous bone tissue. Bone atrophy may be systemic, regional, or local.

atrophy, central papillary, *n* a lesion on the central dorsum of the tongue, possibly due to a fungal infection, not a developmental disorder; it may be raised or flat. Formerly called *median rhomboid glossitis.*

atrophy, diffuse alveolar, *n* See periodontosis.

atrophy, facial, *n* the failure of facial development. If it is bilateral, it may produce brachygnathia; unilateral types, although rare, are more common than the bilateral type. Causes include physical injury, neurovascular disease, and paralysis.

atrophy, gerodontic mucosal **(jerōdon′tik myōōkō′səl),** *n* an oral degeneration in which the tissue of the epithelium in the oral cavity thins and loses some of its vascular structure and elasticity.

atrophy, muscular, *n* a wasting of muscle tissue, especially resulting from lack of use. There are numerous causes for simple atrophy of muscle, such as chronic malnutrition, immobilization, and denervation.

atrophy, of disuse, *n* an atrophy resulting from a lack of function of a tissue, organ, or body part.

atrophy, periodontal, *n* the quantitative degenerative changes that occur in the periodontium of a tooth as a result of disease or disuse. When a

A

tooth loses its antagonist, osteoporotic changes in the supporting bone, an afunctional change in the direction of periodontal fibers, and a narrowing of the periodontal ligament.

atrophy, postmenopausal, n a thinning of the oral mucosa after menopause.

atrophy, pressure, n the tissue destruction and reduction in size as a consequence of prolonged or continued pressure on a local area or group of cells.

atrophy, pressure, by epithelial attachment, n a theoretical type of atrophy. The theory, advanced to explain destruction of gingival fibers during gingival inflammation, states that gingival fiber degeneration is produced by pressure exerted by the proliferating pocket epithelium. It is now generally conceded that proteolytic substances produced in the tissues during inflammation are responsible for gingival fiber destruction; subsequently, the epithelium can proliferate apically.

atrophy, senile, n the atrophy or diminution of all tissues characteristic of advanced age.

atropine (at′rōpēn), *n* an alkaloid that annuls parasympathetic effects and antagonizes the effects of pilocarpine. It acts directly on the effector cells, preventing the action but not the liberation of acetylcholine. It suppresses sweat and other glandular sections.

atropine sulfate, n brand name: Sal-Tropine; *drug class:* anticholinergic; *action:* inhibits muscarinic actions of acetylcholine at postganglionic parasympathetic neuroeffector sites; *uses:* reduction of salivary and bronchial secretions.

attached gingiva, *n* See gingiva, attached.

attachment, *n* **1.** a fastener, connector, associated part. *n* **2.** a mechanical device for retention and stabilization of a dental prosthesis.

attachment, abnormal frenum **(frē′nəm),** *n* the insertions of labial, buccal, or lingual frena capable of initiating or continuing periodontal disease, such as creating diastemata between teeth, limiting lip or tongue movement.

attachment, epithelial (EA), n the epithelial-derived tissue device that connects the junctional epithelium to the tooth surface.

attachment, gingival, n the fibrous attachment of the gingival tissues to the teeth.

attachment, intracoronal, n (precision attachment, slotted attachment). See retainer, intracoronal.

attachment level, clinical (CAL), n the amount of space between attached periodontal tissues and a fixed point, usually the cementoenamel junction. A measurement used to assess the stability of attachment as part of a periodontal maintenance program.

attachment loss, n See loss of attachment (LOA).

attachment, migration of epithelial, n the apical progression of the epithelial attachment along the tooth root.

attachment, orthodontic, n a device, secured to the crown of a tooth, that serves as a means of attaching the arch wire to the tooth.

attachment, parallel, n a prefabricated device for attaching a denture base to an abutment tooth. Retention is provided by friction between the parallel walls of the two parts of the attachment.

attachment, precision, n See retainer, intracoronal.

attachment, slotted, n See retainer, intracoronal.

attack, heart, *n* See thrombosis, coronary.

attending dental professional's statement, *n* a form used to report dental procedures to a third-party payer. The claim form was developed by the American Dental Association. Also called *dental claim form.*

attention, *n* the element of cognitive functioning in which the mental focus is maintained on a specific issue, object, or activity. The length of time of such focus is called *attention span.*

attention deficit hyperactivity disorder (ADHD), *n* a neurologic disorder that manifests itself as excessive movement, irritability, immaturity, and an inability to concentrate or control impulses. It affects learning and skill acquisition.

attenuation (əten′yōōā′shən), *n* **1.** to make thinner, weaker, or less virulent. **2.** the process by which a beam of radiation is reduced in energy when passing through some material.

attrition (ətrish′ən), *n* the normal loss of tooth substance resulting from friction caused by physiologic forces.

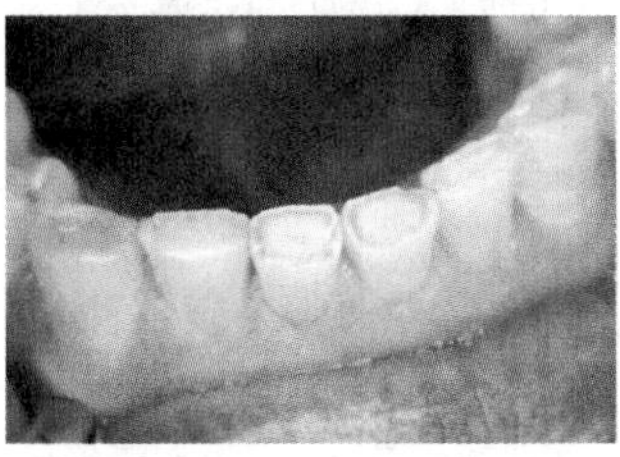

Attrition. (Sapp/Eversole/Wysocki, 2004)

attritional occlusion (ətrish′ənəl əklōō′zhən), *n* See occlusion, attritional.

atypical (ātip′ikəl), *adj* pertaining to deviation from the basic or typical.

Au, *n* See unit, angstrom.

audioanalgesia, *n* the use of music, white noise, or other sounds to decrease the perception of pain. It is commonly used during dental work.

audiogram (ô′dēəgram), *n* a graphic summary of the measurement of hearing loss showing the number of decibels lost at each frequency tested.

audiologist, *n* individual trained to identify, diagnose, measure, and rehabilitate hearing impairments.

audiology (ô′dēol′əjē), *n* the study of the entire field of hearing, including the anatomy and function of the ear; impairment of hearing; and evaluation, education or reeducation, and treatment of persons with hearing loss.

audiometer (ôdēom′ətər), *n* a device for testing hearing; calibrated to register hearing loss in terms of decibels.

audit, *n* **1.** an examination of records or accounts to check accuracy. *n* **2.** a posttreatment record review or clinical examination to verify information reported on claims.

audit of treatment, *n* **1.** an administrative or professional review of a participating dental professional's treatment recommendations (peer audit). *n* **2.** the review of reimbursement claims for service performed (postaudit).

auditory stimuli, *n.pl* in dentistry, the irregularities or deposits on the surface of a tooth that may be detected by ear of both patient and clinician during examination and probing. As an example, the movement of an instrument across clean enamel makes no sound, while calculus and metallic restorations are noisy when scraped.

augmentation (ôg′mentā′shən), *n* **1.** assistance to respiration by the application of intermittent pressure on inspiration. *n* **2.** an increase in size beyond the existing size, such as an implant placed over the mandibular or maxillary ridges.

aura, *n* the brief period of heightened sensory activity that immediately precedes the onset of a seizure. It may be characterized by numbness, nausea, or unusual sensitivity to light, odor, or sound.

aural (ôr′əl), *adj* relating to the ear.

auranofin (ôran′əfin), *n brand name:* Ridaura; *drug class:* gold salt; *action:* specific antiinflammatory action unknown; *uses:* rheumatoid arthritis.

Aureomycin (ô′rēōmī′sin), *n* the brand name for chlortetracycline.

auricle (ô′rikəl), *n* **1.** the oval flap of the external part of the ear. *n* **2.** atrium, the chamber of the heart that receives the blood: on the right, from the general circulation, and on the left, from the pulmonary circulation.

auricular fibrillation (ôrik′yələr fib′rilā′shən), *n* See fibrillation, auricular.

auricular tags, *n* the rudimentary appendages of auricular tissue on the face along the line of union of the first branchial arch.

auriculotemporal syndrome (ôrik′yəlōtem′pərəl), *n* See syndrome, Frey.

aurothioglucose/gold sodium thiomalate (ôr′ōthī′ōglōō′kōs thī′ōmal′āt), *n brand name:* Solganal/Myochrysine; *drug class:* antiinflammatory gold compound; *action:* unknown; may decrease phagocytosis, lysosomal activity, prostaglandin

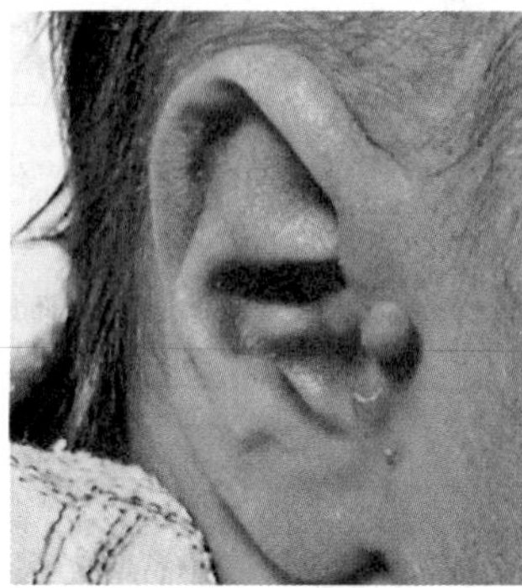

Auricular tags. (Zitelli/Davis, 2002)

synthesis; *uses:* rheumatoid arthritis; juvenile arthritis.

auscultation (ôskultā′shən), *n* the examination procedure of listening for sounds produced by the body to detect or judge an abnormal condition.

auscultatory gap (ôskul′tətōrē), *n* a pause that occurs during the auscultatory method of measuring blood pressure. Noted as the silent period that is present when the sound of systolic pressure diminishes and returns at a lower pressure point. Many errors in recording low blood pressure are attributed to the auscultatory gap.

authorization, *n* a written consent to release protected health information.

autism, *n* a developmental disorder usually appearing in children before the age of 3 that is characterized by communication, behavioral, and sensory impairments, including the inability to interact with others in a socially acceptable manner. The condition may require a special approach when working with the patient as well as when instructing in oral care.

autoantibody, *n* an immunoglobulin produced by the immune system that is directed against one or more of the host's own proteins. Many autoimmune diseases in humans, most notably lupus erythematosus, are caused by such antibodies.

autoclave (ô′tōklāv), *n* a device for effecting sterilization by steam under pressure. It uses steam heated to 121° C (250° F), at 103 kPa (15 psi) above atmospheric pressure, for 15 minutes. The steam and pressure transfer sufficient heat into organisms to kill them.

autogenous (ôtoj′ənəs), *adj* self-originated; springing from within.

autogenous bone graft, *n* See graft, autogenous bone.

autograft, *n* See graft, autogenous.

autograft, free gingival, *n* a procedure in which a graft is attached to an exposed area of a tooth's root. The graft is normally obtained from the palate of the oral cavity.

autoimmune (ô′tōimyōōn′), *adj* the development of an immune response to one's own tissues.

autoimmune disease, *n* May also be called *autoimmune disorder.* See disease, autoimmune, and autoantibody.

autologous (ôtol′əgəs), *adj* in biology, refers to tissues, cells, or proteins that are transplanted from one part of a patient's body to another. In dentistry, autologous bone grafts are used in the reconstruction of the mandible and the reconstruction of alveolar defects prior to dental implants.

automatic condenser, *n* See condenser, mechanical.

automatic mallet, *n* See condenser, mechanical.

automation, *n* the use of a machine designed to follow repeatedly and automatically a predetermined sequence of individual operations. Automation is used extensively in preparing tissue for microscopic examination.

automatism (ôtom′ətiz′əm), *n* a tendency to take extra or superfluous doses of a drug when under its influence.

autonomic, *n* See autonomic nervous system.

autonomic drugs, *n* agents that act on the autonomic nervous system.

autonomic dysreflexia/hyperreflexia **(ôtənom′ik disrēflek′sēə hī′perrəflek′sēə),** *n* an emergent, typically life-threatening, medical condition resulting from a dramatic increase in blood pressure occurring in individuals with traumatic lesions at or above T6. Symptoms may include a throbbing headache, blushing, chills, sweating, stuffy nose, and fidgetiness.

autonomic nervous system (ANS), *n* a subdivision of the efferent peripheral nervous system that regulates involuntary vital function, including the activity of the cardiac muscle, the smooth muscle, and the glands. Has two parts: the sympathetic nervous system, which accelerates heart rate, constricts blood vessels, and raises blood pressure; and the parasympathetic nervous system, which slows heart rate, increases intestinal peristalsis and gland activity, and relaxes sphincters. See also peripheral nervous system.

autonomic nervous system, fibers of, in pulp, n.pl the nerve fibers of the sympathetic autonomic system that enter the pulp tissue and function in regulating blood flow.

autonomic symptoms, n the indications of pathology or trauma, including paleness, sweating, blushing, dilation of pupils, irregular cardiac rhythm, and lack of bladder control.

autopolymer (ô′tōpol′imur), *n* a resin to which certain chemicals have been added to initiate and propagate polymerization without addition of heat.

autopolymer resin, n See resin, autopolymer.

autopolymerization (ô′tōpol′iməriză′shən), *n* (cold-curing), the accomplishment of polymerization by chemical means without external application of heat or light.

autoprothrombin I (ô′tōprōthrom′bin), *n* See factor VII.

autoprothrombin II, *n* See factor IX.

autopsy, *n* a postmortem examination performed to confirm or determine the cause of death.

autoradiography (ô′tōrādēog′rəfē), *n* **1.** a photographic recording of radiation from radioactive material, obtained by placing the surface of the radioactive material in close proximity to a photographic emulsion. *n* **2.** the use of radioactive substances introduced into tissue followed by the placement of a photographic plate on the surface of the tissue preparation, usually employed in cytology and histology.

autosomal dominant disorders (ôtəsō′məl), *n.pl* the genetic disorders that are transmitted by a dominant gene within an autosomal chromosome as opposed to a sex chromosome.

autosomal recessive disorders, *n.pl* the genetic disorders carried by a recessive gene within an autosomal chromosome as opposed to a sex chromosome.

autotransformer, *n* a transformer with a single winding, having a large number of connections, or taps. Used to deliver a precise voltage to the high-tension primary circuit.

autotransplant, *n* See graft, autogenous.

auxiliary, *adj* supporting or assisting; supplementary; secondary.

auxiliary personnel, n.pl a group of dental professionals that work in a dental office or clinic with a dentist includes dental hygienists who are formally trained and may be licensed or certified by state authorities. It also includes dental assistants, laboratory technicians, and other auxiliaries, who may or may not be formally trained, certified, or licensed.

auxiliary wires, n.pl the orthodontic wires that support or augment the action of the main or primary arch wire in an orthodontic appliance. The Begg technique and the segmental technique make frequent and regular use of auxiliary wires.

AV, *n* **1.** the abbreviation for atrioventricular. *n* **2.** the abbreviation for auriculoventricular.

average life (mean life), *n* the average of the individual lives of all of the atoms of a particular radioactive substance; 1.443 times radioactive half-life. See also half-life.

avidin (av′idin), *n* a glycoprotein in nondenatured egg whites (raw) that binds biotin and prevents its absorption, causing biotin depletion.

avitaminosis (āvī′təminō′sis), *n* a disease or condition resulting from a deficiency of one or more vitamins in the diet (e.g., scurvy, resulting from ascorbic acid deficiency, and beriberi, resulting from a thiamine deficiency).

avitaminosis, fat-soluble, n a disease resulting from deficiency of the fat-soluble vitamins (i.e., A, D, E, and K).

avoidance behavior, *n* a conscious or unconscious defense mechanism by which a person tries to escape from unpleasant situations or feelings, such as anxiety and pain.

avoirdupois system (av′ərdəpioz′), *n* See system, avoirdupois.

avulse, *v* to tear off forcibly, as when a tooth is lost in an accident.

avulsed tooth, *n* See tooth, evulsed.

avulsion (əvul′shən), *n* See evulsion.

avulsion, nerve, n See evulsion, nerve.

axial filaments (ak′sēəl), *n.pl* the means of mobility for the spirochete-type bacteria.

axial inclination, *n* See inclination, axial.

axial plane, *n* See plane, axial.

axial wall plane, *n* See plane, axial wall.

axilla, *n* a pyramid-shaped space forming the underside of the shoulder between the upper part of the arm and the side of the chest.

axiopulpal (ak′sēōpul′pəl), *adj* relating to the angle formed by the axial and pulpal walls of a prepared cavity.

axis (ak′sis), *n* **1.** a straight line around which a body may rotate. *n* **2.** the second cervical vertebra, which articulates with the first (atlas) and third cervical vertebrae.

axis, cephalometric, n See axis, Y.

axis, condylar, n an imaginary line through the two mandibular condyles around which the mandible may rotate during a part of the opening movement.

axis, condylar, determination, n the location of the condylar axis by fixing a face-bow rigidly to the mandibular teeth, having the patient open and close the jaws, and recording the most posteriosuperior points of pure rotation with tattoo ink on the outer skin. See also face-bow and hinge-bow.

axis, condyle, n one of three axes of the jaw condyles: (1) the hinge axis, an intercondyle imaginary line across the face through both condyles; whenever either condyle is chosen to be a rotator, it will display (2) a vertical axis, and (3) a sagittal axis. The hinge axis is a moving center for the opening and closing movements. The vertical axis is the center for the horizontal components of orbital movements. The sagittal axis is the center for the vertical components of orbital movements.

axis, hinge, -orbital plane, n a craniofacial plane determined by three tattooed points. Two are located with one on each side of the face at the point of exit through the skin in front of the tragus of the imagined extended rearmost mandibular hinge axis. The third point is located on the right side of the nose at the level of the orbital rim just beneath the pupil when the patient is gazing directly forward. This plane corresponds to the anthropologic Frankfort plane.

axis, horizontal, n See axis, hinge.

axis, long, n an imaginary line passing longitudinally through the center of a body.

axis, mandibular, n See axis, condylar.

axis of preparation, n the path taken by a restoration as it slides on or off the preparation.

axis, opening, n See axis, condylar.

axis, orbital movements of, n.pl the movements projected on the axis-orbital plane in gathering the input data for an articulator.

axis, sagittal, n the imaginary line around which the working condyle rotates in the frontal plane during lateral mandibular movement. The sagittal and vertical axes function concurrently.

axis shift, n the imprecise term used before the nine different directionalized laterotrusions were discovered and named.

axis, vertical, n the imaginary line around which the working condyle rotates in the horizontal plane during lateral mandibular movement. The sagittal and vertical axes function concurrently.

axis, Y, n (cephalometric axis), the angle of a line connecting the sella turcica and the gnathion and related to a horizontal plane. An indicator of downward and forward growth of the mandible.

axon (ak′son), *n* an extension of a nerve cell body that conducts impulses away from the cell. Generally there is only one axon to a cell.

azatadine maleate (əzat′ədēn mā′lēāt), *n brand name:* Optimine; *drug class:* antihistamine; *action:* decreases allergic response by blocking histamine; *uses:* allergy symptoms, rhinitis, chronic urticaria, pruritus.

azathioprine (az′əthīōprēn), *n brand name:* Imuran; *drug class:* immunosuppressant; *action:* inhibits purine synthesis in cells, thereby preventing RNA and DNA synthesis; *uses:* renal transplants to prevent graft rejection, refractory rheumatoid arthritis, bone marrow transplants, glomerulonephritis.

azelaic acid (az′əla′ik), *n brand name:* Azelex; *drug class:* a naturally occurring straight-chain dicarboxylic acid; *action:* has antimicrobial activity against *P. acnes* and *S. epidermidis; use:* topical therapy of mild-to-moderate inflammatory acne vulgaris.

azidothymidine (AZT) (əzid′ōthī′mədēn), *n brand name:* Retrovir; *drug class:* antiviral thymidine analog; *action:* a drug used to lengthen or extend the median incubation period of the human immunodeficiency virus.

azithromycin (əzith′rōmī′sin), *n brand name:* Zithromax; *drug class:* macrolide antibiotic; *action:* binds to 50S ribosomal subunits of susceptible bacteria and suppresses protein synthesis; similar spectrum of activity to erythromycin; *uses:* infections of the upper and lower respiratory tract, uncomplicated skin infections.

AZT, *n* the abbreviation for azidothymidine. See also azidothymidine.

B

B point, *n* See point, B.

Babesia microti, *n.pl* the parasitic protozoan microbes from the Apicomplexa phylum, spread primarily by ticks. They are implicated in babesiosis, a disease with malaria-like manifestations.

babesiosis (bəbē′zēo′sis), *n* a disease caused by *B. microti* that is evidenced by malaria-like symptoms. Also called *babesiasis* or *piroplasmosis.*

baby bottle tooth decay, *n* a dental condition that occurs in children from 1 to 3 years of age as a result of being given a bottle at bedtime, resulting in prolonged exposure of the teeth to milk, formula, or juice with a high sugar content. Dental caries results from the breakdown of sugars to lactic acid and other decay-causing substances. Newer term is early childhood caries.

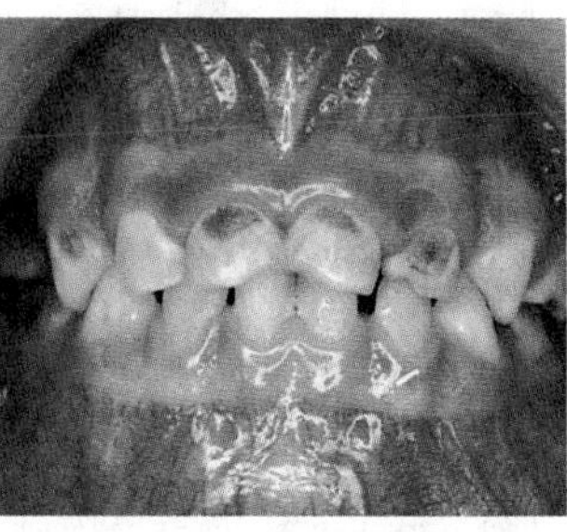

Baby bottle tooth decay. (Zitelli/Davis, 2002)

bacampicillin HCl (bəkam′pəsil′in), *n brand names:* Penglobe, Spectrobid; *drug class:* aminopenicillin; *action:* interferes with cell-wall replication of suspectible organisms; *uses:* respiratory tract, skin, and urinary tract infections; effective for gram-positive cocci.

bacillary dysentery (bas′iler′ē), *n* a gastrointestinal tract infection contracted from food or water contaminated by infected individuals. Also called *shigellosis.* See also *Shigella.*

Bacillus **(bəsil′əs),** *n* a genus of gram-positive, spore-producing bacteria in the family Bacillaceae, order Eubacteriales.

B. anthracis, *n* causes anthrax. The spores of this organism, if inhaled, can cause a pulmonary form; the spores can live for many years in animal products such as hides and wool, as well as in the soil.

B. stearothermophilus **(stēer′ōthurmof′əlus),** *n* a type of biologic spore, the absence of which is tested for to verify proper sterilization of equipment in the dental environment; used with steam autoclave sterilizing or chemical vapor sterilizer methods.

bacitracin, topical, *n brand names:* Baciguent, Bacitin; *drug class:* local antiinfective produced by gram-positive, spore-forming organism of the *B. lichen formis* group; *action:* interferes with bacterial cell-wall function by inhibiting protein synthesis; *uses:* topical for nonserious infections caused by staphylococci and streptococci.

back, *n* the posterior or dorsal portion of the trunk of the body between the neck and the pelvis. The skeletal portion of the back includes the thoracic and lumbar vertebrae and both scapulae. The nerves that innervate the muscles of the back include some branches of the dorsal primary divisions of the spinal nerves, the lateral branches of the dorsal primary division of the middle and lower cervical nerves, and some branches of the ventral primary division of the spinal nerves.

back pain, *n* a pain in the lumbar, lumbosacral, or cervical regions of the back, varying in sharpness and intensity. Causes may include muscle strain or pressure on the root of a nerve.

back-action clasp, *n* See clasp, back-action.

backing, *n* a metal support used to attach a facing to a prosthesis.

baclofen (bak′lōfen′), *n brand name:* Lioresal; *drug class:* central-acting skeletal muscle relaxant; *action:* inhibits both monosynaptic and polysynaptic reflexes in the spinal cord; *uses:* treatment for skeletal muscle spasticity in multiple sclerosis and spinal cord injury.

bacteremia (bak′tirē′mēə), *n* **1.** the presence of bacteria in the bloodstream. It may be transient, intermittent, or continuous. Transient bacteremia may result from dental procedures such as extraction and adult prophylaxis or it may accompany the early phases of many infections. Continuous bacteremia is a feature of endocarditis. *n* **2.** the presence of bacteria in the blood (e.g., as occurs during adult prophylaxis of a patient with the risk of complications due to bacteremia).

bacteria, *n.pl* **1.** small, unicellular microorganisms of the kingdom Monera. The genera vary morphologically, being spheric (cocci), rod-shaped (bacilli), spiral (spirochetes), or comma-shaped (vibrios). *n* **2.** the phylum in which these microorganisms are classified.

bacteria, aerobic, *n.pl* bacteria that require the presence of oxygen to live and grow.

bacteria, anaerobic, *n.pl* bacteria that can survive and grow without the presence of free oxygen in their immediate environment. See anaerobe, facultative.

bacteria, chromogenic (krō′məjen′ik), *n* a microorganism that reacts with the iron in saliva to create a stain on the surface of the teeth. The color of the stain is indicative of the color, or chroma, of the bacteria. E.g., a green stain is caused by bacteria such as *Penicillium* and *Aspergillus.*

bacteria, resident (oral), *n.pl* the microorganisms that are normally in the oral flora of an individual.

bacterial culture, *n* See culture, bacterial.

bacterial spore, *n* a bacteria that, because of its thick outer wall, is easily able to survive in hostile environments otherwise not conducive to bacterial growth and reproduction.

bacterial toxin, *n* any poisonous substance produced by a bacterium. Two general types are common: those formed within the cell (endotoxins) and those formed within the cell and excreted (exotoxins).

bactericide (baktir′isīd), *n* a substance that kills bacteria. See also bacteriophage.

bacteriology, *n* the scientific study of bacteria.

bacteriolytic action (baktir′ēōlit′ik), *n* the breaking down of bacteria by an enzyme or other agent (e.g., by antibacterial factors in saliva).

bacteriophage, *n* any virus that causes lysis of host bacteria.

bacteriostatic (baktir′eōstat′ik), *adj* preventing bacteria from growing and multiplying but possibly not killing them.

Bacteroides **(bak′təroi′dēz),** *n* a genus of *Schizomycetes* with rod-shaped, highly pleomorphic, gram-negative, nonspore-forming obligate anaerobic bacteria.

B. endodontalis **(en′dōdon′təlis),** *n* a strain of *B. melaninogenicus* associated with pulpal infections.

B. forsythus **(forsith′əs),** *n* a recently identified strain found in periodontal pockets.

B. fragilis **(frəjil'is),** *n* the most common and virulent strain, normally found in the oral cavity, upper respiratory system, colon, and genital tract.

B. gingivalis **(jin'jəval'is),** *n* a strain of *B. melaninogenicus* associated with acute periodontitis.

B. intermedius, *n* a strain of *B. melaninogenicus* associated with acute necrotizing ulcerative gingivitis.

B. melaninogenicus **(melaninō-jenikəs),** *n* a small, diplobacillus, also known as *B. melaninogenicum,* found in the oral cavity and pharynx; sometimes associated with periodontitis.

bad-faith insurance practices, *n.pl* **1.** the failure to deal with a beneficiary of a dental benefits plan fairly and in good faith. *n.pl* **2.** an activity that impairs the right of the beneficiary to receive the appropriate benefits of a dental benefits plan or receive them in a timely manner (e.g., evaluating claims based on standards significantly at variance with the standards of the community, failure to investigate a claim for benefits properly, and unreasonably and purposely delaying or withholding payment of a claim).

badge, film, *n* See film badge.

bailment, *n* the delivery of personal property by one person to another in trust for a specific purpose with an expressed or implied contract that after the purpose has been fulfilled the property shall be returned, duly accounted for, or kept until reclaimed.

balance, *n* **1.** equilibrium or harmony. *n* **2.** in dentistry, an occlusal equilibrium or facial esthetic harmony.

balance, acid-base, *n* in metabolism, the balance of acid to base necessary to keep the blood pH level normal (between 7.35 and 7.43).

balance billing, *n* the billing of a patient for the difference between the dental professional's actual charge and the amount reimbursed under the patient's dental benefits plan.

balance sheet, *n* a condensed statement showing the nature and amount of a company's assets, liabilities, and capital on a given date. In dollar amounts the balance sheet shows the assets the company owns, the money it owes, and the ownership interest in the company of its stockholders.

balanced articulation, *n* See occlusion, balanced.

balanced bite, See occlusion, balanced.

balanced occlusion, *n* See occlusion, balanced.

balancing contacts, *n.pl* the contacts of teeth on the side opposite the bolus side. See also contact, balancing.

balancing occlusal surfaces, See surfaces, occlusal, balancing.

balancing side, *n* the side opposite the working side of the dentition or denture.

balloon payment, *n* a final payment larger than the preceding payments when a debt is not fully amortized.

balloon, sinus, *n* a hollow rubber structure expandable with liquid or air that is used to support depressed fractures of the walls of the maxillary sinus.

BANA, *n.pr* an acronym for benzol-arginine napthylamide. See also benzol-arginine naphthylamide.

band, *n* **1.** a cord, tie, chain, or metal collar by which something is bound. *n* **2.** a contrasting strip or strip of material running through or along the edge of a material.

band adapter, *n* See adapter, band.

band, adjustable orthodontic, *n* a band provided with an adjusting screw to permit alteration in size.

band, apron, *n* See apron band.

band, orthodontic, *n* a thin metal ring, usually stainless steel, that secures orthodontic attachments to a tooth. The band, with orthodontic attachments welded or soldered to it, is closely adapted to fit the contours of the tooth and then is cemented into place.

band, pusher, *n* an instrument used to adapt the metal band to the tooth.

band remover, *n* an instrument used to remove bands from the teeth.

band, rubber, *n* See elastic.

band, slip, *n* a band formed when a metal is placed under a load and one grain tends to slip or slide on another.

band, striated **(strī'ātəd),** *n* See striations, muscle.

bandage, *n* a strip of material wrapped about or applied to any body part.

bandage, Barton's, *n.pr* a figure-

B

eight bandage passing below the mandible and around the cranial bone to give upward support to the mandible.

bandage, thyroid, *n* a large bandage consisting principally of a towel applied around the neck that exerts moderate pressure to the anterolateral part of the neck.

bank plan, *n* a financial arrangement made between the dental professional, patient, and bank for financing dental accounts; the bank provides the capital for a rate of interest that enables the patient to pay the dental account over a longer period than would otherwise be possible—usually 12 to 18 months.

bankruptcy, *n* the legal process by which a person, business, or corporation is declared to be insolvent and unable to pay creditors.

bar, *n* a metal segment of greater length than width. See also bar, connector.

bar, anterior palatal, *n* See connector, major, anterior palatal.

bar, arch, *n* any one of several types of wires, bars, and splints conforming to the arch of the teeth and used for the treatment of fractures of the jaws and the stabilization of injured teeth (e.g., *Erich, Jelenko, Niro,* or *Winter*).

bar, buccal, *n* an orthodontic appliance auxiliary consisting of a rigid metal wire extending from the buccal side of the molar band anteriorly.

bar clasp, *n* See clasp, bar.

bar, connector, *n* a connector of greater thickness and reduced width as compared with a platelike connector, which has greater width and is thinner.

bar, fixable-removable cross arch, *n* See connector, cross arch bar splint.

bar, Gilson fixable-removable, *n.pr* See connector, cross arch bar splint.

bar, Kennedy, *n* See connector, minor, secondary lingual bar.

bar, labial, *n* a major connector located labial (or buccal) to the dental arch that joins bilateral parts of a mandibular removable partial denture.

bar, lingual, *n* a major connector located lingual to the dental arch that joins bilateral parts of a mandibular removable partial denture. May also be the orthodontic splinting on the lingual of either the maxillary or mandibular anterior teeth to maintain position of the teeth over time. See also connector, major, lingual bar.

bar, palatal, *n* a major connector that crosses the palate and unites bilateral parts of a maxillary removable partial denture. See also connector, major.

bar, posterior palatal, *n* See connector, major, posterior palatal.

bar, secondary lingual, *n* See connector, minor, secondary lingual bar.

barb-, a combining form used to indicate derivatives of barbituric acid.

barbiturate (bärbich′ŏŏrāt), *n* a derivative of barbituric acid that acts as a sedative or hypnotic. They are controlled substances that have addictive potentials.

barbiturates, ultrashort-acting, *n.pl* drugs administered to bring on rapid anesthesia; e.g., thiopental sodium (Pentathol) and methehexital sodium (Brevital); rapid onset is countered by an abbreviated period of duration.

barium (Ba) (ber′ēəm), *n* a pale yellow, metallic element classified with the alkaline earths.

barium sulfate, *n* a white, finely ground, tasteless powder that is insoluble in water, solvents, and solutions of acids and alkalis; used in radiography as a contrast medium because of its opacity to roentgen rays and as a protective barrier in plaster walls.

barodontalgia (barēōdontal′jēə), *n* sudden, sharp tooth pain that may occur in response to a decrease in atmospheric pressure such as that experienced during flight at high altitudes. Also called *aerodontalgia.*

barosinusitis (bar′ōsī′nəsī′təs), *n* the painful symptoms related to the maxillary sinus resulting from a change in barometric pressure.

barrier, protective, *n* a material of a composition that greatly absorbs radiation (e.g., lead or concrete).

barrier techniques, *n.pl* protocols used in infection control to prevent cross-contamination between health care worker and patient, between patient and health care worker, and between patients. Strict barrier techniques are recommended by the Centers for Disease Control and Prevention (CDC) and the American Dental Association (ADA).

basal (baz′əl), *adj* **1.** describing the minimal functions necessary for life. *adj* **2.** located at or forming the base of a structure. *n* **3.** the fundamental structures from which an organism is derived.

basal bone, *n* portion of the jawbones that forms the body of the maxilla or mandible.

basal lamina, *n* a layer composed of the lamina densa and the lamina lucida. It is an extracellular matrix that lies beneath the epithelium and is believed to inhibit cell migration. The term is usually associated with electron microscopy, whereas the term *basement membrane* is usually associated with light microscopy.

basal layer, *n* See stratum basale.

basal metabolic rate (BMR) **(bā′səl met′əbol′ik),** *n* a type of basal rate, or energy exchange, determined by means of a clinical test of oxygen consumption in a subject who has had a good night's rest, has fasted for 12 to 14 hours, and has been physically, mentally, and emotionally at rest for 30 minutes; usually indicated as a percentage of the normal calorie production per surface area, the normal values ranging between plus and minus 20%.

basal metabolism, *n* See basal metabolic rate.

basal seat, *n* the oral tissues and structures that support a denture.

basal seat area, *n* See area, basal seat.

basal seat outline, *n* an outline on the mucous membrane or on a cast of the entire area that is to be covered by a denture.

basal surface, *n* See surface, basal.

base, *n* **1.** the foundation or support on which something rests; the point of attachment of a part; the principal ingredient of a material. *n* **2.** a compound that yields hydroxyl ions in water solution and causes neutralization of acid to form a salt and water. **3.** the part of a denture that supports the prosthetic teeth and receives support from the oral mucosa, anchoring teeth, or alveolar ridge. See also basic. Opposite: acid.

base, acrylic resin, *n* a denture base made of an acrylic resin.

base, apical (basal arch), *n* the portion of the jawbone that gives support to the teeth.

base, cement, *n* a layer of insulated, sometimes medicated dental cement placed in the deep portions of a cavity preparation to protect the pulp, reduce the bulk of the metallic restoration, or eliminate undercuts in a tapered preparation.

base, denture, *n* **1.** the part of a denture that fits the oral mucosa of the basal seat, restores the normal contours of the soft tissues of the dentulous oral cavity, and supports the artificial teeth. *n* **2.** the portion of a denture that overlies the soft tissue, usually fabricated of resin or combinations of resins and metal.

base, extension (free-end), *n* a unit of a removable prosthesis that extends anteriorly or posteriorly, terminating without end support by a natural tooth.

base, film, *n* a thin, flexible, transparent sheet of cellulose acetate or similar material.

base, mandibular, *n* the body of the mandible, on which the teeth and alveolar tissues are situated.

base, material, *n* a substance from which a denture base may be made (e.g., acrylic resin, vulcanite, polystyrene resin, and metal).

base, metal, *n* the basal surface of a denture constructed of metal (e.g., aluminum, gold, and cobalt-chromium) to which the teeth are attached.

base, plastic, *n* a denture base, baseplate, or record base made of a plastic material.

base, record, *n* See baseplate.

base, shellac, *n* a resinous material adapted to maxillary or mandibular casts to form baseplates.

base, sprue, *n* See crucible former.

base, temporary, *n* See baseplate.

base, tinted denture, *n* a denture base that simulates the coloring and shading of natural oral tissues.

base, trial, *n* See baseplate.

Basedow's disease (baz′ədōz), *n.pr* See goiter, exophthalmic.

baseline, *n* a reference point used to indicate the initial condition against which future measurements are compared.

basement lamina (lam′ənə), *n* the thin layer of noncellular material

B

beneath epithelial cells that is composed primarily of collagen. Also known as the basal lamina.

baseplate, *n* a temporary form representing the base of a denture and used for making maxillomandibular (jaw) relation records, arranging artificial teeth, or facilitating trial placement in the oral cavity.

baseplate, stabilized, *n* a baseplate lined with plastic or other material to improve its adaptation and stability.

baseplate wax, *n* See wax, baseplate.

basic, *adj* having the ability to neutralize acids.

basic life support (BLS), *n* fundamental emergency treatment consisting of cardiopulmonary resuscitation (CPR) or emergency cardiac care (ECC) that is provided until more precise medical treatment can begin.

basic metabolic rate, *n* See basal metabolic rate.

basic services, *n.pl* frequently insurance companies split dental procedures into basic and major categories. Basic services usually consist of diagnostic, preventive, and routine restorative dental services. The plan may provide different deductibles, coinsurance, and maximums for basic versus major services as incentives to good dental care.

basion (bā′sēon), *n* the midline point at the anterior margin of the occipital foramen.

basis, *n* the principal active ingredient in a prescription.

basophil (bā′səfil), *n* See leukocyte.

basophilia (bā′sōfil′ēə), *n* an aggregate of blue-staining granules found in erythrocytes; seen in lead poisoning, leukemia, malaria, severe anemias, and certain toxemias.

basophilic line (bā′sōfil′ik), *n* See line, basophilic.

bass wood interdental cleaner, *n* a triangular strip of wood that can be softened and used to clean a tooth that has little or no interdental papilla.

batch processing, *n* **1.** data processing in which a number of similar input data items are grouped together and processed during a single machine run with the same program. **2.** the processing of a group of instruments through sterilization or disinfection.

Battle's sign, *n* See sign, Battle's.

bayonet (bā′ənet), *n* a binangled instrument, the nib or blade of which is generally parallel to the shaft; resembles a bayonet. See also angle former, bayonet and condenser, bayonet.

beading, *n* the scribing of a shallow groove (less than 0.5 mm in width or depth) on a cast that outlines the major connector. It is used to transfer the design to the investment cast and ensure tissue contact of the major connector.

beam, *n* a stream or approximately unidirectional emission of electromagnetic radiation or particles.

beam, central, *n* the center of the beam of roentgen rays emitted from the tube.

beam, useful, *n* the part of the primary radiation that passes through the aperture, cone, or other collimator.

beclomethasone dipropionate (bek′ləmeth′əsōn dī′prō′pēənāt′), *n brand names:* oral—Beclovent, Vanceril; nasal—Vancenase AQ Nasal, Beconase AQ Nasal; *drug class:* corticosteroid, synthetic; *action:* prevents inflammation by depression of migration of polymorphonuclear leukocytes and fibroblasts and reversal of increased capillary permeability; *uses:* chronic asthma and rhinitis.

beeswax, *n* a wax that melts at low heat and is an ingredient of many dental waxes.

Begg's appliance, *n.pr* See appliance, Begg's.

behavior, *n* the manner in which a person acts or performs; any or all of the activities of a person, including physical action learned and unlearned, deliberate or habitual.

behavior management, *n* the techniques used to control or modify an action or performance of a subject. In dentistry, usually associated with the management of oral hygiene behavior, dietary behavior, or patient behavior under stress.

behavior modification, *n* alterations, changes, or transfers from a socially unacceptable and destructive act to a socially acceptable, nondestructive one. In dentistry, usually associated with oral habits such as finger or thumb sucking, oral cavity breathing, nail biting, and smoking.

behavior therapy, *n* psychotherapy that attempts to modify observable, maladjusted patterns of behavior by the substitution of a new response or set of responses to a given stimulus.

behavioral medicine, *n* a branch of clinical psychology that deals with behavior modification and may involve assertiveness training, aversion therapy, contingency management, operant conditioning, and systemic desensitization.

behavioral sciences, *n.pl* those sciences devoted to the study of human and animal behavior.

Behçet's syndrome (bechets′), *n* See syndrome, Behçet's.

bell stage, *n* the developmental stage of tooth development during which the cup-shaped enamel organ is transformed into a bell-shaped structure. Fourth stage of odontogenesis, in which differentiation occurs to its furthest extent.

Bell's palsy, sign, palsy test, *n.pr* See palsy, Bell's; sign, Bell's; and palsy test, Bell's.

belladonna alkaloids, *n brand name:* Bellafoline; *drug class:* gastrointestinal anticholinergic; *action:* inhibits muscarinic actions of acetylcholine at postganglionic parasympathetic neuron effector sites; *uses:* treatment of peptic ulcer disease and irritable bowel syndrome in combination with other drugs.

Benadryl, *n.pr* brand name for diphenhydramine hydrochloride, an antihistamine with anticholinergic (drying) and sedative side effects.

benazepril (bənā′zəpril′), *n brand name:* Lotensin; *drug class:* angiotensin-converting enzyme (ACE) inhibitor; *action:* selectively suppresses renin-angiotensin-aldosterone system; *uses:* treatment of hypertension, alone or in combination with thiazide diuretics.

Bence Jones protein, *n.pr* See protein, Bence Jones.

Benedict's test, *n.pr* See test, Benedict's.

beneficiary, *n* **1.** a person eligible for benefits under a dental plan. *n* **2.** a person who receives benefits under a dental benefit contract. See also covered person; insured; member; and subscriber.

benefit booklet, *n* a booklet or pamphlet provided to the subscriber that contains a general explanation of the benefits and related provisions of the dental benefits program. Also known as a *summary plan description.*

benefit plan summary, *n* the description or synopsis of employee benefits required by the Employee Retirement Income Security Act (ERISA) to be distributed to employees.

benefits, *n.pl* **1.** the monies paid and discounts applied for various procedures performed. *n.pl* **2.** the dental services or procedures covered by the insurance policy, also known as the *schedule of benefits.*

benign (bēnīn′), *adj* a condition that, untreated or with symptomatic therapy, will not become life threatening. It is used particularly in relation to tumors, which may be benign or malignant. They do not invade surrounding tissues and do not metastasize to other parts of the body. The word is slightly imprecise, as some can, due to mass effect, cause life-threatening complications.

Bennett angle, movement, *n* See angle, Bennett and movement, Bennett.

benzathine penicillin G (ben′zəthēn′), *n* a benzathine salt of natural penicillin that forms a slowly absorbable injectable antibiotic effective against penicillin-susceptible organisms.

benzene, abuse of, *n* an improper, recreational inhaling of the chemical hydrocarbon C_6H_6. It is found in gasoline and adhesives.

benzocaine (topical), *n brand names:* 20% liquid—Anbesol Maximum Strength, Orajel Mouth Aid; 20% gel—Anbesol Maximum Strength, Hurricaine, Orajel Brace-Aid; 10% gel—Denture Orajel, Baby Orajel Nighttime; *drug class:* topical ester local anesthetic; *action:* inhibits conduction of nerve impulses from sensory nerves and is derived from aminobenzoic acid; *uses:* treatment of oral irritation or sores, toothache, and pain caused by dental prostheses, orthodontic appliances, or teething. Mainly used for preanesthetic anesthesia of the oral mucosa. May cause localized allergic reactions and gag reflex if not used properly.

B

benzodiazepine (ben′zōdīaz′əpēn), *n* a drug used to decrease emotional stress, lessen anxiety, and bring about sleep.

benzol-arginine naphthylamide (ben′zolar′gənēn nafthil′əmīd), *n* a bacterial enzyme that mimics the activity of trypsin. It is used as a marker of bacterial growth in dental plaque or in the diagnosis of periodontal disease involving *Bacteroides gingivalis, B. forsythus,* and *Treponema denticola.*

benzonatate (benzon′ətāt′), *n brand name:* Tessalon; *drug class:* antitussive, nonnarcotic; *action:* inhibits cough reflex by anesthetizing stretch receptors in respiratory system; *uses:* nonproductive cough relief.

benzoyl peroxide, *n* **1.** a chemical incorporated into the polymer of resins to aid in the initiation of polymerization. *n* **2.** an antibacterial, keratolytic drying agent prescribed in the treatment of acne.

benztropine mesylate (benz′trō′pēn mes′ilāt′), *n brand names:* Apo-benzotropin, benztropine mesylate; *drug class:* anticholinergic, antidyskinetic; *action:* blocks central acetylcholine receptors; *use:* treatment of Parkinson's disease symptoms.

bepridil HCl (bep′ridil), *n brand names:* Vascor, Bepadin; *drug class:* calcium channel blocker; *action:* inhibits calcium ion influx across cell membrane during cardiac depolarization; *uses:* treatment of stable angina, alone or in combination with propranolol or nitrates.

beriberi (asjike, athiaminosis, endemic multiple neuritis, endemic polyneuritis, hinchazon, inchacao, kakke, loempe, panneuritis endemica, perneiras) (ber′ēber′ē), *n* a nutritional disease resulting from a deficiency of thiamine. Classically it is characterized by multiple neuritis, muscular atrophy, weakness, cardiovascular changes, and progressive edema.

beryllium (Be) (bəril′ēəm), *n* a steel-gray, lightweight metallic element with an atomic number of 4 and an atomic weight of 9.01218. Alloys are used in fluorescent powders. Inhalation of beryllium fumes or particles may cause the formation of granulomas in the lungs, skin, and subcutaneous tissues.

beta cells, *n* See cells, beta.

beta receptors, *n* See receptors, beta.

beta-blocker, non-specific, *n* drug that targets either of the two β-receptors, $β_1$ or $β_2$, of the effector organs, which in turn blocks the sympathetic autonomic nervous system action.

beta-blocker, specific, *n* a drug that specifically blocks either $β_1$ or $β_2$ receptors of the effector organs, which in turn block the sympathetic autonomic nervous system action.

betamethasone (valerate, betamethasone benzoate, betamethasone dipropionate) (bā′təmeth′əsōn), *n brand names:* Uticort, Beben, and others; *drug class:* topical corticosteroid; *action:* interacts with steroid cytoplasmic receptors to induce antiinflammatory effects; possesses antipruritic, antiinflammatory actions; *uses:* treatment of psoriasis, eczema, contact dermatitis, pruritus, and oral ulcerative inflammatory lesions.

betatron (bā′tətron), *n* a machine that produces high-speed electrons through magnetic induction.

betaxolol HCl (batak′səlol), *n brand name:* Kerlone; *drug class:* antihypertensive, selective $β_1$-blocker; *action:* produces fall in blood pressure without reflex tachycardia or significant reduction in heart rate; *uses:* treatment of hypertension.

bethanechol chloride (bəthan′əkol), *n brand names:* Duvoid, Urecholine, Urebeth; *drug class:* cholinergic stimulant; *action:* stimulates muscarinic acetylcholine receptors directly; stimulates gastric motility; *uses:* treatment of postoperative or postpartum urinary retention and neurogenic atony of bladder with retention.

bevel, *n* the inclination that one surface makes with another when not at right angles; in cavity preparation, a cut that produces an angle of more than 90° with a cavity wall.

bevel, cavosurface, *n* the incline or slant of the cavosurface angle of a prepared cavity wall in relation to the plane of the enamel wall.

bevel, contra, *n* blade placement toward the base of the periodontal pocket to separate the sulcular from the external epithelium. Also known as a *reverse,* or *internal, bevel.*

bevel, incisal, *n* the angle of an incisor; it can be less than or greater than 90°.

bevel, instrument, *n* the sloping keen edge of a cutting instrument.

bevel, reverse, *n* See bevel, contra.

BHN, *n.pr* See number, Brinell hardness and test, Brinell hardness.

bias, *n* in statistics, the systematic distortion of a statistic caused by a particular sampling process.

bibulous (bib'yōōlus), *adj* pertaining to absorption; a material's ability to absorb fluids.

bibulous pad (saliva absorber), *n* a permeable cotton pad placed inside the cheek during the application of a sealant to staunch the flow of saliva and keep the treatment field dry.

bicarbonate, *n* a salt resulting from the incomplete neutralization of carbonic acid such as from passing excess carbon dioxide into a base solution.

Bicillin, *n.pr* the brand name for penicillin G benzathine.

bicuspid (bīkus'pid), *n* See premolar.

b.i.d., *adv* a Latin phrase meaning "twice a day"; abbreviation used in writing prescriptions.

bidi, *adj* an abbreviation for "bidirectional": moving or occurring in two, usually opposite, directions.

bidigital palpation (bīdij'itəl), *n* a tactile method of oral examination in which the examiner uses the thumb and forefinger of one hand to rule out abnormalities.

Biermer's anemia (bir'murz), *n.pr* See anemia, pernicious.

bifid (bī'fid), *adj* divided in two.

bifid tongue, *n* See tongue, bifid.

bifid uvula, *n* See uvula, bifid.

Bifidobacterium **(bif'idōbakter'ēəm),** *n* a genus of anaerobic bacteria containing gram-positive rods of highly variable appearance. Pathogenicity for human beings or for animals has not been reported, although these bacteria have been isolated from the feces of infants and older people.

bifurcation (bī'furkā'shən), *n* the division of a tooth's roots into two parts or branches.

biguanides (bīgwan'īdz), *n.pl* orally administered agents used in the treatment of type 2 diabetes, which prevents the liver from breaking down glycogen into glucose and increases the sensitivity body tissues have to insulin. See metformin HCl.

bilateral (bīlat'ərəl), *adj* pertaining to both sides.

bile, *n* an alkaline fluid secreted by the liver that breaks down fat and aids in its absorption in the small intestine. It has a yellow, green, or brown color and a bitter taste. Interference with its flow can result in jaundice.

bilharziasis (bil'härzī'əsis), *n* See schistosomiasis.

biliary atresia (bil'ēərē' ətrē'zhə), *n* a congenital absence or underdevelopment of one or more of the biliary structures, causing jaundice and early liver damage.

bilirubinemia (bil'irōōbinē'mēə), *n* the presence of bilirubin in the blood. It may result from obstruction inside or outside the liver or from increased hemolysis. The total serum bilirubin in an adult is 0.2 to 0.7 mg/100 ml.

bilirubinuria (bil'irōōbinyōō'rēə), *n* the presence of bilirubin in the urine. More often, an excess of bilirubin in the urine resulting from excessive hemolysis.

billing, *n* the procedure of preparing a financial statement.

bimanual palpation, *n* a tactile method of oral examination in which the examiner uses both hands to examine the patient's oral cavity from both the inside and outside at the same time.

bimaxillary (bīmak'silerē), *adj* pertaining to the right and left maxillae; sometimes incorrectly used to refer to the maxillae and mandible.

bimaxillary protrusion, *n* See protrusion, bimaxillary.

bimeter (bīmē'tur), *n* a gnathodynamometer with a central bearing point adjustable to varying heights. See also gnathodynamometer.

Bimler's appliance, *n.pr* See appliance, Bimler's.

B

binangle (bin′anggəl), *n* an instrument having two offsetting angles in its shank. The angles keep the cutting edge or the face of the nib within 3 mm of the axis of the shaft.

binder, *n* a substance, usually sticky, that holds the solid particles in a mixture together, thus aiding in the preservation of the physical form of the mixture.

binding, *n* a reversible combination of various drugs with body constituents such as plasma proteins.

binding site, *n* the location on the surface of a cell or molecule where other cell fragments or molecules attach to initiate a chemical or physiologic action.

binge-eating and purging, *n* a type of anorexia nervosa in which an individual consumes a large amount of food and then forces vomiting or uses enemas, laxatives, or diuretics to avoid additional weight gain.

binocular loupe, *n* See loupe, binocular.

bioburden, *n* the number of bacteria living on a surface before it is sterilized.

biochemistry, *n* the chemistry of living organisms and life processes.

biocidal (bī′ōsī′dəl), *adj* capable of destroying microorganisms.

biocompatible, *adj* compatible with living cells, tissues, organs, or systems, and posing no risk of injury, toxicity, or rejection by the immune system.

biocompatible material, *n* a substance that does not threaten, impede, or adversely affect living tissue.

biodegradability, *n* the natural ability of a chemical substance to be broken down into less complex compounds with fewer carbon atoms by bacteria or other microorganisms.

biodegradable, *adj* the ability to be broken down into smaller, harmless products by way of the action of living organisms.

bioelectrical impedance (bīōelek′trikəl impē′dəns), *n* a method of measuring total body fat that uses electrical current and is based on the premise that lean body mass is a better conductor of electricity than fat. See also body mass index calculation.

bioethics, *n* the study of social and moral issues raised in the field of biology, including medicine and dentistry.

biofeedback, *n* the instrumented process or technique of learning voluntary control over automatically regulated body functions; useful in the treatment of bruxism, temporomandibular joint dysfunction, and pain, and in facilitating anxiety control in the dental setting.

biofeedback, electromyographic (EMG) **(əlek′trômī′ōgraf′ik),** *n* an instrumented process that helps patients learn control over muscle tension levels previously under automatic control; especially useful in treatment of dental disorders such as bruxism, temporomandibular joint dysfunction, tension headaches, and other disorders involving the muscles of mastication. In addition to neuromuscular education, electromyographic type is useful in treating dental phobias and anxiety and facilitating pain control by helping patients learn deep-muscle relaxation techniques.

biofeedback, temperature, *n* an instrumented learning process whereby a patient learns to control temperature of body parts. Training in self-controlled vasodilation (handwarming) technique has been found useful in treating migraine headaches and anxiety in dental patients.

biofilm, *n* a very thin layer of microscopic organisms that covers the surface of an object.

biofilm, bacterial plaque, *n* a thick grouping of microorganisms that are very resistant to antibiotics and antimicrobial agents and that live on gingival tissues, teeth, and restorations, causing caries and periodontal disease; also known as *bacterial plaque biofilm.*

biofilm, dental, *n* See biofilm, bacterial plaque.

biofilm, plaque, *n* See plaque.

biofilm, waterline, *n* a microbial growth that adheres to the waterlines used in dental procedures. Poses a serious risk for immunocompromised individuals.

bioflavonoids (bī′ōflav′ənoidz′), *n.pl* naturally occurring flavone or coumarin derivatives having the activity of so-called vitamin P. Their use in controlling gingival bleeding remains controversial.

bioglass, *n* a fused silica-containing aluminum oxide that presents a surface-reactive glass film compatible with connective and epithelial tissues. Bioglass is used as a surface coating in blade and endosteal implants.

biointegration, *n* a condition that occurs when ceramic implant materials are used and there is no space located between the bone and dental implant.

biologic, *adj* pertaining to biology.

biologic death, *n* the permanent cessation of electrical activity in the central nervous system. Also called brain death.

biologic factors, *n* the variables that influence life and living tissues.

biologic (permucosal) seal, *n* the health-protecting zone between the living soft tissue and the post or implant in patients with full replacement dental work. Works to prevent bacteria and any other health-threatening organisms from breaching healthy tissue.

biologic science, *n* the science that deals with life processes.

biologic value (BV), *n* a number reached by comparing the amount of nitrogen retained with the amount absorbed to aid in determining protein quality.

biologic vector, *n* the live carrier, usually an arthropod, in which an infectious organism matures prior to infecting a receiver.

biologic age, *n* See age, biologic.

biologic width, *n* the combined height of connective tissue and epithelium that isolates the bone from the oral cavity. It is the distance considered necessary for the existence of healthy bone and tissue from the most apical extent of a dental restoration.

biology, *n* the science of life or living matter in all its forms and phenomena.

biomarker, *n* a short-lived radioactive molecule that can be used as a marker to follow a condition or a process.

biomass, *n* the total quantity of living organisms in a particular volume of matter.

biomechanics (bī′ōməkan′iks), *n* See biophysics.

biomedical engineering, *n* a system of techniques in which knowledge of biologic processes is applied to solve practical medical problems and answer questions in biomedical research.

biometrics (bī′ōmet′riks), *n* the science of the application of statistical methods to biologic facts.

bionator (bī′ōnā′tər), *n* a removable orthodontic appliance designed to correct functional and skeletal anteroposterior discrepancies between the maxilla and mandible.

biophysics (bīōfiz′iks), *n* the science dealing with the forces that act on living cells of the body, the relationship between the biologic behavior of living structures and the physical influences to which they are subjected, and the physics of vital processes. Also known as *biomechanics.*

biophysics, dental, *n* the branch of biophysics that deals with the biologic behavior of oral structures as influenced by dental restorations.

biopsy (bī′opsē), *n* the removal of a tissue specimen or other material from the living body for microscopic examination to aid in establishing a diagnosis.

biopsy, aspiration, *n* See aspiration, fine needle (FNA).

biopsy, excisional **(eksizh′ənəl),** *n* the removal of an entire lesion, usually including a significant margin of contiguous normal tissue, for microscopic examination and diagnosis.

biopsy, exploratory, *n* an exploration combined with biopsy to determine method and degree of local extension, usually of bone or deep soft-tissue lesions.

biopsy, incisional **(insizh′ənəl),** *n* the surgical removal of a selected mass of a lesion and adjacent normal tissue for microscopic examination and diagnosis.

biopsy, needle, *n* See aspiration, fine needle (FNA).

biopsy, oral brush, *n brand name:* OralCDx; a noninvasive procedure used to detect early oral cancer during which a sterile brush is rotated against the suspected lesion to obtain a tissue sample.

B

biopsy, punch, *n* biopsy material obtained by use of a punch.

biopsy, shave, *n* a biopsy of skin or mucosal tissue made by removing part or all of a lesion with a scalpel held parallel to the base of the lesion.

bioresorbable, *n* the materials that can be broken down by the body and that do not require mechanical removal, such as sutures or the chlorhexidine chip.

biosynthesis, *n* the formation of a chemical compound by enzymes.

biotechnology, *n* **1.** the study of the relationships between humans or other living organisms and machinery. *n* **2.** the industrial application of the results of biologic research such as recombinant deoxyribonucleic acid (DNA) and gene splicing that permit the production of synthetic hormones or enzymes.

biotin (bīʹətin), *n* See vitamin, biotin.

biotransformation, *n* the chemical and physical changes produced in drugs after they enter the body (e.g., hydrolysis, conjugation).

biperiden lactate, *n brand name:* Akineton; *drug class:* anticholinergic; *action:* centrally acting competitive anticholinergic; *use:* treatment of Parkinson's disease symptoms.

bird face, *n* See brachygnathia; retrognathism.

birth control, *n* **1.** a regimen of one or more actions, devices, or medications followed in order to deliberately prevent or reduce the likelihood of a woman becoming pregnant or giving birth. **2.** oral contraceptives, usually a mixture of a steroid having progestational activity and an estrogen.

birth, premature, *n* a birth in which the child is delivered before it has reached the full period of gestation (37 weeks).

birth weight, *n* the measured heaviness of a baby when born.

bis-, *pref* a prefix meaning that two like or mirror-image moieties are joined together to form a chemical compound.

bisacodyl (bisakʹədil), *n brand names:* Dulcolax, Fleet Bisacodyl, Bisacodyl Uniserts, Fleet Laxative; *drug class:* laxative, stimulant; *action:* acts directly on intestine by increasing motor activity; *uses:* short-term treatment of constipation, and bowel or rectal preparation for surgery or examination.

biscuit, *n* the firing bakes, or stages (referred to as *low, medium,* and *high*), during the fusing of dental porcelain preceding the final, or glaze, bake.

bisecting-angle technique, *n* See angulation, bisecting-angle technique.

bisecting-angle technique, central ray direction for, *n* a technique used when taking a periapical survey where the ray should be directed through the apical third of the targeted teeth. The maxillary apices can be determined by imagining a line from the tragus of the ear to the ala of the nose, which is roughly the level where the apices are located. The manibular apices are located about a half an inch above the bottom of the mandible.

bisecting-angle technique, film placement and position for, *n* a technique when taking a periapical survey that uses the bisecting angle technique in which the film center should be centered on the teeth being radiographed, except for a maxillary canine film, which is arranged slightly farther from the front and center of the jaw; the film should be kept flat as much as possible.

bisecting-angle technique, patient position for, *n* a technique for taking a periapical survey using the bisecting-angle technique in which the patient should be positioned so that their sagittal plane is at a right angle to the floor, and the occlusal plane is parallel to the floor.

bisecting-the-angle error, *n* an error in which the vertical angulation is not well controlled, resulting in either very long or short images. See also distortion, film-fault.

Bismarck brown (Easlick's disclosing agent), *n.pr* one of a variety of dental applications, reveals deposits on the teeth by temporarily coloring them. Characterized by its brown color and licorice flavor.

bismuth (bizʹməth), *n* a reddish, crystalline, trivalent metallic element that in combination with other elements forms salts that are used in the production of many pharmaceutical compounds.

bismuth poisoning, *n* See bismuthosis.

bismuth subsalicylate, *n brand names:* Bisamatrol, Pepto-Bismol; *drug class:* antidiarrheal; *action:* mechanism of action unknown; *uses:* treatment of diarrhea, prevention of diarrhea when traveling.

bismuthia (bizmyōō′thēə), *n* the discoloration of mucous membranes and skin from bismuth poisoning.

bismuthism, *n* See bismuthosis.

bismuthosis (biz′məthō′sis), *n* an acute or chronic bismuth intoxication resulting from the ingestion or injection of bismuth salts. Possible manifestations include albuminuria, exfoliative dermatitis, gastrointestinal disturbances, and stomatitis. Also known as *bismuth poisoning* or *bismuthism.* See also stomatitis, bismuth.

bisoprolol fumarate (bis′ōprō′lol fyōō′mərāt′), *n brand name:* Zebeta; *drug class:* antihypertensive, selective β_1 blocker; *action:* produces fall in blood pressure without reflex tachycardia or significant reduction in heart rate; *uses:* treatment of hypertension as a single agent or in combination.

bisphosphonate (bisfos′fənōt), *n brand names:* Fosamax, Didrone; *drug class:* two classes: the N-containing (atendronate) and non-N-containing (Etidronate); *action:* used to inhibit bone resorption; *uses:* prevention and treatment of osteoporosis, osteitis deformans ("Paget's disease of bone"), bone metastasis (with or without hypercalcemia), multiple myeloma and other conditions that feature bone fragility. Can rarely cause osteonecrosis of the jaw; this may be reason to postpone drug treatment until after dental treatment, as they remain bound to the bone for a prolonged period. Most cases occur in high-dose intravenous types used in cancer patients, but a small proportion happens in patients on oral types. Also called *diphosphonate.* See also osteonecrosis, bisphosphonate-associated (BON).

bisphosphonate-associated osteonecrosis of the jaw (BON), *n* See osteonecrosis, bisphosphonate-associated (BON).

bisulfite, allergy to (bīsul′fāt), *n* a hypersensitive reaction to certain antioxidant substances, such as the preservatives sodium metabisulfite, acetone sodium bisulfite, and sodium or potassium bisulfite, which are used in local anesthetics containing vasoconstrictors.

bite, *n* **1.** the part of an artificial tooth on the lingual side between the shoulder and the incisal edge of the tooth. *n* **2.** an interocclusal record or relationship. See also denture space; distance, interarch; record, interocclusal; and record, maxilloman.

bite, balanced, *n* See occlusion, balanced.

bite block, *n* **1.** in intraoral radiography, a film holder that the patient bites to provide stable retention of the film packet. *n* **2.** an occlusion rim. *n* **3.** a commercially available device, usually made of rubber, which can be used to prop open a patient's oral cavity during a prolonged treatment session.

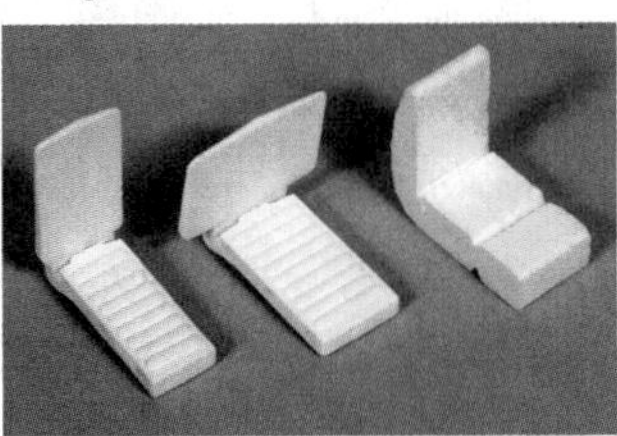

Disposable bite block. (Bird/Robinson, 2005)

bite, close, *n* See distance, small interarch.

bite, closed, *n* **1.** an abnormal overbite. *n* **2.** a decrease in the occlusal vertical dimension produced by factors such as tooth abrasion and loss or failure of eruption of supportive posterior teeth. See also distance, reduced interarch.

bite closing, *n* See dimension, vertical decrease.

bite, convenience, *n* See occlusion, acquired, eccentric.

bite, edge-to-edge, *n* an occlusion in which the incisal edge of the maxillary incisors meets the incisal edge of

B

the mandibular incisors. See also occlusion, edge-to-edge.

bite force, *n* the interocclusal force produced in jaw closure, usually measured in grams or pounds.

bite fork, *n* See fork, face-bow.

bite guard, *n* See guard, bite.

bite guard splint, *n* See splint, acrylic resin bite-guard.

bite, human, *n* a puncture or laceration of tissue caused by human teeth. The markings may be distinctive and useful in forensic pathology to determine the person responsible. Human bite wounds may become infected, requiring antibiotic treatment and tetanus toxoid injection.

bite, locked, *n* See occlusion, locked.

bite marks, *n.pl* the distinctive tooth patterns in a wound that may have forensic or legal implications.

bite, normal, *n* See occlusion, normal.

bite, open, *n* See apertognathia.

bite opening bends, *n.pl* the bends made in maxillary and mandibular light round wires mesial to the molar tubes in orthodontics.

bite plate, *n* See plate, bite.

bite, power, *n* the strength of the closing motion of the mandible.

bite pressure, *n* the pressure produced by jaw closure per unit of area, usually measured in grams per square millimeter. See also pressure, occlusal.

bite raising, *n* See dimension, vertical, increasing occlusal.

bite record, *n* See path, generated occlusal.

bite rest, *n* See position, rest, physiologic.

bite rim, *n* See rim, occlusion.

bite, working, *n* See occlusion, working.

bite mark analysis, *n* See analysis, bite mark.

biteplane (bīt′plān), *n* a removable appliance that covers the occlusal surfaces of the teeth to prevent their articulation.

bite-wing film, *n* See film, bite-wing.

bite-wing radiograph, *n* See radiograph, bite-wing.

biting, cheek, *n* See habit.

biting, lip, *n* See habit.

biting, nail, *n* See habit.

biting pressure, *n* See pressure, occlusal.

biting strength, *n* See strength, biting.

bitolterol mesylate (bitol′ərol mes′ilāt′), *n brand name:* Tornalate; *drug class:* adrenergic beta-2-agonist; *action:* causes bronchodilation; *uses:* treatment or prophylaxis of asthma, bronchitis, bronchospasm.

Black's Classification of Dental Caries and Restorations, *n.pr* a standard classification system used to indicate the location of caries and various methods to restore the tooth. G. V. Black developed this system in the early 1900s.

blackout, *n* the brief impairment of short- and long-term memory occurring during episodes of excessive alcohol consumption or of other substance abuse; consciousness is retained.

blade, *n* See specific instrument parts.

blanching, gingival, *n* See gingival blanching.

Blandin and Nuhn's gland, *n.pr* See gland, Blandin and Nuhn's.

blanket stitch, *n* See suture, blanket.

blastomatoid lesion (blastō′mətoid), *n* an overzealous reactive process that because of tumescence has some features of neoplasia. Specific tissue elements, such as fibroblasts, endothelial cells, osteoblasts, osteoclastic giant cells, or nerves, predominate in a specific lesion to form granuloma pyogenicum, giant cell reparative granuloma, traumatic fibroma, tori, or traumatic neuroma.

Blastomyces dermatitidis **(blastōmī′sēz dur′mətit′ədis),** *n* a species of fungus causing North American blastomycosis.

blastomycosis (blastōmīkō′sis), *n* an infection resulting from the fungus *B. dermatitidis* (North American blastomycosis) or *B. brasiliensis* (South American blastomycosis); characterized by chronic suppurative lesions. The disseminated form is usually fatal.

blastomycosis, South American, *n* a fungous infection that often begins when organisms enter the body through the oral mucosa, producing local ulcers, or through an extraction site, producing papillary lesions. Dissemination leads to granulomatous lesions of the lymph nodes, gastrointestinal tract, liver, and lungs and to

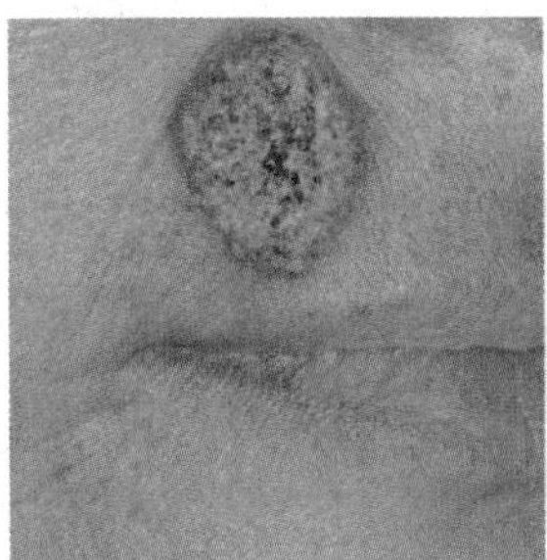

Blastomycosis. (Neville/Damm/Allen/Bouquot, 2002, Courtesy Dr. William Welton)

microabscesses of the skin. The causative agent is *B. brasiliensis.*

bleaching, *n* the use of a chemical oxidizing agent to lighten tooth discolorations. Preferred term is *whitening.* See also agent, whitening.

bleeding, *n* the flowing of blood.

bleeding disorders, *n.pl* hemorrhagic disorders including capillary abnormalities, platelet deficiencies, and blood clotting defects characterized by spontaneous and sometimes uncontrollable bleeding. Consideration before most invasive dental procedures.

bleeding, gingival, *n* See gingival bleeding.

bleeding, occult **(əkult′),** *n* a hemorrhage of such small proportions that the blood can be detected only by chemical test, microscope, or spectroscope.

bleeding points, *n.pl* a series of puncture points made through the gingival tissue; used as a guide for making the gingivectomy incision.

bleeding time, *n* the time required for blood to stop flowing from a tiny wound. Normal bleeding time is from 2 to 6 minutes. Bleeding time is increased in disorders of platelet count, uremia, and ingestion of aspirin and other antiinflammatory medications.

blepharophimosis (blef′ərō′fəmō′sis), *n* a decrease in the size of the palpebral opening without a fusion of the eyelid margins.

blepharoptosis (blef′əroptō′sis), *n* a drooping of the upper eyelid.

blindness, color, *n* defective color vision characterized by decreased ability to detect differences in color. See also achromatopsia.

blindness, color, blue-yellow, *n* a color disability in which the spectrum is seen in reds and greens; a form of protanopia.

blindness, color, red-green, *n* the more common form of color disability, in which the entire spectrum is constituted by yellows and blues; a form of protanopia.

blindness, legal, *n* a condition distinguished by having less than 20/200 vision with the use of eyeglasses to correct vision.

blister, *n* See vesicle or bulla.

blisterform oral lesions, *n* well-defined, fluid-filled lesions in the oral cavity; may appear as pustules, vesicles, or bullae; characterized by elevation above the level of the surface where they are found, blisterform oral lesions are typically see-through and soft. Color varies according to content of blister, which may include blood, serum, mucin, or suppuration; ranges in size from less than 1 cm in diameter to larger than 1 cm in diameter.

Bloch-Sulzberger syndrome (blok-sulz′bergər), *n.pr* See syndrome, Bloch-Sulzberger.

block, *n* **1.** a mental obstacle that prohibits a patient from having favorable responses to the dental professional and suggested treatment plans. **2.** the blocking of sensation like pain to an area. **3.** a large amount of information.

block, data, *n* a physical unit of data that can be conveniently stored by a computer on an input or output device. The block is normally composed of one or more logical records or a portion of a logical record. Synonymous with *physical record.*

block, nerve, *n* See nerve block.

blocking, *n* the process of obstructing or deadening, as a nerve.

blocking agent, *n* See agent, blocking.

blockout, *n* the elimination of undesirable undercut areas on a cast to be used in the fabrication of a removable denture. Also known as *waxout.*

blood, *n* the fluid circulating through the heart, arteries, capillaries, and veins; carries nutrients and oxygen to body tissues.

B

blood alcohol concentration (BAC), *n* the amount of ingested alcohol absorbed into the body's cells and intercellular fluid; measured by a percentage based on milligrams of alcohol per deciliter of blood. The higher the BAC, the greater the physical and mental impairment. Most states have a legal limit of 0.10% (100 mg/dL) or lower for intoxication.

blood, arterial, *n* oxygen-rich blood taken away from the heart through the arteries and used as nourishment for the tissues of the body.

blood-borne pathogens, *n.pl* pathogenic microorganisms that are present in human blood and cause disease in humans.

blood-borne pathogens exposure control plan, *n* a plan that is compliant with Occupational Safety and Health Administration (OSHA) regulations and that explains ways to minimize or eliminate exposure of humans to blood-borne pathogens.

blood-brain barrier, *n* an anatomic-physiologic feature of the brain thought to consist of walls of capillaries in the central nervous system and surrounding glial membranes. It prevents or slows the passage of some drugs, other chemical compounds, radioactive ions, and disease-causing organisms such as viruses from the blood into the nerve tissues of the central nervous system.

blood calcium, *n* the level of calcium in the blood plasma, generally regulated by parathyroid gland activity in conjunction with the degree of calcium ingestion, absorption, use, and excretion. Normal value is 8.5 to 11.5 mg/100 ml of blood serum.

blood cell count, *n* an estimation of the number and types of circulating blood cells (e.g., red blood cells [erythrocytic series], white blood cells, differential).

blood cells, *n.pl* the formed elements of the blood, including red cells (erythrocytes), white cells (leukocytes), and platelets (thrombocytes).

blood chemistry, *n* the determination of the chemical constituents of blood by assay in a clinical laboratory as part of a diagnostic protocol.

blood circulation, *n* the circuit of blood through the body from the heart through the arteries, arterioles, capillaries, venules, and veins and back to the heart.

blood clot, *n* See clot, blood.

blood clotting, *n* the conversion of blood from a free-flowing liquid to a semisolid gel. Within seconds of injury to a blood vessel wall, platelets clump at the site. If normal amounts of calcium, platelets, and tissue factors are present, prothrombin will be converted to thrombin. Thrombin acts as a catalyst for the conversion of fibrinogen to a mesh of insoluble fibrin in which all the formed elements of blood are immobilized. Also called *blood coagulation.*

blood coagulation disorder, *n* a disturbance in the normal clotting mechanism of the blood.

blood, color index of, *n* a figure gained by dividing the hemoglobin percentage by the red blood cell percentage. In most anemias the result is lower than 1, but in pernicious anemia it is characteristically higher than 1.

blood, components of, *n.pl* a cellular fraction consisting of erythrocytes, leukocytes, and platelets, and a noncellular fraction made up of plasma.

blood component transfusion, *n* the administration of one or more elements of blood rather than the whole blood. May include red blood cells, platelets, and other elements.

blood disorders, *n.pl* hematologic dyscrasias that affect the component cells and plasma elements of the blood. They are generally divided into two broad groups: those in which an increase in bulk occurs (e.g., plethora, hydremia, polycythemia) and those in which a decrease in bulk occurs (e.g., anhydremia, dehydration, anemia).

blood dyscrasias (diskrā′zhēəz), *n* the pathologic conditions or disorders such as leukemia or hemophilia in which the constituents of the blood are abnormal or are present in abnormal quantity.

blood gas analysis, *n* the study of gas dissolved in the liquid part of the blood. Blood gases include oxygen, carbon dioxide, and nitrogen, all components of inspired air.

blood glucose level(s), *n* the concentration of sugar (chiefly glucose—"true blood sugar") in the blood. It is usually kept within a narrow range by an interplay of many factors: glycogenolysis, glyconeogenesis, intestinal absorption, insulin, insulin antagonists, and other hormones. In the testing of total reducing substances, the normal range of concentration of fasting blood sugar is 80 to 120 mg/ml; in the testing of true blood sugar, the normal range of concentration is 70 to 100 mg/ml. An unusually low level results in hypoglycemia, whereas an abnormally high level causes hyperglycemia; an important level to monitor in diabetic patients, because changes in insulin levels can adversely affect glucose levels. Many methods of measurement are available, both invasive (finger prick) and noninvasive methods (must be used with traditional blood sampling). See also diabetes mellitus.

blood groups, *n.pl* the division of blood into types on the basis of the compatibility of the erythrocytes and serum of one individual with the erythrocytes and serum of another individual. The groups are immunologically and genetically distinct.

blood pressure, *n* the pressure exerted on the arterial walls by the blood when the heart is in systole (systolic pressure), and the pressure maintained by the elasticity of the arteries when the heart is in diastole (diastolic pressure). A consistent arterial pressure greater than 120 over 80 is considered high and suggestive of hypertensive vascular disease. See also hypertension, systole, diastole.

blood pressure classification, *n* the rating system for blood pressure levels in millimeters of mercury (mm Hg), given as the systolic over the diastolic pressure. Both the systolic and diastolic pressure, if at increased levels, are indicators of concern for cardiovascular problems. Normal is less than 120 over 80; prehypertension is 120-139 over 80-89, stage 1 hypertension is 140-159 over 90-99; stage 2 hypertension is 159 or higher over 99 or higher. See also hypertension.

blood pressure, diastolic, *n* the pressure in the bloodstream when the heart relaxes and dilates, filling with blood. See also blood pressure; blood, pressure, stages; and diastole.

blood pressure, systolic, *n* the pressure exerted on the bloodstream by the heart when it contracts, forcing blood from the ventricles of the heart into the pulmonary artery and the aorta. See also blood pressure; blood, pressure, stages; and systole.

blood pressure cuff, *n* a part of a sphygmomanometer that fits over the patient's arm. It comes in four sizes, for children up to obese adults. It should be made of a nonelastic material, and the cuff used should be about 20% bigger than the arm it fits over—an undersized cuff will cause the blood pressure reading to appear higher than it is in reality, whereas an oversized cuff will cause the reading to appear too low.

blood pressure stages, *n* any of the three stages of hypertension marked by elevated blood pressure. Stage I is 140-159 over 90-99; Stage II is 160-179 over 100-109; Stage III is 180-209 over 110-119.

blood products, *n* the constituents of whole blood such as plasma or platelets that are used in replacement therapy.

blood transfusion, *n* the administration of whole blood or a component such as packed red cells to replace blood lost through trauma, surgery, or disease.

blood urea nitrogen (BUN), *n* the nitrogen in the form of urea in whole blood or serum. Its concentration is a gross measure of renal function. The upper limit of the normal range is 25 mg/100 ml.

blood, venous, *n* the deoxygenated blood that is returned from tissues throughout the body to the heart, then pumped into the lungs for reoxygenation.

blood vessel(s), *n* the network of muscular tubes that carry blood. The kinds of blood vessels are arteries, arterioles, capillaries, venules, and veins.

blood vessels, periodontal ligament, *n.pl* a well-developed vascular system that enters the periodontal ligament and supplies blood to all the regions surrounding the tooth.

blood vessels, pulp, *n.pl* a well-

B

developed vascular system that enters the apical foramen of the tooth and supplies blood to the pulp tissue.

blood, volume index of, *n* the volume of red blood cells divided by the total volume of blood times 100 times the volume percent of packed red blood cells (hematocrit index). A value greater than 1 indicates an abnormally large number or size of erythrocytes.

blower, chip, *n* See syringe, air, hand.

blowpipe, *n* a torch that employs gas-oxygen, or oxygen and acetylene, to melt metal in dental casting and soldering procedures.

blue, methylene (meth′əlēn), *n* **1.** a dye used to color bacteria for microscopic examination. *n* **2.** an aniline dye often used as an antiseptic and topical analgesic in the treatment of lesions of the oral mucosa and skin.

blue nevus, *n* See nevus, blue.

BMR, *n* See basal metabolic rate.

board certification, *n* the examination program that establishes the clinical proficiency of a dental specialist according to the procedures established by the individual specialty certification board under the rules and authority of the Council on Dental Education of the American Dental Association.

board certified, *adj* the status of a dental specialist such as an orthodontist who has become a board diplomate by successfully completing the certification program of the recognized certification board in that area of practice.

board diplomate, *n* a dental specialist who has achieved certification by the recognized certifying board in that specialty, as attested by a diploma from the board.

board eligible, *adj* the status of a dental specialist whose educational qualifications have been verified by acceptance of an application for certification by the recognized certifying board. Board eligibility depends on advanced education in the specialty and timely progress toward completion of the certification procedure. Regular renewal is required to maintain eligibility until the examination is completed.

board qualified, *adj* an unrecognized term used variously and inaccurately to identify any of the stages from educational qualification to certification.

bodily movement, *n* See movement, body.

body, *n* any mass or collection of material.

body burden, *n* the activity of a radiopharmaceutical retained by the body at a specified time after administration.

body dysmorphic disorder (BMD), *n* See disorder, body dysmorphic.

body fluid, *n* a liquid portion of the body such as plasma, lymph, tears, saliva, and urine.

body, foreign, *n* an object or material that is not normal for the area in which it is located.

body height, *n* the overall length of the body from the crown to the bottom of the feet, usually taken in the standing position. Body length refers to the overall length taken in the supine position.

body image, *n* a person's subjective concept of personal physical appearance. The loss of a limb, breast, or tooth may cause psychologic trauma because of unresolved conflict in the change of body image. A distorted body image may be a causal factor in anorexia nervosa and bulimia. See also disorder, body dysmorphic (BDD).

body, ketone, *n* any of the compounds acetoacetic acid, betahydroxybutyric acid, and acetone that are formed in the liver and released in the blood. Elevated levels occur during excessive fat use such as in diabetes or starvation. See also ketoacidosis.

body mass index (BMI) calculation, *n* a method for assessing obesity and determining optimal weight, which involves dividing body weight in kilograms by height in square meters.

body mechanics, *n* the field of physiology that investigates actions and functions of the muscular system relating to body posture maintenance.

body, Schaumann's **(shou′mänz),** *n.pr* a round to oval cytoplasmic inclusion composed of concentric deposits of an amorphous material. Present in the giant cells of sarcoidosis, in beryllium lesions, and sometimes in other giant cells.

body shields, *n.pl* protective coverings patients are sometimes legally required to wear during radiographic examinations; usually a leaded apron containing lead 0.25 mm thick. The protective surface covers the torso and gonads.

body temperature, *n* the level of heat produced and sustained by body processes. Variations and changes in body temperature are major indicators of disease and other abnormalities.

Boeck's disease (bœks), *n.pr* See sarcoidosis.

Boeck's sarcoid, *n.pr* See sarcoidosis.

Bogarad's syndrome, *n.pr* See syndrome, Frey.

Bohn's nodules, *n* See cysts, palatal, of the newborn.

boil (furuncle), *n* a painful skin lesion caused by infection of a hair follicle, characterized by a central core surrounded by inflamed tissue.

boil, gum, *n* See parulis.

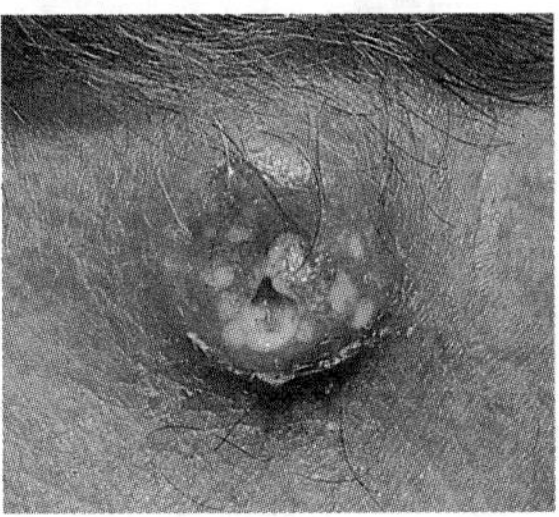

Boil. (Thibodeau/Patton, 2005)

Boley gauge, *n.pr* See gauge, Boley.

Bolton analysis, *n.pr* a computation developed by Wayne Bolton for the evaluation of tooth size discrepancies between maxillary and mandibular arches.

Bolton-nasion plane, *n.pr* See plane, Bolton-nasion.

Bolton plane, *n.pr* See plane, Bolton-nasion.

Bolton point, triangle, *n.pr* See point, Bolton and triangle, Bolton.

bolus (bō′ləs), *n* a mass of food ready to be swallowed or a mass passing through the intestines.

bond, *n* the force that holds two or more units of matter together.

bond, peptide **(pep′tīd),** *n.pl* the linking mechanisms that bind together the amino acid building blocks of proteins.

bond, primary, *n* a chemical bond that requires some change in structure of matter. Primary bonds are ionic, covalent, or metallic.

bond, secondary, *n* a physical bond (sometimes called *van der Waals forces*) that involves weak interatomic attractions such as variations in physical mass or location of electrical charge.

bond strength, *n* the force with which a sealant holds fast to the surface of a tooth.

bonding, *n* an adhesion of orthodontic attachments to the teeth without use of an interposed band.

bonding agent, *n* See agent, bonding.

bonding, chemical, *n* the process of using a chemical in order to form a bond to the structure of the tooth. It is facilitated by the sharing and exchanging of electrons in order to form an arranged structure.

bonding, dentin, *n* the attachment of dental material to the dentin of tooth through various means, and the strength of that attachment.

bonding, direct, *n* an individual placement of attachments on the teeth at the time of adhesion.

bonding, enamel, *v* the process of adhering a coating, or liquid enamel, to the surface of a tooth. It is utilized for various aesthetic and functional reasons, including the repair of caries and chipped or cracked surfaces or to cover exposed roots due to gingival recession. See also sealant, enamel.

bonding, indirect, *n* the positioning of attachments on a dental cast and transfer of them to the teeth en masse for adhesion by means of a molded matrix bone.

bone, *n* **1.** the material of the skeletons of the tissue composing bones. *n* **2.** dense, hard, and slightly elastic connective tissue in which the fibers are impregnated with a form of calcium phosphate similar to hydroxyapatite. **3.** the bones of the human skeleton. *n* **4.** a single element of the skeleton such as a rib or femur.

bone, alveolar **(alvē′ələr),** *n* the specialized bone structure that contains the alveoli or sockets of the teeth and supports the teeth.

bone, alveolar, architecture, *n* the structural pattern of the alveolar bone and its subjacent latticework of supporting bone. The alveolar bone is thin and compact adjacent to the periodontal ligament. The trabecular bone connects and reinforces the individual alveoli. The architecture of a bone is the result of functional stimuli to that bone; the stimuli vary according to type, intensity, and duration.

bone, alveolar, metabolism, *n* the metabolic activity occurring within alveolar bone, which is generally slower than that occurring within metaphyseal bone but more rapid than that of diaphyseal bone.

bone apposition, *n* See bone deposition.

bone augmentation, *n* a procedure used to build or enhance bone. It refers to either bone grafting or bone growing. Bone augmentation materials are classified as osseous, in which bone or bony substitutes are used to form new bone, or osseous conductive, in which these materials provide a platform for regeneration without taking part in actual bone formation.

bone, basal, *n* the part of the mandible and maxilla from which the alveolar process develops.

bone, bundle, *n* the bone forming the immediate bone attachment of the numerous bundles of collagen fibers of the periodontal ligament that have been incorporated into the bone.

bone bur, *n* a drill designed to cut into bone.

bone, cadaver, *n* bone that has been donated for medical purposes from one person to another; used especially in bone grafting procedures. See also allogenic and allografts.

bone calcium content, *n* the amount of calcium stored in bone tissue. Plasma calcium is in constant exchange with the calcium of the extracellular fluid and bones. The parathyroid gland maintains the constancy of the calcium concentration in the plasma. The bones serve as a reservoir of calcium and phosphate to provide for the other needs of the body and supply minerals for deposition in the skeleton.

bone, cancellous (spongy bone, supporting bone, trabecular bone), *n* the bone that forms a trabecular network, surrounds marrow spaces that may contain either fatty or hematopoietic tissue, lies subjacent to the cortical bone, and makes up the main portion of a bone.

bone, cancellous, atrophy of disuse **(kan′seləs),** *n* the wasting of bone tissue occurring with loss of function of a part (e.g., a tooth). The supporting bone assumes an osteoporotic nature, and the marrow remains fatty or hematopoietic.

bone cells, *n.pl* the group includes osteoblasts, osteocytes, osteoclasts, and osteoprogenitor cells.

bone changes, mechanical factors, *n.pl* the pressure and tension forces that play an important role in determining bone structure. Improperly controlled appliances can resorb bone faster than deposition can occur, causing mobile teeth and traumatic occlusion. Poor vascularity is a concomitant cause of undue pressure and tension and may inhibit repair and cause necrosis.

bone chips, *n.pl* the small pieces of cancellous bone generally used to fill in bony defects and precipitate recalcification.

bone, compact, *n* the hard, dense bone composing the outer cortical layer and consisting of periosteal bone, endosteal bone, and haversian systems.

bone conduction, *n* See conduction, bone.

bone crest, *n* the most coronal portion of alveolar bone.

bone cyst, *n* **1.** a vascular cyst eccentrically placed within a bone. *n* **2.** ostitis fibrosa cystica, a parathyroid disorder characterized by cyst formation and the replacement of bone tissue with fibrous connective tissue.

bone defects, angular, *n.pl* the usually localized anomalies that occur in the crestal bone as the result of both periodontal inflammation and occlusive trauma.

bone density, *n* the compactness of bone tissue. The demonstration of bone density by means of radiographs directly depends on the quantity of inorganic salts contained in the bone tissue.

bone deposition, *n* the apposition or formation of new bone as a normal physiologic process.

bone development, *n B* See bone, endochondral, formation; bone formation; and bone, intramembranous, formation.

bone, effect of external radiation to, *n* damage to the bones of adults is most often seen after heavy and localized radiation treatment.

bone, endochondral **(en′dōkon′drəl),** *n* a bone that is developed in relation to antecedent cartilages (e.g., long bones, mandible). See also bone, intramembranous.

bone, endochondral, formation, *n* a replacement of previously formed embryonic cartilage with an adult bony structure. The actual replacement of cartilage by bone is only part of the process, however; much of the bone is laid down directly external to the embryonic cartilage. See also bone, membrane, formation.

bone formation, *n* the deposition of an organic mucopolysaccharide matrix (osteoid) that is subsequently mineralized with calcium salts. See also bone apposition and bone deposition.

bone graft, autogenous **(ôtoj′ənəs),** *n* See graft, autogenous bone.

bone graft, donor site, *n* See donor site.

bone graft, onlay, *n* See graft, onlay bone.

bone graft, recipient site, *n* See recipient site.

bone groove, *n* an osteotomy into or near the crest of the alveolar ridge for placement of an endosteal blade type of implant.

bone groove, canted, *n* an osteotomy sloped to avoid the mandibular canal or keep the implant infrastructure within the medullary confines.

bone, horizontal loss of, *n* a resorption of bone caused by periodontal inflammation in which the bone crest remains even with the cemento-enamel junctions of two adjoining teeth. The condition may be localized or generalized.

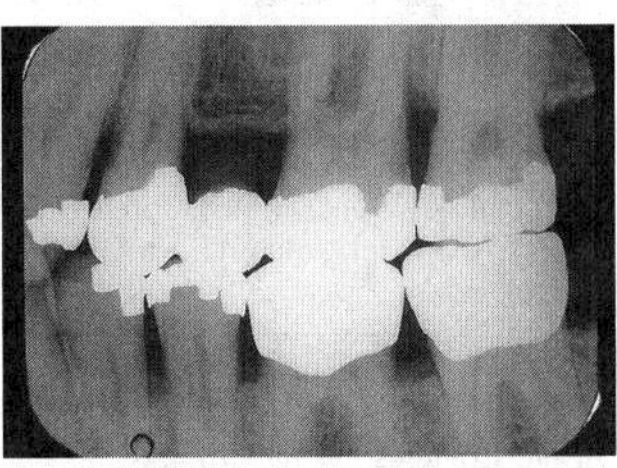

Horizontal bone loss. (Regezi/Sciubba/Pogrel, 2000)

bone, internal reconstruction of, *n* the formation of bone on the tensional side of the periodontal ligament with concurrent resorption from the marrow space; contralaterally, resorption of alveolar bone with apposition from the endosteum in the marrow space.

bone, interproximal, *n* the bone that forms the septa between the teeth; consists primarily of a spongy supporting bone covered by a layer of cortical bone. See also septum, interdental.

bone, intramembranous, *n* a bone developed within a membrane but having no associated cartilage (e.g., parietal, frontal, bones of upper face). See also bone, endochondral.

bone, intramembranous, formation, *n* membrane bone forms directly from the mesenchyme, first as a thin, flattened, irregular bony plate or membrane in the dermis and gradually expanding at its margins and becoming thickened by the deposition of successive layers of additional bone on the inner and outer surfaces. See also bone, endochondral, formation.

bone involvement, *n* changes in the alveolar and supporting bone occurring as a sequel to or accompanying inflammatory or dystrophic disease; usually of a resorptive nature.

bone, lacrimal **(lak′riməl),** *n* the small, fragile, paired facial bone that helps form a part of the orbital wall and also a small part of the nasal cavity. The bone has four borders and

B

two surfaces that articulate with four other facial bones.

bone lamella, *n* bone having the appearance of layers of thin leaves or plates. This appearance is produced by lines representing periods of inactivity of bone formation.

bone, malar (zygomatic bone), frontal process of, *n* a prominence on the zygomatic bone (cheekbone) that forms the anterior lateral orbital wall.

bone, malar (zygomatic bone), maxillary process of **(zī′gəmat′ik mā′lər mak′səler′ē),** *n* a prominence on the zygomatic bone (cheekbone) that forms part of the inferior rim of the orbit and a small part of the orbital wall.

bone, malar (zygomatic bone), temporal process of *n* a prominence on the inferior aspect of the zygomatic bone (cheekbone) that articulates with the zygomatic process of temporal bone to form the zygomatic arch.

bone, marble, *n* See osteopetrosis.

bone marrow, *n* the soft vascular tissue that fills bone cavities and cancellous bone spaces and consists primarily of fat cells, hematopoietic cells, and osteogenetic reticular cells.

bone marrow transplant, *n* the transplantation of bone marrow from healthy donors to stimulate production of formed blood cells. It is used in treatment of hematopoietic or lymphoreticular diseases such as aplastic anemia, leukemia, immune deficiency syndromes, and acute radiation syndrome.

bone membranes, *n.pl* the membrane structures associated with the growth, development, and repair of bone. They include the periosteum, a connective tissue layer adjacent to bone surfaces; periodontal ligament, a modified periosteum associated with tooth structure; and endosteum, a thin layer of connective tissue lining the walls of the bone marrow spaces.

bone, microscopic appearance of, *n* the composition of bone tissue as viewed under a microscope. Microscopically, bone is composed of osteocytes embedded within lacunae in a calcified intercellular matrix. Extending from the lacunae are small canals called canaliculi, which communicate with canaliculi of adjacent lacunae. Through this system of canals, nutrient material reaches the osteocytes and provides avenues for the removal of waste products of metabolism. It is deposited in incremental layers (lamellae) around haversian canals, the lamellae toward the surface of the bone being more or less parallel to it.

bone mineral content, chemistry of, *n* the hardness of bone results from its mineral content in the organic matrix. The minerals (commonly designated as bone salts) and the organic matrix make up the interstitial substance of bone. The bone salts consist essentially of hydroxyapatite ($Ca_{10}[PO_4]_6[OH_2]$), carbon dioxide, and water, with small amounts of other ions.

bone morphogenetic protein (BMP), *n* See protein, bone morphogenetic (BMP).

bone, normal level of, *n* the distance from the interdental bone crest to the cementoenamel junction in healthy teeth, usually 1 to 1.5 mm.

bone, occipital **(əksip′itəl),** *n* the saucer-shaped cranial bone that forms the most posterior part of the skull; the spinal cord passes through the foramen magnum, an opening at its base.

bone onlay, *n* See graft, onlay bone.

bone, perichondrial **(perikon′drēəl),** *n* bone that is deposited in concentric layers around the long shaft of the bone in a manner similar to that of the growth of endochondral bone.

bone, physical properties of, *n* a compact bone has the following physical characteristics: specific gravity, 1.92 to 1.99; tensile strength, 13,000 to 17,000 psi; compressive strength, 18,000 to 24,000 psi; compressive strength parallel to the long axis, 7150 psi; compressive strength at right angles to the long axis, 10,800 psi. These physical characteristics make bone particularly suitable for carrying out its functions of weight bearing, leverage, and protection of vulnerable viscera.

bone rarefaction **(rar′əfak′shən),** *n* a decreased density of bone such as a decrease in weight per unit of volume.

bone recession, *n* See recession, bone.
bone, resorption and repair of, *n* an adaptive physiologic mechanism occurring as long as the individual retains the natural dentition. See also resorption of bone.
bone, resting lines in, *n.pl* the regular lines created by alternating periods of bone formation and rest, giving a tierlike appearance to lamellar bone.
bone, reversal lines in, *n.pl* the irregular lines containing concavities directed away from the bundle bone and serving as histologic indications that resorption has taken place up to that line from the marrow side.
bone sequestrum, *n* See sequestrum.
bone, spongy, *n* See bone, cancellous.
bone support, *n* the amount of alveolar and trabecular bone adjacent to a tooth that can provide attachment, investment, and support for the tooth.
bone, supporting, *n* See bone, cancellous.
bone, supporting, atrophy of disuse, *n* See bone, cancellous, atrophy of disuse.
bone surgery, *n* See surgery, osseous.
bone, thickened margin of, *n* the widening of the crest of the alveolus, primarily on the buccal and lingual aspects, varying from a thick ledge to a "beading" of the bone margin; results in a more or less bulbous contour of the gingival tissue overlying it.
bone, trabecular **(trəbek′yələr),** *n* See bone, cancellous.
bone, vertical loss of, *n* a resorption of bone caused by periodontal inflammation and occlusal trauma in which the bone crest is below the cementoenamel junctions of two adjoining teeth. It can be localized (mainly) or generalized.
bone, vertical plates of the palatine, *n* the thin, oblong-shaped bone with two surfaces and four borders. It helps to form the floor of the orbit, the outer wall of the nasal cavity, and several adjoining structures.
bone volume (mass), age-affecting, *n* decreases that occur in human body bone mass after age 40. Diet and exercise may be contributing factors.
bone wax, *n* See wax, bone.
bone, woven, *n* a character and pattern of bone resulting from the interweaving of broad bands of bone.
bone(s), cranial, *n* the eight bones that make up the skull and protect the brain and include the ethmoid, frontal, occipital, sphenoid, two parietal, and two temporal bones.
bone(s), facial, *n* the 14 bones that include the mandible, maxilla, frontal bones, nasal bones, and zygoma. With the exception of the mandible, maxilla, and vomer bones, the bones of the face occur in pairs, thus accounting for facial symmetry. They provide the framework for the face, serve as entry points for the digestive and respiratory systems, and provide the attachments for the muscles controlling facial expression.
bone(s), horizontal plates of palatine, *n* the bones that form the posterior part of the hard palate and consist of four borders and two surfaces.
Bonwill-Hawley chart, *n.pr* See chart, Hawley.
Bonwill's triangle, *n* See triangle, Bonwill's.
bony crater, *n* a concave resorptive defect in the alveolar crest, usually occurring interdentally.
bony crepitus, *n* See crepitus, bony.
borax, *n* a principal ingredient in casting fluxes. Used in gypsum products as a retardant for the setting reaction and a strengthener for hydrocolloids.
border, *n* a circumferential margin or edge.
border, denture (denture edge, denture periphery), *n* the limit, boundary, or circumferential margin of a denture base.
border, mandibular (mandibular plane), *n* a tangent to the inferior border of the mandible. A line joining point gonion to point gnathion.
border molding, *n* the shaping of an impression material by the manipulation or action of the tissues to determine the denture border position.
border movement, *n* See movement, border.
border seal, *n* the contact of the denture border with the underlying or adjacent tissues to prevent the passage of air or other substances.

B

border structures, *n.pl* the oral structures that bound the borders of a denture.

border tissues, movement, *n* the action of the muscles and other structures adjacent to the borders of a denture.

***Bordetella pertussis* (bor′dətel′ə pertus′is),** *n.pl* the infectious bacteria responsible for whooping cough (pertussis), which is spread from person to person by direct contact with mucosal discharges.

boutons terminaux (bŏŏt′ons ter′-minō), *n.pl* See end-feet.

Bowen's disease, *n.pr* See carcinoma in situ.

box, light, *n* See illuminator.

boxing, *n* the building up of vertical walls, usually in wax, around an impression to produce the desired size and form of the base of the cast.

boxing strip, *n* See strip, boxing.

brace, *n* an orthotic device to support and hold part of the body in the correct position to allow function, such as a leg brace that permits walking and standing. Sometimes used to describe orthodontic appliances.

brachycephalic (brak′isəfal′ik), *adj* descriptive term applied to a broad, round head having a cephalic index of more than 80.

brachydactyly (brā′kēdak′təlē), *n* an abnormal shortness of the fingers, usually associated with some congenital syndrome.

brachygnathia (bird-face, micro-gnathia) (brak′ignā′thēə), *n* marked underdevelopment of the mandible. *adj* brachygnathous. See also retrognathism.

bracing, *n* a resistance to the horizontal components of masticatory force.

bracket, *n* a small metal attachment fixed to a band that serves as a means of fastening the arch wire to the band.

bradycardia (brad′ikär′dēə), *n* an abnormal slowness of the heart as evidenced by a slowing of the pulse rate (less than 50 beats per minute).

bradydiastole (brad′idīas′tōle), *n* an abnormal prolongation of diastole.

bradykinesia (brad′ikinē′zhə), *n* an irregular slowness in motions and reflexes.

bradykinin (brā′dəkī′nin), *n* one of a number of plasma kinins, a potent vasodilator; physiologic mediators of an anaphylactic reaction.

bradypnea (brad′ipnē′ə), *n* an abnormal slowness of breathing.

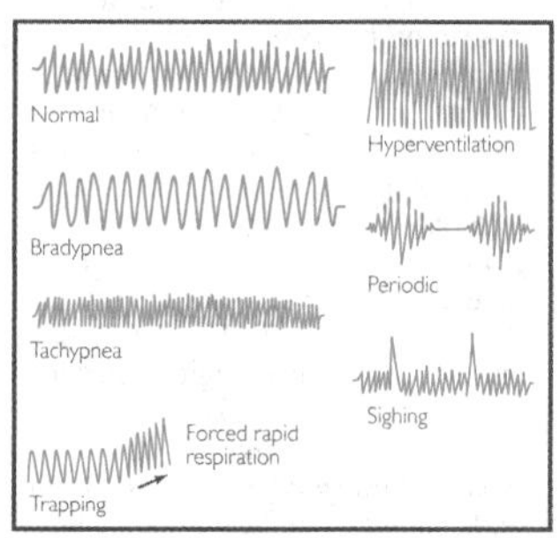

Respiration patterns. (Kinn/Woods, 2007)

Braille (brāl), *n.pr* a printing and writing system using elevated dots to represent letters. The system allows those individuals with limited or no visual ability to read via touch.

brain death, *n* an irreversible form of unconsciousness characterized by a complete loss of brain function while the heart continues to beat.

brain, electrical activity of, *n* the electrical energy that can be observed as waves with electroencephalographic equipment. These rhythms and patterns have been organized into a system that imputes values for the state of health and disease. Electrical evidence of it in the cerebral cortex reveals that different potential patterns are produced by different states of mental activity (e.g., tension, mental work, sleep).

brainstem, *n* the portion of the brain comprising the medulla oblongata, pons, and mesencephalon. It performs motor, sensory, and reflex functions.

branchial nerve, *n* See nerve, branchial.

brand name, *n* a name given to a product by its manufacturer that becomes part of the product's identity.

Branemark technique, *n.pr* See osseointegration.

breach of contract, *n* See contract, breach of.

break-even point, *n* the level of patient visits or net revenues at which the revenues for a period are equal to the expenses incurred in that period.

breath, *n* the air inhaled and exhaled in respiration.

breath, bad (offensive), n See halitosis.

breathing check, *n* a series of steps, based on the pneumonic ABCD (Airway, Breathing, Circulation, Disability), used to determine the respiratory status of a patient in respiratory distress.

breathing, Kussmaul (kōōs′môl), *n.pr* a deep, slow breathing that requires great effort, which often occurs during a diabetic coma.

breathing, oral cavity, *n* the process of inspiration and expiration of air primarily through the oral cavity. It is commonly seen in nasal conditions such as deviated septum, hypertrophied adenoids, and allergies and may produce excessive drying of the oral mucosa with a tendency to gingival hyperplasia and inflammation of mainly the maxillary anterior teeth.

breathing, rescue, *n* an emergency treatment aimed at restoring natural respiration in a person who has stopped breathing in which the rescuer inflates the victim's lungs by breathing air into his or her oral cavity or nose directly or through a ventilation device. The technique may be combined with cardiac compressions if the victim has no pulse.

bregma (breg′mə), *n* the point at which the sagittal and coronary sutures meet.

Breuer's reflex, *n.pr* See reflex, Hering-Breuer.

bridge, *n* a colloquial expression for a fixed partial denture. See also denture, partial, fixed.

bridge, cantilever, n See denture, partial, fixed, cantilever.

bridge, fixed, n See denture, partial, fixed.

bridge, removable, n a colloquial expression for a removable partial denture. See also denture, partial, removable.

bridge splint, n See splint, fixed.

Brill-Symmers disease, *n.pr* See lymphoma, giant follicular.

Brinell hardness number, *n.pr* See number, Brinell hardness.

Brinell hardness test, *n.pr* See test, Brinell hardness.

brittle, friable, *adj* technically a brittle material is one in which the proportional limit and ultimate strength are close together in value. See also ductility.

broach, *n* an instrument with numerous barbs protruding from a metal shaft. It is generally used to engage the dental pulp for extirpation.

broach, barbed, n See broach.

broach holder, n an instrument similar to a pin vise used to hold a broach.

broach, pathfinder, n See broach, smooth.

broach, smooth (pathfinder, pathfinder broach), n an instrument used for locating the opening of a root canal and exploring the canal to determine the accessibility of the root end.

broad spectrum, *adj* indicates that a chemical can be used for its intended function with a wide variety of microbes.

Broders' classification, *n.pr* See index, Broders'.

bromide (brō′mīd), *n* a broad-acting chemical agent used to disinfect surfaces in the dental environment; comes in tablet form and is for use on hard surfaces only.

bromine (brō′mēn), *n* a toxic, red-brown, liquid element of the halogen group. Bromine is widely used in industry, photography, the manufacture of organic chemicals, and pharmaceuticals.

bromism (brō′mizəm), *n* the toxic state induced by excessive exposure to or ingestion of bromine or bromine-containing compounds.

bromocriptine mesylate (brō′-mōkrip′tēn mes′ilāt′), *n brand name:* Parlodel; *drug class:* dopamine receptor agonist, ovulation stimulant; *action:* inhibits prolactin release by activating postsynaptic dopamine receptors; *uses:* treatment of female infertility, Parkinson's disease, amenorrhea.

bromodeoxyuridine (brō′mōdē-oksyur′ədēn), *n* a compound that competes with uridine for incorporation in ribonucleic acid.

bromopnea (brəmop′nēə), *n* See halitosis.

B

brompheniramine maleate (brom′fənē′rəmēn′ mā′lēāt), *n brand names:* Bromphen, Dehist, Veltane; *drug class:* antihistamine, H_1-receptor antagonist; *action:* acts on blood vessels and gastrointestinal and respiratory systems by competing with histamine for H_1-receptor sites; *uses:* treatment of allergy symptoms, rhinitis.

bronchia (brong′kēə), *n.pl* the bronchial tubes smaller than bronchi and larger than bronchioles.

bronchiarctia (brong′kēärk′shēə), *n* the stenosis of a bronchial tube.

bronchiectasis (brong′kēek′təsis), *n* a chronic disease characterized by dilation of the bronchi and bronchioles, clinically recognizable by fetid breath and purulent matter; dilation of the bronchi, either local or general.

bronchiocele (brong′kēōsēl), *n* a dilation or swelling of a branch smaller than a bronchus.

bronchiole (brong′kēōl), *n* a terminal division of a bronchium.

bronchitis, *n* an acute or chronic inflammation of the mucous membranes of the tracheobronchial tree.

bronchium (brong′kēəm), *n* one of the subdivisions of a bronchus.

bronchoalveolar, *adj* referring to both the bronchia and alveoli of the lungs.

bronchoconstriction (brong′kō-kənstrik′shən), *n* the reduction of the caliber of the bronchi.

bronchodilation (brong′kōdī-lā′shən), *n* the dilation of a bronchus; the operation of dilating a stenosed bronchus.

bronchodilator (brong′kōdī-lā′tur), *n* a drug that dilates, or expands, the size of the lumina of the air passages of the lungs by relaxing the muscular walls.

bronchopneumonia (bron′kōnə-mō′nyə), *n* an acute inflammation of the lungs and bronchioles characterized by chills, fever, high pulse and respiratory rates, bronchial breathing, cough with purulent bloody sputum, severe chest pain, and abdominal distension.

bronchoscope, *n* a curved flexible tube for visual examination of the bronchi.

bronchoscopy (bronkos′kəpē′), *n* the visual examination of the tracheobronchial tree using a standard rigid, tubular metal bronchoscope or a narrower, flexible, fiberoptic bronchoscope. Bronchoscopy is used to secure a biopsy, aspirate fluids, and diagnose such conditions as lung abscess, bronchial obstruction, and localized atelectasis.

bronchospasm (brong′kōspaz′əm), *n* a spasmodic contraction of the muscular coat of the bronchial tubes such as occurs in asthma.

bronchostenosis (brong′kōstən-ō′sis), *n* the stenosis of the bronchi; bronchiarctia.

bronchus, *n* the subdivisions of the trachea serving to convey air to and from the lungs.

Brooke's tumor, *n.pr* See epithelioma adenoides cysticum.

brown dental stains, *n* the dark, mottled spots on teeth that may indicate fluorosis; may be caused by a prolonged exposure to a high concentration of fluoride during a crucial time in tooth development.

brown pellicle, *n* See pellicle, brown.

bruise, *n* a contusion or ecchymosis; injury, usually caused by blunt impact, in which the capillaries are damaged, allowing blood to seep into the surrounding tissue. Normally minor but painful. Can be serious, leading to hematoma, or can be associated with serious injuries, including fractures and internal bleeding. Minor ones are easily recognized by their characteristic blue or purple color in the days following the injury.

bruit (brōō′ē), *n* an extracardiac blowing sound heard at times over peripheral vessels; generally denotes cardiovascular disease.

brush, bristle polishing, *n* a polishing brush with natural or synthetic bristles.

brush, clasp, *n* a uniquely conceived tool, made to clean the clasps that connect a prosthesis to the natural teeth. Because the clasps are in a critical and difficult to reach position, the 2- to 3-inch tool features a twisted, tapered brush that removes plaque and other debris.

brush, Dixon bristle, *n* a soft brush used to polish the nonmetal parts of removable dentures.

brush, interdental, *n* a dental brush with an angled orientation whose placement in a plastic base enables enhanced interproximal maneuverability during oral care.

brush, interproximal, *n* See brush, interdental.

brush, polishing, *n* an instrument consisting of natural, synthetic, or wire bristles mounted on a mandrel or in a hub to fit on a lathe chuck; used to carry abrasive or polishing media to polish teeth, restorations, and prosthetic appliances.

brush, wheel polishing, *n* a polishing brush with bristles mounted similar to spokes of a wheel.

brush, wire polishing, *n* a polishing brush with bristles of wire, usually steel or brass.

brushing, *n* See abrasion, denture.

brushing plane, *n* See plane, brushing.

bruxism (bruk′sizəm), *n* the involuntary gnashing, grinding, or clenching of teeth. It is usually an unconscious activity, whether the individual is awake or asleep; often associated with fatigue, anxiety, emotional stress, or fear, and frequently triggered by occlusal irregularities, usually resulting in abnormal wear patterns on the teeth, periodontal breakdown, and joint or neuromuscular problems.

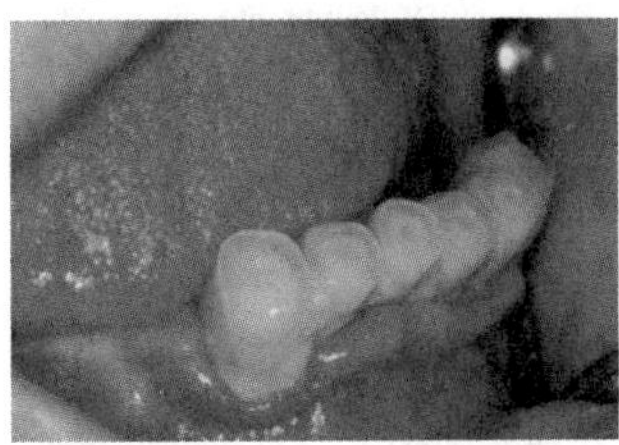

Bruxism. (Courtesy Dr. Charles Babbush)

BSP test, *n* See test, Bromsulphalein.

bubo (byōō′bō), *n* a lymph node that is enlarged as a result of an infection. The process may lead to suppuration; seen in primary syphilis, chancroid, plague, malaria, and other infectious processes.

buccal (buk′əl), *adj* pertaining to or adjacent to the cheek.

buccal aspect, *n* See aspect, buccal.

buccal contour, *n* See contour, buccal.

buccal corridor width **(buk′əl kor′idər),** *n* the negative space between the buccal surface of the maxillary first premolar and the inner point at which the lips join when the patient smiles. It is often stated as a ratio of the inner lip commissure width divided by the distance between the first maxillary premolars.

buccal flange, *n* See flange, buccal.

buccal lymph nodes, *n* See lymph nodes, buccal.

buccal mucosa, *n* See mucosa, oral.

buccal notch, *n* See notch, buccal.

buccal shelf, *n* See shelf, buccal.

buccal splint, *n* See splint, buccal.

buccal surface, *n* See surface, buccal.

buccal tube, *n* See tube, buccal.

buccal vestibule, *n* See vestibule, buccal.

buccinator muscle (buk′sinātər), *n* the muscle consisting of three bands and composing the wall of the cheek between the mandible and the maxilla; it causes the cheek to stay tight to the teeth and the lip corners to pull inward. It is often known as the "cheek muscle."

buccoclusion (buk′ōklōō′zhən), *n* an occlusion in which the dental arch or group of teeth is buccal to the normal position.

buccolingual relationship (buk′ōling′gwəl), *n* See relationship, buccolingual.

buccolingual stress, *n* See stress, buccolingual.

buccoversion (buk′ōvur′zhən), *n* a deviation from the normal line of occlusion toward the cheeks.

buck knife, *n* See knife, buck.

buckling, *n* the crowding of anterior teeth in the dental arch.

buclizine HCl (buk′lizēn), *n brand name:* BucladinS; *drug class:* antihistamine, H_1-receptor antagonist; *action:* acts centrally by blocking chemoreceptor trigger zone; *uses:* treatment for motion sickness.

bud stage of tooth, *n* the second stage in the development of a tooth; it is the result of the proliferation of cells in the basal layer of the oral epithelium.

budesonide (byōōdes′ōnīd′), *n brand names:* Rhinocort Nasal In-

B

haler, Pulmicort; *drug class:* corticosteroid, synthetic; *action:* interacts with steroid cytoplasmic receptors to induce antiinflammatory effects; *uses:* management of symptoms of allergic rhinitis in adults and children; perennial nonallergic rhinitis in adults.

budget plan, *n* a method of financing dental accounts in which arrangements are made for the patient to pay a series of small amounts on an account, usually over a period of 12 to 18 months.

buffer, *n* a substance in a fluid that tends to lessen the change in hydrogen ion concentration that otherwise would be produced by adding acids or alkalis.

buffering capacity, *n* the body's ability to neutralize the acids that play a role in the demineralization of teeth; may be enhanced by eating firmly textured foods, which improve chewing and stimulate the flow of saliva.

bug, *n* an error in a computer program.

bulb, speech, *n* See aid, speech, prosthetic, pharyngeal section.

bulimarexia (bōōlim′ərek′sēə), *n* an eating disorder distinguished by a combination of the symptoms prevalent in both anorexia nervosa and bulimia nervosa; develops primarily in teenage and young adult females.

bulimia (bəlē′mēə), *n* repeated secretive bouts of excessive eating followed by self-induced vomiting, purging, and anorexia, usually accompanied by feelings of guilt, depression, and self-disgust. Oral signs may include dental erosion of the lingual surface of the maxillary anterior teeth.

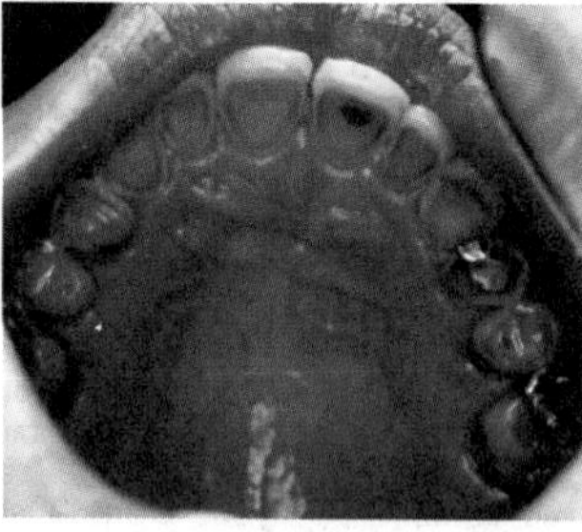

Bulimia. (Sapp/Eversole/Wysocki, 2004)

bulla (bŏŏl′ə), *n* a circumscribed, elevated lesion of the skin containing fluid and measuring more than 5 mm in diameter.

bumetanide (byōōmet′ənīd′), *n* *brand name:* Bumex; *drug class:* loop diuretic; *action:* acts on the loop of Henle to decrease reabsorption of chloride and sodium with resultant diuresis; *uses:* treatment of edema in chronic heart disease, renal disease, pulmonary edema, ascites, and hypertension.

BUN, *n* See blood urea nitrogen.

Bunnell test, *n.pr* See test, Paul-Bunnell.

Bunyaviridae **(bun′yəvir′idā),** *n* a grouping of enveloped, helix-shaped ribonucleic acid (RNA) viruses, implicated in certain forms of encephalitis and sandfly fever.

bupivacaine HCl (local) (byōōpiv′əkān′), *n* *brand names:* Marcaine, Senorcaine; *drug class:* amide local anesthetic; *action:* inhibits ion fluxes across membranes, particularly sodium transport across cell membranes; decreases rise of depolarization phase of action potential; blocks nerve action potential; *uses:* local dental anesthesia, epidural anesthesia, peripheral nerve block, caudal anesthesia.

bupropion (byōō′prō′pēon), *n* *brand names:* Wellbutrin, Zyban; *drug class:* antidepressant; *action:* weak uptake inhibitor of dopamine, serotonin, norepinephrine; mechanism unknown; *uses:* treatment of depression and anxiety disorders; tobacco cessation.

bur, *n* a rotary cutting instrument of steel or tungsten carbide, supplied with cutting heads of various shapes.

bur, carbide, *n* a bur made of tungsten carbide; used at high rotational speeds.

bur, crosscut, *n* a bur with blades slotted perpendicularly to the axis of the bur.

bur, end-cutting, *n* a bur that has cutting blades only on the end of its head.

bur, excavating, *n* a bur used to remove dentin and debris from a cavity.

bur, finishing, *n* a bur with numerous fine-cutting blades placed close together; used to contour metallic restorations.

bur, intramucosal insert base-preparing **(in′trəmyōōkō′səl),** *n* See insert, intramucosal.

bur, inverted cone, n a bur with a head shaped like a truncated cone, the larger diameter being at the terminal (distal) end.

bur, plug-finishing, n See bur, finishing.

bur, round, n a bur with a sphere-shaped head.

bur, straight fissure, n a bur without crosscuts that has a cylindrical head.

bur, tapered fissure, n a bur having a long head with sides that converge from the shank to a blunt end.

burden of proof, *n* in a legal proceeding, the duty to prove a fact or facts in dispute.

Burkitt tumor, *n.pr* See lymphoma, Burkitt.

Burlew wheel, *n.pr* a brand name for an abrasive-impregnated, knife-edged, rubber polishing wheel; used on a mandrel in the dental handpiece to smooth metallic restorations and tooth surfaces.

Burlew wheel, high luster, n a Burlew wheel in which jeweler's rouge or iron peroxide is used as the abrasive agent.

Burlew wheel, midget, n a miniature form of a Burlew wheel.

Burlew wheel, sulci, n See Burlew wheel, midget.

burn, *n* a lesion caused by contact of heat, radiation, friction, or chemicals with tissue. Thermal ones are classified as follows: first degree, by erythema; second degree, by formation of vesicles; third degree, by necrosis of the mucosa or dermis; and fourth degree, by charring into the submucous or subcutaneous layers of the body.

burn, aspirin, n an irregularly shaped, whitish area on the oral mucosa caused by the topical application of acetylsalicylic acid.

burnisher, *n* an instrument shape with rounded edges used to burnish, polish, or work-harden metallic surfaces.

burnisher, ball, n a burnisher with a working point in the form of a ball.

burnisher, beaver-tail, n See burnisher, straight.

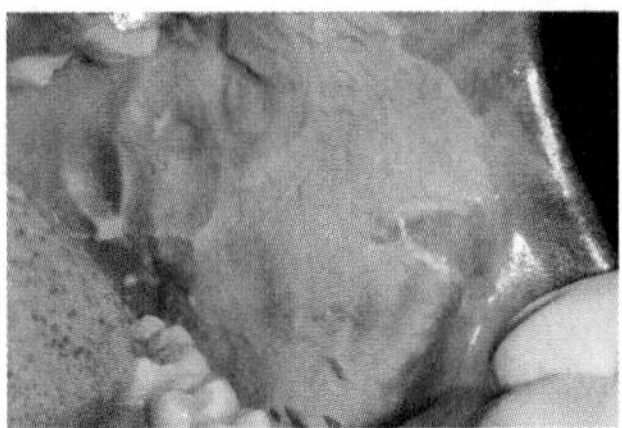

Aspirin burn. (Neville/Damm/Allen/Bouquot, 2002)

burnisher, fishtail, n a burnisher that slightly resembles a fish's tail in shape.

burnisher, straight, n a burnisher that resembles a beaver's tail in shape; the broad, flat blade is smoothly continuous with the shank, meeting it in a slight curve; the edges and the point are smoothly rounded.

burnishing, *n* a process related to polishing and abrading; the metal is moved by mechanically distorting the normal space lattice. Commonly accomplished during the polishing of soft golds.

burnout, *n* the elimination by heat of an invested pattern from a set investment to prepare the mold to receive casting metal.

burnout, high heat, n the use of temperatures higher than 1100° F (593.5° C) to effect wax elimination and prepare the mold to receive casting metal.

burnout, inlay (wax), n the elimination of wax from an invested inlay flask. See also wax elimination.

burnout, job, n the condition of having no energy left to care, resulting from chronic, unrelieved job-related stress and characterized by physical and emotional exhaustion and sometimes by physical illness.

burnout, radiographic, n the excessive penetration of the radiographic beam of an object or part of an object, producing a totally black, or overexposed, area on the radiograph.

burnout, wax, n See burnout, inlay and wax elimination.

business area, *n* the area adjacent to the reception room in which the receptionist conducts the business affairs of the office and directly through which patients must pass to enter and leave the dental office.

business hours (office hours), *n.pl* the hours of the day during which professional, public, and other kinds of business are ordinarily conducted.

business office, *n* the room where the business of the dental practice is conducted.

buspirone HCl (byōōspī′rōn), *n brand name:* BuSpar; *drug class:* antianxiety agent; *action:* unknown; may inhibit 5-HT receptors or dopamine receptors; *use:* management and short-term relief of anxiety disorders.

busulfan (byōōsul′fən), *n brand name:* Myleran; *drug class:* antineoplastic; *action:* changes essential cellular ions to covalent bonding with resultant alkylation, which interferes with biologic function of deoxyribonucleic acid; *uses:* treatment of chronic myelocytic leukemia.

butoconazole nitrate (byōōtəkon′əzōl′ nī′trāt), *n brand name:* Femstat; *drug class:* antifungal; *action:* binds sterols in fungal cell membrane, which increases permeability; *use:* treatment of vulvovaginal infections caused by *Candida.*

butt, *v* to place directly against the tissues covering the residual alveolar ridge; to bring two square-ended surfaces into contact, as a butt joint.

button, *n* the excess metal remaining from the casting and sprue; located at the end of the sprue, opposite the casting.

button, implant, *n* See insert, intramucosal.

buttonhole approach, *n* a method of surgical treatment of a periodontal abscess in which, after an incision is made in the fluctuant abscess, an additional attempt is made to curet the area adjoining the root and the fundus of the abscess through the destroyed portion of the alveolar plate or bone.

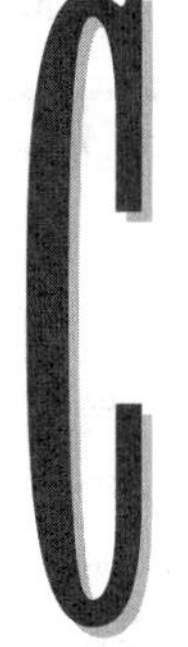

cachexia (kəkek′sēə), *n* the weakness, loss of weight, atrophy, and emaciation caused by severe or chronic disease such as with AIDS.

cachexia, hypophysial, *n* See disease, Simmonds'.

cachexia hypopituitary, *n* See disease, Simmonds'.

cadaver (kədav′ər), *n* a deceased body, most often used in reference to a body used for dissection and study.

cadaverine (kədav′ərēn′), *n* a foul-smelling diamine formed by bacterial decarboxylation of lysine. It is poisonous and irritating to the skin.

cadmium (Cd) (kad′mēəm), *n* a bluish-white metallic element that resembles tin. Cadmium bromide, used in engraving, lithography, and photography, can cause severe gastrointestinal symptoms if ingested.

café-au-lait spots, *n.pl* See spots, café-au-lait.

cafeteria plan, *n* an employee benefits plan in which employees select their medical insurance coverage and other nontaxable fringe benefits from a list of options provided by the employer.

caffeine (kafēn′, kaf′ēin), *n* a white, odorless, bitter compound isolated from tea and coffee that is used as a stimulant of the central nervous system. See also aspirin, phenacetin.

CAGE questionnaire, *n.pr* a four-question survey used to identify potential alcohol dependence. CAGE is an acronym for the four areas identified (felt need to **C**ut back, **A**nnoyance by critics, **G**uilt about drinking, and **E**ye-opening morning drinking).

calcific metamorphosis (of dental pulp), *n* a frequently observed reaction to trauma, characterized by partial or complete obliteration of the pulp chamber and canal.

calcification (kal′sifikā′shən), *n* the process whereby calcium salts are deposited in an organic matrix. The condition may be normal, as in bone and tooth formation, or pathologic.

calcification, dystrophic, *n* the pathologic deposition of calcium salts in necrotic or degenerated tissues.

calcification, ectopic oral, n the displaced accumulation of hardened calcium salts in the oral cavity; stones found in pulp or saliva. See also salivary stone and denticle.

calcification, metastatic, n the pathologic deposition of calcium salts in previously undamaged tissues. This process is caused by an excessively high level of blood calcium, such as in the hyperparathyroid.

calcifying epithelial odontogenic tumor (Pindborg tumor), *n* an uncommon tumor arising from odontogenic epithelium characterized by focal areas of calcification. It has the same age, gender, and site distribution as the ameloblastoma.

calcination (kal'sinā'shən), *n* a process of removing water by heat; used in the manufacture of plaster and stone from gypsum.

calcinosis (kal'sənō'sis), *n* **1.** the deposition of calcium salts in various tissues because of hypercalcemia and tissue degeneration. **2.** the presence of calcification in or under the skin. The condition may occur in a localized (calcinosis circumscripta) or generalized (calcinosis universalis) form.

calcipotriene (kal'sipōtri'ēn), *n brand name:* Dovonex; *drug class:* vitamin D3 derivative (synthetic); *action:* regulation of skin cell production and development; *use:* moderate plaque psoriasis.

calcite, *n* an abrasive agent made from crystallized natural calcium carbonate.

calcitonin (kal'sitō'nin), *n brand names:* Calcitonin, Calcimar, Miacalcin; *drug class:* synthetic polypeptide calcitonins; *action:* inhibits bone resorption, reduces osteoclast function, reduces serum calcium levels in hypercalcemia; *uses:* Paget's disease, postmenopausal osteoporosis, hypercalcemia.

calcitriol (kal'sitri'ol), *n brand name:* Calcijex; *drug class:* vitamin D3 hormone; *action:* increases intestinal absorption of calcium and phosphorus; *uses:* hypocalcemia in chronic renal dialysis and rickets, nutritional supplement.

calcium (Ca) (kal'sēəm), *n* a basic element, with an atomic weight of 40.07, found in nearly all organized tissues. Essential for mineralization of bone and teeth. The normal level of it in the blood is 9 to 11.5 mg/100 ml. A deficiency of it in the diet or in use may lead to rickets or osteoporosis. Overexcretion in hyperparathyroidism leads to osteoporotic manifestations. See also factor IV.

calcium binding protein, n See calmodulin.

calcium, blood, n See blood calcium.

calcium carbonate, n brand names: Maalox Antacid, Rolaids Calcium Rich, Tums E-X; *drug class:* antacid; *action:* neutralizes gastric acidity, supplies calcium; *uses:* antacid, calcium supplement.

calcium carbonate and magnesium hydroxide, n brand name: Rolaids; *drug class:* antacid; *action:* neutralizes gastric acidity; *use:* antacid.

calcium channel blocker, n a drug that inhibits the flow of calcium ions across the membranes of smooth muscle cells. The reduction of calcium flow relaxes smooth muscle tone and reduces the risk of muscle spasms. Calcium channel blockers are used in the prevention and treatment of coronary artery spasms.

calcium, dietary, n the amount of absorbable calcium ingested daily.

calcium fluoride, n a compound that is used as a flux in the manufacture of some silicate cements.

calcium hydroxide, n a white powder that is mixed with water or another medium and used as a base material in cavity liners and for pulp capping.

calcium oxalate, n an insoluble sediment in the urine and urinary calculi.

calcium phosphate, n an odorless, tasteless white powder, the various forms of which are sometimes used as abrasives in dentifrices.

calcium salts, n.pl the calcium present in salivary fluid as phosphates and carbonates. They are believed to form dental calculus on their precipitation from saliva.

calcium sulfate, n See alpha-hemihydrate, beta-hemihydrate, gypsum.

calcium tungstate, n a chemical substance used in crystal form to coat screens; the screens fluoresce when struck by roentgen rays.

calculogenesis (kal′kūlōjen′əsis), *n* the process during which calculus is formed.

calculogenic (kal′kūlōjen′ik), *adj* pertaining to the formation of calculus on tooth surfaces.

C

calculus (dental) (kal′kyələs), *n* a hard deposit on the exposed surfaces of the teeth and any oral prosthesis within the oral cavity. It is composed of calcium phosphate, calcium carbonate, magnesium phosphate, and other elements within an organic matrix composed of plaque, desquamated epithelium, mucin, microorganisms, and other debris. Factor in the initiation and continuation of periodontal disease. The colloquial term is tartar.

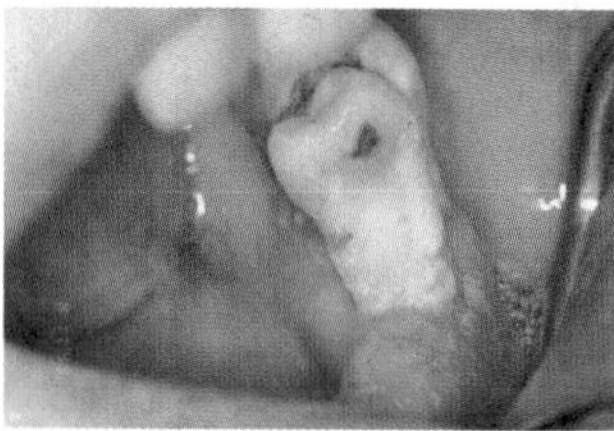

Advanced calculus. (Courtesy Dr. Charles Babbush)

calculus, identification of, by air application, *n* the use of compressed air to dry the periodontium and visualize minimal amounts of calculus, which are otherwise difficult to see, especially subgingivally.

calculus record, *n* a written accounting of the number and distribution of calculus deposits on tooth surfaces that becomes part of the patient's permanent chart and is used to monitor progress and plan treatment.

calculus, subgingival, *n* the calculus deposited on the tooth structure and found apical to the gingival margin within the periodontal pocket. Usually darker and denser than supragingival calculus. Older term is *serumal calculus.*

calculus, supragingival, *n* the calculus deposited on the teeth coronal to the gingival margin. Usually lighter in color (unless stained) and less dense than subgingival calculus. Older term is *salivary calculus.*

calibrated probe, *n* See probe, periodontal.

calibration (kal′əbrā′shən), *n* **1.** the process of comparing a measurement instrument against a verified standard instrument. The US Bureau of Standards maintains the national calibration instruments for weights and measures. **2.** the comparison of procedures between clinicians to achieve a clinical standard.

calibration of radiography unit, *n* See unit, radiography calibration.

Caliciviridae **(kal′isēvir′idā),** *n* a grouping of nonenveloped, 20-sided RNA viruses, and includes the Norwalk gastroenteritis virus.

caliper, axis-orbital, *n* a caliper used to record facial measurements and transfer them to an adjustable articulator. It consists of the following: (1) a hinge-bow, (2) a bite fork covered with compound, (3) an indicator of the axis-orbital plane, (4) an upright rod to hold the orbital indicator in place, (5) a toggle to freeze the bow's base to the bite fork, and (6) a toggle to attach and allow adjustments for the support of the indicator. Also called *hinge-bow transfer recorder.*

Callahan's method, *n.pr* See method, chloropercha.

callus (kal′əs), *n* the tissue near and about the broken fragments of a bone that becomes involved in the repair of the fracture through various stages of exudate, fibrosis, and new bone formation.

calmodulin (kalmoj′əlin), *n* a calcium-binding protein that mediates a variety of biochemical and physiologic processes, including the contraction of muscles and the release of norepinephrine.

calorie, *n* the amount of heat required to raise 1 g of water 1° C at atmospheric pressure, also called gram calorie or small calorie. A great calorie, or kilocalorie, consists of 1000 small calories. The kilocalorie is the unit used to denote the heat expenditure of an organism and the fuel or energy value of food.

calorimetry, *n* the measurement of the amounts of heat radiated and absorbed.

Camper's line, *n.pr* See line, Camper's.

camphorated opium tincture (kam′fərā′təd), *n brand name:* Paregoric; *drug class:* antidiarrheal; *action:* antiperistaltic and analgesic with activity related to morphine content; *use:* diarrhea.

camphorated parachlorophenol (per′əklôr′ōfē′nol), *n* a mixture of 35% parachlorophenol and 65% camphor; used to treat root canals and periapical infections.

***Campylobacter* (kam′pəlōbak′tər),** *n.pr* a microorganism associated with progressive periodontal destruction and refractory forms of periodontitis.

Campylobacter gastroenteritis, *n* a gastrointestinal tract infection with typical symptoms, caused by *C. jejuni* bacteria, the microaerophilic bacteria naturally occurring in humans.

Canadian Dental Hygienists' Association (CDHA), *n.pr* a nonprofit advocacy group established in 1964 representing Canadian dental hygienists nationwide. The CDHA promotes dental standards, releases position statements and safety alerts, and aims to educate the Canadian public on the importance of oral health.

canal, *n* the portion of the root that contains the pulp tissue and is surrounded by dentin.

canal, accessory root, *n* a lateral branching of the main root canal, usually occurring in the apical third of the root. Also called *lateral canal.*

canal, alimentary, *n* the entire digestive route, beginning at the oral cavity and ending at the anus, in which food enters, nourishment is extracted, and waste products are expelled.

canal, branching, *n* See canal, collateral pulp.

canal, calcified, *n* a root canal that has been subjected to calcification, the hardening of decaying of dead soft tissue.

canal, collateral pulp (branching canal), *n* a pulp canal branch that emerges from the root at a place other than the apex.

canal, interdental (nutrient canal), *n* the nutrient channels that pass upward through the body of the mandible. Present as radiolucent lines on radiographs.

canal, mandibular, *n* a channel extending from the mandibular foramen on the medial surface of the ramus of the mandible to the mental foramen. It contains mandibular blood vessels (arteries and veins) and a portion of the mandibular branch of the trigeminal nerve, the incisive nerve, and the inferior alveolar nerve.

canal, nutrient, *n* See canal, interdental.

canal, pulp, *n* the space in the radicular portion of the tooth occupied by the pulp.

canal, root, *n* See canal, pulp.

canal, root, measurements, *n.pl* a technique employing the use of radiographs to determine the length of the root canal.

canaliculus (kan′əlik′yəlus), *n* a small channel that extends from or to the lacunae of bone and cementum and contains filamentous processes of the cells that occupy the lacunae; interconnects with canaliculi extending from neighboring lacunae.

cancellous (kan′seləs), *adj* possessing a permeable, porous structure. Frequently used in conjunction with *bone* to refer to the spongy, typically artery- and vein-rich section at the ends of long bones.

cancer (kan′sur), *n* a malignant neoplasm. The term is sometimes incorrectly used to include any neoplasm, whether benign or malignant. *Carcinoma* and *sarcoma* are more specific terms.

cancer, oral, *n* malignancies indicative of unchecked cell growth that are mainly found in and around the oropharynx, gingiva, floor of the oral cavity, lower lip, and base of the tongue.

cancrum oris (kang′krəm ôr′is), *n* See noma.

***Candida albicans* (kan′didə al′bəkanz),** *n.pr* a budding, yeast-like fungus present in the normal flora of the mucous membrane of the female genital tract and respiratory and gastrointestinal tracts (including the oral cavity) that is capable of assuming a pathogenic role in the production of oral and systemic moniliasis, such as thrush and monilial infection.

candidiasis (kan′didī′əsis), *n* an infection by *C. albicans.* See also moniliasis; thrush.

C

candidiasis, angular cheilitis, n a condition that forms fissures or ulcers radiating from the corners of the oral cavity (commissures) often accompanied by white plaques. Usually observed in elderly patients, although when observed in a young person, it may be an indicator of HIV infection. Candidiasis of the esophagus, trachea, bronchi, or lungs is associated with group IV human immunodeficiency virus (HIV) infection. See also acquired immunodeficiency syndrome (AIDS).

candidiasis, erythematous (atrophic), n a condition that forms smooth red patches on the hard or soft palate, buccal mucosa, or dorsal surface of the tongue.

candidiasis, hyperplastic, n a condition that forms white plaques that cannot be removed by wiping or scraping.

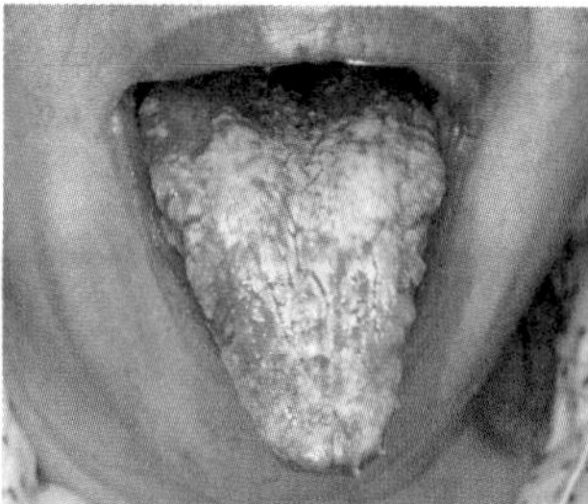

Chronic hyperplastic candidiasis. (Ibsen/Phelan, 2004)

candidiasis, pseudomembranous, n a condition that forms loosely adherent (wipeable), yellowish-white plaques on the oral mucosal surface.

canine (kā'nīn), *n* one of the four pointed teeth situated one on each side of each jaw, distal to the lateral incisor; forms the keystone of the arch. Older term is *cuspid.*

canine eminence **(em'ənəns),** *n* a bony projection that covers the root of the canine tooth on the labial surface of the maxillary arch.

canine fossa, n See fossa, canine.

canine guidance, n a concept of occlusal function in which the canine teeth are assigned a major control role in the excursive movements of the mandible.

canker (kang'kur), *n* See aphtha.

cannabis (kan'əbis), *n* a psychoactive herb derived from the flowering tops of a variety of hemp, *Cannabis sativa.* It is the active ingredient of marijuana. It has been used in the treatment of glaucoma and as an antiemetic in some cancer patients to counter the nausea and vomiting associated with chemotherapy. It is controlled under Schedule I of the Comprehensive Drug Abuse Prevention and Control Act of 1970.

cannula (kan'yələ), *n* a tube for insertion into the body; its caliber is usually occupied by a trocar during the act of insertion.

cannula, nasal, n a small, half-moon shaped plastic tube, the ends of which fit into the nostrils of an individual.

canthus, lateral (kan'thus), *n* a lateral angle between the upper and lower eyelids.

canthus, medial, *n* a medial angle between the upper and lower eyelids.

cantilever bridge (kan'təlē'vər), *n* See denture, partial, fixed, cantilever.

cantilever partial denture, *n* See denture, partial, cantilever fixed.

cap, *n* See crown.

cap stage of tooth, *n* the third period of development in a tooth bud. During this stage, the amorphous cellular structure of the bud takes shape, ultimately resulting in a caplike appearance.

capacity, *n* legal qualification, competency, power, or fitness.

capacity, functional residual, n (normal capacity), the volume of gas in the lungs at resting expiratory level.

capacity, iron-binding, n a measure of the binding capacity of iron in the serum; helps to differentiate the causes of hypoferremia. This capacity tends to increase in iron deficiency and diminishes in chronic diseases and during infection.

capacity, normal, n See capacity, functional residual.

capacity, total lung (TLC), n the volume of air in the lungs at the end of maximal inspiration.

capacity, vital (VC), n the maximum volume of air that can be expired after maximal inspiration.

capillarity (kap′iler′itē), *n* the phenomenon by which a film of fluid is drawn and held between two closely approximating surfaces.

capillary (kap′ilerē), *n* the terminal vessels uniting the arterial with the venous systems of the body. They are organized into extensive branching reticular beds to provide a maximal surface for exchange of fluids, electrolytes, and metabolites between tissues and the vascular system.

capillary attraction, *n* the quality or state that, because of surface tension, causes elevation or depression of the surface of a liquid that is in contact with a solid. Considered to be one of the factors in retention of complete dentures.

capillary disorder, *n* a hemorrhagic disorder caused by increased fragility of the blood vessels that may cause hemorrhages in the skin and mucous membranes

capital budgeting, *n* the process of planning expenditures on assets, the returns of which are expected to extend beyond 1 year.

capitation (kap′ətā′shən), *n* **1.** the practice of dentistry financed by a set fee per person per given period of time. A form of contracted dental care, usually by a corporation, institution, or other group. **2.** a system by which the contracting dental professional, assuming the financial risk, is compensated at a fixed per capita rate, usually on specific, predetermined dental services as appropriate and necessary to eligible subscribers. **3.** a dental benefits program in which a dental professional or dental professionals contract with the program's sponsor or administrator to provide all or most of the dental services covered under the program to subscribers in return for payment on a per capita basis.

capitation fee, *n* a predetermined per-person charge made by the carrier for benefits available under an insurance plan.

capitulum (kəpich′əlum), *n* the European term for a small head, instead of *head* or *condyle.*

capitulum mandibulae, *n* See process, condyloid.

***Capnocytophaga* (kap′nositof′əgə),** *n* a species of gram-negative facultatively anaerobic bacteria belonging to the genus *Capnocytophaga.* It is present in both normal and diseased oral cavities. Possibly associated with periodontal disease.

capnophilic (kap′nōfil′ik), *adj* the ability to thrive in conjunction with carbon dioxide.

capping, direct pulp, *n* an application to the exposed pulp of a drug or material for the purpose of stimulating repair of the injured pulpal tissue.

capping, indirect pulp, *n* a chemical (usually calcium hydroxide) placed over a layer of carious dentin remaining over the potentially exposed pulp to protect the pulp from external irritants.

capping, pulp, *n* the covering of an exposed dental pulp with a material that protects it from external influences.

capsaicin (kapsā′isin), *n brand names:* Zostrix, Capzasin-P, Axsain; *drug class:* topical analgesic for selected pain syndromes; *action:* depletes and prevents reaccumulation of substance P in peripheral sensory neurons; *uses:* neuralgia associated with herpes zoster, rheumatoid arthritis, temporomandibular joint (TMJ) pain.

capsule, joint, *n* a fibrous sac or ligament that encloses a joint and limits its motion. It is lined with synovial membrane.

capsule, temporomandibular joint, *n* See articulation, temporomandibular, capsule.

captopril (kap′təpril), *n brand name:* Capoten; *drug class:* angiotensin-converting enzyme; *action:* dilation of arterial and venous vessels; *use:* hypertension.

carat, *n* a standard of fineness of gold, 24 carats being taken as expressing absolute purity.

carbamazepine (kär′bəmaz′əpēn), *n brand names:* Apo-Carbamazepine, Epitol, Novo Carbamaz; *drug class:* anticonvulsant; *action:* inhibits nerve impulses by limiting influx of sodium ions across cell membrane in motor cortex; *uses:* tonic-clonic complex-partial, mixed seizures, a specific analgesic for trigeminal neuralgia, sometimes used in the treatment of herpes zoster.

C

carbaminohemoglobin, *n* a hemoglobin compounded with CO_2.

carbenicillin (kärben'isil'in), *n* a semisynthetic penicillin that is acid resistant and rapidly absorbed from the small intestine and thus suitable for oral administration.

carbide bur, *n* See bur, carbide.

carbides (kar'bīdz), *n* **1.** in chemistry, carbon binary compounds with strong electron-releasing properties. **2.** mixtures of carbon with at least one heavy metal. E.g., the bur, or metal alloy bit, of a dental drill has a composition of tungsten carbide.

carbohemia (kär'bōhē'mēə), *n* an imperfect oxygenation of the blood.

carbohydrates, *n.pl* a group of organic compounds with the class name saccharides, which are the aldehydric or ketonic derivatives of polyhydric alcohols. Ones such as sugar, starch, cellulose, and gum are generally synthesized by green plants. They constitute the main energy source in the diet and are classified as mono-, di-, tri-, and polysaccharides.

carbohydrate tolerance, *n* See tolerance, carbohydrate.

carbon, *n* a nonmetallic tetravalent element that occurs in pure form in diamonds and graphite. It occurs as a component of all living tissue. Most of the study of organic chemistry focuses on the vast number of carbon compounds.

carbon coated, *adj* a vitreous carbon coating applied to either an endosteal or blade implant to improve tissue compatability.

carbon dioxide, *n* a colorless, odorless gas produced by the complete oxidation of carbon. It is a product of cell respiration and is carried by the blood to the lungs and exhaled. The acid-base balance of body fluids and tissues is affected by the level of it and its carbonate compounds.

carbon monoxide, *n* a colorless, odorless, poisonous gas produced by the combustion of carbon or organic fuels in a limited oxygen supply. It combines irreversibly with hemoglobin, preventing the formation of oxyhemoglobin and reducing the oxygen supply to the tissues.

carbonate, *n* a mineral salt of carbonic acid.

carbonate hydroxyapatite **(kär'bənāt hīdrok'sēap'ətīt),** *n* the composition and crystal structure of hard tissues.

carbonic acid, *n* an unstable acid formed by dissolving carbon dioxide in water. It is the basis of carbonated beverages and contributes the negative ion to carbonate salts.

carbonic anhydrase (kärbon'ik anhī'drās'), *n* an enzyme that plays a role in transferring carbon dioxide from tissue cells to the lungs by turning carbon dioxide into carbonic acid in red blood cells. Also called *carbonate dehydratase.*

Carborundum stone, *n.pr* See stone, Carborundum.

carboxylate, *n* a carboxylic acid salt, ester, or ion.

carboxylation (kärbok'səlā'shən), *n* the chemical process by which a carboxyl group (COOH) is added or displaces a hydrogen atom.

carboxypeptidase (kärbok'sēpep'tidās), *n* an exopeptidase that stimulates the hydrolytic cleavage of the last or second to last peptide bond at the C-terminal end of a peptide or polypeptide.

carcinogen (kärsin'əjen), *n* a substance or agent that causes the development or increases the incidence of cancer.

carcinoma (kär'sinō'mə), *n* a malignant epithelial tumor. Also called *cancer.*

carcinoma, adenoid cystic, *n* a salivary gland malignancy of ductal and myoepithelial cells that may arise in both major and minor salivary glands. Although it grows slowly, perineural invasion and its relentless nature makes long-term survival poor.

carcinoma, basal cell (basal cell epithelioma, rodent ulcer, turban tumor), *n* an epithelial neoplasm with a basic structure resembling the basal cells of the epidermis. It develops from basal cells of the epidermis or from the outer cells of hair follicles or sebaceous glands, particularly the middle third of the face. It rarely, if ever, metastasizes but is locally invasive. It does not arise from oral mucosa. It develops as a plaque that then ulcerates in the center, becoming indurated.

carcinoma, basosquamous, *n* a carcinoma that histologically exhibits both basal and squamous elements. It may occasionally be seen in the oral cavity; considered to have a greater tendency to metastasize than does basal cell carcinoma.

carcinoma, epidermoid **(ep′əder′-moid),** *n* a malignant epithelial neoplasm with cells resembling those of the epidermis. The term *squamous cell carcinoma* is used for intraoral lesions of this nature. See also carcinoma, squamous cell (SCC).

carcinoma, exophytic, *n* a malignant epithelial neoplasm with marked outward growth similar to a wart or papilloma.

carcinoma in situ, *n* a dysplastic epithelial disease involving the skin and mucous membranes and considered to be precancerous. Dysplasia (premature keratinization) is evident, but no invasion has yet occurred.

carcinoma, intraepithelial, *n* See carcinoma in situ.

carcinoma, mucoepidermoid **(myōō′-kōep′əder′moid),** *n* a malignant epithelial tumor of the salivary gland characterized by acini with mucus-producing cells.

carcinoma, squamous cell (SCC), *n* the second most common skin cancer after basal cell carcinoma. It arises from the epidermis or oral mucosa and resembles the squamous cells that comprise most of the upper layers. It may occur on all areas of the body, including the mucous membranes, but is most common in areas exposed to the sun. Risk factors include actinic (sun) damage, alcohol use, and tobacco use.

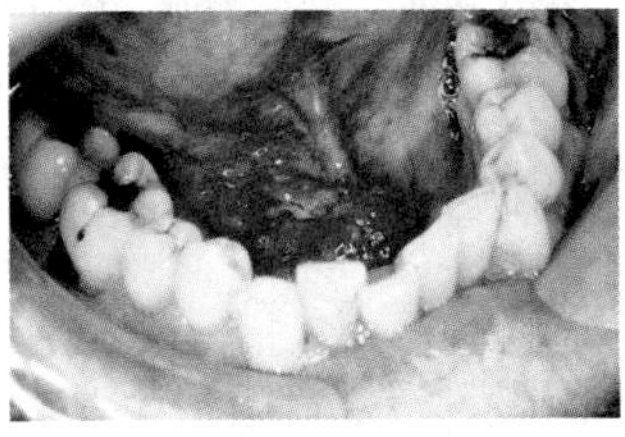

Squamous cell carcinoma. (Sapp/Eversole/Wysocki, 2004)

carcinoma, transitional cell, *n* a malignant tumor arising from a transitional type of stratified epithelium.

carcinoma, verrucous, *n* a squamous cell carcinoma, usually intraoral, that is exophytic and has a papillary appearance. Associated with spit tobacco.

cardia (kär′dēə), *n* the opening between the esophagus and the cardiac portion of the stomach; characterized by the absence of acid cells. Also an archaic term formerly used to describe the heart and the region surrounding it.

cardiac, *adj* relating to the heart.

cardiac arrest, *n* a stopping of heart action; a complete cessation of heart function.

cardiac dysrhythmia **(disrith′mēə),** *n* an irregular or abnormal heartbeat rhythm. Also known as *cardiac arrhythmia.*

cardiac massage, *n* See massage, cardiac.

cardiac output, *n* the volume of blood put out by the heart per minute; the product of the stroke volume and the heart rate per minute.

cardiac pacemaker, *n* See pacemaker.

cardiac surgery, *n* an operative procedure used to treat a disease of the heart or its blood vessels.

cardioinhibitory (kär′dēōinhib′-itôrē), *adj* restraining or inhibiting the movements of the heart.

cardiokinetic (kär′dēōkinet′ik), *adj* exciting the heart; a remedy that excites the heart.

cardiology, *n* the scientific study of the anatomy, normal function, and disorders of the heart.

cardiomyopathy, hypertrophic, *n* a disease of the heart in which the heart is enlarged.

cardiopulmonary, *adj* pertaining to the heart and lungs.

cardiopulmonary resuscitation (CPR), *n* a basic emergency procedure for life support, consisting of mainly manual external cardiac massage and some artificial respiration.

cardiovascular disease (CVD), *n* any one of a number of abnormal conditions that involve dysfunction of the heart and blood vessels, including but not limited to systemic hypertension, atherosclerosis and coronary heart disease, and rheumatic heart disease.

C

cardiovascular system, *n* the network of structures, including the heart and blood vessels, that convey the blood throughout the body.

carditis, *n* an inflammation of the heart muscle tissue. Pericarditis, myocarditis, and endocarditis are types of carditis affecting specific regions of the heart.

care, *n* as a legal term, the opposite of negligence.

care, reasonable, *n* such care as an ordinarily prudent person would exercise under the conditions existing at the time that person is called on to act.

care plan, *n* strategies designed to guide health care professionals involved with patient care. Such plans are patient specific and are meant to address the total status of the patient. Care plans are intended to ensure optimal outcomes for patients during the course of their care.

caregiver, *n* a person providing treatment or support to a sick, disabled, or dependent individual.

caries (ker′ēz), *n* in dentistry, the decay of a tooth. Colloquial term is *cavity.*

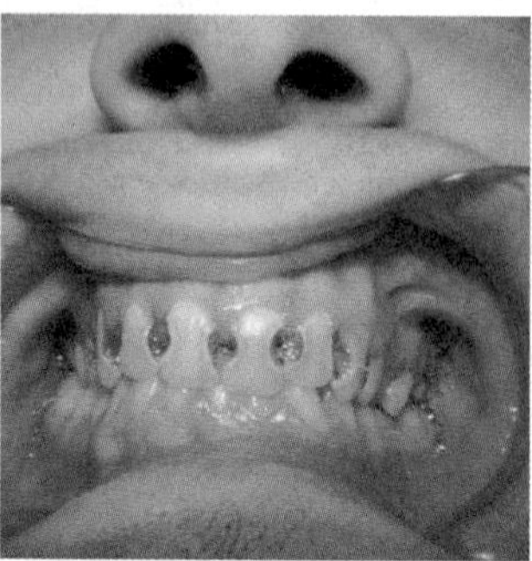

Advanced caries. (Courtesy Dr. Charles Babbush)

caries, arrested, *n* the state existing when the progress of the decay process has halted. It is noted by its dark staining without any breakdown of tooth tissues.

Caries Assessment Tool (CAT), *n.pr* an analysis that examines the risk factors for the development of dental caries in infants and young children. Risk factors such as the environment, family history, and general health can be identified early, thereby reducing a patient's risk for developing dental caries and other diseases of the teeth and gingival tissues.

caries, baby bottle, *n* See caries, early childhood (EEC).

caries, cemental (root surface), *n* the decay of the cementum that occurs as a result of gingival recession and exposure of the root surface. See also caries, cervical (root surface).

caries, cervical (root surface), *n* the decay that appears on the root at the cementoenamel junction or the neck as a result of gingival recession and exposure of the root surface. See also caries, cemental (root surface).

caries, chronic, *n* a form of caries that occurs over time and demands regular dental intervention.

caries, compound, *n* a type of caries that affects two or more surfaces of a tooth.

caries, early childhood (EEC), *n* a form of severe dental decay occurring in young children that is caused by long and frequent exposure to liquids that are high in sugar, such as milk or juice. Because this form can damage the underlying bone structure, it may affect the development of permanent teeth.

caries, enamel, *n* the decay that occurs in the enamel of a tooth because of a fissure or the collection of bacterial plaque. It appears first as white spots, which later darken to brown.

caries, gross, *n* a form of caries with advanced dental decay that is easily seen clinically.

caries, healed, *n* See caries, arrested.

caries, incipient, *n* a decayed part of a tooth in which the lesion is just coming into existence.

caries, nursing, *n* See caries, early childhood (EEC).

caries, pit-and-fissure, *n* See cavity, pit and fissure. See also sealant, enamel.

caries, plaque-related, *n* the caries associated with plaque formation. Most commonly located in the pits and fissures of the teeth, especially the molar and premolar teeth, and along the gingival tissue and also the margins associated with dental restorations.

caries, proximal, *n* decay occurring in the mesial or distal surface of a tooth.

caries, rampant, *n* a suddenly appearing, widespread, rapidly progressing type of caries.

caries, recurrent, *n* the extension of the carious process beyond the margin of a restoration. Also called *secondary caries.*

caries, residual, *n* (residual carious dentin), the decayed material left in a prepared cavity and over which a restoration is placed.

caries, root, *n* tooth decay occurring on a portion of the root that is exposed.

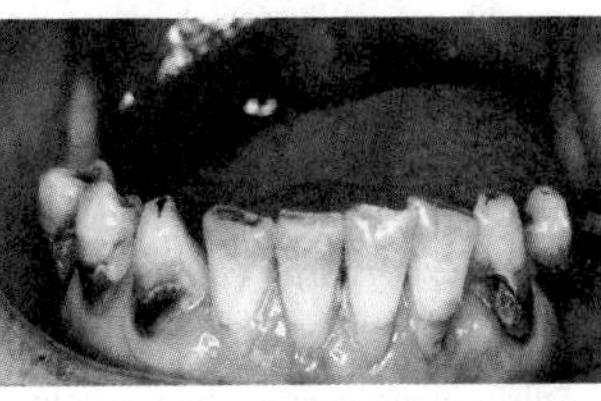

Root caries. (Sapp/Eversole/Wysocki, 2004)

caries, senile (senile decay), *n* older term for the decay noted particularly in the elderly when supporting tissues have receded; occurs in cementum, usually on proximal surfaces of the teeth.

caries, smooth surface, *n* the decay that occurs on the smooth surfaces of the tooth. See also caries, proximal dental and *S. mutans.*

caries, vaccine, *n* a vaccine currently under development to treat dental caries by inoculating against bacteria commonly known to contribute to their formation, particularly *S. mutans.*

cariogenesis (ker′ēōjen′əsis), *n* the process during which cavities develop in teeth.

cariogenic (kerēōjen′ik), *adj* contributing to the advancement of caries. Often used in the context of describing sugary foods.

cariogenic challenge, *n* an episode in which tooth enamel is exposed to acid, a byproduct of cariogenic foods and plaque bacteria.

cariogenicity (ker′ēōjənis′itē), *n* the ability of a substance to induce or potentiate the formation of dental caries.

cariostatic (ker′ēōstat′ik), *adj* pertaining to the oils in fats that provide a protective coating for teeth to keep food particles from sticking and to prevent sugars and acids from entering or leaving plaque. See anticariogenic.

carious (ker′ēus), *adj* pertaining to caries or decay.

carious dentin, *adj* pertaining to caries or decay. See wax, carious.

carisoprodol (ker′īsōprō′dol), *n* *brand names:* Soma, Vanasom; *drug class:* skeletal muscle relaxant, central acting; *action:* nonspecific central nervous system sedation; *uses:* adjunct for relief of muscle spasm in musculoskeletal conditions.

carnauba wax, *n* See wax, carnauba.

carnitine (kar′nətēn′), *n* a compound found naturally in red meat and dairy, as well as in legumes and nuts, this quaternary ammonium compound assists in the movement of fatty acids through the membrane of the mitochondria.

Carnoy's solution, *n.pr* See solution, Carnoy's.

carotene (ker′ətēn), *n* an orange pigment found in carrots, leafy vegetables, and other foods that may be converted to vitamin A in the body.

carotenemia (ker′ətēnē′mēə), *n* excess carotene in the blood, producing a pigmentation of the skin and mucous membranes that resembles jaundice.

carotid (kərot′id), *n* either one of the two main right and left arteries of the neck.

carotid stenosis, *n* the narrowing and hardening of the carotid artery.

carotid triangle, *n* See triangle, carotid.

carpal tunnel syndrome, *n* an irritation and inflammation of the synovials surrounding the tendons controlling the fingers. It is a disabling condition for persons who work with their hands, particularly those engaging in keyboard activities, data management, and instrumentation such as those in the dental office.

carrier, *n* **1.** a person harboring a specific infectious agent without clinical evidence of disease and who serves as a potential source or reservoir of infection for others. May be a healthy or convalescent carrier. *n* **2.** the party of the dental plan contract who agrees to pay claims or provide service. Also called *insurer, underwriter,* and *administrative agent.* See also third party.

carrier, amalgam, *n* an instrument used to carry plastic amalgam to the prepared cavity or mold into which it is to be inserted.

carrier, foil, *n* See foil passer.

carteolol (kär′tēəlol), *n brand name:* Cartrol; *drug class:* nonselective β-adrenergic blocker; *action:* competitively blocks stimulation of β-adrenergic receptors within vascular smooth muscle, decreases rate of sinoatrial (SA) node discharge, increases SA node recovery time; *use:* mild to moderate hypertension.

carteolol HCl, *n brand name:* Ocupress; *drug class:* β-adrenergic blocker; *action:* nonselective β-adrenergic blocking agent, reduces production of aqueous humor by unknown mechanisms; *uses:* chronic open-angle glaucoma, ocular hypertension.

cartilage, *n* a derivative of connective tissue arising from the mesenchyme. Typical hyaline type is a flexible, rather elastic material with a semitransparent, glasslike appearance. Its intercellular substance is a complex protein (chondromucoid) through which is distributed a large network of connective tissue fibers.

cartilage, articular, *n* a thin layer of hyaline cartilage located on the joint surfaces of some bones. Not usually found on articular surfaces of temporomandibular joints, which are covered with an avascular fibrous tissue.

cartilage, condylar **(kar′tlij kon′dələr),** *n* the cartilage containing a rounded articular protrusion, or condyle, present at bone joints. Condylar cartilage of the mandible is a common type.

cartilage, cricoid, *n* the most inferior cartilage of the larynx.

cartilage, Meckel's, *n.pr* the cartilaginous process in the embryo derived from the mesenchymal tissue of the mandibular process.

cartilage, primary, *n* the cartilage formed during fetal development that is not replaced by bone.

cartilage, Reichert's **(rī′kherts),** *n.pr* the cartilaginous process located laterally in the embryonic tympanum; gives rise to styloid processes, stylohyoid ligaments, and lesser horns of hyoid bone.

cartridge, *n* in dentistry, a device of various configuration and composition used with a syringe for the application of anesthetic or other materials to a patient.

caruncle (ker′ungkəl), *n* a small, fleshy growth.

caruncle, sublingual **(subling′gwəl),** *n* See caruncle, submandibular.

caruncle, submandibular (ker′-ungkəl), *n* the opening of the submandibular (Wharton's) duct that opens into the oral cavity on small papillae bilateral to the lingual frenum. See also gland, submandibular salivary.

carvedilol (kär′vədil′ol), *n brand name:* Coreg; *drug class:* nonselective β-adrenergic blocking agent with α-blocking activity; *action:* produces fall in blood pressure without reflex tachycardia or significant reduction in heart rate; *use:* essential hypertension alone or with other antihypertensives.

carver (carving instrument), *n* an instrument used to shape a plastic material such as wax or amalgam.

carver, amalgam, *n* an instrument used to shape plastic amalgam.

carving, *n* the shaping and forming with instruments.

case, *n* the term often incorrectly used instead of the appropriate noun (e.g., *patient, flask, denture, casting*). Case is not synonymous with patient because the latter is more than just the case of situations they present.

case charting, *n* the recording of a patient's status of health or disease.

case dismissal, *n* the technique of illustrating to the patient the results of treatment, usually done during the last appointment of a series.

case history, *n* See history, case.

case management, *n* the monitoring and coordination of treatment rendered to patients with specific diagnoses or requiring high cost or extensive services.

case presentation, n an explanation of dental needs to the patient.

case summary, n enumeration of all the services to be performed for an estimated amount of money.

case-control study, *n* an investigation employing an epidemiologic approach in which previously existing incidents of a medical condition are used in lieu of gathering new information from a randomized population. Control is obtained by comparing known cases of the medical condition with a group of persons who have not developed the medical problem.

cash budget, *n* a schedule showing cash flows (receipts, disbursements, net cash) for a firm over a specified period.

cash cycle, *n* the length of time between the purchase of raw materials and the collection of accounts receivable generated in the sale of the final product.

cash flow, *n* the reported net income of a corporation plus amounts charged off for depreciation, depletion, amortization, and extraordinary charges to reserves, which are bookkeeping deductions not paid out in actual dollars and cents. A measurement tool used in recent years to offer a better indication of the ability of a company to pay dividends and finance expansion from self-generated cash than the conventional reported net income figure.

cassette (kəset′), *n* a light, tight container in which radiographic films are placed for exposure to radiographs; usually backed with lead to eliminate the effect of backscattered radiation.

cassette, cardboard (cardboard film-holder), n a cardboard envelope of simple construction suitable for use in making radiographs on "direct exposure" or "no-screen" types of radiographic films.

cassette, screen-type, n a cassette usually made of metal, with the exposure side of low-atomic-number material, such as Bakelite, aluminum, or magnesium, and containing intensifying screens between which a "screen type" of film or films may be placed for exposure to radiographs.

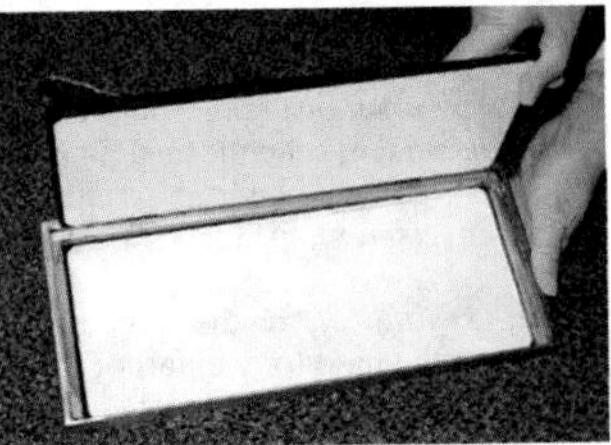

Screen-type cassette. (Bird/Robinson, 2005)

cast, *n* **1.** an object formed by pouring plastic or liquid material into a mold in which it hardens. *v* **2.** to throw metal into an impression to form the casting.

cast, bar splint, n See splint, cast bar.

cast, corrected master, n a dental cast that has been modified by the correction of the edentulous ridge areas as registered in a supplemental, correctable impression.

cast, dental, n a positive likeness of a part or parts of the oral cavity reproduced in a durable hard material.

cast, diagnostic, n a positive likeness of dental structures for the purpose of study and treatment planning.

cast, diagnostic, anatomic portion, n the section of a finished cast that contains the actual impression of the teeth and surrounding tissue. It should account for approximately 65% of the cast's total height.

cast, diagnostic, double-pour method, n a method of forming the base of a cast in which the inverted impression is held against the surface of prereadied stone while the sides and edges of the cast are shaped; eliminates the possibility of inverting the impression before the stone has set. Also called *two-step method.*

cast, diagnostic, implant, n a cast made from a conventional mucosal impression on which the wax trial denture and surgical impression trays are made or selected.

cast, gnathostatic **(nath′ostat′ik),** *n* a cast of the teeth trimmed so that the occlusal plane is in its normal position in the oral cavity when the cast is set on a plane surface. Such casts are used in the gnathostatic technique of orthodontic diagnosis.

C

cast, implant, *n* a positive reproduction of the exposed bony surfaces made in a surgical bone impression and on which subperiosteal implant frame is designed and fabricated.

cast, investment, *n* See cast, refractory.

cast, keying of, *n* the process of forming the base (or capital) of a cast so that it can be remounted accurately. Also referred to as the split-cast method of returning a cast to an articulator.

cast, master, *n* an accurate replica of the prepared tooth surfaces, residual ridge areas, or other parts of the dental arch reproduced from an impression from which a prosthesis is to be fabricated.

cast, mounted, *n* a reproduction of all or part of the oral cavity, which is then attached to a support for ease of display.

cast, preextraction, *n* a cast made before the extraction of teeth. See also cast, diagnostic.

cast, preoperative, *n* See cast, diagnostic.

cast, record, *n* a positive replica of the dentition and adjoining structures, used as a reference for conditions existing at a given time.

cast, refractory, *n* a cast made of materials that can withstand high temperatures without disintegrating and that, when used in partial denture casting techniques, expand to compensate for metal shrinkage.

cast, trimming diagnostic, *n* a set of finishing steps for a study cast in which the bases, posterior borders, sides, heels, and anterior surfaces are smoothed and shaped to ensure a finished product that is attractive, well proportioned, and useful as a diagnostic tool. The treatment is best accomplished using a mechanical model trimmer.

cast, working, *n* an accurate reproduction of a master cast; used in preliminary fitting of a casting to avoid injury to the master cast.

casting, *n* **1.** a metallic object formed in a mold. **2.** forming a casting in a mold.

casting flask, *n* See flask, refractory.

casting machine, *n* a mechanical device used for throwing or forcing a molten metal into a refractory mold.

casting machine, air pressure, *n* a casting machine that forces metal into the mold via compressed air.

casting machine, centrifugal, *n* a casting machine that forces the metal into the mold via centrifugal force.

casting machine, vacuum, *n* a casting machine in which the metal is cast by evacuation of gases from the mold. Atmospheric pressure actually forces metal into the mold.

casting model, *n* See cast, refractory.

casting ring, *n* See flask, refractory.

casting temperature, *n* See temperature, casting.

casting, vacuum, *n* the casting of a metal in the presence of a vacuum. See also casting machine, vacuum.

casting wax, *n* See wax, casting.

Castle's intrinsic factor, *n.pr* See factor, Castle's intrinsic.

castration anxiety (kastrā′shən), *n* **1.** the fantasized fear of injury to or loss of the genital organs. **2.** a general threat to the body image of a person or the unrealistic fear of bodily injury or loss of power or control.

casualty insurance, *n* insurance against loss caused by accidents; usually applied to property but may apply to bodily injury or death from accident.

cat-scratch disease, *n* See disease, cat-scratch.

catabolism (kətab′ōlizəm), *n* the destructive processes (opposite of the anabolic-metabolic processes) by which complex substances are converted into more simple compounds. A proper relation between anabolism and catabolism is essential for the maintenance of bodily homeostasis and dynamic equilibrium.

catabolism of energy, *n* the dissipation of energy in living tissues as work or heat (one phase being metabolism, the other being anabolism).

catabolism of substance, *n* the destructive metabolism; the conversion of living tissues into a lower state of organization and ultimately into waste products.

catalase reaction (kat′əlās), *n* the response of bubbling in the presence of hydrogen peroxide given by blood exudates or transudates.

catalysis (kətal′əsis), *n* the increase

in rate of a chemical reaction, induced by a substance called a *catalyst,* which takes no part in the reaction and remains unchanged.

catalyst (kat′əlist), *n* a substance that induces an increased rate of a chemical reaction without entering into the reaction or being changed by the reaction.

catamenia (kat′əmē′nēə), *n* menses. A term used frequently to designate age at onset of menses.

cataract (kat′ərakt), *n* an abnormal progressive condition of the lens of the eye, characterized by loss of transparency.

catatonia (kat′ətō′nēə), *n* a form of schizophrenia characterized by alternating stupor and excitement. A patient's arms often retain any position in which they are placed.

catecholamine (kat′əkō′ləmēn′), *n* any one of a group of sympathomimetic compounds composed of a catechol molecule and the aliphatic portion of amine. Some catecholamines (epinephrine and norepinephrine) are produced naturally by the body and function as key neurologic chemicals.

catechol-o-methyl transferase (COMT), *n* an enzyme that deactivates epinephrine and norepinephrine.

catgut, *n* a sheep's intestine prepared as a suture and used for ligating vessels and closing soft tissue wounds.

catheter (kath′ətər), *n* a hollow, flexible tube that can be inserted into a vessel or cavity of the body to withdraw or instill fluids.

catheter, balloon-tip, *n* a tube with a balloon at its tip that can be inflated or deflated without removal after insertion.

catheter, indwelling, *n* a catheter left in place in the bladder; usually a type of balloon catheter.

catheterization (kath′ətərizā′shən), *n* the process of introducing a hollow, flexible tube into a blood vessel or body cavity to withdraw or instill fluids.

cathode (kath′ōd), *n* a negative electrode from which electrons are emitted and to which positive ions are attracted. In radiographic tubes, the cathode usually consists of a helical tungsten filament, behind which a molybdenum reflector cup is located to focus the electron emission toward the target of the anode.

cathode ray tube (CRT), *n* a vacuum tube in which a beam of electrons is focused to a small point on a luminescent screen and can be varied in position to form a pattern.

cathode-anode circuit, high-voltage, *n* one of the two electrical circuits required to take radiographs, provides the power to accelerate electrons enough to create radiographic photons.

cation (kat′īon), *n* a positive ion carrying a charge of positive electricity, therefore attracted to the negatively charged cathode.

cationic detergent, See detergent, cationic.

causalgia (kôzal′jə), *n* a postextraction localized pain phenomenon usually characterized by a continuous burning sensation.

causality, *n* a relationship between one event or action that precedes and initiates a second action or influences the direction, nature, or force of a second action. In scientific study, causality must be observable, predictable, and reproducible and thus is difficult to prove.

cause of action, *n* a ground or reason for a legal action; a wrong that is subject to legal redress.

caustic, *adj* destroying living tissue by chemical burning action.

cauterize (kô′tərīz), *v* to sear or burn living tissue in order to stop bleeding; a corrosive agent, hot metal, or electricity may be used.

cavernous sinus (kav′ərnəs), *n* one of a pair of irregularly shaped, bilateral venous channels located below the base of the brain between the sphenoid bone of the skull and the dura mater. Also called *cavernous venus sinus.*

cavernous sinus thrombosis, *n* an infection of the cavernous venous sinus. Increased risk with local anesthesia in the maxillary arch if infection is present ("needle track" infection).

cavitation (kav′itā′shun), *n* the formation and collapse of bubbles in the fluid spray released by a mechanized instrument used for debridement.

cavity, *n* a carious lesion or hole in a tooth.

cavity, access, n See access cavity.

cavity, amniotic, n the space between the developing fetus and the amnion, consisting of amniotic fluid.

cavity, axial surface, n a cavity occurring in a tooth surface in which the general plane is parallel to the long axis of the tooth.

cavity classification, n carious lesions are classified according to the surfaces of a tooth on which they occur (e.g., labial, buccal, occlusal), type of surface (i.e., pit, fissure, or smooth surface), and numerical grouping (G. V. Black's classification).

cavity classification, artificial (G. V. Black), n a classification of cavities.

cavity, complex, n a cavity that involves more than one surface of a tooth.

cavity, compound, n See cavity, complex.

cavity floor, n the base-enclosing side of a prepared cavity. See also cavity, prepared.

cavity, gingival (gingival third cavity), n a cavity occurring in the gingival third of the clinical crown of the tooth (G. V. Black's Class 5).

cavity lining, n the material applied to the prepared cavity before the restoration is inserted to seal the dentinal tubules for protection of the pulp.

cavity medication, n a drug used to clean or treat a cavity before inserting a dressing, base, or restoration.

cavity, nasal, n the two irregular spaces that are situated on either side of the midline of the face, extend from the cranial base to the palate, and are separated from each other by a thin vertical septum. In radiographs it appears over the roots of the maxillary incisors as a large, segmented, radiolucent area. Also called *nasal fossa.*

cavity, pit and fissure, n a cavity that begins in microscopic faults in the enamel. Caused by imperfect closure of the enamel.

cavity preparation, n the orderly operating procedure required to remove diseased tissue and establish in a tooth the biomechanically acceptable form necessary to receive and retain a restoration.

cavity, prepared, n the form developed in a tooth to receive and retain a restoration.

cavity, prepared, floor of, n the flat bottom or enclosing base wall of a prepared cavity; on an axial plane it is called the *axial wall,* and on the horizontal plane it is called the *pulpal wall.*

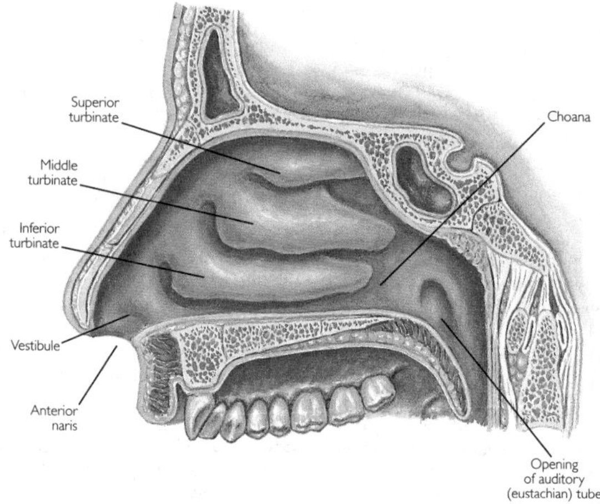

The nasal cavity. (Seidel/Ball/Dains/Benedict, 2006)

cavity, prepared, impression, *n* a negative likeness of a tapered type of prepared cavity.

cavity, proximal, *n* a cavity occurring on the mesial or distal surface of a tooth.

cavity, pulp, *n* the space in a tooth surrounded by the dentin; contains the dental pulp. The part of the pulp cavity within the coronal portion of the tooth is the pulp chamber, and the part found within the root is the pulp canal, or root canal.

cavity, simple, *n* a cavity that involves only one surface of a tooth.

cavity, smooth surface, *n* a cavity formed by decay beginning in surfaces of teeth that are without pits, fissures, or enamel faults.

cavity toilet, *n* G. V. Black's final step in cavity preparation. Consists of freeing all surfaces and angles of debris.

cavity varnish, *n* See varnish, cavity.

cavity wall, *n* See wall, cavity.

cavosurface angle (kā′vōsur′fəs), *n* See angle, cavosurface.

cavosurface bevel, *n* See bevel, cavosurface.

cavosurface margin, *n* See margin, cavosurface.

CBC, *n* the abbreviation for *complete blood cell count,* a procedure in which all the blood cells are counted per cubic millimeter, including a differential counting of the white blood cells (leukocytes).

CD-ROM, *n* the acronym for compact disk/read-only memory. These disks are used to store program information (software) for computer programs. Information and instructions can be retrieved from these disks, but information cannot be added or revised without destruction of the existing data.

CD4 (T4) lymphocyte, *n* an immunologically important white cell that is responsible for cell-mediated immunity. It is the cell invaded by the human immunodeficiency virus and in which the virus replicates itself.

CDC, *n.pr* the acronym for the Centers for Disease Control and Prevention.

cecum (sē′kəm), *n* a cul-de-sac constituting the first part of the large intestine. It forms the junction between the ileum and the large intestine.

cefaclor (sef′əklor), *n brand names:* Ceclor, Ceclor CD; *drug class:* second-generation cephalosporin; *action:* inhibits bacterial cell wall synthesis; *uses:* eradication of gram-negative bacilli from the upper and lower respiratory tract and treatment of urinary tracts and skin infections and otitis media.

cefadroxil (sef′ədrok′səl), *n brand names:* Duricef, Ultracef; *drug class:* first-generation cephalosporin; *action:* inhibits bacterial cell wall synthesis, rendering cell wall osmotically unstable; *uses:* eradication of gram-negative bacilli from the upper and lower respiratory tracts, and treatment of urinary tract and skin infections and otitis media.

cefazolin sodium (sifaz′ələn), *n brand names:* Ancef, Kefzol, Zolicef; *drug class:* first-generation cephalosporin; *action:* inhibits bacterial cell wall synthesis, rendering cell wall osmotically unstable; *uses:* eradication of gram-negative bacilli from the upper and lower respiratory tract, and treatment of urinary tracts, skin, bone, joint, biliary, genital infections, endocarditis, surgical prophylaxis, and septicemia.

cefepime (sef′əpēm), *n brand name:* Maxipime; *drug class:* fourth-generation cephalosporin; *action:* inhibits cell wall synthesis in sensitive organisms and is bactericidal; *uses:* respiratory tract, urinary tract, and skin and other soft tissue infections associated with gram-negative organisms.

cefixime (sef′iksēm′), *n brand name:* Suprax; *drug class:* third-generation cephalosporin; *action:* inhibits bacterial cell wall synthesis, rendering cell wall osmotically unstable; *uses:* uncomplicated urinary tract infections, pharyngitis and tonsillitis, otitis media, acute bronchitis, and acute exacerbations of chronic bronchitis.

cefpodoxime proxetil (sef′podok′-sēm prok′sətil), *n brand name:* Vantin; *drug class:* second-generation cephalosporin; *action:* inhibits bacterial cell wall synthesis, rendering cell wall osmotically unstable; *uses:* upper and lower respiratory tract infections, pharyngitis and tonsillitis, gonorrhea, urinary tract infections, skin structure infections.

cefprozil monohydrate (sef'prōzil mon'ōhī'drāt), *n brand name:* Cefzil; *drug class:* second-generation cephalosporin; *action:* inhibits bacterial cell wall synthesis, which renders cell wall osmotically unstable; *uses:* pharyngitis and tonsillitis, otitis media, secondary bacterial infection of acute bronchitis, skin and skin structure infections.

ceftibuten (sef'tib'yōōtən), *n brand name:* Cedax; *drug class:* third-generation cephalosporin; *action:* causes cell death by attaching to the bacterial membrane wall; *uses:* lower respiratory and urinary tract infections, gynecologic and enteric infections, pharyngitis, tonsillitis, and otitis media caused by susceptible organisms.

cefuroxime axetil (sef'yōōrok'sēm ak'sətil), *n brand name:* Ceftin; *drug class:* second-generation cephalosporin; *action:* inhibits bacterial cell wall synthesis, rendering cell wall osmotically unstable; *uses:* eradication of gram-negative bacilli and gram-positive organisms; treatment of serious lower respiratory tract, urinary tract, skin, and gonococcal infections, septicemia, and meningitis.

celiac sprue (sē'lēak sprōō), *n* a genetic disorder in which the body cannot digest certain gluten proteins found in wheat, barley, rye, and oats. This leads to inflammation and flattening of the wall of the small intestine and a reduction in the body's ability to absorb nutrients. Also known as *celiac disease (CD).*

cell(s), *n* the basic unit of vital tissue. One of a large variety of microscopic protoplasmic masses that make up organized tissues. Each cell has a cell membrane, protoplasm, nucleus, and a variety of inclusion bodies. Each type of cell is a living unit with its own metabolic requirements, functions, permeability, ability to differentiate into other cells, reproducibility, and life expectancy.

cell, beta, *n* any cell that produces insulin in the islets of Langerhans region of the pancreas.

cell, bone-forming, *n.pl* See osteoblast.

cell, central, of the dental papillae, *n* the inner cells of the dental papilla within the concavity of the enamel organ that are the primordium of the pulp.

cell, centrioles of **(sen'trēōls),** *n.pl* cylinder-shaped organelles that contain microtubules. Function is to organize spindle fibers during cell division.

cell, connective tissue, *n* the fibroblast, which for purposes of clarity is characterized by such terms as *perivascular connective tissue cell* or *young connective tissue cell.*

cell count, *n* the number of cells contained in a unit volume; usually refers to red and/or white blood cells in a unit volume of blood.

cell culture, *n* living cells that are maintained in vitro in artificial media of serum and nutrients for the study and growth of certain strains, experiments in controlling diseases, or study of the reaction to certain drugs or agents.

cell cycle, *n* the sequence of events that occur during the growth and division of tissue cells.

cell, cytoplasm of **(sī'tōplazəm),** *n* the aqueous part of the cell in which are suspended all the organelles and inclusions. Site of all metabolic activities in the cell.

cell death, *n* the point in the process of dying at which vital functions have ceased at the cellular level. It precludes the use of tissue or organs as transplant donors.

cell, defense, *n* a cell, mobilized within inflamed, irritated, or otherwise diseased tissue, that acts as a protective element to neutralize or wall off the foreign irritant. Defense cells include plasma cells, polymorphonuclear leukocytes, and the cells of the reticuloendothelial system.

cell, dendritic **(sel dendrit'ik),** *n* the immune cells involved in the activation of T cells and B cells. They are primarily found in exposed tissue such as skin, the lungs, the stomach and intestines, and the membranes of the nose, but they are also found in blood. Not to be confused with dendrites.

cell differentiation, *n* the development of the cells into the various basic cell units of tissue: the epithelial cell and the nerve cell, which arise from the ectodermal tissue layer of the embryo; and the blood, muscle, bone, cartilage, and other connective tissue cells, which arise from the mesodermal tissue of the embryo. The mature tissue cell has many intermediary, transitional forms that are sequential in their development from the primitive, less differentiated anlage cell forms. These intermediary forms are evident clinically in disease in blood dyscrasias, tumors, and inflammation and in health in the normal processes of growth, development, healing, and repair.

cell, endoplasmic reticulum of, *n* See endoplasmic reticulum.

cell, endosteal, *n* a reticular cell that is modified and identified by its location; the endosteum is a condensation of the stroma of the bone marrow.

cell, filaments of, *n.pl* threadlike structures the function of which is to support the cytoskeleton; also integral parts of intercellular junctions.

cell, germ, *n* a cell of an organism the function of which is to reproduce an entity similar to the organism from which the germ cell originated. Germ cells are characteristically haploid.

cell, giant, *n* a large cell frequently having several nuclei.

cell, Golgi complex in, *n* See Golgi apparatus.

cell homeostasis, *n* See homeostasis, cell.

cell, homeostasis of **(hō′mē-ōstā′sis),** *n* See homeostasis, cell.

cell, inclusions of, *n.pl* nonliving bodies, by-products of cellular metabolism present in the cytoplasm.

cell, Langerhans, *n.pr* star-shaped cells of unknown function that appear to be permanent residents of the epithelium.

cell, lysosomes in **(lī′sōsōm),** *n.pl* membranous organelles produced from the Golgi complex; contain hydrolytic enzymes, which aid intracellular digestion.

cell membrane, *n* the outer covering of a cell. The membrane controls the exchange of materials between the cell and its environment.

cell, membrane of, transport through, *n* the movement of biomolecules into and out of cells. See diffusion, osmosis, active transport, phagocytosis.

cell, mesenchymal **(mezen′kəməl),** *n* an embryonic connective tissue cell with an outstanding capacity for proliferation and capable of further differentiation into reticular cells or osteoblasts. When persisting in the adult organism, the cells are usually arranged in loose connective tissue along the small blood vessels or in reticular fibers. They are identified by their location and capacity to differentiate into other cell types, such as smooth muscle cells in the formation of new arteries, phagocytes in inflammatory processes, and bone cells in the formation of new bone tissue.

cell, microtubules of, *n.pl* See microtubule.

cell, mitochondria of, *n.pl* See mitochondria.

cell, mucous, *n* a mucous-secreting cell.

cell, nucleus of, *n* See nucleus.

cell, outer, of the dental papillae, *n* an outer cell of the dental papilla within the concavity of the enamel organ that will differentiate into dentin-secreting cells or odontoblasts.

cell, plasma, *n* a cell of disputed origin (lymphatic versus undifferentiated mesenchymal cell) that is seen in chronic inflammation and certain disease states and tumors but not normally in the circulating blood. The cell is larger than a lymphocyte and has a cartwheel-like, eccentric nucleus with basophilic nuclear chromatin peripherally located. The cells synthesize antibodies (immunoglobulins).

cell, progenitor, *n* a cell that is able to transform into different types of cells through replication and differentiation.

cell, replication, *n* See mitosis.

cell, reticular, *n* a cell of reticular connective tissue, such as in the stroma of the bone marrow, that retains both osteogenic and hematopoietic potencies; it is identified by its location, morphology, potency, and direct origin from mesenchymal cells.

cell, serous, *n* a specialized glandu-

C

lar epithelial cell that produces enzymatic secretions. These cells have a rounded nucleus and special secretory granules, or vesicles, in their cytoplasm. Serous cells include the acinar cells of the salivary glands and pancreas, gastric chief cells, and intestinal Paneth cells.

cell, somatic **(sōmat′ik),** *n* a cell that forms parts of the body, including the cells of the skin, bone, blood, connective tissue, and internal organs. From the Greek word *soma,* meaning "body."

cell, stem, *n.pl* the cells in the bone marrow from which all blood cells originate.

cell, typical, *n* See cell.

cell wall, *n* See cell membrane.

cells, radiosensitivity of, *n* the amount of sensitivity of a particular cell, determined by three factors: cell metabolism—the higher the metabolic rate, the more sensitive; cell differentiation—less mature cells are more sensitive than specialized cells; and mitotic activity—cells are more sensitive when they are dividing or rapidly reproducing.

cell-surface marker, *n* an antigenic area on the surface of a cell that identifies that cell as a particular type.

cellulitis (sel′yōōlī′tis), *n* a diffuse inflammatory process that spreads along fascial planes and through tissue spaces without gross suppuration.

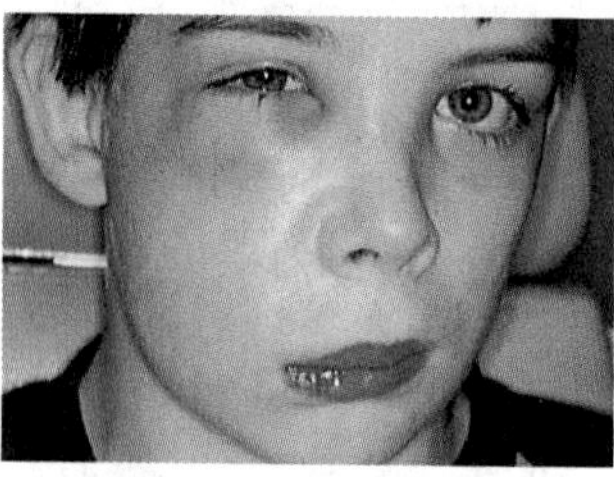

Cellulitis. (Zitelli/Davis, 2002)

celluloid strip, *n* See strip, plastic.

cellulose, *n* the primary component of plant cell walls; provides the fiber and bulk necessary for optimal functioning of the digestive tract.

cellulose, oxidized **(sel′yōōlōs),** *n* cellulose, in the form of cotton, gauze, or paper, that has been more or less completely oxidized.

cement, *n* a material that produces a mechanical interlocking effect on hardening.

cement, acrylic resin dental, *n* a dental cement, dispensed as a powder and a liquid, that is mixed as is any other cement. The powder contains polymethyl methacrylate, a filler, plasticizer, and polymerization initiator. The liquid monomer is methyl methacrylate with an inhibitor and an activator.

cement, copper dental, *n* a zinc phosphate cement to the powder of which has been added a copper oxide.

cement, dental, *n* the materials used in dentistry as luting agents, bases, and temporary restorations. See also cement, acrylic resin dental; cement, zinc.

cement, dental base, *n* an insulating layer of cement placed in the deeper portion of a prepared cavity to insulate the pulp.

cement dressing, *n* a postoperative dressing applied after periodontal surgery.

cement dressing, dental, Kirkland, *n.pr* See dressing, Kirkland cement.

cement, Kryptex dental, *n.pr* See cement, silicophosphate.

cement line, *n* See line, cement.

cement, polycarboxylate, *n* a dental cement used for cementation of cast restorations and orthodontic appliances and as bases. Prepared by mixing a zinc oxide powder with a liquid of polycarboxylic acid.

cement, resin, *n* See resin cement.

cement sealer, *n* a compound used in filling a root canal; it is inserted in a plastic condition, solidifies after placement, and fills any irregularities in the surface of the canal.

cement, silicate, *n* a relatively hard, translucent restorative material used primarily in anterior teeth. Prepared by mixing a liquid and a powder. The powder is an acid-soluble glass prepared by the fusion of CaO, SiO, Al_2O_3, and other ingredients with a fluoride flux. The liquid is a buffered phosphoric acid solution.

cement, silicious dental, *n* See cement, silicate.

cement, silicophosphate **(sil′ikōfos′fāt),** *n* (Kryptex cement), a combination zinc phosphate and silicate cement. Less translucent, less irritating, and less soluble than silicate and stronger than zinc phosphate cement.

***cement, zinc oxide–eugenol dental* (ok′sīd-yōō′jənol),** *n* the least irritating of the cements. The powder is essentially zinc oxide with strengtheners and accelerators. The liquid is basically eugenol.

cement, zinc phosphate, *n* a material used for cementation of inlays, crowns, bridges, and orthodontic appliances; occasionally used as a temporary restoration. Prepared by mixing a powder and a liquid. The powders are composed primarily of zinc oxide and magnesium oxides. The principal constituents of the liquid are phosphoric acid, water, and buffer agents.

cement-retained, *adj* referring to any of several methods for restoring lost or missing teeth by cementing them to a prosthetic attachment anchored in the jaw.

cemental repair, *n* See repair, cemental.

cemental tear, *n* a small portion of cementum forcibly separated, either partially or completely, from the underlying dentin of the root as a result of occlusal force; seen on the tension side in occlusal traumatism.

cementation (sē′mentā′shən), *n* attachment of an appliance or a restoration to natural teeth or attachment of parts by means of a cement.

cementicle (səmen′tikəl), *n* a calcified body sometimes found in the periodontal ligament of older individuals. Degenerated epithelial cells are presumed to form into the calcified body.

cementifying fibroma, *n* See fibroma, ossifying.

cementing line, *n* See line, cemental.

cementoblast (səmen′tōblast), *n* the cell that forms the organic matrix of cementum. Derived from the inner aspect of the dental sac during the initial formation of cementum or from the mesenchymal cell of the periodontal membrane after completion of primary cementogenesis. The cementoblast, trapped within cellular cementum, becomes a cementocyte.

cementoclasia (səmen′tōklā′zhə, -zēə), *n* the destruction of cementum by cementoclasts.

cementocyte (səmen′tōsīt), *n* the cell found within lacunae of cellular cementum; possesses protoplasmic processes that course through the canaliculi of the cementum; derived from cementoblasts trapped within newly formed cementum.

cementoenamel junction (CEJ), *n* See junction, cementoenamel.

cementogenesis (sēmen′tōjen′əsis), *n* the formation of cementum, the calcified connective tissue that covers the roots of teeth, from the epithelial root sheath. See also cementoblast.

cementoid (səmen′toid), *n* the cementum matrix produced by the cementoblasts, which forms the most recent uncalcified layer covering the surface of cementum.

cementoma (sēmentō′mə), *n* (traumatic osteoclasia), an apical lesion associated with the apices of teeth. It may be present as a mass of fibrous connective tissue, fibrous connective tissue with spicules of cementum, or a calcified mass resembling cementum and having few cellular elements.

cementoma, first-state, *n* See fibroma, periapical.

cementopathia (səmen′tōpath′ēə), *n* the concept wherein necrotic, diseased cementum and lack of productivity of cementum are implicated in the causation of periodontitis and periodontosis.

cementum (səmen′tum), *n* a specialized, calcified connective tissue that covers the anatomic root of a tooth, giving attachment to the periodontal ligament.

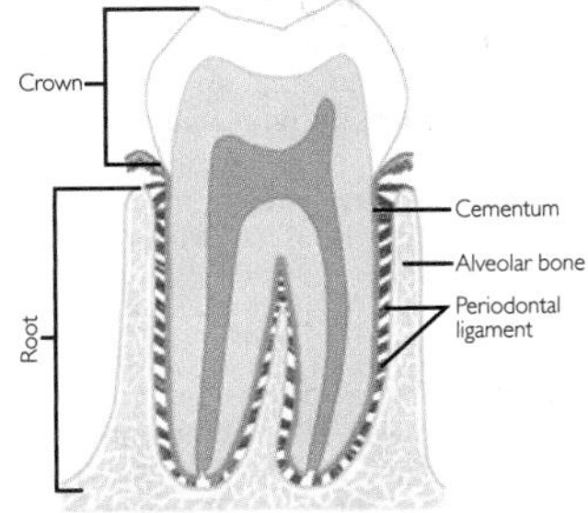

Cementum. (Bath-Balogh/Fehrenbach, 2006)

C

cementum, abnormalities of, *n.pl* includes the reversal lines in the cementum, which represent bone tissue resorption or cementum resorption. Cementicles are calcified epithelial cells found in older persons. Hypercementosis is cementum overgrowth on the roots. See also reversal lines, cementicle, and hypercementosis.

cementum, acellular, *n* the cementum that contains no cementocytes.

cementum, cellular, *n* the portion of the calcified substance covering the root surfaces of the teeth. It is bonelike and contains cementocytes embedded within lacunae, with protoplasmic processes of the cementocytes coursing through canaliculi that anastomose with canaliculi of adjacent lacunae. The lacunae are dispersed through a calcified matrix arranged in lamellar form. It is localized primarily at the apical portion of the root but may deposit over the acellular cementum or serve to repair areas of cemental resorption.

cementum, collagen fibrils of, *n* the fibrils that penetrate the cementum surface and are continuous with the periodontal fibers necessary for tooth support.

cementum, lamellar, *n* the cementum in which layers of appositional cementum are arranged in a sheaflike pattern, the layers of cementum being more or less parallel to the cemental surface and demarcated by incremental lines that represent periods of inactivity of cementum formation.

cementum, necrotic, *n* nonvital cementum that is situated coronal to the bottom of the periodontal pocket.

cementum, properties of, *n.pl* the calcified, avascular connective tissue that is derived from the dental sac and functions in protecting the roots of teeth.

cementum, secondary, *n* the term used to describe all subsequent layers of cementum formed after the primary layer. It may be cellular or acellular.

center of rotation, *n* a point or line around which all other points in a body move.

Centers for Disease Control and Prevention (CDC), *n* the federal facility for disease eradication, epidemiology, and education, headquartered in Atlanta, Georgia.

central bearing, *n* the application of forces between the maxilla and mandible at a single point located as near as possible to the center of the supporting areas of the upper and lower jaws. The purpose is to distribute the closing forces of the jaws evenly throughout the areas of the supporting structures during the registration and recording of maxillomandibular (jaw) relations and the correction of occlusal errors.

central bearing device, *n* a device that provides a central point of bearing or support between upper and lower occlusion rims. It consists of a contracting point attached to one occlusion rim and a plate on the other rim that provides the surface on which the bearing point rests or moves.

central bearing point, *n* See point, central-bearing.

central nervous system (CNS), *n* that portion of the nervous system consisting of the brain and spinal cord. The portion of the nervous system beyond the brain and cord is known as the *peripheral nervous system.*

central occlusion, *n* See occlusion, centric.

central processing unit (CPU), *n* the primary processor of a computer, containing the internal memory unit (memory), arithmetic logic unit (ALU), and input/output control unit (I/O control).

central tendency, *n* the tendency of a group of scores to cluster around a central representative score. The statistics most frequently used for measures of central tendency are the mean, median, and mode.

centric (sen′trik), *adj* (objectionable as a noun) describing jaw and tooth relationships. See also position, centric; relation, centric; occlusion, centric.

centric checkbite, *n* See record, occluding, centric relation.

centric occlusion, *n* See occlusion, centric.

centric position, *n* See position, centric.

centric relation, *n* See relation, centric.

centric stops, *n* the stable points of contact between occluded maxillary and mandibular teeth, located in the central pits, marginal ridges, and buccal and lingual cusps of posterior teeth and the incisals and linguals of anterior teeth.

centrifugal force (sentrif′əgəl), *n* See force, centrifugal.

cephalexin (sef′əlek′sin), *n brand names:* Ceporex, Keftab, Keflex; *drug class:* first-generation cephalosporin; *action:* inhibits bacterial cell wall synthesis, rendering cell wall osmotically unstable; *uses:* removal of gram-negative bacilli from the upper and lower respiratory tracts, urinary tract, and skin; treatment of bone infections and otitis media.

cephalic index (sefal′ik), *n* an anthropometric value based on the ratio between the width and length of the head.

cephalogram (sef′əlōgram), *n* a cephalometric radiograph. On tracings of these films, anatomic points, planes, and angles are drawn that assist in the evaluation of the patient's facial growth and development.

cephalometer (sef′əlom′ətur), *n* See cephalostat.

cephalometer, radiographic, *n* See cephalostat.

cephalometric analysis (sef′əlōmet′rik), *n* See analysis, cephalometric.

cephalometric landmark, *n* See landmark, cephalometric.

cephalometric radiograph, *n* See radiograph, cephalometric.

cephalometric skeletal analysis, *n* an assessment of the facial type of a skeleton; the relationship of the parts to each other, to the skull, and to an estimated "normal."

cephalometric tracing, *n* a tracing of selected structures from a cephalometric radiograph made on translucent drafting paper or film for purposes of measurement and evaluation.

cephalometrics (sef′əlōmet′riks), *n* the scientific study of the measurements of the head.

cephalometry (sef′əlom′ətrē), *n* the measurement of the bony structure of the head using reproducible lateral and anteroposterior radiograms.

cephalophore (sef′əlō′fôr), *n* a cephalostat designed to take in-sequence-oriented facial photographs and gnathostatic models.

cephalosporins (sef′ələspor′ins), *n* semisynthetic derivatives of an antibiotic originally derived from the microorganism *C. acremonium.* They are similar in structure to penicillins.

cephalostat (sef′əlōstat), *n* a head-positioning device that ensures reproducibility of the relations between a radiographic beam, a patient's head, and radiographic film in radiography.

cephradine (sef′rədēn), *n brand name:* Velosef; *drug class:* first-generation cephalosporin; *action:* inhibits bacterial cell wall synthesis, rendering cell wall osmotically unstable; *uses:* removal of gram-negative bacilli and gram-positive organisms from serious respiratory tract, urinary tract, and skin infections and otitis media.

ceramic coating, *n* a thin layer of ceramic material, commonly hydroxyapatite, used to cover dental implants. This typically increases the hardness of the implant and can also make the implant bond more readily with bone.

ceramics, *n* the art of making dental restorations or parts of restorations from fused porcelain.

ceramics, orthoclase, *n* See feldspar.

cerebellum (ser′əbel′um), *n* a major division of the brain, behind the cerebrum and above the pons and fourth ventricle, consisting of a median lobe, two lateral lobes, and major connections through pairs of peduncles to the cerebrum, pons, and medulla oblongata. It is connected with the auditory vestibular apparatus and the proprioceptive system of the body and hence is involved in maintenance of body equilibrium, orientation in space, and muscular coordination and tonus.

cerebral arteries, *n.pl* the arteries to the brain that supply the cerebrum.

cerebral cortex, *n* a thin layer of gray matter on the surface of the cerebral hemisphere, folded into gyri with about two thirds of its area buried in fissures. It integrates higher mental functions, general movement, visceral functions, perception, and behavioral reactions.

C

cerebral hemorrhage, *n* an emergency condition indicated by the rupturing of a blood vessel in the brain and the subsequent bleeding into the tissues of the brain. Type of stroke or cerebrovascular accident (CVA).

cerebral infarction, *n* the blockage of the flow of blood to the cerebrum, causing or resulting in brain tissue death. Blockage may be caused by a thrombosis, an embolism, a vasospasm, or a rupture of a blood vessel. Type of stroke or cerebrovascular accident (CVA).

cerebral ischemia, *n* the reduction or loss of oxygen to the cerebrum; prolonged ischemia may lead to cerebral infarction.

cerebral palsy, *n* See palsy, cerebral.

cerebrospinal fluid, *n* the fluid that flows through and protects the four ventricles of the brain, subarachnoid space, and spinal canal.

cerebrovascular accident, signs and symptoms of, *n* a complete paralysis on one side of the body or various parts (e.g., face, arm, or leg), a diminished capacity to see, speak, swallow, or control saliva, an increase or decrease in sensitivity to touch and pain, and an alteration in mental processes and personality; depends on the degree of involvement and the area of the brain damage.

cerebrum (ser′əbrum, sərē′brum), *n* the largest portion of the brain. Operating at the highest functional level and occupying the upper part of the cranium, it consists of two hemispheres united at the bottom by commissures of large bundles of nerve fibers. As with all parts of the nervous system, each part of it has highly specific functions (e.g., a specific outer cortical area controls voluntary mastication, whereas certain inner subcortical areas are involved in involuntary jaw posture).

cerium, *n* a ductile, gray rare-earth element. Cerium oxalate is used as a sedative, an antiemetic, and an antitussive. Cerium oxide is used in dental porcelains to stimulate the natural fluorescence found in human dental enamel.

certificate holder, *n* **1.** the person, usually the employee, who represents the family unit covered by the dental benefits program; other family members are referred to as *dependents.* **2.** generally refers to a subscriber of a traditional indemnity program. **3.** in reference to the program for dependents of active-duty military personnel, the certificate holder is called the *sponsor.* See also subscriber. Synonyms: subscriber, enrollee.

certificate of eligibility, *n* an official identification card or similar document issued to program beneficiaries as evidence of entitlement to services.

certificate of insurance, *n* a statement issued to a group member describing in general terms the policy provisions for eligibility, deductibles, coinsurance, allowances, and maximums. Used in lieu of issuing copies of the group or master contract to each individual employee member of an insured group.

certification, *n* a process by which an individual, institution, or educational program is evaluated and recognized as meeting certain predetermined criteria and standards.

certified dental assistant (CDA), *n* a person who has completed the Certification Board of the American Dental Assistant Association (ADAA).

cervical (sur′vikəl), *adj* relating to the neck, or cervical line, of a tooth.

cervical appliance, *n* See appliance, cervical.

cervical convergence, *n* See convergence, cervical.

cervical fibers, *n* See nerve fibers.

cervical line, *n* See junction, cementoenamel.

cervical ridge, *n* See ridge, cervical.

cervical third, *n* an inferior part of the horizontal divisions in the tooth's crown.

cervical triangle, posterior, *n* See triangle, cervical, posterior.

cervical vertebrae, *n* the first seven segments of the vertebral column that defines the neck.

cervical chain (lymph nodes), *n* one of three serially linked groups of lymph nodes located in the neck, including the superficial, deep, and posterior chains.

cervical collar, *n* a leaded device positioned over the throat roughly midway between the chin and collarbones. Used because extended expo-

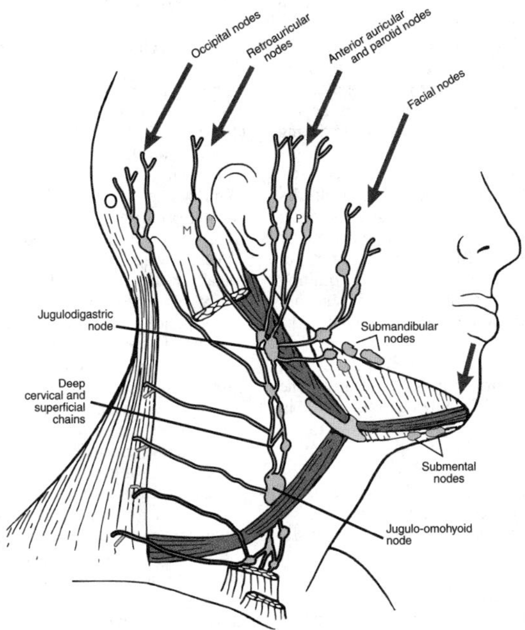

Lymphatic drainage of the face. (Liebgott, 2001)

sure of the thyroid gland to radiographs can cause thyroid cancer. See also apron, lead.

cervical lymphadenectomy (limfad′ənek′tōmē), *n* See neck dissection.

cesium (sē′zēəm), *n* an alkali metal element used in photoelectric cells and television cameras.

cestode (ses′tōd), *n* a tapeworm that resides in the small intestine or other vital organs (including the brain). It can be passed on to humans through contaminated or improperly cooked meats, including fish. Symptoms of infection, when they occur, are similar to mild food poisoning.

cetirizine HCl, *n brand names:* Reactine, Zyrtec; *drug class:* antihistamine; *action:* competitive antagonist for peripheral H_1 receptors; *uses:* treatment of symptoms of seasonal allergic rhinitis, perennial allergic rhinitis, chronic urticaria.

cetylpyridinium chloride (sē′tilpir′idin′ēum), *n* an antiinfective agent used as a topical disinfectant and as a preservative in prepared pharmaceutical compounds.

Chagas' disease (chäg′əs), *n.pr* a parasitic disease caused by *Trypanosoma cruzi* transmitted to humans by the bite of bloodsucking insects.

chalazion forceps (kəlā′zēon), *n* See forceps, chalazion.

chalk, *n* an abrasive agent made from compact calcite.

chamber, *n* an enclosed area.

chamber, air-equivalent ionization, *n* a chamber in which the materials of the wall and electrodes produce ionization essentially similar to that produced in a free-air ionization chamber.

chamber, air-wall ionization, *n* an ionization chamber with walls of material of low atomic number, having the same effective atomic number as atmospheric air.

chamber, extrapolation ionization **(ekstrap′əlā′shən ī′ənīzā′shən),** *n* an ionization chamber with electrodes of which the spacing can be adjusted and accurately determined to permit extrapolation of its reading to zero chamber volume.

chamber, free-air ionization, *n* an ionization chamber in which a delimited beam of radiation passes between the electrodes without striking them or other internal parts of the equipment. The electric field is maintained perpendicular to the electrodes in the collecting region; as a result the ionized volume can be accurately determined from the dimensions of the collecting electrode and limiting diaphragm. This is the basic standard instrument for dosimetry within the range of 5 to 400 kV.

chamber, ionization **(ī′ənīzā′shən),** *n* an instrument for measuring the quantity of ionizing radiation, in terms of the charge of electricity associated with ions produced within a defined volume of air.

chamber, monitor ionization, *n* an ionization chamber used for checking the constancy of performance of the roentgen-ray apparatus.

chamber, pocket ionization, *n* a small, pocket-sized ionization chamber used for monitoring radiation exposure of personnel. Before use it is given a charge, and the amount of discharge is a measure of the quantity of radiation received.

chamber, pulp, *n* (pulp cavity), the space occupied by the pulp.

chamber, relief, *n* a recess in the impression surface of a denture created to reduce or eliminate pressure from the corresponding area of the oral cavity.

chamber, standard ionization, *n* See chamber, ionization, free-air.

chamber, suction, *n* See chamber, relief.

chamber, thimble ionization, *n* a small cylindrical or spherical chamber, usually with walls of organic material.

chamber, thin-wall ionization, *n* an ionization chamber having walls so thin that nearly all secondary corpuscular rays reaching them from external materials can penetrate them easily.

chamber, tissue-equivalent ionization, *n* a chamber in which the walls, electrodes, and gas are selected to produce ionization essentially equivalent to the characteristics of the tissue under consideration.

chamfer (cham′fər), *n* in extracoronal cavity preparations, a marginal finish that produces a curve from an axial wall to the cavosurface.

chancre (autochthonous ulcer) (shang′kur), *n* the primary lesion of syphilis, located at the site of entrance of the spirochete into the body, occurring about 3 weeks after contact. It begins as a papule and then develops into a clean-based shallow ulcer. Secondary infection may produce suppuration. Has the appearance of a buttonlike mass because of the contiguous induration and rolled border. Weeping characteristics also are present.

chancre of lip, *n* the primary lesion of syphilis that often appears as an ulcerated or crusted, indurated lesion with a brownish or copper-colored weeping base when located on the lip, which contains *T. pallidum.*

chancre, soft, *n* See chancroid.

chancroid (shang′kroid), *n* (soft chancre), a sexually transmitted disease caused by *H. ducreyi.* It is characterized by a soft chancre that is a necrotic draining ulcer similar to a chancre but without characteristic induration. A regional bubo may occur.

channel, *n* a definite furrow, groove, or tubelike passage.

channel, vascular, *n* a blood or lymph vessel through which inflammatory infiltrate and periodontitis proceed from a localized superficial area to involve the deeper structures of the periodontium.

Chantix (chan′tiks), *n* the brand name for the prescription drug verenicline, which is prescribed to aid in the cessation of smoking. Chantix provides minimal nicotine effects to ease symptoms of withdrawal and blocks the impact of nicotine if the user resumes smoking.

character, *n* one of a set of elementary symbols that may be arranged in groups to express information. They may include the decimal digits 0 to 9, the letters A to Z, punctuation marks, operation symbols, and any other single symbol that a computer may read, store, or write.

characteristics, acquired, *n.pl* environmentally influenced attributes that manifest after birth.

characteristics, sex, *n.pl* **1.** the primary sex characteristics are those organs concerned with reproduction such as the gonads and genitalia. **2.** secondary sex characteristics include differences in voice range and timbre, muscularity, and distribution of hair and adipose tissue.

charcoal, *n* a carbonized reduction of wood used as fuel and as an adsorptive substance to cleanse the air; it is used in some medical products.

Charcot's joint, *n.pr* See joint, Charcot's.

charges, *n.pl* the financial obligation made to a patient's account for services rendered, usually on a quoted fee for explicit services provided.

charlatan (shar′lətən), *n* a quack, a person who pretends to have skills or knowledge that he or she does not possess.

Charles' law, *n* See law, Charles'.

chart, *n* a sheet of paper or pasteboard that presents a graphic representation of a condition or state.

chart, Bonwill-Hawley, *n.pr* See chart, Hawley.

chart, dental, *n* a diagrammatic chart of the teeth on which the findings from the clinical and radiographic examinations are recorded.

chart, Hawley, *n.pr* (Bonwill-Hawley chart), graded outlines of dental arch sizes based on the mesiodistal diameters of the six anterior teeth.

chart, health, *n* See chart, history.

chart, history, *n* forms and records for obtaining a thorough medical and oral history combined with a complete record of findings that enable the practitioner to gather and have on hand the necessary records to render total patient care.

chart, tooth, *n* See chart, dental.

Charters' method, *n.pr* See method, Charters'.

charting, *n* the tabulation of the progress of a disease; the compilation of a clinical record.

charting, computerized, *n* an automated method for documenting a patient's dental health, utilizing such computer innovations as voice activation and mouse-activated software to ensure accuracy and save time.

charting symbols, *n.pl* commonly accepted notations that are made to the patient's chart to indicate the condition, position, and restorative history of individual teeth.

Chayes' attachment (shāz), *n.pr* believed to be the first internal precision attachment. See also attachment, intracoronal.

Cheadle's disease (chēdls), See scurvy, infantile.

check key, *n* a device used to maintain accuracy while interchanging semiadjustable articulators.

checkbite, *n* See record, interocclusal.

checkbite, centric, *n* See record, interocclusal, centric and record, maxillary.

checkbite, eccentric, *n* See record, interocclusal, eccentric.

checkbite, lateral, *n* See record, interocclusal.

checkbite, protrusive, *n* See record, interocclusal, protrusive.

cheek, *n* the fleshy area on each side of the face below the eye and between the ear, nose, and oral cavity.

cheek biting, *n* the chewing of one's cheek (buccal mucosa) because of malocclusion, oral habit, or lack of coordination in the chewing cycle. Can result in trauma to the area.

cheilion (kīlē′ən), *n* the corner of the oral cavity.

cheilitis, actinic (solar cheilitis) (kīlī′tis aktin′ik), *n* crusting, desquamation, ulceration, atrophy, and inflammation of the lips, especially the lower lip, caused by chronic exposure to the elements and actinic rays of sunlight.

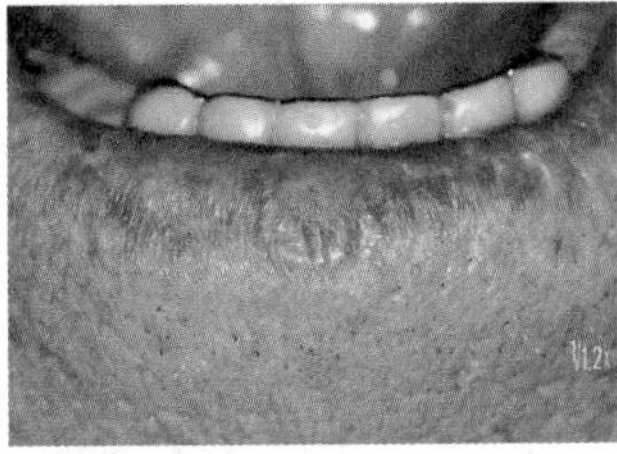

Actinic cheilitis. (Regezi/Sciubba/Pogrel, 2000)

cheilitis, cigarette paper, *n* focal areas of inflammation of the lips caused by cigarette paper sticking to the surface and injury produced by efforts to remove it.

***cheilitis, glandularis apostematosa* (glan′jəlar′is apəstem′ətō′sə),** *n* chronic diffuse nodular enlargement of the lower lip associated with purulent inflammatory hyperplasia of the mucous glands and ducts. Rare; unknown etiology.

cheilitis, solar, *n* See cheilitis, actinic.

cheiloplasty (kī′əplastē), *n* corrective surgery or restoration of the lips.

cheilorraphy (kīlôr′əfē), *n* surgical repair of a congenital cleft lip.

cheilosis, actinic (kīlō′sis aktin′ik), *n* a diffuse degenerative change of the lower lip as a result of sun damage, which may result in cancer and present with white/red patches or nonhealing ulcers, without a distinct border.

cheilosis, angular, *n* See perleche.

cheilotomy (kīlôt′əmē), *n* incision into or excision of a part of the lip.

chelating agents, *n.pl* chemical compounds used to bind or inactivate metal poisons in the body.

chelation (kēlā′shən), *n* chemical reaction of a metallic ion (e.g., calcium ion) with a suitable reactive compound (e.g., ethylenediamine tetra-acetic acid) to form a compound in which the metal ion is tightly bound.

chelation therapy, *n* the use of a chelating agent to bind firmly and sequester metallic poisons.

chemamnesia (kem′amnē′zhə, -zēə), reversible amnesia produced by a chemical or drug.

Chemclave, *n.pr* the brand name for chemical vapor sterilizer that uses a mixture of alcohols, ketones, formaldehyde, and water heated to approximately 127°C under a pressure of at least 20 pounds per square inch. American Dental Association accepted. See also sterilization, chemical.

chemical cure, *n* a type of treatment in which a chemical process begins when the ingredients are completely mixed. The setting time depends on temperature and any added accelerator.

chemical dependence, *n* psychologic or physical reliance on any number of drugs, both legal and illegal, prescription and over the counter. The individual may experience withdrawal symptoms if the chemical is no longer taken into the body.

chemical solutions, darkroom, *n.pl* developer, fixer and distilled water use to mix the chemicals for processing radiographic films.

chemically induced, *adj* initiating biologic action or response by the introduction of a chemical.

chemistry, *n* the science dealing with the elements, their compounds, and the molecular structure and interactions of matter.

chemoreceptor (kē′mōrēsep′tər), *n* a specialized sensory end organ adapted for excitation by chemical substances (e.g., olfactory and gustatory receptors) or specialized sense organs of the carotid body that are sensitive to chemical changes in the bloodstream.

chemotaxis (kē′mōtak′sis), *n* a response involving movement that is positive (toward) or negative (away from) to a chemical stimulus.

chemotaxis, leukocyte, *n* the phagocytic activity of neutrophils and monocytes in response to chemical factors released by invading microorganisms.

chemotherapeutic agent, *n* See agent, chemotherapeutic.

chemotherapy, *n* a cancer treatment method that uses chemical agents to modify or destroy cancer cells; dental patients who are undergoing chemotherapy may have increased needs for certain nutrients and the treatment may affect the oral cavity. See also agent, chemotherapeutic.

chemotherapy, local, for gingivitis, *n* the treatment of gingivitis with a topical antibiotic agent.

chenodiol (kē′nōdī′ol), *n brand name:* Chenix; *drug class:* anticholelithic; *action:* increases amount of bile acids in relation to cholesterol; *use:* dissolving gallstones.

cherubism (familial intraosseous swelling) (cher′əbiz′əm), *n* **1.** a fibroosseous disease of the jaws of genetic nature. The swollen jaws and raised eyes give a cherubic appearance; multiple radiolucencies are evident on radiographic examination. **2.** a familial form of fibrous dysplasia characterized by unilateral or, more often, bilateral swelling of the jaws in children. See also dysplasia, fibrous.

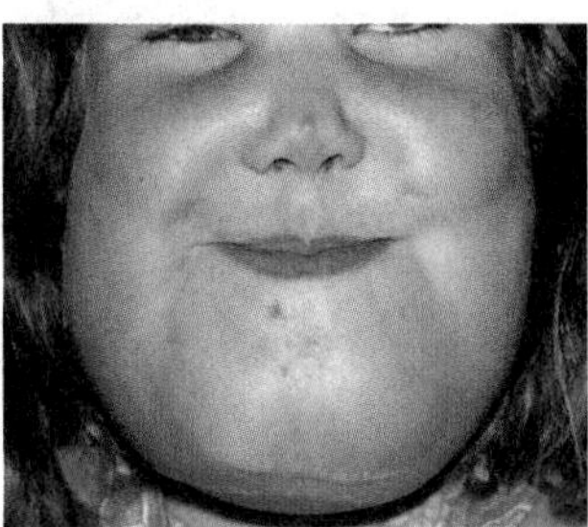

Cherubism. (Regezi/Sciubba/Pogrel, 2000)

chest pain, *n* a physical complaint that requires immediate diagnosis and evaluation. It may be symptomatic of cardiac disease such as angina pectoris, myocardial infarction, or pericarditis or disease of the lungs and its linings. It also may be referred from the gastrointestinal tract or elsewhere. The differential diagnosis of chest pain is a crucial element of medical practice. See also angina pectoris.

chew-in record, functional, *n* the method by which the patient's occlusal paths in the wax patterns are recorded to be used in making restorations. In making the grooves and ridges in the wax patterns directly, the patient is asked to make right-and-left and fore-and-aft sliding occlusal strokes to generate the paths of the opposite prominences. See also path, generated occlusal.

chewing, *n* the movements of the mandible during mastication; controlled by neuromuscular action and limited by the anatomic structure of the temporomandibular joints. See also mastication.

chewing cycle, *n* See cycle, chewing.

chewing force, *n* See force, chewing.

chewing tobacco, *n* See smokeless tobacco.

Cheyne-Stokes reflex, *n.pr* See respiration, Cheyne-Stokes.

Cheyne-Stokes respiration, *n.pr* See respiration, Cheyne-Stokes.

chi square (kī), *n* a nonparametric statistic used with discrete data in the form of frequency count (nominal data) or percentages or proportions that can be reduced to frequencies. Used to determine differences between categories (e.g., yes-no; visits dental office every 6 months, 1 year, 2 years, 5 years); compares the observed results with the expected results to determine significant differences. May be used with many categories of response.

chickenpox, *n* See varicella.

child, *n* **1.** a person of either gender between the time of birth and adolescence, or puberty. **2.** in the law of negligence and in laws for the protection of children, a term used as the opposite of *adult* (generally under the age of puberty) without reference to parentage and distinction of gender.

child abuse, *n* the physical, sexual, or emotional maltreatment of a person under 18 years of age. Child abuse occurs predominantly with children under 3 years of age. Symptoms include bruises and contusions, medical record of repeated trauma, radiographic evidence of fractures, emotional distress, and failure to thrive.

child neglect, *n* a form of child abuse in which proper care is denied or withheld.

chin, *n* the raised triangular extension of the anterior portion of the mandible below the lower lip. It is formed by the mental protuberance of the mandible.

chin cup, *n* See cup, chin.

chip, *n* a logic element containing electronic circuit components, both active and passive, embedded in a cohesive material of any shape.

chip blower, *n* See syringe, air, hand.

chiropractic, *n* a branch of the healing arts dealing with the nervous system and its relationship to the spinal column and interrelationship with other body systems in health and disease. The primary spinal and paraspinal structural derangements with which chiropractors are concerned are known as *chiropractic subluxations.* Treatment is referred to as *chiropractic adjustment.*

chisel, *n* an instrument modeled after a carpenter's chisel intended for cutting or cleaving hard tissue. The cutting edge is beveled on one side only; the shank may be straight or angled.

chisel, contra-angle (binangle chisel), *n* a chisel-shaped, binangled, paired cutting instrument whose blade meets the shank at an angle greater than 12°.

chisel, posterior, *n* See chisel, contra-angle.

chisel, Wedelstaedt, *n.pr* a chisel with a blade that is continuous with the shank, has no constricting neck, curves rather than angles into the shank, and is available in varying widths.

***Chlamydia* (kləmid′ēə),** *n.pr* a genus of microorganisms that live as intercellular parasites and have a number of properties in common with gram-negative bacteria. Two species have been identified; both are pathogenic.

***C. psittaci* (sit′əsē),** *n.pr* an organism that infests birds and causes a type of pneumonia in humans (psittacosis).

***C. trachomatis* (trəkō′mətis′),** *n.pr* an organism that lives in the conjunctivae of the eye and the epithelium of the urethra and cervix and is responsible for conjunctivitis, lymphogranuloma venereum, and trachoma.

chloral hydrate (klor′əl hī′drāt), *n brand names:* Aquachloral Supprettes, Novo-chlorhydrate; *drug class:* sedative-hypnotic chloral derivative, controlled substance schedule IV, schedule F; *action:* produces central nervous system depression; *uses:* sedation, treatment of insomnia, anesthesia adjunct.

chlorambucil (kloram′byəsil′), *n brand name:* Leukeran; *drug class:* antineoplastic alkylating agent; *action:* inhibits enzymes that allow synthesis of amino acids in proteins; *uses:* chronic lymphocytic leukemia, Hodgkin's disease, breast carcinoma, ovarian carcinoma.

chloramine solution, *n* See solution.

Chloramphenicol, *n* a broad-spectrum antibacterial and antirickettsial agent that should be reserved for serious infections in which other agents are ineffective.

chlordiazepoxide HCl, *n brand names:* Librium, Novopoxide; *drug class:* benzodiazepine antianxiety; *action:* produces central nervous system depression; *uses:* short-term management of anxiety, acute alcohol withdrawal, preoperatively for relaxation.

chlorhexidine (CHX) gluconate, *n brand names:* Peridex, PerioGard; *drug class:* antiinfective oral rinse; *action:* absorbed by tooth surfaces, dental plaque, and oral mucosa; sustained reduction of plaque organisms; *uses:* as a rinse as a part of treatment of periodontal disease, irrigation during periodontal procedures, and possibly as an aseptic prerinse before dental procedures.

chloride shift (klôr′īd), *n* the exchange of a chloride ion for a bicarbonate ion across the enthrocyte membrane as part of the buffering system in the blood. It accounts for the greater chloride content of venous erythrocytes than arterial erythrocytes.

chlorine, *n* a yellowish-green gaseous element of the halogen group. It has a strong, distinctive odor that is irritating to the respiratory tract and is poisonous if ingested or inhaled. It occurs mainly as a compound of sodium chloride. It is used as a bleach and disinfectant. Chlorine compounds are used in solvents, cleaning fluids, and chloroform and formerly in general use as an anesthetic.

chlorine dioxide, *n* an oxidizing agent used in oral care to decrease amounts of volatile sulfur compounds that may cause halitosis.

chloroform, *n* a nonflammable, volatile liquid that was the first inhalation anesthetic to be discovered. It is no longer in general use because of its inherent risk factors and low margin of safety.

chloroformization (klôr′əfôrm′izā′shən), *n* the administration of chloroform.

Chloromycetin, *n.pr* the brand name for chloramphenicol. See also chloramphenicol.

chloropercha (klôr′ōpur′chə), *n* a solution obtained by mixing various amounts of chloroform with gutta-percha.

chloropercha method, *n* See method, chloropercha.

chlorophyll (klôr′ōfil), *n* the pigment required for photosynthesis in plants.

chlorophyllin (klôr′əfilin), *n* any one of a number of products resulting from the reaction of certain decomposition products of chlorophyll with copper and other metallic ions.

chloroquine HCl/chloroquine phosphate, *n brand names:* Aralen HCl, Aralen Phosphate; *drug class:* antimalarial; *action:* inhibits parasite replication; *uses:* malaria, rheumatoid arthritis, amebiasis.

chlorothiazide (klor′əthī′əzīd′), *n brand name:* Diuril; *drug class:* thiazide diuretic; *action:* acts on distal tubule by increasing excretion of water, sodium chloride, potassium; *uses:* edema and hypertension, diuresis.

chlorotrianisene, *n brand name:* TACE; *drug class:* nonsteroidal synthetic estrogen; *action:* required for the development, maintenance, and adequate function of the female reproductive system; decreases release of gonadotropin-releasing hormone, inhibits ovulation, and helps maintain bone structure; *uses:* prostatic cancer, menopause, female hypogonadism, atrophic vaginitis.

chlorpheniramine maleate (klor′fənir′əmēn′mā′lēāt), *n brand names:* Chlor-Trimeton, Novo-pheniram; *drug class:* antihistamine H_1-receptor antagonist; *action:* acts on blood vessels, gastrointestinal system, respiratory system by competing with histamine for H_1-receptor site;*uses:* relief of allergy symptoms, rhinitis.

chlorphensin carbamate, *n brand name:* Maolate; *drug class:* skeletal muscle relaxant, central acting; *action:* unknown; may be related to sedative properties; does not directly relax muscle or depress nerve conduction; *use:* adjunct for relieving pain in acute, painful musculoskeletal conditions.

chlorpromazine HCl, *n brand name:* Thorazine; *drug class:* antipsychotic; *action:* blocks neurotransmission at dopaminergic synapses in the cerebral cortex, hypothalamus, and limbic system; *uses:* psychotic disorders, mania, schizophrenia, anxiety, intractable hiccups, nausea, vomiting, preoperatively for relaxation, behavioral problems in children.

chlorpropamide, *n brand names:* Apo-Chlorpromide, Diabinese; *drug class:* antidiabetic, first generation sulfonylurea; *action:* causes functioning beta cells in pancreas to release insulin, leading to drop in blood glucose levels; *uses:* stable type 2 diabetes mellitus.

chlortetracycline (klôr′tetrəsī′klēn), *n* (Aureomycin) a broad-spectrum antibiotic possessing bacteriostatic properties of some value in the treatment of disease produced by large viruses (the psittacosis and lymphogranuloma inguinale groups).

chlorthalidone, *n brand names:* Novothalidone, Apo-Chlorthalidone, Thalitone; *drug class:* diuretic with thiazide-like effects; *action:* acts on distal tubule by increasing excretion of water, sodium, chloride, potassium; *uses:* edema, hypertension, diuresis, chronic heart disease.

chlorzoxazone, *n brand names:* Paraflex, Parafon Forte DSC; *drug class:* skeletal muscle relaxant, central acting; *action:* depresses multisynaptic pathways in the spinal cord; *use:* adjunct for relief of muscle spasm in musculoskeletal conditions.

choice of path of placement, *n* See placement, choice of path of.

cholagogue (kō′ləgog), *n* a substance that stimulates emptying of the gallbladder and flow of bile.

cholera (kôl′erə), *n* an acute bacterial infection of the small intestine characterized by severe diarrhea and vomiting, muscular cramps, dehydration, and depletion of electrolytes. The disease is spread by water and food that have been contaminated by feces of infected persons. The cholera vibrio produce an exotoxin, cholera toxin (choleragen), that stimulates the secretion of electrolytes and water into the small intestine, draining body fluids and weakening the patient. A vaccine is available.

choleretic (kō′ləret′ik), *n* a substance that stimulates production of bile by the liver.

cholestasis (kō′ləstā′sis), *n* the interruption in the flow of bile through any part of the biliary system from the liver to duodenum.

C

cholesteatoma (kəles′tēətō′mə), *n* a cystic mass composed of epithelial cells and cholesterol that is found in the middle ear and occurs either as a congenital defect or as a serious complication of chronic otitis media.

cholesterol (kəles′tərôl), *n* a lipid common to all animal, but not plant, cells. As a sterol, it contains the cyclopentanophenanthrene nucleus. High levels are found in nerve tissue, atheromas, gallstones, and cysts. Normally 140 to 220 mg are present in 100 ml of blood.

cholestyramine, *n brand names:* Questran, Cholybar; *drug class:* antilipemic; *action:* absorbs, combines with bile acids to form insoluble complex that is excreted through the feces; lowers cholesterol levels; *uses:* primary hypercholesterolemia, pruritus associated with biliary obstruction, diarrhea caused by excess bile acid, digitalis toxicity, xanthomas.

choline, *n* a nutrient essential for cardiovascular and brain function and for cellular membrane composition and repair. Classified as an essential nutrient by the Food and Nutrition Board of the Institute of Medicine (USA). Adequate intakes (AI) have been established.

choline salicylate, *n brand name:* Arthropan; *drug class:* salicylate analgesic; *action:* inhibits prostaglandin synthesis by interfering with cyclooxygenase need for biosynthesis; *uses:* relief of mild to moderate pain from fever, arthritis, juvenile rheumatoid arthritis.

cholinergic (parasympathomimetic) (kō′linur′jik), *adj* producing or simulating the effects of acetylcholine.

cholinergic blocking agent, *n* See agent, blocking, cholinergic.

cholinergic crisis, in myasthenia gravis, *n* a medical condition resulting from an administration of too much anticholinesterase, indicated by an immediate increase in muscle weakness, excessive secretion of pulmonary matter, diarrhea, and cramps.

cholinesterase (kō′lines′tərās), *n* an esterase that hydrolyzes acetylcholine. It is an enzyme that is widely distributed throughout the muscles, glands, and nerves of the body and that converts acetylcholine into choline and acetic acid.

cholinolytic (kō′linōlit′ik), *n/adj* See anticholinergic.

chondrodysplasia punctata (kon′drōdisplā′shə punkta′tə), *n* an inherited form of dwarfism characterized by skin lesions, radiographic epiphyseal stippling, and a pug nose. Two types are most often seen: a benign type marked by mild asymmetric limb shortening that is transmitted by an autosomal dominant gene and a lethal type with marked proximal limb shortening that is transmitted by an autosomal recessive gene.

chondroectodermal dysplasia (Ellis-van Creveld syndrome) (kon′drōek′tōdur′məl displā′zhə), *n* a syndrome characterized by the following tetrad: (1) bilateral polydactyly; (2) chondrodysplasia of the long bones resulting in acromelic dwarfism; (3) anomalies of the teeth, nails, hair, and maxillary and mandibular region anteriorly; and (4) heart malformation.

chondroitin (kondroit′ən), *n* a mucopolysaccharide present in the intercellular substance or matrix of connective tissue, particularly cartilage.

chondroiton sulfate (kondrō′itin, kondroi′tin), *n* a mucopolysaccharide contained in skin, bones, teeth, and cartilage.

chondroma (kondrō′mə), *n* a benign tumor of cartilage. However, many chondrosarcomas arise in preexisting chondromas.

chondromyxosarcoma (kon′drōmik′sōsärkō′mə), *n* See chondrosarcoma.

chondrosarcoma (kon′drōsärkō′mə), *n* a malignant neoplasm composed of cartilage-like tissue.

chondrosarcoma, mesenchymal (mezen′kĭməl), *n* a malignant cartilage tumor primarily found in younger adults, usually located in or near the jaw.

chorda tympani nerve (kor′də tim′pənē), *n* a nerve branch of the facial nerve that passes through the tympanic cavity to join the lingual branch of the mandibular nerve; it conveys taste sensation from the anterior two thirds of the tongue and

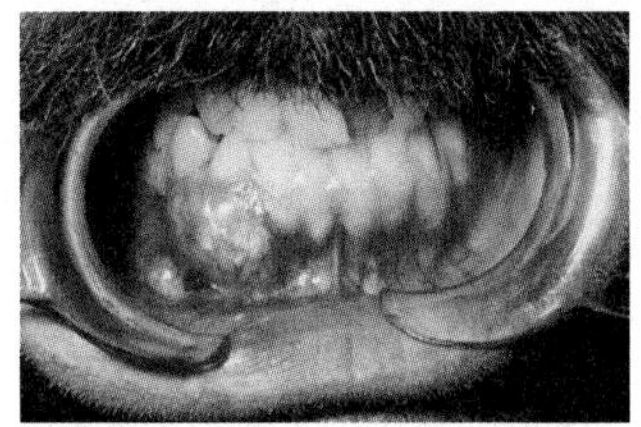

Chondrosarcoma. (Sapp/Eversole/Wysocki, 2004)

carries parasympathetic preganglionic fibers to the submandibular and sublingual salivary glands.

chorea (St. Vitus' dance) (kôrē′ə), *n* a disorder of the central nervous system resulting in purposeless, involuntary athetoid (writhing) movements of the muscles of the face and extremities. It may be associated with or follow rheumatic fever (Sydenham's chorea), hysteria, senility, or infections, or it may be a hereditary disorder (Huntington's chorea).

choriamnionitis (kor′ēōam′nēōnī′tis), *n* an inflammatory reaction in the amniotic membranes caused by bacteria or viruses in the amniotic fluid.

Christian's disease, *n.pr* See disease, Hand-Schüller-Christian.

Christmas disease, *n.pr* See hemophilia B.

chroma, *n* a measurement of color saturation or the degree of color pureness. A color that is identified with a high chroma hue is almost completely free of white.

chromatin (krō′mətin), *n* the genetic material present in the nucleus, consisting of DNA and associated proteins, seen as irregular clumps in quiescent cells.

chromatography, *n* any one of several processes for separating and analyzing various gaseous or dissolved chemical materials according to differences in their absorbency with respect to a specific substance.

chromium, (Cr), *n* a hard, brittle, metallic element with an atomic number of 24 and an atomic weight of 51.996. Chromium strongly resists corrosion and is used extensively to plate other metals and as an alloy to harden steel. Stainless steels are more than 10% chromium.

chromium-cobalt-molybdenum, *n* a stainless alloy used in interosseous implants for dental prostheses.

chromogenic (krō′mōjen′ik), *adj* pertaining to color production.

chromosomal, *adj* relating to chromosome, or a configuration within the cell's nucleus that contains a linear thread of DNA that conveys genetic data.

chromosomes (krō′məsōms), *n* the small, dark-staining, and more or less rod-shaped bodies situated in the nucleus of a cell. At the time of cell division, chromosomes divide and distribute equally to the daughter cells. They contain genes arranged along their length. The number of chromosomes in the somatic cells of an individual is constant (the diploid number), whereas just half this number (the haploid number) appears in germ cells.

chromosome aberration, *n* a rearrangement of chromosome parts as a result of breakage and reunion of broken ends.

chronic, *adj* characterized by a long, slow course, as opposed to *acute.*

chronic pulmonary emphysema, *n* a condition in which breathing is made difficult by an accumulation of mucus in the bronchioles and a loss of elasticity in the lungs.

chronology, *n* the arrangement of events in a time sequence, usually from the beginning to the end of an event.

chylomicrons (kī′lōmī′kronz) *n.pl* the tiny lipoproteins of approximately 2% protein that convey dietary fat throughout the body.

cicatricial pemphigoid (sikətrishəl pem′figoid′), *n* See pemphigoid, benign mucous membrane.

cicatrix (sik′ətriks) (scar), *n* the result of healing by secondary intention; characterized microscopically by excessive collagenation of the granulation tissue.

cicatrization (sikətrizā′shən), *n* the conversion of granulation tissue into scar tissue.

ciclopirox olamine (sik′lōpē′roks) (topical), *n brand name:* Loprox; *drug class:* topical antifungal; *action:* interferes with fungal cell membrane; *uses:* tinea cruris, tinea corporis, tinea pedis, tinea versicolor, cutaneous candidiasis.

ciliophora protozoa (sil′ēof′ôrə), *n* the only human ciliate parasite *(Balantidium coli)* implicated in a type of dysentery and contracted from fecal contamination of water supplies.

cimetidine (simet′idēn′), *n brand names:* Tagamet, Apo-Cimetidine; *drug class:* H_2-histamine receptor antagonist; *action:* inhibits histamine at H_2-histamine receptor site in parietal cells, which inhibits gastric acid secretion; *uses:* short-term treatment of duodenal and gastric ulcers by the control of hyperacidity.

cineradiography (sin′irā′dēog′rəfē), *n* the making of motion pictures by means of roentgen rays and image intensification. Studies are used for diagnosis and research purposes. Speech patterns can be studied during the process of phonation; the action of the tongue, jaws, and palate can be studied during mastication and deglutition.

cingulum (sing′gyūlum), *n* the portion of the incisor teeth and canines, occurring on the lingual surface, that forms a convex protuberance at the cervical third of the anatomic crown.

cingulum modification, *n* the alteration of the lingual form of an anterior tooth to provide a definite seat for the support of a rest unit of a removable partial denture.

cinoxacin (sinok′səsin), *n brand name:* Cinobac; *drug class:* urinary tract antibacterial; *action:* interferes with deoxyribonucleic acid replication; *use:* urinary tract infections.

ciprofloxacin, *n brand name:* Cipro; *drug class:* fluoroquinolone antiinfective; *action:* a broad-spectrum bactericidal agent that inhibits enzyme deoxyribonucleic acid (DNA) gyrase needed for replication of DNA; *uses:* adult urinary tract infection, uncomplicated gonorrhea, typhoid fever; effective against some periodontal organisms.

circuit voltmeter, *n* the device on the radiograph machine that records the line voltage on the circuit prior to the voltage being augmented by the transformer. Also may be used to measure the kilovoltage produced by the action of the transformer.

circuits, in radiograph machine, *n.pl* a radiograph machine contains two circuits, the low-voltage filament circuit and the high-voltage cathode-anode circuit. The low-voltage circuit uses a step-down transformer to form an electron cloud by heating up the filament. The high-voltage circuit uses a step-up transformer to increase the current enough to accelerate the electrons to the point that they create radiographic photons.

circular compression, *n* the compacting or pressing together of an object with equal circumventing force.

circulation, *n* the movement of blood through blood vessels.

circulation, peripheral, *n* the passage of fluids, electrolytes, and metabolites through the walls of terminal vessels of the vascular tree into and out of the tissue spaces.

circulation, pulmonary, *n* the circulation of venous blood from the right ventricle of the heart to the lungs and back to the left atrium of the heart.

circulation, systemic, *n* the circulation of oxygenated blood from the left ventricle of the heart to the various tissues and of venous blood back to the right atrium of the heart.

circulatory system, *n* the system for the circulation of blood, consisting of the heart, arteries, arterioles, capillaries, venules, and veins.

circumferential fibers, *n.pl* See fibers, circular.

circumferential probing, *n* an examination technique in which the probe remains in the sulcus or periodontal pockets while it is "walked" around the oral cavity; prevents excessive trauma to the gingiva that can occur from repeated probe insertion and withdrawal.

circumferential wiring, *n* See wiring, circumferential.

cirrhosis (sirō′sis), *n* a chronic degenerative disease of the liver in which blood flow is restricted and metabolic and detoxification functions are impaired or destroyed. Cirrhosis is most commonly the result of chronic alcohol abuse.

cisapride (sis′əprīd′), *n brand name:* Propulsid; *drug class:* oral prokinetic; *action:* enhancement of acetylcholine release; *uses:* symptomatic treatment and prophylaxis of nocturnal heartburn caused by gastroesophageal reflux disease.

cisplatin (sisplat'in), *n* an antineoplastic prescribed in the treatment of a wide variety of neoplasms such as metastatic testicular, prostatic, and ovarian tumors.

citric acid, *n* a white, crystalline, organic acid freely soluble in water and alcohol. It can be extracted from citrus fruits or through a fermentation of sugars. It is a key intermediary in metabolism. See also citric acid cycle.

citric acid cycle, *n* a sequence of enzymatic reactions involving the metabolism of carbon chains of sugars, fatty acids, and amino acids to yield carbon dioxide, water, and high-energy phosphate bonds. Also called *Krebs' citric acid cycle* or *tricarboxylic acid cycle.*

citrin (sit'rin), *n* See factor, platelet 1.

civil action, *n* a noncriminal legal action.

civil law, *n* a statutory law, as opposed to common law or judge-made law (such as case law). The Dental Practice Act in every state is a civil law.

claim, *n* **1.** in a juridic sense, a demand of some type made by one person or another. **2.** a request for payment under a dental benefits plan. **3.** a statement listing services rendered, the dates of services, and itemization of costs. Includes a statement signed by the beneficiary and treating dental professional that services have been rendered. The completed form serves as the basis for payment of benefit.

claim form, *n* the form used to file for benefits under a dental benefits program; includes sections for the patient and the dental professional to complete.

claimant, *n* a person who files a claim for benefits. May be the patient or the certificate holder.

claims payment fraud, *n* the intentional manipulation or alteration of facts submitted by a treating dental professional, resulting in a lower payment to the beneficiary or the treating dental professional than would have been paid if the manipulation had not occurred.

claims reporting fraud, *n* the intentional misrepresentation of material facts concerning treatment provided and charges made to cause a higher payment.

claims review, *n* **1.** in dental prepayment, the routine examination by a carrier or intermediary of the claim submitted to it for payment or predetermination of benefits; may include determination of eligibility, coverage of service, and plan liability. **2.** in quality assurance, examination by organizations of claims as part of a quality review or use review process.

clamp, *n* a device used to effect compression or retention.

clamp, cervical, *n* See clamp, gingival.

clamp, Ferrier 212 gingival, *n.pr* a purposely unbalanced gingival rubber dam clamp for retracting gingival tissue from the field of operation. It must be stabilized to position with modeling compound.

clamp, gingival, *n (cervical clamp),* a rubber dam clamp intended to retract gingival tissues.

clamp, Hatch gingival, *n.pr* an adjustable gingival rubber dam clamp.

clamp, root rubber dam, *n* a clamp with jaws designed to fit on the root surfaces of a tooth; usually used for the retention of a rubber dam.

clamp, rubber dam **(rubber dam retainer),** *n* a device made of spring metal and used to retain a rubber dam in place or improve the operating field by isolating it from the oral environment.

clarithromycin, *n brand name:* Biaxin; *drug class:* macrolide antibiotic; *action:* binds to 50S ribosomal subunits of susceptible bacteria and suppresses protein synthesis; *uses:* treatment of mild to moderate infections of the upper and lower respiratory tracts, otitis media, acute maxillary sinusitis.

Clark's rule, *n.pr* See rule, Clark's.

clasp, *n* an extracoronal direct retainer of a removable partial denture, usually consisting of two arms, a retentive arm and a reciprocal arm, joined by a body that may connect with an occlusal rest.

clasp, Adams, *n.pr* a formed wire clasp of modified arrowhead design using the buccomesial and disto-

C

proximal undercuts of a tooth for retention.

clasp, arm, *n* the clasp extensions, usually from minor connectors, that provide retention, reciprocation, or stabilization.

clasp, arm, fatigue of, *n* a situation in which the retentive arm of a clasp metal has undergone flexure at the same point repeatedly, and fracture has resulted. Tapering the clasp arm tends to distribute the flexure and reduce such tendency to fracture.

clasp, arm, reciprocal, *n* an arm of a clasp, usually at or occlusal to the height of contour, located in such a manner as to reciprocate any force arising from an opposing clasp arm on the same tooth.

clasp, arm, retentive (retention terminal), *n* a clasp arm that is flexible and engages the infrabulge area at the terminal end of the arm.

clasp, arrowhead, *n* a wire clasp, for retention of removable appliances, whose active elements are in the shape of an arrowhead and engage the mesioproximal and distoproximal undercuts on the buccal aspects of adjacent teeth.

clasp, back-action, *n* a clasp that originates on one surface of a tooth and traverses the suprabulge area to another surface, where it is supported by an occlusal rest; it then continues to encircle the tooth on the third surface, where it terminates in the infrabulge area beyond the opposite angle of the tooth surface where it originated.

clasp, bar, *n* a clasp with arms that are bar-type extensions from major connectors or from within the denture base; the arms pass adjacent to the soft tissues and approach the point of contact on the tooth in a cervicoocclusal direction.

clasp, bar, arm, *n* a clasp arm that originates from the denture base or from a major or minor connector. It consists of the arm, which traverses but does not contact the gingival structures, and a terminal end, which approaches its contact with the tooth in a cervicoocclusal direction.

clasp, cast, *n* a clasp made of an alloy that has been cast into the desired form and retains its crystalline structure.

clasp, circumferential **(sərkum′fəren′shəl),** *n* a clasp that encircles more than 180° of a tooth, including opposite angles, and usually contacts the tooth throughout the extent of the clasp, at least one terminal being in the infrabulge area (cervical convergence).

clasp, circumferential arm, *n* a clasp arm that has its origin in a minor connector and follows the contour of the tooth approximately in a plane perpendicular to the path of placement of the removable partial denture.

clasp, combination, *n* a clasp that employs a wrought-wire retentive arm and a cast reciprocal or stabilizing arm. A clasp that employs a bar type of retentive arm and a cast reciprocal or stabilizing arm.

clasp, continuous, *n* a secondary lingual bar.

clasp design, *n* the determination of the shape and construction of a clasp with its position outlined on the cast.

clasp, embrasure **(embrā′zhur),** *n* a clasp used where no edentulous space exists. It passes through the embrasure, using two occlusal rests, and clasps the two teeth with circumferential clasps that have a common body.

clasp flexibility, *n* the property of a clasp that enables it to be bent without breaking and to return to its original form. Factors that affect the flexibility of a retentive clasp arm are its length, diameter, cross-section form, structure, and the alloy of which it is made.

clasp flexure, *n* See flexure, clasp.

clasp, formed, *n* See clasp, wrought.

clasp, mesiodistal **(mez′ēədis′təl),** *n* a type of clasp that embraces the distolingual and mesial surfaces of a tooth and takes its retention in either or both mesial and distal undercuts.

clasp, reciprocal, circumferential arm, *n* an arm of a clasp located in such a manner as to reciprocate any force arising from an opposing clasp arm on the same tooth.

clasp, retentive circumferential arm (retention terminal), *n* a circumferential clasp arm that is flexible and engages the infrabulge area at the terminal end of the arm.

clasp, Roach, *n* See clasp, bar.

clasp, stabilizing circumferential arm, n a circumferential clasp arm that is rigid and contacts the tooth at or occlusal to the surveyed height of contour.

clasp, stress-breaking action of, n the relief for the abutment teeth from all or part of torquing occlusal forces; partially achieved by having a retentive arm of maximum flexibility that will provide adequate retention.

clasp, wrought (formed clasp), n a clasp made of an alloy that has been drawn into various forms of wire.

classification, *n* the systematic arrangement according to characteristics of groups or classes.

classification, Angle's, n See Angle's classification of malocclusion (modified).

classification, Broders', n See index, Broders'.

classification, cavity, n See cavity, classification.

classification, Kennedy, n See Kennedy classification.

classification of habits, n a compilation of orofacial habits that may be a factor in the etiology of periodontal disease. Habit neuroses include lip biting, cheek biting, biting of foreign objects, and abnormal tongue pressure against the teeth. Occupational ones include thread biting, musician's habits, holding nails in the oral cavity, etc. Miscellaneous ones include thumb sucking, pipe smoking, incorrect toothbrushing habits, cracking nuts with the teeth, and oral cavity breathing.

classification of motion, n a classification system that identifies the extent of involvement of the body in completing a dental motor task.

classification of partial dentures, n grouping of partially edentulous situations based on various conditions (e.g., location of the edentulous space, location of remaining teeth, position of direct retainers, and ability of oral structures to support a partial denture).

classification of periodontal diseases, n the division of periodontal diseases into: (1) gingival disease; (2) chronic periodontitis; (3) aggressive periodontitis; (4) periodontitis as a manifestation of a systemic disease; (5) necrotizing periodontal diseases; (6) abscesses of the periodontium; (7) periodontitis associated with endodontic lesions; and (8) development of acquired deformities and conditions.

classification of pockets, n the division of periodontal pockets into two classes: (1) suprabony and (2) infrabony, according to the number of osseous walls (i.e., three osseous walls, two osseous walls, one osseous wall). See also pocket.

clavicle (klav′ikəl), *n* a long, curved, horizontal bone just above the first rib, forming the ventral portion of the shoulder girdle. It articulates medially with the sternum and laterally with the scapula.

cleansing, biomechanical, *n* the process of cleaning and shaping a root canal with endodontic instrumentation in conjunction with irrigating solutions.

cleansing solution, *n* See solution, cleansing.

clearance, *n* **1.** a condition in which moving bodies may pass without hindrance. **2.** removal from the blood by the kidneys (e.g., urea or insulin) or by the liver (e.g., certain dyes).

clearance, interocclusal **(in′ter-əklōō′səl),** *n* the difference in the height of the face when the mandible is at rest and when the teeth are in occlusion. This is determined by measuring the amount of space between the maxillary and mandibular teeth when the mandible is in the position of physiologic rest. The difference between the rest vertical dimension and the occlusal vertical dimension of the face, as measured in the incisal area. See also distance, interocclusal.

clearance, occlusal **(əklōō′səl),** *n* a condition in which the mandibular teeth may pass the maxillary teeth horizontally without contact or interference.

clearance time, *n* the time taken for a cariogenic exposure to pass from the oral cavity; depends largely upon type of food ingested, efficiency of the lips, teeth, and tongue, and the amount of saliva present in an individual's oral cavity.

cleat (klēt), *n* a fixed point of anchorage, usually in the form of a metal spur or loop embedded in the acrylic resin base of a Hawley retainer or soldered onto an arch wire, to which a rubber dam elastic or other device is attached during orthodontic tooth movement.

C

cleft (kleft), *n* a longitudinal fissure of opening.

cleft, facial, n the fissures along the embryonal lines of the junction of the maxillary and lateral nasal processes; usually extend obliquely from the nasal ala to the outer border of the eye (canthus).

cleft, gingival, n a cleft of the marginal gingiva; may be caused by many factors, such as incorrect toothbrushing, a breakthrough to the surface of pocket formation, or faulty tooth positions, and may resemble a V-shaped notch.

cleft lip, n a congenital anomaly of the face caused by the failure of fusion between embryonic maxillary and medial nasal processes.

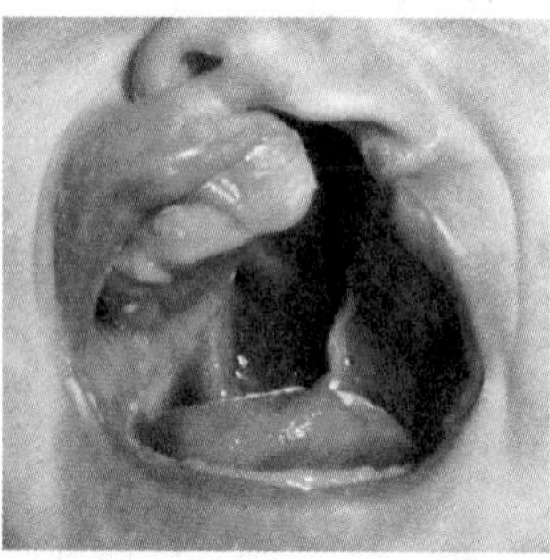

Cleft lip and palate. (Zitelli/Davis, 2002)

cleft, occult, n See submucous cleft.

cleft, operated, n (postoperative cleft), a cleft that has been surgically repaired.

cleft palate, n a congenital anomaly of the oral cavity caused by the failure of fusion between the embryonic palatal shelves.

cleft palate, alveolar graft, n a bone graft placed at the site of a hard palate cleft before teeth have an opportunity to erupt through the gingiva tissue. It creates the architecture necessary for normal eruption of the maxillary teeth and provides support for adjacent teeth. It may also eliminate the need for prosthetic intervention in the future.

cleft palate, hard palate graft, n a bone graft used to block the oronasal passage in order to facilitate breathing in children with hard palate clefts.

cleft palate prosthesis, n See prosthesis, cleft palate.

cleft, postoperative, n See cleft, operated.

cleft, Stillman's, n the small fissures extending apically from the midline of the gingival margin in teeth subjected to trauma. Although these clefts may be found in traumatism, they are not necessarily diagnostic of occlusal trauma.

cleft, submucous, n See submucous cleft.

cleft, unoperated, n a cleft of the palate that has not been surgically repaired.

cleidocranial dysostosis, *n* See dysostosis, cleidocranial.

clemastine fumarate (klem′əstēn′ fyōō′mərāt′), *n brand names:* Tavist, Tavist-1; *drug class:* antihistamine, H_1-receptor antagonist; *action:* acts on blood vessels and gastrointestinal and respiratory systems by competing with histamine for H_1-receptor sites; *uses:* allergy symptoms, rhinitis, angioedema, urticaria.

clenching (klen′ching), *n* the nonfunctional, forceful intermittent application of the mandibular teeth against the maxillary teeth. It can become habitual and cause damage to the periodontium.

cleoid (klē′oid), *n* a carving instrument having a blade shaped like a pointed spade or claw, with cutting edges on both sides and tip.

clicking, *n* a sound sometimes associated with the functioning of the temporomandibular joint; also the sound made by poorly fitting dentures.

clidinium bromide (klindin′ēəm brō′mīd), *n brand name:* Quarzan; *drug class:* gastrointestinal anticholinergic; *action:* inhibits muscarinic actions of acetylcholine at postganglionic parasympathetic neuroeffector sites; *use:* treatment of peptic ulcer disease in combination with other drugs.

climacteric (klīmak′tərik, klī′mak-ter′ik), *n* the period during which women gradually lose their reproductive capabilities as a result of aging. Also used as an adjective to describe this period.

climate, occlusal, *n* the new occlusal relationship and environment produced by occlusal adjustment, orthodontic tooth movement, or a periodontal prosthesis.

clindamycin HCl/clindamycin palmitate HCl (klin′dəmī′sin pal′-mətāt′), *n brand names:* Cleocin, Dalacin C.; *drug class:* lincomycin-derivative antiinfective; *action:* binds to 50S subunit of bacterial ribosomes, suppresses protein synthesis; *uses:* infections caused by staphylococci, streptococci, pneumococci, topically for acne, bacterial vaginosis.

clinic, table, *n* a display or demonstration of a topic, limited in scope, for transmitting information to a small number of persons at a time.

clinical, *adj* pertaining to a clinic, direct patient care, or materials used in the direct care of patients.

clinical attachment level (CAL), n a measurement to determine periodontal health; consists of the distance in millimeters that exists between the edge of the enamel of a tooth to the gingival tissue that is adherent to its root, its epithelial attachment.

clinical crown, n See crown, clinical.

clinical crown:clinical root ratio, n See ratio, clinical crown:clinical root.

clinical death, n a defined time at which bodily functions have ceased and are unable to be revived. In many instances, the definition of clinical death applies to circumstances where brain activity ceases despite the continuance of body functions.

clinical diagnosis, n See diagnosis, clinical.

clinical medicine, n the aspect of medicine that deals with direct patient care.

clinical protocol, n the detailed outline of the steps to be followed in the treatment of a patient.

clinical trials, n organized studies to provide large bodies of clinical data for statistically valid evaluation of treatment.

clinical trial, *n* a trial based upon the scientific method in which a control group and a test group are compared over time in order to study a single, differing factor.

clinician, *n* a licensed dental professional who provides preventative, therapeutic, and educational services that promote oral health.

clinoidale (klinoid′al), *n* the most superior point on the contour of the anterior clinoid.

clioquinol (klē′ōkwin′ol), *n brand name:* Vioform; *drug class:* topical antifungal; *action:* topically to treat angular cheilitis.

clobetasol propionate (klōbā′təsol′ prō′pēənāt′), *n brand names:* Dermovate, Temovate, Temovate Emollient Cream; *drug class:* topical corticosteroid group I potency; *action:* possesses antipruritic and antiinflammatory properties; *uses:* psoriasis, exzema, contact dermatitis.

clock system, *n* **1.** system in which the dental instrument and the sharpening tool are held in such a way that the optimum angle required for sharpening is achieved. **2.** the seating position for a clinician (and/or assistant) to facilitate instrumentation.

clocortolone pivalate (klōkor′təlōn piv′əlāt′), *n brand name:* Cloderm; *drug class:* topical corticosteroid, group III medium potency; *action:* possesses antipruritic and antiinflammatory properties; *uses:* psoriasis, eczema, contact dermatitis, pruritus.

clofibrate (klōfī′brāt), *n brand names:* Abitrate, Atromid-S, Claripex, Novofibrate; *drug class:* antihyperlipidemic; *action:* inhibits biosyntheis of VLDA and LDL, which are responsible for triglyceride development; increases excretion of neutral steroids; *use:* hyperlipidemia types III, IV, V.

clomiphene citrate (klō′məfēn′ sit′-rāt), *n brand names:* Clomid, Serophene, Milphene; *drug class:* nonsteroidal ovulatory stimulant; *action:* binds to estrogen receptors, resulting in increase of LH and FSH release from pituitary; *use:* female infertility.

clomipramine (klōmip′rəmēn′), *n brand name:* Anafranil; *drug class:* tricylic antidepressant; *action:* inhibits both norepinephrine and serotinin (5-HT) uptake in brain; *uses:* obsessive-compulsive disorder, panic disorder, neurogenic pain.

clonazepam (klōnaz′əpam′), *n brand names:* Klonopin, Rivotril; *drug class:* anticonvulsant, benzodiazepine derivative, controlled substance schedule IV; *action:* inhibits spike-wave formation; *uses:* akinetic myoclonic seizures.

clonic (klon′ik), *n* the alternating pattern of releasing and tightening a muscle.

clonidine HCl/clonidine transdermal, *n brand names:* Catpres, Dixarit, Catapres-TTS; *drug class:* antihypertensive, central α-adrenergic agonist; *action:* inhibits sympathetic vasomotor center in central nervous system; *uses:* hypertension, nicotine withdrawal, vascular headache.

clonus (klō′nəs), *n* an alternating muscular spasm and relaxation in rapid succession.

clorazepate dipotassium (klor′əzepāt′ dī′pətas′ēəm), *n brand names:* Tranxene, Gen-Xene, Apo-Chlorazepate, Tranxene-SD; *drug class:* benzodiazepine, controlled substance schedule IV; *action:* produces central nervous system depression; *uses:* anxiety, acute alcohol withdrawal.

closed bite, *n* See bite, closed.

closed panel, *n* **1.** in a prepayment plan, a group of dental professionals sharing office facilities who provide stipulated services to an eligible group for a set premium. For beneficiaries of plans using closed panels, choice of dental professionals is limited to panel members. Dentists must accept any beneficiary as a patient. **2.** a closed-panel dental benefits plan exists when patients eligible to receive benefits can receive them only if services are provided by dental professionals who have signed an agreement with the benefits plan to provide treatment to eligible patients. As a result of the dental professional reimbursement methods characteristic of a closed-panel plan, only a small percentage of practicing dental professionals in a given geographic area are typically contracted by the plan to provide dental services.

closed procedure, *n* the reduction of a fracture of the jaw or placement of an implant without surgical flap retraction.

closed reduction, for jaw fracture, *n* a process by which the broken portions of the jaw are approximated and stabilized without surgically opening the mucosal covering. The fixation of the reestablished approximation of the parts is accomplished with preformed bars attached to the teeth with ligatures or elastic bands.

***Clostridium* (klostrid′ēəm),** *n* a genus of spore-forming anaerobic bacteria of the Bacillaceae family.

***C. bifermentans* (bī′fermen′təns),** *n* causes gaseous gangrene.

***C. botulinum* (boch′əlī′nəm),** *n* causes botulism.

***C. perfringens* (perfrin′jəns),** *n* the main cause of gas gangrene in humans; also causes food poisoning, cellulitis, and wound infections.

***C. tetani* (tet′ənē′),** *n* causes tetanus.

closure, *n* the act or condition of being brought together or closed up.

closure, adjustive arcs of, *n.pl* the arcs of jaw closure found in deflective malocclusion caused by an intercusping of the teeth that does not coincide with a centrically related jaw closure.

closure, arcs of mandibular, *n.pl* the circular or elliptic arcs created by closure of the mandible.

closure, centric path of, *n* the path traversed by the mandible during closure when its associated neuromuscular mechanism is in a balanced state of tonus.

***closure, velopharyngeal* (vē′lōfərin′jēəl),** *n* the closure of nasal air escape by the knee-action elevation of the soft palate and contraction of the posterior pharyngeal wall.

closure, voluntary arcs of, *n.pl* jaw closure directions consciously made by a patient.

clot, *n* coagulated blood, plasma, or fibrin.

clot, blood, *n* a coagulum formed of blood of a semisolidified nature. See also clotting factors.

clotrimazole (klōtrim′əzōl′), *n brand names:* Lotrimin, Canesten, Gyne-Lotrimin, Mycelex-7, Mycelex Troches; *drug class:* inidazole antiinfective; *action:* interferes with fungal

DNA replication; *uses:* tinea pedis, tinea cruris, tinea corporis, tinea versicolor, and *C. albicans* infection of the oral cavity, pharynx, vulva, and vagina.

clotting factors, *n.pl* the chemical and cellular constituents of the blood responsible for the conversion of fibrinogen into a mesh of insoluble fibrin causing the blood to coagulate or clot.

cloxacillin sodium (klok′səsil′in), *brand names:* Apo Cloxi, Cloxapen, Novo-cloxin, Tegopen; *drug class:* penicillinase-resistant penicillin; *action:* interferes with cell-wall replication of susceptible organisms; *uses:* effective for gram-positive cocci when penicillinase-producing organisms are the confirmed pathogens.

clozapine (klō′zəpēn′), *n brand name:* Clozaril; *drug class:* antipsychotic, atypical; *action:* interferes with binding of dopamine at D_1 and D_2 receptors; acts as adrenergic, cholinergic, histaminergic, and serotonergic antagonist; *uses:* management of psychotic symptoms in schizophrenic patients for whom other antipsychotics have failed.

clubbing (pulmonary osteoarthropathy), *n* a deforming enlargement of the terminal phalanges of the fingers. It is usually acquired and may be associated with certain cardiac and pulmonary diseases.

cluster, *n* in epidemiology, a composite of confirmed cases of a disease, defect, or disability that occur in close proximity to one another with regard to time or space.

cluster analysis, *n* a complex statistical technique of data analysis of numeric scale scores, producing clusters of variables related to one another.

cluster headache, *n* See histamine headache.

clutch, *n* a device made for gripping the teeth in a dental arch, to which face-bows or tracing devices may be attached rigidly enough to behave in space relations during the movements as if they were jaw outgrowths.

CMV, *n* the abbreviation for *cytomegalovirus.* See also cytomegalovirus.

coagulating current, *n* See current, coagulating.

coagulation (kōag′ūlā′shən), *n* causing a liquid to solidify; clotting.

coagulation time, *n* See time, coagulation.

coal tar, *n* an extract of coal used in combination with other compounds for the treatment of chronic skin diseases, such as eczema and psoriasis. Also a derivative of tobacco smoke that may act as an irritant and carcinogen.

coalescing (kōəles′ing), *n* a joining or fusing of parts.

coaptation (kō′aptā′shən), *n* the bringing together of two parts so as to create a seamless alignment.

coated tongue, *n* See tongue, coated.

coating, enteric (enter′ik), *n* a tablet covering that resists the action of the fluids and enzymes in the stomach but dissolves readily in the upper intestine.

coating material, *n* a biologically acceptable, usually porous nonmetal applied over the surface of a metallic implant with the expectation that tissue ingrowth will occur in the pores. Often a carbon polymer or ceramic substance.

cobalamin, *n* See vitamin, cobalamin.

cobalt-chromium alloy, *n* See alloy, cobalt-chromium.

cocaine (C, Cadillac, Charlie, coke, freebase, gold dust, joy powder, snow), abuse of, *n* the illegal recreational use of cocaine hydrochloride or one of its derivatives. Medically prescribed for its anesthetic properties. Psychologic addiction may result from continued, compulsive use, typically by sniffing, injecting, applying topically, or smoking. Complications can occur with the concomitant use of it and epinephrine in the dental office. See also crack cocaine.

***Coccidioides immitis* (koksid′ēoid′ēz im′itəs),** *n* a dust-borne fungus endemic to the wind-blown desert dust of southwest United States. It is the chief culprit in coccidioidomycosis. Appears microscopically as uniformly scattered small ovals.

coccidioidomycosis (koksid′ēoid′ōmīkō′sis), *n* an infectious fungal disease caused by the inhalation of spores of the bacterium *C. immitis,* which is carried on windborne dust particles. Although endemic in the southeastern United States, it is considered among the opportunistic infections that are indicators of AIDS.

C

code, *n* **1.** a system of recording information by symbols so that only selected people will know the meaning. Used also to conserve space. **2.** a systematic statement.

code of ethics, *n* a series of principles used as a guide in assisting a dental professional to fulfill the moral obligations of professional dental practice.

codeine (kō′dēn), *n* a crystalline alkaloid, morphine methyl ether that is used as an analgesic and antitussive. It is a controlled substance.

codeine sulfate/codeine phosphate, *n* generic codeine; *drug class:* narcotic analgesic, controlled substance schedule II, Canada N; *action:* depresses pain impulse transmission in central nervous system by interacting with opioid receptors; *uses:* mild-to-moderate pain, nonproductive cough.

coding, *n* writing instructions for a computer either in machine language or nonmachine language.

Coecal (kō′kôl), *n* the brand name for dental stone (hydrocal).

coefficient, absorption, *n* See absorption coefficient.

coefficient of thermal expansion, *n* See expansion, thermal coefficient.

coefficient, phenol, *n* the ratio of potency of a given germicide to that of phenol under standard conditions.

coenzyme (kōen′zīm), *n* a nonprotein substance, such as a B-complex vitamin, that combines with enzymes to assist in the catabolic process.

coenzyme A (CoA), *n* an important metabolite in the citric acid cycle. Although not a true enzyme, it plays a significant role in the transfer of acetyl groups and the metabolism of acids and amino acids.

cofactor V, *n* See factor VII.

cognition (cognish′ən), *n* the higher mental processes, including understanding, reasoning, knowledge, and intellectual capacity.

cognitive (cog′nitiv), *adj/n* pertaining to the mental processes of knowing, perceiving, or being aware; an expression of intellectual capacity.

cognitive domain, *n* area of study that deals with the processes and measurable results of study, as well as the practical ability to apply intelligence.

cognovit note (kognō′vit), *n* a written authority of a debtor granting entry of a judgment against the debtor if the amount set forth in the note is not paid by the debtor when due. A cognovit note sets aside every defense that the maker of the note may otherwise have had.

cohere (kōhēr′), *v* to stick together, to unite, to form a solid mass.

coherent (Thompson/unmodified) scattering (kōhēr′ənt), *n* the dispersing of low-energy radiographs without losing photon energy, caused by elastic collision.

cohesion (kōhē′zhən), the ability of a material to adhere to itself.

cohesive, *n* the capability to cohere or stick together to form a mass.

cohort, *n* in statistics, a collection or sampling of individuals who share a common characteristic, such as the same age or sex.

cohort study, *n* a scientific study that focuses on a specific subpopulation, such as children born on a certain date in a specific environment.

coinsurance, *n* **1.** a means of sharing, dividing, or splitting the cost of dental services between the dental plan and the insured patient. A common division is 80/20. This means the insurance company will pay 80% of the cost of the dental service and that the patient will pay 20%. Percentages vary and may be applied to scheduled or usual, customary, and reasonable fee plans. **2.** a provision of a dental benefits program by which the beneficiary shares in the cost of covered services, generally on a percentage basis. **3.** the percentage of a covered dental expense that a beneficiary must pay (after the deductible is paid). A typical coinsurance arrangement is one in which the third party pays 80% of the allowed benefit of the covered dental service and the beneficiary pays the remainder of the charged fee. Percentages vary and may apply to a table of allowance plans; usual, customary, and reasonable plans; and direct reimbursement programs.

coinsurance clause, *n* a provision in

an insurance contract stipulating that the insurer will pay a specified share of dental expenses covered by the plan.

coitus (kō′itus), *n* the act of sexual intercourse.

col (kôl), *n* a depression in the gingival tissue of the interdental papilla apical to the contact.

colchicine (kol′chəsēn′), *n* generic colchicine; *drug class:* antigout agent; *action:* inhibits deposition of ureate crystals in soft tissues; *uses:* gout, gouty arthritis, to arrest progression of neurologic disability in multiple sclerosis.

cold, clinical applications of, *n.pl* the clinical uses of cold to treat cold injury such as frostbite, relieve pain in burn injury, relieve pain in severe and acute inflammation (pulpitis), and relieve pain and swelling in contusions, abrasions, and sprains. See also heat, applied, and cold.

cold, physiologic effects of, *n* in reference to application of cold to a local area, marked vasoconstriction followed by vasodilation and edema. In extreme exposure the effects include a significant drop in temperature on the surface and a lesser drop in deeper tissue layers, depending on the degree of cold and duration of application; decreased phagocytosis; a decrease in local metabolism; and analgesia to varying degrees of anesthesia of the part exposed to cold.

cold sore, *n* See herpes labialis.

cold welding, *n* See welding, cold.

cold work, *n* a deformation of the space lattice of metals by mechanical manipulation at room temperature. The process alters certain properties (e.g., ductility).

cold-curing resin, *n* See resin, autopolymer.

colestipol HCl (kəles′təpol), *n brand name:* Colestid; *drug class:* antihyperlipidemic; *action:* absorbs, combines with bile acids to form insoluble complex that is excreted through feces; loss of bile acids lowers cholesterol levels; *uses:* primary hypercholesterolemia, xanthomas, digitalis toxicity, pruritus caused by biliary obstruction, diarrhea caused by bile acids.

colic (kôl′ik), *n* a sharp visceral pain resulting from torsion, obstruction, or smooth muscle spasm of a hollow or tubular organ, such as a ureter or an intestine.

colitis (kəlī′tis), *n* an inflammatory condition of the large intestine. Most of the diseases of this group are of unknown origin.

collagen (kol′əjin), *n* an intercellular constituent of connective tissue and bone consisting of bundles of tiny reticular fibrils, most noticeable in the white, glistening, inelastic fibers of tendons, ligaments, and fascia.

collagenase (kol′əjənās′), *n* an enzyme capable of depolymerizing collagen, found in some microorganisms and believed to contribute to periodontal disease.

collapse, *n* a state of extreme prostration and depression with failure of circulation; abnormal falling in of the walls of any part or organ; with reference to a lung, an airless or fatal state of all or part of the lung.

collar, *n* the small part of the root of a tooth that is a part of an artificial tooth (denture).

collective bargaining, *n* the negotiations between organized labor and employers on matters such as wages, hours, working conditions, and health and welfare programs.

collimating film holder (kol′əmā′ting), *n* a stainless steel holder for radiographic film that provides rectangular lining-up (collimation) of the radiographic beam; useful when employing the paralleling technique for periapical survey. May also be called *precision film holder.*

collimation (kol′imā′shən), *n* in radiology, collimation refers to the elimination of the peripheral (more divergent) portion of a useful radiographic beam by means of metal tubes, cones, or diaphragms interposed in the path of the beam. See also diaphragm.

collimation, rectangular, *n* a method for minimizing a patient's exposure to unnecessary radiation during treatment by using a rectangular position-indicating device (PID) to reduce the size of the radiation beam.

collimator (kol′imātur), *n* a diaphragm or system of diaphragms made of an absorbent material and designed to define the dimensions and direction of a beam of radiation.

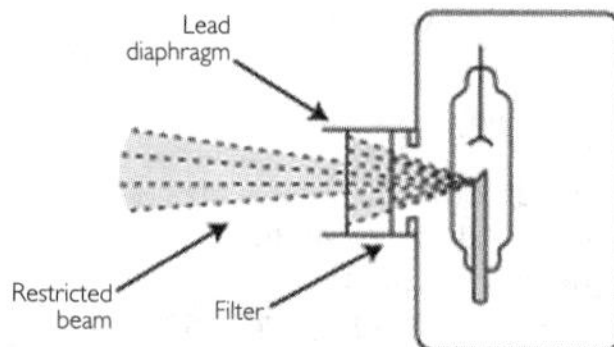

Collimation of a radiographic beam. (Frommer/Stabulas-Savage, 2005)

collision tumor, *n* See tumor, collision.

colloid (kol′oid), *n* a suspension of particles in a dispersion medium. The particles generally range in size from 1 to 100 mm. Hydrocolloids and silicate cements are examples of dental colloids.

colon, *n* the body of the large intestine between the cecum and rectum.

color blindness, *n* See blindness, color.

color, temper, *n* the color produced by the thickening of the oxide coating on carbon steel as temperature is increased. Used as an indication of the degree of tempering.

coloring, extrinsic, coloring from without, as in the application of color to the external surface of a prosthesis.

coloring, intrinsic, *n* coloring from within. The incorporation of pigment within the material of a prosthesis.

Coloumb per kilogram (C/kg) (kōō′lōm pur kil′əgram), *n* the unit of measurement for radiation exposure from the French Système International d'Unités; can be converted to the traditional Roentgen (R) by the formula 1 R = 2.58×10^{-4} C/kg.

coma (kō′mə), *n* a state of unconsciousness from which the patient cannot be aroused, even by powerful stimulation. It is gradual in onset, prolonged, and not spontaneously reversible.

coma, diabetic, n the state of unconsciousness accompanying severe diabetic acidosis. It may develop from lack of insulin, surgical complications, or disregard of dietary restrictions. Premonitory symptoms include weakness, anorexia, dry skin and oral cavity, drowsiness, abdominal pain, and fruity breath odor. Late symptoms are coma, air hunger, low blood pressure, tachycardia, dehydration, soft and sunken eyeballs, glycosuria, hyperglycemia, and a high level of ecetoacetic acid. See also shock, insulin.

comatose (kō′mətōs), *adj* relating to the state of being unconscious and unable to wake.

combination clasp, *n* See clasp, combination.

command, *n* the portion of a computer-related instruction that specifies the operation to be performed. A term used with hardware operations.

comminution of food, *n* See food, comminution of.

Commission on Dental Accreditation (CODA), *n.pr* the body responsible for accrediting dental education programs. Sponsored by the American Dental Association and established in 1975, the Commission establishes quality standards and conducts program reviews to ensure that an educational program seeking accreditation meets these standards.

commissure (kəmish′ur), *n* the corners of the oral cavity.

common deductible, *n* a deductible amount that is common to the dental and another health insurance policy (usually a major medical policy). In a major medical policy with a $100 common deductible, once $100 of medical or dental expense has been incurred under either policy or both, no further deductible is required.

common law, *n* a judge-made law, as contrasted with statutory law. This body of law originated in England and was in force at the time of the American Revolution; modified since that time on a case-by-case basis in the courts.

communicable disease, *n* a disease transmitted from one person or animal to another directly or by vectors.

communicable period, *n* the period when the infectious agent that causes a communicable disease may be transmitted to a susceptible host, such as in diseases that initially involve the mucous membrane (e.g., diphtheria and scarlet fever). The period of communicability is from the time of exposure to the disease until termination of the carrier state, if one develops.

communication, *n* the technique of conveying thoughts or ideas between two people or groups of people.

communication, privileged, n the class of communications between persons who stand in a confidential or fiduciary relationship to each other that the law will not permit to be divulged in court. Examples of confidential relationships are those of psychiatrist and patient and attorney and client. Confidentiality of communications depends on the law in each state.

community dentistry, *n* a branch, discipline, or specialty of dentistry that deals with the community and its aggregate dental or oral health rather than that of the individual patient. Formal recognition of dental professionals engaged in community dentistry is through the American Board of Public Health Dentistry. See dental public health.

community health aides, *n.pl* the paraprofessionals who assist in the treatment or support of patients (in their residential setting) within the patient's community environment.

Community Periodontal Index of Treatment Needs (CPITN), *n.pr* an assessment tool used to establish periodontal treatment priorities for individual children and adults or groups.

compact, *v* to form by uniting or condensing particles with the application of pressure (e.g., the progressive insertion and welding of foil and the building up of plastic amalgam in a preparation).

compacter (kompak′tər), *n* a rotary instrument used in the McSpadden endodontic technique to condense the guttapercha cone into the root canal.

compaction (kompak′shən), *n* the act of compacting or the state of being compact.

compensating curve, *n* See curve, compensating.

compensation, *n* the monetary reward for rendering a service; insurance providing financial return to employees in the event of an injury that occurs during the performance of their duties and that prohibits work. Compulsory in many states.

compensation, unemployment, n insurance covering the employee so that compensation may be provided for loss of income as a result of unemployment.

competence, *n* a measure of the degree of a person's ability to cope with all aspects of the environment.

competent, *adj* having legal capacity, ability, or authority.

compiler, *n* a computer program that translates a high-level language program into a corresponding machine instruction. The program that results from compiling is a translated and expanded version of the original program.

complaint, *n* an ailment, problem, or symptom disclosed by the patient.

complaint, chief (CC), n the main symptom or reason for which the patient seeks treatment. The most troublesome ailment, problem, or symptom.

complement (kom′pləment), *n* one of 11 complex, enzymatic serum proteins. In an antigen-antibody reaction, complement causes lysis. Complement is also involved in anaphylaxis and phagocytosis.

complement fixation, n an immunologic reaction in which an antigen combines with an antibody and its complement, causing the complement factor to become inactive, or "fixed."

complement-fixation test (C-F test), n a serologic test in which complement fixation is detected, indicating the presence of a particular antigen. The Wassermann test for syphilis is a C-F test, used to detect amebiasis, Rocky Mountain spotted fever, trypanosomiasis, and typhus.

complemental air, *n* See volume, inspiratory reserve.

complete blood count, *n* See count, blood, complete.

complete denture, *n* See denture, complete.

complex, *n* a combination of a number of things; the sum or total of various things.

complex, craniofacial, n the bones and surrounding soft structure of the cranium and face.

complex odontoma, n See odontoma, complex.

C

complex, orofacial, n referring to the dentition and surrounding structures.

compliance (komplī′əns), *n* **1.** the fulfillment by the patient of the health care professional's recommended course of treatment. **2.** the fulfillment of oversight criteria and/or standards of care necessary for licensure, certification, and accreditation.

complication (kom′plikā′shən), *n* a disease or injury that develops during the treatment of an earlier disorder. An example is a bacterial infection acquired by a person weakened by a viral infection.

component(s), *n* a part or element.

component, A, n See factor II.

component of force, n See force, component of.

component of partial denture, n See denture, partial, components of.

component, salivary, n See lysozyme.

component, thromboplastic cellular (TCC), n See factor, platelet, 3.

composite, *n* in dentistry, material made from mixture of resin and silica used in tooth-colored fillings and other restorative work. It was created as an alternative to metallic fillings, which were much more visible due to their dark coloring. Also known as a *resin matrix.*

composite cement, n a dental adhesive made of colloidal silica powder combined with the matrix monomer dimethacrylate.

composite odontoma, n See odontoma, compound.

composite resin, n See resin, composite.

composites, hybrid, n.pl resins made from a combination of macrofill and microfill particles that are generally considered easy to polish and highly resistant to fracture and wear. They may be used for either anterior or posterior applications. See also resin, composite and resin-filled.

composites, macrofilled, n.pl strong resins made from small particles filled with either glass or quartz. They may be difficult to polish. See also resin, composite and resin-filled.

composites, microfilled, n.pl filled resins made from finely ground silica used for anterior esthetic restorations because they polish well and retain their shine. See also resin, composite and resin-filled.

compound, *n* **1.** a combination of elements held together in a well-defined pattern by chemical bonds. In pharmacy, a mixture of drugs. **2.** a thermoplastic substance used as a nonelastic impression material.

compound A, B, E, F, S, n See corticoid, adrenal.

compound cone, n a compound in the form of a cone or pyramid; used for impressions of individual preparations.

compound, impression (modeling compound), n See compound.

compound, intermetallic, n a compound of two metals in which the metals are only partially soluble in one another; exhibits a homogeneous grain structure, but the atoms do not intermingle randomly in all proportions.

compound, modeling, n See compound, impression.

compound, phenolic, n a mouthwash made from essential oils in combination with alcohol that is available over the counter and approved by the American Dental Association for use in controlling plaque and gingivitis. Also called *essential oils mouthrinses.*

compound tracing stick, n a compound dispensed in stick form.

compound, tray, n a compound similar to impression compound but with less flow and more viscosity when soft and more rigidity when chilled.

comprehensive dental care, *n* the coordinated delivery of the total dental care required or requested by the patient.

comprehensive health care, *n* the coordinated delivery of the total health care required or requested by the patient.

comprehensive orthodontic therapy, *n* a coordinated approach to improvement of the overall anatomic and functional relationships of the dentofacial complex, as opposed to partial correction with more limited objectives such as cosmetic improvement. Usually but not necessarily uses fixed orthodontic attachments as a part of the treatment appliance. Includes treatment and adjunctive procedures, such as extractions, maxillofacial surgery, other dental services, nasopharyngeal surgery, and speech therapy, directed at malrelationships within the entire dentofacial complex. Optimal care requires periodic evaluation of patient needs, especially during the growing years. Treatment is most effective when begun in the primary or mixed dentitions and accomplished in successive phases as the face matures. Active correction in the adult dentition can usually be accomplished in one phase.

compressed gas cylinders, *n.pl* the color-coded storage cylinders containing either nitrous oxide (light blue) or oxygen (green or white) under pressure; used in controlled combination to induce conscious sedation.

compression, *n* the act of pressing together or forcing into less space.

compression molding, n See molding, compression.

compression of tissue, n See tissue, displaceability.

compressive strength, *n* See strength, compressive.

compromise (käm′prəmīz′), *n* an arrangement arrived at, in or out of court, for settling a disagreement on terms considered by the parties to be fair.

Compton scatter radiation, *n.pr* the incidental radiation that is energized enough to break an electron bond, but instead strikes a weak bond. The leftover energy then continues in an altered direction.

compulsion (kəmpul′shən), *n* a repetitive, stereotyped, and often trivial motor action, the performance of which is compelled even though the person does not wish to perform the act. Oral habits such as bruxism and clenching may become compulsions.

computed tomography (CT) (tōmog′rəfē), *n* a radiographic body scanning technique in which thin or narrow layer sections of the body can be imaged for diagnostic purposes. The technique uses a computer-linked radiographic machine to focus the radiographs on a particular section of the body to be viewed.

computer, *n* a device capable of accepting data in the form of facts and figures, manipulating them in a prescribed way, and supplying the results of these processes as meaningful information. This device usually consists of input and output devices, storage, arithmetic and logic units, and a control unit. Usually an automatic, stored-program machine is implied.

computer, digital, n a computer that operates on discrete data by performing arithmetic and logic processes on them.

computer graphics, n the use of computers to create illustrations or designs.

computer imaging, n in general, a branch of computer science that works with digital images. In surgical terms, the production of hypothesized postprocedural images, e.g., to show a patient what his face will look like after cosmetic surgery; also called digital imaging.

computer language, n the vocabulary and syntax of a set of symbols that are used to instruct a computer on what to do (e.g., Java, Ada, or C++).

computer literacy, n a functional knowledge of the use and application of computers, from word processing to data management.

computer output microfilm (COM), n a system that allows a computer user to produce microfilm copies of computer output. The COM unit operates independently of the CPU and is therefore called an *off-line* device. Output from computer processing is recorded on generic media and later recorded on microfilm.

computer simulation, n the use of computers to replicate a mechanical or biologic function.

computer-aided design (CAD), *n* the use of computers to assist a draftsman, architect, or artist in the creation of drawing, illustration, or other visual art. Along with this is computer-assisted design/computer-assisted manufacturer (CAD-CAM).

computer-controlled local anesthetic delivery system (CCLAD), *n* a computer-driven arrangement of software, hardware, and dental implements used to administer anesthetic injections in which the amount of drug and injection speed are predetermined by a software-driven motor. The injection itself is manually applied.

C

concanavalin A (kon′kənav′əlin), *n* a hemagglutinin, isolated from the meal of the jack bean, that reacts with polyglucosans in the blood of mammals, causing agglutination. It has been used to stimulate T-cell production.

concavity, *n* **1.** the condition of being concave. *n* **2.** a concave surface, such as a depression on the surface of an organ or tissue.

conceal, *v* to hide; secrete; withhold from the knowledge of others.

conchae, inferior nasal (kong′kē infē′rēr nā′zəl), *n* the most inferior of the three concha, or scroll-shaped bones, that protrude from the lateral wall of the nasal cavity.

concise, *n.pr* the brand name for diacrylate resin adhesives used in composite restorations and for bonding orthodontic appliances to the enamel.

concrescence (känkres′əns), *n* the union of two teeth after eruption, by the fusion of their cementum surfaces.

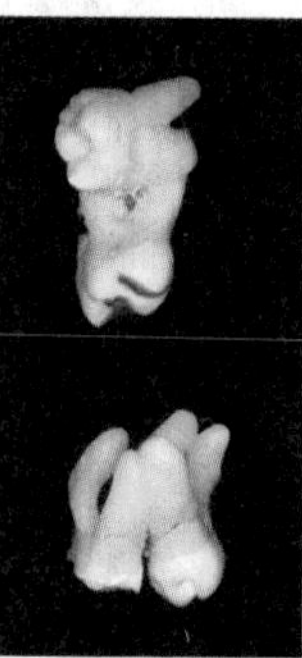

Concrescence. (Sapp/Eversole/Wysocki, 2004)

condensation (kän′densā′shən), *n* a commonly used term for the insertion and compression or compaction of dental materials into a prepared cavity. Compaction is a more accurate term than condensation. See also compaction.

condenser (kənden′sur), *n* (formerly called *plugger*), an instrument or device used to compact or condense a restorative material into a prepared cavity. Its working end is called the *nib,* or *point;* the end of the nib is termed the *face*. The face may be smooth or serrated.

condenser, amalgam (amalgam plugger), *n* an instrument used to condense plastic amalgam.

condenser, automatic, *n* See condenser, mechanical.

condenser, back-action, *n* a condenser with the shank bent into a U shape so that the condensing force is a pulling motion rather than the usual pushing force.

condenser, bayonet, *n* a condenser in which the offset of the nib and the approximately right-angled bends in the shank permit a better line of force for condensation of direct filling gold. There are many variations in angles, length, and diameter of the nib.

condenser, electromallet (McShirley's electromallet), *n* an electromechanical device for compacting direct filling gold. Frequency of blows may be varied from 200 to 3600 strokes/min; the intensity of the blow is controlled electronically.

condenser, foil, *n* a condenser used to compact direct-filling gold.

condenser, foot, *n* a foil condenser with the nib shaped like a foot.

condenser, hand, *n* an instrument that compacts material, the force being applied by the muscular effort of the clinician with or without supplementary force from a mallet in the hand of the assistant.

condenser, Hollenback, *n.pr* See condenser, pneumatic.

condenser, long-handled foil, *n* a hand condenser of varied design for compacting gold foil.

condenser, mechanical, *n* (automatic mallet), a device to supply an automatically controlled blow for condensing restorative material. It may be spring activated, pneumatic, or electronically controlled.

condenser, parallelogram **(par′əlel′əgram′),** *n* a condenser the face of which is shaped like a rectangle or parallelogram.

condenser, pneumatic (Hollenback condenser) **(nōōmat′ik),** *n* a pneumatic mechanical device developed by George M. Hollenback to supply a compacting force. The force is delivered by controlled pneumatic pressure. Blows are variable in intensity, with speed variable up to 300 strokes/min.

condenser point, *n* See point, condenser.

condenser, round, *n* a condenser the face of which has a circular outline.

condenser, stepping, *n* the orderly movement of a condenser point over the surface of gold foil or amalgam during its placement and compaction.

condensing force, *n* See force, condensing.

condensing osteitis, *n* See osteitis, condensing.

condensor (spreader), *n* an instrument used in filling a root canal to compress the filling material in a lateral direction.

conditioner, *n* **1.** an additive substance used to increase the effectiveness of another substance. **2.** a substance added to enamel that improves a sealant's ability to adhere.

conditioning, *n* a form of learning based on the development of a response or set of responses to a stimulus or series of stimuli.

conduct, dishonorable, *n* conduct that mars the character and lessens the reputation; conduct that is shameful, disgraceful, base.

conduction, *n* the carrying of sound waves, heat, light, nerve impulses, and electricity.

conduction, air, *n* the process of transmitting sound waves to the cochlea by way of the outer and middle ear. In normal hearing, practically all sounds are transmitted in this way, except those of the hearer's own voice, which are transmitted partly by bone conduction.

conduction, bone, *n* the transmission of sound waves or vibrations to the cochlea by way of the bones of the cranium.

conduction, impulse, *n* the conduction of an impulse along the nerve fiber, accompanied by an alteration of the electrical potential of the fiber tissue and an exchange of electrolytes across the nerve fiber membrane.

conductivity, *n* the capacity for conduction; ability to convey.

conductivity, electrical, *n* the ability of a material to conduct electricity. Metals are usually good conductors, and nonmetals are poor conductors.

conductivity, thermal, *n* the ability of a material to transfer heat. Thermal conductivity is of great importance in dentistry, where a low thermal conductivity is desirable in restorative material and a high thermal conductivity is desirable when soft tissue is covered.

condylar (kän′dilur), *adj* pertaining to the mandibular condyle.

condylar axis, *n* See axis, condylar.

condylar cartilage, *n* See cartilage, condylar.

condylar guide, *n* See guide, condylar.

condylar guide inclination, *n* See guide, condylar, inclination.

condyle (kän′dīl), *n* the rounded surface at the articular end of a bone. Also called *capitulum.*

condyle head, *n* a redundant term—the word *condyle* means *head.* See also condyle.

condyle, lateral path, *n* the path of the condyle in the glenoid fossa when a lateral mandibular movement is made.

condyle, mandibular, *n* the articular process of the mandible; the condyloid process of the mandible.

condyle, neck of, *n* See process, condyloid, neck of.

***condyle, occipital* (kän′dīl oksip′itl),** *n* the rounded projection that joins with the bones of the vertebrae located at the base of the occipital bone. It permits the head to rotate and flex.

condyle, orbiting, *n* See orbiting condyle.

condyle path, *n* the path traveled by the mandibular condyle in the temporomandibular joint during the various mandibular movements.

condyle, protrusive path, *n* the path of the condyle when the mandible is moved forward from its centric position.

condyle, rod, *n* See rod, condyle.

condyle, rotating, *n* the condyle on the side of the bolus formation, or the one that is braced and placed and rotated while the bolus is being chewed.

condylectomy (kän′dilek′tōmē), *n* the surgical removal of a condyle.

C

condyloid process (kon′dloid′), *n* See process, condyloid.

condyloplasty (kon′dəlōplas′tē), *n* a surgical procedure to alter the shape of the condyle to remove the effects of degenerative disease.

condylotomy (kän′dilot′ōmē), *n* a surgical division through, without removal of, a condyle; or removal of a portion, usually the articular surface, of a condyle.

cone, *n* **1.** a geometric shape with a circular base tapering evenly to an apex. **2.** a solid substance, usually guttapercha or silver, having a tapered form similar in length and diameter to a root canal; used to fill the space once occupied by the pulp in the root of the tooth. **3.** an accessory device on a dental radiograph machine, designed to indicate the direction of the central axis of its radiographic beam and to serve as a guide in establishing a desired source-to-film distance.

cone distance, n the distance between the focal spot and the outer end of the cone; usually expressed in inches or centimeters. Modern dental roentgen-ray units usually have cone distances of from 5 to 20 inches (12.5 to 50 cm).

cone, long, n a tubular "cone" designed to establish an extended anode-to-skin distance, usually within a range of from 12 to 20 inches (30 to 50 cm).

cone, sharpening, n a tapered or straight cylindrical stone that is used primarily to sharpen the curvature of dental instruments. See also stone, Arkansas and stone, Carborundum.

cone, short, n a conical or tubular "cone" having as one of its functions the establishment of an anode-to-skin distance of up to 9 inches (22.5 cm).

cone socket handles, *n.pl* the hand-held parts of instruments that may be separated from the working ends in order to replace or exchange individual parts by screwing them together.

cone-cut, *n* a technical error in the radiograph-taking process in which the position-indicating device is improperly aligned, causing the film to be incompletely covered by the radiation beam.

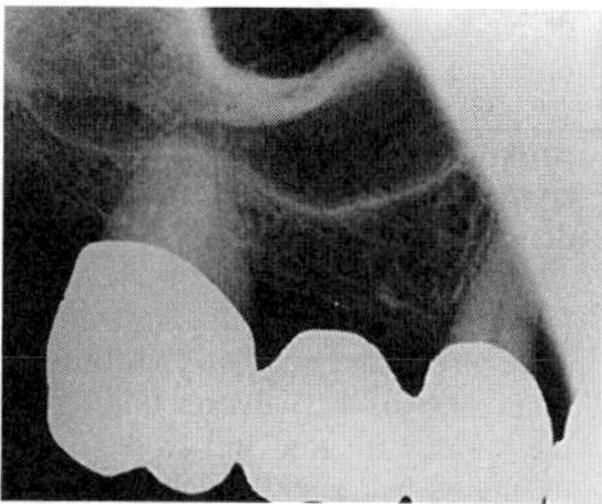

Cone cutting. (Frommer/Stabulas-Savage, 2005)

confidence interval, *n* a statistical device used to determine the range within which an acceptable datum would fall. Confidence intervals are usually expressed in percentages, typically 95% or 99%.

confidential, *adj* pertaining to information that is only shared with those directly responsible for patient care.

confidentiality, *n* the nondisclosure of certain information except to another authorized person.

confusion, *n* a mental state characterized by disorientation regarding time, place, or person that causes bewilderment, perplexity, lack of orderly thought, and inability to act decisively or perform the activities associated with daily living.

congenital, *adj* present at birth and usually developed in utero.

congestion, *n* See hyperemia.

congestive heart failure (kənjes′tiv), *n* an abnormal condition characterized by circulatory congestion (retention of fluids) caused by cardiac or kidney disorders. It usually develops chronically in association with the retention of sodium and water by the kidneys. The acute form may result from myocardial infarction of the left ventricle.

conjugate (kon′jəgāt′), *v* **1.** to unite. **2.** the product of conjugation.

conjugation (kon′jəgā′shən), *n* in biochemistry, the union of a drug or toxic substance with a normal constituent of the body, such as glucuronic acid, to form an inactive product that is then eliminated.

conjunctiva (kon′junktī′və), the mucous membrane lining the inner surfaces of the eyelids and anterior part of the sclera.

conjunctivitis (kon′junktivī′təs), *n* an inflammation of the conjunctiva, caused by bacterial or viral infection, allergy, or environmental factors. Also called *pinkeye.*

connective tissue, *n* See tissue, connective.

connector, *n* the part of a partial denture that unites its components.

connector, anterior palatal major, *n* a major connector uniting bilateral units of a maxillary removable partial denture. It is a thin metal plate that is located in the anterior palatal region.

connector bar, *n* See bar, connector.

connector, cross-arch bar splint, *n* a removable cross-arch connector used to stabilize weakened abutments that support a fixed prosthesis by attachment to teeth on the opposite side of the dental arch. It can be removed by the dental professional but not by the patient.

connector, lingual bar major, *n* a type of connector used to unite the right and left components of a mandibular removable partial denture and occupy a position lingual to the alveolar ridge.

connector, linguoplate major **(ling′-wōplāt′),** *n* a major connector formed by the extension of a metal plate from the superior border of the regular lingual bar, across gingivae, and onto the cingulum of each anterior tooth.

connector, major, *n* a metal plate or bar (e.g., lingual bar, linguoplate, palatal bar) used to join the units of one side of a removable partial denture to those located on the opposite side of the dental arch.

connector, minor, *n* the connecting link between the major connector or base of a removable partial denture and other units of the restoration, such as direct and indirect retainers and rests.

connector, nonrigid, *n* a connector used where retainers or pontics are united by a joint permitting limited movement. It may be a precision or a nonprecision type of connector.

connector, posterior palatal major, *n* (posterior palatal bar), a major transpalatal connector located in the posterior palatal region. It is used when the anterior palatal bar alone is insufficient to provide the necessary rigidity.

connector, rigid, *n* a connector used where retainers or pontics are united by a soldered, cast, or welded joint.

connector, saddle, *n* See connector, major.

connector, secondary lingual bar major (Kennedy bar), *n* often called a *continuous clasp* or *Kennedy bar.* It rests on the cingulum area of the lower anterior teeth and serves principally as an indirect retainer and/or stabilizer for weakened anterior lower teeth.

connector, subocclusal, *n* a nonrigid connector positioned gingival to the occlusal plane.

consanguinity (kon′sangwin′itē), *n* a hereditary or "blood" relationship between persons, by virtue of having a common parent or ancestor.

conscious, *adj* pertaining to the state of mind in which an individual is able to breathe on his or her own and to respond to verbal commands and physical prompts.

conscious sedation, *n* a state of sedation in which the patient remains aware of his or her person, surroundings, and conditions but without experiencing pain or anxiety.

consciousness, *n* a state in which the individual is capable of rational response to questioning and has all protective reflexes intact, including the ability to maintain a patent airway.

consent, *n* the concurrence of wills; permission.

consent, express, *n* consent directly given by voice or in writing.

consent, implied, *n* consent made evident by signs, actions, or facts, or by inaction or silence.

consideration, *n* inducement to make a contract. It may be a benefit to the promisor or a loss or detriment to the promisee. Consideration must be regarded as such by both parties.

Consolidated Omnibus Budget Reconciliation Act (COBRA), *n.pr* legislation relative to mandated benefits for all types of employee benefits plans. The most significant aspects within this context are the requirements for continued coverage for employees and their dependents for 18 months who would otherwise lose coverage (30 months for dependents in the event of an employee's death).

C

consonant, *n* a conventional speech sound produced, with or without laryngeal vibration, by certain successive contractions of the articulatory muscles that modify, interrupt, or obstruct the expired airstream to the extent that its pressure is raised.

consonant, semivowel, n consonants that are like vowels both perceptually and physiologically.

constipation, *n* a difficulty passing stools or incomplete or infrequent passage of hard stools.

constituent (kənstich′ūənt), *n* a part of the whole; component.

constitution, *n* the general makeup of the body as determined by genetic, physiologic, and biochemical factors. An individual's constitution may be markedly influenced by environment.

constriction (kənstrik′shən), *n* an abnormal closing or reduction in the size of an opening or passage of the body.

construction, single denture, *n* the making of one maxillary or mandibular denture as distinguished from a set of two complete dentures.

consultant, *n* a professional or nonprofessional person who, by virtue of special knowledge of professional or nonprofessional aspects of a dental practice, is sought out for advice and training.

consultation, *n* a meeting of persons to discuss or decide an issue.

consultation, patient, n a meeting among a dental professional, patient, and other interested persons for the purpose of discussing the patient's dental needs, proposing treatment, making business arrangements, making appointments, and giving referrals.

consultation, professional, n a joint deliberation by two or more dental professionals and/or health care professionals to determine the diagnosis, treatment, or prognosis for a particular dental patient.

consumer, *n* one who may receive or is receiving dental service; the term is also used in health care legislation and programs as a reference to someone who is never a practitioner or is not associated in any direct or indirect way with the supplying or provision of dental services.

contact, *n* the act of touching or meeting.

contact, balancing, n the contact established between the maxillary and mandibular dentures at the side opposite the working side (anteroposteriorly or laterally) for the purpose of stabilizing the dentures.

contact, deflective occlusal, n (cuspal interference), a condition of tooth contacts that diverts the mandible from a normal path of closure to centric jaw relation or causes a denture to slide or rotate on its basal seat. See also contact, interceptive occlusal.

contact, faulty, n imperfections in the contact between adjacent teeth. Often leads to food impaction between the teeth, with subsequent initiation or perpetuation of periodontal lesions.

contact, initial, n the first meeting of opposing teeth on elevation of the mandible toward the maxillae.

contact, interceptive occlusal, n an initial contact of teeth that interferes with the normal movement of the mandible. See also contact, deflective occlusal.

contact, premature, n See deflective occlusal and contact, interceptive.

contact, working, n a contact of the teeth made on the side of the dental arch toward which the mandible has been moved.

contagious (kəntā′jus), *adj* capable of being transmitted from one person to another by direct or indirect contact.

contaminated, *v* **1.** made radioactive by the addition of small quantities of radioactive material. **2.** made contaminated by adding infective or radiographic materials. **3.** an infective surface or object.

contamination, radioactive, *n* the deposition of radioactive material in any place where it is not desired, and particularly where its presence may be harmful or may constitute a radiation hazard.

contingent (kəntin′jənt), *adj* dependent for effect on something that may or may not occur.

continuant (kəntin′yōōənt), *n* a speech sound in which the speech organs are held relatively fixed during the period of production.

continuing education, *n* postgraduate study offered either in an institution of higher learning by groups with an organized dental program or by individuals who are especially qualified in certain areas. Required by most state licensing boards for license renewal for dental professionals. Credit accumulates for special qualifications to join special interest groups.

continuing education unit (CEU), *n* educational classes or experiences for licensed dental professionals that extend, update, or renew their knowledge of practices in their field. Some classes may be required for relicensing. Usually, one CEU equals 1 clock hour of instruction.

continuous bar retainer, *n* See retainer, continuous bar.

continuous clasp, *n* See retainer, continuous bar.

continuous loop wiring, *n* See wiring, continuous loop.

contour (kon′tōōr), *n* the external shape, form, or surface configuration of an object.

contour, anatomic height of **(an′ə-tom′ik),** *n* a line encircling a tooth to designate its greatest convexity.

contour, buccal, *n* the shape of the buccal aspect of a posterior tooth. It normally has occlusocervical convexity, with its greatest prominence at the gingival third of the clinical buccal surface.

contour, gingival, *n* the shape of the natural or artificial gingiva as it approximates the natural or artificial tooth.

contour, height of, *n* the greatest convexity of a tooth viewed from a predetermined position.

contour, proximal **(prok′səməl),** *n* the form of the mesial or distal surface of a tooth.

contour, restoration, *n* the restoration of a proper contour where surfaces of teeth have been destroyed by disease processes or excessive wear.

contour, tooth, *n* a shape of a tooth that is essential to a healthy gingival unit because it enables the bolus of food to be deflected from gingival margins during mastication.

contouring, occlusal, *n* the correction, by grinding, of gross disharmonies of the occlusal tooth form (e.g., uneven marginal ridges, plunger cusps, extruded teeth, malpositioned teeth) to establish a harmonious occlusion and protect the periodontium of the tooth.

contouring pliers, *n* See pliers, contouring.

contra-angle (kän′trə-ang′gəl), *n* more than one angle. An instrument having two or more offsetting angles such that the end of the instrument is kept within 3 mm of the axis of the shaft.

contraception, *n* a process or technique for the prevention of pregnancy by means of a medication, device, or method that blocks or alters one or more of the processes of reproduction in such a way that sexual union can occur without impregnation.

contract, *n* **1.** an agreement based on sufficient consideration between two or more competent parties to do or not to do something that is legal. **2.** a legally enforceable agreement between two or more individuals or entities that confers rights and duties on the parties. Common types of contracts include (1) those contracts between a dental benefits organization and an individual dental provider to provide dental treatment to members of an alternative benefits plan. These contracts define the dental provider's duties both to beneficiaries of the dental benefits plan and the dental benefits organization, and usually define the manner in which the dental provider will be reimbursed; and (2) contracts between a dental benefits organization and a group plan sponsor. These contracts typically describe the benefits of the group plan and the rates to be charged for those benefits.

contract, breach of, *n* the failure, without legal excuse, to perform an obligation or duty in a contract.

contract dentist/dental professional, *n* a practitioner who contractually agrees to provide services under special terms, conditions, and financial reimbursement arrangements.

contract dentistry, *n* **1.** the providing of dental care under a specific set of guidelines and for a specific set of individuals under an accepted written agreement by the patient, dental professional, and employer. **2.** the practice of dentistry whereby the dentist/

dental professional enters into a written agreement with either patients or an employer to provide dental care for a set group of people.

contract, express, *n* a contract that is an actual agreement between the parties, with the terms declared at the time of making, being stated in explicit language either orally or in writing.

contract fee schedule plan, *n* a dental benefits plan in which participating dental professionals agree to accept a list of specific fees as the total fees for dental treatment provided.

contract, implied, *n* a contract not evidenced by explicit agreement of the parties but inferred by the law from the acts and circumstances surrounding the transactions.

contract, open-end, *n* **1.** a contract that permits periodic reevaluation of the dental plan during the contract year. If indicated by the reevaluation, dental services may be deleted or added to achieve a balance between the premium and cost of service provided. **2.** a contract that sets no dollar limits on the total services to be provided to beneficiaries but does list the particular services that will be included in the plan.

contract practice, *n* a type of dental practice in which an employer or third-party administrator contracts directly with a dental professional or group of dental professionals to provide dental services for beneficiaries of a plan. See also closed panel.

contract term, *n* the period, usually 12 months, for which a contract is written.

contraction (kəntrak′shən), *n* **1.** a shortening, shrinkage, or reduction in length or size. **2.** a condition in which teeth or other maxillary and mandibular structures, such as the dental arch, are nearer than normal to the median plane.

contraction, concentric muscle, *n* an unresisted ordinary shortening of muscle.

contraction, eccentric muscle, *n* an increase in muscle tonus during lengthening of the muscle. Eccentric contraction occurs when muscles are used to oppose movement but not to stop it (e.g., the action of the biceps in lowering the forearm gradually and in a controlled manner). Eccentric contractions are called *isotonic,* because the muscle changes length.

contraction, isometric muscle **(ī′sōmet′rik),** *n* an increase in muscular tension without a change in muscle length, as in clenching the teeth.

contraction, isotonic muscle **(ī′sōton′ik),** *n* an increase in muscular tension during movement without resistance (either lengthening or shortening), as in free opening and closing of the jaws.

contraction, metal, *n* the shrinkage associated with the congealing of a metal from its molten state to a solid after having been cast. See also expansion, thermal.

contraction, muscle, *n* the development of tension in a muscle in response to a nerve stimulus.

contraction, muscle, changes in striation bands, *n.pl* alterations in bands of striated muscle during contraction. Striated muscle is composed of a darker A band and a lighter I band. Both these alternating bands develop tension during contraction but not to the same degree. In isometric contraction (clenched teeth), the sarcomere muscle unit remains unchanged in length, whereas the A band (the darker band) actually shortens and the I band (the lighter band) lengthens. When a muscle is passively stretched, such as when the mandible is opened by gravity, the A band lengthens relatively more than the I band, and during isotonic contraction, almost all the shortening is in the A segment. It is thus concluded that the contractile properties are not the same throughout the sarcomere, which is the unit of contractility. It is suggested that the darker A band has a greater concentration of contractile substance than the I band and that, in addition to contractile elements, the I band contains elastic noncontractile elements that constitute a series of elastic components throughout the fibril. Thus there is, throughout a fiber, an arrangement of dark, contractile components alternating with lighter, elastic components.

contraction, muscle, chemical factors in, *n.pl* the chemical constituents and action involved in the contraction of muscle fibers. Muscle is a structure with working units built up largely from two proteins, actin and myosin, which appear to be organized into separate filaments running longitudinally through the muscle fibers. Neither type of filament runs continuously along the length of the fiber, although the effect is that of a continuous structure. The filaments are organized into a succession of groupings of one type of fiber. Each group is arranged in a regular palisade to overlap the next group of fibers, which are similarly arranged in palisades. This gives a banded appearance to the fiber. The thicker filaments contain myosin and are restricted to the A bands, where they give rise to a higher density and double refraction. The thinner filaments contain actin and extend to either side of the Z band, which is at the center of the I band. When the muscle contracts or is stretched, the two groups of filaments slide past each other like the alternating units of a sliding gate. The controlled sliding motion is presumably brought about through the mediation of oblique cross links between the filaments. These cross links are the structural expression of the biochemical interaction between actin and myosin. The chemical substance that initiates the interaction between these fibrils is adenosine triphosphate (ATP). The final effect of the interaction between ATP, myosin, and actin is to enable the two types of filaments to crawl past each other to create the shortened state of the muscle.

contraction, postural muscle **(pos′-churəl),** *n* the maintenance of muscular tension (usually isometric muscular contraction) sufficient to maintain posture.

contraction, premature ventricular (PVC), *n* an extra heartbeat caused by premature contractions of the heart's ventricles resulting in palpitations, or a skipped beat, followed by a more pronounced beat.

contraction, smooth muscle, mechanism of, *n* the mechanisms that regulate the functions of smooth muscle fibers. These regulatory mechanisms vary and are affected principally by two methods. First, the parasympathetic and sympathetic nerve fiber endings of the autonomic nervous system form a reticulum around the muscle cells before entering them. The action of these fibers is antagonistic; they act directly on the muscle cell, not on each other. Examples of the structures principally under the control of the autonomic nerve mechanism are the blood vessels and the pilomotor fibers. Second, the selection response to rhythmic activity associated with the automaticity of a viscus or other organ depends on local or hormonal factors. An example of this mechanism is the function of the uterus under the control of the estrogenic hormone.

contraction, static muscle, *n* the contraction in which opposing muscles contract against each other and prevent movement. Fixation action of a muscle in a static contraction is termed *isometric,* because it develops tension without changing length.

contractor, independent, *n* one who, exercising an independent employment, contracts to do a piece of work according to the conditions of the contract and without being subject to control except as to the result of the work.

contracture (kəntrak′chər), *n* a permanent shortening, or contraction, of a muscle.

contraindication (kon′trəin′dikā′-shən), *n* any symptom or circumstance indicating the inappropriateness of a form of treatment otherwise advisable. This is further divided into the concepts of absolutes and relative contraindications.

contralateral (kon′trəlat′ərəl), *adj* originating from or affecting the opposite side of the body.

contrast, radiographic (radiographic image), *n* the differences in photographic or film density produced on a radiograph by structural composition of the object radiographed or by varying amounts of radiation.

contrast, radiographic, long-scale, *n* an increased number of gradations of gray between the blacks and whites on a radiograph. Higher kilovoltages increase the scale of contrast.

C

contrast, radiographic, media, *n* See radiograph, contrast media.

contrast, radiographic, short-scale, *n* a minimum number of gradations of gray between the blacks and whites on a radiograph. Lower kilovoltages decrease the scale of contrast.

contrast, subject, *n* See contrast, radiographic.

contributory negligence, *n* See negligence, contributory.

contributory plan, *n* a method of payment for group insurance coverage in which part of the premium is paid by the employee and part is paid by the employer or union.

contributory program, *n* a dental benefits program in which the enrollee shares in the monthly premium of the program with the program sponsor (usually the employer). Generally done through payroll deduction.

control group, *n* the group of participants in a clinical study who do not receive the drug or treatment being studied against which the reactions of individuals in the experimental group may be compared. See also controlled clinical trial.

control, stress, *n* a method used to diminish or remove the stress load generated by occlusal contact, whether the contact is functional in origin or the result of a habit cycle.

controlled clinical trial, *n* a research strategy that calls for two samples: an experimental sample of patients receiving a pharmaceutical, and a second sample of control patients receiving a placebo. Neither the patient nor the researcher knows which is receiving the pharmaceutical and which the placebo.

controlled substance, a drug as defined in the five categories of the federal Controlled Substances Act of 1970. The categories, or schedules, cover opium and its derivatives, hallucinogens, depressants, and stimulants.

controlled-release therapeutic systems, *n* a drug or hormone delivery system that releases predetermined amounts of drug or hormone into the body over a specified period.

contusion (kəntōō′zhən), *n* a bruise that is usually produced by impact from a blunt object and that does not cause a break in the skin.

convenience form, *n* See form, convenience.

convergence, cervical, *n* the angle formed between the cervicoaxial inclination of a tooth surface on one side and a diagnostic stylus of a dental cast surveyor in contact with the tooth at its height of contour.

conversion privilege, *n* the right of an individual covered by a group dental insurance policy to continue having coverage on a direct payment basis when association with the insured group is terminated.

converter, rotary, *n* a motor generator set or unit that, when operated by one type of current, produces another (e.g., the conversion of alternating to direct current).

convertin, *n* See thromboplastin, extrinsic.

convex (konveks′), *adj* having a surface that curves outward.

convulsion (kənvul′shən), *n* an intense seizure.

coolant (kōō′lənt), *n* air or liquid directed onto a tooth, tissue, or restoration to neutralize the heating effect of a rotary instrument.

Cooley's anemia, *n.pr* See thalassemia major.

Cooley's trait, *n.pr* See thalassemia minor.

Coolidge filament transformer, tube, *n.pr* See transformer, Coolidge.

coordination, *n* the harmonious functioning of body systems.

coordination of benefits clause, *n* **1.** a provision in an insurance contract that when a patient is covered under more than one group dental plan, benefits paid by all plans will be limited to 100% of the actual charges after each deductible has been satisfied. **2.** COB: a method of integrating benefits payable under more than one plan. Benefits from all sources should not exceed 100% of the total charges.

Copal resin (kōpəl), *n.pr* brand name for a mixed resin of diverse plant origin used in cavity varnishes. Its effectiveness in protecting the pulp from the phosphoric acid in dental cements is questioned.

copayment, *n* the beneficiary's share of the dental professional's fee after the benefits plan has paid.

cope, *n* the upper half of a flask in the casting art; hence also the upper, or cavity, side of a denture flask.

coping (thimble) (kō′ping), *n* a thin metal covering or cap over a prepared tooth.

coping, parallel, n a casting placed over an implant abutment to make it parallel to other natural or implant abutments.

coping, transfer, n a covering or cap, made of metal, acrylic resin, or other material used to position a die in an impression.

copolymer (kōpäl′imur), *n* a polymerization of two or more monomers that have slightly different chemical formulas. Used in dentistry to impart certain desirable physical properties such as flow.

copolymerization (kōpäl′iməriză′shən), *n* the formation of a copolymer.

copper, *n* a malleable, reddish-brown metallic element. It is a component of several important enzymes in the body and is essential to good health. A deficiency is rare, because only 2 to 5 mg daily are necessary, and that amount is easily obtained in a normal diet.

coprolalia (kop′rōlā′lēə), *n* the uncontrollable vocalization of obscene or offensive words.

coproporphyria (kop′rōpôr′fir′ēə), *n* the presence of an abnormal concentration of coproporphyrin in the urine. Normal values range from 70 mg to 250 mg/day. An increased amount of coproporphyrin III occurs in the urine in clinical lead poisoning, exposure to lead without clinically apparent symptoms, infections, malignant disease, alcoholic cirrhosis, after ingestion of small amounts of ethanol, and normally in some individuals.

coproporphyrin (kop′rəpor′firin), *n* a nitrogenous organic substance normally excreted in the feces as a breakdown of bilirubin.

cord(s), *n* a long, rounded organ or body.

cord, spinal, n the central nervous system cord contained in the vertebral column. It is essential to the regulation and administration of various motor, sensory, and autonomic nerve activities of the body. Through its pathways it conducts impulses from the extremities, trunk, and neck to and from the higher centers and to consciousness. It thus provides for simple reflexes, has control over visceral activities, and participates in the conscious activities of the body.

cord, vocal, the membranous structures in the throat that produce sound; the thyroarytenoid ligaments of the larynx. The inferior cords are called the *true vocal cords,* and the superior cords are called the *false vocal cords.*

core, *n* the central part. A section of a mold, usually of plaster, made over assembled parts of a dental restoration or construction to record and maintain the relationships of the parts so that the parts can be reassembled in their original positions. Also called a *laboratory core.*

core, amalgam, n the foundational replacement of the badly mutilated crown of a tooth whose purpose is to provide a rigid base for retention of a cast crown restoration. The core may be retained by undercuts, slots, pins, or the pulp chamber of an endodontically treated tooth.

core, cast, n a metal casting, usually with a post in the canal or a root, designed to retain an artificial crown.

core, composite, n a composite resin buildup to provide retention for a cast crown restoration.

core, laboratory, a section of a mold, usually of plaster, made over assembled parts of a dental restoration or construction to record and maintain the relationships of the parts so that the parts can be reassembled in their original positions.

cornea (kor′nēə), *n* the transparent anterior part of the eye.

cornification (kor′nifikā′shən), *n* the conversion of epithelium to a hornlike substance. *Keratinization* is a more specific term. See also keratin.

cornu (kôr′nōō), *n* a bony projection.

coronal, *adj* pertaining to the crown portion of teeth.

C

coronary angioplasty, percutaneous transluminal, *n* a surgical technique designed to improve circulation. It involves the insertion of a balloon-carrying catheter into a blood vessel of the heart that is clogged with plaque, then alternately inflating and deflating the balloon several times to flatten the plaque against the arterial walls and reestablish the free flow of blood. Also called *balloon angioplasty* or *coronary dilation.*

coronary artery bypass, *n* an open-heart surgery in which a section of a blood vessel is grafted onto one or more of the coronary arteries to improve the blood supply to the muscles of the heart.

Coronaviridae **(kôrō′nəvir′idā),** *n.pl* a family of enveloped, helical, airborne RNA viruses responsible for some respiratory and gastrointestinal diseases. It can also be contracted from unsanitary equipment or from human carriers.

coronoid notch, *n* See notch, coronoid.

coronoid process, *n* See process, coronoid.

coronoidectomy (kor′ōnoidek′tōmē), *n* the surgical removal of the coronoid process of the mandible.

corporate dentistry, *n* **1.** the dental care provided for a specific group of employees within a single business under a contract arrangement or on a salaried basis, with costs borne by the corporation. **2.** a company-owned-and-operated dental care facility that provides services to employees and sometimes dependents.

corpus callosum (kor′pəs kəlō′-səm), *n* the largest commissure of the brain connecting the cerebral hemispheres.

corpuscle(s) (kor′pusəl), *n* a small body, mass, or organ.

corpuscle, blood, *n* a formed element in the blood. See also erythrocyte, leukocyte, lymphocyte, monocyte.

corpuscle, Golgi's, *n.pr* a small, spindle-shaped proprioceptive endorgan located in tendons and activated by stretch.

corpuscle, Krause's, *n.pr* the bulboid encapsulated nerve endings located in mucous membranes and activated by cold.

corpuscle, Meissner's, *n.pr* the medium encapsulated nerve endings found in the skin and activated by light touch.

corpuscle, Merkel's, *n.pr* the specialized sensory nerve endings located in the submucosa of the oral cavity and activated by light touch.

corpuscle, Pacini's, *n.pr* the large sensory nerve endings, scattered widely in subcutaneous tissues, joints, and tendons and activated by deep pressure.

corpuscle, Ruffini's, *n.pr* the specialized sensory nerve organs in the skin and mucous membranes for perceiving heat. Temperature variations of less than 5°C are not readily received by these end organs.

corrected master cast, *n* See cast, master, corrected.

correction, occlusal, *n* the fixing of malocclusion, by whatever means is employed, including the elimination of disharmony of occlusal contacts.

corrective, *n* a prescription ingredient designed to compensate for or nullify specific undesirable effects of the principal pharmaceutical agent and the adjuvant.

correlation, *n* a statistical procedure used to determine the degree to which two (or more) variables vary together. Correlation does not suggest a cause-effect relationship but only the degree of parallelism or concomitance between the variables, the cause of which may be unknown. The *Pearson product-moment correlation (r)* is the most frequently used, and this coefficient is used unless another is specified.

correlation, coefficient number **(kō′əfish′ənt),** *n* the result of statistical computation that indicates the strength of the tendency of two or more variables to vary concomitantly. The coefficient is expressed in fractions (that is, r = 80), ranging from 21 to 11, and indicates the magnitude of the relationship between the variables. Perfect direct correspondence is expressed by 11; perfect inverse correspondence by 21; complete lack of correspondence by 0. Fractional values are not read as percents.

correlation, linear, *n* a correlation in

which the regression line, the line that best describes the relationship between the two variables, is a straight line, so that for any increase in the magnitude of one variable there will be a proportional change in the magnitude of the other variable.

correlation, multiple, *n* a complex correlation procedure in which scores on two or more variables are combined to predict scores on another variable, called the *dependent variable.*

correspondence, *n* written or typed communication between two individuals or groups of individuals.

corrosion, *n* an electrolytic or chemical attack of a surface. Usually refers to the attack of a metal surface.

cortex, *n* the outer layer of an organ or other structure.

cortex, adrenal, *n* the outer layer of the adrenal gland, the site of secretion of the adrenocortical hormones.

cortex, cerebral, *n* the outer gray matter of cerebrum, where many of the higher functions, such as volition, consciousness, conceptualization, and sensation, are carried out.

cortical, *adj* pertaining to or consisting of a cortex.

corticalosteotomy (kôr′tikəlos′tēot′ōmē), *n* an osteotomy through the cortex at the base of the dentoalveolar segment, which serves to weaken the resistance of the bone to the application of orthodontic forces.

corticoid, adrenal (kôr′tikoid), *n* an adrenal corticosteroid hormone (e.g., 11-dehydrocorticosterone [compound A], corticosterone [compound B], 11-deoxycorticosterone [cortexone, DOC], cortisone [compound E], cortisol [compound F], 11-desoxycortisol [substance S], aldosterone, androgen, progesterone, estrogen, and many other inactive steroids). See also aldosterone, androgen, corticosterone, cortisone, estrogens, hydrocortisone, and progesterone.

corticosteroid (kôr′tikōstir′oid), *n* See steroid, adrenocortical.

corticosterone (Kendall's compound B) (kôr′tikōstir′ōn, kôr′tikos′tərōn), *n* an adrenal corticosteroid hormone necessary for the maintenance of life in adrenalectomized animals; protects against stress, influences muscular efficiency, and influences carbohydrate and electrolyte metabolism.

corticotropin (kôr′tikōtrō′pin), *n* a purified preparation of adrenocorticotropic hormone derived from the pituitary gland of animals. See also ACTH.

cortisol, *n* See hydrocortisone.

cortisone (17-hydroxy-11-dehydrocorticosterone, Kendall's compound E) (kor′tisōn′), *n* a hormone produced by the adrenal cortex; a glucocorticoid, 17-hydroxy-11-dehydrocorticosterone; useful in the treatment of rheumatoid arthritis, lupus erythematosus, and some allergic conditions. Has marked antiinflammatory properties. Excess production or administration produces signs of hyperadrenocorticalism (Cushing's syndrome) with hyperlipemia and obesity hyperglycemia and edema.

cortisone acetate, *n brand name:* Cortone; *drug class:* gluocorticoid, short acting; *action:* decreases inflammation by suppression of macrophage and leukocyte migration, reduces capillary permeability; *uses:* inflammation, severe allergy, adrenal insufficiency, collagen, and respiratory and dermatologic disorders.

corundum, *n* See emery.

Corynebacterium **(kor′ənēbakter′ēəm),** *n* a common genus of rod-shaped, curved bacilli. The most common pathogenic species are *C. acnes,* commonly found in acne lesions, and *C. diphtheriae,* the cause of diphtheria.

cosmetic orthodontics, *n* limited orthodontic therapy for the purpose of improving appearance, such as the closing of an unsightly diastema between maxillary incisors that presents no other handicap.

cost containment, *n* the features of a dental benefits program or of the administration of the program designed to reduce or eliminate certain charges to the plan.

cost share, *n* the share of health expenses that a beneficiary must pay, including the deductibles, copayments, coinsurance, and charges over the amount reimbursed by the dental benefits plan.

cost-benefit analysis, *n* the comparative study of the service or production costs of a service or item and its value to the subject.

cost-effective, *n* the minimal expenditure of dollars, time, and other elements necessary to achieve the health care result deemed necessary and appropriate.

Costen's syndrome, *n.pr* See syndrome, Cushing's.

cotherapist, *n* in oral health care, a designation for the relationships among patient, dental hygienist, and dental professional in securing the patient's regular treatment.

cotinine (kō′tinēn), *n* a substance that remains in body fluids after nicotine has been used. Presence of this chemical in body fluids is considered proof of recent nicotine use. It is currently being studied for its possible contribution to a range of oral diseases.

cotton, absorbent, *n* the fibers or hairs of the seed of cultivated varieties of *Gossypium herbaceum,* so prepared that the cotton readily absorbs liquid.

cotton pliers, *n* See pliers, cotton.

cough, *n* a sudden, noisy expulsion of air from the lungs. See also mechanism, cough.

cough, gander, *n* the characteristic clanging, brassy cough of tracheal obstruction.

Council on Dental Therapeutics, *n.pr* an appointed council within the Division of Scientific Affairs of the American Dental Association directed to study, evaluate, and disseminate information with regard to dental therapeutic agents, their adjuncts, and dental cosmetic agents that are offered to the public or profession.

counseling, *n* the act of providing advice and guidance to a patient or the patient's family.

count, blood, complete, *n* the determination of the number of red blood cells (erythrocytes), white blood cells, and platelets in an accurately measured volume of blood. It usually includes the quantity of hemoglobin per cubic millimeter of blood. A normal red blood count is 4 to 5.5 million cells/cubic mm of blood.

count, differential white blood cell, *n* the determination of the number of each type of white blood cell in the peripheral blood. The relative count is obtained by counting the number of each type of cell in every 100 cells. The results are expressed in percentages. The normal figure for neutrophils is 60% to 70%, lymphocytes 20% to 35%, monocytes 2% to 8%, basophils 0% to 1%, and eosinophils 2% to 4%.

count, platelet, *n* the determination of the number of platelets in a cubic millimeter of blood. The normal count is 200,000 to 500,000.

count, reticulocyte (rətik′yəlōsīt), *n* the number of reticulocytes in the circulating blood, giving some indication of bone marrow activity. The number is increased after acute blood loss and after recovery from anemia. The number is decreased in anemias associated with defective red cell or hemoglobin production (nutritional, endocrine, toxic, or displacement anemias). The normal range is 0.5% to 1.5% of the erythrocytes.

count, white blood cell, *n* the determination of the number of white blood cells in an accurately measured volume of blood. The normal value is from 4000 to 9000 per cubic millimeter of blood.

counter, *n* a device for enumerating ionizing events.

counter, Geiger-Muller (G-M counter, Geiger counter), *n.pr* a highly sensitive gas-filled device that measures radiation.

counter, proportional, *n* a gas-filled radiation detection tube in which the pulse produced is proportional to the number of ions formed in the gas by the primary ionizing particle.

counter, scintillation **(sintəlā′shən),** *n* a combination of phosphor, photomultiplier tube, and associated circuits for counting the light emissions that are produced in the phosphor.

counterdie (koun′tərdī), *n* the reverse image of a die, usually made of a softer and lower-fusing metal than the die. It is used to swage metal, wax, or other material over a die. See also die.

counterirritant, *n* an irritant that blocks perception of pain by diverting attention to the sensation that it produces.

coverage, *n* **1.** benefits available to an individual covered under a dental benefits plan. **2.** See denture coverage.

coverage year, *n* the 12-month period over which deductibles and maximum benefits apply for each person.

cover screw, *n* a screw placed on the superior part of a dental implant immediately after it is placed in the bone, completely covering the top of the implant and sealing it off from bone and other debris during the healing and integration period. The screw is removed at the beginning of the next phase of the implant process, when the abutment that will hold the new tooth is placed.

covered charges, *n.pl* the charges for services rendered or supplies furnished by a dental professional that qualify as covered services and are paid for in whole or in part by the dental benefits program. May be subject to deductibles, copayments, coinsurance, annual or lifetime maximums, or table of allowances, as specified by the terms of the contract.

covered person, *n* an individual who is eligible for benefits under a dental benefits program.

covered services, *n.pl* the services for which payment is provided under the terms of the dental benefits contract.

Coxiella burnetii **(kok′sēel′ə),** a species that causes Q fever in man. From the genus of filterable bacteria of the order *Rickettsiales.*

Coxsackie A disease (koksak′ē), *n* See herpangina.

crack cocaine, *n* a street drug made by chemically converting cocaine hydrochloride to a form that can be smoked. Smoking crack is a faster, more direct way of getting cocaine into the brain. The narcotic effect of smoking crack cocaine is faster and more intense than it is when injected, inhaled, or ingested. No medical application exists for crack cocaine. See cocaine.

cracked tooth syndrome, *n* a transient acute pain in a tooth experienced occasionally while chewing. Difficult to locate and reproduce. Likely to occur among individuals who crack nuts and crush ice with their teeth, and among popcorn eaters. Usually a vertical crack or split in the tooth extends across a marginal ridge through the crown and into the root, involving the pulp. Visible by transilluminated light or with the use of disclosing dyes.

cranial base, *n.pl* the bones forming the base of the skull. In cephalometric analysis, defined by the angle formed by a line drawn basion to point S (sella turcica) and from point S to point N (frontonasal suture).

cranial nerves, *n* See nerves, cranial.

cranial prosthesis (krānēəl prosthē′sis), *n* an artificial replacement for a portion of the skull.

cranial sutures, *n.pl* the fibrous joints between the bones of the cranium, some of which are fused in adults.

craniofacial (krā′nēōfā′shəl), *adj* pertaining to the portion of the skull that contains the face and brain.

craniofacial anomalies **(ənom′əlēs),** *n.pl* congenital malformations of the skull and face, frequently associated with genetically transmitted syndromes.

craniofacial dysostosis **(krā′nēōfā′shəl dis′ostō′sis),** *n* See dysostosis, craniofacial.

craniofacial templates, *n.pl* a series of cephalometric tracings of normal faces by age, sex, and race by which variations in the facial form of a patient can be determined and a treatment objective arranged.

craniometry (krā′nēom′ətrē), *n* the study of the measurements of the skull.

craniopharyngioma (krā′nēōfərin′jēō′mə), *n* a tumor histologically identical to ameloblastoma that arises from remnants of the craniopharyngeal duct.

craniosynostosis (krā′nēōsin′ostō′sis), *n* premature fusion of the cranial sutures resulting in a malformed head, which may lead to an increase in intracranial pressure and consequential brain damage.

craniotabes (kra′nēōtā′bēz), *n* a soft, yielding skull; shallow pitting and thinning of skull bones of infants as a result of congenital syphilis or rickets.

craniotomy, *n* a surgical opening into the skull, performed to relieve intracranial pressure, to control bleeding, or to remove a tumor.

cranium, *n* the skull that covers and protects the brain.

C

crater formation, *n* a circular depression or pit in the surface of a tissue or body part, such as in cancer of the skin. Also seen in the formation of interdental depressions in the gingival tissues or subjacent bone; often associated with the destructive effects of necrotizing periodontal disease.

cratered, *adj* the condition of having one or more pits, depressions, or hollows (often found on tissues and caused by ulcers).

crazing of plastic teeth, *n* the small cracks appearing on the surface of plastic teeth induced by the release of internal stress.

creatine kinase (krē′ətēn′ kī′nās′), *n* an enzyme in muscle, brain, and other tissues that catalyzes the transfer of a phosphate group from adenosine triphosphate to creatine, producing adenosine diphosphate and phosphocreatine.

creatinine (krēat′ənēn′), *n* a substance formed from the metabolism of creatine, commonly found in blood, urine, and muscle tissue.

credential, license by, *n* the establishment of a license to practice in one state or province based on licensing history from another state or province with comparable regulations and requirements. Also called *reciprocity.*

credit rating, *n* the evaluation of a person's responsibility toward meeting financial obligations.

creditor, *n* a person to whom a debt is owed.

crenation of tongue, *n* scalloping along the lingual periphery of the tongue caused by the tongue lying against the lingual surface of the mandibular teeth.

creosote, N.F. XI (wood creosote), *n* a mixture of phenols obtained from wood tar and occasionally used to treat root canals.

crepitus (krep′itus), *n* a crackling sound such as that produced by the rubbing together of fragments of a fractured bone or by air moving in a tissue space.

crepitus, bony, *n* the crackling sound noted during auscultation; also the sensation noted during palpation when the fragments of a fractured bone are rubbed together.

crest, *n* a projecting ridge or structure.

crest, alveolar, *n* See bone crest.

crest, gingival, *n* the coronal margin of the gingival tissue.

crest module, *n* the portion of a two-piece metal dental implant designed to hold the prosthetic component in place and to create a transition zone to the load-bearing implant body.

CREST syndrome, *n* See syndrome, CREST.

crestal resorption (kres′təl rēsôrp′shən), *n* bone resorption at the border or crest of the dental alveolus. This bone loss follows tooth extraction and may result from periodontal infection or through the use of heavy orthodontic forces.

cretin, *n* a thyroid-deficient dwarfed individual with mental subnormality.

cretinism (krē′tənizəm) (congenital hypothyroidism), *n* See hypothyroidism.

crevice, gingival, *n* See gingival, crevice.

crevicular fluid (krevik′yōōlur), *n* an older term for a clear, usually unnoticeable fluid that can serve as a defense mechanism against infection by carrying antibodies and other substances between the connective tissue and sulcus or pocket. Also called *gingival sulcus fluid* or *sulcular fluid.*

crib, Jackson, *n.pr* a removable orthodontic appliance retained in position by crib-shaped wires.

crib, lingual, *n* an orthodontic appliance consisting of a wire framework suspended lingually to the maxillary incisor teeth; used to obstruct thumb and tongue habits.

crib splint, *n* See splint, crib.

cribriform plate (krib′rəform′), *n* **1.** the aveolar bone that forms the tooth socket and to which the periodontal ligament is attached (radiographically presents as the lamina dura). **2.** the horizontal plate of the ethmoid bone that is perforated with foramina for the olfactory nerves.

cricoid cartilage (krī'koid), *n* See cartilage, cricoid.

cricoidynia (krī'koidī'nēə), *n* pain in the cricoid cartilage.

cricothyrotomy (krī'kōthīrot'əmē), *n* an incision between the cricoid and thyroid cartilages for the purpose of maintaining a patent airway.

cri-du-chat syndrome (krē'-dōō-shä'), *n* See syndrome, cri-du-chat.

criminology, the study of crime, the people who commit crimes, and penal codes used to deter crime and punish criminals.

crisis, adrenal, an acute adrenocortical insufficiency, with clinical manifestations of headache, nausea, vomiting, diarrhea, confusion, costovertebral angle pain, circulatory collapse, and coma. May occur in relation to stress of dental or medical procedures in patients with latent adrenal disease or in patients who have undergone prior ACTH or cortisone therapy, especially without control or termination of therapy.

crisis, thyroid, *n* a complication occurring after thyroidectomy, or before or during other surgical procedures where even mild hyperthyroidism is present. It is characterized by tachycardia, a high temperature, nervousness, and occasionally delirium.

cristobalite (kristō'bəlīt), *n* a form of crystalline silica used in dental casting investments because of its relatively high capacity for thermal expansion and resistance to breaking down by heat.

criteria (krītēr'ēə), *n.pl* predetermined rules or guidelines for dental care, developed by dental professionals relying on professional expertise, prior experience, and the professional literature, with which aspects of actual instances of dental care may be compared. *Explicit* criteria are predetermined, specific, and measurable; *implicit* criteria are implied or understood but not directly expressed.

critical care, *n* See intensive care.

cromolyn sodium (krō'məlin' sō'dēəm), *n brand names:* Intal, Nasalcrom, Rynacrom; *drug class:* antiasthmatic; *action:* stabilizes the membrane of the sensitized mast cell, preventing release of chemical mediators; *uses:* allergic rhinitis, severe perennial bronchial asthma, exercise-induced bronchospasm.

cross linkage, *n* See polymerization, cross.

cross-arch bar splint, *n* See connector.

cross-arch bar splint connector, *n* See connector, cross-arch bar splint.

cross-arch splinting, *n* See splinting, cross-arch.

crossbite, *n* an occlusion with the line of occlusion of the mandibular teeth anterior and/or buccal to the maxillary teeth. See also occlusion, crossbite.

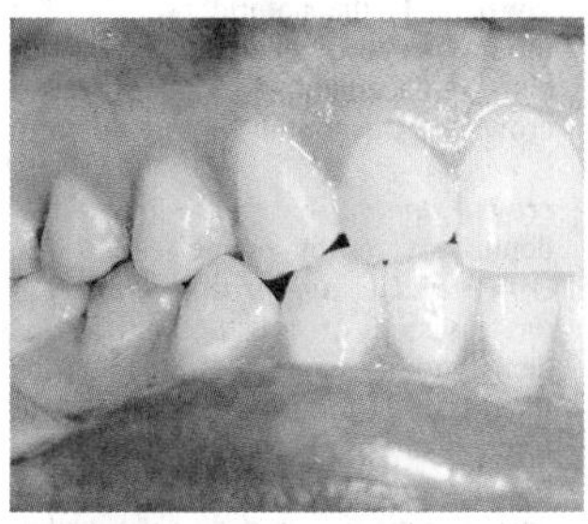

Crossbite. (Bird/Robinson, 2005)

crossbite, anterior, *n* the primary or permanent maxillary incisors locked lingual to mandibular incisors.

crossbite, posterior, *n* the primary permanent maxillary posterior teeth in lingual position in relation to the mandibular teeth.

cross-contamination, *n* the transfer of an infection directly from one person to another or indirectly from one person to a second person via a fomite.

cross-examination, *n* the questioning of a witness by the party against whom he or she has been called and examined.

cross-infection, *n* the transmission of a communicable disease from one person to another because of a poor barrier protection.

cross-resistance, *n* See resistance, cross-.

cross-section form, *n* See clasp, flexibility of.

cross-sectional study, *n* the scientific method for the analysis of data gathered from two or more samples at one point in time.

cross-tolerance, *n* See tolerance, cross-.

crotch, furcation, *n* the point at which the root of a tooth forks into two or more branches.

Crouzon disease (krōōzonz′), See syndrome, Crouzon.

Crouzon syndrome, *n.pr* See syndrome, Crouzon.

crowding, *n* **1.** in dentistry, when the dental arch length is less than the mesial distal width of the teeth intended to occupy it. **2.** malocclusion characterized by inadequate arch circumference to accommodate the teeth in proper alignment.

crown, *n* **1.** the natural portion of a tooth covered by enamel. **2.** an artificial replacement for the natural crown of the tooth. Colloquial term is *cap.*

crown, anatomical, *n* the portion of dentin covered by enamel.

crown and bridge prosthodontics, *n* the division of prosthodontics that deals with crown restorations and the fixed type of tooth-borne partial denture prosthesis. See also prosthodontics, fixed.

crown, artificial, *n* a dental prosthesis restoring the anatomy, function, and esthetics of part or all of the coronal portion of the natural tooth.

crown, ceramic, *n* one of several materials that can make up a crown, which can be combined with other components such as porcelain or metal to improve long-term crown function.

crown, cervical aspect **(ser′vikəl),** *n* the clinical view of a crown from its most narrow angle of insertion into the gingival tissues.

crown, clinical, *n* **1.** the portion of enamel visibly present in the oral cavity. **2.** the portion of a tooth that is occlusal to the deepest part of the gingival sulcus.

crown, complete, *n* a restoration that reproduces the entire surface anatomy of the clinical crown and fits over a prepared tooth stump.

crown, crown veneer, *n* a restoration that reproduces the total clinical coronal surface contour of the tooth. Colloquial term is *veneers.*

crown, dowel, *n* a restoration that replaces the entire coronal portion of a tooth and derives its retention from a dowel extending into a treated (filled) root canal.

crown, extraalveolar clinical **(ek′strəalvē′ələr),** *n* the portion of a tooth that extends occlusally or incisally from the junction of the tooth root and the supporting bone.

crown, faced, *n* See crown, veneered metal.

crown, full, restoration, *n* an individual tooth prosthesis encompassing the entire prepared clinical crown. See also crown, complete veneer.

crown, gold, *n* a metal variety of crown using gold.

crown, jacket, *n* See crown, complete.

crown lengthening, *n* a surgical procedure to remove marginal gingival tissues to expose more of the crown of the tooth to facilitate a reconstructive or operative procedure.

crown, partial, *n* a restoration that covers three or more, but not all, surfaces of a tooth.

crown, porcelain-faced, *n* an artificial crown that makes use of porcelain inlayed in or veneered onto the labial or buccal surface.

crown, porcelain jacket, *n* a type of crown composed of porcelain mixed with metal, commonly used for its appearance and tooth-bonding properties.

crown, stainless steel, *n* a preformed steel crown used for the restoration of badly broken-down primary teeth and first permanent molars. Also used as a temporary restoration of fractured permanent incisors.

crown, temporary, *n* a short-term crown placed on a tooth while the final impression of the permanent crown is being cast.

crown, three-quarter, *n* a term frequently used to designate a partial veneer crown.

crown, veneered metal, *n* a complete crown that has one or more surfaces prepared for and covered by a tooth-colored substance such as porcelain or resin.

crown-implant ratio, *n* See ratio, crown-implant.

crown-root ratio, *n* the relation of the clinical crown to the clinical roots of the teeth—an important consideration in diagnosis, prognosis, and treatment planning.

crown-rump length, *n* the length of an embryo, fetus, or newborn as measured from the crown of the head to the prominence of the buttocks.

Crozat appliance, *n.pr* See appliance, Crozat.

CRT, *n* the abbreviation for cathode-ray tube.

crucible (kroo′sibəl), *n* a vessel or container that will withstand high heat and is used for melting or holding material.

crucible crushing strength, n See strength, compressive.

crucible former (sprue base), n the stand or base into which a sprued pattern is placed. It establishes the shape or form of the hollowed-out end of the investment in the casting ring, which will receive the molten metal on its course through the sprue hole. See also sprue former.

crust, *n* a hard-coating surface layer composed of coagulated tissue fluid and blood products mixed with epithelial and inflammatory cells covering a lesion formed by the rupture of a bulla, vesicle, or pustule.

(sodium aluminum fluoride [Na_3AlF_6]), cryolite (krī′ōlīt), *n* a fluoride often used as a flux in the manufacture of silicate cements.

cryosurgery (krī′ōsur′jərē), *n* the use of subfreezing temperature to destroy tissue. Cryosurgery is used to cause the edges of a detached retina to heal, to remove cataracts, and in the treatment of Parkinson's disease.

cryotherapy (krī′ōther′əpē), *n* a use of cryosurgery in the treatment of cutaneous tags, warts, actinic keratosis, and dermatofibromas. The agent is usually liquid nitrogen, applied briefly with a sterile cotton-tipped applicator.

cryptococcosis (krip′tōkäkō′sis), *n* a fungal infection from the organism *C. neoformans,* found primarily in pigeon feces. It often affects individuals with weakened or compromised immune systems.

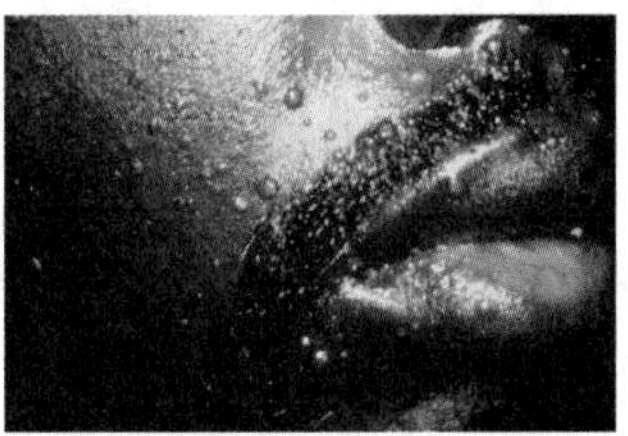

Cryptococcosis. (Neville/Damm/Allen/Bouquot, 2002, Courtesy Dr. Catherine Flaitz)

cryptogenic (krip′tōjen′ik), *n* a condition distinguished by an unknown cause.

crystal(s), *n* a naturally produced solid. The ultimate units of the substance from which it was formed are arranged systematically.

crystal, fluorapatite **(flŏŏrap′ətīt),** *n* the crystalline structure that occurs after hydroxyapatite changes into fluorapatite as a result of the tooth being exposed to fluoride.

crystal gold, n See gold, mat.

crystal, silver halide **(hal′īd),** *n* the silver compounds, usually silver bromide and silver iodide, that are impregnated in the photographic emulsion of film. These compounds, when acted on by actinic rays, are disintegrated, with the formation of metallic silver in a finely divided state. The photographic image results when the film is subjected to processing.

crystallization, *n* the production or formation of crystals, either by cooling a liquid or gas to a solid state or by cooling a solution until the solute precipitates as a crystalline deposit.

cubital (kū′bitəl), *adj* pertaining to the forearm.

cubitus (kū′bitus), *n* the forearm.

cuboid (kū′boid), *adj* (cuboidal), resembling a cube in form.

cuboidal, *adj* See cuboid.

cue, *n* a stimulus that determines or may prompt the nature of a person's response.

cultural characteristics, *n.pl* See culture 2.

cultural diversity, *n* a population consisting of two or more cultural groups.

culture, *n* **1.** the growth of microorganisms or other living cells on artificial media. **2.** a set of learned values, beliefs, customs, and behavior that is shared by a group of interacting individuals.

culture, bacterial, n the bacterial growth on or in an artificial medium. The medium used may be selective for a given type or genus of organism

C

C

(e.g., tomato juice agar for lactobacilli).

culture, endodontic, *n* the growth of microorganisms obtained from root canals or periapical tissues.

culture, endodontic medium, *n* a type used for endodontic cultures.

culture medium, *n* a type used for cultivating bacteria.

cumulative, *adj* increasing in effect.

cup, chin, *n* **1.** an orthopedic device that directs a posterior and/or vertical force to the mandible, through the attachment of a cup fitting over the chin to a headcap. **2.** a drug used to cause muscle relaxation during anesthesia by blocking acetylcholine at the neuromuscular and synaptic junctions.

cure, *n* **1.** the successful treatment of a disease or wound. **2.** a procedure or reaction that changes a plastic material to a hard material (e.g., vulcanization and polymerization). See also process.

curet, (curette) (kyŏŏret′), *n* a periodontal or hand instrument having a sharp, spoon-shaped working blade; used for debridement. It is available in many sizes and shapes; used for root planing and gingival curettage, both surgically and nonsurgically.

curet, area-specific, *n* any of a number of curets designed for use on specific tooth surfaces. It may feature an elongated shank or shortened blade.

curet, mini-bladed, *n* a small dental instrument employed in the surgical removal of unwanted materials, useful in getting at narrow or closed-off areas of the teeth and oral cavity.

curet, nonsurgical Gracey, *n* an instrument used for removal of subgingival deposits and root debridement.

curet, nonsurgical Langer, *n* an instrument that has combined features of the Gracey curet and universal curet.

curet, nonsurgical rigid, *n* an instrument made with a rigid shank that is stronger and aids in removal of tenacious deposits.

curet, nonsurgical universal, *n* an instrument designed to permit access to all surfaces of the tooth without the need to change instruments during deposit removal or root planing.

curet, universal, *n* an instrument used on subgingival sufaces. It has a blade with an unbroken cutting edge that curves around the toe and a flat face that is set at a 90° angle to the lower shank.

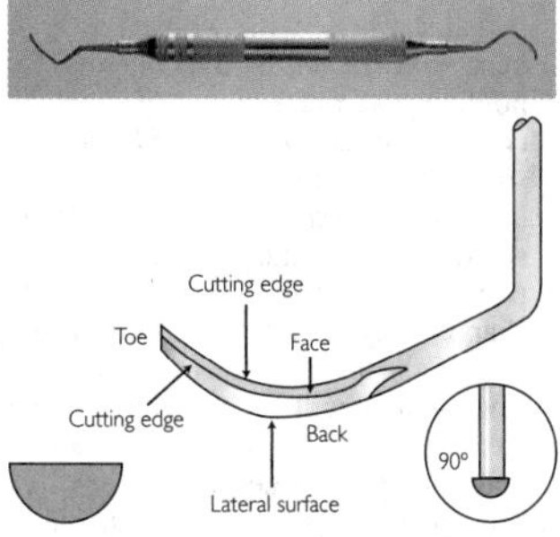

Universal curet. (Boyd, 2005)

curettage (kyŏŏ′rətäzh′), *n* the scraling with a curet.

curettage, angle for gingival, *n* an angle between 45° and 90° at which the curet should be held against the gingiva to clean out a pocket effectively. See also curettage, subgingival.

curettage, apical, *n* (apoxesis), the curettement of diseased periapical tissue without excision of the root tip. See also curettage, subgingival.

curettage, gingival, *n* See curettage, subgingival.

curettage, gingival, closed, *n* See curettage, subgingival.

***curettage, inadvertent* (kyŏŏ′rətazh′ in′ədver′tənt),** *n* the accidental removal of the gingival tissues with typical surgical instrument usage.

curettage, infrabony pocket, *n* the enucleation, by means of suitable instrumentation, of the inflammatory soft tissue elements lying within and surrounding the crest of an infrabony resorptive defect; also includes the debridement and planing of the root surface of the pocket.

curettage, root (root planing), *n* the debridement and planing to smoothness of the root surface of a tooth to eliminate deposits on the root.

curettage, subgingival, *n* the process of debridement of the epithelial attachment, the ulcerated and entire (pocket) epithelium, and subjacent inflamed and altered gingival tissues. The procedure is no longer recommended for the health of the periodontium.

curette, *n* See curet.

curie (kyŏŏ′rē), a measurement of radioactivity produced by the disintegration of unstable elements. The curie is that quantity of a radioactive nuclide in which the number of disintegrations per second is 3.700 times 10^{-10}. Because the curie is a relatively large unit, the millicurie (0.00 curie) and the microcurie (one-millionth of a curie) are more often used. The curie is based on the number of nuclear disintegrations and not on the number or amount of radiations emitted.

curing, *n* the act of polymerization.

curing, denture, *n* See denture curing.

curing light, *n* a blue light held by the dental professional to harden photopolymerized sealants of tooth-colored restorations, the process of which takes approximately 20 to 60 seconds; special protective glasses or shields must be used by the dental professional and patient to protect against retinal damage from the light.

current, *n* a measure of the number of electrons per second that pass a given point on a conductor.

current, alternating, *n* a current that alternately changes its direction of flow. It usually consists of 60 complete cycles/sec.

current, coagulating, *n* an electrical current, delivered by a needle, ball, or other variously shaped points, that coagulates tissue.

current dental terminology (CDT), *n* a listing of descriptive terms and identifying codes developed by the American Dental Association (ADA) for reporting dental services and procedures to dental benefits plans.

current, direct, *n* an electrical current in which the electron flow is in only one direction.

current, galvanic, *n* a direct current created by a battery.

current procedural terminology (CPT), *n* a listing of descriptive terms and identifying codes developed by the American Medical Association (AMA) for reporting practitioner services and procedures to medical plans and medicare.

current, saturation, *n* the maximum current in a roentgen-ray tube that fully uses all electrons that are available at the cathode for the production of roentgen rays.

curriculum, *n* a course of study; the linked series of academic courses leading to mastery of a discipline.

cursor, *n* the pointer on a PC monitor or other display that indicates where the next character will be entered.

curvature, occlusal, *n* See curve of occlusion.

curve, *n* a nonangular deviation from a straight line or surface.

curve, alignment, *n* See alignment.

curve, anti-Monson, *n.pr* See curve, reverse.

curve, compensating, *n* the curvature of alignment of the occlusal surfaces of the teeth that is developed to compensate for the paths of the condyles as the mandible moves from centric to eccentric positions. A means of maintaining posterior tooth contacts on the molar teeth and providing balancing contacts on dentures when the mandible is protruded. Corresponds to the curve of Spee of natural teeth.

curve, dose-effect, *n* a curve relating the dose of radiation with the effect produced.

curve, dose-response, *n* a graphical representation of the relationship between dosage (x-axis) and degree of response (y-axis); used to determine the effective dose of any given drug.

curve, milled-in, *n* See path, milled-in.

curve, Monson **(mon′sən),** *n.pr* the curve of occlusion, described by Monson, in which each cusp and incisal edge touch or conform to a segment of the surface of a sphere 8 inches (20 cm) in diameter, with its center in the region of the glabella. See also curve, compensating.

curve of occlusion (occlusal curvature), *n* **1.** a curved occlusal surface that makes simultaneous contact with the major portion of the incisal and occlusal prominences of the existing teeth. **2.** the curve of a dentition on which the occlusal surfaces of the teeth lie. See also curve, reverse.

curve of Spee, *n.pr* **1.** an anatomic curvature of the occlusal alignment of teeth, beginning at the tip of the mandibular canine, following the buccal cusps of the natural premolars and molars, and continuing to the anterior border of the ramus, as described by von Spee. **2.** the curve of the occlusal surfaces of the arches in vertical dimension, brought about by a dipping downward of the mandibular premolars, with a corresponding adjustment of the maxillary premolars.

curve of Wilson, *n.pr* the curvature of the cusps, as seen from the front view. The curve in the mandibular arch is concave, whereas the one in the maxillary arch is convex.

curve, reverse, *n* a curve of occlusion that is convex upward when viewed in the frontal plane.

curve, sine, *n* the wave form of an alternating current, characterized by a rise from zero to maximum positive potential, then descending below zero to its maximum negative value, and then rising to its maximum positive potential, to fall to zero again.

curve, survival, *n* a curve obtained by plotting the number or percentage of organisms surviving at a given time against a given dose of radiation. A curve showing the percentage of individuals surviving at different intervals after a particular dosage of radiation.

Cushing's syndrome, *n.pr* See syndrome, Cushing's.

cusp (kusp), *n* a notably pointed or rounded eminence on or near the masticating surface of a tooth.

cusp, angle, *n* See angle, cusp.

cusp-fossa relations **(kusp fos′ə),** *n.pl* the organic relations between a stamp cusp and its fossa.

cusp height, *n* the shortest distance between the deepest part of the central fossa of a posterior tooth and a line connecting the points of the cusps of the tooth.

cusp, shoeing, *n* See restoration of cusps.

cusp, talon, *n* an extra well-defined cusp that may be found on the lingual surfaces of the anterior teeth.

cusp tips, *n* the points on the occlusal surface of the molars, premolars, or canines that are used for tearing or chewing.

cuspal interference, *n* See contact, deflective occlusal.

cuspid (kus′pid), *n* See canine.

cuspidor (kus′pədor), *n* a fixture provided on some dental operating units into which patients can expectorate. In current practice, most operating fields are kept clear of saliva by high-volume suction saliva ejectors.

customary fee, *n* the fee level determined by the administrator of a dental benefits plan from actual submitted fees for a specific dental procedure to establish the maximum benefit payable under a given plan for that specific procedure. See also fee, usual and fee, reasonable.

cutaneous (kūtā′nēus), *adj* relating to the skin. Tests of cutaneous hypersensitivity may be indicators of malnutrition and are useful in determining a patient's readiness for surgery.

cuticle (kyōō′tikəl), *n* the outer layer of the skin. Also, a layer that covers the free surface of an epithelial cell.

cuticle, primary, *n* **1.** the transitory remnants of the enamel organ and oral epithelium covering the enamel of a tooth after eruption. *Synonym:* Nasmyth's membrane. **2.** is believed to be the last substance formed by ameloblasts, mediating the attachment of ameloblasts to the enamel.

cuticle, secondary, *n* **1.** the second cuticle formed when the ameloblasts are replaced by the oral epithelium. It then covers the primary cuticle on the enamel and is the only cuticle on the cementum. **2.** a keratinized pedicle found between the gingival epithelium and the surface of a tooth.

cuticula dentis (kūtik′ūlə den′tis), *n* See cuticle, primary.

cutting edge, *n* the edge of a periodontal instrument formed where the lateral side and face of the instrument meet.

cutting instrument, *n* See instrument, cutting.

CVA, *n* See accident, cerebrovascular.

cyanocobalamin (sī′ənō′kōbal′əmin), *n* (vitamin B_{12}), *brand names* (some): Alpha Redisol, Betalin-12, Cobex; *drug class:* Vitamin B_{12} water-soluble vitamin; *action:* needed for adequate nerve functioning, protein and carbohydrate metabolism, normal growth, red blood cell development, and cell reproduction; *uses:* vitamin B_{12} deficiency, pernicious anemia, hemolytic anemia, hemorrhage, and renal and hepatic diseases.

cyanosis (sī'ənō'sis), *n* a characteristic bluish tinge or color of the skin and mucous membranes associated with reduction in hemoglobin brought about by inadequate respiratory change (5 gm/100 ml are necessary for color to be perceptible).

cyclamate (sī'kləmāt'), *n* a noncaloric artificial sweetening agent used in conjunction with saccharin; presently banned by the FDA because of its carcinogenic potential.

cycle, chewing, *n* a complete course of movement of the mandible during a single masticatory stroke.

cycle, masticating, *n* the three-dimensional patterns of mandibular movements formed during the chewing of food.

cyclic AMP cycloheximide (sī'klōhek'səmīd'), *n* a cyclic nucleotide formed from adenosine triphosphate by the action of adrenyl cyclase. Known as the "second messenger," it participates in the action of catecholamines, vasopressin, adrenocorticotropic hormone, and many other hormones.

cyclic neutropenia (nōō'trəpē'nēə), *n* a hereditary disease primarily afflicting young children and infants; characterized by flulike symptoms (weakness, tenderness in the pharynx, aching head, and fever) as well as stomatitis, periodontitis, and gingivitis; cycles every 3 to 4 weeks with painful lesions and damage to the alveolar bone; should be medicated with antibiotics prior to any oral surgery.

cyclizine HCl/cyclizine lactate, trade (sīkləzēn lak'tāt), *n brand name:* Marezine; *drug class:* antiemetic, antihistaminic, anticholinergic; *action:* may act centrally on vomiting center, also antagonizes histamine peripherally; *uses:* motion sickness, prevention of postoperative vomiting.

cyclobenzaprine HCl (sīklōben'zəprēn'), *n brand name:* Cycoflex, Flexeril; *drug class:* skeletal muscle relaxant, centrally acting tricyclic; *action:* has actions similar to those of tricyclic antidepressants; *uses:* adjunct for relief of muscle spasm and pain in musculoskeletal conditions.

cyclophosphamide (sīklōfos'fəmīd'), *n brand names:* Cytoxan, Neosar, Procytox; *drug class:* antineoplastic alkylating agent; *action:* alkylates DNA, RNA; inhibits enzymes that allow synthesis of amino acids in proteins; *uses:* Hodgkin's disease; lymphomas; leukemia; cancer of female reproductive tract, lung, prostate; multiple myeloma; neuroblastoma; retinoblastoma; Ewing's sarcoma.

cycloserine (sī'klōserēn), *n brand name:* Seromycin Pulvules; *drug class:* antitubercular; *action:* inhibits cell wall synthesis, analog of D-alanine; *uses:* pulmonary tuberculosis.

cyclosporine (sī'klōspor'ēn), *n brand name:* Sandimmune; *drug class:* immunosuppressant; *action:* produces immunosuppression by inhibiting lymphocytes; *uses:* to prevent rejection of tissues and/or organ transplants.

cyclothymia (sī'klōthī'mēə), *n* See psychosis, manic-depressive.

cyclotron (sī'kləträn), *n* a device for accelerating charged particles to high energies by means of an alternating electrical field between electrodes placed in a constant magnetic field.

cylinder, glass, *n* one of several components forming the cartridge, a fundamental component of the anesthesiologist's kit; its cylindrical body contains the volume and content of the anesthesia.

cylindroma (sil'indrō'mə), *n* **1.** an obsolete term for an adenoid cystic carcinoma. See carcinoma, adenoid cystic. **2.** a benign adnexal neoplasm of skin that most often occurs on the scalp.

cyproheptadine HCl (sī'prōhep'tədēn'), *n brand name:* Periactin; *drug class:* antihistamine H_1 receptor antogonist; *action:* acts on blood vessels, gastrointestinal and respiratory systems by competing with histamine for H_1 receptor site; *uses:* allergy symptoms, rhinitis, pruritus, cold urticaria.

cyst (sist), *n* a pathologic space in bone or soft tissue containing fluid or semifluid material and, in the oral regions, almost always lined by epithelium.

cyst, aneurysmal bone **(an′yəriz′-məl),** *n* a nonmalignant osteolytic lesion expanding a long bone or within a vertebra in which the space, filled with blood, is networked with fibrous tissue containing multinucleated giant cells.

cyst, apical periodontal, *n* See cyst, periapical.

cyst, branchial, *n* (branchial cleft cyst), a soft-tissue cyst usually seen on the lateral side of the neck, arising from epithelial illusions within the cervical lymph nodes. Microscopic examination shows the epithelial lining of stratified squamous epithelium surrounded by lymphoid tissue.

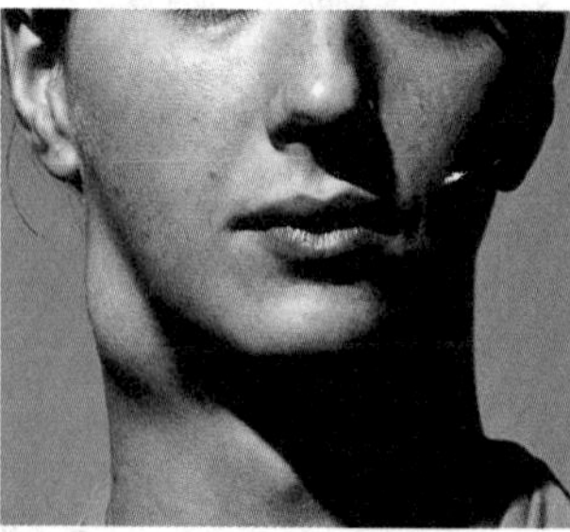

Branchial cyst. (Regezi/Sciubba/Pogrel, 2000)

cyst, calcifying odontogenic (Gorlin cyst), *n* a cyst arising from odontogenic epithelium, with abundant production of keratin-containing ghost cells and areas of dystrophic calcification. This lesion has a predilection for young adults.

cyst, dental, *n* See cyst, periodontal.

cyst, dental lamina **(lam′ənə),** *n* See cyst, eruption.

cyst, dentigerous **(dentij′ərəs),** *n* an epithelium-lined sac filled with fluid or semifluid material that surrounds the crown of an unerupted tooth or odontoma.

cyst, dentoalveolar, *n* See cyst, periodontal.

cyst, dermoid **(der′moid),** *n* an epithelium-lined sac with one or more skin appendages (hair follicles, sweat glands, sebaceous glands) in its wall. It may be found in the floor of the oral cavity. This lesion should not be confused with the teratomatous dermoid cyst of the ovary.

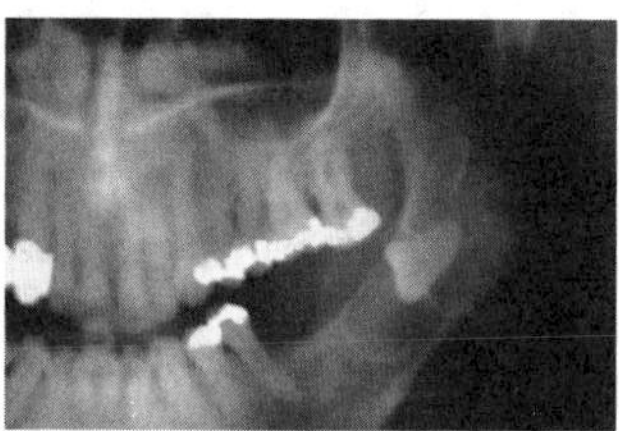

Dentigerous cyst. (Courtesy Dr. Charles Babbush)

cyst, developmental, *n* a pathologic fluid sac that may be caused by infection or disease. See also cyst, dentigerous and cyst, odontogenic.

cyst, epidermoid **(ep′əder′moid),** *n* a fluid-filled, epithelium-lined sac thought to arise from hair follicles of the skin.

cyst, eruption, *n* a dentigerous cyst that causes a clinically evident bulging of the overlying alveolar ridge.

cyst, extravasation, *n* See cyst, traumatic.

cyst, fissural, *n* a cyst that arises from the enslaved epithelium in maxillary suture lines caused by fusion of the embryonic processes of the facial bones.

cyst, follicular **(fəlik′yələr),** *n* See cyst, dentigerous.

cyst, gingival, of the adult, *n* a rare gingival cyst, usually painless, that originates on dental laminar rests. It is usually categorized as an extraosseous instance of a lateral periodontal cyst.

cyst, gingival, of the newborn, *n* a keratin-filled benign cyst on the alveolar mucosa that is common among newborn infants. Similar to palatal cysts of the newborn.

cyst, globulomaxillary **(globyəlō-mak′səler′ē),** *n* thought to have been a developmental fissural cyst arising in the area between the nasal process and maxillary process. It is now believed that all these lesions are actually other odontogenic cysts, such as odontogenic keratocysts or lateral periodontal cysts.

cyst, Gorlin, *n* See cyst, calcifying odontogenic (Gorlin cyst).

cyst, hemorrhagic **(hem′əraj′ik),** *n* an extravasation cyst or lesion; traumatic bone cyst or lesion. This is not a true cyst but is probably a defect in the bone produced by trauma and repair. It appears as a definite radiolucent area with a sharply marked radiopaque border. It contains air and is lined by a thin endosteum. See also cyst, solitary bone.

cyst, incisive canal, *n* See cyst, nasopalatine.

cyst, indefinite bone, *n* See cyst, traumatic.

cyst, lateral, *n* See cyst, periodontal.

cyst, lateral periodontal (botryoid odontogenic cyst), *n* a noninflammatory cyst found in the tooth-generating tissue on the lateral surface of the root of a tooth.

cyst, median palatal, *n* an epithelium-lined sac containing fluid; appears as a radiolucency in the midline of the palate. It is of developmental origin.

cyst, multilocular **(mul′tilok′yələr),** *n* a follicular cyst containing many loculi, or spaces, and not associated with a tooth.

cyst, nasoalveolar **(nā′zōalvē′ələr),** *n* a fluid-containing sac lined by epithelium and located at the ala of the nose. A developmental cyst, it may simulate a nasal or periapical abscess.

cyst, nasopalatine duct **(nā′zōpal′ətīn),** *n* a cyst arising within the nasopalatine canal. Radiographically it may appear as a heart-shaped radiolucency between the maxillary central incisors. Histologically it may show mucous cells and nerve bundles in addition to a lining of stratified squamous or respiratory epithelium. The incisive canal cyst and the cyst of the papilla incisiva are the recognized subtypes.

cyst, nonodontogenic, *n* a soft tissue abnormality that may develop in any number of locations within the oral cavity but is not directly associated with a tooth.

cyst, odontogenic, *n* an epithelium-lined sac produced from the tooth-forming tissues (e.g., primordial, dentigerous, and periodontal cysts).

cyst, palatal, of the newborn, *n* a common developmental cyst found on the hard palates of most infants. It is small, white, and filled with keratin. Called Epstein's pearls when found on the midline of the palate, and Bohn's nodules when found elsewhere on the palate, though both types are the same.

cyst, periapical, *n* a cyst that has a fibrous connective tissue wall and a lining of stratified squamous epithelium and that is attached to the apex of the root of a tooth with a nonvital pulp or a defective root canal filling.

cyst, periodontal (dental root cyst, dentoalveolar cyst, lateral cyst, periapical cyst), *n* an epithelium-lined sac containing fluid usually found at the apex of a pulp-involved tooth. Lateral types occur less frequently along the side of the root.

cyst, primordial **(prīmor′dēəl),** *n* an epithelium-lined sac containing fluid and appearing as a radiolucency in the jaws. It is derived from an enamel organ before any hard tissue is formed.

cyst, radicular (periapical cyst, root end cyst) **(rədik′yələr),** *n* See cyst, periapical.

cyst, residual, *n* an odontogenic cyst that remains within the jaw after the removal of the tooth with which it was associated. May be radicular or follicular.

cyst, root end, *n* See cyst, periapical.

cyst, simple bone, *n* a diseased bone cavity that forms around the roots of teeth, easily identifiable during radiologic exam. Of uncertain origin. Previously known as traumatic bone cyst and solitary bone cyst.

cyst, soft tissue, *n* a broad classification of oral abnormalities that may include blisterlike obstructions of salivary glands and growths in the thyroglossal tract, lymph nodes, and epithelial cells on the floor of the oral cavity.

cyst, soft tissue developmental, *n* a pathologic fluid sac that occurs in mucous membranes or other soft tissue of the body, as opposed to those occurring in bone or teeth. See also cyst, thyroglossal duct and cyst, lateral cervical.

cyst, solitary bone, *n* See cyst, simple bone.

cyst, thyroglossal duct **(thī′rō-glos′əl,** *n* an epithelium-lined sac containing fluid formed in portions of the incompletely involuted thyroglossal duct, which connects the primitive pharynx with the tongue in embryonic life. These cysts may appear in the midline at any region from the subhyoid to the base of the tongue.

cyst, traumatic bone, n See cyst, simple bone.

cystadenoma (sist′adənō′mə), *n* an adenoma with the development of cystic spaces caused by dilation of acinar or ductal structures.

cystadenoma, papillary, lymphomatosum (Warton's tumor), n a benign salivary gland tumor that consists of numerous cystic spaces lined by a double layer of epithelium. A dense aggregate of lymphocytes containing germinal centers surrounds the cystic spaces.

cysteine (sis′təēn′), *n* a nonessential amino acid found in many proteins in the body.

cystic fibrosis (sis′tik fībrō′sis), *n* an inherited disorder of the exocrine glands, causing those glands to produce abnormally thick secretions of mucus, elevation of sweat electrolytes, increased organic and enzymatic constituents of saliva, and overactivity of the autonomic nervous system.

cystinuria (sis′tinyŏŏ′rēə), *n* a hereditary defect caused by the dysfunctional reabsorption of the amino acid cystine into the kidneys; it results in regular, abnormally high levels of cystine in urine.

cystostomy (sistos′təmē), *n* creating a surgical opening into the urinary bladder or gallbladder.

cytochrome (sī′təkrōm′), *n* one of a class of hemoproteins that act as electron transport. Cytochromes are classified as *a, b, c,* and *d.*

cytokine (sī′təkīn′), *n* a nonantibody protein, such as lymphokine. Cytokines are released by a cell population on contact with a specific antigen. Cytokines act as intercellular mediators in the generation of immune response.

cytologic smear (sī′təloj′ik), *n* the product of a diagnostic technique where cells are scraped off the surface of a lesion found in the oral cavity. The gleaned cells are then examined under a microscope for indications of a variety of diseases. Considered a preliminary diagnostic test, it is not used to detect more serious conditions that require deeper tissue samples.

cytology (sītol′əjē), *n* the study of the anatomy, physiology, pathology, and chemistry of a cell.

cytology, exfoliative, n the study of desquamated cells.

cytomegalic inclusion disease, *n* See disease, salivary gland.

Cytomegalovirus (CMV), *n* a visceral disease virus, a member of the group of herpesviruses having special affinity for the salivary glands. Considered one of the indicator infections of AIDS.

cytoskeleton, *n* the intracellular filaments that serve to support or stiffen cells.

cytosol, *n* the totality of the intracellular substance exclusive of mitochondria and endoplasmic reticulum components.

cytotoxicity (sī′tōtoksis′itē), *n* a description of the extent of the destructive or killing capacity of an agent. Most often used to describe the character of immune activity or toxicity of certain drugs that limit the development of cancer cells.

cytozyme (sī′tōzīm), *n* See thromboplastin.

D

d-lysergic acid diethylamide (LSD) (lisur′jik as′id dīeth′əlam′id), *n* a hallucinogenic street drug taken to induce a perceived state of euphoria, freedom, and control.

daily food requirements, *n* actively teaching patients proper nutrition, personal diet analysis, reasonable portion sizes, and how to choose foods from the Food Guide Pyramid to enjoy overall good health.

Dalton's law, *n* See law, Dalton's.

dam, a barrier to the passage of moisture or saliva.

dam, post-, n See seal, posterior palatal.

dam, rubber, *n* a thin sheet of latex rubber used to isolate a tooth or teeth and keep them dry during a dental procedure.

dam, rubber, punch, *n* a hand-punch instrument with progressively larger openings, used to make a hole(s) in the rubber dam.

damages, *n.pl* compensation or indemnity that may be recovered in the courts by any person who has suffered loss, detriment, or injury to person, property, or rights through the unlawful act or negligence of another.

damages, compensatory, *n.pl* a sum that compensates the injured party for injury only.

damages, exemplary (punitive damages) **(igzem′plərē),** *n.pl* damages awarded to the plaintiff over those that will barely compensate for property loss. Such compensation may be awarded when the wrong done to the plaintiff involves violence, malice, or fraud by the defendant. The object is to provide compensation for mental suffering or loss of pride. It may be employed as punishment of the defendant.

damages, nominal, *n.pl* a small sum awarded to a plaintiff in an action in which there is no substantial loss or injury to be compensated but in which the law still recognizes a technical invasion of rights or a breach of the defendant's duty. Also awarded in cases in which, although there has been a real injury, the plaintiff's evidence is not sufficient to show its amount.

damages, punitive, *n.pl* See damages, exemplary.

danazol (dan′əzol′), *n brand name:* Danocrine; *drug class:* androgen, α-ethinyl testosterone derivative; *action:* decreases FSH and LH output; *uses:* endometriosis, prevention of hereditary angioedema, fibrocystic breast disease.

dantrolene sodium (dantrōlēn), *n brand name:* Dantrium; *drug class:* skeletal muscle relaxant, direct acting; *action:* interferes with intracellular release of calcium necessary to initiate contraction; *uses:* spasticity in multiple sclerosis, stroke, spinal cord injury, cerebral palsy, malignant hyperthermia.

dapsone (DDS) (dap′sōn), *n brand name:* Avlosulfon; *drug class:* leprostatic, antibacterial; *action:* bactericidal and bacteriostatic against *M. leprae;* may also be immunosuppressant; *uses:* leprosy and dermatitis herpetiformis.

Darier's disease, *n.pr* See disease, Darier's.

darkroom, *n* a completely lightproof room or cubicle that is used in the processing of photographic, medical, and dental films. See also safe light.

darkroom, features of, *n* a darkroom for developing radiographic films, should be absolutely devoid of white light, as well as chemicals or dust that could damage the film while it is being processed; a filtered safe light of less than 15 watts should be the only light in the room.

Darvon, *n.pr* the brand name for propoxyphene hydrochloride, a mild, centrally acting narcotic analgesic agent.

data, *n.pl* facts and figures; data are processed and interpreted to yield information.

data aggregation **(ag′grəgā′shən),** *n* a collection of protected health information used to conduct data analysis relating to the health care operations of the entity.

database, *n* an organized collection of data. A medical database is all the information that exists in the practice at any time.

data processing, *n* the collection of data, processing of the data to obtain usable information, and communication of this usable information.

data set, *n* a hardware device that converts digital pulses (square waveform) into modulated frequencies (sinusoidal wave) for transmission, a process called modulation. It also converts modulated frequencies into voltage pulses, a process called demodulation. Also called *modem.*

daughter (decay product), *n* **1.** a nuclide formed from the radioactive decay of another nuclide called the parent. **2.** after meiosis, one parent cell produces four daughter cells. These cells have half the number of chromosomes found in the original parent cell and, with crossing over, are genetically different.

day sheet, *n* a form that permits

systematic record keeping of treatment of patients and of monies received and spent.

Day's syndrome, *n.pr* See syndrome, Riley-Day.

daylight loader method, *n* method for developing radiographic films without a darkroom, using a flexible apparatus that allows you to insert your hands into a dark space without admitting any light. Insert the exposed radiographic film in the daylight loader compartment and remove the protective packets. With ungloved hands, process the film, touching only the edges.

D

DDC, *n* the abbreviation for dideoxycytidine. See dideoxycytidine.

DDI, *n* the abbreviation for dideoxyinosine. See dideoxyinosine.

dead space, *n* See space, physiologic dead space, and anatomic dead space.

deaf, *adj* without usable hearing.

deafen, *v* to make deaf; to cause the loss of all usable hearing.

deafness (def′nes), *n* a condition characterized by a partial or complete loss of hearing.

deafness, central, n impaired hearing caused by interference with cerebral auditory pathways or in the auditory centers in the brain (e.g., cerebrovascular accidents and other degenerative brain diseases). Hearing aids are of little benefit.

deafness, conduction **(kənduk′shən),** *n* See deafness, transmission.

deafness, nerve, n impaired hearing caused by pathologic conditions in the auditory nerve or the hair cells of the organ of Corti in the inner ear (e.g., high-tone deafness, which comes with age; damage to the organ of Corti by noise; or a tumor of an auditory nerve). Hearing aids are usually of little benefit.

deafness, transmission (conduction deafness), n impaired hearing caused by interference with passage of sound waves through the external ear (e.g., interference caused by wax) or middle ear (e.g., interference caused by otitis media, aerotitis media, or otosclerosis). May be characterized by greater interference with hearing of low tones. Hearing aids that amplify may be helpful.

deaminated (dēam′inātəd), *adj* pertaining to α-amino acids that have undergone the chemical alteration that removes ammonia (NH_3) from glutamate.

deamination (dēam′inā′shun), *n* a chemical alteration of α-amino acids that removes ammonia (NH_3) from glutamate.

deanesthesiant (dē′anəsthē′zē-ənt), *n* anything that will arouse a patient from a state of anesthesia.

death (deth), *n* **1.** the cessation of life; the stoppage of life beyond the possibility of resuscitation. *n* **2.** the cause or occasion of loss of life. *n* **3.** the total absence of activity in the brain and central nervous system, the cardiovascular system, and the respiratory system as observed and declared by a physician or other legally authorized agent.

death, brain, n in addition to the generally accepted definition of death, some states, either by statute or court decision, have added a "brain death" definition to the law, applicable when there has been an irreversible cessation of brain function.

death certificate, n the signed affidavit that life has ceased, giving the time, place, and cause of death. It is required by law to be filed in the proper local or regional geopolitical office.

debility (debil′itē), *n* weakness; lack of strength; asthenia.

debonding, *n* a procedure by which brackets and bonding resin are removed and the surface of the tooth is restored to its previous condition.

debridement (dabrēd′mənt), *n* the removal of foreign material and/or devitalized tissue from the vicinity of a wound.

debridement, epithelial (deepithelization), n See curettage, subgingival.

debridement, nonsurgical periodontal, n the removal of deposits on the tooth surface. See also scaling.

debris (debrē′), *n* foreign material or particles loosely attached to a surface. In dentistry, food deposits (Materia alba) or cellular matter on a surface, such as a tooth or its roots.

debt, *n* a sum of money due by agreement; the contract may or may not be express and does not necessarily set the precise amount to be paid.

debug, *v* to locate and correct any errors (bugs) in a computer program.

decalcification (dēkal′sifikā′shən), *n* an older term for the loss or removal of calcium salts from calcified tissues. Newer term is *demineralization.*

decarboxylation (dē′karbok′səlā′shən), *n* a chemical reaction involving the removal of a molecule of carbon dioxide from carboxylic acid.

decay, *v* to decompose.

decay, dental, n See caries.

decay product, n See daughter.

decay, radioactive, n the disintegration of the nucleus of an unstable nuclide by the spontaneous emission of charged particles and/or photons.

decay, senile, n See caries, senile dental.

decayed teeth, indices and scoring methods for, *n.pl* See index, DEF and index, DMF.

deceleration (dēsel′ərā′shən), *n* a decrease in the speed or velocity of an object or reaction.

decibel (des′ibel), *n* a logarithmic ratio unit that indicates by what proportion one intensity level differs from another.

deciduous (dēsid′ūəs), *adj* that which will be shed (exfoliated). Older term pertaining specifically to the first dentition. Preferred term is *primary.*

deciduous dentition, n See dentition, primary.

deciduous teeth, n See teeth, primary.

decision-making, *n* the process of coming to a conclusion or making a judgment.

decision-making, evidence-based, n a type of informal decision-making that combines clinical expertise, patient concerns, and evidence gathered from scientific literature to arrive at a diagnosis and treatment recommendations. See also evidence-based care.

decision-making, statistical, n a type of formal decision-making that proceeds from a hypothesis to a conclusion by incorporating such techniques as statistical inference and significance, probability analysis, literature review, sampling, and discussion.

decision tree, *n* an algorithm or a formal stepwise process used in coming to a conclusion or making a judgment.

declaration and provision for affairs, *n* a systematic statement of the affairs and estate of a person, in which all assets and property are listed.

D

decompensate, *n* the development or worsening of a mental disorder.

decompression, *n* **1.** a technique used to readapt an individual to normal atmospheric pressure after exposure to higher pressures, as in diving. *n* **2.** the removal of pressure caused by gas or fluid in a body cavity such as the stomach or intestinal tract.

decompression, nerve, n the release of pressure on a nerve trunk by surgical widening of the bony canal.

decontamination, *n* the process of making a person, object, or environment free of microorganisms, radioactivity, or other contaminants.

deductible (diduk′təbəl), *n* **1.** a stipulated sum the covered person must pay toward the cost of dental treatment before the benefits of the program go into effect. The deductible may be annual or payable only once and may vary in amount from program to program. *n* **2.** the amount of dental expense for which the beneficiary is responsible before a third party will assume any liability for payment of benefits. Deductible may be an annual or one-time charge and may vary in amount from program to program. See also family deductible.

deductible amount, n the portion of dental care expense the insured must pay before the plan's benefits begin.

deductible clause, n a provision in an insurance contract stipulating that the insurer will pay only that amount that is in excess of a specified amount.

deductive reasoning, *n* the ability to distill the pertinent facts and details of a situation from a wider body of evidence and generalizations.

deep bite, *n* See overbite.

deep sensibility, See sensibility, deep.

D

deepithelization (dēep'ithē'lizā'shən), *n* See debridement, epithelial.

DEF rate, See rate, DEF.

defamation (def'əmā'shən), *n* the act of detracting from the reputation of another. The offense of injuring a person's reputation by false and malicious statements.

default, *n* **1.** an omission of that which should be done. *v* **2.** to fail to fulfill an obligation or a promise.

defecation, *n* the elimination of feces from the digestive tract through the rectum.

defect, *n* **1.** the absence of some legal requisite. **2.** an imperfection.

defect, atrial septal, n a congenital defect in the heart that is often present from birth. It is sometimes referred to as a "hole" in the heart and is caused by the unsuccessful closure of the septum between the atria of the heart. The failure of the septum to close properly leaves a hole between the right and left atria.

defect, operative, n the incomplete repair of bone after root resection or periapical curettage.

defect, osseous, n a concavity in the bone surrounding one or more teeth, resulting from periodontal disease.

defect, speech, n deviation of speech that is outside the range of acceptable variation in a given environment.

defective, mentally, *adj* a mentally subnormal individual. A person in whom a basic nervous system defect may be assumed because of social and intellectual deficiencies (e.g., persons afflicted with microcephaly, hydrocephalus, or mongolism).

defendant, *n* the party against whom relief or recovery is sought in a lawsuit.

defense, *n* the reasons, in law or fact, offered by the defendant in a legal proceeding as to why the plaintiff should not prevail.

defense cell, n See cell, defense.

defense mechanism, n an unconscious, intrapsychic reaction that offers protection to the self from threatening or stressful situations. Defense mechanisms may be useful to diminish anxiety and facilitate coping behaviors, or may be harmful because of denying, displacing, isolating, or repressing anxiety and preventing useful coping responses.

defibrillation (dēfib'rilāshən), *n* the arrest of fibrillation, usually that of the cardiac ventricles. An intense alternating current is briefly passed through the heart muscle, throwing it into a refractory state.

defibrillator (dēfib'rilā'tur), *n* a device for defibrillating the ventricles of the heart.

defibrillator, automatic external (AED), n a mobile electric device attached to the abdomen or chest that terminates erratic heartbeat by shock, thereby restoring the normal cardiac rhythm.

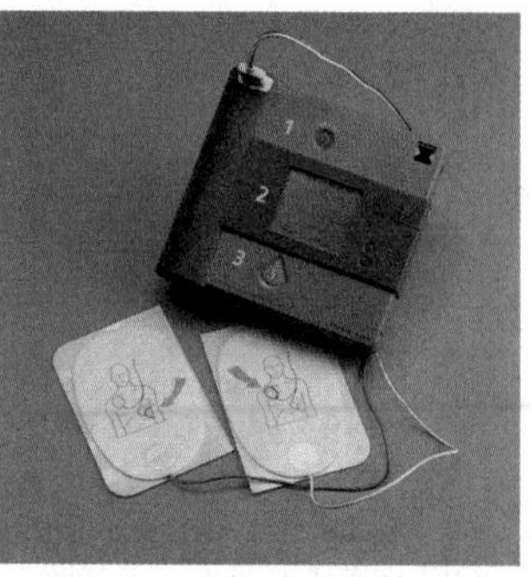

Automatic external defibrillator.
(Sanders, 2007)

deficiency, *n* a lack or defect.

deficiency, ac-globulin, n See parahemophilia.

deficiency, dietary, n an inadequate amount of food intake or an insufficiency of any of the food elements necessary for proper nutrition.

deficiency, mineral, n a form of nutritional deficiency produced by the inadequate ingestion, absorption, use, and/or overexcretion of essential inorganic elements such as calcium, magnesium, and phosphorus.

deficiency, nicotinic acid **(nik'ətin'ik),** *n* a deficiency of nicotinic acid in the diet, resulting in acute erythematous stomatitis, papillary atrophy of the tongue, and ulcerative gingivitis.

deficiency, nutritional, n See deficiency, dietary.

deficiency, plasma thromboplastic

antecedent **(throm'bōplas'tik),** *n* See hemophilia C.

deficiency, protein, *n* a malnutritive state produced by inadequate ingestion, absorption, use, or overexcretion of essential protein elements. Degenerative lesions produced in the periodontium include osteoporosis of the alveolar and supporting bone and disappearance of fibroblasts and connective tissue fibers of the periodontal membrane.

deficiency, PTA, *n* See hemophilia C.

deficiency, salivary **(sal'əvar'ē),** *n* an insufficiency in the amount of saliva produced by the salivary glands. The lack of saliva production can result in dry mouth (xerostomia), caries, and infection of the oral cavity.

deficiency, vitamin A, gingival hyperplasia in, *n* the hyperplastic and hyperkeratotic gingival changes occurring with decreased ingestion, diminished absorption, faulty use, or overexcretion of vitamin A. E.g., in diabetes mellitus, the liver often cannot effectively convert carotene to vitamin A.

definition (image), *n* the property of projected images relating to their sharpness, distinctness, or clarity of outline. Penumbra width is a measure of definition. See also resolution.

definitive care, *n* the completion of recommended treatment.

deflective occlusal contact, *n* See contact, deflective occlusal.

deformation (dē'fôrmā'shən), *n* a distortion; a disfigurement.

deformation, elastic, *n* the change in shape of an object under an applied load from which the object can recover or return to its original unloaded state when the load is removed.

deformation, inelastic, *n* a deformation occurring when a material is stressed beyond its elastic limit.

deformation, permanent, *n* a deformation occurring beyond the yield point so that the structure will not return to its original dimensions after removal of the applied force.

deformity, *n* a distortion or disfigurement of a portion of the body; may be congenital, familial, hereditary, acquired, pathologic, or surgical.

deformity, gingival, *n* a deviation from the normal gingival topographic and architectural pattern.

degassing (dēgas'ing), *adj* related to degasification, the process by which dissolved gas is removed from water or other liquid solutions.

degeneration, ballooning, *n* a condition seen in vesicles of viral origin in which epithelial cells are washed from the vesicle wall. The cells swell and their nuclei undergo amitotic division, resulting in multinucleated giant cells that may be seen floating in vesicular fluid.

degeneration, basophilic granular, See basophilia.

degenerative joint disease, *n* See osteoarthritis.

degloving (dēgluv'ing), *n* an intraoral surgical exposure of the bony mandibular anterior region. This procedure can be performed in the posterior region if necessary.

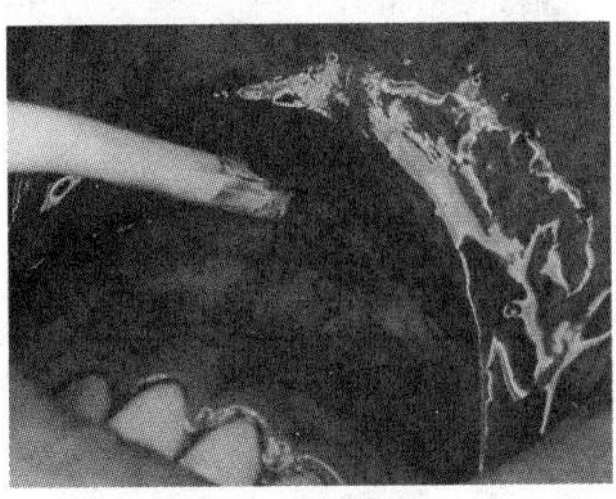

Degloving injury. (Zitelli/Davis, 2002)

deglutition (dē'glootish'ən), *n* (swallowing), a succession of muscular contractions from above downward or from the front backward; propels food from the oral cavity toward the stomach. The action is generally initiated at the lips; it proceeds back through the oral cavity, and the food is moved automatically along the dorsum of the tongue. When the food is ready for swallowing, it is passed back through the fauces. Once the food is beyond the fauces and in the pharynx, the soft palate closes off the nasopharynx, and the hyoid bone and larynx are elevated upward and forward. This action keeps food out of the larynx and dilates the esophageal opening so that the food may be passed quickly toward the stomach by peristaltic contractions. The separation between the voluntary and involuntary characteristics of this wave of contractions is not sharply defined. At birth the process is already well established as a highly coordinated activity, i.e., the swallowing reflex.

degradation (deg′rədā′shən), *n* the reduction of a chemical compound to a less complex compound.

degrees of freedom (df), *n.pl* a statistic, based on the number of observations and groups in a study, that is necessary to determine statistical significance. One looks up the degrees of freedom and the significance level in a table of significance values to determine if the magnitude of the value obtained is significant. Used with the t-test, chi square, analysis of variance, and correlation.

dehiscence (dēhis′əns), *n* a fissural defect in the facial alveolar plate extending from the gingival margin apically.

dehiscent mandibular canal, *n* a condition caused by bone resorption that leaves the mandibular canal without a covering or roof of bone.

dehydration (dē′hīdrā′shən), *n* **1.** the removal of water (e.g., from the body or tissue). *n* **2.** a decrease in serum fluid coupled with the loss of interstitial fluid from the body. It is associated with disturbances in fluid and electrolyte balance.

dehydration of gingivae, *n* the drying of gingival tissue, leading to a lowered tissue resistance, which can result in gingival inflammation; seen in mouth breathing. See also breathing, mouth and oral cavity.

dehydrogenase (dē′hīdroj′ənās′), *n* an oxidoreductase class (EC 1) enzyme that induces the transportation of electrons or hydrogen from a donor, which usually indicates the dehydrogenase, to an acceptor compound.

delayed expansion, *n* See expansion, delayed.

delict (dilikt′), *n* a wrong or an injury; an offense; a violation of public or private obligation.

delinquent (deling′kwent), *n* pertaining to a debt or claim that is due and unpaid at the time due.

delirium (delir′ēəm), *n* a condition of mental excitement, confusion, and clouded sensorium, usually accompanied by hallucinations, illusions, and delusions; precipitated by toxic factors in diseases or drugs.

delirium tremens (DT), *n* See alcohol withdrawal delirium.

Delta Dental Plan, *n.pr* an active member organization of the Delta Dental Plans Association (a not-for-profit organization), formed and guided by state dental societies to provide prepaid dental care to the public on a group basis.

delusion, *n* a persistent, aberrant belief or perception held inviolable by a person despite evidence to the contrary.

demand, *n* in economics, refers to the buying of services or goods; in dental care, generally denotes the active request for and purchase of dental care services.

demeclocycline HCl (dem′əklōsī′klēn), *n brand name:* Declomycin; *drug class:* tetracycline; *action:* inhibits protein synthesis, phosphorylation in microorganisms; *uses:* uncommon gram-positive or gram-negative bacteria or both, protozoa.

dementia (dimen′shə), *n* a progressive, organic mental disorder characterized by chronic personality disintegration, confusion, disorientation, stupor, deterioration of intellectual capacity and function, and impairment or control of memory, judgment, and impulses (e.g., senile psychosis, also associated with AIDS).

Demerol (dem′ərôl), *n.pr* the brand name for meperidine hydrochloride.

demilune, serous (dem′ēloon sēr′əs), *n* a half-moon-shaped body of serous cells located on the surface of some mucoserous acini in salivary glands.

demineralization, *n* a measurable decrease in the level of inorganic salts or minerals such as bone or enamel. Older term is *decalcification.*

demography (dimog′rəfē), *n* the study of populations, particularly the size, distribution, and characteristics of members of population groups. Demographic techniques are employed in the long-term continuing study of the residents of Framingham, Massachusetts, by the National Institutes of Health.

demurrer (dēmur′ər), *n* an admission of the facts charged by the opponent while maintaining that those facts are legally insufficient to establish liability.

demyelinate (dēmī′əlināt), *n* the process of removing or damaging the myelin sheath surrounding a nerve.

denasality (dēnəzal′itē), *n* the quality of the voice when the nasal passages are obstructed, preventing adequate nasal resonance during speech.

dendrite (den′drīt), *n* **1.** the fingerlike projections formed during the solidification of crystalline materials. *n* **2.** a branched, treelike protoplasmic process of a neuron that carries nerve impulses toward the cell body. See also axon.

denervation (de′nurvā′shən), *n* the sectioning or removal of a nerve to interrupt the nerve supply to a part.

dens evaginatus (denz ivaj′ənātəs), *n* See dens in dente.

dens in dente (denz in den′tā), *n* (older terms: *dens invaginatus, gestant odontoma),* an anomaly of the tooth found mainly in maxillary lateral incisors; characterized by invagination of the enamel, giving a radiographic appearance that suggests a "tooth within a tooth."

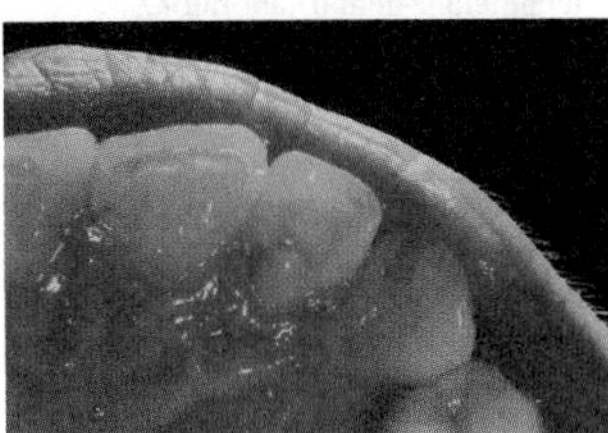

Dens in dente. (Bird/Robinson, 2005)

dens invaginatus (denz invajinä′təs), *n* See dens in dente.

Densite (den′sīt), *n.pr* the brand name for a form of α-hemihydrate with a low setting expansion and greater hardness; used for dies, models, and casts; sometimes referred to as a Class II stone.

densitometer (den′sitom′ətur), *n* an instrument for determining the degree of darkening of developed photographic or radiographic film, based on the use of a photoelectric cell to measure the light transmission through a given area of the film.

density, *n* the concentration of matter, measured by mass per unit volume.

density, radiographic, *n* the degree of darkening of exposed and processed photographic or radiographic film, expressed as the logarithm of the opacity of a given area of the film.

D

dental, *adj* relating to the teeth.

dental abutment, *n* See abutment.

dental alloy, *n* See alloy.

dental amalgam, *n* See amalgam.

dental ankylosis **(ang′kəlō′sis),** *n* See tooth, ankylosed.

dental anxiety, *n* See anxiety.

dental arch, *n* See arch, dental.

dental articulator, *n* See articulator.

dental assistant, *n* See assistant, dental.

dental auxiliary, *n* See auxiliary personnel.

dental benefits organization, *n* an organization offering a dental benefits plan. Also known as dental plan organization.

dental benefits plan, *n* the plan entitles covered individuals to specified dental services in return for a fixed, periodic payment made in advance of treatment. Such plans often include the use of deductibles, coinsurance, or maximums to control the cost of the program to the purchaser.

dental benefits program, *n* the specific dental benefits plan being offered to enrollees by the sponsor.

dental biofilm, *n* See biofilm, dental.

dental bonding, *n* See bonding.

dental calculus, *n* See calculus.

dental care, *n* the treatment of the teeth and their supporting structures.

dental care for children, *n* See pedodontics.

dental caries, *n* See caries.

dental caries susceptible, *n* See susceptible.

dental cavity lining, *n* See cavity lining.

dental cement, *n* See cement, dental.

dental cementum, *n* See cementum.

dental chart, *n* See chart, dental.

dental clinic, *n* See clinic.

dental cooperative, *n* a dental facility organized to provide dental services for the benefit of subscribers and not for profit. There is no discrimination as to who may subscribe, and each subscriber has equal rights and voice in the control of the cooperative. The operation of the cooperative usually rests with a lay board of directors elected by subscribers.

D

dental deposit, *n* See calculus.

dental dysfunction, *n* See dysfunction, dental.

dental enamel, *n* See enamel.

dental enamel, hypoplastic, *n* See hypoplasia.

dental engine, *n* See engine, dental.

dental equipment, *n* See equipment.

dental fissure, *n* See fissure.

dental fistula, *n* See fistula.

dental floss, *n* a waxed or plain thread of nylon or silk used to clean the interdental areas; an aid in oral physiotherapy. Shredproof Teflon expanded polytetrafluoroethylene (ePTFE), ultra-high-molecular-weight polyethylene (UHMWPE), or nylon flosses are still believed to be the best materials for removing plaque from the teeth.

dental fluorosis, *n* See fluorosis, dental.

dental geriatrics, *n* See geriatrics.

dental granuloma, *n* See granuloma, dental.

dental handpiece, *n* See handpiece.

dental health services, *n* the sum of the diagnostic, preventive, consultative, supportive, and therapeutic dental care offered by the dental profession or that portion provided a member of a dental health plan.

dental health surveys, *n* the use of questionnaires and oral examinations of a target population to determine the need or demand for dental care or the opinions or attitudes of patients or consumers.

dental history, *n* See history.

dental hygiene armamentarium, *n* See armamentarium.

dental hygiene diagnostic model, *n* one of four approaches to patient care. Its purpose is to arrive at a plan for recommended treatment by the systematic use of six steps that cover the major aspects of care, from initial inquiry to problem solving to patient education.

dental hygiene instrumentarium, *n* See instrumentarium.

dental hygiene process model, *n* one of four approaches to patient care, characterized by the documentation of a patient's expressed needs as they relate to a range of possible causes. Patient is questioned about various areas of concern, including overall health care.

dental hygienist, *n* See hygienist, dental.

dental identification, *n* the process of establishing the unique characteristics of teeth and dental work of an individual, leading to the identification of an individual by comparison with the person's dental charts and records. Used in forensic dentistry.

dental implant, *n* See implant.

dental impression material, *n* See impression.

dental instrument, *n* See instruments.

dental insurance, *n* a policy that insures against the expense of treatment and care of dental disease and accident to teeth.

***dental jurisprudence* (jur′isprū′dəns),** *n* the application of the principles of law as they relate to the practice of dentistry. See also jurisprudence, dental.

dental laboratory technician, *n* See technician, dental laboratory.

dental lamina, *n* See lamina, dental.

dental material, *n* See material, dental.

dental model, *n* See model.

dental neglect, *n* the purposeful denial of the minimum amount of oral health care or maintenance required to sustain functioning periodontium and teeth. The caretaker may exhibit a disregard for the patient's health and may focus primarily on pain relief for the patient. It is considered a warning sign of possible child or elder abuse.

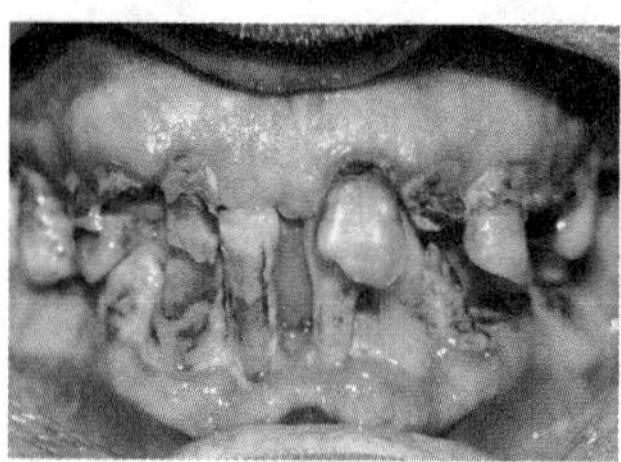

Dental neglect. (Christensen, 2002)

dental occlusion, *n* See occlusion.

dental papilla, *n* See papilla.

dental pathology, *n* that branch of dentistry that deals with all aspects of dental disease. See also pathology.

dental perioscopy **(per′ēos′kəpē),** *n* See endoscopy, periodontal.

dental pin, *n* See pin.

dental plan, *n* an organized method for the financing of dental care.

dental plaque, *n* See plaque.

dental porcelain, *n* See porcelain, dental.

dental prepayment, *n* a system for budgeting the cost of dental services in advance of their receipt.

dental prophylaxis, *n* See prophylaxis.

dental prosthesis, *n* See prosthesis.

dental prosthetic restoration, *n* See prosthesis, dental.

dental public health, *n* may also be called *public health dentistry.* The science and art of preventing and controlling dental diseases and promoting dental health through organized community efforts. It is that form of dental practice that serves the community as a patient rather than the individual. It is concerned with the dental health education of the public, with applied dental research, and with the administration of group dental care programs as well as prevention and control of dental diseases on a community basis. See community dentistry.

dental pulp, *n* See pulp.

dental pulp capping, *n* See capping, pulp.

dental pulp cavity, *n* See cavity, pulp.

dental pulp exposure, *n* See exposure.

dental record, *n* a confidential document containing the clinical and financial data of the dental patient, including the patient's identity, pertinent history, medical and dental conditions, services rendered, and charges and payments made.

dental research, *n* the formal scientific study of issues related to dentistry.

dental review committee, *n* a group of dental professionals and administrative personnel that reviews questionable dental claims and can suggest policy decisions regarding dental care.

dental sac, *n* a portion of the tooth germ consisting of ectomesenchyme surrounding the outside of the enamel organ, which produces the periodontium of a tooth. Older term is *dental follicle.*

dental scaling, *n* See scaling.

dental sealant, *n* See sealant.

dental senescence, *n* See senescence, dental.

dental service corporation, *n* a legally constituted, not-for-profit organization that negotiates and administers contracts for dental care. Delta Dental and Blue Cross/Blue Shield corporations are two such organizations.

dental service, hospital, *n* **1.** the location of the dental facility within a hospital. *n* **2.** the array of dental procedures offered within a hospital setting.

dental splint, *n* See splint, dental.

dental staff, *n* the personnel employed or engaged by the dental professional to conduct the assignable professional and management functions of the dental clinic, office, or practice.

dental stone, *n* See stone, dental.

dental tape, *n* See tape, dental.

dental technician, *n* See technician.

dental unit, *n* See unit, dental.

dentate (den′tāt), *adj* having teeth.

denticle (den′tikəl), *n* (endolith, pulp nodule, pulpstone), a calcified body found in the pulp chamber of a tooth; it may be composed either of irregular dentin (true denticle) or an ectopic calcification of pulp tissue (false denticle).

dentifrice (toothpaste) (den′təfris′), *n* a pharmaceutical compound used in conjunction with the toothbrush to clean and polish the teeth. Contains a mild abrasive, a detergent, a flavoring agent, a binder, and occasionally deodorants and various medicaments designed as caries preventives (e.g., antiseptics).

dentifrice abrasion, *n* See abrasion, dentifrice.

dentifrice, anticalculus **(an′tēkal′kyələs),** *n* a commercially available toothpaste, gel, or powder formulated to inhibit the development of new calculus and which contains, among other ingredients, either pyrophosphate or zinc. It has no effect on existing calculus.

dentifrice, calculus-control, n See dentifrice, anticalculus.

dentifrice, cosmetic, n a dentifrice, or solution, applied to a toothbrush or other cleaning device in order to remove tooth deposits such as stain and plaque. It has an effect on teeth appearance over the short term.

dentifrice, flavoring agents, n an additive in liquid, powder, or paste oral hygiene products designed to enhance the product's taste. Flavors tend to be mint and are derived primarily from essential oils.

dentifrice, foaming agents in, n the detergents or surfactants that generate foam. These nontoxic, chemically compatible ingredients also serve to remove unwanted matter from dental surfaces, make teeth feel smoother, and break down stains and deposits.

dentifrice, therapeutic **(den′təfris ther′əpū′tik),** *n* a material or substance, such as mouthwash, prompting physical changes that positively influence dental health.

dentigerous cyst, *n* See cyst.

dentin (den′tin), *n* the portion of the tooth that lies subjacent to the enamel and cementum. Consists of an organic matrix on which mineral (calcific) salts are deposited; pierced by tubules containing the processes of the odontoblasts that line the pulpal chamber and canal. It is of mesodermal origin. Older term is *dentine.*

dentin bonding agent, n a tissue compatible adhesive that adheres to dentin.

dentin, carious, n the dentin that is involved in or affected by the carious process.

dentin dysplasia, n See dysplasia, dentinal.

dentin eburnation **(ē′burnā′shən),** *n* a change in carious teeth in which the decayed dentin assumes a hard, brown, polished appearance and becomes arrested.

dentin, globular, n part of dentinal matrix consisting of completely fused and calcified globules of predentin.

dentin, hereditary opalescent **(ō′pəles′ənt),** *n* See dentinogenesis imperfecta.

dentin, hyperesthesia of **(hī′pəristhē′zhə),** *n* an excessive sensibility of dentin.

dentin, interglobular, n the incompletely calcified dentinal matrix present between the calcified globules.

dentin, intertubular, n the dentin present between the dentinal tubules.

dentin irritation (tertiary dentin, reparative dentin), n the dentin formed in response to an injury or irritant.

dentin, mantle, n the outer portion of dentin bordering the enamel or cementum of the tooth.

dentin, primary, n a type of dentin, made of straight dentinal tubules, that develops until the apical foramen of the root of the tooth is fully formed.

dentin, residual carious, n See caries, dental, residual.

dentin, sclerotic, n See dentin, transparent.

dentin, secondary, n the dentin formed or deposited on the walls of pulp chambers and canals subsequent to the complete formation of the tooth; caused by certain metabolic disturbances that result in irritation and stimulation of the odontoblasts to renewed activity.

dentin, transparent (sclerotic dentin) **(sklərot′ik),** *n* dentin formed as a defense mechanism in reaction to various stimuli. Dental tubules are obliterated by deposits of calcium salts that are harder and denser than normal dentin. This dentin appears transparent in ground sections.

dentin wall, n the portion of the wall of a prepared cavity that consists of dentin.

dentinal (den′tənəl), *adj* pertaining to the dentin.

dentinal dysplasia, n See dysplasia, dentinal.

dentinal fluid, n the tissue fluid in the dentinal tubule that surrounds the odontoblastic process.

dentinal permeability, n the degree to which fluids can pass through intact dentin.

dentinal tubule, n a microscopic tube within dentin that spreads outward from the tooth's center. It carries dentinal fluid.

dentine, *n* See dentin.

dentinocemental junction (DCJ) (dentin′ōsēmen′təl), *n* See junction, dentinocemental.

dentinoenamel junction (DEJ) (den′tinōinam′əl), *n* See junction, dentinoenamel.

dentinogenesis imperfecta (den′tinōjen′əsis), *n* (hereditary opalescent dentin) **1.** a disturbance of the dentin of genetic origin; characterized by early calcification of the pulp chambers and root canals, marked attrition, and an opalescent hue to the teeth. *n* **2.** a localized form of mesodermal dysplasia affecting the dentin of the tooth. It may be hereditary and may be associated with osteogenesis imperfecta. *n* **3.** a hereditary condition associated with a defect in dentin formation; the enamel remains normal.

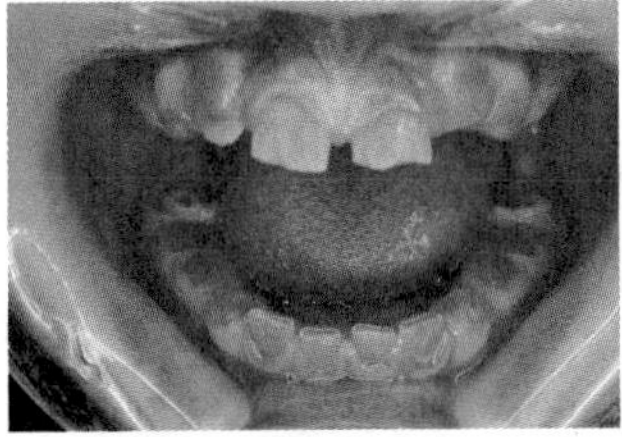

Dentinogenesis imperfecta.
(Regezi/Sciubba/Jordan, 2008)

dentinoma (den′tinōmə), *n* an odontogenic tumor composed of regular or irregular dentin.

dentist, *n* a person who is qualified by training and licensed by a state or region to diagnose and treat abnormalities of the teeth, gums, and underlying bone, including conditions caused by disease, trauma, and heredity. Required training consists of 2 to 4 years in an undergraduate college, a satisfactory score on a Dental Aptitude Test, and 4 years at an American Dental Association–accredited dental college. After completing dental college, a dentist is awarded a degree of either Doctor of Dental Surgery (D.D.S.) or Doctor of Dental Medicine (D.M.D.); the two degrees are equivalent.

dentistry, *n* the evaluation, diagnosis, and/or treatment (nonsurgical, surgical, or related procedures) of diseases, disorders, and/or conditions of the oral cavity, maxillofacial area, and/or the adjacent and associated structures and their impact on the body; provided by dental professionals, within the scope of his/her education, training, and experience, in accordance with the ethics of the profession and applicable law.

dentistry, forensic, *n* See jurisprudence, dental.

dentistry, four-handed, *n* the technique of chairside operating in which four hands are kept busy working in the oral cavity simultaneously.

dentistry, neuromuscular **(ner′ōmus′kyələr),** *n* a subdiscipline of dentistry concerned with correcting alignment problems at the temporomandibular joint. This branch of dentistry focuses primarily on caring for the muscles, nerves, and other tissue as opposed to teeth and bones.

dentistry, operative, *n* the branch of oral health service concerned with operations to restore or reform the hard dental tissues (e.g., operations necessitated by caries, trauma, and impaired function, and for improvement of appearance).

dentistry, preventive, *n* a subdiscipline of dentistry concerned with preventing cavities and other dental disorders and preserving healthy teeth and gingival tissues.

dentistry, prosthetic, *n* See prosthodontics.

dentistry, psychosomatic **(sī′kəsōmat′ik),** *n* a type of dentistry that concerns itself with the mind-body relationship.

dentistry, washed-field, *n* the constant flushing of the operative field with an irrigant (usually water) and the evacuation of the washing (debris) from the oral cavity by vacuum airstream. See also technique, hydroflow.

dentition (dentish′ən), *n* the natural teeth in position in the dental arches.

dentition, artificial, *n* the artificial substitutes for the natural dentition. See also denture.

dentition, deciduous, *n* See dentition, primary.

dentition, mixed, *n* the teeth in the jaws after the eruption of some of the permanent teeth but before all the primary teeth are exfoliated. This period usually begins with the eruption of the first permanent molars and ends with the exfoliation of the last primary tooth. Also called the transitional dentition. See also ugly duckling stage.

dentition, permanent (secondary dentition, permanent teeth), *n* the 32 teeth of adulthood that either replace or are added to with the shedding (exfoliation) of the primary teeth.

dentition, primary, *n* the 12 teeth present that erupt first and are usually replaced by the permanent teeth. This term is currently preferred over *deciduous.*

dentition, prognosis of, *n* an evaluation by the dental professional of the prospect of recovery from dental disease, combined with a forecast of the probability of maintaining the dentition and its associated structures in function and health.

dentition, secondary, *n* See dentition, permanent.

dentition, transitional, *n* See dentition, mixed.

dentoalveolar surgery (den′tō-alvē′əlur), *n* the category of oral surgery concerned with the extraction of teeth and the repair or restructuring of supporting bone. See also exodontics.

dentoform (den′tōform′), *n* See typodont.

dentogenesis (den′tōjen′əsis), *n* formation of the connective tissue, dentin, from odontoblasts during the development of the tooth. See also dentin.

dentogingival junction (DGJ), *n* See junction, dentogingival.

dentulous (dent′yooləs), *adj* (dentulism), having the natural teeth present in the oral cavity. Opposite term: *edentulous.*

denture, *n* an artificial substitute for missing natural teeth and adjacent tissues.

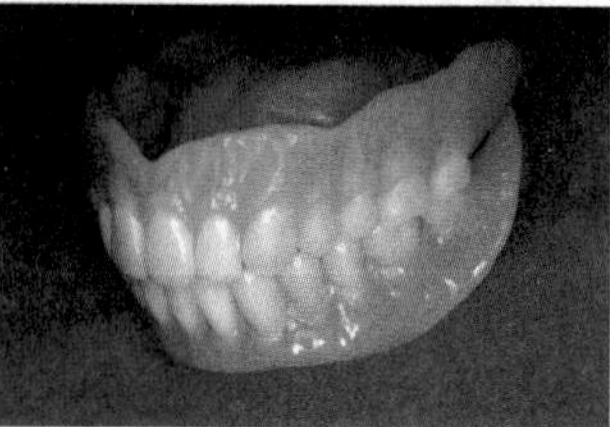

Denture. (Courtesy Dr. Charles Babbush)

denture, acrylic resin, *n* a denture made of acrylic resin.

denture adhesive, *n* a pliable, self-adjusting product used to hold a dental prosthesis in position. Also referred to as an *adherent.*

denture, artificial, *n* See denture.

denture, basal surface of (impression surface of denture, foundation surface of denture), *n* the part of a denture base that is shaped to conform to the basal seat for the denture.

denture-bearing area, *n* See area, basal seat.

denture, bilateral partial, *n* a dental prosthesis that supplies teeth and associated structures on both sides of a semiedentulous arch.

denture brush, *n* a brush designed especially for cleaning dentures.

denture characterization, *n* a modification of the form and color of the denture base and teeth to produce a more lifelike appearance.

denture, complete (complete dental prosthesis), *n* a dental prosthesis that replaces all the natural dentition and associated structures of the maxillae or mandible. It may be supported solely by the mucosa or attached to implants in the alveolar process.

denture, complete, lower, *n* a prosthetic replacement of all the teeth in the mandibular dental arch.

denture, complete, upper, *n* a prosthetic replacement of all the teeth in the maxillary dental arch.

denture, coping, *n* See overdenture.

denture coverage, *n* the extent to which the oral tissue is covered by the denture base.

denture curing, *n* the process by which the denture base materials are hardened in a denture mold to the form of a denture. See also process.

denture delivery, *n* See denture placement.

denture deposits, *n* these deposits range in degree of severity and ease of removal. They first appear as easily dissolved food matter or mucin, can progress to dental plaque or yeast infection, and in severe cases can result in the formation of calculus, a deposit that requires professional intervention to remove.

denture design, *n* a planned visualization of the form and extent of a denture.

denture dislodging force, *n* See force, denture dislodging.
denture, duplicate, *n* a second denture intended to be a copy of the first denture.
denture edge, *n* See border, denture.
denture engraving tool, *n* a tool used to permanently inscribe the patient's name on the flange of his or her dental prosthesis for identification purposes.
denture esthetics, *n* See esthetics, denture.
denture, finish of, *n* the final perfection of the form of the polished surfaces of a denture.
denture flange, *n* See flange.
denture foundation, *n* the portion of the oral structures that supports the complete or partial denture base under occlusal load. See also area, basal seat.
denture foundation, surface of, *n* See denture, basal surface of.
denture, full, *n* improper term. See denture, complete.
denture, heel of, *n* See distal end.
denture, immediate (immediate-insertion denture), *n* a removable dental prothesis constructed for placement immediately after removal of the remaining natural teeth.
denture, implant, *n* a denture that gains its support, stability, and retention from a substructure that is implanted under the soft tissues of the basal seat of the denture and is in contact with bone.
denture, implant, substructure, *n* See substructure, implant.
denture, implant, superstructure, *n* See superstructure, implant.
denture, impression surface of, *n* See denture, basal surface of.
denture, inclusion markers, *n* the temporary labels affixed to the impression surface of the denture for identification during processing.
denture, insertion, *n* See denture, placement.
denture, interim **(in'terəm),** *n* a dental prosthesis that is to be used for a short interval of time.
denture liner, *n* a resin used to coat the tissue surface of a dental prosthesis to restore or improve the conformation of the prosthesis to the tissue; generally used to improve the retention of the denture.
denture, maintenance of, *n* an important part of prosthodontic treatment and a major factor in the longevity of the service that the restoration can be expected to give.
denture, metal base, *n* a denture with a base of gold, chrome-cobalt alloy, aluminum, or other metal.
denture, model, wax, *n* See denture, trial.
denture overlay, *n* a complete denture that is supported by both tooth and mucosa. Remaining teeth are used to provide additional stability to the denture.
denture packing, *n* See packing, denture.
denture, partial (partial dental prosthesis), *n* a prosthesis that replaces one or more, but less than all, of the natural teeth and associated structures.
denture, partial, cantilever **(kan'təlē'vər),** *n* See denture, partial, cantilever fixed.
denture, partial, cantilever fixed, *n* a fixed dental prosthesis that has one or more abutments at one end of the denture supporting pontic(s) at its other end.
denture, partial, components of, *n* the units that compose a removable partial denture (e.g., the base, the artificial teeth, direct and indirect retainers, major and minor connectors).
denture, partial, construction of, *n* the science and technique of designing and constructing partial dentures.
denture, partial, extension, *n* a removable partial denture that is retained by natural teeth at one end of the denture base segments only; a portion of the functional load is carried by the residual ridge.
denture, partial, fixed, *n* a tooth-borne partial denture that is intended to be permanently attached to the teeth or roots that furnish support to the restoration.
denture, partial, removable, *n* a partial denture that can be readily placed in the oral cavity and removed by the wearer.
denture, partial, temporary, *n* See denture, partial, treatment.
denture, partial, tissue-borne, *n* a removable partial denture that is not supported entirely by the natural teeth.

D

denture, partial, tooth-borne, *n* a partial denture that is supported entirely by the teeth that bound the edentulous area covered by the base.

denture, partial, tooth-borne/tissue-borne, *n* a partial denture that gains support from both an abutment tooth or teeth and from the structures of the edentulous area covered by the base.

denture, partial, treatment (temporary partial denture), *n* a dental prosthesis used for the purpose of treating or conditioning the tissues that are needed to support and retain a denture base.

denture, partial, unilateral **(ū′nəlat′ərəl),** *n* a dental prosthesis that restores lost or missing teeth on one side of the arch only.

denture periphery, *n* See border, denture.

denture placement, *n* the act of inserting a dental prosthesis into the place in a patient's oral cavity for which it was designed. Also called *denture delivery* or *denture insertion.*

denture, polished surface of, *n* the portion of the surface of a denture that extends in an occlusal direction from the border of the denture and includes the palatal surface. It is the part of the denture base that is usually polished and includes the buccal and lingual surfaces of the teeth.

denture processing, *n* See processing, denture.

denture, provisional **(prōvizh′ənəl),** *n* a prosthetic appliance to be used for a short period for reasons of esthetics, function, or occlusal support; more commonly referred to as a temporary, interim, or transitional denture. A provisional denture is usually an immediate denture and is most often employed in the maxillary arch.

denture repair, *n* the restoration of a broken or damaged dental prosthesis.

denture retention, *n* See retention, denture.

denture-sore oral cavity, *n* See oral cavity, denture-sore.

denture space, *n* the space between the residual ridges and the cheeks and tongue that is available for dentures. See also distance, interarch.

denture stability, *n* See stability, denture.

denture, stomatitis, *n* See oral cavity, denture-sore.

denture supporting area, *n* See area, basal seat.

denture supporting structure, *n* See structure, denture supporting.

denture, temporary, *n* a denture intended to serve for a very short time in a temporary or emergency situation.

denture, tooth-mucosa-supported, *n* See denture.

denture, transitional, *n* a removable partial denture that serves as a temporary prosthesis to which teeth will be added as more teeth are lost and that will be replaced after postextraction tissue changes have occurred. A transitional denture may become an interim denture when all the teeth have been removed from the dental arch.

denture, trial (wax model denture), *n* a temporary denture, usually made of wax on a baseplate, that is used for checking jaw relation records, occlusion, and the arrangement and observation of teeth for esthetics.

denture cleanser, *n* a variety of products designed to safely remove stains, deposits, and debris from the surfaces of dental prostheses, by means of immersion or brushing with a denture brush and paste, toothpaste, or powder.

denture cleanser, alkaline hypochlorite (hī′pōklôr′īt), *n* a chemical ingredient used in some solutions to clean removable oral prostheses. The active ingredient is dilute sodium hypochlorite. It effectively removes food, stains, and plaque, and is readily available in household bleach; it has a strong lingering scent and may damage prostheses.

denture cleanser, alkaline peroxide, *n* a light-duty denture cleaner; active ingredient is typically sodium perborate or sodium percarbonate. Comes in tablet or powder form; when combined with water, it creates bubbles. Does not effectively deal with calculus or darker staining.

denture cleanser, dilute acid, *n* a chemical containing inorganic acids as its active ingredient; used to clean prosthetic dental appliances in an immersion regimen. Solutions range include 3% to 5% hydrochloric acid or a combination of phosphoric and hydrochloric acids. Regular use of dilute acids can damage any metal on the prosthetic device.

denture cleanser, enzyme, n an agent that is sometimes added to immersion cleaning solutions, which works by weakening polysaccharides and plaque proteins.

denturist (den′chərist), *n* a person other than a dental professional (usually a technician) who engages in the practice of dentistry that is usually limited to making and fitting complete or partial dentures. Dental practice acts vary in allowing this.

denudation (den′yoodā′shən), *n* stripping bare; the process of removing the outer (epithelial) layer by surgery or disease.

deoxyribonucleic acid (DNA) (dēok′sērī′bōnooklā′ik), *n* See DNA.

deoxyribonucleic acid (DNA) probes, *n* a nucleic acid fragment labeled with a radioisotope that is complementary to a sequence in another nucleic acid fragment that will bind to it and thus identify it. It is used as a diagnostic tool to identity the species of microbe involved in an infectious process such as refractory periodontal disease.

dependence, physical, *n* the level of substance abuse at which disagreeable or severe physiologic symptoms will occur if use of the substance is suddenly terminated.

dependency, *n* the state of being dependent.

dependency, drug, n a psychologic craving for, habituation to, or addiction to a chemical substance; the term replaces *drug addiction,* which emphasizes physiologic craving.

dependency, emotional, n an emotional need manifested by a marked and habitual inclination to rely on another for comfort, support, guidance, and decision making; the tendency to seek help from others in making decisions or in carrying out difficult actions; the need to be mothered, loved, taken care of, emotionally supported. In extreme cases such persons lose their ability to function independently.

dependents, *n.pl* the spouse and children of a subscriber, as defined in a contract. Under some contracts, parents or other members of the family may be beneficiaries.

deplaquing, *n* the removal of plaque from the tooth's surface or the gingival tissues.

depletion, salt (dēplē′shən), *n* a condition resulting from inadequate water intake, low intake of sodium and chlorides in the alimentary tract, and secretion of sweat and urine. The most significant of these losses are the gastrointestinal fluid losses resulting from vomiting, diarrhea, and fistulas.

depolarization (dēpō′ləriză′shən), *n* a neutralization of polarity; the breaking down of polarized semipermeable membranes, as in nerve or muscle cells in the induction of impulses.

deponent (dipō′nənt), *n* one who gives under oath testimony reduced to writing.

deposit, bismuth, *n* See stomatitis, bismuth.

deposit, calcareous, *n* See calculus.

deposition (dep′ōzish′ən), *n* the evidence given by a witness under interrogation, oral or written, and usually written down by an official person and intended to be used in the trial of an action in court.

deposits, assessment of, *n* the examination of the teeth for evidence of calculus and debris, which, if not removed, may lead to caries and/or periodontal infection.

deposits, nonmineralized (soft), *n.pl* the soft deposits, consisting of acquired pellicle, plaque, and debris, that accumulate on tooth surfaces and within the gingival sulcus or periodontal pockets. If left unattended, will harden into calculus and may lead to caries and/or periodontal disease.

depot (dē′pō), *n* in physiology, the site of accumulation, deposit, or storage of body products not immediately or actively involved in metabolic processes (e.g., a fat depot).

depreciation, *n* the charges against earnings to write off the cost, less salvage value, of an asset over its estimated useful life. It is a bookkeeping entry and does not represent any cash outlay, nor are any funds earmarked for the purpose. There are three classic methods of applying depreciation: straight line, sum of the year's digits, and double declining balance.

depressant (dēpres′ənt), *n* a medicine that diminishes functional activity.

D

depressed oral lesions, *n.pl* lesions characterized by their subsurface appearance and nonuniform shape. They may be classified as either erosions, which are considered superficial (i.e., having a depth of less than 3 mm), or the more frequently occurring ulcers, which may be up to 3 mm in depth. Ulcers may be the result of elevated lesions that have burst, and vary in appearance, with centers being yellow to gray, while the borders are typically red.

depression (dēpresh′ən), *n* **1.** a decrease of functional activity. *n* **2.** a pitted area on a tooth or other anatomic surface.

depression, developmental, *n* depression seen in a defined region on a tooth.

depression, mandible, *n* the lowering of the mandible caused by rotational movement of the temporomandibular joint.

depression, postpartum, *n* a moderate to severe form of depression that occurs in women beginning approximately 2 to 3 weeks after childbirth as a result of physical and psychologic factors. Symptoms include fatigue, loss of appetite, and lack of enthusiasm for everyday activities.

depression, psychologic, *n* a clinical syndrome of neurotic or psychotic proportions, consisting of lowering of mood tone (feelings of painful dejection), difficulty in thinking, and psychomotor retardation. As commonly used, depression ordinarily refers only to the mood element, which would be more appropriately labeled dejection, sadness, gloominess, despair, or despondency. Many such patients lack motivation and concern for their oral health or dental needs.

derivative (dēriv′ətiv), *n* a chemical substance that is the result of a chemical reaction.

dermal undergloves, *n* an additional pair of protective hand coverings, worn to protect sensitive skin from the latex or nonlatex material of the outer glove.

dermatalgia (durmətal′jēə), *n* pain, burning, and other sensations of the skin unaccompanied by any structural change; probably caused by some nervous disease or reflex influence.

dermataneuria (dur′matənŏŏrēə), *n* a derangement of the nerve supply of the skin, causing disturbance of sensation.

dermatitis (durmətī′tis), *n* an inflammation of the skin.

dermatitis, allergic contact, *n* the reaction of the skin to direct contact with a specific antigen. Poison ivy rash is a common example of an allergic contact dermatitis.

dermatitis, atopic **(ātō′pik),** *n* an atopic eczema characterized by the distinctive phenomenon of atopy, a familial related allergic response associated with IgE antibody.

dermatitis, contact, *n* a delayed type of induced sensitivity (allergy) of the skin with varying degrees of erythema, edema, and vesiculation, resulting from cutaneous contact with a specific allergen. It is an occupational hazard in dentistry.

dermatitis herpetiformis **(hərpet′iformis),** *n* dermatitis characterized by grouped, erythematous, papular, vesicular, pustular, or bullous lesions occurring in various combinations, often accompanied by vesicobullous and ulcerative lesions of the oral mucosa.

dermatitis infectiosa eczematoides (Engman's disease), *n* a pustular eczematous eruption that frequently follows or occurs coincidentally with some pyogenic process.

dermatitis, occupational, *n* a contact dermatitis associated with allergens found in the workplace.

dermatitis, radiation, *n* an inflammation of the skin resulting from a high dose of radiation. The reaction varies with the quality and quantity of radiation used and is usually transitory.

dermatitis, seborrheic **(seb′ərē′ik),** *n* a chronic inflammatory skin disease that can affect the scalp, face, ears, armpits, breasts, and groin. Its symptoms include moist, greasy, or dry scaling and patches of yellowish

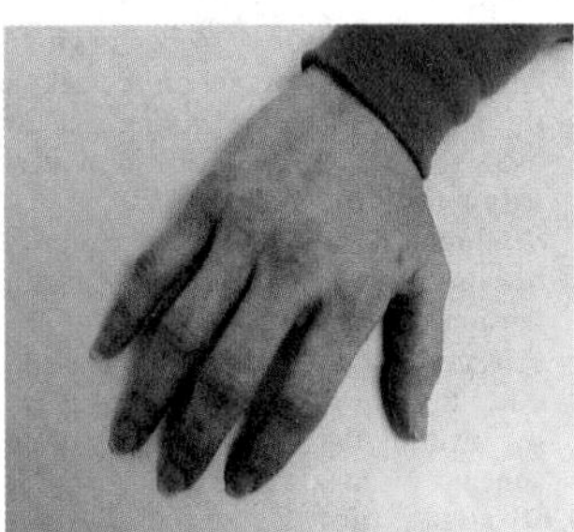

Dermatitis. (Bird/Robinson, 2005)

crust. Although the cause is unknown, it can be treated with selenium sulfide shampoos, topical antibiotics, and topical and oral corticosteroids.

dermatoglyphics (dur′mətōglif′iks), *n* the study of the skin ridge patterns on fingers, toes, palms of hands, and soles of feet. The patterns are used as a basis of identification (fingerprinting).

dermatology, *n* the study of the skin, including the anatomy, physiology, and pathology of the skin and the diagnosis and treatment of skin disorders.

dermatoma (dur′mətō′mə), *n* a circumscribed thickening or hypertrophy of the skin.

dermatome (dur′mətōm′), *n* **1.** an instrument for cutting thin slices or layers of skin for grafting or for sequentially removing small lesions. **2.** dermatologic regions of sensory innervation supplied by particular posterior root spinal nerves.

dermatomyositis (dur′mətōmī′-ōsī′tis), *n* (polymyositis, dermatomucosomyositis) a form of collagen disease related to scleroderma and lupus erythematosus. The skin lesions are diffuse erythematous desquamations or rashlike lesions. The skin symptoms are related to a variety of patterns of myositis.

dermatophyte (dərmat′əfīt′), *n* fungi that cause parasitic skin disease.

dermatosclerosis (dur′mətōsklərō′sis), *n* See scleroderma.

dermatosis (dur′mətō′sis), *n* a disease of the skin.

dermis (dur′mis), *n* the layer of skin just below the epidermis consisting of vascular connective tissue.

dermoid cyst, *n* See cyst, dermoid.

desaturation (dēsat′yərā′shən), *n* the conversion of a saturated compound such as stearin into an unsaturated compound such as olein by the removal of hydrogen.

desensitization (dēsen′sitizā′shən), *n* **1.** a condition of insusceptibility to infection or an allergen; established in experimental animals by the injection of an antigen that produces sensitization or an anaphylactic reaction. After recovery, a second injection of the antigen is made, bringing about no reaction and thus producing desensitization. *n* **2.** a reduction in dentin hypersensitivity by the addition of medicaments to the exposed dentin surface.

desensitization, psychologic, *n* the deliberate exposure of an individual to imagined or actual emotionally stressful experiences to treat phobias and other related conditions.

desiccate (des′ikāt), *n* to dry by chemical or physical means; e.g., electrocoagulation can produce desiccation in tissues.

desiccation (des′ikā′shən), *n* an excessive loss of moisture; the process of drying up. See also electrocoagulation.

design, *v* **1.** to plan or delineate by drawing the outline of a proposed prosthesis. *n* **2.** the graphical and artistic representation of a plan.

designer drugs, *n.pl* the synthetic organic compounds that are designed as analogs of illicit drugs and have the same narcotic or other dangerous effects.

desipramine HCl (dəsip′rəmēn), *n* *brand names:* Norpramin, Petrofrane; *drug class:* antidepressant, tricyclic; *action:* inhibits both norepinephrine and serotonin (5-HT) uptake in the brain; *use:* depression.

desmins (dez′minz), *n.pl* α-amino acids, usually lysine and norleucine, condensed through their sidechains rather than through the α-amino and carboxyl groups. They copolymerize with vimentin to form constituents of connective tissue.

desmolysis (desmol′isis), *n* the destruction and disintegration of connective tissue. Some authorities associate this desmolytic process with the destruction of connective tissue lying between the enamel and oral epithelium, which thus permits proliferation of the oral epithelium and fusion of enamel and oral epithelium.

D

desmopressin acetate (des′mōpres′ən as′ətāt), *n brand name:* Stimate; *drug class:* synthetic antidiuretic hormone; *action:* promotes reabsorption of water by action on renal tubular epithelium; *uses:* primary nocturnal enuresis, hemophilia A with factor VIII levels of less than 5%, von Willebrand disease, and neurogenic diabetes insipidus.

desmosomes, *n.pl* See epithelium, desmosomes of.

desonide (des′ənīd′), *brand names:* DesOwen, Tridesilon; *drug class:* topical corticosteroid, group IV low potency; *actions:* possesses antipruritic, antiinflammatory actions; *uses:* psoriasis, eczema, contact dermatitis, pruritus.

desoximetasone (desok′sēmet′əsōn), *n brand names:* Topicort, Topicort LP; *drug class:* topical corticosteroid, group II potency (0.25%), group III potency (0.05%); *action:* interacts with steroid cytoplasmic receptors to induce antiinflammatory effects; *uses:* psoriasis, eczema, contact dermatitis, pruritus.

desquamation (des′kwəmā′shən), *n* a naturally occurring process in which the outer layer of skin or mucosa cells is sloughed off.

detector, radiation, *n* See radiation detector.

detention, *n* restraint; custody; confinement.

detergent (dētur′jənt), *n* a cleanser. Also applied in a more specific sense to chemicals that possess surface-active properties in water and whose solutions are therefore able to wet surfaces that are normally water repellent, thereby assisting in the mechanical dispersion and emulsification of fatty or oily material and other substances that soil the surface.

detergent, anionic, *n* a detergent in which the cleansing action resides in the anion. Soaps and many synthetic detergents are anionic.

detergent, cationic, *n* a detergent in which the cleansing action resides in the cation. Many are strong germicides (e.g., those that contain quaternary ammonium compounds).

detergent, nonionic, *n* a cleanser that acts by depressing the surface tension of water but does not ionize.

detergent, synthetic, *n* a cleanser, other than soap, that exerts its effect by lowering the surface tension of an aqueous cleansing mixture.

detoxicate (dētok′sikāt), *v* See detoxify.

detoxify, *v* (detoxicate), to remove the toxic quality of a substance.

detritus (det′ritus), *n* the fragments or scraps that cling to teeth, gingival tissues or other oral surfaces.

deuterium (dootēr′ēəm), a stable isotope of the hydrogen atom, used as a tracer. Also called *heavy hydrogen.* Deuterium oxide, or heavy water, is formed from an isotope of hydrogen, which has twice the weight of ordinary hydrogen (hence the name).

developed countries, *n.pl* the countries with an economic base built largely on manufacturing and technology rather than agriculture. Although the need for medical and dental care may not differ from undeveloped to developed countries, the effective demand does vary. They have the available health professionals, the economic base to support the purchase of health care, and an informed public.

developer, *n* a chemical solution that converts the invisible (latent) image on a film into a visible one composed of minute grains of metallic silver.

developer stain, *n* See film fault, black spots.

developing countries, *n.pl* the countries in transition from an agrarian economy to a manufacturing- and technology-based economy.

developing, time-temperature method, *n* the procedure of developing dental films; a solution of fixed temperature is used, and the films are immersed in the solution for a specific length of time.

developing, visual method, *n* the procedure of developing dental films by placing the films in the developing solution and holding them from time to time before a safelight. Correct development has occurred when the film becomes so dark that it is difficult to distinguish between tooth and bone structure.

development, *n* the process by which an individual reaches maturity.

development hyperactivity, *n* a condition distinguished by continuous movement, restlessness, impetuosity, excitability, and a short span of attention. Also called *hyperkinesis.*

developmental biology, *n* the study of life processes occurring during growth and maturation.

developmental disabilities (DD), *n.pl* the pathologic conditions that have their origin in the embryology and growth and development of an individual. DDs usually appear clinically before 18 years of age. The limitations of physiologic or mental function usually persist throughout life.

deviation (dē′vēā′shən), *n* the turning from a regular course; deflection.

device, scavenging (skav′ənjing), *n* a device that collects and removes exhaled nitrous oxide during the administration of nitrous oxide and oxygen for sedation. The device is recommended by the American Dental Association to avoid occupational exposure to the gas.

devital tooth, See tooth, pulpless.

dexamethasone/dexamethasone acetate/dexamethasone sodium phosphate (dek′səmeth′əsōn), *n brand names:* Decadron, Hexadrol, Oradexan; *drug class:* glucocorticoid, long-acting; *action:* decreases inflammation by suppression of macrophage and leukocyte migration, reduces capillary permeability; *uses:* inflammation, allergies, neoplasm, cerebral edema, shock, collagen disorders.

dexamethasone/dexamethasone sodium phosphate, *n brand name:* Decaderm; *drug class:* synthetic topical corticosteroid; *action:* interacts with steroid cytoplasmic receptors to induce antiinflammatory effects; *uses:* corticosteroid-responsive dermatoses; oral ulcerative inflammatory lesions.

dexchlorpheniramine maleate (deks′klorfənir′əmēn′ mălēāt), *n brand names:* Dexchlor, Poladex TD; *drug class:* antihistamine; *actions:* acts on blood vessels, gastrointestinal system, respiratory system by competing with histamine for H_1 receptor sites; decreases allergic response by blocking histamine; *uses:* allergy symptoms, rhinitis, pruritus, contact dermatitis.

dextran (dek′stran), *n* ($C_6H_{10}O_5$) a water-soluble polymer of glucose of high molecular weight. A purified form, having an average molecular weight of 75,000, is used in a 6% concentration in isotonic sodium chloride solution to expand plasma volume and maintain blood pressure in emergency treatment of hemorrhagic and traumatic shock.

dextro-, *adj/comb* the prefix designating that an aqueous solution of a substance rotates the plane of polarized light to the right. See also isomers, optical.

dextroamphetamine sulfate (dek′strōamfet′əmēn′ sul′fāt), *n brand names:* Dexedrine, Oxydess II; *drug class:* amphetamine, Controlled Substance Schedule II; *action:* increases release of norepinephrine and dopamine in the cerebral cortex to the reticular activating system; *uses:* narcolepsy, attention deficit disorder with hyperactivity.

dextromethorphan hydrobromide (dek′strōməthor′fan hī′drōbrō′-mīd), *n brand names:* Benylin DM, Robitussin Pediatric, Vicks Formula 44; *drug class:* antitussive, nonnarcotic; *action:* depresses cough center in medulla; *use:* nonproductive cough.

dextrorotatory (dek′strōrō′tətôrē), *adj* turning the plane of polarization, or rays of polarized light, to the right.

dextrose (dek′strōs), *n* dextrorotatory glucose, a monosaccharide occurring as a white, crystalline powder; colorless and sweet.

diabetes (dīəbē′tēz), *n* a deficiency condition involving carbohydrate metabolism and characterized by increased urination.

diabetes, bronzed, *n* the combination of hemochromatosis and diabetes mellitus. The skin takes on a bronzed appearance as a result of the deposition of an iron-containing pigment in the skin.

D

diabetes, gestational **(jestāshənəl),** *n* the term describing patients who acquire glucose intolerance when pregnant.

diabetes insipidus **(insip′idəs),** *n* **1.** a metabolic disturbance characterized by marked urinary excretion and great thirst but no elevation of sugar in the blood or urine. *n* **2.** a pituitary dysfunction characterized by an insufficient output of antidiuretic hormone, leading to polyuria and polydipsia.

diabetes, juvenile, *n* an older term for diabetes mellitus occurring in children and adolescents, usually of a more severe and rampant nature than diabetes mellitus in adults, with consequent difficulty of regulation. Now considered a form of type 1 diabetes mellitus.

diabetes mellitus **(mel′ətəs),** *n* a metabolic disorder caused primarily by a defect in the production of insulin by the islet cells of the pancreas, resulting in an inability to use carbohydrates. Characterized by hyperglycemia, glycosuria, polyuria, hyperlipemia (caused by imperfect catabolism of fats), acidosis, ketonuria, and a lowered resistance to infection. Periodontal manifestations if blood sugar is not being controlled may include recurrent and multiple periodontal abscesses, osteoporotic changes in alveolar bone, fungating masses of granulation tissue protruding from periodontal pockets, a lowered resistance to infection, and delay in healing after periodontal therapy. See also blood glucose level(s).

diabetes mellitus, amputation, *n* a great number of limb amputations are caused by diabetes, especially amputations of the feet; blood infections in the feet can go unnoticed by the patient because of a lack of feeling caused by diabetic neuropathy.

diabetes mellitus, type 1, *n* diabetes that usually includes patients requiring the administration of insulin to prevent ketosis. Previously called *insulin-dependent (IDDM), juvenile-onset diabetes, brittle diabetes,* and *ketosis-prone diabetes.*

diabetes mellitus, type 2, *n* diabetes that includes patients who can maintain proper blood sugar levels within the administration of insulin. Previously called *non–insulin-dependent (NIDDM), maturity-onset diabetes, adult-onset diabetes, ketosis-resistant diabetes,* and *stable diabetes.*

diabetes, phlorizin **(flor′əzin),** *n* a condition of glycosuria caused by inhibition of phosphorylation of phlorizin. It is not related to an endocrine disturbance.

diabetic (dī′əbet′ik), *adj* of or pertaining to diabetes.

diabetic ketoacidosis (DKA) **(kē′-tōas′idō′sis),** *n* a diabetic coma; an acute, life-threatening complication of uncontrolled diabetes mellitus in which urinary loss of water, potassium, ammonium, and sodium results in hypovolemia, electrolyte imbalance, extremely high blood glucose levels, and the breakdown of free fatty acids causing acidosis. Causes "fruity" or acetone breath. See also acetone breath.

diabetic nephropathy **(nəfro′pəthē′),** *n* the negative effects on the kidneys or renal system caused by diabetes mellitus. The condition may necessitate dialysis or kidney transplant.

diabetic neuropathy, *n* the complications to the nervous system that can be caused by diabetes mellitus, some of which may necessitate amputation or result in oral or facial symptoms.

diabetic retinopathy **(ret′inop′əthē),** *n* the complication to the eye that can be caused by diabetes mellitus, some of which may result in blindness.

diadochokinesia (dīad′əkōkīnē′zēə, -zhə), *n* the act or process of repeating at maximum speed a simple cyclical, reciprocating movement such as raising and lowering of the mandible or protrusion and retracting the tongue.

diagnose, *v* to distinguish irregularities and other issues of concern based upon a patient's examination and interview.

diagnosis, *n* the translation of data gathered by clinical and radiographic examination into an organized, classified definition of the conditions present.

diagnosis, clinical, *n* the determination of the specific disease or diseases involved in producing symptoms and signs by examination of the patient and use of analogy.

diagnosis, dental hygiene, *n* the professional determination of a dental hygienist, including evaluation and recommendation, regarding a patient's personal hygienic needs.

diagnosis, differential, *n* the process of identifying a condition by differentiating all pathologic processes that may produce similar lesions.

diagnosis, final, *n* the diagnosis arrived at after all the data have been collected, analyzed, and subjected to logical thought. Treatment may be necessary in some instances before the final diagnosis is made.

diagnosis, laboratory, *n* a diagnosis made from chemical, microscopic, microbiologic, immunologic, or pathologic study of secretions, discharges, blood, or tissue sections.

diagnosis, oral, *n* the identification of the cause of a dental disease or abnormality.

diagnosis, radiographic, *n* a limited term used to indicate those radiologic interpretations that cannot be verified or disproved by clinical examination.

diagnosis-related group (DRG), *n* a system of classifying hospital patients on the basis of diagnosis consisting of distinct groupings. A DRG assignment to a case is based on the patient's principal diagnosis, treatment procedures performed, age, gender, and discharge status.

diagnosis, surgical, *n* a surgical incision into a body part or the excision of a lesion for the purpose of determining the cause or nature of an illness.

diagnostic cast, *n* See cast, diagnostic.

diagnostic equilibration (ikwil′əbrā′shən), a measuring method of determining and recording on dentodes the amount and direction that interfering cusps deflect the closure direction of the mandible, as can be seen in mountings.

diagnostic error, *n* a mistake in judgment regarding the cause of an illness.

diagnostic imaging, *n* the use of radiographic, sonographic, and other technologies to create a graphic depiction of the body part(s) in question.

diagnostic services, *n.pl* the imaging and laboratory capabilities available for determining the cause of an illness.

diagnostic wax-up, *n* a process in which wax is applied to a model of the patient's teeth to simulate the procedure and results of planned reconstruction, repair, or enhancement.

dialysis (dīal′isis), *n* a type of filtration used to separate smaller molecules from larger ones contained in a solution. The molecular solution is placed on one side of a semipermeable membrane and water on the other side. The smaller molecules pass through the membrane into the water; the larger molecules are retained in the solution.

dialysis, kidney, artificial, *n* See kidney dialysis, artificial.

diamond, *n* a crystalline carbon substance, the hardest natural substance known, used industrially and in dentistry for cutting and grinding.

diamond particles, *n.pl* the elements of a diamond polishing paste that are used to bring out the natural luster of porcelain surfaces.

diaphoresis (dī′əfərē′sis), *n* excessive sweating.

diaphragm (dī′əfram), *n* **1.** a musculotendinous partition that separates the thorax and abdomen. *n* **2.** a metal barrier plate, often of lead, pierced with a central aperture so arranged as to limit the emerging, or useful, beam of roentgen rays to the smallest practical diameter for making radiographic exposures. See also collimation; collimator; distance, cone.

diaphragm, lead, *n* a collimating device with a small opening, designed to limit the size of the outgoing x-ray beam. It is usually made of lead one-eighth of an inch thick and located between the position-indicating device and the radiographic tube itself.

diaphragm, Potter-Bucky, See grid, Potter-Bucky.

diaphysis (diaf′isis), *n* the shaft of a long bone.

diarrhea (dī′ərē′ə), *n* a condition with the frequent passage of loose, watery stools. The stool may also contain mucus, suppuration, blood, or excessive amounts of fat. It is usually a symptom of some underlying disorder. See antidiarrheals.

diarthrosis (dī'ärthrō'sis), *n* See synovial joint.

diastema (dī'əstē'mə), *n* an abnormal space between two adjacent teeth in the same dental arch. The gap between the maxillary central incisors is very noticeable.

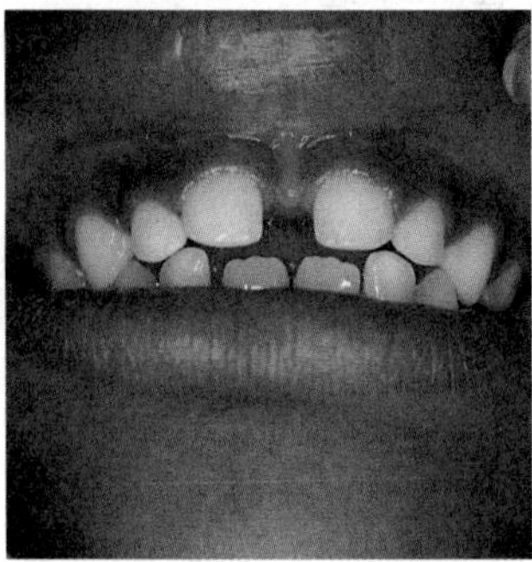

Diastema. (Zitelli/Davis, 2002)

diastole (dīas'təlē), *n* **1.** the rhythmic period of relaxation and dilation of a chamber of the heart during which it fills with blood. *n* **2.** the period after the contraction of the heart muscle, during which the aorta releases the potential energy stored in its elastic tissue. The energy is converted into kinetic energy and sustains the pressure necessary for steady flow of blood in the vessels. The pressure measured at this period is the lowest attained during the cardiac pumping cycle and is called the *diastolic pressure.* The normal pressure in the adult is approximately 120/80 mm Hg (systolic/diastolic) and increases with age from 128/85 at 45 years of age to 135/89 at 60 years of age. See also blood pressure classification.

diathermy (di'əthur'mē), *n* a generalized rise in tissue temperature produced by a high-frequency alternating current between two electrodes. The temperature rise is produced without causing tissue damage.

diathesis (dīath'əsis), *n* a tendency, based on body makeup or constitutional, hereditary, or acquired states of the body, that causes a predisposition or susceptibility to disease.

***diathesis, hemorrhagic* (hem'əraj'ik),** *n* a condition that may be caused by defects in the coagulation mechanism, blood vessel wall, or both.

diazepam (dīaz'əpam'), *n brand name:* Valium; *drug class:* benzodiazepine, anxiolytic Controlled Substance Schedule IV; *action:* produces CNS depression by acting on parts of the limbic system and the thalamus and hypothalamus, inducing a calming effect; *uses:* management of short-term anxiety disorders and relief of symptoms of anxiety, short-term relief of skeletal muscle spasm, acute alcohol withdrawal.

Dick's test, *n* See test, Dick's.

diclofenac (dīklō'fənak'), *n brand names:* Cataflam, Voltaren; *drug class:* nonsteroidal antiinflammatory; *action:* inhibits prostaglandin synthesis; *uses:* acute and chronic rheumatoid arthritis, osteoarthritis, ankylosing spondylitis.

dicloxacillin sodium (dīklok'səsil'ən), *n brand names:* Dycill, Dynapen, Pathocil; *drug class:* penicillinase-resistant penicillin; *action:* interferes with cell wall replication of susceptible organisms; *uses:* infections caused by penicillinase-producing *Staphylococcus.*

dicyclomine HCl (dīsī'kləmēn'), *n brand names:* Antispas, Dibent; *drug class:* GI anticholinergic; *action:* inhibits muscarinic actions of acetylcholine at postganglionic parasympathetic neuroeffector sites; *uses:* peptic ulcer disease in combination with other drugs; infant colic.

didanosine (dīdan'əsin'), *n brand name:* Videx; *drug class:* synthetic antiviral; *action:* converted by cellular enzymes that act as antimetabolites to inhibit HIV replication; *uses:* advanced HIV infections in adults and children who have been unable to use zidovudine or who have not responded to treatment with zidovudine.

dideoxycytidine (dī'dēok'sēsī'tidēn'), *n* See Zalcitabine.

dideoxyinosine (dī'dēok'sēin'əsēn'), *n* See didanosine.

die, *n* the positive reproduction of the form of a prepared tooth in any suitable hard substance, usually in metal or specially prepared (improved) artificial stone.

die, lubricant, *n* a material applied to a die to serve as a separating medium so that the wax pattern will not adhere to the die but may be withdrawn from it without sticking.

die, stone, *n* a positive likeness in artificial (dental) stone; used in the fabrication of a dental restoration.

die, waxing, *n* a mold into which wax is forced for the production of standardized wax patterns.

dienestrol (dīˈənesˈtrol), *n brand name:* Ortho Dienestrol; *drug class:* nonsteroidal synthetic estrogen; *action:* needed for adequate functioning of female reproductive system; affects release of pituitary gonadotropins, inhibits ovulation; *uses:* atrophic vaginitis, kraurosis vulvae.

diet, *n* **1.** the food and drink consumed by a given person from day to day. Not all the diet is necessarily used by the body. For this reason, diet and nutrition must be differentiated. *v* **2.** to eat according to a plan.

diet, alkaline, *n* a diet that is basic in reaction; produced by the addition of alkaline salts, including sodium bicarbonate.

diet, cariogenic, *n* the intake of food that is heavy in refined carbohydrates and other food stuffs that support the growth of caries-producing bacteria.

diet, lysine-poor, *n* a diet deficient in lysine, an essential amino acid. All the essential amino acids must be present in the diet; should one or more be absent, proper use of the others cannot occur. Periodontal changes described in experimental animals with lysine deficiency include osteoporosis of supporting bone and disintegration and failure of replacement of periodontal fibers.

dietary carbohydrates, *n* the amount of simple and complex sugars consumed; the physical character of the diet. It may tend to produce or modify periodontal disease.

dietary fiber, *n* a generic term for nondigestible chemical substances found in plant cell walls. Foods high in dietary fiber are fruits, green leafy vegetables, root vegetables, and whole-grain cereals and bread.

dietary history, *n* See analysis, dietary.

dietary reference intakes (DRIs), *n.pl* a set of nutritional guidelines concerning the intake of vitamins and minerals from food rather than supplements.

dietetics, *n* the science of applying nutritional principles to the planning and preparation of foods and the regulation of the diet in relation to both health and disease.

diethylpropion HCl (dīethˈəl-prōˈpēən), *n brand names:* Tenuate Dospan, Ten-Tab; *drug class:* anorexant, amphetamine-like analog Controlled Substance Schedule IV; *action:* exact mechanism of appetite suppression is unknown; may have an effect on the satiety center of the hypothalamus; *use:* exogenous obesity.

diethylstilbestrol (dīethˈilstilbesˈtrôl), *n* an estrogenic substance, $C_{18}H_{20}O_2$, that has an estrogenic activity considered to be greater than that of estrone. Useful in treating menopausal symptoms and occasionally used in the therapy of chronic desquamative gingivitis associated with artificial or natural menopause.

dietitian, registered (dī-ətishˈən), *n* an individual who meets the requirements of the American Dietetic Association (ADA) including possession of a bachelor's degree in dietetics or nutrition, a passing grade on the registration exam, and a demonstrated commitment to continuing education through updated courses taken annually.

difenoxin HCl with atropine sulfate (difˈənokˈsin atˈrəpēnˈ sulˈfāt), *n brand name:* Motofen; *drug class:* antidiarrheal Controlled Substance Schedule IV; *action:* inhibits gastric motility by acting on mucosal receptors responsible for peristalsis; *uses:* acute nonspecific diarrhea and acute exacerbations of chronic functional diarrhea.

differential force, *n* a term sometimes used to describe the design and application of an orthodontic appliance to distribute the reciprocal forces of the appliance over significantly different root areas with the objective of eliciting a differential response.

difficult eruption, See teething.

D

diffusibility (difūz'ibil'itē), *n* capable of being diffused.

diffusion (difū'zhən), *n* a property of ions or molecules of a solute that permits them to pass through a membrane or to intermingle by rapid or gradual permeation with the molecules of a solvent.

diffusion barrier, *n* a thin layer of material placed between two other materials to prevent one from corrupting the other.

diffusion, facilitated, *n* an absorption process during which only certain recognized molecules are allowed to pass into the receiving area.

diflorasone diacetate (dif'lorəsōn dīas'ətāt), *n brand names:* Florone, Maxiflor, Psorcon; *drug class:* topical corticosteroid, group II high potency; *action:* possesses antipruritic, antiinflammatory actions; *uses:* psoriasis, eczema, contact dermatitis, pruritus.

diflunisal (dīfloo'nəsal'), *n brand name:* Dolobid; *drug class:* salicylate derivative, nonsteroidal antiinflammatory; *action:* inhibits prostaglandin synthesis; *uses:* mild to moderate pain, symptoms of rheumatoid arthritis and osteoarthritis.

digestion, *n* the conversion of food into absorbable substances in the GI tract.

digit, *n* **1.** a single symbol or character representing a quantity. *n* **2.** a finger or toe.

digit sucking, *n* an oral habit, usually referred to as *finger* or *thumb sucking,* that is not unusual in preschool children. Prolonged, persistent, or vigorous sucking into the transition dentition period can cause tooth displacement malocclusions.

digital, *adj* **1.** involving the use of the fingers. *adj* **2.** a means of data storage in which information is converted to numeric strings. *adj* **3.** using alphanumeric characters to display data, as opposed to analog, which uses the relative position of needles or "hands" (as with a clock) against a background scale.

digital massage, *n* a manual technique developed to increase blood flow to the area of the oral cavity where dentures are worn. The technique involves a moderate, pulse-squeeze movement with the index finger and the thumb over the affected region.

digitalization (dij'italizā'shən), *n* the administration of digitalis in sufficient amount by any of several types of dosage schedules to build up the concentration of digitalis glycosides in the body of a patient.

digitoxin (dij'itok'sin), *n brand names:* Crystodigin, Digitaline; *drug class:* cardia glycoside; *action:* inhibits the formation of sodium-potassium ATPase, which makes more calcium available for contractile proteins; *uses:* congestive heart failure (CHF), atrial fibrillation, paroxysmal atrial flutter, atrial tachycardia.

digoxin (dijok'sin), *n brand names:* Lanoxicaps, Lanoxin, Novadigoxin; *drug class:* cardiac glycoside; *action:* acts by inhibiting the sodium-potassium ATPase, which makes more calcium available for contractile proteins; *uses:* CHF, atrial fibrillation, atrial flutter, paroxysmal atrial tachycardia.

dihydrotachysterol (DHT) (dīhī'drōtəkis'tərol), *n brand names:* DHT Intensol, Hytakerol; *drug class:* vitamin D analog; *action:* increases intestinal absorption of calcium, increases renal tubular absorption of phosphate; *uses:* nutritional supplement, rickets, hypoparathyroidism, postoperative tetany.

dihydroxyaluminum sodium carbonate (dīhī'drok'sēəloo'mənəm), *n brand name:* Rolaids; *drug class:* antacid; *action:* neutralizes gastric acidity; *use:* antacid.

dilaceration (dīlas'ərā'shən), *n* a severe angular distortion in the root of a tooth or at the junction of the root and crown. It results from trauma during tooth development.

Dilantin enlargement, *n.pr* See hyperplasia, gingival, Dilantin.

Dilantin gingival hyperplasia, *n.pr* See hyperplasia, gingival, Dilantin.

Dilantin sodium (dīlan'tin sō'dēəm), *n.pr* the brand name for diphenylhydantoin sodium.

dilation (dīlā'shən), *n* the act of stretching or dilating.

diltiazem HCl (diltī'əzem), *n brand names:* Cardizem, Cardizem SR, Cardizem CD; *drug class:* calcium channel blocker; *action:* inhib-

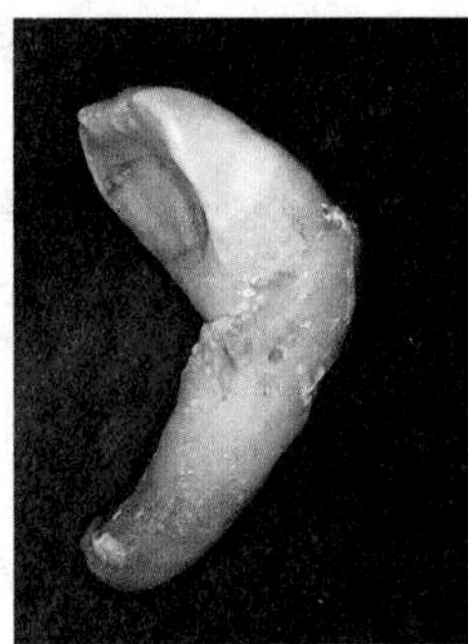

Dilaceration. (Sapp/Eversole/Wysocki, 2004)

its calcium ion influx across cell membrane during cardiac depolarization; produces relaxation of coronary vascular smooth muscle, dilates coronary arteries, slows SA/AV node conduction; *uses:* chronic stable angina pectoris, coronary artery spasm, hypertension.

diluent (dil′ūənt), *n* an agent that dilutes the strength of a solution or mixture; medication that dilutes any of the body fluids.

dilute (diloot′, dīloot′), *v* to make weaker the strength of a solution or mixture.

dimenhydrinate (dī′menhī′drināt), *n brand names:* Calm-X, Dimentabs, Dinate, Dramamine; *drug class:* antihistamine, H_1 receptor antagonist; *actions:* acts on blood vessels and gastrointestinal and respiratory systems by competing with histamine for H_1 receptor sites; decreases allergic response by blocking histamine; *uses:* motion sickness, nausea, vomiting.

dimension, vertical, *n* **1.** a vertical measurement of the face between any two arbitrarily selected points that are conveniently located one above and one below the oral cavity, usually in the midline. *n* **2.** the vertical height of the face with the teeth in occlusion or acting as stops. See also relation, vertical.

dimension, vertical, decrease, n a decrease of the vertical distance between the mandible and the maxillae by modifications of teeth or the positions of teeth or occlusion rims, or through alveolar or residual ridge resorption.

dimension, vertical, increase, n an increase of the vertical distance between the mandible and the maxillae by modifications of teeth or the positions of teeth or occlusion rims.

dimension, vertical, occlusal, n the vertical dimension of the face when the teeth or occlusion rims are in contact in centric occlusion.

dimension, vertical, rest, n the vertical dimension of the face with the jaws in the rest relation.

dimension, vertical, rest, decrease, n may or may not accompany a decrease in occlusal vertical dimension. It may occur without a decrease in occlusal vertical dimension in patients with a preponderant activity of the jaw-closing musculature, as in chronic gum chewers or patients with muscular hypertension.

dimension, vertical, rest, increase, n may or may not accompany an increase in occlusal dimension. It sometimes occurs after the removal of remaining occlusal contacts, perhaps as a result of the removal of noxious reflex stimuli.

dimensional stability, *n* See stability, dimensional.

dimethyl sulfoxide (dīmeth′əl sulfok′sīd), *n* an antiinflammatory agent and organic solvent.

dimethylbenzene (dīmeth′ilben′zēn), *n* See xylene.

diopter magnification (dīop′tər mag′nifikā′shən), *n* an optical feature that allows an enlarged, focused view of a small area.

diphenhydramine HCl (dīfenhī′drəmēn), *n brand names:* Benadryl, Sominex Formula 3; *drug class:* antihistamine, H_1 receptor antagonist; *action:* acts on blood vessels and gastrointestinal and respiratory systems by competing with histamine for H_1-receptor sites; decreases allergic response by blocking histamine; *uses:* allergy symptoms, rhinitis, motion sickness, antiparkinsonism, nighttime sedation, infant colic, nonproductive cough.

diphenoxylate HCl with atropine sulfate (dī′fenok′səlāt′ at′rəpēn sul′fāt), *n brand names:* Lofrol, Logene, Lomotil, Lonox; *drug class:* antidiarrheal (opioid with atropine) Controlled Substance Schedule V;

D

action: inhibits gastric motility by acting on muscosal receptors responsible for peristalsis; *use:* simple diarrhea.

diphenylhydantoin sodium (dīfen′ilhīdan′tōin), *n* (Dilantin sodium), a drug used for the control of convulsive grand mal and petit mal epileptic seizures; often associated with the production of a profuse gingival hyperplasia. See also phenytoin sodium.

diphtheria (difthir′ēə), *n* an acute disease caused by *C. diphtheriae* resulting in swelling of the pharynx and larynx with fever. Vaccination is available.

dipivefrin HCl (dīpiv′əfrin), *n brand name:* Propine; *drug class:* adrenergic agonist; *action:* converted to epinephrine with decreased aqueous production and increased outflow; *use:* open-angle glaucoma.

diplococci, morphologic form of (dip′lōkôk′ē môr′fəloj′ik), *n.pl* the uniformly scattered pairs of half ovals, resembling shoeprints, which are characteristic of the diplococci bacteria.

diplomate (dip′ləmāt′), *n* a dental specialist who has achieved certification by the recognized certification board in that specialty, as attested by a diploma from the board.

diplopia (diplō′pēə), *n* seeing a single object as two images. May occur after fracture of the bony orbital cavity as a result of displacement of the globe of the eye inferiorly.

dipyridamole (dīpir′idəmol′), *n brand name:* Persantine; *drug class:* platelet aggregation inhibitor; *action:* specific action unclear; inhibits ability of platelets to aggregate; *uses:* prevention of transient ischemic attacks (TIA), inhibition of platelet aggregation to prevent myocardial reinfarction, prevention of coronary bypass graft occlusion with aspirin.

dipyrone (dī′pirōn), *n* an analgesic, antiinflammatory, and antipyretic agent that is rarely used because of a high incidence of agranulocytosis.

direct (dīrekt′), *adj* relating to any restorative procedure performed directly on a tooth without the use of a die (e.g., a wax pattern formed in the prepared cavity), silver amalgam, or one of the powdered, granular, or foil golds compacted into a prepared cavity.

direct access storage device, *n* a device used for storage of direct access files. It could be a magnetic disk or diskette units.

direct billing, *n* a process whereby the dental professional bills a patient directly for his or her fees.

direct gold, *n* any of the forms of pure gold that may be compacted directly into a prepared cavity to form a restoration.

direct pulp capping, *n* See capping, pulp, direct.

direct reimbursement, *n* a self-funded program in which the individual is reimbursed based on a percentage of dollars spent for dental care provided, allowing the beneficiary to seek treatment from the dental professional of his or her choice.

direct retainer, *n* See retainer, direct.

direct retention, *n* See retention, direct.

direct supervision, *n* a circumstance of treatment in which the dental professional must be present on the premises to diagnose, authorize, and approve all work performed on the patient by the members of the dental staff.

director, *n* **1.** a person elected by shareholders at the annual meeting to establish company policies. The directors appoint the president, vice presidents, and all other operating officers. Directors decide, among other matters, if and when dividends shall be paid. **2.** the manager of an institution, office, or clinic.

directory, *n* **1.** an organized list of names, organizations, or other data bases for ease of retrieval or reference. *n* **2.** the listing of files in a computer storage system.

dirithromycin (dīrith′rōmī′sin), *n brand name:* Dynabac; *drug class:* macrolide antibiotic; *action:* binds to 50S ribosomal subunits of susceptible bacteria to inhibit bacterial growth; *uses:* treatment of secondary bacterial infection of acute bronchitis, community-acquired pneumonia, streptococcal pharyngitis, and uncomplicated skin and skin structure infections.

disability, *n* the inability to function in the normal or usual manner; examples of an outcome measure are days missing from work or lessened productivity.

disability, denial of, *n* a symptom in which patients deny the existence of a disease or disability. Denial by these patients is a nonrealistic attempt to maintain their predisease status. These patients regard ill health and disability as an imperfection, a weakness, and even a disgrace.

disaccharide (dīsak′ərīd), *n* a general term for simple carbohydrates (sugars) formed by the union of two monosaccharide molecules. Sucrose is the most common disaccharide sugar.

disarticulation (dis′ärtik′ūlā′shən), *n* the amputation or separation of joint parts, as in hemimandibulectomy, with inclusion of the condyloid process of the mandible.

disc of temporomandibular joint, *n* a plate of fibrous tissue that divides the joint into an upper and lower synovial cavity. The disc is attached to the articular capsule and moves forward with the condyle in free opening and protrusion. Also called *meniscus.* See also articulation, temporomandibular.

discharge, *v* **1.** to release; liberate; annul; unburden. To cancel a contract; to make an agreement or contract null and void. *n* **2.** a substance that exudes from an opening.

discharge, purulent, *n* See suppuration.

discharge summary, *n* the clinical notes written by the discharging physician or dental professional at the time of releasing a patient from the hospital or clinic, outlining the course of treatment, the status at release, and the postdischarge expectations and instructions.

disclosing solution, *n* a material, usually some form of dye, applied to the teeth to stain plaque on the surfaces of teeth. It is used to help patients identify plaque in their own oral cavities. See also plaque.

disclosing solution, two-tone, *n* a type that stains older plaque blue and newer plaque red.

disclosure, *n* a release of information.

disclusion (diskloo′zhən), *n* a separation of the occlusal surfaces of the teeth directly and simply by opening the jaws, or indirectly in excursions by the anterior teeth.

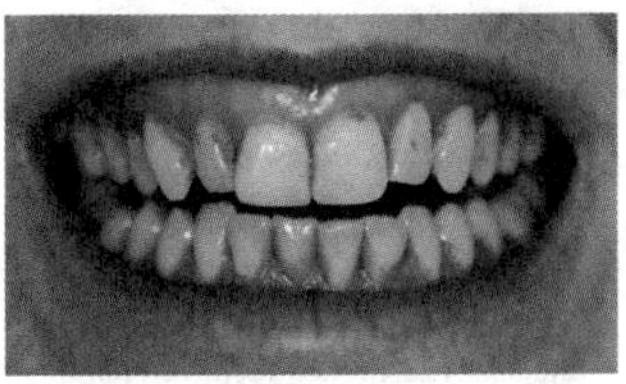

Disclosing solution. (Courtesy Dr. David Nunez)

discoid (dis′koid), *n* a carving instrument with a blade of circular form that has a cutting edge around the entire periphery.

discoloration, enamel, *n* See tetracycline.

discoloration, gingival, *n* See gingival discoloration.

discoplasty (dis′kōplas′tē), *n* the surgical shaping or contouring of the meniscus of the temporomandibular joint.

discount, *n* **1.** an allowance or deduction made from a gross sum. *v* **2.** to reduce the amount of a professional fee.

discrimination, legal, *n* a situation that leads one to treat unequally or unfairly on the basis of race, gender, national origin, religion, or handicap.

discrimination, tactile, *n* the ability to perceive two simultaneous touch stimuli; two-point discrimination. When the distance between the two stimuli is diminished to the point where only one stimulus is perceived, a value is determined for the two-point discrimination capacity of a special part. When patients are anesthetized by local agents, they have diminished tactile sense and frequently bite their lips rather severely without being aware of it. Thus patients should be instructed not to eat or chew until the "numbness" has completely gone and full tactile sense has returned.

disease(s) (dizēz′), *n* a definite deviation from the normal state characterized by a series of symptoms. Disease may be caused by developmental disturbances, genetic factors, metabolic factors, living agents, or physical, chemical, or radiant energy, or the cause may be unknown.

disease, Adams-Stokes (Adams-Stokes syndrome), *n.pr* a disease characterized by a slow and perhaps irregular pulse, vertigo, syncope, occasional pseudoepileptic convulsions, and Cheyne-Stokes respirations.

disease, adaptation (adaptation syndrome), *n* the metabolic disorders occurring as a result of adaptation or resistance to severe physical or psychologic stress. See also syndrome, general adaptation.

disease, Addison's, *n.pr* a chronic adrenocortical insufficiency caused by bilateral tuberculosis, aplasia, atrophy, or degeneration of the adrenal glands. Symptoms include severe weakness, weight loss, low blood pressure, digestive disturbances, hypoglycemia, lowered resistance to infection, and abnormal pigmentation (bronze color of the skin, with associated melanotic pigmentation of the oral mucosa, especially of the gingival tissues).

disease, adrenocortical, *n* the disorders of adrenocortical function, giving rise to Addison's disease, Cushing's syndrome, adrenogenital syndrome, and primary aldosteronism.

disease, Albers-Schönberg, *n.pr* See osteopetrosis.

disease, autoallergic, *n* See disease, autoimmune.

disease, autoimmune (autoallergic disease, autoimmunization syndrome, chronic hypersensitivity), *n* a disease that is believed to be caused in part by reactions of hypersensitivity of the host tissue (antigens). Includes various hemolytic anemias, idiopathic thrombocytopenias, rheumatoid arthritis, systemic lupus erythematosus, glomerulonephritis, scleroderma, Hashimoto's thyroiditis, and Sjögren's syndrome.

disease, Barlow's, *n.pr* See scurvy, infantile.

disease, Basedow's, *n.pr* See goiter, exophthalmic.

disease, Behçet's, *n.pr* See syndrome, Behçet's.

disease, Besnier-Boeck-Schaumann, *n.pr* See sarcoidosis.

disease, bleeder's, *n* See hemophilia.

disease, blood, *n* a disease affecting the hematologic system (e.g., anemia, leukemia, agranulocytosis purpura, infectious mononucleosis). Such a disease often results in lesions of the oral structures, particularly the mucosal surfaces.

disease, Bowen's, *n.pr* See carcinoma in situ.

disease, Brill-Symmers, *n.pr* See lymphoblastoma, giant follicular.

disease, brittle bone, *n* See osteogenesis imperfecta.

disease, Caffey's, *n.pr* See hyperostosis, infantile cortical.

disease, Cannon's, *n.pr* See nevus, white sponge.

disease, cardiac, *n* a disease affecting the heart.

disease, cat-scratch, *n* a granulomatous disease caused by *B. henselae* that occurs at the site of a scratch or bite of a house cat. Local lesions occur at the site of injury with a regional adenitis that is out of proportion to the primary lesion occurring within 1 to 3 weeks. Systemic symptoms of infection may occur. Diagnosis is confirmed by serologic tests.

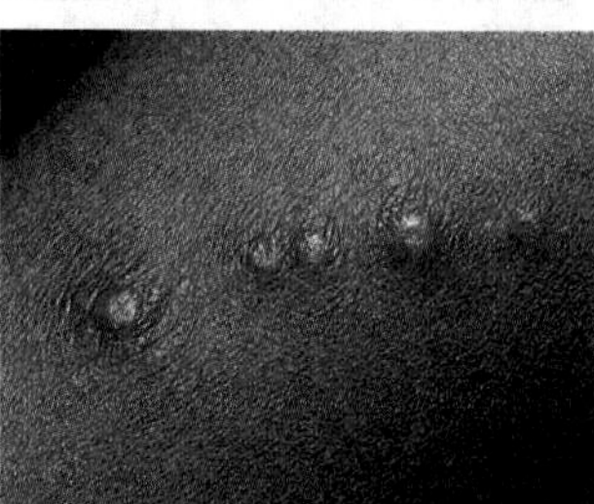

Cat-scratch disease. (Zitelli/Davis, 2002)

disease, celiac, *n* See celiac sprue.

disease, Cheadle's, *n.pr* See scurvy, infantile.

disease, Christmas, *n.pr* See hemophilia B.

disease, chronic hypersensitivity, *n* See disease, autoimmune.

disease, chronic obstructive pulmonary (COPD), *n* a disease marked by decreased expiratory flow rates resulting in increased total lung capacity. Patients with this condition are prone to acute respiratory failure from infections or general anesthesia.

disease, collagen (group disease, vis-

ceral angiitis) **(kol′əjin),** *n* a group of diseases affecting the collagenous connective tissue of several organs and systems. These diseases have similar biochemical structural alterations and include rheumatic fever, scleroderma, rheumatoid arthritis, systemic lupus erythematosus, periarteritis, and serum sickness.

diseases, communicable, *n* a disease that may be transmitted directly or indirectly to a well person or animal from an infected person or animal. A disease with the capacity for maintenance by natural modes of spread (e.g., by contact, by airborne routes, through drinking water or food, by arthropod vectors).

disease, congenital, *n* a disease present at birth, or, more specifically, one that is acquired in utero.

disease, Coxsackie A, *n.pr* See herpangina.

disease, Crouzon, *n.pr* See syndrome, Crouzon.

disease, Cushing's, *n.pr* hypercortisolism that results from an adrenal or pituitary neoplasm. The term *Cushing's syndrome* refers to hypercortisolism that is not related to an endogenous process.

disease, cytomegalic inclusion, generalized, *n* See disease, salivary gland.

disease, Darier's (keratosis follicularis), *n.pr* an apparently genetic dermatologic disease that also involves mucous membranes. The oral lesions are whitish papules of the gingiva, tongue, or palate. It is characterized histologically by the presence of corps ronds.

disease, deficiency, *n* a disturbance produced by lack of nutritional or metabolic factors. Used mainly in reference to avitaminosis.

disease, degenerative joint, *n* See osteoarthritis.

disease, dermatologic, *n* a disease affecting the skin; often accompanied by pathologic manifestations of various mucosal surfaces (e.g., the oral mucosa, genital mucosa, conjunctiva).

disease, end-stage, *n* the last phase of an illness, at which point the patient's life is gravely endangered.

disease, Engman's, *n.pr* See dermatitis infectiosa eczematoides.

disease, exanthematous **(eg′zanthē′mətəs),** *n* a group of diseases caused by a number of viruses but having as a prominent feature a skin rash (e.g., smallpox, chickenpox, cowpox, measles, rubella).

disease, familial, *n* a disease occurring in several members of the same family. Often used to mean members of the same generation and occasionally used synonymously with hereditary disease.

disease, Feer's, *n.pr* See erythredema polyneuropathy and acrodynia.

disease, fibrocystic (mucoviscidosis) **(fī′brōsis′tik mū′kōvis′idō′sis),** *n* a hereditary defect of most of the exocrine glands in the body, including the salivary glands. The secretion of the affected mucous glands is abnormally viscous.

disease, fifth, *n* a viral infection caused by the human parvovirus B19; spread via the upper respiratory tract, this virus impacts on children more strongly than adults. Also called *erythema infectiosum.*

disease, Fordyce's, *n.pr* See Fordyce granules.

disease, functional, *n* a disease that has no observable or demonstrable cause.

disease, Gaucher's **(gôshāz′),** *n.pr* a constitutional defect in the metabolism of the cerebroside kerasin. This glycoprotein accumulates in the reticuloendothelial system and leads to splenomegaly, hepatomegaly, lymph node enlargement, and bone defects.

disease, graft-versus-host (GVHD), *n* a potentially deadly condition resulting from allogenically transplanted hematopoietic cells that reject host cells in the transplant recipient. In early stages, this condition may result in lichenoid and erosive lesions on the oral mucosa.

disease, Graves', *n.pr* See goiter, exophthalmic.

disease, hand-foot-and-mouth (aphthous fever, epidemic stomatitis, epizootic stomatitis) **(af′thəs),** *n* primarily a disease of animals caused by a filterable virus that may be transmitted to humans and that occasionally produces symptoms. The human form is characterized by fever, nausea, vomiting, malaise, and ulcer-

D

ative stomatitis. Skin lesions consisting of vesicles may appear, usually on the palms of the hands and soles of the feet. Spontaneous regression usually occurs within 2 weeks.

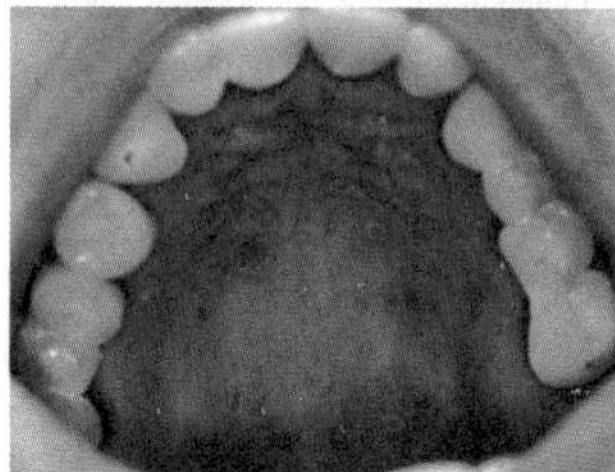

Hand, foot, and mouth disease. (Regezi/Sciubba/Pogrel, 2000)

disease, Hand-Schüller-Christian (chronic disseminated histiocytosis X), *n.pr* a type of cholesterol lipoidosis characterized clinically by defects in membranous bones, exophthalmos, and diabetes insipidus.

disease, Hansen's, *n.pr* See leprosy.

disease, heart, *n* an abnormal condition of the heart (organic, mechanical, or functional) that causes difficulty.

disease, heart, arteriosclerotic, *n* a variety of functional changes of the myocardium that result from arteriosclerosis.

disease, heart, congenital, *n* a defective formation of the heart or of the major vessels of the heart.

disease, heart, ischemic **(iskē′mik),** *n* a heart condition in which an inadequate supply of oxygenated blood reaches the heart, resulting in damage to the heart muscle; it is usually caused by atherosclerosis, a buildup of fatty plaque deposits in the main coronary arteries that leads to narrowing or hardening of the arteries. Symptoms include chest pain or discomfort (angina pectoris), ventricular fibrillation, heart attack (myocardial infarction), or sudden death. Also known as *coronary artery disease* and *coronary heart disease.*

disease, heart, rheumatic, *n* a scarring of the endocardium resulting from involvement in acute rheumatic fever. The process most often involves the mitral valve.

disease, heart, thyrotoxic **(thī′rōtok′sik),** *n* cardiac failure occurring as the result of hyperthyroidism or its superimposition on existing organic heart disease. Thyrotoxicosis is an important cause of auricular fibrillation.

disease, hemoglobin C, *n* a disease resulting from an abnormal hemoglobin (hemoglobin C); occurs primarily in African Americans and causes a mild normochromic anemia, target cells, and vague, intermittent arthralgia.

disease, hemolytic, of newborn, *n* a hemolysis caused by isoimmune reactions associated with Rh incompatibility or with blood transfusions in which there is an incompatibility of the ABO blood system. Several forms of the disease occur: erythroblastosis fetalis, congenital hemolytic disease, icterus gravis neonatorum, and hydrops fetalis.

disease, hemophilioid **(hēməfil′ēoid),** *n* a hemophilic states (conditions) that clinically resemble hemophilia (e.g., parahemophila, hemophilia B [Christmas disease]).

disease, hemorrhagic, of newborn **(hem′əraj′ik),** *n* a hemorrhagic tendency in newborn infants occurring usually on the third or fourth day of life; believed to be caused by defects of prothrombin and factor VII, resulting from a deficiency of vitamin K.

disease, hereditary, *n* a disease transmitted from parent to offspring through genes. Three main types of mendelian heredity are recognized: dominant, recessive, and sex-linked.

disease, hidebound, *n* See scleroderma.

disease, Hodgkin, *n.pr* See lymphoma, Hodgkin.

disease, hypersensitivity, *n* See disease, autoimmune.

disease, iatrogenic **(īat′rəjen′ik),** *n* a disease arising as a result of the actions or words of a health care professional.

disease, idiopathic **(id′ēōpath′ik),** *n* a disease in which the etiology is not recognized or determined.

disease, infectious, *n* the pathologic alterations induced in the tissues by the action of microorganisms and/or their toxins. Some infectious diseases involving the oral tissues are herpes zoster, herpetic gingivostomatitis, moniliasis, syphilis, and tuberculosis.

disease, inflammatory neoplastic, *n* See granuloma; tumor, inflammatory.

disease, kissing, *n* See mononucleosis, infectious.

disease, Langerhans cell (Langerhans cell histiocytosis), *n* a group of three diseases identified by an abundance of Langerhans cells—eosinophils combined with histiocytic cells. See also disease, Letterer-Siwe; disease, Hand-Schüller-Christian; and granuloma, eosinophili.

disease, Letterer-Siwe **(sē′vā),** *n.pr* (acute disseminated histiocytosis X, nonlipid histiocytosis, nonlipid reticuloendotheliosis), a fatal febrile disease of unknown cause occurring in infants and children; characterized by focal granulomatous lesions of the lymph nodes, spleen, and bone marrow. Results in enlargement of the lymph nodes, spleen, and liver, defects of the flat and long bones, anemia, and sometimes purpura.

disease, lipoid storage (lipoidosis, reticuloendothelial granuloma) **(lip′oid ritik′yəlōen′dōthē′lēəl gran′yəlō′mə lipoidō′sis),** *n* group of diseases in which lipid substances accumulate in the fixed cells of the reticuloendothelial system. Included are Gaucher's disease, Niemann-Pick disease, and the Hand-Schüller-Christian disease complex. Other storage diseases include lipochondrodystrophy (gargoylism) and cerebral sphingolipidosis.

disease, Lobstein's, *n.pr* See osteogenesis imperfecta.

disease, macrovascular, *n* a disease of the large blood vessels, including the aorta, and coronary arteries. Fatty plaque buildup and thrombosis formation in these vessels may lead to a myocardial infarction, cerebral infarction, and circulation problems in the limbs. It is often a complication of long-term diabetes.

disease, Marie's, *n.pr* See acromegaly.

disease, Mediterranean, *n.pr* See thalassemia major.

disease, metabolic bone, *n.pl* the diseases of the bone which may be attributed to cellular changes or to nutritional deficiencies/excesses brought on by dietary imbalances. These include hyperparathyroidism, osteoporosis, osteomalacia, rickets, and the many diseases associated with an abnormal abundance of Langerhans cells.

disease, Mikulicz' **(mik′ūlich′əz),** *n.pr* a benign hyperplasia of the lymph nodes of the parotid or other salivary glands and/or the lacrimal glands.

disease, Moeller's, *n.pr* See scurvy, infantile.

disease, molecule, *n* a disease associated with genetically determined abnormalities of protein synthesis at the molecular level.

disease, muscle, *n* the pathologic muscle tissue changes that can lead to disease. Such changes reveal few structural alterations, and the highly differentiated contents of muscle fibers tend to react as a whole. The pathologic features that distinguish one muscle disease from another are the age and character of changes within a muscle, distribution of those changes within one or several muscles, presence of inflammatory cells and parasites, and coexistence of pathologic changes in other organs. Muscles undergo a number of degenerative changes. There are alterations in the striation in certain pathologic states caused by cloudy swelling, granular degeneration, waxy or hyaline degeneration, and other cellular modifications such as multiplication of the sarcolemmic nuclei and phagocytosis of muscle fibers.

disease, neuromuscular, *n* a condition in which various areas of the central nervous system are affected; results in dysfunction or degeneration of the musculature and disabilities of the organ.

disease, Niemann-Pick **(nē′män),** *n.pr* a congenital, familial disorder occurring mainly in Jewish female infants that terminates fatally before the third year and is characterized by the accumulation of the phospholipid sphingomyelin in the cells of the reticuloendothelial system.

disease, oral, hereditary, *n* the heritable defects of oral and paraoral structures (excluding the dentition) without generalized defects; includes ankyloglossia, hereditary gingivofi-

D

bromatosis, and possibly cleft lip and cleft palate. Many oral and paraoral defects are associated with generalized defects (e.g., Peutz-Jeghers, Franceschetti, Ehlers-Danlos, Pierre Robin, and Sturge-Weber syndromes; hemorrhagic telangiectasia; Crouzon's disease; sickle cell disease; acatalasemia; white spongy nevus; xeroderma pigmentosum; gargoylism; neurofibromatosis; familial amyloidosis; and achondroplasia).

disease, oral manifestations of systemic, *n* the lesions in association with systemic disease, often influenced by the local environmental factors within the oral cavity.

disease, organic, *n* a disease in which actual structural changes have occurred in the organs or tissues.

disease, Osler's, *n.pr* See erythremia.

disease, Owren's, *n.pr* See parahemophilia.

disease, Paget's, of bone (osteitis deformans), *n.pr* a bone disease characterized by thickening and bowing of the long bones and enlargement of the skull and maxillae. It is represented radiographically by a cotton-wool appearance of the bone and microscopically by a mosaic bone pattern with so-called reversal lines. Hypercementosis and loosening of the teeth may be significant manifestations. Increased serum alkaline phosphatase may be an early finding.

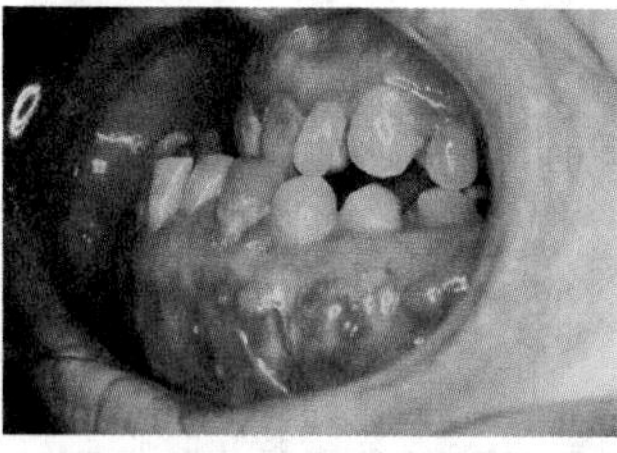

Paget's disease of the bone. (Regezi/Sciubba/Jordan, 2008)

disease, Parkinson's, *n.pr* a progressive neurologic disorder for which there is no known cure that is thought to be the result of neuron degeneration in the section of the brain controlling spontaneous movement and balance. The disease causes postural changes, tremors, muscle rigidity, and weakness. Oral manifestations include difficulty in swallowing and excess salivation.

disease, periodic, *n* See disorder(s), periodic.

disease, periodontal **(per′ēōdon′təl),** *n* a disturbance of the periodontium. Diseases affecting the periodontium include aggressive and necrotizing types, as well as gingivitis. Etiologic factors may be local or systemic or may involve an interplay between the two. Periodontal diseases may be involved in increasing the risk and course of systemic diseases.

disease, periodontal, etiologic factors of, *n.pl* the local and systemic factors, singly or in combination, that initiate periodontal lesions.

disease, periodontal, local factors of, *n.pl* the environmental conditions within the oral cavity that initiate, enable, or alter the course of diseases of the periodontium (e.g., calculus, diastemata between teeth, food impaction, prematurities in the centric path of closure, and tongue habits).

disease, peripheral vascular, *n* a disease of arteries, veins, and/or lymphatic vessels.

disease, pink, *n* See acrodynia.

disease, Pott's, *n.pr* a spinal curvature (kyphosis) resulting from tuberculosis.

disease progression, *n* the course of the disease within a patient/host from onset to resolution.

disease, psychosomatic **(sī′kōsōmat′ik),** *n* a disease that appears to have been precipitated or prolonged by emotional stress; manifested largely through the autonomic nervous system. Various conditions may be included (e.g., certain forms of asthma, dermatosis, migraine headache, and hypertension). See also disorder, psychophysiologic, autonomic, and visceral.

disease, Quincke's, *n.pr* See edema, angioneurotic.

disease, Rendu-Osler-Weber **(ron′doo),** *n.pr* See telangiectasia, hereditary hemorrhagic.

disease, rheumatic, *n* See rheumatism.

disease, rickettsial **(riket′sēəl),** *n* a disease caused by microorganisms of the order Rickettsiales (e.g., Rocky Mountain spotted fever, rickettsialpox, typhus, and Q fever).

disease, Riga-Fede **(rē′gə-fā′də),** an ulceration of the lingual frenum of infants caused by abrasion by natal or neonatal teeth.

disease, Sainton's, *n.pr* See dysplasia, cleidocranial.

disease, salivary gland (generalized cytomegalic inclusion), *n* a generalized infection in infants caused by intrauterine or postnatal infection with a cytomegalovirus of the group of herpesviruses. Manifestations include jaundice, purpura, hemolytic anemia, vomiting, diarrhea, chronic eczema, and failure to gain weight.

disease, Schüller's **(shü′lerz),** *n.pr* See osteoporosis.

disease, Selter's, *n.pr* See acrodynia.

disease, sex-linked, *n* a hereditary disorder transmitted by the gene that also determines sex (e.g., hemophilia).

disease, sickle cell, *n* a hematologic disorder caused by the presence of an abnormal hemoglobin (hemoglobin S) that permits the formation or results in the formation of sickle-shaped red blood cells. Two forms of the disease occur: sickle cell trait and sickle cell anemia. See also anemia, sickle cell; trait, sickle cell.

disease, Simmonds' (pituitary cachexia, hypophyseal cachexia, hypopituitary cachexia), *n.pr* a panhypopituitarism resulting from destruction of the pituitary gland, usually from hemorrhage or infarction.

disease, Sturge-Weber-Dimitri (encephalotrigeminal angiomatosis), *n.pr* See angiomatosis, Sturge-Weber.

disease susceptibility, *n* the degree to which a patient or host is vulnerable to a disease.

disease, Sutton's, *n.pr* See periadenitis mucosa necrotica recurrens.

disease, Swift's, *n.pr* See acrodynia.

disease, systemic, *n* a disease involving the whole body.

disease, Takahara's **(tä′kəhä′rəz),** *n.pr* a form of rare progressive oral gangrene occurring in childhood and seen only in Japan. Apparently related to a congenital lack of the enzyme catalase (acatalasemia). Characterized by a mild to severe form of a peculiar type of oral gangrene that may develop at the roots of the teeth or the tonsils. Loss of teeth occurs, with necrosis of the alveolar bone. Patients become symptom free after puberty.

disease, transmissible, *n* a disease capable of being transmitted from one individual to another; a disease capable of being maintained in successive passages through a susceptible host, usually under experimental conditions such as by injection. See also disease, communicable.

disease transmission, *n* the method by which a disease is passed from one patient or host to another. The three most common methods of transmission are direct contact, aerosols, and vectors, such as insects.

disease, Vaquez' **(väkēz′),** *n.pr* See erythremia.

disease vectors, *n.pl* the intermediary hosts that carry the disease from one species to another, such as mosquitoes, ticks, and rabid animals.

disease, von Recklinghausen's, *n.pr* See hyperparathyroidism; osteitis; generalized fibrosa cystica; and neurofibromatosis.

disease, von Recklinghausen's, of bone **(fōn rek′linghouzenz),** *n.pr* See hyperparathyroidism; osteitis fibrosa cystica.

disease, von Recklinghausen's, of skin, *n.pr* See neurofibromatosis.

disease, von Willebrand's **(fōn vil′ebränts),** *n.pr* an inherited blood coagulation disorder attributed to a deficiency or malfunction of factor VIII. It may cause prolonged or excessive gingival bleeding.

disease, Weil's (epidemic jaundice) **(vīlz),** *n.pr* an acute febrile disease caused by *Leptospira icterohaemorrhagiae* or *L. canicola.* Manifestations include fever, petechial hemorrhage, myalgia, renal insufficiency, hepatic failure, and jaundice.

disease, Werlhof's **(verl′hofs),** *n.pr* See purpura, thrombocytopenic.

diseases, demyelinating **(dēmī′elənā′ting),** *n* the diseases that have in common a loss of myelin sheath, with preservation of the axis cylinders (e.g., multiple sclerosis, Schilder's disease).

diseases, dental, hereditary, *n.pl* the heritable defects of the dentition without generalized disease, which

D

include amelogenesis imperfecta, dentinogenesis imperfecta, dentinal dysplasia, localized and generalized hypoplasia of enamel, peg-shaped lateral incisors, familial dentigerous cysts, missing teeth, giantism, and fused primary mandibular incisors. Dental defects occurring with generalized disease include dentinogenesis imperfecta with osteogenesis imperfecta, missing teeth with ectodermal dysplasia, enamel hypoplasia with epidermolysis bullosa dystrophica, retarded eruption with cleidocranial dysostosis, missing lateral incisors with ptosis of the eyelids, missing premolars with premature whitening of the hair, and enamel hypoplasia in vitamin D–resistant rickets.

diseases, group, *n* See disease, collagen.

disharmony, occlusal (əkloo′səl), *n* a phenomenon in which contacts of opposing occlusal surfaces of teeth are not in harmony with other tooth contacts and with the anatomic and physiologic controls of the mandible. See also contact, deflective occlusal; contact, interceptive occlusal; and malocclusion.

disinfect (dis′infekt′), *v* to destroy pathogenic microorganisms.

disinfectant (dis′infek′tənt), *n* a chemical intended to destroy most pathogenic microorganisms. Does not cause sterilization.

disinfectant, alcohol, *n* an unaccepted method of sterilization. Although ethanol and isopropanol both have cleansing properties when used on the skin, they are insufficient as sterilizers.

disinfectant, chlorine dioxide, *n* a chemical disinfectant that can be used for 24 hours once it is activated. It can corrode some steel tools.

disinfectant holding solution, *n* an antimicrobial liquid into which an object can be temporarily placed while awaiting sterilization.

disinfection, *n* the process of destroying pathogenic organisms or rendering them inert.

disinfection, full oral cavity, *n* a procedure used to reduce active periodontal disease, usually completed within a certain short time frame.

disintegration, induced nuclear, *n* the disintegration resulting from artificial bombardment of a material with high-energy particles such as alpha particles, deuterons, protons, neutrons, or gamma rays.

disintegration, nuclear, *n* a spontaneous nuclear transformation (radioactivity) characterized by the emission of energy or mass from the nucleus. When numbers of nuclei are involved, the process is characterized by a definite half-life.

disk, *n* a thin, flat, circular object.

disk, abrasive, *n* a disk with abrasive particles attached to one or both of its surfaces or its edge.

disk, diamond, *n* a disk of steel with diamond chips bonded to its surface.

disk, garnet, *n* a disk with particles of garnet as the abrading medium.

disk, Joe Dandy, *n.pr* the brand name for a separating disk. See also disk, separating.

disk, lightning, *n* a steel separating disk.

disk, Merkel's, *n.pr* See corpuscle, Merkel's.

disk, pack, *n* a set of circular magnetic surfaces mounted coaxially on a shaft for computer storage of files. Can be used for storage of serial or direct access files.

disk, polishing, *n* a disk with an extremely fine abrasive; used to finish and polish a surface.

disk, safe-side, *n* a separating disk with abrasive on one side only; the other side is smooth.

disk, sandpaper, *n* an abrasive disk with sandpaper as the abrading medium.

disk, separating, *n* a disk of steel or hard rubber.

disk, storage, *n* a storage device that uses magnetic recording on flat, rotating disks.

disking, *v* the act of grinding or reducing the superficial surface of the tooth with an abrasive material.

dislocation, *n* the displacement of any part, especially a bone or bony articulation.

dislodgment, *n* the movement or removal of a prosthesis from its established position.

disopyramide (dīsōpir′əmīd′), *n brand name:* Norpace CR; *drug class:* antidysrhythmic (Class IA); *action:* prolongs action potential duration and effective refractory period;

uses: PVCs, ventricular tachycardia, atrial flutter, atrial fibrillation.

disorder(s), *n* derangement of function.

disorder, bipolar, *n* a major mood disorder characterized by alternating periods of mania or elation and depression. Formerly called *manic-depressive disorder.*

disorder, body dysmorphic (BBD) (dismôr′fik), *n* a mental disorder in which an otherwise physiologically healthy person obsesses about an imaginary physical defect.

disorder(s), coagulation, *n* any one of the hemorrhagic diseases caused by a deficiency of plasma thromboplastin formation (deficiency of antihemophilic factor, plasma thromboplastic antecedent, Hageman factor, Stuart factor), deficiency of thrombin formation (deficiency of prothrombin, factor V, factor VII, Stuart factor), and deficiency of fibrin formation (afibrinogenemia, fibrinogenopenia).

disorder, conversion, *n* uncontrolled change or loss of control of physical function due to a mental, not physical, need or conflict.

disorder, cumulative trauma, *n* a disorder of the musculature and skeleton after repetitive strain injuries to muscles, tendons, joints, bones, and nerves.

disorder, panic, *n* a disorder marked by repeated panic attacks and fear, which interrupts normal functioning.

disorder(s), periodic, *n.pl* a variety of disorders of unknown cause that have in common periodic recurrence of manifestations. Such disorders are usually benign, resist treatment, often begin in infancy, and occasionally have a hereditary pattern. Included are periodic sialorrhea, neutropenia, arthralgia, fever, purpura (anaphylactoid purpura), edema (angioneurotic edema), abdominalgia, and periodic parotitis (recurrent parotitis).

disorder, pervasive developmental, *n* a disorder of behavioral and sensory impairment that generally appears during infancy or early childhood and continues to affect the individual's ability to communicate and interact with others throughout his or her life. See also autism.

disorder(s), platelet, *n.pl* a hemorrhagic disease caused by an abnormality of the blood platelets (e.g., thrombocytopenia, thrombasthenia).

disorder, posttraumatic stress, *n* a condition characterized by acute or recurring anxiety which has been brought about as the result of experiencing a traumatic event, such as a natural disaster, automobile accident, terrorist attack, military combat, rape, physical torture, or childhood sexual abuse. Symptoms may include flashbacks, nightmares, mild to severe depression, and panic attacks.

disorder(s), psychophysiologic, autonomic, and visceral, *n* the standard psychiatric nomenclature for what are commonly known as psychomotor disorders. The disorders are disturbances of visceral function, secondary to chronic attitude and long-continued reaction to stress. These disorders may occur in any organ innervated by the autonomic nervous system, since overactivity or underactivity of that system as a result of stress appears to trigger the disorder. See also disease, psychosomatic.

disorder(s), visual, *n.pl* disorders that may result from injury or disease to the eyeball and its adnexa, the retina, or the cornea (e.g., contusions of the orbit and eyelids, opacities of the lens, corneal scars, vascular changes to the retina). These peripheral disorders are effective in causing partial or total loss of vision in one or both eyes. They are simple, concrete, and fundamental. One sees or one does not see, and gray visions are generally quantitative differences that affect the perception of light and shadow and color and form. They may also result from injury or disease to the optic tract fibers, optic chiasma, cerebral pathways, and visual cortex in the occipital region of the cerebrum. These are qualitative deviations from normal, and the symptoms include visual field defects such as tubular vision found in hysteria, complete blindness in one or both eyes as a result of optic nerve injury, and hemianopsia, in which vision may be lost in one half of the visual field of one or both eyes. Others include night and day blindness, color blindness, and the serious visual agnosia that results from trauma, tumor, or vascular disorders in the visual cortex of the cerebrum.

disorder(s), cognitive impairment, n.pl the mental disorders distinguished by a limitation of mental functions (e.g., memory, comprehension, and judgment).

D

disorder(s), dissociative, n.pl the mental disorders distinguished by the psychologically induced, distinct partition of separate mental functions from normal behavior or consciousness (e.g., dissociative amnesia and depersonalization disorder).

disorder(s), factitious **(faktish′əs),** *n.pl* the mental disorders distinguished by the self-induced creation of artificial physical or mental symptoms to assume the role of a sick individual.

disorder(s), feeding, n.pl conditions distinguished by an inability to eat sufficiently, a continual need to consume abnormal items of food or substances lacking nutrients, or frequent vomiting episodes without any indications of a gastrointestinal infection.

disorder(s), impulse control, n.pl the mental disorders distinguished by an uncontrollable tendency to commit an unplanned behavior (e.g., pathologic gambling, kleptomania, and pyromania).

disorder(s), sexual, n.pl disorders of sexual performance or desire, which may include sexual dysfunction, feelings of discomfort about one's gender, and perverse sexual urges or activities. Also called paraphilia.

disorder(s), sleep, n.pl conditions characterized by a disruption in normal sleeping patterns, which may be the result of serious medical conditions, including breathing difficulties or thyroid disorders, or external factors such as stress or substance abuse. Manifestations include insomnia, sleep apnea, and narcolepsy.

disorder(s), somatoform **(sō′matəform′),** *n.pl* disorders characterized by symptoms that seem to suggest the presence of an illness, but for which there is no physical proof. Often may be attributed to unresolved emotional conflicts. Types include conversion disorder, hypochondriasis, body dysmorphic disorder, and pain disorder.

disorder(s), substance-related, n.pl conditions or illnesses that may be directly attributed to overuse of drugs, alcohol, nicotine, or caffeine and may also include nutritional deficiencies, cardiovascular disease, oral lesions, liver disease, and sleep disorders.

disorder(s), tic, n.pl conditions characterized by involuntary and sometimes violent muscle spasms, including Tourette's syndrome and chronic motor or vocal tic disorders.

disprove, *v* to refute or to prove false by affirmative evidence to the contrary.

dissection, neck, *n* the removal of the lymph nodes and contiguous tissues from a primary site in the mandibular or maxillofacial area as treatment of neoplastic cells that have involved the regional cervical lymphatic system.

disseminated intravascular coagulation (DIC) (disem′ənātəd in′trəvas′kyələr kōag′yəlā′shən), *n* a grave coagulopathy resulting from the overstimulation of clotting and anticlotting processes in response to disease or injury, such as septicemia, acute hypotension, poisonous snake bites, neoplasms, and severe trauma.

dissociation, *n* the psychologically induced, distinct partition of separate mental functions (e.g., identity, memory, and awareness) from normal behavior or consciousness.

dissociative fugue (fūg), *n* a sudden departure from a home or workplace without any ability to recall personal history or identity.

dissolve, *v* to terminate, cancel, annul, disintegrate. To release the obligation of anything, as to dissolve a partnership.

distal (dis′təl), *adj* away from the median sagittal plane of the face and following the curvature of the dental arch.

distal end, adj the most posterior part of a removable dental restoration or denture flange.

distance, *n* the measure of space intervening between two objects or two points of reference.

distance, cone, n the distance between the focal spot and the outer end of the cone; usually expressed in inches or centimeters. Modern dental roentgen-ray units usually have cone distances of from 5 to 20 inches (12.5 to 50 cm).

distance, interarch (interridge distance), n the vertical distance between the maxillary and mandibular arches under conditions of vertical relations that must be specified.

distance, interocclusal (interocclusal gap, free-way space), n the distance between the occluding surfaces of the maxillary and mandibular teeth when the mandible is in its physiologic rest position. This can be determined by calculating the difference between the rest vertical dimension and the occlusal vertical dimension of the face.

distance, interridge, n See distance, interarch.

distance, large interarch, n a large distance between the maxillary and mandibular arches.

distance, long (extended) cone, n the distance is usually 14 to 20 inches (35 to 50 cm). See also cone, long.

distance, object-film, n the distance, usually expressed in centimeters or inches, between the object being radiographed and the cassette or film.

distance, operator, n See positions at the chair.

distance, short cone, n a focal-skin distance of 9 inches (22.5 cm) or less; usually refers to the distance as determined by the cone supplied by the manufacturer of the basic radiograph unit.

distance, small interarch, n a small distance between the maxillary and mandibular arches.

distance, target-film (anode-film distance, focal-film distance), n the distance between the focal spot of the tube and the film; usually expressed in inches or centimeters.

distention, *n* a state of dilation.

distoclusion (dis′tōkloo′zhən), *n* the mandibular teeth occluding distal to their normal relationship to the maxillary teeth, as in an Angle Class II malocclusion. It can present either bilaterally or unilaterally.

distomolar (dis′tōmō′lər), *n* a supernumerary (fourth) molar located posterior to the third molar.

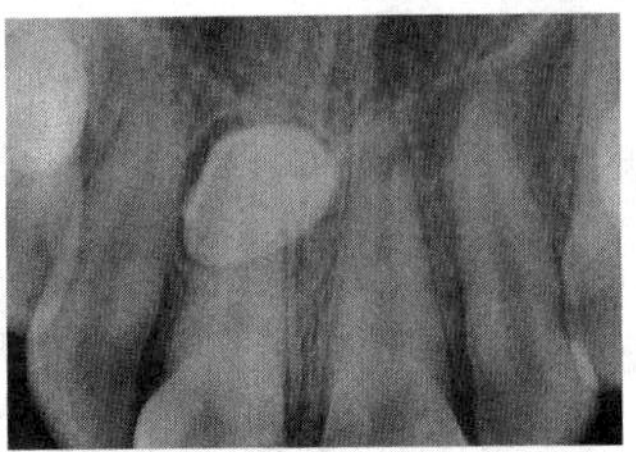

Distomolar. (Courtesy Dr. Charles Babbush)

distortion, *n* **1.** a deviation from the normal shape or condition. *n* **2.** a modification of the speech sound in some way so that the acoustic result only approximates the standard sound and is not accurate. *n* **3.** a twisting or deformation. A loss of accuracy in reproduction of cavity form.

distortion, film-fault, n an imperfection in the size or shape of a film image by either magnification, elongation, or foreshortening.

distortion, horizontal, n a disproportional change in size and shape of the image in the horizontal plane as a result of oblique horizontal angulation of the radiographic beam.

distortion, magnification, n a proportional enlargement of a radiographic image. It is always present to some degree in oral radiography but is minimized with extended focal-film distances.

distortion, vertical (foreshortening), n a disproportional change in size, either elongation or foreshortening, caused by incorrect vertical angulation or improper film placement.

distoversion (dis′tōver′zhən), *n* the placement of a tooth farther than normal from the median plane or midline.

distraction, *n* the placement of teeth or other maxillary or mandibular structures farther than normal from the median plane.

distraction osteogenesis (DO) (distrak′shən os′tēəjen′isis), *n* a surgical process in which two bony segments are gradually separated so new soft tissue and bone will form between them. There are three periods to this process: latency, distraction, and consolidation.

D

disturbances, occlusal, *n.pl* the derangements in the patterns of occlusion.

disulfiram (dīsul′fəram′), *n brand name:* Antabuse; *drug class:* aldehyde dehydrogenase inhibitor; *action:* blocks oxidation of alcohol at acetaldehyde stage; *uses:* chronic alcoholism (as adjunct).

ditch (ditching), *n* the undesirable loss of tooth substance in the region of a restoration margin (usually gingival).

ditching, *n* See ditch.

diuretic (dī′yəret′ik), *n* **1.** a drug that increases the formation of urine. *adj* **2.** pertaining to the increased formation of urine. Used mainly in the initial treatment of hypertension (high blood pressure).

diuretic, loop, *n* a high-potency therapeutic agent used to control hypertension by exerting influence on the loop of Henle in order to facilitate the removal of surplus water and sodium from the body. See furosemide.

diurnal (dīur′nəl), *adj* relating to or happening in the daytime or portion of the day that is light.

diverticulitis, *n* an inflammatory pouching of the intestinal wall.

dizziness, *n* a sensation of faintness or an inability to maintain normal balance in a standing or seated position. A patient who experiences it should be carefully lowered to a safe position on a bed, chair, or floor because of the danger of injury from falling. See also syncope.

DMF index rate, *n* See rate, DMF index.

DNA, *n* an acronym for deoxyribonucleic acid. A type of nucleic acid that contains genetic instructions for the development of cellular life forms. Capable of replicating itself and of producing another type of nucleic acid known as RNA.

DNA, bacterial, *n* the DNA specific to a bacterial strain.

DNA fingerprinting, *n* the use of DNA analysis to identify a subject from blood or other suitable tissue.

DNA probe, *n* See deoxyribonucleic acid probes.

DO cavity, *n* a cavity on the distal and occlusal surfaces of a tooth. See also cavity, Class 2.

doctor, *n* a learned person; one qualified in a science or art; one who has received the highest academic degree in a particular field. See also dentist and physician.

documentation, *n* the permanent recording of information properly identified as to time, place, circumstances, and attribution.

docusate calcium/docusate potassium/docusate sodium (dok′usāt), *n brand names:* Colace, Correctol Extra Gentle, Sulfalax; *drug class:* laxative; *action:* increases water, fat penetration in intestine; allows for easier passage of stool; *uses:* stool softener.

dolichocephalic (dol′ikōsəfal′ik), *adj* pertaining to a long and narrow head (with a cephalic index below 75).

dolor (dō′lôr), *n* pain.

donor site, *n* the portion of the body from which an organ or tissue is removed for transplant or grafting.

donor tissue, *n* the tissue contributed by a donor to be used in tissue or organ transplant.

dopa (dō′pə), *n* an amino acid derived from tyrosine that occurs naturally in plants and animals. It is a precursor of dopamine, epinephrine, and norepinephrine.

dopamine (dō′pəmēn′), *n* a sympathomimetic catecholamine used in the treatment of shock, hypotension, and low cardiac output.

dope, *n* a colloquial term denoting a drug taken temporarily or habitually without medical cause and that is intended to alter mood.

dornase alfa (dor′nās al′fə), *n brand name:* Pulmozyme; *drug class:* recombinant human deoxyribonuclease (DNase); *action:* reduces sputum viscosity; *uses:* cystic fibrosis; reduces incidence of pulmonary infection, improves pulmonary function.

dorsal (dôr′səl), *adj* pertaining to the back or to the posterior part of an organ.

dorsum sellae (dôr′səm sel′ē), *n* the most posterior point on the internal contour of the sella turcica.

dosage (dō′səj), *n* the amount of a medicine or other agent administered for a given case or condition.

dose, *n* **1.** the quantity of drug necessary to produce a desired effect. *n* **2.** the total radiation delivered to a specified area or volume or to the whole body. See also dose, radiation-absorbed.

dose, absorbed (D), *n* the amount of energy imparted by ionizing particles to unit mass of irradiated material at a place of interest. The unit of absorbed dose is the rad (100 ergs/Gm).

dose, air, *n* a radiographic dose delivered at a point in free air; expressed in roentgens. It consists only of the radiation of the primary beam and the radiation scattered from surrounding air; does not include backscatter from radiated matter (e.g., tissue).

dose, booster, *n* the portion of an immunizing agent given at a later time to stimulate the effects of a previous dose of the same agent.

dose, cumulative **(kū′myələtiv),** *n* the total accumulated dose resulting from a single or repeated exposure to radiation of the same region or of the whole body. If used in area monitoring, it represents the accumulated radiation exposure over a given period.

dose, depth, *n* the absorbed dose of radiation imparted to matter at a particular depth below the surface, usually expressed as "percentage depth dose." See also dose, percentage depth.

dose, distribution, *n* a representation of the variation of dose with position in any region of an irradiated object. The dose distribution may be measured using detectors small enough to avoid disturbing the distribution, or it may be calculated and expressed in mathematical form.

dose, doubling, *n* the amount of ionizing radiation, absorbed by the gonads of the average person in a population over a period of several generations, that will result in a doubling of the current rate of spontaneous mutations.

dose, effect curve, *n* See curve, dose effect.

dose, equivalent (DE), *n* the product of absorbed dose and modifying factors, namely the quality factor (QF), distribution factor (DF), and any other necessary factors. The unit of dose equivalent is the rem (rads times qualifying factors).

dose, erythema **(erəthē′mə),** *n* the dose of radiation necessary to produce a temporary redness of the skin. This dose varies with the quality of radiation.

dose, exit, *n* the absorbed dose delivered by a beam of radiation at the surface through which the beam emerges from a phantom or patient.

dose, exposure, *n* See exposure.

dose, fractionation, *n* a dose given by a number of shorter exposures over a longer period than would be required if the dose was given by a continuous exposure in one session at the same dose rate.

dose, gonadal, *n* the dose of radiation absorbed by the gonads.

dose, integral (integral absorbed dose, volume dose), *n* the total energy absorbed by a part or object during exposure to radiation. The unit of integral dose is the gram rad (100 ergs/gm).

dose, lethal, *n* **1.** the amount of a drug that would prove fatal to the majority of persons. *n* **2.** the amount of radiation that will be or may be sufficient to cause the death of an organism.

dose, maintenance, *n* the quantity of drug necessary to sustain a normal physiologic state or a desired blood or tissue level of drug.

dose, maximum permissible (MPD), *n* the maximum relative biologic effect dose that the body of a person or specific parts thereof shall be permitted to receive in a stated period. In most instances, for the roentgen rays used in dental radiography, it is satisfactory to consider the RBE dose in rems numerically equal to the absorbed dose in rads and the absorbed dose in rads numerically equal to the exposure dose in roentgens. See also dose, weekly permissible.

dose, median effective (ED50), *n* a dose that, under standard conditions, is effective in 50% of a randomly selected group of subjects.

dose, median lethal (LD50), *n* the amount of ionizing radiation required to kill, within a specified period, 50% of the individuals in a large group or population of animals or organisms.

D

dose, minimum lethal (MLD), *n* the minimal amount of a drug that will kill an experimental animal.

dose, percentage depth, *n* the ratio (expressed as a percentage) of the absorbed dose at a given depth in an irradiated body, to the absorbed dose at a fixed reference point on the central ray, usually the surface-absorbed dose.

dose, priming, *n* a quantity several times larger than the maintenance dose; used at the initiation of therapy to rapidly establish the desired blood and tissue levels of the drug.

dose, protraction **(prōtrak′shən),** *n* a method of radiation administration delivered continuously over a relatively long period at a relatively low dosage rate.

dose, radiation, *n* the amount of energy absorbed per unit mass of tissue at a site of interest. Note: This definition limits the use of "dose" to conform with the 1962 recommendations of the International Commission on Radiological Units and Measurements (ICRUM). The following terms therefore become obsolete but will be found in this dictionary under the general heading of exposure: air dose, cumulative dose, exposure dose, and threshold dose.

dose, radiation-absorbed (rad), *n* the unit of absorbed dose, with a value of 100 ergs per gram.

dose, rate, *n* the time rate at which radiation dose is applied, expressed in either roentgens per unit time or rads per unit time.

dose, safely tolerated (STD), *n* the dose that can be safely tolerated without producing serious acute toxicity.

dose, skin, *n* See dose, surface-absorbed.

dose, subantimicrobial **(sub′antēmīkrō′bēəl),** *n* the quantity of medication to be taken at one time for purposes other than the elimination of disease-causing microorganisms.

dose, surface-absorbed, *n* the absorbed dose delivered by a radiation beam at the point where the central ray passes through the superficial layer of the phantom or patient.

dose, therapeutic, *n* a quantity several times larger than the maintenance dose; used in vitamin therapy in which a marked deficiency exists.

dose, threshold, *n* the minimum dose that will produce a detectable degree of any given effect.

dose, tissue, *n* the dose absorbed by a tissue or tissues in a region of interest.

dose, tolerance, *n* See dose, maximum permissible.

dose, toxic, *n* the amount of a drug that causes untoward symptoms in the majority of persons.

dose, transit, *n* a measure of the primary radiation transmitted through the patient and measured at a point on the central ray at some point beyond the patient.

dose, U.S.P, *n* See dose, median effective (ED50); dose, lethal.

dose, volume, *n* See dose, integral.

dose, weekly permissible, *n* a dose of ionizing radiation accumulated in 1 week and of such magnitude that, in view of present knowledge, exposure at this weekly rate for an indefinite period of time is not expected to cause appreciable bodily injury during a person's lifetime.

dosimetry (dōsim′etrē), *n* the accurate and systematic determination of the amount of radiation to which an animal or person has been exposed during a given period.

dovetail (dov′tāl), *n* a widened or fanned-out portion of a prepared cavity, usually established deliberately to increase the retention and resistance form.

dovetail, lingual, *n* a dovetail established as a step portion, with lingual approach, in some Class 3 and Class 4 preparations; used to supplement the retentions and resistance form.

dovetail, occlusal, *n* a dovetail established at the terminal of the occlusal step of a proximal cavity.

dowel, *n* a post or pin, usually made of metal, fitted into a prepared root canal of a natural tooth to improve retention of a restoration.

Down syndrome, *n* a congenital condition characterized by varying degrees of mental retardation and multiple developmental defects. It is most commonly caused by the presence of an extra chromosome 21. It is also called *trisomy 21* and *trisomy G* *syndrome.* The term *mongolism* is no longer used.

downcoding (doun'kō'ding), *n* a practice of third-party payers in which the benefits code has been changed to a less complex or lower cost procedure than was reported.

downtime, *n* the time interval during which a device is malfunctioning or inoperative.

doxazosin mesylate (doksā'zōsin mes'ilāt'), *n brand name:* Cardura; *drug class:* peripheral α-adrenergic blocker; *action:* peripheral blood vessels are dilated, peripheral resistance lowered; *uses:* hypertension.

doxepin HCl, *n brand name:* Sinequan; *drug class:* antidepressant, tricyclic; *action:* inhibits both norepinephrine and serotonin (5-HT) reuptake in synapses in brain; *uses:* major depression, anxiety.

doxepin (topical) (dok'səpin), *n brand name:* Zonolon; *drug class:* topical antipruritic (tricyclic antidepressant); *action:* antipruritic mechanism unknown; has antihistaminic activity; also produces drowsiness; *uses:* pruritus associated with eczema, atopic dermatitis, lichen simplex chronicus.

doxycycline hyclate (dok'sisī'klēn hī'klāt), *n brand names:* Doryx, Doxy-Caps, Vibra-Tabs; *drug class:* tetracycline, broad-spectrum anti-infective; *action:* inhibits protein synthesis, phosphorylation in microorganisms; *uses:* syphilis, chlamydia trachomatis, gonorrhea, lymphogranuloma venereum, uncommon gram-negative and gram-positive organisms, necrotizing ulcerative gingivostomatitis.

drachm (dram), *n* See dram.

draft, *n* See draw.

drag, *n* the lower, or cast, side of a denture mold or flask, to which the cope is fitted. The base of the cast is embedded in plaster or stone, with the remainder of the denture pattern exposed to be engaged by the plaster or stone in the cope (the upper part of the flask).

drain, *n* **1.** a substance that provides a channel for release or discharge from a wound. *v* **2.** to release or remove a fluid substance.

drain, cigarette, *n* See drain, Penrose.

drain, Penrose (cigarette), *n.pr* a thin-walled rubber tube through which a piece of gauze has been pulled.

drainage, *n* the placement or creation of a pathway from a deep lesion to the surface of the body to provide an avenue for the body to expel the byproducts of an infection or inflammation.

dram (drachm), *n* a unit of weight that equals the eighth part of the apothecaries' ounce. Symbol ʒ.

draught (draft), *n* See draw.

draw (draft, draught), *n* the taper or divergence of the walls of a preparation for insertion of a cemented restoration.

dressing, chemically cured, *n* a protective covering that contains the ingredients and accelerator necessary to initiate a chemical process upon application to a wound.

dressing, Coe-pak, *n.pr* the brand name of a commonly used chemical-cured dressing that is easy to place and remove. It is available as a pliable paste.

dressing, collagen (kol'əjin), *n* a protective covering made of natural materials that are particularly suited for application over moist or bleeding wounds.

dressing, Kirkland cement, *n.pr* a surgical dressing applied to the tissues after periodontal surgery; consists of zinc oxide, tannic acid, and powdered rosin, admixed with a liquid composed of lump rosin, sweet almond oil, and eugenol.

dressing, PerioCare, *n.pr* the brand name of a commonly used chemical-cured dressing that provides comfortable protection and is easy to apply and remove; available as a pliable paste-gel.

dressing, postoperative surgical, *n* a surgical cement dressing applied to the teeth and tissues after surgical periodontal therapy. Possesses supportive, protective, hemostatic, analgesic, and other properties.

dressing, pressure, *n* a protective covering applied with pressure on top of a wound in order to stop bleeding or to hold a tissue flap or graft in place.

D

dressing, Ward's, *n.pr* See Ward's Wonderpack.

DRG, *n* the abbreviation for diagnosis-related group.

drift, *n* See tooth, drifting.

drill, *n* a cutting instrument for boring holes by rotary motion.

drill, bibevel **(bībev′əl),** *n* a drill with two flattened sides and the end cut in two beveled planes.

drill, spear-point, *n* a drill with a tri-beveled, or threeplaned, point.

drill, trephine **(trifīn′),** *n* a surgical drill with a hollow cutting head used to remove a circular section of bone or other tissue; also used to remove failed dental implants.

drill, twist, *n* a drill with one or more deep spiral grooves that extend from the point to the smooth part of the shaft.

drilling, *n* a colloquial term for boring a hole into a tooth with a rotary cutting instrument during cavity preparation. See preparation, cavity.

drip, *n* the continuous slow intravenous introduction of fluid containing nutrients or drugs.

droperidol (drōper′ədol), *n* a butyrophenone drug used in neuroleptanalgesia and preanesthetic medication.

droplet spread, *n* transmission of an infection through the projection of oral and nasal secretions by coughing, sneezing, or talking.

dropsy (drop′sē), *n* See anasarca.

drowning, *n* asphyxiation because of submersion in a liquid.

drug(s), *n* a substance used in the prevention, cure, or alleviation of disease or pain or as an aid in some diagnostic procedures.

drug absorption, *n* See absorption, drug.

drug abuse, *n* an excessive or improper use of drugs, especially through self-administration for nonmedical purposes. This term has increased significance because of the enactment of the Comprehensive Drug Abuse Prevention and Control Act of 1970, which replaces the Harrison Narcotic Act. See also substance abuse.

drug combinations, *n.pl* the use of drugs together to enhance the properties of both to the benefit of the patient.

drug dependence, *n* a physical or psychologic state in which a person displays withdrawal symptoms if drug use is halted suddenly; can lead to addiction.

Drug Enforcement Administration (DEA), *n.pr* the federal agency charged with monitoring use and abuse of narcotics. It provides the drug schedules used to determine the addiction potential of dental drugs.

drug hypersensitivity, *n* an allergic reaction that occurs after exposure to a suspect medication. It may manifest with a fever or rash and in severe cases, organ damage or death. It is classified as (1) immediate or occurring rapidly after exposure, or (2) delayed or occurring several days after exposure.

drug idiosyncrasy **(id′ēōsing′krəsē),** *n* an adverse drug reaction that occurs in a small number of persons and presents no correlation to dosage or means of therapy.

drug interaction, *n* a modification of the effect of a drug when administered with another drug. The effect may be an increase or a decrease in the action of either substance, or it may be an adverse effect that is not normally associated with either drug.

drug resistance, *n* the capacity of a microorganism to build a tolerance to a drug.

drug stability, *n* the length of time a drug retains its properties without loss of potency; usually referred to as shelf life.

drug therapy, *n* the use of a drug in the treatment of a patient with a specific disease or illness.

drug tolerance, *n* the body's ability to increasingly withstand the effects of the substance being used, thereby requiring larger quantities of said substance in order to bring about the desired result.

drug toxicity, *n* the critical or lethal reaction to an erroneous dosage of a medication. Drug toxicity may occur due to human error or intentional overdose in the case of suicide or homicide.

drugs, antibiotic, *n.pl* the chemical compounds obtained from certain living cells of lower plant forms, such as bacteria, yeasts, and molds, and from synthesis. They are antagonistic to certain pathogenic organisms and have a lethal effect on them.

drugs, antimicrobial, *n.pl* the drugs, mainly penicillin and its derivatives, used to combat viral, fungal, and parasitic infections.

drugs, antiseptic, *n.pl* the chemical compounds used to reduce the number of microorganisms in the oral cavity.

drugs, autonomic, *n.pl* the drugs that mimic or block the effects of stimulation of the autonomic nervous system.

drugs, desensitizing, *n.pl* the agents used to diminish or eliminate sensitivity of teeth, especially the dentin, to physical, chemical, thermal, or other irritants (e.g., strontium chloride, silver [ammoniacal] or potassium nitrate, sodium fluoride, formalin, zinc chloride). See hypersensitivity, dentin.

drugs, endodontic, *n.pl* the drugs used in treating the dental pulp and dental periapical tissues.

drugs, nonofficial, *n.pl* the drugs that are not listed in the United States Pharmacopeia (U.S.P.) or the National Formulary (N.F.).

drugs, official, *n.pl* the drugs listed in the U.S.P. or N.F.

drugs, officinal **(ōfis′inəl),** *n.pl* drugs that may be purchased without a prescription. More commonly called *over-the-counter (OTC) drugs.*

drugs, over-the-counter (OTC), *n.pl* the drugs that may be purchased without a prescription. Sometimes called nonlegend drugs because the label does not bear the prescription legend required on all drugs that may be dispensed only on prescription.

drugs, parasympathetic **(par′əsim′pəthet′ik),** *n.pl* the belladonna alkaloids that inhibit glandular secretions of the nose, oral cavity, pharynx, and bronchi. This is the main reason for using atropine and scopolamine for preanesthetic or preprocedural medication.

drugs, parasympatholytic **(per′əsim′pəthōlit′ik),** *n.pl* the drugs that block nerve impulses passing from parasympathetic nerve fibers to postganglionic neuroeffectors.

drugs, parasympathomimetic **(per′əsim′pəthōmimet′ik),** *n.pl* the drugs that have an effect similar to that produced when the parasympathetic nerves are stimulated.

drugs, proprietary **(prəprī′iter′ē),** *n.pl* the drugs that are patented or controlled by a private organization or manufacturer.

drugs, psychoactive **(sī′kōak′tiv),** *n.pl* the drugs or other agents that have the capacity to become habit forming because of their influence on mood, behavior, or conscious thought; may be therapeutic or recreational.

drugs, sympathetic, *n.pl* the agents that imitate the sympathetic autonomic nervous system actions. They usually cause raised levels of alertness and anxiety. Various types are used in dentistry as vasoconstricters in conjunction with local anesthetics. See also adrenergic agents.

dry field, *n* the isolation of a surgical or operating field from body fluids such as saliva and blood. A dry field is essential in the placement of some enamel sealants and restorative fillings.

Dry-foil, *n.pr* the brand name for tinfoil that is supplied with an adhesive powder or coating on one side.

dry heat, *n* a method of sterilization of suitable instruments using a well-calibrated and time-controlled convection oven.

dry ice, *n* a solid form of carbon dioxide, with a temperature of about −140° F.

dry socket, *n* See socket, dry and osteitis.

drying, for sealant application, *n* the removal of moisture from the affected area prior to applying a sealant.

DSM-IV ***(Diagnostic and Statistical Manual of Mental Disorders),*** *n* a publication of the American Psychiatric Association that classifies mental conditions.

dual choice (dual option), *n* the federal legislation that requires employers to give their employees the option to enroll in a local health maintenance organization rather than in the conventional employer-sponsored health program.

dual impression technique, *n* See technique, impression, dual.

duct, *n* a small passage such as in glandular tissue.

duct, Bartholin's, n See duct, sublingual.

duct, intercalated, n a duct that is connected to an acinus of the salivary glands. See also acinus.

duct, nasopalatine **(nā'zōpal'ətīn),** *n* See cyst, nasopalatine.

duct, parotid, n the duct of the parotid gland; it passes lateral to the masseter muscle and enters the oral cavity through the buccal tissues adjacent to the maxillary first and second molars. Older term is *Stenson's duct.*

duct, Stensen's, n.pr See duct, parotid.

duct, striated, n a part of the ductal system to which the intercalated ducts are connected in the lobules of the salivary gland.

duct, sublingual **(subling'gwəl),** *n* the duct associated with sublingual salivary gland. Located on the floor of the oral cavity, inferior to the tongue. Older term is *Bartholin's duct.*

duct, submandibular, n the excretory duct of the submandibular glands; opens into the oral cavity at the sublingual caruncle on the floor of the mouth, posterior to the mandibular incisor teeth. Older term is *Wharton's duct.*

duct, Wharton's, n.pr See duct, submandibular.

ductility (duktil'itē), *n* the property of a material that allows permanent deformation under tension without rupture. It is measured as a percentage increase in length on rupture compared with original length and is termed percentage elongation, or elongation.

due process, *n* the rules governing the fair practice of law. Due process dictates that everyone is equal in the eyes of the law, and it also states that the law must be fair and clearly stated to prevent arbitrary actions by the state.

Duke's test, *n.pr* See test, Duke's.

duodenal ulcer, *n* a peptic ulcer located in the duodenum. See also ulcer, peptic.

duodenum (doo'ədē'nəm), *n* the first, shortest, and most fixed portion of the small intestine. The duodenum courses from the pyloric valve of the stomach and terminates in a junction with the jejunum at the duodenojejunal flexure.

duplication, *n* the procedure of accurately reproducing a cast or other object.

duplication impression, n See duplication.

dust-borne organisms, *n.pl* the organisms, including pathogens, which enter an inhabited space attached to dust particles and contaminate the contents of the inhabited space or the respiratory tracts of the inhabitants.

duty, *n* that which is due from a person; that which a person owes to another; an obligation.

DVD, *n* the acronym for digital versatile disk or digital video disk. A high-density compact disk for storing large amounts of data, especially high-resolution audio-video material.

dwarf, pituitary (pitoo'iterē), *n* an individual who is of small stature as a result of a deficiency of growth hormones. Such dwarfs usually are well proportioned.

dwarfism, *n* deficient growth and development leading to small stature and often skeletal deformity. It may be associated with ovarian agenesis, pituitary insufficiency, mongolism, progeria, rickets, renal disease, dietary deficiency, achondroplasia, cleidocranial dysostosis, osteogenesis imperfecta, microcephaly, hydrocephaly, sexual precocity, and delayed adolescence.

dyclonine hydrochloride (dī'klənēn), *n* a ketone-type liquid topical anesthetic agent that may be applied with a cotton swab or used as a mouthrinse.

dye, occlusal registration, *n* a water-soluble dye used as an aid in locating occlusal contacts. A valuable aid in effecting fine adjustments in the final phases of the selective grinding procedure.

dyes, plaque detection, *n.pl* See disclosing solution.

dyes, treatment, *n.pl* the dyes used in medicine and dentistry in the treatment of diseased states, the most useful of which are the rosaniline dyes (e.g., gentian violet, crystal violet) and the fluorescein dyes (e.g., Mercurochrome), which possess antiseptic and protective properties.

dynamic relation, *n* See relation, dynamic.

dyphylline (dī′fəlin), *n brand names:* Dilor, Dyflex, Lufyllin; *drug class:* Xanthine derivative; *action:* relaxes smooth muscle of respiratory system by blocking phosphodiesterase; *uses:* bronchial asthma, bronchospasm in chronic bronchitis, COPD, emphysema.

dysarthria (disärth′rēə), *n* a speech impediment brought on by emotional distress, paralysis, or muscle spasticity.

dysautonomia, familial (dis′ôtōnō′mēə), *n* See syndrome, Riley-Day.

dyscrasia (diskrā′zhə, -zēə), *n* **1.** a morbid condition, especially one that involves an imbalance of component elements. *n* **2.** an abnormal composition of the blood, such as that found in leukemia and anemia.

dysdiadochokinesia (dis′dīad′ōkōkinē′zhə, -zēə), *n* a disturbance of musculoskeletal function. There is a disorganization in the reciprocal innervation of agonists and antagonists and a loss of the ability to stop one act in terms of rate, magnitude, and the direction of movement and immediately to follow it with another act diametrically opposite (e.g., alternately elevating and depressing the mandible). Another example is observed in the inappropriate use of the tongue during mastication when it is necessary to change, reverse, and modify the energy and direction of movement.

dysentery (dis′ənter′ē), *n* an inflammation of the intestine, especially of the colon, that may be caused by chemical irritants, bacteria, protozoa, or parasites. It is characterized by frequent and bloody stools and severe abdominal pain.

dysesthesia (dis′esthē′zhə, -zēə), *n* an impairment of the senses, especially the sense of touch. No sensation is painful with dysesthesia.

dysfunction (disfunk′shən), *n* (malfunction), an abnormality or impairment of function or the inability of a body, organ, or organ system to perform normally.

dysfunction, dental, *n* an abnormal functioning or impairment of the functioning of the dental organ.

dysfunction, endocrine, *n* an abnormality in the function of an endocrine gland, either by hypofunction or hyperfunction of the secretory elements of the gland.

dysfunction, immune, *n* a reduction in the function of the immune system most often associated with chronic fatigue syndrome (CFIDS), which causes prolonged periods of debilitating fatigue.

dysgeusia (disgyoo′zēə), *n* an abnormal or impaired sense of taste.

dysgnathia (disnā′thēə), *n* the abnormalities that extend beyond the teeth and include the maxilla, the mandible, or both. See also anomaly, dysgnathic.

dyskeratosis (dis′kerətō′sis), *n* an irreversible alteration in the maturation of stratified squamous epithelium. Refers to an increase of abnormal mitosis, individual cell keratinization, epithelial pearls within the spinous layer, loss of polarity of the cells, hyperchromatism, nuclear atypia, and basilar hyperplasia.

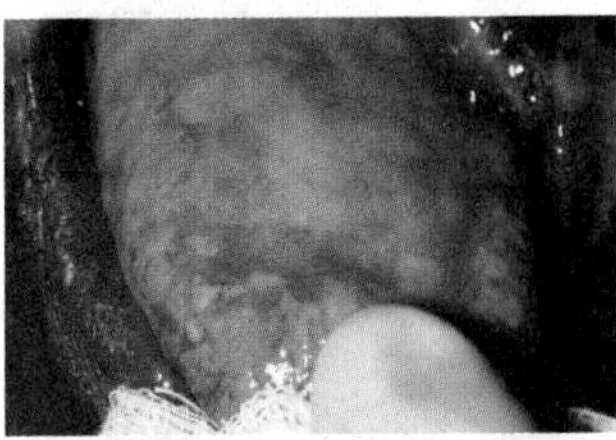

Dyskeratosis. (Neville/Damm/Allen/Bouquot, 2002)

dyslexia (dislek′sēə), *n* an impairment of the ability to read. These persons often reverse letters and words, cannot adequately distinguish the letter sequences in written words, and have difficulty determining left from right.

dyslipidema (dislip′idēmə), *n* a state characterized by irregular or elevated quantities of lipids or lipoproteins in the blood. Dyslipidemia can be the result of genetic predisposition or lifestyle issues such as poor diet.

dysmenorrhea (dis′menərē′ə), *n* painful menstruation.

dysmetria (dismē′trēə), *n* the loss of ability to gauge distance, speed, or power of movement associated with muscle function; e.g., the patient is unable to control the force of closure and strikes the opposite occluding teeth with greater vigor than necessary.

dysmorphism (dismôr′fizəm), *n* an aberration of form.

D

dysostosis (disostō′sis), *n* defective ossification.

dysostosis, cleidocranial **(klī′dōkrā′nēəl),** *n* (Sainton's disease), See dysplasia, cleidocranial.

dysostosis, craniofacial, *n* See syndrome, Crouzon.

dysostosis, mandibulofacial (Treacher-Collins syndrome), *n* a developmental disturbance of the cranial bones and hypoplasias of the upper part of the face. The mandibular body is underdeveloped, but the ramus is hyperplastic. The teeth are crowded and malposed.

dysostosis multiplex, *n* See syndrome, Hurler's.

dyspepsia, *n* a vague feeling of epigastric discomfort, felt after eating. It is not a distinct condition but may be a sign of underlying intestinal disorder, such as peptic ulcer, gallbladder disease, or chronic appendicitis. The symptoms usually increase during periods of stress.

dysphagia (disfā′jēə), *n* difficulty in swallowing. It may be caused by lesions in the oral cavity, pharynx, or larynx; neuromuscular disturbances; or mechanical obstruction of the esophagus (e.g., dysphagia of Plummer-Vinson syndrome [sideropenic dysphagia], peritonsillar abscess, Ludwig's angina, and carcinoma of the tongue, pharynx, larynx).

dysphoria (disfôr′ēə), *n* a feeling of discomfort or restlessness. See also euphoria.

dysplasia (displā′zhə), *n* **1.** a developmental abnormality. See also dysplasia, dentinal. *n* **2.** the reversible, regressive alteration in adult cells, seen as alterations in their size, shape, orientation, and functions; leads to change in tissue architecture and is related to chronic inflammation or protracted irritation. **3.** an abnormality of development. *n* **4.** a disharmony between component parts.

dysplasia, anteroposterior (anteroposterior facial dysplasia), *n* an abnormal anteroposterior relationship of the maxillae and mandible to each other or to the cranial base.

dysplasia, cementoosseous, *n* a fairly common benign fibroosseous lesion (BFOL) that appears in the jawbone. They appear on radiographic examinations as highly visible areas of mixed radiolucent/radiopaque bone. The three categories of cementoosseous dysplasia are focal, periapical, and florid. Such lesions are easily diagnosed with radiographic examination and do not require a biopsy, which can damage adjacent bone tissue.

dysplasia, cleidocranial **(klī′dōkrā′nēəl),** *n* (Sainton's disease), a familial disease or congenital disorder characterized by failure to form, or retarded formation of, the clavicles; delayed closure of the sutures and fontanels; and delayed eruption of teeth, with formation of supernumerary teeth. It is characterized by underdevelopment of the maxillae, agenesis or aplasia of the clavicle, abnormalities in other skeletal bones and muscles, and irregularities of the dentition. The syndrome may be mutational or transmitted on an autosomal dominant basis.

dysplasia, craniofacial, *n* a disharmony between the cranium and the face.

dysplasia, dentinal, *n* a genetic disturbance of the dentin characterized by early calcification of the pulp chambers and root canals and by root resorption. It is differentiated from dentinogenesis imperfecta by the latter's characteristics of attrition and relative freedom from root resorption.

dysplasia, dentofacial, *n* a disharmony between teeth and bones of the face (e.g., crowding and spacing).

dysplasia, ectodermal **(ek′tōdur′məl),** *n* a group of diseases characterized by failure to form two or more ectodermal derivatives. Sweat glands and teeth may be missing (anhidrosis and hypodontia, respectively), and there may be scant hair, faulty fingernails, and malformation of the iris.

dysplasia, enamel, *n* a development abnormality of enamel tissue.

dysplasia, fibroosseous, *n* See dysplasia, fibrous.

dysplasia, fibrous (fibroosseous dysplasia), *n* a metabolic disturbance characterized by replacement of the bone marrow with fibrous tissue and slow, progressive remolding and enlargement of the bone. It may be monostotic (limited to one bone) or polyostotic (present in many bones). McCune-Albright syndrome shows polyostotic fibrous dysplasia and other symptoms. See also syndrome, McCune-Albright.

dysplasia, focal osseous, *n* See fibroma, periapical.

***dysplasia, maxillomandibular* (mak′sōmandib′yələr),** *n* a disharmony between one jaw and the other.

***dysplasia, osseous* (os′ēəs),** *n* a chronic reaction of the bone to injury characterized by replacement of the bone marrow with fibrous connective tissue, unilateral enlargement of the maxillae or mandible, and characteristic radiographic findings. It is similar or identical to monostotic fibrous dysplasia and ossifying fibroma.

***dysplasia, polyostotic fibrous* (pol′ēostot′ik fī′b′rəs),** *n* the disease of fibrous dysplasia occurring in more than one bone. See also dysplasia, fibrous; osteofibroma; and syndrome, Albright's.

dyspnea (dispnē′ə), *n* difficult, labored, or gasping breathing; inspiration, expiration, or both may be involved.

dystonia (distō′nēə), *n* a disorder or lack of tonicity.

dystrophy (dis′trōfē), *n* a state of faulty nutrition. Often used to refer to the results of faulty nutrition, that is, wasting away.

E

e-antigen, *n* a peptide present in blood infected with the hepatitis B virus. The e-antigen is indicative of an actively reproducing hepatitis B virus and probable liver damage.

E space, *n* the net difference between the combined mesiodistal width of the primary canine, primary first molar, and primary second molar and that of the permanent canine, first premolar, and second premolar. In the mandible the mean leeway space is 3.4 mm, and in the maxilla it is 1.9 mm. Also called *leeway space.*

Eames' technique (ēmz), *n* See technique, Eames'.

early-onset, *adj* describes a condition that has occurred before the normally prescribed time. E.g., early-onset Alzheimer's refers to the presence of Alzheimer's disease in persons younger than the age of 65, the average age of onset.

earnings report, *n* a statement issued by a company showing its earnings or losses over a given period. The earnings report lists the income earned, expenses, and net result. Also called *income statement.*

Eastman Interdental Bleeding Index (EIBI), *n.pr* an assessment tool used to determine the extent of interdental inflammation based on bleeding that occurs within 15 seconds after a wooden cleaning stick is inserted between the teeth.

eating disorders, *n.pl* a group of dysfunctional behaviors of nutrition, including anorexia, bulimia, or cravings for such nonfood items as ice, clay, or starch.

EBIT, *n* the abbreviation for **earnings before interest and taxes.**

eburnation (ē′burnā′shən), *n* an increase in bony density into an ivory-like mass. See also osteitis, condensing and dentin eburnation.

eccentric (eksen′trik), *n* **1.** a deviation from the normal or conventional. *adj* **2.** away from the central or reference position.

eccentric checkbite, *n* See record, interocclusal, eccentric.

eccentric jaw relation, *n* See relation, jaw, eccentric.
eccentric occlusion, *n* See occlusion, eccentric.
eccentric position, *n* See position, eccentric.

ecchymosis (ek′imō′sis), *n* a discoloration of mucous membranes caused by a diffuse extravasation of blood. See also bruise.

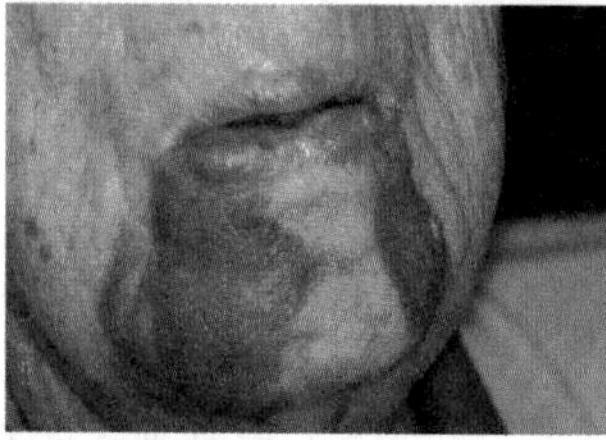

Ecchymosis. (Courtesy Dr. Charles Babbush)

echocardiogram, *n* a visual representation, produced through ultrasound waves, of the heart's structure and movement.

echocardiography (ek′ōkar′dēog′rəfē), *n* a diagnostic procedure for studying the structure and motion of the heart using ultrasonic waves that pass through the heart and are reflected backward, or echoed, when they pass from one type of tissue to another.

echolalia (ek″ola′leə), *n* an uncontrollable reiteration of a word or phrase recently stated by another individual.

echoviruses (ECHO virus), *n.pl* an enteric pathogen associated with fever and mild respiratory disease; sometimes may produce an aseptic meningitis.

ecology, *n* the study of the interaction between living organisms and their environment.

econazole nitrate (topical), *n* *brand name:* Ecostatin; *drug class:* local antifungal; *action:* interferes with fungal cell membrane, which increases permeability, leaking of cell nutrients; *uses:* tinea pedis, tinea cruris, tinea corporis, tinea versicolor, cutaneous candidiasis.

economics, *n* in dentistry, a broad term that covers all the business aspects of dental practice.

ecosystem, *n* the sum total of all living and nonliving things that support the chain of life events within a particular area.

ectoderm (ek′tədurm), *n* the outermost of the three primary cell layers of an embryo. The ectoderm gives rise to the nervous system, the organs of special sense, the epidermis, and epidermal tissues such as fingernails, hair, and skin glands.

ectodermal dysplasia (ek′tədurməl displā′zhə), *n* See dysplasia, ectodermal.

ectomesenchyme (ek′tōmez′ənkīm), *n* a mass of tissue consisting of neurocrest cells present in the early formation of an embryo. It eventually forms the hard and soft tissues of the neck and cranium.

ectomorph (ek′tōmôrf), *n* a constitutional body type (Sheldon's classification) characterized by long, fragile bones and a highly developed nervous system.

ectopia lentis, *n* a displacement of the lens of the eye.

ectopic (ektop′ik), *adj* occurring outside the expected or usual location; displaced.
ectopic eruption, *n* See eruption, ectopic.

ectropion (ektrō′pēon), *n* an eversion, or rolling outward, of the eyelid margin.

eczema (ek′zəmə), *n* an inflammatory skin disease characterized by vesiculation, inflammation, watery discharge, and the development of scales and crusts. The large variety of types can be distinguished according to location and causal agent.

ED50, *n* See dose, median effective.

edema (edē′mə), *n* the accumulation of fluid in the tissues or in the peritoneal or pleural cavities. Primary factors favoring edema are increased capillary hydrostatic pressure (increased venous pressure), decreased osmotic pressure of plasma (hypoproteinemia), decreased tissue tension and lymphatic drainage, increased osmotic pressure of tissue fluids, and increased capillary permeability. Additional renal and hormonal factors are important. Clinical manifestations may consist of a steady weight gain or localized or generalized swelling.

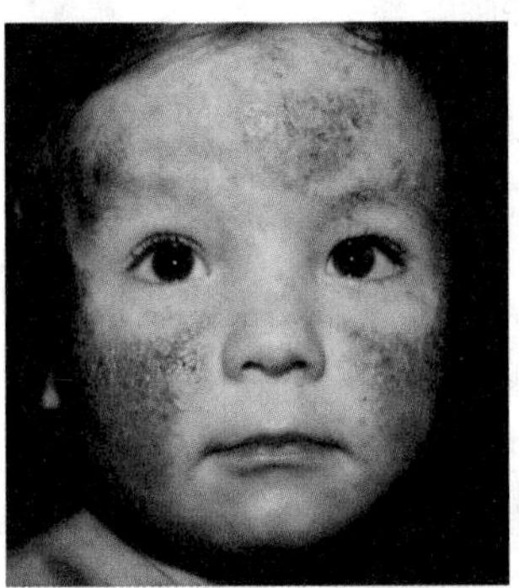

Eczema. (Zitelli/Davis, 2002)

edema, angioneurotic **(an′jēōner-to′ik),** *n* See angioedema.

edema, cardiac, *n* an edema caused by venous congestion in association with congestive heart failure; tends to appear first in such dependent parts as the legs.

edema, dependent, *n* an edema that changes its position with the posture of dependent parts (e.g., edema of the legs in progressive heart failure).

edema of glottis **(glot′is),** *n* an edema caused by fluid accumulation in the soft tissues of the larynx. The condition, usually inflammatory, may result from an infection, injury, allergy, or inhalation of toxic substances.

edema, periorbital **(per′ēor′bitəl),** *n* an edema of the eyelids in association with local injury, allergic reactions, hypoproteinemia, trichinosis, and myxedema.

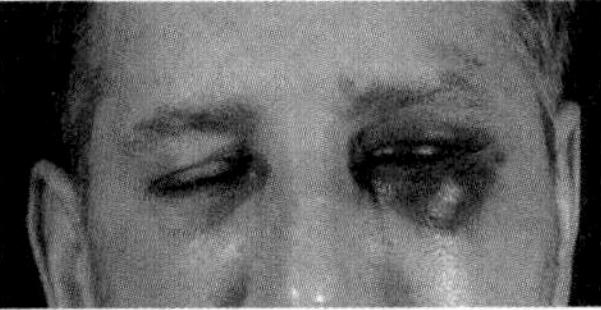

Periorbital edema. (Courtesy Dr. Charles Babbush)

edema, pitting, *n* a persistent indentation of the skin when pressure is applied to an edematous area.

edentulism (ēden′tūlizəm), *n* the condition of being edentulous, without teeth.

edentulous (ēden′tūləs), *adj* without teeth; lacking teeth.

edge strength, *n* See strength, edge.

edge-to-edge bite, *n* See occlusion, edge-to-edge.

edge-to-edge occlusion, *n* See occlusion, edge-to-edge.

edgewise appliance, *n* See appliance, edgewise.

EDP, *n* the abbreviation for **electronic data processing.**

Edtac, *n* the brand name for a chelating agent used to soften calcified tissue.

education, *n* the act or process of imparting or acquiring knowledge, skill, or judgment.

education, continuing, *n* education that occurs after the completion of a course of study leading to a degree. Usually taken in short (1- to 2-day) courses covering a specific topic or procedure.

education dental, *n* the formal education necessary to become qualified to practice dentistry; typically 4 years of full-time study in an accredited school of dentistry.

education of patient, *n* effective communication between the dental professional and the patient concerning dentistry and the principles of treatment and prevention. The procedure of increasing the patient's knowledge of the oral cavity and its care to the point where the reasons for proposed dental services are understood.

education, predental, *n* the formal education necessary to qualify for placement in a dental curriculum, typically 4 years of full-time study at the baccalaureate level.

educational status, *n* the level of education and skill obtained within a discipline or profession, usually referred to as a generalist or specialist in a discipline.

effect, *n* the result of an action.

effect, heel (anode heel effect), *n* the variation of intensity over the cross section of a useful radiographic beam, caused by the angle at which radiographs emerge from beneath the surface of the focal spot, which causes a differential attenuation of photons composing the useful beam.

effect of external radiation on bone, *n* See osteoradionecrosis.

effect of function on bone, n See law, Wolff's.

effect, photoelectric, n the process by which radiographic images are produced when the energy of an incident photon is absorbed as the result of bound electron ejection.

effect, wedging, n an effect produced by food impaction that forces the teeth apart.

effective half-life, *n* See life, radioactive.

effectiveness, *n* the degree to which action(s) achieves the intended health result under normal or usual circumstances.

effector (ēfek′tur), *n* **1.** a motor or secretory nerve ending in an organ, gland, or muscle; consequently called an *effector organ. n* **2.** an on-the-job organ of the body that responds to stimulations asking for corrections. Antonym: receptor.

efferent (ef′ərənt), *adj* conveying away from a center toward the periphery.

efferent nerves, n.pl See nerves, efferent.

efficacy (ef′ikəsē), *n* the ability to provide a clinically measurable effect, preferably beneficial.

efficiency, *n* the operation of a dental practice in such a way that both business and professional services are performed in a minimal amount of time without sacrificing quality of work, sympathetic attitude, and kindliness.

eH, *n* the symbol for oxidation-reduction potential, which is regarded as a significant factor in the protection of the body against anaerobic bacteria. The eH of living tissue of pH level 7.4 is about 0.12 volt.

Ehlers-Danlos syndrome (ā′lurz-dan′lus), *n.pr* a hereditary disorder of connective tissue, marked by hyperplasticity of skin, tissue fragility, and hypermotility of joints. Minor trauma may cause a gaping wound with little bleeding. Sprains, dislocations, and synovial effusions are common. See also syndrome, Ehlers-Danlos.

EIA, *n* the abbreviation for **enzyme immunoassay;** better known as ELISA for enzyme-linked immunosorbent assay, used to detect the presence of HIV antibody to HIV in the blood.

Eikenella corrodens **(īkənelə kərod′ənz),** *n.pr* a gram-negative, rod-shaped, facultatively anaerobic bacteria that is part of the normal flora of the oral cavity but may become an opportunistic pathogen in immunocompromised patients.

ejector (ijektər), *n* by common usage, a device used to remove debris and fluids by negative pressure. Another term is *aspirator.* See also aspirator.

ejector, saliva, n a device (containing a removable tip) that is attached to a vacuum supply to remove saliva from a dental field of operation.

ejector, saliva, tip, n a removable tip, made of metal, glass, rubber, plastic, or a combination of these, that is attached to a saliva ejector and bent to fit over lower teeth and reach the floor of the oral cavity.

elastic, *adj* referring to property of a solid substance that permits recovery of its shape after a deformation resulting from force application.

elastic deformation, n See deformation, elastic.

elastic impression, n See impression, elastic.

elastic, intermaxillary, n See elastic, maxillomandibular.

elastic, intramaxillary, n an elastic band used within either the maxillary or mandibular arch.

elastic limit, n See limit, elastic.

elastic, maxillomandibular, n an elastic band used between the maxillary and mandibular dentitions.

elastic memory, n **1.** the property of a material such as wax that enables it, after being warmed, bent, and cooled, to return to its original form upon rewarming. *n* **2.** a rubber plastic band used to apply force to the teeth.

elasticity (ilastis′itē), *n* the quality or condition of being elastic.

elasticity, modulus of, n (Young's modulus) a measurement of elasticity obtained by dividing stress below the proportional limit by its corresponding strain value. A measure of stiffness.

elastomer (ēlas′tōmur), *n* a soft, rubberlike material; synthetic rubber. A rubber base impression material (e.g., silicone, mercaptan).

elastosis (ē′lastō′sis), *n* a degeneration of the elastic tissues; found particularly in the lips and associated with senile or actinic cheilitis.

elastosis, senile, n a dermatologic disease that results from degeneration of the elastic connective tissue.

elder abuse, *n* the infliction of physical, sexual, or emotional trauma on an elder.

elderly, *adj* used to describe a person who is beyond middle age and approaching old age. Also called *senior citizens.* See also geriatric dentistry.

electroanesthesia (ilek′trōanesthē′zēə, -zhə), *n* local or general anesthesia induced by electric current.

electrocardiography (ilek′trōkar′dēog′rəfē), *n* a method of recording electrical activity generated by the heart muscle.

electrochemistry, *n* chemical reactions that elicit electrical potentials, and electrical potentials that initiate chemical reactions.

electrocoagulation (ēlek′trōkōag′yōōla′shən), *n* the use of electrically generated heat to destroy tissue by coagulation necrosis. Usually a platinum wire electrode or loop is used.

electroconvulsive therapy, *n* the induction of a brief convulsion by passing an electric current through the brain for the treatment of affective disorders, especially in patients resistant to psychoactive drug therapy.

electrode (ēlek′trōd), *n* an instrument with a point or a surface from which a current can be discharged into or received from the body of a patient or a solution.

electrodiagnosis, *n* the diagnosis of disease or injury by applying electric stimulation to various nerves and muscles.

electroencephalograph (EEG) (ēlek′trōensef′əlōgraf), *n* an instrument for recording the electrical activity of the brain.

electrogalvanism (galvanism) (ēlektrōgal′vənizəm), *n* the flow of electric current between two different metals in an electrolyte solution. Dissimilar metals used in different intraoral restorations.

electrolyte (ēlek′trōlīt), *n* a solution that conducts electricity by means of its ions.

electrolyte affinity, n the attraction of the electrolytes in the body to the different fluid compartments of the intracellular and extracellular environments. Sodium is the predominant cation in the extracellular fluid; potassium is the predominant cation within the cells; chlorine and bicarbonate are the predominant anions in the plasma and interstitial fluids; and phosphates and proteins are the main anions in the cells.

electrolyte balance, fluid and, n See fluid and electrolyte balance.

electrolyzer (ionizer) (ēlek′trōlīzur), *n* an electric apparatus designed for use in a root canal to break down a treatment chemical into its various ions by direct current. See also electrosterilizer.

electromallet, McShirley's, *n* See condenser, electromallet.

electrometer (ēlektrom′ətur), *n* an electrostatic instrument for measuring the potential difference between two points. In radiology, electrometers are used to measure changes in the potential of charged electrodes resulting from ionization occasioned by radiation.

electromyography (ēlek′trōmīog′rəfē), *n* the detection, recording, and interpretation of electric voltage generated by the skeletal muscles.

electron (e) (ēlek′tron), *n* a negatively charged elementary particle constituent in every neutral atom, with a mass of 0.000549. (Particles with an equal but opposite charge are called *positrons.*)

electron beam, n See electron stream.

electron stream, n (electron beam, cathode ray, cathode stream), a stream of electrons emitted from the negative electrode (cathode) in a roentgen-ray tube; their bombardment of the anode gives rise to the roentgen rays.

electronic, *adj* pertaining to the application of that branch of science that deals with the motion, emission, and behavior of currents of free electrons, especially in vacuum, gas, or phototubes and special conductors or semiconductors. Contrasted with *electric,* which pertains to the flow of large currents in wires only.

electronic knife, n See knife, electronic.

electrophoresis, *n* the movement of charged suspended particles through a liquid medium in response to changes in an electric field.

electroplating, *n* plating by electrolysis. Impressions are plated in dentistry to form metalized working dies.

electropolishing, *n* the removal of a minute layer of metal by electrolysis to produce a bright surface.

electrosection (ilek′trōsek′shən), *n* an incision created by electrosurgery, ideally by using a fully rectified, alternating high-frequency current and producing minimal cellular injury.

electrosterilization (ilek′trōster′əlizā′shən), *n* medication of a prepared root canal by use of electrolysis of the medicament.

electrosterilizer, *n* an electric apparatus designed for use in root canal treatment for the electrolysis of a halide, such as sodium iodide, to release iodine in the cleaned root canal for the purpose of destroying residual organisms. See also electrolyzer.

electrosurgery, *n* the use of electrically generated energy from high-frequency alternating currents to cut or alter tissue within definite limits.

element, *n* a simple substance that cannot be decomposed by chemical means and is made up of atoms that are alike in their peripheral electronic configuration and chemical properties but differ in their nuclei, atomic weights, and radioactive properties.

elephantiasis (el′əfəntī′əsis), *n* a chronic disease caused by filariasis of the lymph channels with resultant inflammation and blockage. The term is also used for hypertrophy of tissues from other causes (e.g., gingival elephantiasis).

elephantiasis gingivae, n See fibromatosis gingivae.

elevated oral lesions, *n.pl* lesions occurring above the surface of the oral mucosa, categorized as either blisterform (bulla, pustule, or vesicle) or nonblisterform (nodules, tumors, plaques, or papules).

elevator, *n* an instrument used to raise or lift something.

elevator, dental, n one of a variety of blades used for engaging teeth and roots to remove them from their alveoli.

elevator, malar, n an instrument used to elevate or reposition the zygomatic bone.

elevator, periosteal, n a thin blade used to lift periosteum from bone.

eligibility date, *n* the date an individual and dependents become eligible for benefits under a dental benefits contract. Often referred to as *effective date.*

eligibility rules, *n.pl* the conditions that define who may be entitled to dental benefits, when persons first become entitled to such benefits, and any provisions that determine how long an individual remains entitled to benefits.

eligible person, *n* See beneficiary.

ELISA, *n* the abbreviation for **enzyme-linked immunosorbent assay** used to detect the presence of HIV antibody to HIV in the blood. See also EIA.

elixir (ēlik′sur), *n* a pleasantly flavored, sweetened hydroalcoholic solution of a drug intended for oral administration.

elliptocytosis (ēlip′tōsītō′sis), *n* (ovalcytosis, oval cell anemia), a hereditary anomaly in which the red blood cells are elliptical, or oval shaped, and are predisposed to hemolysis.

elongation (ē′lônggā′shən), *n* the process or condition of increasing in length before breaking; indicates ductility (e.g., of a metal).

elongation, percent, n **1.** the increase in length of a material after fracture in tension. *n* **2.** a mechanical test usually employed to measure ductility.

emaciation (imā′shēā′shən), *n* an excessive leanness caused by disease or lack of nutrition.

e-mail (electronic mail), *n* the exchange of computer-stored messages by telecommunication.

embedded, *adj* referring to a tooth, root tip, or foreign body that is covered in bone.

embolism (em′bəlizəm), *n* the clogging of a blood vessel by matter, such as a clot, air, or oil, that is carried by the bloodstream to some point where the lumen of the blood vessel narrows. This is the opposite of thrombosis, in which the clotting mechanism is organized in situ.

embolism, air, *n* See aeroembolism.

embolus (em′bəlus), *n* a blood clot or other material that travels in the bloodstream and then lodges in a blood vessel and obstructs circulation.

embrasure (embrā′zhər), *n* the small triangle-like spaces between the curved proximal surfaces of the teeth. Embrasure spaces provide an escape route for food to pass during chewing.

embrasure, buccal, *n* an embrasure that opens toward the cheeks.

embrasure clasp, *n* See clasp, embrasure.

embrasure hook, *n* an extension of a removable partial denture into the embrasure above the contact area between two adjacent teeth, which resists movement in a cervical direction.

embrasure, interdental, *n* the spaces formed by the interproximal contours of adjoining teeth, beginning at the contact area and extending lingually, facially, occlusally, and apically.

embrasure, labial, *n* an embrasure that opens toward the lips.

embrasure, lingual, *n* an embrasure that opens toward the tongue.

embrasure, occlusal, *n* an embrasure that opens toward the occlusal surface or plane.

embryo (em′brēō), *n* an organism in the earliest stages of development; the stage between the time of implantation of the fertilized ovum until the end of the seventh or eighth week of gestation.

embryoblast layer (em′breoblast″), *n* a group of cells near the embryonic axis of the blastocyst that develop into the embryo.

embryology (em′brēol′əjē), *n* the study of the origin, growth, development, and function of an organism from fertilization to birth.

embryonic period (em″breon′ik pe′reod), *n* the stage between the second and eighth week of embryonic development, during which differentiation of organs and organ systems occurs.

emergence profile, *n* the axial contour of a tooth or crown as it relates to the adjacent soft tissue.

emergency, *n* an unforeseen occurrence or combination of circumstances that calls for immediate action or remedy; pressing necessity.

emergency cart/kit, *n* a portable container holding all the equipment and medicines that one would need to assist a patient in case of a medical crisis.

emergency medicine, *n* a branch of medicine concerned with the diagnosis and treatment of conditions resulting from trauma or sudden illness.

emergency prevention, *n* the procedures necessary to avoid creating a life-threatening crisis for a patient.

emergency training, *n* the system of imparting knowledge and skills to be used in case of an accident or an unforeseen occurrence.

emergency treatment, *n* treatment that must be rendered to the patient immediately for the alleviation of the sudden onset of an unforeseen illness or injury that, if not treated, would lead to further disability or death.

emergency treatment, burns, *n* the immediate, urgent care given to a burn victim to stabilize the individual until further medical assistance can be found.

emergency treatment, cortical deficiency, *n* the immediate, urgent care given to an individual experiencing adrenal crisis to stabilize that individual until further medical assistance can be found.

emergency treatment, facial fractures, *n* the immediate, urgent care given to a patient with facial fractures to stabilize the individual until further medical assistance can be found.

emergency treatment, heart failure, *n* the immediate, urgent care given to a patient experiencing heart failure to stabilize the individual until further medical assistance can be found.

emery (em′ərē), *n* an aluminum-based abrasive agent. Two types are aluminum oxide and levigated alumina. Emery is not suitable for pol-

E

ishing dental enamel. Also called *corundum.*

emesis (em′əsis), *n* the sudden expulsion of gastric contents through the esophagus into the pharynx. The act is partly voluntary and partly involuntary. See also vomiting.

emetic (əmet′ik), *n* a drug that induces vomiting.

emetine hydrochloride (em′ətēn), *n* an alkaloid, $C_{29}H_{40}N_2O_4$ 2HCl, regarded as a protozoacide and formerly used in the treatment of periodontitis and amebic dysentery.

EMF, *n* the abbreviation for **erythrocyte-maturing factor.**

emigration, *n* movement of erythrocytes or leukocytes through the walls of the vessels that carry them.

eminence, retromylohyoid (em′inəns, ret′rōmī′lōhī′oid), *n* the distal end of the lingual flange of a mandibular denture. It occupies the retromylohyoid space.

eminenectomy (em′inenek′tōmē), *n* the operative removal of the anterior articular surface of the glenoid fossa.

emollient (ēmi′lēənt), *n* an agent that is soothing to the skin or mucous membrane; makes the skin softer or smoother.

emotion, *n* a complex feeling or state (affect) accompanied by characteristic motor and glandular activities; feelings; mood.

emotional, *adj* describing a person experiencing an emotion; manifesting emotional behavior, rather than logical, rational behavior; describing a person who is easily or excessively given to emotion.

empathy, *n* the quality of putting oneself into the psychologic frame of reference of another, so that the other person's feeling, thinking, and acting are understood and to some extent predictable. A desirable trust-building characteristic of a helping profession. It is embodied in the sincere statement, "I understand how you feel." Empathy is different from sympathy in that to be empathetic one understands how the person feels rather than actually experiencing those feelings, as in sympathy.

emphysema (em′fizē′mə), *n* **1.** a swelling caused by air in the tissue spaces. In the oral and facial regions it may be caused either by air introduced into a tooth socket or gingival crevice with the air syringe, or by blowing of the nose. *n* **2.** a permanent dilation of the respiratory alveoli.

employee, *n* a person who, under the direction and control of the employer, performs services for remuneration.

Employee Retirement Income Security Act (ERISA), *n.pr* a federal act, passed in 1974, that established new standards and reporting and disclosure requirements for employer-funded pension and health care benefits programs. To date, self-funded health care benefit plans operating under ERISA have been held to be exempt from state insurance laws. This exemption is currently under review.

employer-sponsored plan, *n* a program supported totally or in part by an employer or group of employers to provide dental benefits for employees. The plan may be administered directly by the employer or another person or group under a contractual arrangement. Part of the cost may be borne by the employee.

employment, *n* **1.** to be engaged in work for hire. *n* **2.** use of a specific tool or technique in the accomplishment of a task.

empyema (em′pīē′mə, em′pēē′mə), *n* the presence of suppuration in a cavity, hollow organ, or space (e.g., the pleural cavity).

emulsifier (imul′səfīər), *n* an agent such as gum arabic or egg yolk used to suspend droplets of oil in a water-based solution. An agent to maintain any element or particle in suspension within a fluid medium.

emulsion (ēmul′shən), *n* a colloidal dispersion of one liquid in another. See also suspension.

emulsion, digestive, *n* the suspension of fat globules, usually in the bile acid of the small intestine, and their resulting breakdown into smaller particles as part of the digestive process. See also emulsifiers.

emulsion, double, *n* a suspension of sensitive silver halide salts impregnated in gelatin and coated on both sides of a radiographic film base.

emulsion, silver, *n* a suspension of

sensitive silver halide salts impregnated in gelatin and used for coating photographic plates and radiographic films.

emulsion, single, *n* a suspension of sensitive silver halide salts impregnated in gelatin and coated on only one side of a radiographic film base.

enalapril maleate (enal′əpril mālēāt), *n brand names:* Vasotec, Vasotec IV; *drug class:* angiotensin-converting enzyme (ACE) inhibitor; *action:* selectively suppresses renin-angiotensin-aldosterone system; inhibits ACE; prevents conversion of angiotensin I to angiotensin II, leading to dilation of arterial and venous vessels; *uses:* hypertension, heart failure adjunct.

enamel (inam′əl), *n* **1.** the hard, glistening tissue covering the anatomic crown of the tooth. It is composed mainly of hexagonal rods of hydroxyapatite, sheathed in an organic matrix (approximately 0.15%) and oriented with their long axes approximately at right angles to the surface. *n* **2.** the outermost layer or covering of the coronal portion of the tooth that overlies and protects the dentin.

enamel bonding, *v* See bonding, enamel.

enamel hypocalcification **(hī′pōkal′səfikā′shən),** *n* a hereditary condition in which the enamel of the tooth has formed without adequate amounts of mineralization, leaving the surface of the tooth brittle and often stained.

enamel lamellae **(ləmel′ē),** *n.pl* the incompletely calcified, microscopic structures present in the enamel. They may extend to the dentinoenamel junction and beyond.

enamel matrix, *n* the mineral structure of enamel, secreted by ameloblasts.

enamel, mottled, *n* See fluorosis, chronic endemic dental.

enamel, opacity, (white spot) **(ōpas′itē),** *n* a visibly lighter area on a tooth's surface; may be caused by fluorosis, or demineralization.

enamel organ, *n* the part of a developing tooth germ that produces enamel.

enamel pearl, *n* See pearl, enamel.

enamel spindles, *n.pl* tubular projections from the dentinoenamel junction into the enamel, caused by penetration by odontoblasts before the junction is formed.

enamel tufts, *n.pl* the brush-shaped projections from the dentinoenamel junction into the enamel, caused by crystallization defects.

enamel epithelium, *n* See epithelium, enamel.

enameloma, *n* See pearl, enamel.

enanthem (enan′thəm), *n* See enanthema.

enanthema (enanthem) (en′anthē′mə), *n.pl* lesions involving the mucous membrane.

encephalitis (ensef′əlī′tis), *n* an inflammatory condition of the brain.

encounter form, *n* a document or record used to collect data about given elements of a patient visit to a dental office or similar site that can become part of a patient record or be used for management purposes or for quality review activities.

end organ, *n* the expanded termination of a nerve fiber in muscle, skin, mucous membrane, or other structure.

end organ, proprioceptor, *n.pl* the sensory end organs, located mainly in the muscles, tendons, and labyrinth, that provide information on the movements and position of the body. Four specific end organs are the muscle spindles; Golgi corpuscles, stimulated by tension; Pacini's corpuscles, stimulated by pressure; and bare nerve endings, stimulated by pain.

end organ, sensory, *n* the sensory nerve fibers that end peripherally as either unmyelinated fibers or special structures called receptors. Receptors are situated in the skin, mucous membranes, muscles, tendons, joints, and other structures and also in such special sense organs as those for vision, hearing, smell, and taste. The receptors are organized into a system that relates them to the environment: exteroceptors, interoceptors, and proprioceptors.

end points, *n.pl* **1.** the preestablished steps that, when completed, mark the achievement of a treatment goal. *n.pl* **2.** the clinical indications that a specific infectious condition has been lessened or eliminated altogether.

end section, *n* the distal portion of a twin-wire labial arch wire, consisting of a tube in which the anterior section of the labial arch is engaged.

end-bulb, *n* See end-feet.

end-feet (boutons terminaux, end-bulb), *n.pl* the small, terminal enlargements of nerve fibers that are in contact with the dendrites or cell bodies of other nerve cells; the synaptic endings of nerve fibers.

E

end-plate, *n* the terminal fibers of the motor nerves to the voluntary muscles. The nerve endings lose their myelin sheaths as they enter the sheaths of striated muscle fibers, at which point they ramify across the muscle fiber like the roots of a tree.

end-plate, motor, *n* the end-plate by which impulses from nerves are transmitted to the muscle fibers. It is a modification of the sarcolemma and is continuous with it. The end-plate potential generated by the nerve impulse activates the muscle impulse.

end-stage disease, *n* See disease, end-stage.

end-to-end bite, *n* See occlusion, edge-to-edge.

end-to-end occlusion, *n* See occlusion, edge-to-edge.

endemic, *adj* peculiar to a specific location or region, or within a specific group of people.

ending, *n* a termination; the point at which something is concluded.

ending, annulospiral, *n* a nerve ending, associated with an intrafusal muscle fiber, that is stimulated by a stretch impulse resulting from the extension of a muscle. The ending is in the form of a gradual spiral around the length of the intrafusal muscle fiber in the muscle spindle and is connected to the coarse myelinated fibers.

ending, flower spray, *n* a sensory nerve ending that is attached to the distal end of an intrafusal muscle fiber and that is stimulated when the muscle fiber contracts, pulling on the nerve ending.

ending, free nerve, *n* the peripheral terminal of the sensory nerve.

endocarditis, bacterial (en′dō-kahrdī′tis), *n* an inflammation of the heart (endocardium) valves and lining of the heart as a result of a bacterial infection. The term *subacute (SBE)* is no longer used. See also endocarditis, infective and premedication, antibiotic.

endocarditis, infective, *n* a bacterial infection of the heart valves. It may occur in normal or compromised valves. An increasing occurrence of the disease has been documented in those with prosthetic valve replacements, known as *prosthetic valve endocarditis (PVE).*

endocardium (en′dōkär′dēəm), *n* the innermost lining and connective tissue bed of the heart's chambers. It consists of smooth muscle cells, elastin, and collagen fibers.

endochondral bone, *n* See bone, endochondral.

endocrine (en′dōkrin′), *adj* refers to either the gland that secretes directly into the systemic circulation or the substance secreted.

endocrine disease, *n* an abnormal condition caused by some malfunction of an endocrine gland.

endocrine system, *n* the interrelated nature of the physiologic function of endocrine glands.

endocrinology (en′dōkrinol′əjē), *n* the study of the anatomy, physiology, biochemistry, and pathology of the endocrine system and the treatment of endocrine problems.

endodontally involved (en′dō-don′təlē), *adj* pertaining to disease of the dental pulp and dental periapical tissues.

endodontic implant, *n* a metallic implant extending through the root canal into the periapical bone structure to increase support and retention of the tooth.

endodontic techniques, *n.pl* procedures used in pulpless teeth or teeth that are to be made pulpless.

endodontics (en′dōdon′tiks), *n* the branch of dentistry that is concerned with the morphology, physiology, and pathology of the dental pulp and periradicular tissues. Its study and practice encompass the basic and clinical sciences, including biology of the normal pulp; the etiology, diagnosis, prevention, and treatment of diseases and injuries of the pulp; and associated periradicular conditions.

endodontist (en′dōdon′tist), *n* a dental professional who practices endodontics as a specialty.

endodontology (en′dōdontol′ōjē), *n* (endodontia, pulp canal therapy, root canal therapy), the division of dental science that deals with the causes, diagnosis, prevention, and treatment of diseases of the dental pulp and their sequelae.

endogenous (endoj′ənəs), *adj* originating within.

endolith (en′dōlith), See denticle.

endometrium, *n* the uterine mucous membrane lining.

endonuclease (en′dōnoo′klēās′), *n* an enzyme (nuclease) that cleaves polynucleotides at interior bonds, producing polynucleotide or oligonucleotide fragments.

endophthalmitis (en′dofthəlmī′-tis), *n* an inflammation of the tissues of the eyeball.

endophytic (en″dofit′ik), *adj* growing inward or on the inner surface of a structure.

endoplasmic reticulum (ER), *n* an extensive network of membrane-enclosed tubules in the cytoplasm of a cell.

endorphins (endor′fins), *n.pl* substances produced in the brain and pituitary gland that reduce pain sensations by binding to receptors in the nervous system. The three endorphins, called alpha-, beta-, and gamma-endorphin, are subsequences of the 91-amino-acid peptide hormone, beta-lipotropin.

endoscopy, *n* the visualization of the interior of organs and cavities of the body with an illuminated, flexible optical tube.

endoscopy, gastrointestinal, *n* the visualization of the interior of the stomach and intestines with an illuminated, flexible optical tube.

endoscopy, periodontal, *n* the use of a small fiber-optic endoscope attached to a specially designed dental instrument, such as an explorer, showing subgingival deposits in a magnified view.

endosseous (endos′ēəs), *adj* refers to any object, such as a dental implant, placed or contained within a bone.

endosteal, *n* a thin membrane of cells that line the bone's mandullary cavity.

endosteal implants, *n.pl* See implants, endosteal.

endosteum (endos′tēəm), *n* a thin layer of connective tissue that lines the walls of the bone marrow cavities and haversian canals of compact bone and covers the trabeculae of cancellous bone. It has both osteogenic and hematopoietic potencies and, like the periosteum, takes an active part in the healing of fractures.

endothelioma (en′dōthē′lēō′mə), *n* See sarcoma, Ewing's.

endothelium (en′dōthē′lēəm), *n* the layer of simple squamous epithelial cells that line the heart, the blood and lymph vessels, and the serous cavities of the body.

endotoxin (en′dōtok′sin), *n* a nondiffusible lipid polysaccharide-polypeptide complex formed within bacteria (some gram-negative bacilli and others); when released from the destroyed bacterial cells, endotoxin is capable of producing a toxic manifestation within the host.

endotracheal (en′dōtrā′kēəl), *adj* describes placement of an object within the trachea, or windpipe. E.g., an endotracheal tube is placed in the trachea and acts as an artificial airway.

Endur, *n.pr* the brand name for a two-paste diacrylate resin adhesive used as a bonding agent in orthodontics.

enema, *n* a procedure in which a solution is introduced into the rectum for cleansing or therapeutic purposes.

energy, *n* the capacity for doing work.

energy, atomic, *n* the energy that can be liberated by changes in the nucleus of an atom.

energy binding, *n* the energy represented by the difference in mass between the sum of the component parts and the actual mass of the nucleus of an atom.

energy dependence, *n* the characteristic response of a radiation detector to a given range of radiation energies or wavelengths as compared with the response of a standard free-air chamber. Emulsions also show energy dependence.

energy excitation, *n* the energy required to change a system from its ground state to an excited state. With each excited state there is associated a different excitation energy. See also excitation.

energy ionizing, *n* the average energy lost by ionizing radiation in producing an ion pair in a gas. (For air, ionizing energy is approximately 33 V.)

energy kinetic, *n* the energy possessed by a mass because of its motion.

energy nuclear, *n* See energy, atomic.

energy photon (hv), *n* the electromagnetic energy in the form of photons, with a value in ergs equal to the product of their frequency in cycles per second and Planck's constant (E-hv).

energy potential, *n* the energy inherent in a mass because of its position with reference to other masses.

energy radiant, *n* the energy of electromagnetic waves, such as radio waves, visible light, radiographs, and gamma rays.

enflurane (en′flŏŏrān), *n* a nonflammable anesthetic gas belonging to the ether family, used for induction and maintenance of general anesthesia.

engine, dental, *n* an electric motor that, by means of a continuous-cord drive over pulleys, activates a handpiece that holds a rotary instrument.

engineering, dental, *n* the application of physical, mechanical, and mathematical principles to dentistry.

Engman's disease See dermatitis, infectiosa eczematoides.

enkephalin (enkef′əlin), *n* one of two pain-relieving pentapeptides produced in the body.

enlargement, *n* an increase in size.

enlargement, Dilantin, *n.pr* See hyperplasia, gingival, Dilantin.

enlargement, idiopathic, *n* gingival enlargement, of unknown causation, clinically characterized by a firm, rounded thickening of the attached gingival tissues and histologically characterized by connective tissue hyperplasia.

enlargement, parotid **(pərot′id),** *n* a swelling of the parotid glands observed most frequently in those with anorexia and bulimia.

enolase (e′nolās), *n* an enzyme characterized by its crystalline structure and role in carbohydrate utilization.

enostosis (en′ostō′sis), *n* a bony growth located within a bone cavity or centrally from the cortical plate. See also osteoma.

enoxacin (enok′səsin), *n brand name:* Penetrex; *drug class:* fluoroquinolone antiinfective; *action:* a broad-spectrum bactericidal agent that inhibits the enzyme deoxyribonucleic acid (DNA) gyrase, needed for replication of DNA; *uses:* uncomplicated urethral or cervical gonorrhea, uncomplicated and complicated urinary tract infections.

enrollee, *n* an individual covered by a benefit plan. See also beneficiary.

Entamoeba gingivalis **(en′təmē′bə),** *n* a genus of protozoan found in the oral cavity; repeatedly, but not conclusively, associated with the initiation and continuation of periodontitis.

enteral (en′tərəl), *adj* directly into the gastrointestinal tract; pertains to tube feedings that may be necessary when a patient cannot ingest food orally.

enteric coating (enter′ik), *n* See coating, enteric.

enteritis (en′tərī′tis), *n* an inflammation of the mucosal lining of the small intestine.

Enterobacter cloacae **(en′tərōbak′tər klōā′sē),** *n.pr* a common species of bacteria found in human and animal feces, dairy products, sewage, soil, and water. It is rarely the cause of disease.

Enterobacteriaceae **(en′tərōbak′tir′ēā′sēē′),** *n.pr* a family of aerobic and anaerobic bacteria that includes both normal and pathogenic enteric microorganisms such as *Escherichia, Klebsiella, Proteus,* and *Salmonella.*

Enterobius vermicularis **(en′tərō′bēəs vərmik′yəlar′is),** *n* a parasitic worm that resides in the large intestine, more commonly found in children, which may cause pruritis in the anal region. It can be contracted from contact with fomites or by ingesting or inhaling immature forms of the worm. Also called *pinworm.*

enterococcus (en′tərō′kok′əs), *n* any *Streptococcus* bacterium that inhabits the intestinal tract.

entropion (entrō′pēon), *n* the inversion, or infolding, of the eyelid margin.

entry, port of, *n* the point on the body through which infectious microorganisms may enter, such as the eyes, nose, respiratory tract, or open wound.

enucleate (enoo′klēāt), *v* to remove a lesion in its entirety.

enunciation (inun′sēā′shən), *n* an auxiliary function of teeth, particularly those in the anterior sector of the dental arch; the formation of sounds as in speech.

enuresis (enūrē′sis), *n* involuntary urination (e.g., during general anesthesia, at night).

environment (envī′rənment, envī′urnment), *n* the aggregate of all the external conditions and influences affecting the life and development of an organism.

environment, extracellular, *n* the external, or interstitial, environment provided and maintained for the tissue cells.

environment, oral, *n* all oral conditions present and their influences.

environmental health, *n* the various aspects of substances, forces, and conditions in and about a community that affect the health and well-being of the population.

environmental pollutants, *n.pl* the substances and conditions, including noise, that adversely affect the health and well-being of the people within a community.

environmental pollution, *n* the presence of substances and conditions that adversely affect the health and well-being of people within a community; usually substances in the air and water supply.

Environmental Protection Agency (EPA), *n.pr* a federal agency charged with the approval and overseeing of the use and disposal of hazardous materials. Workplace management of hazardous materials falls under the jurisdiction of the Occupational Safety and Health Administration (OSHA).

EPA registered, *adj* indicates that an object or substance has been approved by the Environmental Protection Agency.

environmental tobacco smoke (ETS/passive smoke), *n* the gaseous by-product of burning tobacco products, including but not limited to commercially manufactured cigarettes and cigars; contains toxic elements harmful to the health of adults and children exposed to it. Also called *secondhand smoke.*

enzyme (en′zīm), *n* a protein substance that acts as a catalyst to speed up metabolic and other processes involving organic materials. Some enzymes function within cells; others function in the extracellular fluids and tissue spaces and organs. They are active in all major tissue functions, such as cellular respiration, muscle contraction, digestive processes, and energy consumption, and are produced intracellularly.

enzyme-linked immunosorbent assay (ELISA), *n* a species-specific serologic laboratory procedure used to identify microorganisms infecting or inhabiting a tissue or organ system. Its dental use is in the identification of pathogens involved in periodontal disease.

eosin (e′osin), *n* one of a pair of dyes used to color tissue samples to augment visibility under a microscope. The dyes are rose-colored, causing the cytoplasm to appear pink.

eosinophil (ē′əsin′əfil), *n* See leukocyte, eosinophilic.

eosinophilia (ē′əsin′əfil′ēə), *n* an absolute or relative increase in the normal number of eosinophils in the circulating blood. Various limits are given (e.g., absolute eosinophilia if the total number exceeds 500 mm^3) and relative if greater than 3% but total less than 500 mm^3. It may be associated with skin diseases, infestations, hay fever, asthma, angioneurotic edema, adrenocortical insufficiency, and Hodgkin disease.

eosinophilic granuloma, *n* See granuloma, eosinophilic.

EPA, *n.pr* See Environmental Protection Agency.

ephebodontics (əfe″bodon′tiks), *n* adolescent dentistry. See also pedodontics.

ephedrine sulfate (ifed′rin sul′fāt), *n brand name:* generic; *drug class:* adrenergic, mixed direct and indirect effects; *action:* causes increased contractility and heart rate by acting on β-receptors in heart; also acts on α-receptors, causing vasoconstriction in blood vessels; *uses:* shock, increased perfusion, hypotension, bronchodilation.

E

ephelis (əfē′lis), *n* (freckle) a circumscribed macular collection of pigment in the epidermis or oral mucosa. An increased amount of melanin pigment is seen in the region of the basal layer of cells.

epicanthic fold (ep′ikan′thik), *n* a characteristic crease in the eyelid; seen in persons with Down syndrome.

epicondylitis (ep′ikon′dəlī′tis), *n* a painful repetitive strain injury of the elbow characterized by inflammation or lesions in the muscles or tendons where they attach to the bone. Often known as "tennis elbow" when it affects the outside of the joint or "golfer's elbow" when it affects the inside of the joint.

epidemic, *adj* spreading rapidly and widely among many individuals in a single location or region; illnesses labeled epidemic are those that occur beyond normal expectations and are usually traceable to a single source.

epidemiologic survey, *n* See research, epidemiologic survey.

epidemiology (ep′idē′mēol′əjē), *n* the science of epidemics and epidemic diseases, which involve the total population rather than the individual. The aim of epidemiology is to determine those factors in the group environment that make the group more or less susceptible to disease.

epidemiology, indices in, *n.pl* the data collection tools that aid in the measurement and evaluation of disease indicators and conditions; classification systems featuring numbered scales against which a specific population may be compared.

epidermis (ep′ider′mis), *n* the superficial, avascular layers of the skin.

epidermoid cyst, *n* a common, benign, variable, subcutaneous swelling lined by keratinizing epithelium and filled with a cheesy material composed of sebum and epithelial debris.

epidermolysis bullosa (ep′idurmol′isis), *n* a disease of the skin characterized by bullae, vesicles, cysts, and, often, associated mandibular enlargement. See also syndrome, Goldscheider's and syndrome, Weber-Cockayne.

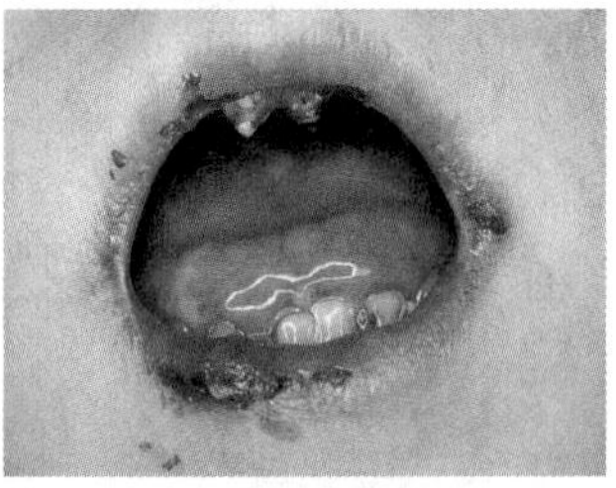

Epidermolysis bullosa. (Regezi/Sciubba/Jordan, 2008)

epiglottis (ep′iglot′is), *n* an elastic cartilage, covered by mucous membrane, that forms the superior part of the larynx and guards the glottis during swallowing.

epilepsy (ep′ilep′sē), *n* a group of neurologic disorders characterized by recurrent episodes of convulsive seizures, sensory disturbances, abnormal behavior, and loss of consciousness. Most epilepsy is of an unknown etiology but may be associated with cerebral trauma, brain tumors, vascular disturbances, or chemical imbalance. Drugs used in the treatment of symptoms (e.g., hydantoin sodium, diphenylhydantoin sodium) may promote gingival hyperplasia.

epiloia (epiloi′ə), *n* See syndrome, Bourneville-Pringle.

epinephrine (ep′inef′rin), *n* a hormone secreted by the adrenal medulla that stimulates hepatic glycogenolysis, causing an elevation in the blood sugar, vasodilation of blood vessels of the skeletal muscles, vasoconstriction of the arterioles of the skin and mucous membranes, relaxation of bronchiolar smooth muscles, and stimulation of heart action. Used in local anesthetics for its vasoconstrictive action to prolong the anesthesia action, provide hemostasis, and reduce systemic complications.

epinephrine/epinephrine bitartrate/ epinephrine HCl, n brand names: EpiPen Jr., Bronkaid Mist, Primatene Mist; *drug class:* adrenergic agonist, catecholamine; *action:* β1- and β2-agonist, causing increased levels of cAMP, producing bronchodilation and cardiac stimulation; *uses:* acute asthmatic attacks, hemostasis, bronchospasm, anaphylaxis, allergic reactions, cardiac arrest, vasopressor. Recommended for the dental office or clinic emergency kit. See EpiPen.

EpiPen, *n.pr* the brand name for an autoinjector containing epinephrine, used to treat severe allergic reactions. Dose is fast-acting and can be self-administered.

epiphysis (epif′isis), *n* the terminal portion of a long bone. The epiphysis is separated from the diaphysis during growth by a cartilaginous zone that serves as a growth center. Once ossification unites the epiphysis with the diaphysis, growth is completed.

epispinal (epispī′nəl), *adj* located on the spinal column.

epistaxis (ep′istak′sis), *n* (nosebleed) bleeding from the nose.

epithelial (ep′ithē′lēəl), *adj* pertaining to the epithelium.

epithelial attachment (EA), n See attachment, epithelial.

epithelial cells, n.pl cells that form the epithelial tissue that lines both the inner and outer surfaces of the body; serve a protective function and also aid in absorption and secretion.

epithelial cuff, attached, n the band of gingival tissue that is located around the tooth's margin.

epithelial cuff, implant, n the band of tissue that is constricted around an implant abutment post.

epithelial desquamation, anesthetic **(des′kwəmā′shən),** *n* the ulceration and shedding of oral epithelial tissue that occurs as the result of prolonged exposure to topical anesthesia.

epithelial inclusion, n the bits of epithelial tissue introduced into bone crypts during perforation osteotomies. See also osteotomy, perforation.

epithelial layers, n the number and type of layers present in epithelium.

epithelial rests of Malassez **(maləsə′),** *n* the remnants of Hertwig's epithelial root sheath within the periodontal ligament.

epithelioma (ep′ithē′lēō′mə), *n* an epithelial neoplasm.

epithelioma adenoides cysticum, n multiple trichoepitheliomas.

epithelioma, basal cell, n See carcinoma, basal cell.

epithelium (ep′ithē′lēəm), *n* the layer of cells that lines a body cavity; cells may be ciliated or unciliated, and may be squamous (flat, scale-like), cuboidal (cube-shaped), or columnar (column-shaped).

epithelium, basement membrane of, n See membrane, basement.

epithelium, desmosomes of **(dez′-mosōmz′),** *n* an electronmicroscopic finding of intercellular bridges that serve to attach adjacent epithelial cells to each other.

epithelium, enamel, inner, n the innermost layer of cells (ameloblasts) of the enamel organ that deposit the organic matrix of the enamel on the crown of the developing tooth. Also the innermost layer of Hertwig's epithelial root sheath.

epithelium, enamel, outer, n the outermost layer of cells of the enamel organ. It is separated from the inner enamel epithelium in the area of the developing crown by the stratum intermedium and stellate reticulum and lies immediately adjacent to the inner enamel epithelium in the area of the developing root.

epithelium, enamel, reduced, n combined enamel epithelium; the remains of the enamel organ after enamel formation is complete. After eruption of the tip of the crown, that part of the combined epithelium remaining on the enamel surface is called the *epithelial attachment.*

epithelium, gingival, n a stratified squamous epithelium consisting of a basal layer; it is keratinized or parakeratinized.

epithelium, hyperplastic, n an increase in thickness, with alterations in structure, produced by proliferation of cellular elements of epithelium.

epithelium, oral, n the epithelial covering of the oral mucosa. Composed of stratified squamous epithelium of varying thickness and varying degrees of keratinization.

epithelium, pocket, *n* the epithelium that lines the periodontal pocket. Its most prominent characteristics are the presence of hyperplasia and ulceration.

epithelium, pseudostratified **(soo′-dōstrat′ifīd),** *n* a type of epithelium in which there appears to be several layers (or strata) of cells, but all cells actually are resting on the base layer. Often ciliated and occurs only in mucosa.

epithelium, squamous **(skwā′məs),** *n* a type of epithelium consisting of flat, scalelike cells.

epithelium, stratified squamous, *n* the variety of epithelium covering the oral mucosa and dermal surfaces; composed of layers of cells oriented parallel to the surface. The various layers of cells in order from basement membrane to surface are stratum germinativum, stratum spinosum (prickle cell layer), and stratum lucidum (in dermal epithelium). The gingival epithelium generally exhibits some degree of keratinization, variable from parakeratinization to orthokeratinization within the layers of the stratum granulosum (granular layer) and stratum corneum (keratin layer).

epithelium, sulcal, *n* the stratified squamous epithelium forming the covering of the soft tissue wall of the gingival sulcus, or crevice. Extends from the gingival margin to the line of attachment of the epithelium to the tooth surface.

epithelialization (epithelization) (ep′əthē′lēəlizā′shən), *n* the natural act of healing by secondary intention; the proliferation of new epithelium into an area devoid of it but that naturally is covered by it.

epizootic fever (ep′izōot′ik), *n* another name for foot and mouth disease in cloven-foot animals; also known as aphthous fever; caused by a type of coxsackievirus, uncommon in the United States. The disease in humans is characterized by malaise, fever, headache, itchy skin, and a sensation of xerostomia despite heavy salivation. Vesicles appear in the oral cavity, around the lips, and on the hands and feet. Oral vesicles and ulcers resolve within approximately 10 days.

epoxy resin (ēpok′sē, əpok′sē), *n* See resin, epoxy.

Epstein's pearls, *n.pr* white, ricelike, keratin-filled lesions of the midline hard palate mucosa. See also cyst, palatal, of the newborn.

Epstein-Barr virus (EBV), *n.pr* a herpesvirus associated with Burkitt's lymphoma and reported in cases of infectious mononucleosis; more recently reported to be associated with AIDS.

epulis (epū′lis), *n* a tumor (tumescence) of the gingiva.

epulis, congenital of newborn, *n* a raised or pedunculated lesion located on the anterior gingivae of the newborn. It is histologically similar to granular cell myoblastoma. See also myoblastoma, granular cell.

epulis fissuratum **(fisŏŏrat′əm),** *n* a curtainlike fold of excess tissue associated with the flange of a denture. Also called *inflammatory fibrous hyperplasia, redundant tissue.*

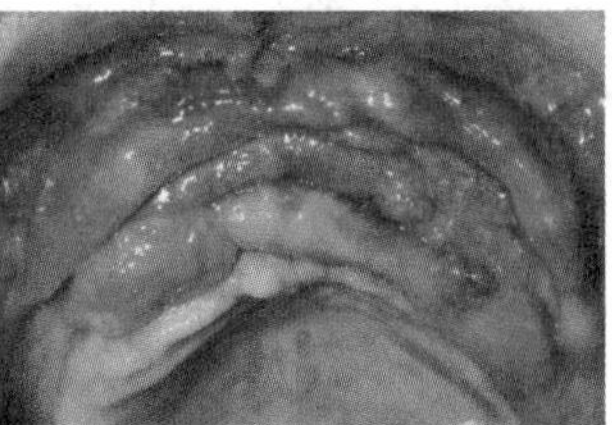

Epulis fissuratum. (Neville/Damm/Allen/Bouquot, 2002)

epulis, giant cell, *n* See granuloma, giant cell reparative, peripheral.

epulis granulomatosa **(gran′yəlō′mətō′sə),** *n* a tumorlike mass of red, easily bleeding, infected granulation tissue that occurs as a result of exuberant reparative phenomena. Seen arising from tooth sockets or is associated with exfoliating necrotic bone. See granulation tissue.

equal protection, *n* clause set out in the Fourteenth Amendment of the U.S. Constitution that dictates that state governments cannot pass or enforce any laws based solely on a specific classification of person by race, gender, religion, ethnicity, or age.

equilibration (ēkwil′ibrā′shən), *n* the act of placing a body in a state of equilibrium.

equilibration diagnostic, n See diagnostic equilibration.

equilibration, mandibular, n the act or acts performed to place the mandible in a state of equilibrium.

equilibration, occlusal, n the modification of occlusal forms of teeth by grinding, with the intent of equalizing occlusal stress and of harmonizing cuspal relations in function.

equilibration of mounted casts, n an equilibration of the occlusion of mounted casts made of a patient for the purpose of observing and recording what must be done to adjust the natural occlusion.

equilibration, proper, n See proper equilibration.

equilibrator (ēkwil′ibrātur), *n* an instrument or device used in achieving or maintaining a state of equilibrium.

equilibrium (ē′kwilib′rēəm), *n* a state of balance between two opposing forces or processes.

equilibrium, functional, n the state of homeostasis within the oral cavity existing when biologic processes and local environmental factors, including the forces of mastication, are in a state of balance.

equilibrium, juvenile occlusal **(joo′vənīl əkloo′səl),** *n* one of the six eruptive phases of dentition, and the first of three postfunctional stages of eruption of the entire dentition. It occurs at or near adolescence when permanent teeth continue to erupt into the oral cavity in response to the vertical growth of the ramus.

equipment, *n* the nonexpendable items used by the dental staff in the office in the performance of professional duties.

equity, *n* a free and reasonable claim or right; fairness; impartiality. The money value of a property or of an interest in a property in excess of claims or liens against it; a risk interest or ownership right in property.

equivalent, *n* a state where there is an equal in force, value, measure, or effect; corresponding in function.

equivalent, aluminum, n the thickness of pure aluminum affording the same radiation attenuation, under specified conditions, as the material or materials being considered.

equivalent, concrete, n the thickness of concrete having a density of 2.35 g/cm^3 that would afford the same radiation attenuation, under specified conditions, as the material or materials being considered.

equivalent, lead, n the thickness of pure lead that would afford the same radiation attenuation, under specified conditions, as the material or materials being considered.

erbium (Er) (ur′bēəm), *n* a rare earth, metallic element with an atomic number of 68 and an atomic weight of 167.26.

erg (urg), *n* a unit of energy equal to the energy consumed by 1 dyne acting through 1 cm, which is equal to 10^{-7} joule.

ergoloid mesylate (ur′gōloid mes′ilāt′), *n brand names:* Hydergine LC, Gerimal; *drug class:* ergot alkaloids; *action:* may increase cerebral metabolism and blood flow; *uses:* senile dementia, Alzheimer's dementia, primary progressive dementia.

ergonomics, *n* the study of workplace design and the physical and psychologic impact it has on workers. It is about the fit between people, their work activities, equipment, work systems, and environment to ensure that workplaces are safe, comfortable and efficient and that productivity is not compromised.

ergotamine tartrate (ur′got′əmēn tar′trāt), *n brand names:* Ergomar, Ergostat; *drug class:* α-adrenergic blocker; *action:* constricts by direct action vascular smooth muscle in peripheral and cranial blood vessels, relaxes uterine muscle; *uses:* vascular headache (migraine or histamine), cluster headache.

ergotoxine (ur′gōtox′in), *n* a potent alkaloid that paralyzes the motor and secretory nerves of the sympathetic system but has no effect on the inhibitory or parasympathetic nerves.

ERISA, *n.pr* the acronym for the **Employee Retirement Income Security Act of 1974.** See also Employee Retirement Income Security Act.

erosion (ērō′zhən), *n* the chemical or mechanicochemical destruction of tooth substance, the mechanism of which is incompletely known, which leads to the creation of concavities of many shapes at the cementoenamel junction of teeth. The surface of the cavity, unlike dental caries, is hard and smooth.

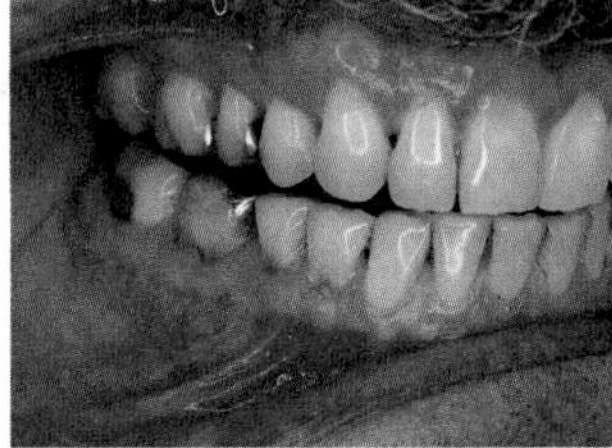

Erosion. (Ibsen/Phelan, 2004)

error, *n* a violation of duty; a fault; a mistake in the proceedings of a court in matters of law or of fact.

error, legal, *n* a mistaken judgment or incorrect belief as to the existence or effect of matters of fact, or a false or mistaken conception or application of the law.

error, numerical, *n* the amount of loss or precision in a quantity; the difference between an accurate quantity and its calculated approximation. Errors occur in numerical methods; mistakes occur in programming, coding, data transcription, and operating; malfunctions occur in computers and are caused by physical limitations of the properties of materials.

error of measurement, *n* the deviation of an individual score or observation from its true value, caused by the unreliability of the instrument and the individual who is measuring.

error, sampling, *n* any mistake in drawing a sample that keeps it from being unrepresentative; selection procedures that are biased; error introduced when a group is described on the basis of an unrepresentative sample.

error, variance, *n* that part of the total variance caused by anything irrelevant to a study that cannot be experimentally controlled.

eruption (erup′shən), *n* the migration of a tooth in the alveolar process of the maxilla or mandible into the oral cavity.

eruption, active, *n* the movement of a developing tooth from its area of development in the jaw into the oral cavity to become part of the dental arch.

eruption, continuous, *n* the normal occlusal progression of teeth noted throughout a lifetime.

eruption cyst, *n* a dentigerous cyst that causes a clinically evident bulging of the overlying alveolar ridge. See also cysts, eruption.

eruption, delayed, *n* the failure of the teeth to erupt from the gingival tissues at the usual developmental time. Often associated with hypothyroidism or impaction.

eruption, ectopic **(ektop′ik),** *n* the abnormal direction of tooth eruption, most common to mandibular first and third molars, which sometimes leads to abnormal resorption of the adjacent tooth.

eruption, forced, *n* the manual, forced eruption of a tooth that has failed to erupt naturally.

eruption hematoma, *n* an eruption cyst that is blood-filled, visualized as a bluish purple area of elevated tissue of the overlying alveolar ridge.

eruption, lingual, *n* the eruption of permanent teeth on the lingual side of primary teeth that have not yet been exfoliated.

eruption, passive, *n* an increasing length of the clinical crown often seen with aging and in the absence of clinical evidence of inflammation.

eruption sequestrum **(erup′shən səkwes′trēəm),** *n* a needlelike piece of calcified tissue that is located over the gingival tissues of an erupting tooth.

eruption, surgical, *n* the surgical removal of tissues covering an abnormally unerupted tooth to allow its natural progress into position.

eruptive gingivitis, *n* See gingivitis, eruptive.

erysipelas (er′isip′ələs), *n* an infectious skin disease characterized by redness, swelling, vesicles, bullae, fever, pain, and lymphadenopathy. It is caused by a species of group A β-hemolytic streptococci.

Erysipelothrix **(er″əsip′əlothriks″),** *n* a gram-positive bacterium that does not produce spores and has cell walls.

erythema (er′ithē′mə), *n* a patchy, circumscribed, or marginated macular redness of the skin or mucous membranes caused by hyperemia or inflammation.

erythema, linear gingival (LGE) **(er′əthē′mə lin′ēer jin′jəvəl),** *n* the thin bands of severe erythema noted in the marginal gingiva. Sometimes present in people with AIDS.

erythema multiforme complex, *n* an acute, inflammatory dermatologic disease of uncertain etiology (although occasionally related to drug administration), characterized by erythematous macules, papules, vesicles, and bullae that appear on the skin and not infrequently on the oral mucosa. See also syndrome, Stevens-Johnson.

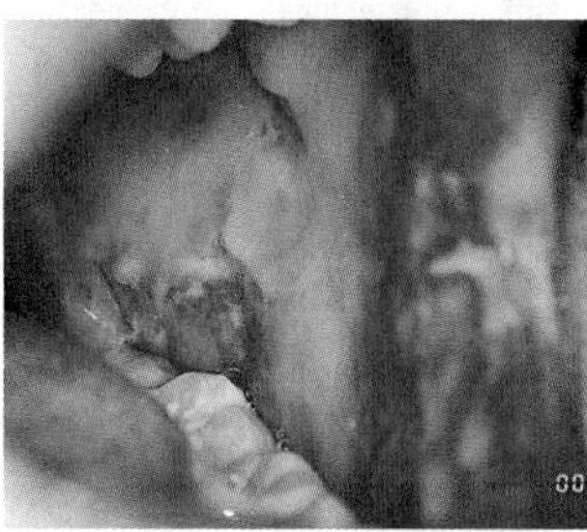

Erythema multiforme. (Daniel/Harfst/Wilder, 2008)

erythema infectiosum, *n* See disease, fifth.

erythematous/atrophic *Candida* (er′əthem′ətəs ātrō′fik kandē′də), *n* a skin disease characterized by patches of smooth, red tissue on the tongue, palate, or oral mucosa. Most commonly seen in people with AIDS.

erythredema polyneuropathy (ərith′redē′mə pol′ēnūrop′əthē), *n* See acrodynia.

erythremia (er′ithrē′mēə), *n* (Osler's disease, polycythemia rubra, polycythemia vera, primary polycythemia, Vaquez' disease) a myeloproliferative disease characterized by a marked increase in the circulating red blood cell mass. Erythremia may represent a neoplastic growth of erythropoietic tissue. Neutrophilia, thrombocytopenia, and splenomegaly are common. Manifestations include plethora, vertigo, headache, and thrombosis.

erythrityl tetranitrate (ərith′ritəl tetrənī′trāt), *n brand name:* Cardilate; *drug class:* organic nitrate; *action:* causes relaxation of vascular smooth muscle; decreases preload/afterload, which is responsible for decreasing left ventricular end diastolic pressure; systemic vascular resistance; improved exercise tolerance; *uses:* chronic stable angina pectoris, prophylaxis of angina pain.

erythroblastosis fetalis (ərith′rōblastō′sis fētal′is), *n* an excessive destruction of red blood cells begun before or shortly after birth in the fetus or newborn. It may be caused by an Rh factor reaction. After birth the skin is yellow, and the teeth may be markedly discolored.

Erythrocin, *n.pr* the brand name for erythromycin.

erythrocyte (ərith′rōsīt), *n* a red blood cell; a nonnucleated, circular, biconcave, discoid, hemoglobin-containing, oxygen-carrying formed element circulating in the blood.

erythrocyte count, *n* the number of red blood cells per cubic millimeter of blood.

erythrocyte indices, *n.pr* the standard values of red blood cell numbers, morphologic characteristics, and behavior in comprehensive hematologic laboratory testing.

erythrocyte sedimentation rate (ESR), *n* the rate at which red blood cells settle in a pipette of unclotted blood, measured in millimeters per hour. It is used as an index of inflammation.

erythrocytosis (ərith′rōsītō′sis), *n* (secondary polycythemia) an increased circulating red blood cell mass resulting from compensatory effort to meet reduced oxygen content. May be seen in persons living at high altitudes, as well as in persons with emphysema, pulmonary insufficiency, and heart failure.

erythromycin (ərith′rōmī′sin), *n* an antibiotic produced by a strain of *S. erythroeus,* only slightly effective against β-hemolytic streptococci (viridans group), and upper and lower respiratory tract, skin, and soft tissue infections of mild to moderate severity. It is no longer recommended by the American Heart Association and the American Dental Association for treatment of bacterial endocarditis in patients hypersensitive to penicillin.

erythromycin base (et al.), *n brand names:* E-mycin, Ery-Tab (et al.); *drug class:* macrolide antibiotic; *action:* binds to 50S ribosomal subunits of susceptible bacteria and suppresses protein synthesis; *uses:* infections caused by *N. gonorrhoeae;* mild to moderate respiratory tract, skin, soft tissue infections caused by *S. pneumoniae, C. diphtheriae, B. pertussis;* syphilis; Legionnaire's disease; *H. influenzae.*

erythroplakia (ərith″ropla′keə), *n* a flat red patch or lesion of unknown etiology on the oral or pharyngeal surfaces.

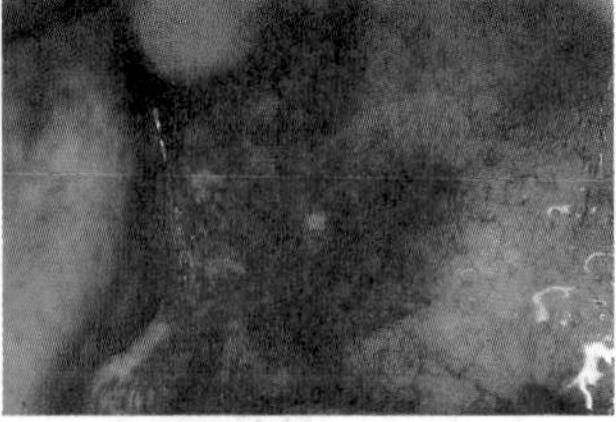

Erythroplakia. (Regezi/Sciubba/Pogrel, 2000)

erythroplasia of Queyrat (ərith′rōplā′zhə əv kərat′, kārī′), *n.pr* a form of intraepithelial carcinoma. The oral lesions are usually seen as plaques with a bright, velvety surface.

erythropoiesis (ərith′rōpoiē′sis), *n* the process in which red blood cells are formed.

erythrosin (ərith′rosēn), *n* a red dye used to reveal plaque deposits on teeth; administered in both tablet and liquid form. See also disclosing solution.

escharotic (es′kīrot′ik), *n* a caustic or corrosive agent that has the strength to burn tissue.

Escherichia coli (E. coli) **(eshərik′ēə kō′lī),** *n.pr* a species of coliform bacteria normally present in the intestines and common in water, milk, and soil can become a pathogen at other body sites.

esculin (es′kəlin), *n* a glucoside from horse-chestnut bark; used as a sunburn protective.

esophageal atresia (isof′əjē′əl ətrē′zhə), *n* an abnormal esophagus that ends in a blind pouch or narrows to a thin cord and thus fails to provide a continuous passage to the stomach. It is usually a congenital anomaly.

esophageal stenosis (isof′əjē′əl stənō′sis), *n* a narrowing or restriction of the lumen of the esophagus that slows or impedes the passage of fluid and foods from the oral cavity to the stomach.

esophagitis (isof′əjītis), *n* an inflammation of the mucosal lining of the esophagus caused by infection or irritation of the mucosa by reflux of gastric juice from the stomach.

esophagus (isof′əgəs), *n* the muscular canal extending from the pharynx to the stomach.

essence (es′ens), *n* an alcoholic solution of an essential oil.

essential oil, *n* See oil, essential.

essentials oils mouthrinses, *n.pl* mouthwashes made from thymol, menthol, eucalyptol, and methylsalicylate in combination with alcohol that are available over the counter for use in controlling plaque and gingivitis. See also mouthwash.

estate, *n* one's interest in land or other property.

estate planning, *n* a detailed, written-out plan (usually arrived at with the advice of estate counselors) in which all the financial affairs of the dental professional are clearly stated and provisions are made for alterations when changing conditions warrant it.

estazolam (estaz′olam), *n brand name:* ProSom; *drug class:* benzodiazepine, sedative-hypnotic, Controlled Substance Schedule IV in United States; *action:* produces central nervous system depression by interaction with benzodiazepine receptor; *use:* insomnia.

ester (es′tur), *n* a compound formed from alcohol and an acid.

ester linkage, *n* the bonding between fatty acids and glycerol that characterizes true fats.

esterase (es′tərās), *n* an enzyme that catalyzes the hydrolysis of an ester into its alcohol and acid.

esterified estrogens, *n.pl brand names:* Estabs, Estratab, Menest;

drug class: synthetic estrogen; *action:* required for development, maintenance, and adequate function of female reproductive system by increasing synthesis of deoxyribonucleic acid, ribonucleic acid, and selected proteins; decreases release of gonadotropine-releasing hormone; inhibits ovulation and helps maintain bone structure; *uses:* menopause, breast cancer, prostatic cancer, hypogonadism, ovariectomy, primary ovarian failure.

esthetic zone, *n* the visible area seen upon full smile, including the teeth, gingiva, and lips.

esthetics (esthet′iks), *n* (aesthetics) the branch of philosophy dealing with beauty, especially with the components thereof; i.e., color and form.

esthetics, dentistry, *n* the skills and techniques used to improve the art and symmetry of the teeth and face to enhance the appearance as well as the function of the teeth, oral cavity, and face.

esthetics, denture, *n* the cosmetic effect, produced by a denture, that affects the desirable beauty, charm, character, and dignity of the individual.

esthetics, denture base, *n* the esthetically proper tinting, contouring, and festooning of the gingival tissue portion of a denture base.

esthetics, gingival tissue (gingival tissue esthetics), *n* See esthetics, denture base.

estimate, *n* the anticipated fee for dental services to be performed.

estimated average requirement (E.A.R.), *n* the accepted standard level of nutrients that an average person requires. The basis for the Recommended Daily Allowance is established by the U.S. government.

estoppel (estop′əl), *n* a preclusion, in law, that prevents a person from alleging or denying a fact because of his or her own previous act or allegation.

estradiol benzoate (es′trədī′ol ben′zōāt), *n* a topical steroid (β-estradiol-3-benzoate) with estrogenic activity, useful in the treatment of lesions produced by diminution of bodily production of estrogens. Experimental administration to aged laboratory mice has resulted in an increased downgrowth of epithelial attachment along the root surface of teeth and subsequent production of periodontal disease.

estradiol/estradiol cypionate/estradiol valerate, *n brand names:* Deladiol, Depogen, Estro-Cyp, Estra-LA; *drug class:* estrogen; *action:* increases synthesis of deoxyribonucleic acid, ribonucleic acid, and selected proteins, decreases release of gonadotropin-releasing hormone, inhibits ovulation, and helps maintain bone structure; *uses:* menopause, prostatic cancer, atrophic vaginitis, kraurosis vulvae, hypogonadism, ovariectomy, primary ovarian failure.

estradiol transdermal system, *n brand names:* Esbrand, Climera; *drug class:* estrogen; *action:* increases synthesis of deoxyribonucleic acid, ribonucleic acid, and selected proteins; decreases release of gonadotropin-releasing hormone; inhibits ovulation and helps maintain bone structure; *uses:* menopause, prostatic cancer, abnormal uterine bleeding, hypogonadism, ovariectomy, osteoporosis.

estrin (es′trin), *n* the generic term for the ovarian estrogens estriol, estrone, and estradiol.

estrogens (es′trōjenz), *n.pl* the collective term for substances capable of producing estrus. The term also applies to the estrogenic hormones in women. Estriol is the principal estrogen found in the urine of pregnant women and in the placenta. Synthetic estrogens include diethylstilbestrol, hexestrol, and ethinyl estradiol.

etch, acid, *v* See acid etching.

etching, *n* a process used to decalcify the superficial layers of enamel as a step in the application of sealants or bonding agents in preventive dentistry and orthodontics. The agent of choice is phosphoric acid in concentrations of 30% to 40%.

ethacrynate sodium/ethacrynic acid (eth′əkrin′āt), *n brand name:* Edecrin Sodium; *drug class:* loop diuretic; *action:* acts on loop of Henle by increasing excretion of chloride, sodium; *uses:* pulmonary edema, edema in congestive heart failure, liver disease, nephrotic syndrome, ascites, hypertension.

ethambutal HCl (ētham′byootol), *n brand name:* Myambutol; *drug* *class:* antitubercular; *action:* inhibits ribonucleic acid synthesis, decreases tubercle bacilli replication; *uses:* pulmonary tuberculosis, as adjunct.

ethane (eth'ān), *n* a constituent of natural and "bottled" gases.

ether, diethyl (ē'thər, dīeth'il), *n* (ethyl ether, ether $[C_2H_5]2O$) a volatile ether used as an anesthetic that causes excellent muscle relaxation with minimal effect on blood pressure, pulse rate, and respiration. It is irritating to the respiratory passages and produces nausea.

ether, divinyl (ē'thər, dīvī'nəl), *n* (divinyl oxide $[CH_2{:}CH]_2O$) a highly volatile, unsaturated ether that is a rapid-acting anesthetic without the aftereffect of nausea produced by diethyl ether.

etherization (ē'therizā'shən), *n* the administration of ether to produce anesthesia.

ethics (eth'iks), *n* **1.** the science of moral obligation; a system of moral principles, quality, or practice. *n* **2.** the moral obligation to render to the patient the best possible quality of dental service and to maintain an honest relationship with other members of the profession and mankind in general.

ethics, dental, *n* See ethics, professional.

ethics, professional, *n* the principles and norms of proper professional conduct concerning the rights and duties of health care professionals themselves and their conduct toward patients and fellow practitioners, including the actions taken in the care of patients and family members.

ethinyl estradiol (eth'inil es'trədī'ol), *n brand names:* Estinyl; *drug class:* nonsteroidal synthetic estrogen; *action:* affects release of pituitary gonadotropins, inhibits ovulation, promotes adequate calcium use in bone structure; *uses:* menopause, prostatic cancer, breast cancer, postmenopausal osteoporosis.

ethionamide (eth'ēon'əmīd'), *n brand name:* Trecator-SC; *drug class:* antitubercular; *action:* bacteriostatic against Mycobacterium tuberculosis; may inhibit protein synthesis; *uses:* pulmonary, extrapulmonary tuberculosis when other antitubercular drugs have failed.

ethnic group, *n* a population of individuals organized around an assumption of common cultural origin.

ethosuximide (eth'ōsuk'səmīd'), *n brand name:* Zarontin; *drug class:* anticonvulsant; *action:* suppresses spike wave formation in absence seizures (petit mal); decreases amplitude, frequency, duration, spread of discharge in minor motor seizures; *uses:* absence seizures (PM).

ethotoin (eth'ətō'ən), *n brand name:* Peganone; *drug class:* hydantoin derivative anticonvulsant; *action:* inhibits spread of seizure activity in motor cortex; *uses:* generalized tonic-clonic or complex-partial seizures.

ethyl acetate, abuse of (eth'əl as'ətāt), *n* the recreational, often compulsive inhaling of the fumes of a liquid solvent, especially those found in paint thinners. See also huffing.

ethyl aminobenzoate (eth'əl əme"noben'zoāt), *n* an ester-type anesthetic agent formulated for surface application as a liquid, gel, ointment, or spray; the most widely used topical numbing agent.

ethyl chloride (eth'il klôr'īd), *n* (C_2H_5Cl) a colorless liquid that boils between 12° and 13° C. It acts as a local, topical anesthetic of short duration through the superficial freezing produced by its rapid vaporization from the skin. Ethyl chloride is used occasionally in inhalation therapy as a rapid, fleeting general anesthetic, comparable to nitrous oxide but somewhat more dangerous.

ethylene (eth'ilēn), *n* (olefiant gas, CH_2CH_2) a colorless gas of slightly sweet odor and taste; used as an inhalation anesthetic.

ethylene oxide sterilization, *n* a process that uses gas to sterilize instruments, equipment, and materials that would otherwise be damaged by heat or liquid chemicals. Effective at room temperature. Requires between 10 and 16 hours to be effective. Gas must penetrate the material. The gas is highly toxic and must be vented before opening the sealed sterilizing unit. Sterilized materials must also be well aerated before using.

etidocaine HCl (local), *n brand names:* Duranest, Duranest MPF; *drug* *class:* amide, local anesthetic; *action:* inhibits ion fluxes across membranes, particularly sodium transport across cell membrane; decreases rise of depolarization phase of action potential; blocks nerve action potential; *uses:* local dental anesthetic, peripheral nerve block, caudal anesthetic, central neural block, vaginal block.

etidronate disodium (ē′tədrō′nāt dīsō′dēəm), *n* *brand name:* Didronel IV; *drug class:* antihypercalcemic; *action:* decreases bone resorption and new bone development (accretion); *uses:* Paget's disease, heterotopic ossification, hypercalemia of malignancy.

etiology (ē′tēol′əjē), *n* **1.** causative factors. *n* **2.** the factors implicated in the causation of disease. *n* **3.** the study of the factors causing disease.

etiology, local factors, *n* the environmental influences that may be implicated in the causation or perpetuation of a disease process.

etiology, systemic factors, *n* generalized biologic factors that are implicated in the causation, modification, or perpetuation of a disease entity. Within the oral cavity, the actions of the systemic factors are modified by interaction with local factors.

etodolac (ētō′dəlak), *n* *brand name:* Lodine; *drug class:* nonsteroidal antiinflammatory; *action:* inhibits prostaglandin synthesis by interfering with cyclooxgenase, which is needed for biosynthesis; *uses:* mild to moderate pain, osteoarthritis.

Eubacterium **(ū′baktē′rēəm),** *n.pr* a genus of anaerobic, non–spore-forming, nonmotile bacteria containing straight or curved gram-positive rods that usually occur singly, in pairs, or in short chains. They usually metabolize carbohydrates and may be pathogenic.

eugenol (yōō′jənol), *n* **1.** an allyl guaiacol obtainable from oil of cloves. Used with zinc oxide in a paste for temporary restorations, bases under restorations, and impression materials. Believed to have a palliative effect on dental pulp and possibly a limited germicidal effect. *n* **2.** a colorless or pale yellow liquid obtained from clove oil; has a clove odor and pungent, spicy taste. Used as the liquid portion of zinc oxide and eugenol cements and in toothache medications.

eugnathia (ūnā′thēə), *n* the normal or proper relationship of the jaws to each other.

euphoria (ūfôr′ēə), *n* a sense of well-being or normalcy. Pleasantly mild excitement.

euphoric (ūfôr′ik), *n* a substance that produces an exaggerated sense of well-being.

eupnea (ūpnē′ə), *n* a situation with easy or normal respiration.

europium (yŏŏrō′pēəm), *n* a rare earth metallic element with an atomic number of 63 and an atomic weight of 151.96.

eustachian tube (ūstā′shən), *n* a tube, lined with mucous membrane, that joins the nasopharynx and the middle ear cavity, allowing equalization of the air pressure in the middle ear with atmospheric pressure. Also called the *auditory tube.*

Eutectic Mixture of Local Anesthetics (EMLA) (ūtek′tik), *n* a topical anesthetic made from equal parts of lidocaine and prilocaine that is applied as a cream on unbroken skin, then covered with an occlusive dressing, to kill pain prior to venipuncture, intramuscular injections, intravenous cannulation, or minor skin procedures. See lidocaine HCl (topical), prilocaine hydrochloride.

euthanasia (ū′thənā′zhə), *n* an act of deliberately bringing about the death of a person who is suffering from an incurable disease or condition; also called *mercy killing.* Active euthanasia is illegal in most jurisdictions; passive euthanasia, or the withholding of some life support systems, has legal standing in some jurisdictions.

euthyroidism (ūthī′roidizəm), *n* a state of normal thyroid function.

evacuation system, *n* a centralized vacuum system connected to each dental operating unit, used to keep the oral cavity clear of water, saliva, blood, and debris, generally operating at a high volume, high velocity, and low pressure.

evaluation, *n* to make a judgment or appraisal of a condition or situation. In dentistry, used to describe the clinical judgment of a patient's dental health or an appraisal of staff performance.

evaluation studies, n.pl the control study of the comparative value of different treatment modalities or medications.

Evans blue, *n.pr* a diazo dye used for the determination of the blood volume on the basis of the dilution of a standard solution of the dye in the plasma after its intravenous injection.

E

evidence, *n* the proof presented at a trial by the parties through witnesses, records, documents, and concrete objects for the purpose of inducing the court or jury to believe their contentions.

evidence, radiographic, n the shadow images depicted in radiographs.

evidence-based care, *n* a philosophy of treatment that relies on up-to-date, germane research as its foundation.

Evipal (ē′vipĭl), *n.pr* the brand name for **hexobarbital,** a rapid-acting barbiturate.

Evipal sodium, n the brand name for **hexobarbital sodium.** An ultrashort-acting barbiturate of the N-methyl type whose pharmacologic actions, from a clinical standpoint, are essentially similar to thiopental (Pentothal).

evoked potential, *n* an electrical response in the brainstem or cerebral cortex that is elicited by a specific stimulus. This property of the brain may be used to monitor brain function during surgery.

evulsed tooth (ivul′st), *n* See tooth, evulsed.

(avulsion), n the sudden tearing out, or away, of tissue as a result of a traumatic episode.

evulsion, nerve, *n* the operation of tearing a nerve from its central origin by traction.

evulsion, tooth, *n* the displacement of a tooth from its alveolar housing; may be partial or complete.

Ewing's sarcoma, *n.pr* See sarcoma, Ewing's.

Ewing's tumor, *n.pr* See sarcoma, Ewing's.

examination, *n* **1.** inspection; search; investigation; inquiry; scrutiny; testing. *n* **2.** the inspection or investigation of part or all of the body to measure and evaluate the state of health or disease. The examination may include visual inspection, percussion, palpation, auscultation, and measurement of mobility as well as various laboratory and radiographic procedures.

examination, anteroposterior extraoral radiographic, n an examination in which the film is placed at the posterior direction with the rays passing from the anterior to the posterior direction to record images.

examination, bite-wing intraoral radiographic, n radiography in which an intraoral radiograph records on a single film the shadow images of the outline, position, and mesiodistal extent of the crowns, necks, and coronal third of the roots of both the maxillary and mandibular teeth and alveolar crests.

examination, body section extraoral radiographic, n (tomogram), a radiographic procedure of various internal layers of the head and body accomplished by the synchronized movement of the roentgen-ray tube and film in parallel planes but in opposite directions from each other. Also known as *tomography, laminagraphy, planigraphy,* and *stratigraphy.*

examination, bregmamentum extraoral radiographic **(breg′məmen′təm),** *n* radiography in which the film is placed beneath the chin, with the rays directed downward through the junction of the coronal and sagittal sutures (bregma) to the chin (mentum).

examination, cephalometric extraoral radiographic **(sef′əlōmet′rik),** *n* See cephalometric radiography.

examination, clinical, n **1.** the visual and tactile scrutiny of the tissues of and surrounding the oral cavity. *n* **2.** the formal testing of the dental professional student to determine whether his or her skills meet or exceed established standards.

examination, complete, n a methodical, complete assessment of an individual involving basic and supplementary procedures as well as evaluation of the plan for preventive care.

examination, extradental intraoral radiographic, n an examination in which the film is placed between the teeth and the tissue of the cheek or lip for the exploration or localization of the internal structures of these tissues.

examination, extraoral radiographic, *n* an examination of the oral and paraoral structures by exposing films placed extraorally, in contrast to intraorally.

examination, gingival, *n* the observation of the primary visual symptoms of periodontal disease, including color changes; changes in surface texture; deviations from normal contour and structure, tissue tone, and vitality; presence or absence of clefts; and the position of attachment.

examination, intraoral, *n* an examination of all the structures contained within the oral cavity.

examination, intraoral radiographic, *n* the examination of the oral and paraoral structures by exposing films placed within the oral cavity.

examination, lateral facial extraoral radiographic, *n* an examination by means of a lateral head film.

examination, lateral head extraoral radiographic, *n* an examination in which the film is placed parallel to the sagittal plane of the head.

examination, lateral jaw extraoral radiographic, *n* an examination in which the film is placed adjacent to the mandible.

examination, limited, *n* an assessment typically conducted during an emergency situation for the management of a critical medical condition.

examination, mental extraoral radiographic, *n* an examination in which the film is placed beneath the chin, and the radiation is directed through the long axis of the mandibular central incisors while the oral cavity is open.

Examination, National Board Dental Hygiene, *n.pr* See National Board Dental Hygiene Examination.

examination, oblique occlusal intraoral radiographic, *n* an exploratory examination of the maxillae or mandible using an occlusal type of film placed between the teeth. The rays are directed obliquely downward or upward (usually 60° to 75° in the vertical plane) and parallel to the sagittal plane.

examination, panoramic extraoral radiographic, *n* a curved, single-film radiography in which the beam source and film rotate in a synchronized manner about the head, exposing oral structures sequentially with simultaneous exposure of corresponding areas of the film.

examination, periapical intraoral radiographic, *n* the basic intraoral examination, showing all of a tooth and the surrounding periodontium.

examination, posteroanterior extraoral radiographic, *n* an examination in which the film is placed anteriorly, with the rays passing from the posterior to the anterior direction.

examination, profile extraoral radiographic, *n* a lateral head examination to show the profile of bone and soft tissue outline. It uses a decrease in milliampere seconds or an increase in target-film distance for recording the soft tissue image.

examination, radiographic, *n* **1.** the production of the number of radiographs necessary for the radiologic interpretation of the part or parts in question. *n* **2.** the study and interpretation of radiographs of the oral cavity and associated structures.

examination, stereoscopic extraoral radiographic, *n* a radiographic examination used in conjunction with a stereoscope for localization. Exposures of two films are made, with identical placement of each film adjacent to the part in question and with a different angulation for each exposure.

examination, temporomandibular extraoral radiographic, *n* an examination in which the film is placed adjacent to the area to be examined, with the rays directed through a point that is 2.5 inches (6.25 cm) above the tragus of the opposite external ear, with a vertical angulation of 15° and a horizontal angulation of 5° downward. Various other techniques and angulations are used, including laminagraphy, in examining this area.

examination, true occlusal topographic intraoral radiographic, *n* the radiography of the maxillae or mandible using an occlusal type of film placed between the teeth, with the rays directed at right angles to the plane of the film or through the long axis of the teeth adjacent to the part in question.

E

examination, Waters extraoral radiographic, n.pr the posteroanterior examination of the paranasal sinuses. The film is placed in contact with the nose and chin, with the rays directed at right angles to the plane of the film.

excavator (eks'kəvātur), *n* an instrument used to remove diseased tissue from teeth and to prepare the resulting cavity for treatment. Such instruments include hoes, curettes, and angle formers.

excavator, spoon, n a paired hand instrument intended primarily to remove carious material from a cavity.

excess, *n* more than is necessary, useful, or specified.

excess, marginal, n a condition in which the restorative material extends beyond the prepared cavity margin.

excess overhang, n a gingival margin excess.

excipient (eksip'ēənt), *n* an ingredient included in a pharmaceutical preparation for the purpose of improving its physical qualities. See also binder; filler; and vehicle.

excision (eksizh'ən), *n* the act of cutting away or taking out.

excision, local, n an excision limited to the immediate area of the lesion in question.

excision, radical, n an excision involving not only the lesion in question but also anatomic parts remote from the site.

excision, wide, n an excision involving the lesion in question and immediately adjacent anatomic structures.

excitant (eksīt'ənt), *n* an agent that stimulates the activity of an organ.

excitation (eksītā'shən), *n* the addition of energy to a system, thereby transferring it from its ground state to an excited state.

exclusions, *n.pl* the dental services not covered under a dental benefits program.

exclusive provider organization (EPO), *n* a dental benefits plan that provides benefits only if care is rendered by institutional and professional providers with whom the plan contracts (with some exceptions for emergency and out-of-area services).

excursion, lateral, *n* the movement of the mandible from the centric position to a lateral or protusive position.

execute, *v* to finish; accomplish; fulfill. To carry out according to certain terms.

exercise, *n* the performance of physical activity for the purpose of conditioning the body, improving health, or maintaining fitness or as a means of therapy for correcting a deformity or restoring the organs and bodily function to a state of health.

exercise, myotherapeutic, *n* See therapy, myofunctional.

exercise prosthesis, *n* See prosthesis, exercise.

exertion, *n* vigorous action, a great effort, a strong influence.

exfoliation (eksfō'lēā'shən), *n* the physiologic loss of the primary dentition. Also called *shedding.*

exhalation (ekshəlā'shən), *n* giving off or sending forth in the form of vapor; expiration.

exhaustion (egzôs'chən), *n* the loss of vital and nervous power from fatigue or protracted disease.

exhibit (egzib'it), *n* a paper, document, or object presented to a court during a trial or hearing as proof of facts, or as otherwise connected with the subject matter, and which, on being accepted, is marked for identification and considered a part of the case.

exit, port of, *n* the means by which infectious microorganisms may leave the body, such as secretions of mucus, blood, saliva, or other fluids.

exocrine (ek'sokrin), *adj* exuding outside the body, from a duct.

exocytosis (ek'sōsītō'sis), *n* the active transport of material from a vesicle out into the extracellular environment.

exodontics (ek'sōdon'tiks), *n* the science and practice of removing teeth from the oral cavity as performed by dental professionals.

exogenous (eksoj'ənəs), *adj* originating or caused by aspects external to a body.

exophthalmos (ek'softhal'mōs), *n* an abnormal protrusion of the eyeball. It is characteristic of toxic (exophthalmic) goiter.

exophytic (ek"sofit'ik), *adj* developing externally.

exostosis (pl. exostoses) (ek′sos-tō′sis), *n* (hyperostosis) a bony growth projecting from a bony surface.

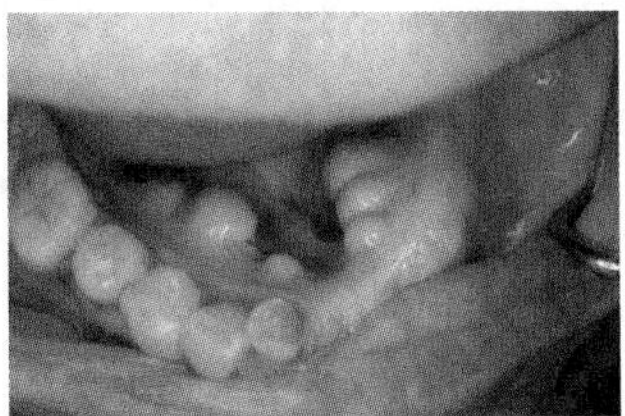

Mandibular tori exostosis. (Courtesy Dr. Charles Babbush)

exotoxin (ek′sōtoksin), *n* the toxic material formed by microorganisms and subsequently released into their surrounding environments.

expanded duty auxiliary, *n* a person trained (and possibly licensed or certified) to carry out dental procedures more complex than the responsibilities usually delegated to dental auxiliaries.

expanded polytetrafluoroethylene (ePTFE) (ekspan′did pol′ētet′rə-flŏŏr′ōeth′əlēn), *n* a stretched polymer of tetrafluoroethylene that allows passage of fluids but not cells; it is used as a nonabsorbable suture material and in guided tissue and bone regeneration as a nonresorbable membrane.

expansile infrastructure endosteal implant (ikspan′sil in′frəstruk′chər endos′tēəl), *n* an intraosseous implant device designed to enlarge or open after its insertion into the bone to provide retention.

expansion, *n* an increase in extent, size, volume, or scope.

expansion, delayed (secondary expansion), *n* **1.** an expansion occurring in amalgam restorations as a result of moisture contamination. *n* **2.** an expansion exhibited by amalgam that has been contaminated by moisture during trituration or insertion.

expansion, dental arch, *n* the therapeutic increase in circumference of the dental arch by buccal or labial movement of the teeth.

expansion, hygroscopic, *n* an expansion, caused by absorption of water during setting of an investment, used to compensate for the shrinkage of metal from the molten to the solid state.

expansion, secondary, *n* See expansion, delayed.

expansion, setting, *n* an expansion that occurs during the setting or hardening of materials such as amalgam and gypsum products.

expansion, thermal, *n* an expansion caused by heat. Thermal expansion of the mold is one of the important factors in achieving adequate compensation for the contraction of cast metal when it solidifies.

expansion, thermal coefficient, *n* a number indicating the amount of expansion caused by each degree of temperature change. The rate of change in restorative materials and tooth substance should be relatively the same.

experience rating, *n* a determination of the premium rate for a particular group partially or wholly on the basis of that group's own experience. Age, sex, use, and costs of services provided determine the premium.

experiment, *n* a trial or special observation made to confirm or disprove something doubtful; an act or operation undertaken to discover some unknown principle or effect or to test, establish, or illustrate some suggested or known truth.

experimental group, *n* the group of participants in a clinical study who receive the actual drug or treatment being studied. See also controlled clinical trial.

expert, *n* a person who has special skill or knowledge in a particular subject, such as a science or art, whether acquired by experience or study; a specialist.

expert system, *n* a computer program that follows a logical pathway or algorithm to a conclusion in a manner that mimics what an expert in the field would follow.

expert testimony, *n* the sworn statements of a person with special knowledge about a subject under consideration by a court of law.

expert witness, *n* a person who has special knowledge of a subject about which a court requests testimony to educate the court and the jury in the subject under consideration.

E

expiration (ek′spərā′shən), *n* **1.** the act of breathing forth or expelling air from the lungs. *n* **2.** a cessation.

expiration date, n **1.** the date on which a dental benefits contract expires. *n* **2.** the date an individual ceases to be eligible for benefits. **3.** the date that the Food and Drug Administration (FDA) requires pharmaceutical manufacturers to provide on all their products. For the majority of drugs sold in the United States, these dates range from 12 to 60 months from the date they are manufactured.

explanation of benefits, *n* a written statement to a beneficiary, from a third-party payer, after a claim has been reported, indicating the benefits and charges covered or not covered by the dental benefits plan.

exploration, *n* **1.** an examination by touch, either with or without instruments. E.g., a carious lesion is explored with a special explorer, but the mucobuccal fold may be explored with the finger. *n* **2.** the process of examination of a surface, with or without the use of instruments, to determine the condition or the surface depth of a defect or other similar diagnostic parameters.

explore, *v* to investigate.

explorer, *n* a dental instrument with a slender head that is honed to a fine point, used to conduct a tactile examination and appraisal of pits and fissures, carious lesions, root surfaces, and margins of restoration.

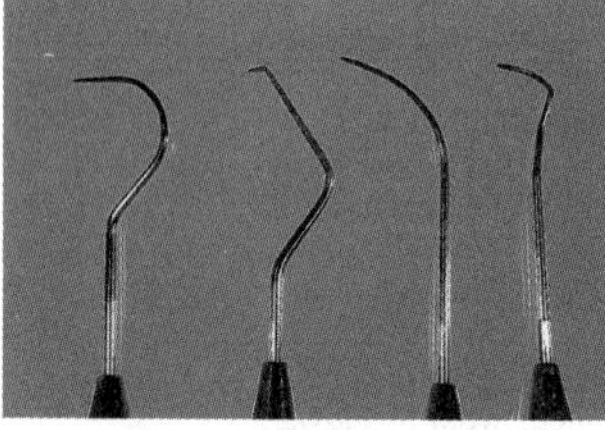

Explorers. (Darby/Walsh, 2003)

explorer, 11/12-type, n a type with a paired working end and long lower shank whose specially angled tip design makes it suited for use in either shallow depressions or deep pockets.

explorer, cowhorn, n a type so named because of the shape of its shank that is used to examine teeth for calculus, caries, and restoration margins. Also called *pigtail explorer.*

explorer, curved shank, n a type used to examine proximal tooth surfaces for calculus and caries, which, because of its arc, allows easier access to back teeth.

explorer, Orban No. 20, n.pr a type that is used to detect calculus, caries, lesions, and cemental changes on the subgingival surfaces of a tooth.

explorer, pigtail, n See explorer, cowhorn.

explorer, pocket, n See explorer, Orban No. 20.

explorer, sickle, n a hand-activated assessment tool, so named because of the distinctive shape of its shank, that is used to examine fissures and the surfaces of natural teeth, restorations, and sealants; not suited for exploration inferior to the gingival margin.

explorer, straight, n a type with an unpaired working end and short lower shank that is used to examine caries inferior to the gingival margin and in restorations with irregular margins; not suited to detecting calculus inferior to the gingival margin.

explorer, TU-17, n.pr a type that is used to detect calculus, caries, lesions, and cemental changes on the subgingival surfaces of a tooth; may be adapted for use on selected supragingival surfaces.

explorers, paired, n.pl two identical explorers with contralateral curves that are used to examine opposite tooth surfaces superior to the gingival margin; mirrored-image explorers.

explosion, *n* a violent, noisy outbreak caused by a sudden release of energy.

exposure (ikspō′zhər), *n* uncovering: subjection to viewing or radiation.

exposure, accidental pulp, n a pulp exposure unintentionally created during instrumentation.

exposure, air, n the radiation exposure measured in a small mass of air under conditions of electronic equilibrium with the surrounding air, i.e., excluding backscatter from irradiated parts or objects.

***exposure, cariogenic* (karēōjen′ik),** *n* an incident in which teeth come into contact with foods that tend to create a favorable environment for development of dental caries.
exposure, carious pulp, *n* a pulp exposure occasioned by extension of the carious process to the pulp chamber wall.
exposure, chronic, *n* a radiation exposure of long duration, either continuous (protraction exposure) or intermittent (fractionation exposure); usually referring to exposure of relatively low intensity.
exposure, cumulative, *n* the total accumulated exposure resulting from repeated radiation exposures of the whole body or of a particular region.
exposure, double, *n* the two superimposed exposures on the same radiographic or photographic film.
exposure, entrance, *n* an exposure measured at the surface of an irradiated body, part, or object. It includes both primary radiation and backscatter from the irradiated underlying tissue or material.
***exposure, erythema* (erəthē′mə),** *n* the radiation exposure necessary to produce a temporary redness of the skin. The exposure required varies with the quality of the radiation to which the skin is exposed.
exposure incident, *n* an event in which a health care professional's potential for infection is heightened after coming into contact with a patient's blood, body fluids, mucous membranes, or broken skin.
exposure, mechanical pulp, *n* See exposure, pulp, surgical.
exposure, parenteral, *n* exposure of the internal systems of the body due to the puncturing of the skin by a needle or other sharp instrument.
exposure, protraction, *n* the continuous exposure to radiation over a relatively long period at a low exposure rate.
exposure, pulp, *n* an opening through the wall of the pulp chamber uncovering the dental pulp.
exposure, radiographic, *n* a measure of the x or γ radiation to which a person or object, or part of either, is exposed at a certain place, this measure being based on its ability to produce ionization. The unit of x- or γ-radiation exposure is the roentgen (R).
exposure, radiographic, entrance (surface), *n* the radiation exposure measured at the external surface of a person or thing that has been irradiated. Measurement includes both backscatter radiation from the exposed tissues and primary radiation.
exposure rate, output, *n* the exposure to radiation at a specified point per unit of time, usually expressed in roentgens per minute.
exposure, surface, *n* See exposure, entrance.
exposure, surgical pulp, *n* (mechanical pulp exposure) the pulp exposure created intentionally or unintentionally during instrumentation.
exposure, threshold, *n* the minimum exposure that will produce a detectable degree of any given effect.
exposure time, *n* the time during which a person or object is exposed to radiation, expressed in one of the conventional units of time.

express, *v* to state distinctly and explicitly and not leave to inference; to set forth in words.

exsufflation (ek′suflā′shən), *n* the forced discharge of the breath.

extension, *n* **1.** an enlargement in boundary, breadth, or depth. *n* **2.** the process of increasing the angle between two skeletal levers having end-to-end articulation with each other; the opposite of flexion.
extension base, *n* See base, extension.
extension for prevention, *n* a principle of cavity preparation promoted by G.V. Black. To prevent the recurrence of decay, he advocated extension of the preparation into an area that is readily polished and cleaned. The philosophy is no longer used in dentistry.
extension base, gingiva, attached, *n* a gingival extension operation; a surgical technique designed to broaden the zone of attached gingiva by repositioning the mucogingival junction apically.
extension base, groove, *n* the enlargement of a cavity preparation outline to include a developmental groove.

extension base of benefits, *n* an extension of eligibility for benefits for covered services, usually designed to ensure completion of treatment commenced before the expiration date. Duration is generally expressed in terms of days.

extension base, ridge, *n* an intraoral surgical operation for deepening the labial, buccal, or lingual sulci.

extenuate (iksten′ūāt′), *v* to lessen; to mitigate.

external oblique line (ōblēk′), *n* See line, external oblique.

external pin fixation, *n* See appliance, fracture.

external traction, *n* See traction, external.

exteroceptors (ek′stərōsep′turz), *n.pl* the sensory nerve end receptors that respond to external stimuli; located in the skin, oral cavity, eyes, ears, and nose.

extirpation, pulp (ek′sturpā′shən), *n* See pulpectomy.

extracellular (eks″trəsel′ulər), *adj* taking place outside of a cell.

extracellular matrix, *n* an amorphous or structured substance produced by cellular activity that lies within the tissue but outside the cell.

extracoronal (ek′strəkôr′ōnəl), *adj* pertaining to that which is outside, or external to, the body of the coronal portion of a natural tooth.

extracoronal retainer, *n* See retainer, extracoronal.

extract, *n* a concentrate obtained by treating a crude material, such as plant or animal tissue, with a solvent, evaporating part or all of the solvent from the resulting solution, and standardizing the resulting product.

extraction, *n* the removal of a tooth from the oral cavity by means of elevators and/or forceps.

extraction, serial, *n* the extraction of selected primary teeth over a period of years (often ending with removal of the first premolar teeth) to relieve crowding of the dental arches during eruption of the lateral incisors, canines, and premolars.

extraoral, *adj* literally, outside the oral cavity. See also anchorage, extraoral.

extraoral anchorage, *n* orthodontic force applied from a base outside the oral cavity. See also anchorage.

extrapolate (ekstrap′ōlāt), *v* to infer values beyond the observable range from an observed trend of variables; to project by inference into the unexplored.

extrasystole (ek′strəsis′tōlē), *n* a heartbeat occurring before its normal time in the rhythm of the heart and followed by a compensatory pause.

extravasation (ekstrav′əzā′shən), *n* the escape of a body fluid out of its proper place (e.g., blood into surrounding tissues after rupture of a vessel, urine into surrounding tissues after rupture of the bladder).

extremity (ikstrem′itē), *n* an arm or a leg; the arm may be identified as an upper extremity, and the leg as a lower extremity.

extrinsic (ikstrin′sik), *adj* originating outside; not inherent or essential.

extroversion (ek′strəvur′zhən), *n* a tendency of the teeth or other maxillary structures to become situated too far from the median plane.

extrude, *v* to elevate; to move a tooth coronally.

extrusion (ikstroo′zhən), *n* the movement of teeth beyond the natural occlusal plane that may be accompanied by a similar movement of investing tissues. See also eruption, continuous.

extubate (eks′toobāt), *v* to remove a tube, usually an endotracheal anesthesia tube or a Levin gastric suction tube.

extubation (eks′toobā′shən), *n* the removal of a tube used for intubation.

exudate (eks′ōōdāt), *n* the outpouring of a fluid substance, such as exudated suppuration or tissue fluid.

exudate, purulent **(eks′ōōdāt pyür′ələnt),** *n* pus or suppuration that exudes from the gingival tissues and contains a mixture of enzymes, dead tissue, bacteria, and leukocytes, primarily neutrophils.

exudates, gingival, *n* the outpouring of an inflammatory exudate from the gingival tissues.

exudation (eks′oodā′shən), *n* See exudate.

eye, *n* one of a pair of organs of sight, contained in a bony orbit at the front of the skull.

eye, assessment of, *n* an examination of the eyes—which includes an observation of pupil size, sclera color, the relative location of the eyeball, and use of corrective eyeware—to determine the presence of disease.

eye-ear plane, n See plane, Frankfort horizontal.

eye loupes, *n* the low-magnification lenses that allow the wearer to visualize small details, such as the teeth and oral cavity.

eye wash station, *n* a cleansing receptacle set apart for the purpose of emergencies in which the eyes must be quickly flushed with water.

eyeglass, postmydriatic (pōst″-mid″reat′ik), *n* a disposable protective eyewear made of pliable plastic material, handed out by ophthalmologists to patients whose pupils have been dilated during a mydriatic examination.

eyelids, *n.pl* a moveable fold of thin skin over the eye. The orbicularis oculi muscle and the oculomotor nerve control the opening and closing of the eyelid.

eyewear, protective, *n* **1.** the goggles or safety glasses that are worn to protect the eyes from dust and debris while using dental powders or trimmers in the preparation of a study cast. *n* **2.** the goggles or safety glasses worn to protect the dental care worker or the patient from accidental eye exposure to blood or other body fluids, or to prevent accidental injury from dental instruments. Pediatric patients or patients with sensitive eyes may be given shaded glasses or goggles to protect the eyes from the brightness of the dental examination lamp.

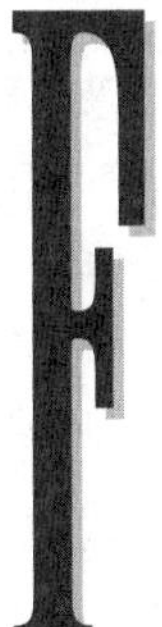

fabrication (fab′rikā′shən), *n* the construction or making of a restoration.

face, *n* the front of the head from the chin to the brow, including the skin and muscles and structures of the forehead, eyes, nose, oral cavity, cheeks, and jaws.

face, changeable area of, n the part of the face from the nose to the chin.

face form, n See form, face.

face, instrument blade, n See instrument blade face.

face shield, n.pl a type of protective eyewear sometimes used by oral health care workers in place of safety glasses. Although intended to cover the face completely for high-spatter treatments such as polishing and scaling, they may have limited impact resistance and should not be considered a replacement for protective breathing masks.

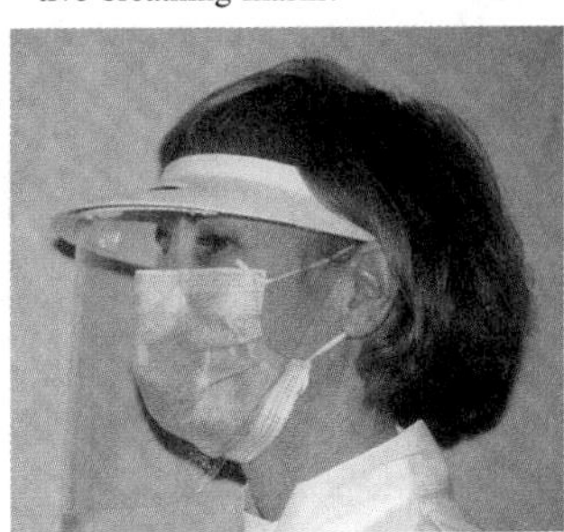

Face shield. (Bird/Robinson, 2005)

face-bow, *n* a caliper-like device that is used to record the relationship of the maxillae to the temporomandibular joints (or opening axis of the mandible) and to orient the casts in this same relationship to the opening axis of an articulator.

face-bow adjustable axis, n See face-bow, kinematic.

face-bow, kinematic (hinge-bow) **(kinəmat′ik),** *n* a face-bow attached to the mandible with caliper ends (condyle rods) that can be adjusted to permit the accurate location of the axis of rotation of the mandible.

facet (fas'et), *n* a flattened, highly polished wear pattern, as noted on a tooth.

facial angle, *n* an anthropomorphic expression of the degree of protrusion of the lower face, assessed by the measured inclination of the facial plane in relation to the Frankfort horizontal reference plane.

facial artery, *n* one of a pair of tortuous arteries that arise from the external carotid arteries, divide into four cervical and five facial branches, and supply various organs and tissues in the head. The cervical branches of the facial artery are the ascending palatine, tonsillar, glandular, and submental. The facial branches are the inferior labial, superior labial, lateral nasal, angular, and muscular.

facial asymmetry (āsim'ətrē), *n* the variation in the configuration of one side of the face from the other when viewed in relation to a projected midsagittal line.

facial bones, *n.pl* the bones of the face, which include the frontal, nasal, maxillary, zygomatic, and mandibular bones.

facial cleft, *n* See cleft, facial.

facial expression, *n* the use of the facial muscles to communicate or to convey mood.

facial injuries, *n.pl* trauma to the face and its associated structures, most frequently from traffic accidents, contact sports, and domestic conflicts.

facial muscles, *n* See muscles, facial.

facial nerve, *n* See nerve, facial.

facial neuralgia, *n* See neuralgia, trigeminal.

facial pain, *n* See pain, facial.

facial profile, *n* the sagittal outline of the face. There are three distinct forms: mesognathic, prognathic, and retrognathic.

facial tic, *n* any repetitive spasmodic and involuntary contraction of groups of facial muscles.

facies (fā'shēēs), *n.pl* the features, general appearance, and expression of a face.

facilitation (fəsilətā'shən), *n* the reinforcement of a lower level nerve stimulus by a higher level nerve stimulus. Thus a reflex that cannot be elicited by a subliminal impulse may be reinforced by an additional stimulus from a higher center. The combined effect of the two stimuli may cause a reflex response.

facsimile (faksim'ilē), *n* a true copy that preserves all the markings and contents of the original.

fact, *n* a thing done; an event or a circumstance; an actual occurrence.

factitious (faktish'us), *adj* false or self-manufactured.

factor(s), *n* a constituent, element, cause, or agent that influences a process or system; a gene; a dietary substance.

factor I (fibrinogen, profibrin), *n* See fibrinogen.

factor II (prothrombin, component A, prothrombase, prothrombin B, thrombogen, thrombozyme), *n* considered the only essential precursor of thrombin.

factor III (thromboplastin [tissue], thrombokinase, cytozyme [platelet], thrombokinin [blood], thromboplastic protein), *n* See thromboplastin.

factor IV (calcium, Ca^{++}), *n* ionized and/or bound calcium, generally required for the coagulation of blood, although some early phases of coagulation and the thrombin-fibrinogen reaction can take place without calcium.

factor V (labile factor, proaccelerin, accelerin, acceleration factor, cofactor of thromboplastin, component A of prothrombin, plasma ac-globulin, plasma prothrombin conversion factor [PPCF], prothrombinase, prothrombin accelerator, prothrombin conversion accelerator I, thrombogen, thrombogene, proaccelerinaccelerin system), *n* a factor apparently necessary for the formation of a prothrombin-converting substance in blood and tissue extracts—i.e., intrinsic and extrinsic prothrombin activators. A deficiency results in parahemophilia (hypoproaccelerinemia).

factor VI, *n* term formerly used to indicate an intermediate product in the formation of thromboplastin and also used synonymously with accelerin and activated factor V. It has no designation at present.

factor VII (stable factor, serum prothrombin conversion accelerator [SPCA], proconvertin, autoprothrombin I, cofactor V, component B of prothrombin, cothromboplas-

tin, kappa factor, precusor of serum prothrombin conversion accelerator [pro-SPCA], prothrombin conversion factor, prothrombin converting factor, prothrombin conversion accelerator II, proconvertinconvertin system, prothrombinogen, serozyme, stable factor), *n* a factor that accelerates the conversion of prothrombin to thrombin in the presence of factors III, IV, and V; a serum factor necessary for the formation of extrinsic prothrombin activator.

factor VII deficiency, *n* a deficiency associated with a lack of vitamin K. A deficiency may be congenital, or it may be acquired in liver disease, or from prothrombinopenic agents used in anticoagulation therapy; it results in a prolonged (quantitative) one-stage prothrombin time test.

factor VIII (antihemophilic factor [AHF], antihemophilic globulin, antihemophilic globulin A, antihemophilic factor A, plasma thromboplastin factor [PTF], plasmokinin, platelet cofactor I, prothrombokinase, thrombocatalysin, thrombocytolysin, thrombokatilysin, thromboplastic plasma component [TPC], thromboplastinogen), *n* a factor essential for the formation of blood thromboplastin. A deficiency results in classic hemophilia (hemophilia A); the clotting time is prolonged, and thromboplastin and prothrombin conversion is diminished.

factor IX (Christmas factor, plasma thromboplastin component [PTC], antihemophilic factor B, antihemophilic globulin B, autoprothrombin II, beta prothromboplastin, plasma factor X, plasma thromboplastin factor B [PTF-B], platelet cofactor II), *n* a factor that is active in the formation of intrinsic blood thromboplastin. A deficiency results in Christmas disease (hemophilia B), which is caused by a decrease in the amount of thromboplastin formed.

factor X (Stuart-Prower factor, Stuart factor, Prower factor), *n* a factor influencing the yield of intrinsic (plasma) thromboplastin. A deficiency results in a prolonged one-stage prothrombin time. Brain tissue or Russell's viper venom are used to test for thromboplastin deficiency.

factor XI (plasma thromboplastin antecedent [PTA], antihemophilic factor C, PTA factor, plasma thromboplastin factor C [PTF-C]), *n* a factor related to intrinsic (plasma) thromboplastin activation, which occurs when blood is exposed to a foreign surface.

factor XI deficiency, *n* a deficiency caused by an autosomal recessive gene resulting in a hemorrhagic tendency. See also hemophilia C.

factor XII (Hageman factor, antihemophilic factor D, clot-promoting factor, fifth plasma thromboplastin precursor, glass factor), *n* a factor the absence of which results in a long clotting time and abnormal prothrombin consumption and thromboplastin generation tests when tests are carried out in glass tubes. No abnormal bleeding tendency occurs with a deficiency of the factor.

factor XIII, *n* a coagulation factor present in normal plasma that acts with calcium to produce an insoluble fibrin clot. Also called *fibrinase* or *fibrin stabilizing factor.*

factor XIII deficiency, *n* a deficiency caused by a deficiency of vitamin E.

factor, acceleration, *n* See factor V.

factor, antihemophilic (AHF), *n* See factor VIII.

factor, antihemophilic A, *n* See factor VIII.

factor, antihemophilic B, *n* See factor IX.

factor, antihemophilic C, *n* See factor XI.

factor, antihemophilic D, *n* See factor XII.

factor, antipernicious, *n* See vitamin B_{12}.

factor, C (contact factor, contact activation product, third thromboplastic factor), *n* a coagulation accelerator product formed by the interaction of active factor XII and factor XI.

factor, Castle's intrinsic (intrinsic factor), *n.pr* a factor produced by the gastric mucosa and possibly the duodenal mucosa, and considered to be responsible for the absorption of vitamin B_{12}. See also anemia, pernicious.

factor, Christmas, *n* See factor IX.

factor, clot-promoting, *n* See factor XII.
factor, clotting, *n* the "trace" proteins (excluding calcium) present in normal blood in such small amounts (except fibrinogen) that their presence is usually established by deductive reasoning and by genetic and biochemical characteristics. They are associated with thromboplastic activity and the conversion of prothrombin to thrombin.
factor, contact, *n* See factor C.
factor, environmental, *n* the local conditions that modify tissue response (e.g., narrow interdental spaces, saddle areas, attachment of frenula, oblique ridges).
factor, erythrocyte-maturation (EMF), *n* See vitamin B complex.
factor, etiologic, *n* the element or influence that can be assigned as the cause or reason for a disease or lesion.
factor, extrinsic, *n* See vitamin B complex.
factor, familial, *n* a characteristic derived through heredity.
factor, glass, *n* See factor XII.
factor, glucocorticoid, *n* See hormone, "S."
factor, Hageman, *n* See factor XII.
factor, Hr, *n* blood factors that are reciprocally related to the Rh factors. They are present in agglutinogens when the corresponding Rh factor is absent from the gene.
factor, hyperglycemic, *n* See glucagon.
factor, hyperglycemic-glycogenolytic, *n* See glucagon.
factor, intrinsic, *n* See factor, Castle's intrinsic.
factor, kappa, *n* See factor VII.
factor, labile, *n* See factor V.
factor, local, *n* the limited factors that include dental plaque, bacterial toxins and irritants, calculus, food impaction, and other surface and locally placed irritants that are capable of injuring the periodontium.
factor, pellagra-preventive, *n* See acid, nicotinic.
factor, plasma prothrombin conversion (PPCF), *n* See factor V.
factor, plasma thromboplastin (PTF), *n* the substances with thromboplastic activity contributed by the plasma. Included are the antihemophilic factor, Christmas factor, plasma thromboplastin antecedent, and Hageman factor. See also factor VIII.
factor, plasma thromboplastin, A (PTF-A), *n* See factor VIII.
factor, plasma thromboplastin, B (PTF-B), *n* See factor IX.
factor, plasma thromboplastin, C (PTF-C), *n* See factor XI.
factor, plasma thromboplastin, D (PTF-D), *n* this factor is considered by some to be a fourth plasma substance with thromboplastic activity; not well characterized.
factor, plasma, X, *n* See factor IX.
factor, platelet, *n* a substance on or in the surface of blood platelet necessary for coagulation in the absence of extravascular thromboplastic substances.
factor, platelet, 1, *n* either factor V or a factor with factor V activity; absorbed on platelets and accelerates conversion of prothrombin to thrombin.
factor, platelet, 2, *n* a substance that accelerates the conversion of fibrinogen to fibrin.
factor, platelet, 3, *n* a substance associated with thromboplastin generation activity.
factor, platelet, 4, *n* an antiheparin factor.
factor, prothrombin conversion, *n* See factor VII.
factor, prothrombin-converting, *n* See factor VII.
factor, Prower, *n.pr* See factor X.
factor, psychosomatic, *n* the psychic, mental, or emotional factors that play a role in determining the initiation, course, and extent of a physical process, either directly or indirectly. Psychosomatic factors have been implicated in bruxism, clenching, and other oral habits.
factor, PTA (plasma thromboplastin antecedent factor), *n* See factor XI.
factor, reparative, *n* the ability of the tissues to heal or regenerate when they have been subjected to injury or disease.
factor, Rh, *n* the agglutinogens of red blood cells responsible for isoimmune reactions such as occur in erythroblastosis fetalis and incompatible blood transfusions.
factor, spreading, *n* an enzyme that

increases the permeability of ground substance.

factor, stable, n See factor VII.

factor, Stuart, n.pr See factor X.

factor, Stuart-Prower, n.pr See factor X.

factor, third thromboplastic, n See factor C.

facultative (fak′əltātiv), *adj* pertaining to an organism's ability to survive under different or varying environmental conditions.

faculty, *n* **1.** a normal physiologic function or natural ability of a living organism. **2.** an ability to do something specific, such as learn languages or to perceive and distinguish sensory stimuli. **3.** a mental ability or power. **4.** the group of people who teach within an institution of learning.

FAD, *n* abbreviation for *flavinadenine dinucleotide.*

failure, *n* a deficiency; an inefficiency as measured by some legal standard; an unsuccessful attempt.

failure to thrive, n the abnormal retardation of the growth and development of an infant resulting from conditions that interfere with normal metabolism, appetite, and activity.

faint, *n* a state of syncope, or swooning.

false light, *n* a misleading fashion in which a person is depicted before the public that a reasonable person finds offensive and damaging.

falsify, *v* to forge; to give a false appearance to anything, as to falsify a record.

famciclovir (famsī′klōvēr), *n brand name:* Famvir; *drug class:* antiviral; *action:* converted to active metabolite, peniciclovir triphosphate, which inhibits viral DNA synthesis and replication; *uses:* acute herpes zoster (shingles) infection.

family, *n* **1.** a group of people related by heredity, such as parents, children, and siblings. The term is sometimes broadened to include related by marriage or those living in the same household, who are emotionally attached, interact regularly, and share concerns for the growth and development of the group and its individual members. **2.** a category of animals or plants situated on a taxonomic scale between order and genus. **3.** the legal definition varies, depending on the jurisdiction and purpose for which the term is defined.

family counseling, n a program that consists of providing information and professional guidance to members of a family concerning specific health matters.

family deductible, n a deductible that is satisfied by combined expenses of all covered family members. A plan with a $25 deductible may limit its application to a maximum of three deductibles, or $75, for the family, regardless of the number of family members.

family dentistry, n the branch of dentistry that is concerned with the diagnosis and treatment of dental problems in people of either sex and at any age. Family dental professionals were formerly known as *general practitioners,* and therefore family dentistry does not constitute one of the specialty areas of dentistry.

family history, n a part of the medical history process; practitioner should ask patient about history of diseases or serious illness in family to determine if the patient might be predisposed to certain illnesses.

family membership, n a membership that includes spouses and/or dependents.

family unit, n an insured group member and dependents who are eligible for benefits under a dental care contract; an accounting unit.

famotidine (fəmō′tədēn′), *n brand names:* Pepcid, Pepcid IV; *drug class:* H_2-histamine receptor antagonist; *action:* inhibits histamine at H_2 receptor site in parietal cells, which inhibits gastric acid secretion; *uses:* short-term treatment of active duodenal ulcer, gastric ulcer, and heartburn.

fascia (pl. fasciae), *n* the fibrous connective tissue of the body that may be separated from other specifically organized fibrous structures such as the tendons, the aponeuroses, and the ligaments. Fascia generally covers and separates muscles and muscle groups.

fascia masseteric-parotid **(fash′ēə mas′iter′ik-pərot′id),** *n* the fascia that covers the masseter, a cheek muscle that closes the jaw. Also known as the *masseteric fascia.*

fascial, *adj* relating to the fascial.

fasciitis (fəsī′tis), *n* a tumorlike growth occurring in subcutaneous tissues in the oral cavity, usually in the cheek. A benign lesion sometimes mistaken for fibrosarcoma, fasciitis consists of young fibroblasts and numerous capillaries. It grows rapidly and may regress spontaneously.

fast, *v* to abstain from ingesting food for a specific period, usually for diagnostic, therapeutic, or religious purposes.

F

fast-set powder, *n* an irreversible, hydrocolloid material used to make impressions of a patient's dentition; this alginate material has a working time of 1.25 minutes and a setting time of 1 to 2 minutes (as opposed to a working time of 2 minutes and a setting time of 4.5 minutes with a normal-set powder).

fast green, *n* a green dye used to reveal plaque deposits on teeth; consists of F. D. & C. Green No. 3 in concentrations of either 5% or 2.5%.

fat, *n* **1.** a substance composed of lipids or fatty acids and occurring in various forms or consistencies ranging from oil to tallow. **2.** a type of connective tissue containing stored lipids.

fat embolism **(em′bəliz′əm),** *n* a circulatory condition characterized by the blocking of an artery by an embolus of fat that enters the circulatory system after the fracture of a long bone, or less commonly, after traumatic injury to fatty tissue or to a fatty liver.

fatal outcome, *n* a consequence that results in death. The course of a disease that results in the death of the patient.

fate, *n* a synonym for the more modern term *biotransformation.* See also biotransformation.

fatigue, *n* a condition of cells or organs under stress, resulting in a diminution or loss of an individual's capacity to respond to stimulation.

fatigue, dental materials, *n* dysfunction due to damage caused by recurring use or stress.

fatigue, muscle, *n* a peripheral phenomenon caused by the failure of the muscle to contract when stimuli from the nervous system reach it. Occurs when muscle activity exceeds tissue substrate and oxygenation capacity.

fatigue strength, *n* the ability of a material to withstand repeated stress. In dental work, the fatigue strength of materials used in fillings and dentures is an important consideration because patients will repeatedly stress their fillings and dentures when eating.

fatty acid, *n* an organic acid produced by the hydrolysis of neutral fats.

fauces (fô′sēz), *n* the archway between the pharyngeal and oral cavities; formed by the tongue, anterior and posterior tonsillar pillars, and soft palate.

faucial pillars (fô′shəl), *n.pl* the vertical folds of tissue created by muscles that create the fauces, which surround the palatine tonsils.

FDA, *n.pr* the abbreviation for the Food and Drug Administration. See also Food and Drug Administration.

F. D. & C., *n* See Food, Drug, and Cosmetic Act.

fear, *n* an emotion, generally considered negative and unpleasant, that is a reaction to a real or threatened danger; fright. Fear is distinguished from anxiety, which is a reaction to an unreal or imagined danger.

febrile (feb′rəl), *adj* pertaining to or characterized by an elevated body temperature. A body temperature of over 100° F is commonly regarded as febrile.

feces (fē′sēz), *n* the waste or excrement from the digestive tract that is formed in the intestine and expelled through the rectum. It consists of water, food residue, bacteria, and secretions of the intestines and liver.

Fede's disease, See disease, Riga-Fede.

Federal Tort Claims Act, *n.pr* a statute passed in 1946 that allows the federal government to be sued for the wrongful action or negligence of its employees. The act, for most purposes, eliminates the doctrine of governmental immunity, which formerly prohibited or limited the bringing of suit against the federal government.

Fédération Dentaire Internationale (F. D. I.) Two-Digit System (fā′dāräsyōN dôNter′ eN′ternäs′yōnäl′), *n.pr* a recognized method used to identify and designate permanent and primary and deciduous teeth within the oral cavity. The first digit represents the quadrant number (1–4) starting with the maxillary right quadrant, moving around the maxillary arch to the left, then down and back to the right, and ending with the mandibular right quadrant. The second digit represents each tooth in the quadrant, numbered distally from the midline. Also called the *International System.*

fee, *n* the compensation for services rendered or to be rendered; payment for professional services.

fee, customary, n a fee is customary if it is in the range of the usual fees charged by dental professionals of similar training and experience for the same service within the specific and limited geographic area (i.e., the socioeconomic area of a metropolitan area or of a county).

fee-for-service plan, n a plan providing for payment to the dental professional for each service performed rather than on the basis of salary or capitation fee.

fee, reasonable, n a fee is considered reasonable if, in the opinion of a responsible dental association's review committee, it is the usual and customary fee charged for services rendered, considering the special circumstances of the case in question.

fee schedule, n **1.** a list of maximum dollar allowances for dental procedures that apply under a specific contract. **2.** a list of the charges established or agreed to by a dental professional for specific dental services.

fee, usual, n the fee customarily charged for a given service by an individual dental professional to a private patient.

feedback, *n* the constant flow of sensory information back to the brain. When feedback mechanisms are deficient because of sensory deprivation, motor function becomes distorted, aberrant, and uncoordinated.

Feer's disease (fārz), *n.pr* See erythredema polyneuropathy.

felbamate, *n brand name:* Felbatol; *drug class:* anticonvulsant; *action:* anticonvulsant action is unclear; *uses:* alone or as an adjunct therapy in partial seizures.

feldspar (feld′spär), *n* a crystalline mineral of aluminum silicate with potassium, sodium, barium, or calcium—$NaAlSi_3O_8$ or $KA_1Si_3O_8$. Feldspar melts over a range of 1,100°F to 2,000°F (593.5°C to 1093.5°C). An important constituent of dental porcelain.

feldspar, orthoclase ceramic, n a clay found in large quantity in the solid crust of the earth. It acts as a filler and imparts body to the fused dental porcelain.

felodipine (fəlō′dəpēn′), *n brand names:* Plendil, Renedil; *drug class:* calcium channel blocker; *action:* inhibits calcium ion influx across cell membrane during cardiac depolarization; produces relaxation of coronary vascular smooth muscle; dilates coronary arteries; decreases SA/AV node conduction; *uses:* essential hypertension, alone or with other antihypertensives, chronic angina pectoris.

felony, *n* a crime declared by statute to be more serious than a misdemeanor and deserving of a more severe penalty. Conviction usually requires imprisonment in a penitentiary for longer than 1 year.

felypressin (fel′ipres′in), *n brand name:* Octapressin; an ingredient that may be added to a local anesthetic for the purpose of constricting blood vessels. It helps to contain the anesthetic in a specific area by reducing systemic absorption, decreasing blood flow, and prolonging effectiveness. It is not available in the United States.

Fen-Phen (fen′-fen′), *n* a combination of fenfluramine hydrochloride and phentermine hydrochloride, two stimulants, which promotes weight loss by reducing appetite. It is no longer available due to its damaging of the heart's valves. Thus it is important for a patient who has a history of using this medication to get a cardiac screening to check for risk of bacterial endocarditis. See also fenfluramine hydrochloride and phentermine hydrochloride.

fenestration, in alveolar plate, (fenestrā′shən, alvē′ələr), *n* a round or oval defect or opening in the alveolar cortical plate of bone over the root surface.

F

fenfluramine HCl (fenflŏŏr'əmēn'), *n brand name:* Pondimin; *drug class:* nonamphetamine anorexiant, Controlled Substance Schedule IV; *action:* influences serotonin pathways in the central nervous system; anorexic mechanisms unknown; *use:* exogenous obesity. See also Fen-Phen.

fenoprofen calcium, *n brand name:* Nalfon; *drug class:* nonsteroidal anti-inflammatory; *action:* inhibits prostaglandin synthesis by interfering with cyclooxygenase needed for biosynthesis; *uses:* mild to moderate pain, osteoarthritis, rheumatoid arthritis, acute gout, dysmenorrhea.

fentanyl transdermal system (fen'tənil transdur'məl), *n brand name:* Duragesic 25, 50, 75, 100 Transdermal Patches; *drug class:* narcotic analgesic, Controlled Substance Schedule II; *action:* interacts with opioid receptors in the central nervous system to alter pain perception; *uses:* management of chronic pain when opioids are necessary.

fermentable, *adj* the ability to undergo a chemical reaction in the presence of an enzyme that results in the creation of either acid or alcohol; in the oral cavity, the ability to create acid in plaque.

fermentation, *n* a chemical change that is brought about in a substance by the action of an enzyme or microorganism, especially the anaerobic conversion of foodstuffs to certain products such as acetic fermentation, alcoholic fermentation.

Ferrier's separator (fer'ēurz), *n.pr* See separator, Ferrier's.

ferritin (fer'itin), *n* the compound iron-appoferritin, which is produced in the intestine and stored primarily in the liver, spleen, and bone marrow. It eventually becomes a component of hemoglobin and can be measured to estimate the body's iron levels.

ferromagnetic (fer'ōmagnet'ik), *adj* pertaining to substances that exhibit unusually strong magnetic properties; ironlike substances.

ferrous fumarate/ferrous gluconate/ferrous sulfate, *n brand names:* Femiron, Feostat; *drug class:* hematinic, iron preparation; *action:* replaces iron stores needed for red blood cell development; *uses:* iron-deficiency anemia, prophylaxis for iron deficiency in pregnancy.

fertility, *n* the ability to reproduce.

ferule (fer'əl), *n* a protective ring (usually of metal) around a natural tooth root used to join an artificial crown. Also spelled *ferrule.*

festoon(s) (festoon'), *n* a carving in the base material of a denture that simulates the contours of the natural tissues being replaced by the denture.

festoon, gingival, *n* the distinct rounding and enlargement of the margins of the gingival tissue found in early gingival involvement.

festoons, McCall's, *n.pr* enlargements of the gingival margins that may be associated with occlusal trauma.

festooning (festoon'ing), *n* the process of carving the base material of a denture or denture pattern to simulate the contours of the natural tissues to be replaced by the denture.

fetal alcohol syndrome (FAS), *n* a set of congenital psychologic, behavioral, cognitive, and physical abnormalities that tend to appear in infants whose mothers consumed alcoholic beverages during pregnancy. It is characterized by typical craniofacial and limb defects, cardiovascular defects, and increased levels of retarded development.

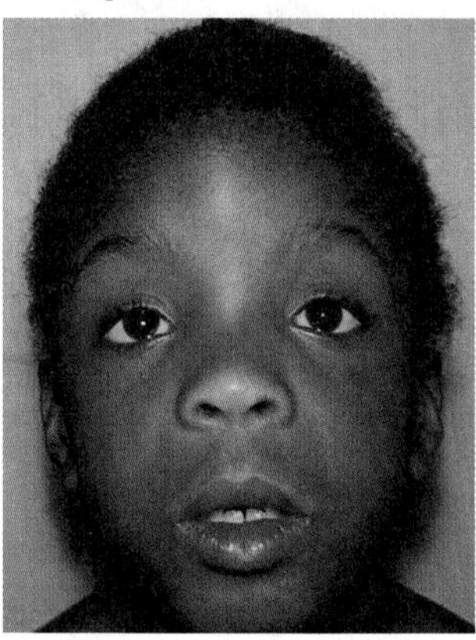

Fetal alcohol syndrome. (Zitelli/Davis, 2002)

fetal period, *n* the stage between the third and ninth months of in utero human development, during which there is growth of preformed structures.

fetor ex ore (fē′tôr eks ō′rē), *n* See halitosis.

fetor oris (fē′tôr ō′ris), *n* bad breath. See also halitosis.

fetus (fē′təs), *n* the structure present during the fetal period of prenatal development derived from the enlarged embryo.

fever (pyrexia) (pīrek′sēə), *n* an elevation of the body temperature.

hand-foot-and-mouth fever, aphthous, *n* See disease.

fever, cat-scratch, *n* See disease, cat-scratch.

fever, hay, *n* rhinitis and conjunctivitis resulting from allergy; frequently caused by allergy to pollens.

fever, of unknown origin, *n* the persistent elevation of body temperature without an identifiable cause.

fever, rheumatic **(roomat′ik),** *n* a severe, apparently infectious disease produced by hemolytic streptococci organisms or associated with their presence in the body; characterized by upper respiratory tract inflammation, cervical lymphadenopathy and lymphadenitis, polyarthritis, cardiac involvement, and subcutaneous nodules. The disease may be produced by an autoantibody reaction.

fever, scarlet (scarlatina), *n* an acute disease caused by a specific type of *Streptococcus* organism and characterized by a rash and strawberry tongue.

fever, uveoparotid (Heerfordt's syndrome, uveoparotitis) **(ū′vēōpərot′id),** *n* **1.** a disease characterized by inflammation of the parotid gland and of the uveal regions of the eye. **2.** the firm, nodular enlargement of the parotid glands, uveitis, and cutaneous lesions may be present. Considered to be a form of sarcoidosis. **3.** a syndrome consisting of sarcoidosis affecting the parotid glands, inflammation of the lacrimal glands, and inflammation of the uveal tract of the eye.

fever blister, *n* See herpes labialis.

fiber(s), *n* an elongated, threadlike structure of organic tissue.

fibers, A-alpha nerve, *n.pl* the large-diameter nerve fibers that connect into the substantia gelatinosa of the dorsal horns of the spinal cord before synapsing with the central transmission of the dorsal horn. A-alpha fibers are associated with the "gate-control" theory of pain.

fibers, A-beta nerve, *n.pl* the large-diameter nerve fibers that are mechanoreceptors for pressure occurring in both the pulp and periodontal ligament, necessary to operate the gate mechanism.

fibers, A-delta nerve, *n.pl* the small-diameter nerve fibers that are mechanoreceptors for pain occurring in both the pulp and the periodontal ligament, necessary to operate the gate mechanism.

fibers, adrenergic **(ad′rəner′jik),** *n.pl* the nerve fibers, including most of the postganglionic sympathetic fibers, that transmit their impulses across synapses or neuroeffector junctions through the local release of the neurohormone, more recently identified as *norepinephrine* and formerly designated *sympathin.*

fibers, alveolar, *n.pl* the collagen fibers of the periodontal ligament that extend from the alveolar bone to the intermediate plexus, where their terminations are interspersed with the terminations of the cemental group of fibers.

fibers, alveolar crest, *n.pl* the collagen fibers of the periodontal ligament that extend from the cervical area of the tooth to the alveolar crest.

fibers, alveolgingival, *n.pl* the collagen fibers of the periodontal ligament that extend from the alveolar crest into the gingiva.

fibers, apical, *n.pl* the collagen fibers of the periodontal ligament radiating apically from tooth to bone.

fibers, association, *n.pl* the extensions of nerve cells that are neither efferent nor afferent neurons but furnish a pathway of connection between them.

fibers, bundle, *n.pl* the gathering together of collagen fibers in a group, particularly the collagen fiber bundles of the periodontal ligament.

fibers, C nerve, *n.pl* the small-diameter nerve fibers that are mechanoreceptors for pain occurring in both the pulp and the periodontal ligament, necessary to operate the gate mechanism.

fibers, cemental, *n.pl* the collagen fibers of the periodontal ligament extending from the cementum to the zone of the intermediate plexus, where their terminations are interspersed with the terminations of the alveolar group of periodontal fibers.

fibers, circular, *n.pl* the collagen fibers in the free gingiva that encircle the tooth in a ringlike fashion.

fibers, collagen, *n.pl* white fibers composed of collagen. The most conspicuous part of connective tissue, including the gingivae and periodontal ligament. Some fibers are distributed haphazardly throughout the connective tissue ground substance, and others are arranged in coarse bundles that exhibit a distinct orientation. Characterized by its hydroxyproline and hydroxylysine content.

fiber, crestal, *n* a group of collagen fibers of the periodontal ligament extending from the cervical area of the tooth to the alveolar crest.

fibers, dentogingival, *n.pl* the fan-shaped fibers of the periodontal ligament that emerge from the supraalveolar connective tissue; composed of circular, dentogingival, dentoperiosteal, and transseptal (interdental) fiber groups.

fibers, dentoperiosteal, *n* the part of the fibers of the periodontal ligament that emerge from the supraalveolar part of the cementum of the tooth and pass outward beyond the alveolar crest in an apical direction into the mucoperiosteum of the attached gingiva.

fibers, gingival, *n* the group of fibers of the periodontal ligament that belong to the gingival and supraalveolar connective tissue; composed of circular, dentogingival, dentoperiosteal, and transseptal fiber (interdental) groups.

fibers, horizontal, *n.pl* the collagen fibers of the periodontal ligament that extend horizontally from the cementum to the alveolar bone.

fibers, interradicular, *n.pl* the collagen fibers of the periodontal ligament noted in multirooted teeth that extend from the cementum to the bone between the roots.

fiber, myelinated nerve **(mī′ələnā′təd),** *n* a nerve fiber inside or outside the brain that is covered with an insulating medullary sheath along which are located nodes of Ranvier that facilitate as relay points the speed of nerve impulses over that of an equivalent nonmedullated fiber.

fibers, nerve, *n.pl* See fiber, myelinated nerve, and fiber, nonmedullated nerve.

fibers, nonmedullated nerve **(non′med′əlā′təd),** *n* a nerve fiber not covered by an insulating medullary sheath that is thus exposed to other tissue fluids and their respective electric potentials. In nonmedul-

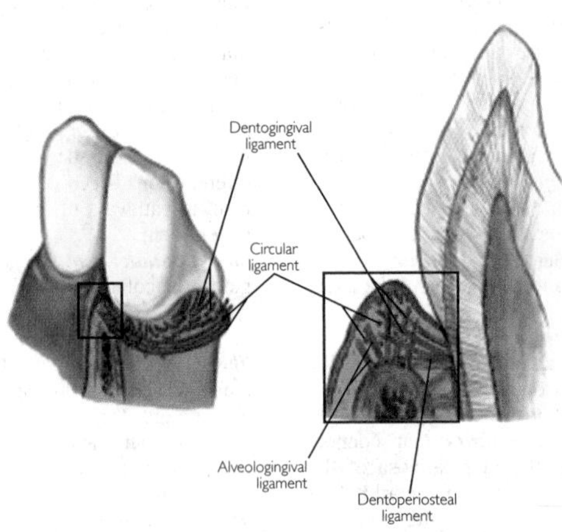

Gingival fibers. (Bath-Balogh/Fehrenbach, 2006)

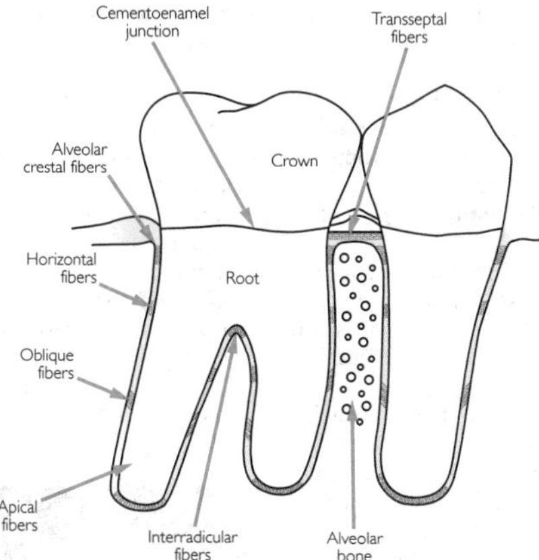

Tissues and fibers of the gingiva and attachment apparatus. (Daniel/Harfst/Wilder, 2008)

lated fibers, the impulse is relayed from point to contiguous point. Most of the nonmedullated fibers are within the substance of the central nervous system, and the distances between the cells are short.

fibers, oblique, *n* the group of collagen fibers in bundle arrangement in the periodontal ligament that are obliquely situated, with insertions in the cementum, and that extend more occlusally in the alveolus.

fibers, periodontal, *n* See ligament, periodontal.

fibers, principal, *n.pl* the numerous bundles of collagen fibers arranged in groups that function as the mode of attachment of the tooth to the alveolus and form the periodontal ligament.

fibers, Sharpey's, *n.pr* the collagen fibers of the periodontal ligament that become incorporated into the cementum or alveolar bone.

fibers, transseptal, *n.pl* a part of the collagen fibers of the periodontal ligament that extends from the supraalveolar cementum of one tooth horizontally through the interdental attached gingiva above the septum of the alveolar bone to the cementum of the adjacent tooth. Also called *interdental fibers.*

fiberoptic light, *n* a miniaturized light source that uses the property of flexible fiberglass strands to conduct light over long distances with little or no distortion; used in intraoral application, such as a light attached directly to the dental handpiece.

fiberoptics (fībərop′tiks), *n* the technical process by which an internal organ or cavity can be viewed, using glass or plastic fibers to transmit light through a special tube designed to magnify and reflect an image of the surface of the internal region under observation.

fibrillation (fib′rilā′shən), *n* a local quivering of muscle fibers.

fibrillation, atrial, *n* a cardiac arrhythmia caused by disturbed spread of excitation through atrial musculature.

fibrillation, auricular **(ôrik′ūlur),** *n* an uncoordinated, independent contraction of the heart that results in marked irregularity of heart action.

fibrillation, ventricular, *n* an uncoordinated, independent contraction of the ventricular musculature resulting in cessation of cardiac output.

fibrinogen (fībrin′əjən) (factor I, profibrin), *n* a soluble plasma protein (globulin) that is acted on by thrombin to form fibrin. The normal level is 200 to 400 mg/100 ml in plasma. Coagulation is impaired if the concentration is less than 100 mg/100 ml. Another form called *tissue fibrinogen,* which has the power of clotting the blood without the presence of thrombin, occurs in body tissues.

fibrinokinase (fī′brinōki′nās) (fibrinolysokinase, lysokinase), *n* an activator of plasminogen found in many animal tissues.

fibrinolysin (fī′brinol′isin), *n* See plasmin.

fibrinolysis (fī′brinol′isis), *n* the continual process of fibrin decomposition during the removal of small fibrin clots by the action of enzyme fibrinolysin.

fibrinolysokinase, *n* See fibrinokinase.

fibrinolytic agents, *n.pl* agents that decrease the breakdown of fibrin.

fibroblast (fī′brōblast), *n* a cell found within fibrous connective tissue, varying in shape from stellate (young) to fusiform and spindle shaped. Associated with the formation of collagen fibers and intercellular ground substance of connective tissue.

fibroblast, of periodontal ligament, n a cell that plays an important role in formation and remodeling of fibrous matrix and intercellular substance.

fibroblastoma (fī′brōblastō′mə), *n* a tumor arising from an ordinary connective tissue cell or fibroblast. The tumor may be a fibroma or a fibrosarcoma.

fibroblastoma, neurogenic, n See neurofibroma.

fibroblastoma, perineural, n See neurilemoma and neurofibroma.

fibrocystic disease, *n* See disease, fibrocystic.

fibroma (fībrō′mə), *n* a benign mesenchymal tumor composed primarily of fibrous connective tissue.

fibroma, ameloblastic, n a mixed tumor of odontogenic origin characterized by the simultaneous proliferation of both the epithelial and mesenchymal components of the tooth germ without the production of hard structure.

fibroma, calcifying, n See fibroma, ossifying.

fibroma, cementifying, n an intrabony lesion not associated with teeth, composed of a fibrous connective tissue stroma containing foci of calcified material resembling cementum; a rare odontogenic tumor composed of varying amounts of fibrous connective tissue with calcified material resembling cementum. Central lesion of the jaws.

fibroma, desmoplastic **(dez′məplas′tik),** *n* a fibrous bone tumor, usually benign, found most commonly in children and young adults.

fibroma, irritation, n a localized peripheral, tumorlike enlargement of connective tissue caused by prolonged local irritation and usually seen on the gingiva or buccal mucosa.

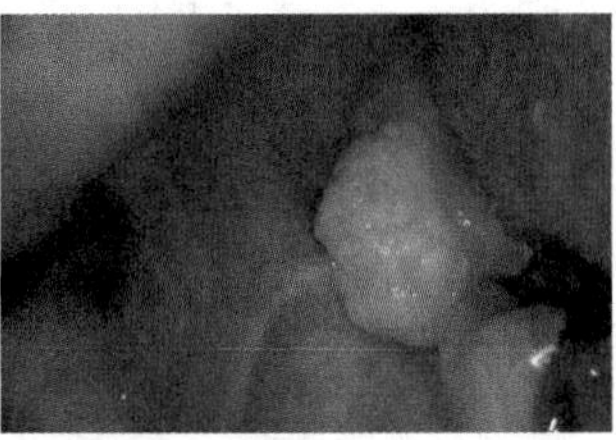

Irritational fibroma. (Courtesy Dr. Charles Babbush)

fibroma, neurogenic, n See neurilemoma; neurofibroma.

fibroma, odontogenic, n a central odontogenic tumor of the jaws, consisting of connective tissue in which small islands and strands of odontogenic epithelium are dispersed. A mesodermal odontogenic tumor composed of active dense or loose fibrous connective tissue; contains inactive islands of epithelium.

fibroma, ossifying, n a benign neoplasm of bone characterized by unilateral swelling and fibroblastic and osteoblastic activity in marrow spaces. An aggressive variant of this lesion has been described and is termed juvenile ossifying fibroma or juvenile active ossifying fibroma.

fibroma, periapical (benign periapical fibroma, fibrous dysplasia, first-state cementoma, focal osseous dysplasia, traumatic osteoclasia), n a benign connective tissue mass formed at the apex of a tooth with a normal pulp.

fibroma, peripheral odontogenic, n a fibrous connective tissue tumor associated with the gingival margin and believed to originate from the periodontium. Often contains areas of calcification. Localized form of fibromatosis gingivae.

fibroma, peripheral ossifying, *n* a type of reactive gingival growth that appears most commonly in teenagers and young adults. They can be surgically removed, but rate of recurrence is high.

fibroma, with myxomatous degeneration, *n* See fibromyxoma.

fibromatosis (fī′brōmətō′sis), *n* a gingival enlargement believed to be a hereditary condition that is manifested in the permanent dentition and characterized by a firm hyperplastic tissue that covers the teeth. Differentiation between this and diphenylhydantoin (Dilantin) hyperplasia is based on a history of drug ingestion.

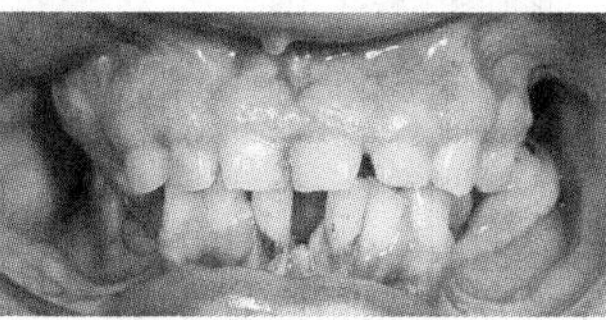

Fibromatosis. (Ibsen/Phelan, 2004)

fibromatosis gingival, *n* a generalized enlargement of the gingivae caused by an overproduction of collagen. May be idiopathic, inherited, or associated with a syndrome.

fibromatosis, idiopathic, *n* See fibromatosis gingival.

fibromyalgia (fī′brōmīal′jēə), *n* a debilitating chronic syndrome characterized by diffuse or specific muscle, joint, or bone pain; fatigue; and a wide range of other symptoms, as well as tenderness on palpation at various sites.

fibromyxoma (fī′brōmiksō′mə) (fibroma with myxomatous degeneration), *n* a fibroma that has certain characteristics of a myxoma; a fibroma that has undergone myxomatous degeneration. Combination of both fibrous and myxomatous elements.

fibro-osseous (fīb′rō-os′ēəs), *adj* composed of bony and fibrous tissue. Often associated with lesions of the jaw.

fibropapilloma (fī′brōpap′ilōmə), *n* See fibroma, irritation.

fibrosarcoma (fī′brōsärkō′mə), *n* a malignant mesenchymal tumor, the basic cell type being a fibroblast. Most fibrosarcomas are locally infiltrative and persistent but do not metastasize.

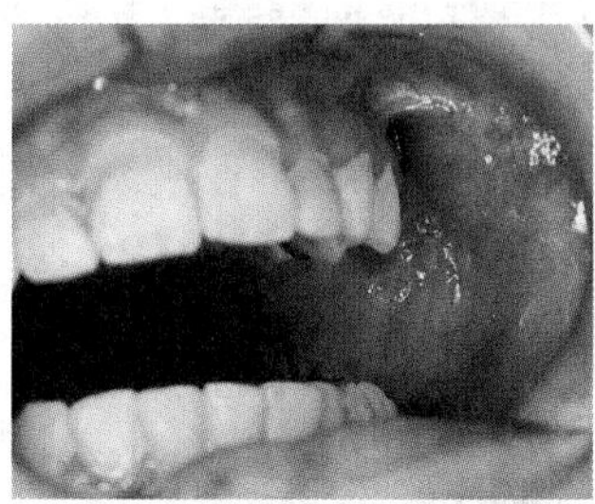

Fibrosarcoma. (Regezi/Sciubba/Jordan, 2008)

fibrosarcoma, odontogenic, *n* an extremely rare malignant form of odontogenic fibroma.

fibrosis (fībrō′sis), *n* **1.** the process of forming fibrous tissue, usually by degeneration (e.g., fibrosis of the pulp). The process occurs normally in the formation of scar tissue to replace normal tissue lost through injury or infection. **2.** an abnormal condition in which fibrous connective tissue spreads over or replaces normal smooth muscle or other normal organ tissue. Fibrosis is most common in the heart, lung, peritoneum, and kidney.

fibrosis, diffuse hereditary gingival, *n* an uncommon form of severe gingival hyperplasia considered to be of genetic origin. The tissue is pink, firm, dense, and insensitive and has little tendency to bleed.

fibrosis, hereditary gingival, *n* an uncommon form of severe gingival hyperplasia that may begin with the eruption of the deciduous or permanent teeth and is characterized by a firm, dense, pink gingival tissue with little tendency toward bleeding.

fibrotomy (fībrô′təmē), *n* an orthodontic surgical procedure in which the gingival fibers around a tooth are severed in order to prevent the orthodontically corrected tooth from relapsing.

fibrous dysplasia, *n.pl* See dysplasia, fibrous.

F

fibrous encapsulation (fīb′rəs enkap′səlā′shən), *n* the fibrous connective tissue layer that forms between the implant and surrounding bone as the final stage in the healing process.

fiduciary (fidoo′shēerē), *n* a person who has a duty to act primarily for another's benefit, as a trustee. Also, pertaining to the good faith and confidence involved in such a relationship.

field, *n* an area, region, or space.

field block, *n* See block, field.

field, operating, *n* the area immediately surrounding and directly involved in a treatment procedure (e.g., all the teeth included in a rubber dam application for the restoration of a single tooth or portions thereof).

field, radiation, *n* the region in which radiant energy is being propagated.

fifth disease, *n* an infectious disease primarily found in children that is caused by transmission of the human parvovirus B19 through the upper respiratory tract. Symptoms include fever and a skin rash that begins on the cheeks and spreads to other body surfaces. Also called *erythema infectiosum.*

filament, *n* an individual manufactured toothbrush bristle.

filament, curved, *n* a single toothbrush bristle, manufactured to bend with the curve of the dental surface, designed to assist contact with the gingival line when used at a 45° angle.

filament, end rounded, *n* refers to the manufactured shaping of an individual toothbrush bristle with an exceptionally rounded tip designed to protect teeth and gums during brushing.

filamentous bacilli, morphologic form of (filəmen′təs bəsil′ē), *n* the clustered strands of narrow filaments, rounded at one end and tapered at the other, which are characteristic of the filamentous bacilli.

file, *n* **1.** a metal tool of varying size and form with numerous ridges or teeth on its cutting surfaces; may be push-cut or pull-cut; used for smoothing or dressing down metals and other substances. **2.** a collection of records; an organized collection of information directed toward some purpose such as patient demographic data. The records in a file may or may not be sequenced according to a key contained in each record. *v* **3.** to reduce by means of a file.

file, gold, *n* a file designed for removing surplus gold from gold restorations; may be pull-cut or push-cut.

file, Hirschfeld-Dunlop, *n.pr* a periodontal file used with a pull stroke for the removal of calculus; available in various angulations for approach to different surfaces of teeth.

file, periodontal, *n* an instrument with multiple, angled cutting edges used to roughen the surface of a smooth calculus deposit before removal with a curet.

file, root canal, *n* a small metal hand instrument with tightly spiraled blades used to clean and shape the canal.

file, sharpening, *n* a difficult honing procedure requiring special tools designed to address the file's numerous parallel ridges.

file-access safeguards, *n.pl* the methods of limiting certain users' access to particular data.

filing, *n* the act of using a file to shape or smooth an object, usually metal.

filled resin, *n* See resin, composite.

filled sealant, *n* See resin, composite and resin-filled.

filled teeth, indices and scoring methods for, *n.pl* See index, DEF and index, DMF.

filling, *n* a material used to fill a space. See also restoration.

filling, dental, *n* a colloquial term for restoration.

filling, "ditched," *n* the marginal failure of amalgam restorations caused by fracture of either the material or the tooth structure itself in that area.

filling, material, *n* See material, filling.

filling, postresection, *n* See filling, retrograde.

filling, retrograde (postresection filling, retrograde obturation), *n* a restoration placed in the apical portion of a tooth root to seal the apical portion of the root canal.

filling, root canal, *n* material placed in the root canal system to seal the space previously occupied by the dental pulp.

filling, technique, *n* See technique, filling.

filling, treatment, *n* a temporary filling, usually of a sedative nature, used to allay sensitive dentin before the final restoration of the cavity.

film, *n* a thin, flexible, transparent sheet of cellulose acetate or similar material coated with a light-sensitive emulsion.

film badge, *n* a pack of radiation-sensitive film used for the detection and approximate measurement of radiation exposure for personnel-monitoring purposes; the badge may contain two or three films of differing sensitivity, and it may contain a filter that shields part of the film from certain types of radiation.

film base, *n* See base, film.

film, bite-wing (interproximal film) (BWX), *n* See examination, bite-wing, intraoral radiographic and radiograph, bite-wing.

film emulsion, *n* See emulsion, silver.

film fault, *n* a defective result in a radiograph; usually caused by a chemical, physical, or electrical error in its production.

film fault, black spots, *n.pl* the spots caused by dust particles or developer on the films before development; also caused by outdated (expired) film.

film fault, blurred, *n* a fault caused by film movement during exposure, bent film during exposure, double exposures, or flowing of emulsion during processing in excessively warm solution.

film fault, clear radiographic, *n* the result of treating the film with fixer before developing or by excessive washing. The problem can be prevented by following appropriate procedures.

film fault, dark, *n* a fault caused by overexposure of the film to radiation, film fog from extended development, accidental exposure to light (light leaks in film packet or dark room), or an unsafe darkroom light.

film fault, distorted, *n* See distortion, film-fault.

film fault, dyschroic fog, *n* a fogging of the radiograph, characterized by the appearance of a pink surface when the film is viewed by transmitted light and a green surface when the film is seen by reflected light. It usually is caused by an exhaustion of the acid content of the fixing solution (incomplete fixation).

film fault, fogged, *n* a fault caused by stray radiation, use of expired film, or an unsafe darkroom light.

film fault, light, *n* a fault caused by underexposure, underdevelopment (expired or diluted developing solution), development in temperatures that are too cold, or accidental use of a wrong film speed.

film fault, reticulation, *n* a network of corrugations produced because of an excessive difference in temperature between any two of the three darkroom solutions.

film fault, roller marks on, *n.pl* the dark lines on films caused by contaminated chemicals in automatic film processing units. Prevented by cleaning and replenishing the developer and fixer solutions regularly.

film fault, stained, *n* a fault caused by contaminated solutions, improper rinsing, exhausted solutions, improper washing, contamination by improper handling of the emulsions during or after processing, or film hangers containing dried fixer on the clips.

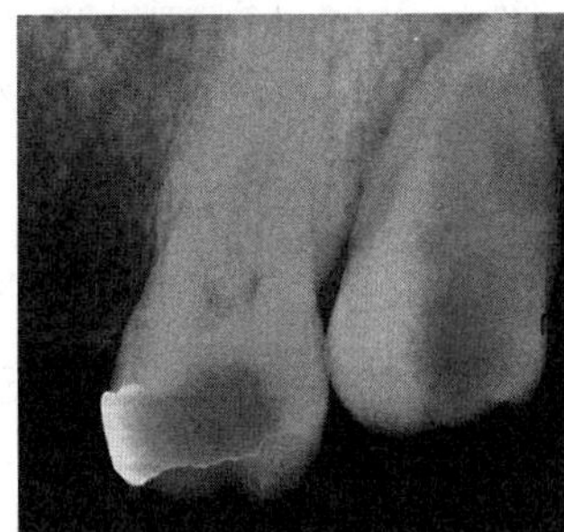

Stain of the film fixer. (Frommer/Stabulas-Savage, 2005)

film fault, static electricity, *n* an image in the emulsion that has the appearance of lightning. Caused by rapid opening of the film pocket or transfer of static electricity from the technician to the film.

film fault, white spots, *n* a fault caused by air bubbles clinging to the emulsion during development or by fixing solution spotted on the emulsion before development.

film hanger, *n* an instrument or device for holding radiographic film during processing procedures.

F

film holder, cardboard, *n* See cassette, cardboard.

film image, *n* the shadow of a structure as depicted on a radiographic or photographic emulsion.

film immersion method, *n* a procedure for processing radiographic films involving submerging the films in a sodium hypochlorite solution for anywhere between 30 seconds and 5 minutes. The solution should be 5.25% sodium hypochlorite.

film, interproximal, *n* See film, bitewing.

film mounting, *n* the placement of radiographs in an orderly sequence on a suitable carrier for illumination and study.

film packet, *n* a small, lightproof, moisture-resistant, sealed paper or plastic envelope containing a radiographic film (or two radiographic films) and a lead-foil backing designed for use in making intraoral radiographs.

film placement, *n* the positioning of the radiographic film to receive the image cast by the roentgen rays.

film processing, *n* a chemical transformation of the latent image, produced in a film emulsion by exposure to radiation, into a stable image visible by transmitted light. The usual procedure is basically a selective reduction of affected silver halide salts to metallic silver grains (development), followed by the selective removal of unaffected silver halide (fixation), washing to remove the processing chemicals, and drying.

film, processing, acids in, *n* the chemicals that arrest the process of film development and also neutralize leftover developer.

film processing, automatic, *n* a fast and efficient method of processing in which the film is mechanically transferred from the developer to the fixer, is washed, and finally is dried.

film processing, rapid, *n* the use of high-speed chemicals or elevated temperatures to reduce processing time.

film speed (film sensitivity), *n* the amount of exposure to light or roentgen rays required to produce a given image density. It is expressed as the reciprocal of the exposure in roentgens necessary to produce a density of 1 above base and fog; films are classified on this basis in six speed groups, between each of which is a twofold increase in film speed.

film thickness, *n* the thickness of a layer of material, particularly in reference to dental cements. In standardization tests, film thickness is the minimal thickness or layer obtained under a specific load.

film, radiographic, *n* older term was *x-ray.* See survey, radiographic.

Filoviridae (fī′lōvir′idā), *n* a major virus family, to which both the Marburg and Ebola viruses belong. Viruses in this family have a single-stranded RNA molecular structure with complex symmetry.

filter, *n* a material placed in the useful beam to absorb preferentially the less energetic (less penetrating) radiations. See also filtration.

filter, added, *n* a filter added to the inherent filter.

filter, compensating, *n* a filter designed to shield less dense areas so that a more uniform image quality will be produced.

filter, inherent, *n* the filtration introduced by the glass wall of the radiographic tube, any oil used for tube immersion, or any permanent tube enclosure in the path of useful beam.

filter, orange, *n* the recommended safelight filter for darkroom illumination when processing intraoral film only. Also called *filter type ML-2.*

filter, red, *n* the recommended safelight filter for darkroom illumination when processing either intraoral or extraoral film. Also called filter type GBX-2.

filter, total, *n* the sum of inherent and added filters.

filtration (filtrā′shən), *n* the use of absorbers for the selective attenuation of radiation of certain wavelengths from a useful primary beam of x-radiation.

filtration, built-in, *n* the filtration put into effect by nonremovable absorbers deliberately built into the tube-head assembly to increase the inherent beam filtration.

filtration, external, *n* the action of absorbers external to the tube-head assembly, consisting of added filtration plus the attenuating effect of materials of which any closed-end cone such as a pointer cone may be made. See also filter, added.

financial management, *n* the management or control of the money or cash flow of a business or enterprise.

financial support, *n* the funding of a project to assist in its accomplishment.

finasteride, *n brand name:* Proscar; *drug class:* synthetic steroid; *action:* competitive inhibitor of 5-α-reductase, which converts testosterone to 5-α-dihydrotestosterone; *use:* symptomatic benign prostatic hyperplasia.

findings, radiographic (roentgenographic findings), *n* the recorded radiographic evidence of normal and deviated anatomic structures.

fineness, *n* a means of grading alloys with regard to gold content. The fineness of an alloy is designated in parts per thousand of pure gold, pure gold being 1000 fine.

finger, *n* any one of the five digits of the hand.

finger, clubbed, *n* a condition seen in hypertrophic osteoarthropathy where the base angle between the base of the fingernail and adjacent dorsal surface of the terminal phalanx is obliterated and becomes 180 degrees or greater. The base of the nail projects downward, and the area of nail is increased.

finger positions, *n.pl* the positions of the fingers when operating; refers not only to the fingers grasping the instrument but also to the fingers used for rests, support, and holding the tissues out of the way.

finger rest, *n* an integral part of instrumentation, in which the fingers of the working hand rest on the teeth, adjacent tissues, and fingers of the opposing hand to improve control of the working stroke of an instrument by providing a fulcrum for movement of the working fingers and instruments.

finger rest, reinforced, *n* the position of the fingers that provides additional force to the instrument by allowing the thumb of the nondominant hand to be placed on the handle or shank of the instrument while the index (first) finger of the nondominant hand is placed on the adjacent tooth.

finger rest, substitute, *n* the position of the fingers used when the customary resting point on an adjacent tooth is inhibited by a missing or inadequately supported tooth. The substitute finger rest may be the dental arch or a gauze sponge or cotton roll packed into the appropriate area.

finger rest, supplementary, *n* the position of the fingers that provides additional support by allowing the index (first) finger of the dominant or instrument hand to rest on the index finger of the nondominant hand when it is placed on the occlusal surface of the adjacent teeth.

finger strut, *n* a bar or similar component of the infrastructure of a subperiosteal or endosteal implant that projects from it, being attached at only one side.

finger sucking, *n* the habit of sucking the finger (or thumb) for oral gratification. It is normal in infants and young children as a comforting device, especially when tired or hungry. If the habit persists beyond the eruption of the permanent teeth, it may cause a malocclusion of the anterior teeth.

finger sweep, *n* a method whereby one uses fingers to remove a foreign object from the oral cavity of an unconscious individual. Finger sweeps should not be performed on small children unless one can clearly see the object.

fingerspelling, *n* the manipulation of fingers into different positions, usually based on the manual alphabet, to represent letters of the alphabet.

finish line, *n* See line, finish.

finish, satin, *n* the degree of finish of a polished surface that has been made very smooth but without a high sheen.

finishing and polishing, *n* the removal of excess restoration material from the margins and contours of a restoration, and polishing of the restoration.

finishing stones, *n.pl* the abrasive stones of varying shapes (flame, round, or pear) used to smooth the surfaces of a restoration.

finishing strip, *n* See strip, abrasive.

F

Firmicutes **(fur′mikūts),** *n.pl* a major category of disease-causing bacteria with many subgroups, to which the *Streptococcus* and *Staphylococcus* varieties belong. A gram-positive type of bacteria that has cell walls.

firmness, *n* a term used to describe the relative flexibility of toothbrush bristles; determined by bristle thickness and height. See also stiffness.

firmware, *n* a special type of permanent program that takes the place of or accomplishes the function of traditional hardware components. Firmware is loaded into the equipment, either at the time it is manufactured or later, by the person installing the equipment or the person using it.

first aid, *n* the immediate care that is given to an injured or ill person before treatment by medically trained personnel.

first surgical stage (subperiosteal), *n* the operation performed to obtain a direct bone impression.

fission (fish′ən), *n* the splitting of a nucleus into two fragments. Fission may occur spontaneously or may be induced artificially. In addition to the fission fragments, particulate radiation energy and gamma rays are usually produced during fission.

fission, nuclear, products, n.pl the elements (nuclides) or compounds resulting from nuclear fission.

fission products, n.pl the nuclides produced by the fission of a heavy-element nuclide.

fissure, *n* a deep groove or cleft; commonly the result of the imperfect fusion of the enamel or adjoining dental lobes.

fissure, gingival, n See cleft, gingival.

fissure, inferior orbital, n the opening between the maxilla and the greater wing of the sphenoid bone through which the inferior ophthalmic vein, infraorbital artery, and infraorbital and zygomatic nerves travel.

fissure, pterygomaxillary **(ter′igōmak′səlerē),** *n* the most posterior point in the anterior contour of the maxillary tuberosity.

fissured tongue, *n* See tongue, fissured.

fistula (fis′tyoolə), *n* an abnormal tract connecting two body surfaces or organs or leading from a pathologic or natural internal cavity to the surface. The tract may be lined with epithelium.

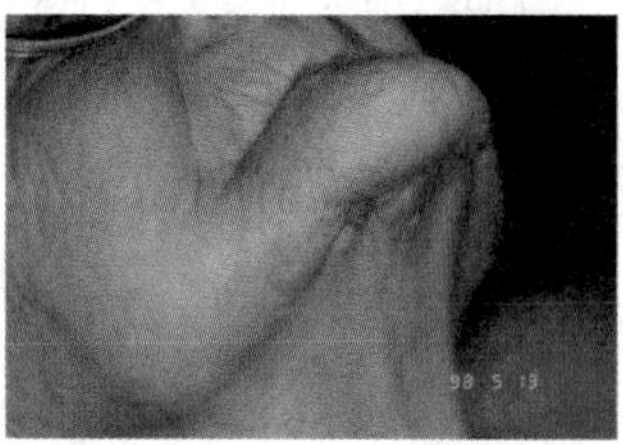

Fistula. (Courtesy Dr. Charles Babbush)

fistula, alveolar, n See parulis.

fistula, arteriovenous, n See shunt, arteriovenous.

fistula, branchial, n a fistula associated with a branchial cyst; usually seen on the lateral surface of the neck.

fistula, dental, n See parulis.

fistula, of lip, n a congenital malformation in which there is a deep pit or fistula on the mucosa of the lip; often bilateral and usually found on the lower lip.

fistula, oroantral, n an opening between the maxillary sinus and the oral cavity, most often through a tooth socket. See also fistula.

fistula, orofacial, n an opening between the cutaneous surface of the face and the oral cavity.

fistula, oronasal, n an opening between the nasal cavity and the oral cavity.

fistula, salivary, n an opening between a salivary duct and/or gland and the cutaneous surface or into the oral cavity through other than the normal anatomic pathway.

fit, *n* an adaptation of any dental restoration. An adaptation of a denture to its basal seat, a clasp to a tooth, an inlay to a cavity preparation.

fix, *v* to make firm, stable, immovable; to place in a desired position and hold there. In dentistry, to secure in position, usually by means of cementation, a prosthesis such as a crown or a fixed partial denture.

fixation (fiksā′shən), *n* the act or result of fixing, such as being bound or limited in position or relationship.

fixation, biphase pin, *n* See appliance, fracture.

fixation, elastic band, *n* the stabilization of fractured segments of the jaws by means of intermaxillary or maxillomandibular elastic bands applied to splints or appliances.

fixation, external pin, *n* See appliance, fracture.

fixation, intermaxillary, *n* See fixation, maxillomandibular.

fixation, intraosseous, *n* the reduction and stabilization of fractured bony parts by direct fixation to one another with surgical wires, screws, pins, and/or plates.

fixation, mandibulomaxillary, *n* See fixation, maxillomandibular.

fixation, maxillomandibular (mandibulomaxillary fixation), *n* a retention of fractures of the maxillae or mandible in the functional relations with the opposing dental arch through the use of elastic wire ligatures and interdental wiring and/or splints.

fixation, nasomandibular, *n* a mandibular immobilization, especially for edentulous jaws, using mandibulomaxillary splints, circummandibular wiring, and intraoral interosseous wiring through the nasal process of the maxillae.

fixation, of elements by the skeleton, *n* the fixation of many elements for long periods in the bone matrix as a result of a special affinity of the elements for the matrix. Recent work with radioactive isotopes has firmly established the concept of the skeleton as a dynamic system. In addition to the changes in structure and distribution of the bone mineral mediated by cellular activity, every ionic grouping in the mineral is capable of replacement.

fixation, osseous, *n* the immobilization of fractured bony segments.

fixation, radiographic, *n* in film processing, the chemical removal of all the undeveloped salts of the film emulsion, so that only the developed (reduced) silver will remain as a permanent image.

fixation, restorative, *n* the act of securing in position, usually by means of cementation, some treatment appliance such as a crown or fixed partial denture so that it cannot be removed.

fixation, Roger-Anderson pin, *n.pr* an appliance used in extraoral fixation of mandibular fractures and prognathisms. See also appliance, fracture.

fixative (fik′sətiv), *n* **1.** a substance used to bind, glue, or stabilize. **2.** a substance used to preserve gross or histologic specimens of tissue for later examination.

fixed appliance system, *n* See prosthesis, fixed expansion and prosthodontics, fixed.

fixed costs, *n.pl* the costs that do not change to meet fluctuations in enrollment or in use of services (e.g., salaries, rent, business license fees, and depreciation).

fixed fee schedule, *n* a list of specified fees for services that will be paid to dental professionals participating in a dental plan.

fixed partial denture, *n* See denture, partial, fixed.

fixed premium, *n* a specified amount charged for insurance that is not changed by such factors as family size or initial year versus maintenance year of dental care coverage. Also called *set premium.*

fixed removable, *n* an artificial restoration fixed to an implant that can only be removed by the dental professional.

fixer, *n* the chemicals used in the final step of film processing that remove the unaffected silver halide particles from the developed film.

fixer stains on film, *n.pl* See film fault, stained.

flabby tissue, *n* See tissue, hyperplastic.

flaccid (flas′id, flak′sid), *adj* being in a relaxed or flabby state, as in a flail-like condition or paralysis of a muscle.

flag, *n* **1.** a type of indicator used for identification. **2.** a label that signals the occurrence of some medical condition ("red flag").

flagella (fləje′lə), *n.pl* hairlike projections that extend from some unicellular organisms and aid in their movement.

flagellates (flaj′əlāts), *n.pl* one of four phyla of parasitic protozoa, also called *Mastigophora.* They can cause diseases such as enteritis, urethritis, vaginitis, and Chagas' disease by means of drinking water contamination, vaginal discharge, and bug bite.

F

flange (flanj), *n* the part of the denture base that extends from the cervical ends of the teeth to the border of the denture.

flange, buccal, n the portion of the flange of a denture that occupies the buccal vestibule of the oral cavity and that extends distally from the buccal notch.

flange, contour of, n the topographic design of the flange of a denture.

flange, labial, n the portion of the flange of a denture that occupies the labial vestibule of the oral cavity.

flange, lingual, n the portion of the flange of a mandibular denture that occupies the space adjacent to the residual ridge and next to the tongue.

flange-guide appliance, *n* an appliance (prosthesis) with a lateral vertical extension designed to direct a resected mandible into centric occlusion.

flap(s), *n* a sheet (or sheets) of soft tissue partially or totally detached to gain access to structures underneath or to be used in repairing defects in an adjacent or a remote part of the body.

flap, envelope, n the mucoperiosteal tissue retracted from a horizontal linear incision (as along the free gingival margin), with no vertical component of the incision.

flap, lingual tongue, n a flap used to repair a fistula of the hard palate, which combines the raising of a palatal flap to form the floor of the nose with a flap taken from the back or edge of the tongue to form the palatal surface.

flap, mucoperiosteal, n a flap of mucosal tissue, including the periosteum, reflected from a bone.

flap, pedicle, n a stalk-shaped attachment to a flap.

flap, periodontal, n a portion of periodontal tissue partially removed for deposit removal or for removing a pocket by rearranging the soft tissue; also useful for gaining access to the alveolar bone.

flap, sliding, n a flap that is advanced from its original location in a direction away from its base, to close a defect.

flap, V-Y, n a flap in which the incision is shaped like a V and after closure like a Y, to lengthen a localized area of tissue. See also flap, Y-V.

flap, Y-V, n a flap in which the incision is shaped like a Y and after closure like a V, to shorten a localized area of tissue. See also flap, V-Y.

flash, *n* the excess material that is squeezed out of the mold (e.g., during packing of a denture by compression technique).

flash, proximal-gingival, n an overhang that may occur inside the matrix band when a proximal wedge is positioned improperly or not used at all; more likely to occur on concave proximal surfaces.

flask, *n* a metal case or tube used in investing procedures.

flask, casting, n See flask, refractory.

flask, closure, n the procedure of bringing the parts of a flask together to form a complete mold.

flask, crown, n a small, sectional, metal, boxlike case in which a sectional mold of plaster of paris or artificial stone is made for the purpose of compressing and curing plastics on small dental restorations.

flask, denture, n a sectional, metal, boxlike case in which a sectional mold of plaster of paris or artificial stone is made for the purpose of compressing and curing dentures or other resinous restorations.

flask, final, closure, n the last closure of a flask before curing and after trial packing the mold with a denture base material.

flask, injection, n a special flask designed to permit the filling of the mold after the flask is closed or to permit the addition of denture base material to that in the flask after the flask is closed.

flask, refractory (casting flask, casting ring), *n* a metal tube in which a refractory mold is made for casting metal dental restorations or appliances.

flask, trial, closure, *n* a preliminary closure made for the purposes of eliminating excess denture base or other plastic material and of ensuring that the mold is completely filled.

flasking, *n* the act of investing a pattern in a flask. The process of investing the cast and a wax denture in a flask preparatory to molding the denture base material into the form of the denture.

***Flavobacterium* (flā′vōbaktē′rēəm),** *n* a genus of aerobic to facultatively anaerobic, nonsporeforming, motile, and nonmotile bacteria. These organisms characteristically produce yellow, orange, red, or yellow-brown pigments. They are found in soil and fresh and salt water; some species are pathogenic.

flavonoids (flā′vənoidz′), *n.pl* a group of substances containing the plant pigment flavone. There is no known requirement for them. They have a constrictor effect on the capillary bed and decrease permeability of blood vessels. Some beneficial effects of flavonoids have been described in the treatment of bruises, contusions, and sprains. Also known as *bioflavonoid.*

flavoxate HCl, *n brand name:* Urispas; *drug class:* antispasmodic; *action:* relaxes smooth muscles in urinary tract; *uses:* relief of nocturia, incontinence, suprapubic pain, dysuria.

flecainide acetate, *n brand name:* Tambocor; *drug class:* antidysrhythmic (Class IC); *action:* decreases conduction in all parts of the heart with greatest effect on His-Purkinje system; *uses:* life-threatening ventricular dysrhythmias, sustained supraventricular tachycardia.

flexibility, *n* the property of elastic deformation under loading.

flexible benefits, *n.pl* a benefits program in which an employee has a choice of credits or dollars for distribution among various benefit options (e.g., health and disability insurance, dental benefits, child care, pension benefits). See also cafeteria plans and flexible spending account.

flexible spending account, *n* an employee reimbursement account primarily funded with employee-designated salary reductions. Funds are reimbursed to the employee for health care (medical and/or dental), dependent care, and/or legal expenses and are considered a nontaxable benefit.

flexion (flek′shən), *n* the bending of a joint between two skeletal members to decrease the angle between the members; opposite of extension.

flexion-extension reflex, *n* See reflex, flexion-extension.

flexure (flek′shur), *n* the quality or state of being flexed.

flexure, clasp, *n* the flexure of a retentive clasp arm to permit passage over the surveyed height of contour, thus permitting the seating or removal of the clasp.

flexure, mandibular, *n* the change in shape of the mandible caused by the pterygoid muscles contracting during opening and protrusion movements.

floater, *n* one or more spots that appear to drift in front of the eye, caused by a shadow cast on the retina by vitreous debris.

floor of cavity, *n* See cavity floor.

flora (flôr′ə), *n.pl* the bacteria living in various parts of the alimentary canal.

flora, fusospirochetal, *n.pl* the microorganisms *F. fusiforme* and *B. vincentii.* Present in most individuals as normal inhabitants of the oral cavity. Believed by some to be the primary and by others the secondary cause of acute necrotizing ulcerative gingivitis (ANUG).

flora, normal oral, *n.pl* the varying types of bacteria that are usually present in the oral cavity.

flora, oral, *n.pl* the microorganisms inhabiting the oral cavity. They are usually saprophytic in nature and live together in a symbiotic relationship. Some are potentially pathogenic, assuming a pathologic role when adverse local or systemic factors such as increased body temperature influence the symbiotic balance of the microorganic flora.

floss, *n* a waxed or unwaxed string or tape used to remove plaque from the interproximal and contact areas of the teeth. Its regular and proper use is essential to good oral hygiene and prevention of both dental caries and periodontal disease.

floss cleft, *n* a narrow gap created in the gingival tissues between the teeth by floss that is repeatedly positioned incorrectly so that it presses against the gingiva.

F

floss cuts, prevention of, *n* the patient care information centered around the protection of injury to the gingival tissues, particularly the col. Instruction includes careful attention to the angle and thickness of floss used, as well as proper flossing technique.

floss, expanded PTFE dental, *n* one of three varieties of filament-based dental hygiene tools; consists of a waxy artificial chemical called politetrafluoroetilene; tends to resist shredding and breaking.

floss, tape, *n* thicker floss.

floss, tufted dental, *n* a floss made from alternating sections of traditional thin fiber and thicker tufted fiber that is especially suited to removing plaque from teeth separated by wide spaces.

flossing, *n* the mechanical cleansing of interproximal tooth surfaces with stringlike, waxed or unwaxed dental floss or tape.

flossing aids, *n.pl* the commercially available devices designed to make flossing easier and more effective, particularly in places that are tight or difficult to reach. These include plastic holders and threaders.

flow, *n* to move in a manner similar to a liquid stream.

flow, dental material, *n* the continued deformation or change in shape under a static load, as with waxes and amalgam.

flow, traffic, *n* the pattern of office personnel and patient movement from one area within the office to another.

flowchart, *n* a graphic representation of a sequence of operations using symbols to represent the operations. Flowcharts often symbolize the most important steps of the process without detailing the algorithm of the way the work is to be performed.

flowmeter, *n* a physical device for measuring the rate of flow of a gas or liquid, such as with nitrous oxide.

fluconazole (flookon′əzōl), *n brand name:* Diflucan; *drug class:* antifungal; *action:* inhibits ergosterol biosynthesis; *uses:* oropharyngeal candidiasis, urinary candidiasis, cryptococcal meningitis, vaginal candidiasis.

fluctuation (fluk′choowā′shən), *n* a wavelike motion produced in soft tissues in response to palpation or percussion. Fluctuation is caused by a collection of fluids or exudates in the tissues.

flucytosine (floosī′təsēn′), *n brand name:* Ancobon; *drug class:* antifungal; *action:* converted to fluorouracil after entering fungi, which inhibits DNA and RNA synthesis; *uses: Candida* infections.

fludrocortisone acetate (floo′drōkor′tisōn′ as′ətāt), *n brand name:* Florinef Acetate; *drug class:* glucocorticoid, mineralocorticoid; *action:* promotes increased reabsorption of sodium and loss of potassium from renal tubules; *uses:* adrenal insufficiency, salt-losing adrenogenital syndrome.

fluid (floo′id), *n* a liquid or gaseous substance.

fluid, crevicular, *n* a clear, usually unnoticeable fluid that can serve as a defense mechanism against infection by carrying antibodies and other therapeutic substances between the connective tissue and sulcus or pocket. Also called *gingival sulcus fluid* or *sulcular fluid.*

fluid delivery, *n* the continual fluid stream of an ultrasonic instrument, either over or through the vibrating tip, which is necessary to maintain a stable instrument temperature throughout a procedure.

fluid, dentinal, *n* the fluid content within the dentinal tubules of the dentin of the tooth.

fluid, lacrimal, *n* a watery secretion of the lacrimal gland, commonly called tears. The fluid is secreted into the lacrimal lake, an area located between the eyeball and the upper eyelid. It helps bathe the sensitive cornea. Tearing can result from eye irritation, or during periods of emotional distress.

fluid, synovial, *n* the small amount of fluid occurring in normal joints. Its principal function is to lubricate the joint surfaces and nourish the articular cartilage, such as in the temporomandibular joint.

fluid, total body, *n* all the fluids contained in the body. There are two main types: the intracellular fluid, which is contained totally within the cells, and the extracellular fluid, which is contained entirely outside the cells.

fluid wax, *n* See wax, fluid.

flumazenil (floo′mazənil′), *n brand name:* Romazicon; *drug class:* benzodiazepine receptor antagonist; *action:* antagonizes actions of benziodiazepines on the central nervous system; *use:* reversal of sedative effects of benzodiazepines.

flunisolide (floonis′əlīd′), *n brand name:* Oral INH aerosol, AeroBid; *drug class:* synthetic glucocorticoid; *action:* long-acting synthetic adrenocorticoid with antiinflammatory activity; *use:* rhinitis (seasonal or perennial).

fluocinonide (floo′əsin′ənīd′), *n brand names:* Licon, Lidex, Lidex-E; *drug class:* topical corticosteroid; *action:* interacts with steroid cytoplasmic receptors to induce antiinflammatory effects; possesses antipruritic, antiinflammatory actions; *uses:* psoriasis, eczema, contact dermatitis, pruritus, oral lichen planus lesions.

fluorapatite (flôrap′ətīt), *n* a member of the family of minerals that make up the basic structure of bones and teeth; basically a hydroxapatite form in which fluoride ions replace hydroxyl ions.

fluorapatite crystal **(kris′təl),** *n* the crystalline structure that occurs after hydroxyapatite changes into fluorapatite as a result of the tooth being exposed to fluoride.

fluorescein (flôres′ēin), *n* in dentistry, a dye applied to teeth to reveal plaque. In ophthalmology, it is used to discover corneal lesions.

fluorescence (flәres′əns), *n* the emission of radiation of a particular wavelength by certain substances as the result of absorption of radiation of a shorter wavelength.

fluorescent screen, *n* See screen, intensifying.

fluorhydroxyapatite (flôr′hīdrok′sēap′ətīt), *n* a member of the family of minerals that make up the basic structure of bones and teeth. It is formed when small amounts of fluoride and teeth mineral react. When higher concentrations of fluoride are involved, the result is the formation of calcium fluoride.

fluoridate (flôr′idāt), *v* to add fluoride to a water supply.

fluoridated salt, *n* a compound of sodium chloride with fluoride added; not considered as effective as fluoridated water.

fluoridation, *n* **1.** the process of adding fluoride to a public water supply to reduce dental caries. **2.** the use of a fluoride to prevent caries and promote remineralization; may be by means of communal water supplies; oral hygiene preparations for home use; or topical applications.

fluoride(s) (flŏŏr′īd), *n* a salt of hydrofluoric acid, commonly sodium or stannous (tin).

fluoride dietary supplements, *n.pl* the orally administered nutritional additives of the chemical fluoride; often taken by individuals without regular access to a fluoridated water supply; available as chewable tablets, drops, pills, and in combination with vitamin supplements. See also fluoride drops.

fluoride drops, *n* a supplemental liquid form of the chemical fluoride. They can be administered to children from 6 months to 3 years of age but are not usually recommended because most children are exposed to normal levels of fluoride in their water systems at home and school and in their beverages.

fluoride, stannous, *n* a compound of tin and fluorine used in dentifrices to prevent caries.

fluoride tablets/lozenges, *n.pl* the supplemental forms of the chemical fluoride. Tablets must be chewed, and lozenges must be held in the oral cavity until dissolved in order to benefit from the fluoride's contact with the teeth.

fluoride toxicity, n poisoning as a result of ingesting too much fluoride. Symptoms range from upset stomach to death.

fluoride varnish, n a topical resin containing fluoride that is thinly applied to the tooth surface and used as a preventive treatment for caries. Can also be used as a desensitizing agent to treat dentinal hypersensitivity by temporarily blocking dentinal tubules.

F

fluorides, topical, n.pl the salts of hydrofluoric acid (usually sodium or tin salts) that may be applied in solution to the exposed dental surfaces to prevent dental caries and promote remineralization. They can be applied by trays or mouthrinses or by techniques such as paint-on.

fluorides, topical, paint-on technique, n a professionally administered procedure in which the exposed dental surfaces are coated with a fluoride solution or gel or varnish to prevent caries and promote remineralization.

fluorine (flŏŏr′ēn), *n* an element of the halogen family and the most reactive of the nonmetals. Its atomic number is 9, and its atomic weight is 19. Small amounts of sodium fluoride added to the public water supply will reduce the incidence of dental caries, particularly among children. Excessive amounts of fluoride can mottle tooth enamel and cause osteosclerosis. Acute fluoride poisoning can cause death.

fluoroscope (flôr′əscōp), *n* a device consisting of a fluorescent screen mounted in a metal frame covered with lead glass. In the presence of a roentgen ray, the screen glows in direct proportion to the intensity of the remnant x-radiation, producing visual impressions of the densities traversed.

fluorosis (flərō′sis), *n* an enamel hypoplasia caused by the ingestion of excess fluoride during the time of enamel formation. General term for chronic fluoride poisoning.

fluorosis, chronic endemic dental (mottled enamel), n an enamel defect caused by excessive ingestion of fluoride, possibly in the water supply (usually 2 to 8 ppm) during the period of tooth calcification. Affected teeth appear chalky white on eruption and later turn brown.

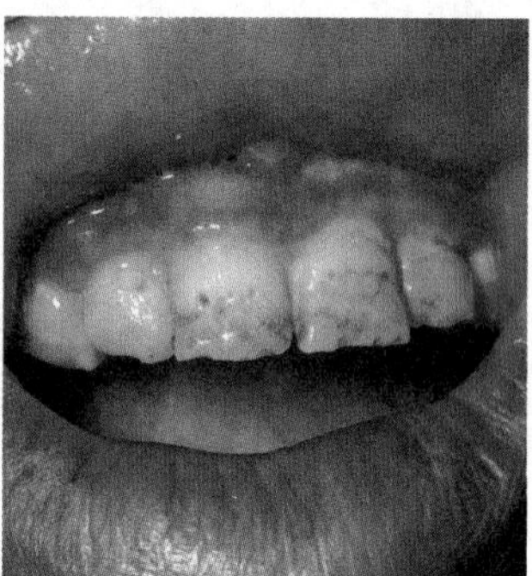

Fluorosis. (Courtesy Dr. Charles Babbush)

fluorosis, dental, n an abnormal condition resulting from the ingestion of too much fluoride, causing a white or brown mottled appearance to the enamel of developing teeth.

fluorosis, index of dental, n a classification system for determining the presence and severity of chronic fluoride poisoning in which the enamel on individual teeth is rated against a 0 to 4 scale with 0 representing normal enamel and 4 severely damaged enamel. This index may be used by communities to adjust the levels of fluoride in their water systems.

fluorouracil (topical) (flŏŏr′əyŏŏr′əsil), *n brand names:* Efudex, Fluoroplex; *drug class:* topical antineoplastic; *action:* inhibits synthesis of DNA and RNA in susceptible cells; *uses:* keratosis, basal cell carcinoma.

Fluothane, *n.pr* the brand name for halothane.

fluoxetine (flŏŏok′sətēn′), *n brand name:* Prozac; *drug class:* antidepressant; *action:* inhibits CNS neuron uptake of serotonin but not norepinephrine; *use:* depressive disorders.

fluoxymesterone (flŏŏok′sēmes′tərōn′), *n brand names:* Android-F, Halotestin; *drug class:* androgenic anabolic steroid, Controlled Substance Schedule III; *action:* increases weight by building body tissue; increases potassium, phosphorus, chloride, nitrogen levels;

increases bone development; *uses:* impotence from testicular deficiency, hypogonadism, breast engorgement, palliative treatment of female breast cancer.

fluphenazine decanoate/fluphenazine enanthate/fluphenazine HCl (floofen′əzēn′ dec′anō′āt), *n brand names:* Decanoate, Moditen, Prolixin Enanthate; *drug class:* phenothiazine antipsychotic; *action:* blocks neurotransmission at dopaminergic synapses in the cerebral cortex, hypothalamus, and limbic system; *uses:* psychotic disorders, schizophrenia.

flurandrenolide (flŏŏr′andren′əlīd), *n brand names:* Cordran, Cordran SP; *drug class:* topical corticosteroid, group III medium potency; *action:* possesses antipruritic, antiinflammatory actions; *uses:* corticosteroid-responsive dermatoses, pruritus.

flurazepam HCl (flŏŏraz′əpam), *n brand name:* Dalmane; *drug class:* benzodiazepine, sedative-hypnotic, Controlled Substance Schedule IV; *action:* produces central nervous system depression by interaction with benzodiazepine receptor to facilitate action of inhibitory neurotransmitter γ-aminobutyric acid (GABA); *uses:* insomnia.

flurbiprofen (flŏŏrbip′rəfen), *n brand name:* Ansaid; *drug class:* nonsteroidal antiinflammatory; *action:* inhibits prostaglandin synthesis by interfering with cyclooxygenase needed for biosynthesis; possesses analgesic, antiinflammatory, antipyretic properties; *uses:* acute, long-term treatment of rheumatoid arthritis, osteoarthritis.

flurbiprofen sodium, *n brand name:* Ocufen; *drug class:* nonsteroidal antiinflammatory ophthalmic; *action:* inhibits enzyme system necessary for biosynthesis of prostaglandins, inhibits miosis; *uses:* inhibition of intraoperative miosis, corneal edema.

flush, *n* **1.** a blush or sudden reddening of the face and neck caused by vasodilation of small arteries and arterioles. **2.** a sudden, subjective feeling of heat. **3.** a sudden, rapid flow of water or other liquid.

flutamide (floo′təmīd′), *n brand name:* Eulexin; *drug class:* antineoplastic; *action:* interferes with testosterone at cellular level, inhibits androgen uptake; *uses:* metastatic prostatic carcinoma, stage D2 in combination with LHRH agonistic analogs (leuprolide).

fluticasone propionate (flŏŏtik′əsōn prō′pēənāt′), *n brand name:* Cutivate (topical), Flonase (nasal spray); *drug class:* synthetic corticosteroid, medium potency; *action:* interacts with steroid cytoplasmic receptors to induce antiinflammatory effects; possesses antipruritic, antiinflammatory actions; *uses:* topical for inflammation of corticosteroid-responsive skin disorders; spray for seasonal and perennial allergic rhinitis.

fluting (floo′ting), *n* the elongated developmental depressions along the root branches of tooth root surfaces of certain teeth.

flutter, *n* a quick, irregular motion.

fluvastatin sodium (floo′vəstat′ən sōdēəm), *n brand name:* Lescol; *drug class:* cholesterol-lowering agent; *action:* inhibits HMG-CoA reductase enzyme, which reduces cholesterol synthesis; *uses:* adjunct in primary hypocholesterolemia (types IIa and IIb).

fluvoxamine maleate (flōōvak′səmēn′ mā′lēāt), *n brand name:* Luvox; *drug class:* antidepressant; *action:* selectively inhibits reuptake of serotonin in central nervous system neurons; *uses:* obsessive-compulsive disorder.

flux, *n* a substance or mixture used to promote fusion, especially the fusion of metals or minerals. Used principally in dentistry as an inclusion in ceramic materials and in soldering and casting metals.

flux, casting, *n* a flux that increases fluidity of the metal and helps to prevent oxidation.

flux, ceramic, *n* a flux used in the manufacture of porcelain and silicate powders.

flux, reducing, *n* a flux that contains powdered charcoal to remove oxides.

flux, soldering, *n* a ceramic material such as borax, boric acid, or a combination, in paste, liquid, or granular form; used to keep metallic parts clean while they are being heated during a soldering procedure. It is a solvent for metallic oxides and will flow over the parts to be soldered at temperatures well below the fusion temperature of solder, but it becomes separated from the solid metal by the molten solder.

FMIA, *n.pr* See angle, Frankfort-mandibular incisor.

focal infection, *n* the site or origin of an infectious process. Endodontically treated teeth have frequently been accused of being the source of septicemias, often without justification. See also infection, focal.

F

focal spot, *n* See spot, focal.

focal-film distance, *n* See distance, target-film.

focus group, *n* a demographic target group of people used to gather opinions or data descriptive of the population represented by the sample selected.

fog (fogging), *n* See film fault, fogged.

fog, chemical, *n* See film fault.

fog, dyschroic, *n* See film fault, dyschroic fog.

fog, light, *n* See film fault.

fog, radiation, *n* the film darkening caused by radiation from sources other than intentional exposure to the primary beam; e.g., film may be exposed to scatter radiation, or accidental exposure may occur if stored film is not protected from radiation.

foil, *n* a very thin, flexible sheet of metal, usually gold, platinum, or tin.

foil, adhesive, *n* a tin foil that is covered on one side with powdered gum arabic or karaya gum.

foil assistant, *n* See foil holder.

foil, cohesive gold, *n* a gold foil that has been annealed or had a surface so completely pure so that it will cohere or weld at room temperature.

foil, corrugated gold, *n* a gold foil made by burning gold foil sheets between paper in the absence of air.

foil cylinder, *n* a cylinder of gold foil formed by repeatedly folding a sheet of foil into a narrow ribbon, which is then rolled into cylindrical form.

foil, gold (fibrous gold), *n* pure gold that has been rolled and beaten from ingots into a very thin sheet. Thickness usually varies from 1/40,000 inch (No. 2 foil) to 1/20,000 inch (No. 4 foil). Classified as cohesive, semicohesive, or noncohesive. One of the oldest restorative materials, the most permanent if used properly, and the yardstick by which all others are measured. It is compacted or condensed into a retentive cavity form piece by piece, using this metal's property of cold welding.

foil holder (foil assistant), *n* an instrument used to retain a foil pellet in place while it is being condensed or to retain a bulk of gold while additions to it are made.

foil, noncohesive gold, *n* a gold foil that will not cohere at room temperature because of the presence on its surface of a protecting or contaminating coating. If the coating is a volatile substance, such as ammonia, the foil may be rendered cohesive by heating or annealing it to remove the protection.

foil passer (foil carrier), *n* a pointed or forked instrument used to carry pellets of gold foil through an annealing flame or from the annealing tray to the prepared cavity for compaction.

foil pellet, *n* See pellet, foil.

foil, platinized gold **(plat′ənīzd),** *n* a form rolled or hammered from a "sandwich" made of platinum placed between two sheets of gold; used in portions of foil restorations where greater hardness is desired.

foil, platinum, *n* pure platinum rolled into extremely thin sheets. A precious-metal foil whose high fusing point makes it suitable as a matrix for various soldering procedures; also suitable for providing the internal form of porcelain restorations during fabrication.

foil, tin, *n* a base-metal foil used as a separating material, or protective covering (e.g., between the cast and denture base material during flasking and curing procedures).

folate (fō′lāt), *n* a form of folic acid that helps transport single carbon units between molecules.

fold, *n* a doubling back of a tissue surface.

fold, mucobuccal (mucobuccal reflection), *n* the depth of the oral mucosa from the mandible or maxillae to the cheek.

fold, mucolabial, *n* the depth of the oral mucosa from the mandible or maxillae to the lip.

fold, sublingual, *n* the crescent-shaped area on the floor of the oral cavity following the medial wall of the mandible and tapering toward the molar regions.

folder, *n* a heavy paper envelope in which the patient's records are kept.

folic acid, *n* vitamin B_9, a water-soluble B vitamin needed for erythropoiesis, increases red blood cell, white blood cell, and platelet formation in megaloblastic anemias. It functions as a coenzyme with vitamin B_{12} and C in the breakdown and utilization of proteins and in the formation of nucleic acids. It is prescribed for use during pregnancy (helps prevent neural tube defects) and for megaloblastic or macrocytic anemia caused by folic acid deficiency, liver disease, alcoholism, hemolysis, and intestinal obstruction.

folic acid analog, *n* an antimetabolite drug used as an antineoplastic agent in the treatment of malignant cell growths.

follicle (dental), *n* See dental sac.

follicles, *n* the masses that are embedded in a meshwork of reticular fibers within the lobules of the thyroid gland. See also thyroid gland.

follicular cyst, *n* an odontogenic cyst that arises from the epithelium of a tooth bud and dental lamina.

follow-up, *n* the process of monitoring the progress of a patient after a period of active treatment.

fomite (fomes) (fō′mīt, fō′mēz), *n* a nonliving object that may carry germs. An inanimate source of disease, such as a drinking glass used by an infected person.

Fones's method, *n.pr* See method, Fones's.

food, *n* the ingested solids and liquids that supply the body with nutrients and energy.

food additives, *n.pl* substances that are added to foods to prevent spoilage, improve appearance, enhance the flavor or texture, or increase the nutritional value.

Food and Drug Administration (FDA), *n.pr* an agency of the Department of Health and Human Services responsible for the enforcement of the Federal Food, Drug, and Cosmetic Act and other statutes as assigned.

food, comminution of **(kom′inoo′-shən),** *n* the reduction of food into small parts.

food debris, *n* the particles of food remaining in the oral cavity after eating, which collect in tooth crevices and between the teeth and may contribute to the formation of dental caries. See also materia alba.

Food Drug and Cosmetic Act (FD & C), *n.pr* legislation passed in 1906 dealing with import and export activity as well as the enforcement of packaging and labeling requirements of all food, drug, and cosmetic commerce within the United States.

food frequency checklist, *n* a tool used by individuals to determine how often they are ingesting certain types of foods. Consists of a list of various foods from all food groups and a grid allowing for a range of answers, from never to five or more times per day. See also diet.

food gorging, *n* the rapid ingestion of large amounts of food; stuffing; in bulemia, gorging is alternated with purging as a weight-maintenance regimen.

Food Guide Pyramid, *n.pr* a graphic list issued and endorsed by the U.S. Departments of Agriculture and Health and Human Services; outlines recommendations for a healthy, balanced diet. Through the illustration of a three-dimensional triangle, it divides daily diet choices according to recommended frequency of ingestion.

food impaction, *n* See impaction, food.

food, physical character of, *n* the consistency, as the firmness, viscosity, or density, of food substances. Soft, adhesive, and nonabrasive foods tend to cling to the teeth, which may lead to calculus formation, whereas coarse foods leave little debris and create a frictional effect on the tissues, thus cleansing them.

food record, *n* a manually recorded history of an individual's dietary intake over a 24-hour period; subsequently analyzed by a dental hygienist in order to help correct any nutritional imbalances.

F

foramen (fərā′mən), *n* **1.** a natural opening in a bone or other structure. **2.** a natural opening in the root, usually at or near the apical end.

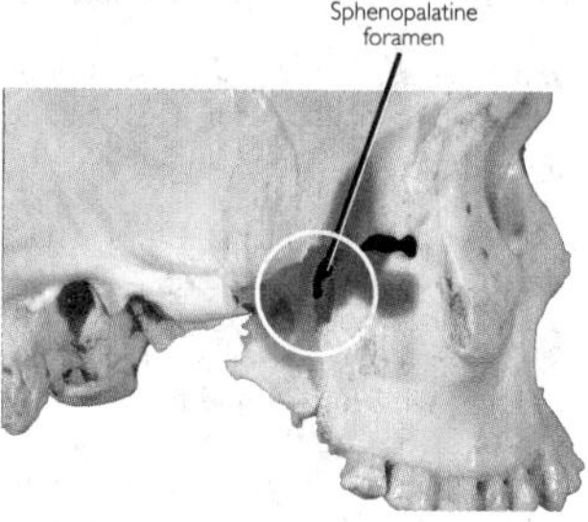

Foramen. (Liebgott, 2001)

foramen, apical **(fərā′mən ā′pikəl),** *n* the opening entryway at the root's apex, from which the blood vessels and nerves radiate out to the rest of the tooth. Often located within a range of several millimeters of the precise anatomic high point of the root.

foramen cecum **(fərā′mən sē′kum),** *n* a small, pit-like depression in the dorsal surface of the tongue where the median lingual sulcus meets the lingual tonsil.

foramen, greater palatine, *n* a small opening of the hard palate located near the second and third molars in which the palatine vessels and greater palatine nerve travel.

foramen, incisive **(insī′siv),** *n* (nasopalatine foramen), **1.** the opening of the incisive (nasopalatine) canal marked by the incisive papilla. **2.** the foramen, or opening, in the midline of the palate in the region where the premaxilla and maxillae join, which is situated palatal to the maxillary central incisors; contains branches of the right and left nasopalatine vessels and nerve.

foramen, infraorbital, *n* a small opening in the maxilla at the terminal end of the infraorbital canal. Its location can be roughly approximated by mapping the intersection of an imaginary straight line drawn between the eyes and the nose.

foramen, lingual, *n* a small opening that can be present in the midline of the mandible through which an artery connecting to the sublingual right and left lingual arteries travels. Cannot be noted radiographically.

foramen magnum, *n* an opening in the occipital bone through which the spinal cord enters the spinal column.

foramen, mandibular, *n* an opening on the medial aspect of the vertical ramus of the mandible approximately midway between the mandibular and gonial notches; may be located posterior to the middle of the ramus. It carries interior alveolar vessels and the inferior alveolar nerve.

foramen, mental, *n* an opening on the lateral aspect of the body of the mandible inferior to the apices of the mandibular second or first premolar. The mental vessels and nerve pass through this foramen to travel through the mandibular canal to supply the lip. In edentulous mandibles, the bone may have been resorbed, so that it is in such a position that the denture base will cover it.

foramen, nasopalatine, *n* See foramen, incisive.

foramen, ovale **(ōvāl′),** *n* **1.** an oval-shaped opening located between the two atria of a developing fetal heart. **2.** an oval-shaped opening located in the sphenoid bone in which travels the mandibular nerve, emissary veins, accessory meningeal artery, and otic ganglion.

foramen, rotundum **(rōtun′dəm),** *n* a round opening located in the sphenoid bone in which travels the maxillary nerve.

force, *n* any application of energy, either internal or external to a structure; that which initiates, changes, or arrests motion.

force and stress, *n* the pressure forcibly exerted on the teeth and on their investing and supporting tissues that is detrimental to tissue integrity. In occlusal trauma, the production of lesions of the attachment apparatus depends on an interrelationship of the strength, duration, and frequency of the application of the force.

force, centrifugal, *n* a force that tends to recede from the center.

force, chewing, *n* the degree of force applied by the muscles of mastication during the mastication of food.

force, component of, *n* **1.** one of the factors from which a resultant force may be compounded or into which it may be resolved. **2.** one of the parts of a force into which it may be resolved.

force, condensing, *n* **1.** the force required to compress gold-foil pellets, facilitating their cohesion, to fabricate or build up a gold-foil restoration. **2.** the force required to compact or condense a plastic material (e.g., amalgam, wax).

force, constant, *n* a continuous force or pressure applied to the teeth.

force, counter-dislodgement, *n* pressure that comes into play when food is evenly distributed in the oral cavity so that contact between the maxillary and mandibular teeth is equalized on both sides during mastication.

force, denture-dislodging, *n* an influence that tends to displace a denture from its intended position on supporting structures.

force, denture-retaining, *n* an influence that tends to maintain a denture in its intended position on its supporting structures.

force, electromotive, *n* the difference in potential in a roentgen-ray tube between the cathode and anode; usually expressed in kilovolts.

force, intermittent, *n* a force or pressure (applied to the teeth) that is alternated with a period of passiveness or rest.

force, line of, *n* the direction of the power exerted on a body.

force, masticatory, *n* the force applied by the muscles attached to the mandible during mastication.

force, occlusal (occlusal load), *n* **1.** the result of muscular forces applied on opposing teeth. **2.** the force transmitted to the teeth and their supporting structures by tooth-to-tooth contact or through a bolus of food or other interposed substance.

force, shear, *n* commonly employed as a calculation of the physical stress a material can bear, it refers to the type of force that is expressed parallel to the face of an object.

force, tensile, *n* the type of force manifested in an extension of an object itself. A stretched rubber band is an example of tensile force.

forced expiratory volume (FEV), *n* the volume of air that can be forcibly expelled in a fixed time after full inspiration.

forceps (for′seps), *n* **1.** a colloquial term for an instrument used for grasping or applying force to teeth, tissues, or other objects, such as when they are extracted. **2.** an instrument used for grasping and holding tissues or specific structures.

forceps, bone, *n* the force used for grasping or cutting bone.

forceps, chalazion, *n* a thumb forceps with a flattened plate at the end of one arm and a matching ring on the other. Originally used for isolation of eyelid tumors. It is useful for isolation of lip and cheek lesions, such as a mucocele, to facilitate removal.

forceps, dental extracting, *n* forceps used for grasping teeth.

forceps, hemostatic, *n* an instrument for grasping blood vessels to control hemorrhage.

forceps, insertion, *n* See forceps, point.

forceps, lock, *n* See forceps, point.

forceps, Magill, *n.pr* a tongs-shaped tool used to remove objects from the oral cavity.

forceps, mosquito, *n* a small hemostatic forceps.

forceps, point (lock forceps, insertion forceps), *n* a device used in filling root canals that securely holds the filling cones during their placement.

forceps, rubber dam clamp, *n* forceps whose beaks are designed to engage holes in the rubber dam retainer to facilitate its placement, adjustment, or removal.

forceps, suture, *n* See needle holder.

forceps, thumb, *n* the forceps used for grasping soft tissue; used especially during suturing.

forceps, tissue, *n* a thumb forceps; an instrument with one or more fine teeth at the tip of each blade for controlling tissues during surgery, especially during suturing.

Fordyce granules (for′dīs gran′ūlz), *n.pr* small, elevated, yellowish areas on the oral mucosa and lips that occur in more than 80% of the population. They are the result of ectopic sebaceous glands and are not considered abnormal.

F

Fordyce's spots, *n.pr* See Fordyce granules.

forecasting, *n* the attempt to predict the future on the basis of expert opinion, market research, trend projection, leading indicators, and other modalities.

forehead, *n* the portion of the face directly above the orbits and extending posteriorly/superiorly to the hairline or crown of the head.

foreign body, *n* an object or substance found in the body in an organ or tissue in which it does not belong under normal circumstances, such as a bolus of food in the trachea or a particle of dust in the eye. See also body, foreign.

forensic (fəren′sik), *adj* pertaining to the law or to legal proceedings.

forensic anthropology, n the use of anatomic structures and physical characteristics to identify a subject for legal purposes.

forensic dentistry, n the use of dental characteristics for the purpose of identifying a subject for legal purposes. See also jurisprudence, dental.

foreshortening, *n* See distortion, vertical.

forging, *n* working or shaping heated metal.

fork, face-bow, *n* the part of the face-bow assembly used to attach an occlusion rim or transfer record of maxillary teeth to the face-bow proper.

form, *n* the configuration, shape, or particular appearance of anything.

form, acquaintance, n a registration sheet for new patients on which data (e.g., the patient's name and address) are recorded and that contains a statement of the policies of the specific dental professional's office or clinic and the responsibilities of the office or clinic to the patient.

form, anatomic, n the natural shape of a part.

form, anatomic charting, n one of three types of manually recorded dental documentation, features a graphic template displaying a representation of each tooth, as well as the roots and gingival tissues. Design provides for note taking associated with each tooth. The form becomes part of the patient's legal health records and is useful for planning patient care and ascertaining legal questions regarding treatment, and is relied upon for patient identification in the event of an emergency. See also form, examination.

form, arch, n the shape of the dental arch. See also arch, dental.

form, convenience, n the modifications necessary, beyond basic outline form, to facilitate proper instrumentation for the preparation of the cavity or insertion of the restorative material; also the placing of starting points or slight undercuts to retain the first portions of restorative material while succeeding portions are placed.

form, examination, n the written documentation recording the thorough assessment of the oral cavity and surrounding structures. The form should include patient history and

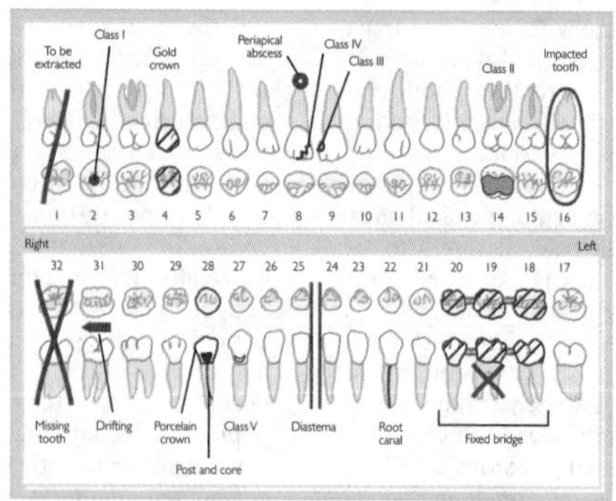

Anatomic charting form. (Bird/Robinson, 2005)

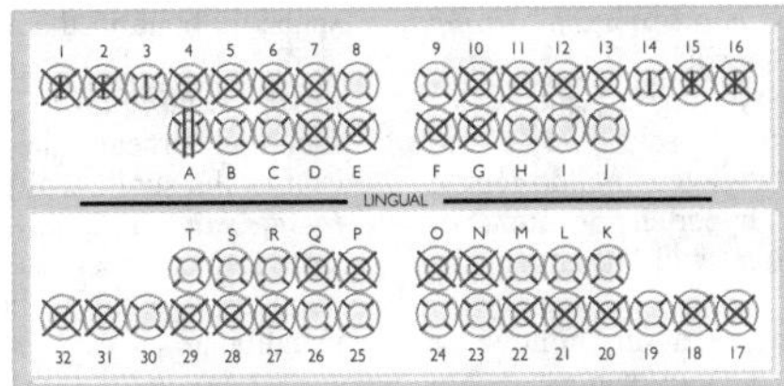

Geographic charting form. (Bird/Robinson, 2005)

descriptions of observed abnormalities of visible characteristics. Also called *record form.*

form, face, *n* the outline form of the face from an anterior frontal view.

form, functional, *n* the shape that permits optimal performance.

form, geographic charting, *n* one of three types of manually recorded dental documentation, describes each tooth by either a number or a letter within a quadrant. The gingival tissues and roots of the teeth are not included, making this chart unsuitable for periodontal assessment.

form, message, *n* a checklist form, by means of which dental office staff can quickly make a record of telephone communications for the dental staff to look at later.

form, occlusal, *n* the form of the occlusal surface of a tooth, a row of teeth, or dentition.

form, outline, *n* the shape of the area of the tooth surface included within the cavosurface margins of a prepared cavity.

form, posterior tooth, *n* the distinguishing contours of the occlusal surface of the various posterior teeth.

form, registration, *n* a form used to gather personal (nonprofessional) data about a patient.

form, resistance, *n* the shape given to a prepared cavity to enable the restoration and remaining tooth structure to withstand masticatory stress.

form, retention, *n* the provision made in a cavity preparation to prevent displacement of the restoration.

form, root, *n* the shape of the root of the tooth. It is capable of being modified by such factors as resorption and cemental apposition.

form, tooth, *n* the characteristics of the curves, lines, angles, and contours of various teeth that permit their identification and differentiation.

formaldehyde (formal'dəhīd'), *n* a toxic, pungent water-soluble gas used in the aqueous form as a disinfectant, fixative, or tissue preservative.

formalin (for'məlin), *n* a clear aqueous solution of formaldehyde. A 37% solution is used to fix and preserve tissues for histologic and pathologic study.

format, *n* a predetermined computer arrangement of characters, fields, lines, page numbers, punctuation marks, and the like.

former, angle, *n* See angle former.

former, crucible, *n* See sprue former.

former, sprue, *n* See sprue former.

formocresol (for'mōkres'ol), *n brand name:* Buckley's Formo Cresol; a compound consisting of formaldehyde, cresol, glycerin, and water used in vital pulpotomy of primary teeth and as a temporary intracanal medicament during root canal therapy.

fortified (fôrtə'fīd), *adj* containing additives more potent than the principal ingredient.

forward protrusion, *n* See protrusion, forward.

foscarnet sodium/phosphonoformic acid (foskär'nət sōdēəm fos'fōnōfor'mik), *n brand name:* Foscavir; *drug class:* antiviral; *action:* antiviral activity is produced by selective inhibition at the pyrophosphate binding site on virus-specific DNA polymerases, inhibits replication of all known herpesviruses; *uses:* CMV retinitis in AIDS, acyclovir-resistant herpes zoster in HIV-infected patients.

Foshay's test, *n.pr* See test, Foshay's.

fosinopril (fosin'ōpril), *n brand name:* Monopril; *drug class:* angiotensin-converting enzyme (ACE) inhibitor; *action:* selectively suppresses renin-angiotensin-aldosterone system; *uses:* hypertension alone or in combination with thiazide diuretics.

fossa(e) (fos'ə), *n* a pit, hollow, or depression on a tooth or bone.

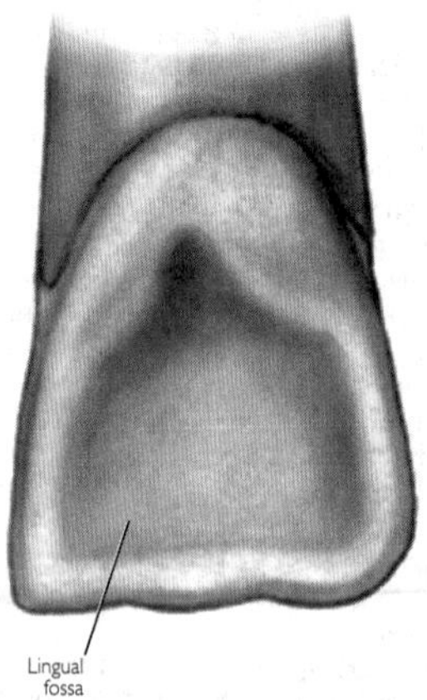

Fossa. (Bath-Balogh/Fehrenbach, 2006)

fossa, articular, n a concave structure situated adjacent to the articular eminence on the temporal bone of the skull. Also known as the *mandibular fossa.*

fossa, canine, n the fossa in the canine maxilla superior to the apex of the canine tooth.

fossa, depth of, n on the occlusal table, the distance from the top of the shorter cusp downward into the bottom of the fossa.

fossa, lateral, n a shallow, concave area of peritoneum on the rear wall of the abdominal cavity, bordered by the lateral umbilical fold and the inguinal ligament.

fossa, mental, n a depression located between the alveolar and mental ridges of the roots of the incisors.

fossa, nasal, n See cavity, nasal.

fossa, pterygopalatine **(ter'igōpal'ətīn),** *n* a depression located between the maxilla and the sphenoid bone in the anatomy of the skull.

fossa, sublingual, n a depression found underneath the tongue, adjacent to the sublingual glands.

fossa, submandibular, n a depression found underneath the internal oblique ridge, which houses the submandibular salivary gland.

foundation, *n* **1.** a charitable organization usually established to allocate private funds to worthy projects or to provide other services. **2.** in dentistry, any device or material added to a remaining tooth structure to enhance the stability and retention of an overlying cast restoration. May be a pin retainer of amalgam, plastic cement, or a casting.

four-handed dentistry, *n* See dentistry, four-handed.

fovea, palatine (fō'vēə), *n* a small depression at the junction between the hard and soft palates; plays a role in the gag reflex.

Fox scissors, *n.pr* See scissors, Fox.

Fox's knife, *n.pr* See knife, Goldman-Fox.

fractionation (frak'shənā'shən), *n* **1.** the separation of a substance into its basic constituents. **2.** the process of isolating a pure culture by sucessive culturing of a small portion of a colony of bacteria. **3.** the process of isolating different components of living cells by centrifugation. **4.** the process of administering a dose of radiation in smaller units over time to minimize tissue damage.

fracture, *n* a break or rupture of a part. In the oral region, fracture is most often seen in teeth and bones.

fracture, avulsion, n the loss of a section of bone.

fracture, blow-out, n a fracture involving the orbital floor, its contents, and the superior wall of the maxillary antrum, in which orbital contents are incarcerated in the fracture area, producing diplopia.

fracture, bulk, n a fracture or failure in the amalgam of a restoration. An improperly finished restoration by the dental professional, poor cavity design, or improper loading of the restoration can lead to a bulk fracture.

fracture, cementum, n the tearing of

fragments of the cementum from the tooth root.

fracture, clasp, *n* failure of a clasp arm because of stresses that have exceeded the elastic limit of the metal from which the arm was made.

fracture, closed reduction of, *n* a reduction and fixation of fractured bones without making a surgical opening to the fracture site.

fracture, comminuted, *n* a fracture in which the bone has several lines of fracture in the same region; a fracture in which the bone is crushed and splintered.

fracture, compound, *n* a fracture in which the bony structures are exposed to an external environment.

fracture, craniofacial dysjunction (transverse facial fracture), *n* a complex fracture in which the facial bones are separated from the cranial bones; a LeFort III fracture.

fracture, dislocation, *n* a fracture of a bone near an articulation, with dislocation of the condyloid process.

fracture, fissured, *n* a fracture that extends partially through a bone, with no displacement of the bony fragments.

fracture fixation, *n* the fractured fragments of bone are stabilized in close proximation to promote healing.

fracture, greenstick, *n* a fracture in which the bone appears to be bent; usually only one cortex of the bone is broken.

***fracture, Guérin's* (gāraz′),** *n.pr* a LeFort I fracture of the facial bones in which there is a bilateral horizontal fracture of the maxillae.

fracture, impacted, *n* a fracture in which one fragment is driven into another portion of the same or an adjacent bone.

fracture, indirect, *n* a fracture at a point distant from the primary area of injury caused by secondary forces.

fracture, intraarticular, *n* a fracture of the articular surface of the condyloid process of a bone.

fracture, intracapsular, *n* a fracture of the condyle of the mandible occurring within the confines of the capsule of the temporomandibular joint.

fracture, LeFort, *n.pr* a transverse fracture involving the orbital, malar, and nasal bones.

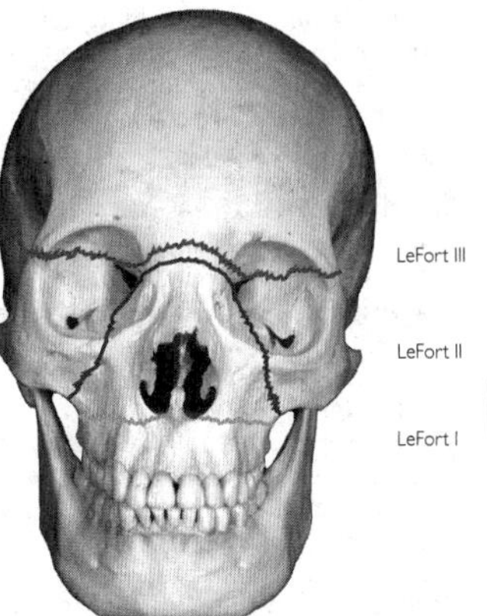

LeFort classifications. (Liebgott, 2001)

fracture, midfacial, *n* fractures of the zygomatic, maxillary, nasal, and associated bones.

fracture, pyramidal, *n* a fracture of the midfacial bones, with the principal fracture lines meeting at an apex in the area of the nasion; a LeFort II fracture.

fracture, root, *n* a microscopic or macroscopic cleavage of the root in any direction.

fracture, simple, *n* a linear fracture that is not in communication with the exterior.

fracture, stress, *n* **1.** a type of stress usually occuring from sudden, strong, violent, endogenous force, such as a simple fracture of the fibula in a runner. **2.** the fracture of metallic parts as a result of fatigue of prolonged or frequent stress.

fracture, tooth, *n* a traumatic injury to a tooth that manifests itself as a chip, crack, or break. Manifestations may also include dislocation or complete displacement of a tooth.

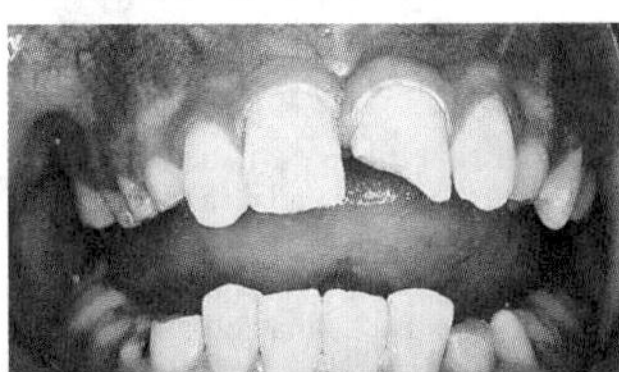

Tooth fracture. (Daniel/Harfst/Wilder, 2008)

F

fracture toughness, *n* the quality of the material used for brackets that indicates its ability to withstand applied force without cracking.

fracture, transverse facial, *n* See fracture, craniofacial dysjunction.

fragilitas ossium (frajil′ētəs os′ēəm), *n* See osteogenesis imperfecta.

fragment, *n* a broken or disconnected part of a larger whole, such as a tooth or root.

F

frail elderly, *n.pl* older persons (usually over the age of 75 years) who are afflicted with physical or mental disabilities that may interfere with the ability to independently perform activities of daily living.

frame, *n* a structure, usually rigid, designed to give support or attachment to a part, or to immobilize a part.

frame, implant, *n* See substructure, implant.

frame, occluding **(ōkloo′ding),** *n* a device for relating casts to each other for the purpose of arranging teeth or for use in making an index of the occlusion of dentures; an articulator. See also articulator.

frame, rubber dam, *n* See holder, rubber dam.

framework, *n* the skeletal metal portion of a removable partial denture around which and to which the remaining units are attached.

franchise dentistry, *n* **1.** the practice of dentistry under a brand name, the rights of which have been purchased from another dental professional or dental practice. Under a franchise license agreement, the franchiser may use the brand name, marketing products, and treatment techniques for a sum of money, as long as certain rules and regulations of the franchise are adhered to. **2.** a system for marketing a dental practice, usually under a brand name, where permitted by state laws. In return for a financial investment or other consideration, participating dental professionals may also receive the benefits of media advertising, a national referral system, and financial and management consultation.

Francisella **(fransĭsel′ə),** *n* a type of gram-negative eubacteria with cell walls. It requires oxygen to survive.

F. tularensis **(too″ləren′sis),** *n.pl* the bacteria that causes the circulatory disease tularemia, which can be contracted via contaminated food or drink, physical contact, spray, or bug bite. Symptoms include fever, headache, swelling of the lymph nodes, and other pain or discomfort.

Frankel appliance, *n.pr* See appliance, Frankel removable orthodontic.

Frankfort horizontal plane, *n.pr* See plane, Frankfort horizontal.

Frankfort-mandibular incisor angle, *n.pr* See angle, Frankfort-mandibular incisor.

F-ratio (F-test), *n* a value used in determining whether the difference between two variables is statistically significant or stable. A larger variance is divided by a smaller variance, both of which are the results of analysis of variance procedures. The value for F is looked up in a table that shows the probability of occurrence of a ratio of this size.

fraud, *n* an intentional perversion of truth for the purpose of inducing another, in reliance on it, to part with something valuable or to surrender a legal right; deliberate deception; deceit; trickery.

fraudulent concealment, *n* the deliberate attempt to withhold information or to conceal an act to avoid contractual responsibility. Fraudulent concealment as applied to health care providers arises when a treating doctor conceals from an aggrieved patient that a previous treating doctor may have committed malpractice.

freckle, *n* See ephelis.

free gingiva, *n* See gingiva, free.

free gingival groove, *n* See groove, gingiva, free.

free gingival margin, *n* See margin, gingival.

free mandibular movement, *n* See movement, mandibular, free.

free radical, *n* a compound with an unpaired electron or proton. It is unstable and reacts readily with other molecules.

free-end, *n* See base, extension.

free-way space, *n* See distance, interocclusal.

freedom of choice, *n* a provision in a dental benefits program that permits the insured to choose any licensed dental professional to provide his/her dental care and receive full benefits under the program.

freeze drying, *n* the freezing of heat-sensitive liquid materials in a vacuum to preserve the characteristics of the substrate and remove the volume of water or liquid by sublimation.

fremitus (frem′itus), *n* the palpable vibrations of nonvascular origin that can be noted by placing the hand on the chest. See also thrill.

frenal pull, charting (frē′nəl), *n* notations made to a patient's chart concerning evidence of the forces exerted by frenums, both on the maxillary and mandibular arches.

frenectomy (frənek′tōmē), *n* **1.** the excision of a frenum. **2.** the surgical detachment and/or excision of a frenum from its attachment into the mucoperiosteal covering of the alveolar processes. Other term: *frenotomy.*

frenoplasty (frē′nōplas′tē), *n* a correction of an abnormal frenum by repositioning it.

frenotomy (frənot′əmē), *n* the cutting of a frenum; posibly the release of ankyloglossia (tongue-tie), although this is not the preferred method of treatment. More common term: *frenectomy.*

frenotomy, traumatic **(frənot′əmē trəmat′ik),** *n* a laceration of an oral frenum, usually the maxillary labial frenum, due to trauma. Most commonly seen in children.

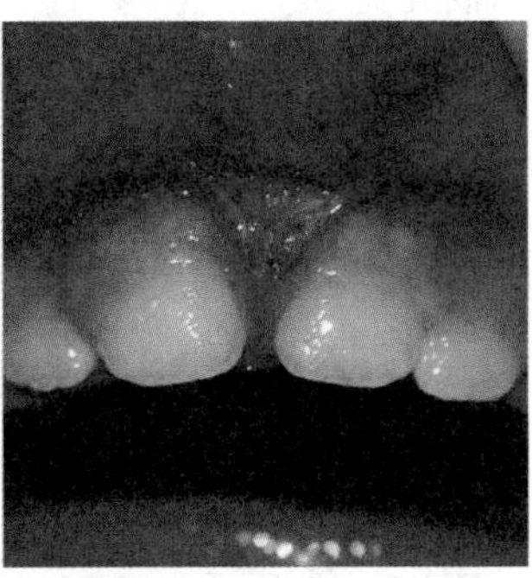

Traumatic frenectomy. (Courtesy Dr. Beth Schulz-Butulis)

frenulum (fren′ūlum). *n* See frenum.

frenum (frē′num), *n* a vertical band of oral mucosa that attaches the cheeks and lips to the alveolar mucosa of the mandibular and maxillary arches, limiting the motions of the lips and cheeks. Older term: *frenulum.*

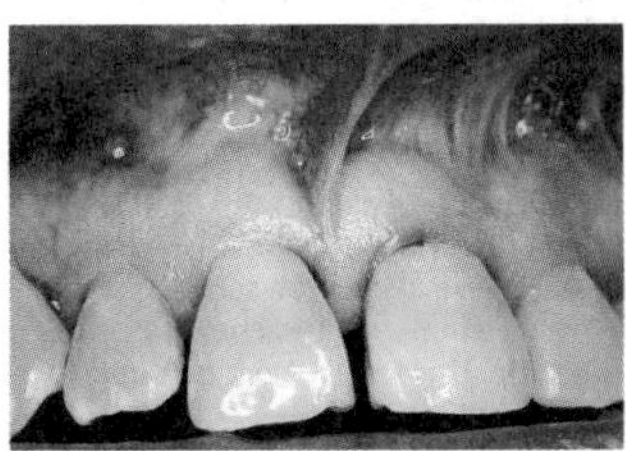

Frenum. (Newman/Takei/Klokkevold/Carranza, 2006)

frenum, abnormal (enlarged labial frenum), *n* a labial frenum appearing to be unusually heavy, broad, or attached too near the crest of the ridge that may be an etiologic factor in periodontal disease involving the marginal gingivae.

frenum, buccal, *n* the vertical band(s) of oral mucosa connecting the residual alveolar ridge to the cheek in the premolar region. They exist in both the maxillary and mandibular arches and separate the labial vestibule from the buccal vestibule.

frenum, enlarged labial, *n* See frenum, abnormal.

frenum, labial, *n* the vertical band of oral mucosa connecting the lip of the residual alveolar ridge near the midline of both the maxillary and mandibular arches.

frenum, lingual, *n* the vertical band of oral mucosa connecting the tongue with the floor of the oral cavity and the alveolar or residual alveolar ridge. See ankyloglossia.

frequency, *n* the number of cycles per second of a wave or other periodic phenomenon.

frequency polygon, *n* a graphic representation of a frequency distribution constructed by plotting each frequency above the score or midpoint of a class interval laid out on a base line and connecting the points so plotted by a straight line.

Frey syndrome (frī), *n.pr* See syndrome, Frey.

F

friable (frī′əbəl), *adj* brittle or fragile; easily damaged.

fricative (frik′ətiv), *n* a speech sound made by forcing the airstream through such a narrow opening that audible high-frequency air currents or vibrations are set up.

friction, *n* the resistance to movement as one object is moved across the other, usually creating heat.

Friedman's test (frēd′mənz), *n.pr* See test, pregnancy.

fringe benefits, *n.pl* the benefits, other than wages or salary, provided by an employer for employees (e.g., health insurance, vacation time, disability income).

frit (frit), *n* a partly or wholly fused porcelain that has been plunged into water while hot. The mass cracks and fractures, and from this "frit," dental porcelain powders are made.

frontal, *adj* in anatomy, referring to the body's frontal plane or to the forehead or frontal bone.

frontal (PA) cephalometric radiograph, *n* a cephalometric radiograph made with the subject facing the film (posteroanterior [PA] view); the axis between the ears is parallel to the film and perpendicular to the radiographic beam.

frontal bone, *n* a single cranial bone that forms the front of the skull from above the orbits posteriorly to a junction with the parietal bones at the coronal suture.

frontal lobe, *n* the largest of five lobes constituting each of the two cerebral hemispheres. The frontal lobe lies beneath the frontal bone. The frontal lobe significantly influences personality and is associated with the higher mental activities, such as planning, judgment, and conceptualizing.

frontal sinus, *n* See sinus(es), frontal.

frozen sections, *n* a histologic section of tissue that has been frozen by exposure to dry ice.

fructose (fruk′tōs), *n* a yellowish-to-white, crystalline water-soluble levorotatory ketose monosaccharide that is sweeter than sucrose and is found in honey, several fruits, and combined in many disaccharides and polysaccharides. Also called *fruit sugar* and *levulose.*

fructose intolerance, *n* an inherited disorder marked by an absence of enzymes needed to metabolize fructose. Symptoms include sweating, tremors, confusion, and digestive distress with vomiting, and failure of infants to grow.

fulcrum, extraoral (fo͝ol′krəm), *n* a stabilizing support point outside the oral cavity against which the hand or finger is placed for leverage during a dental procedure in order to ensure precise control of the instrument; usually the chin or cheek.

fulcrum, intraoral, *n* a stabilizing support point within the oral cavity against which a finger is placed for leverage during treatment in order to ensure precise control of the instrument; usually a tooth that is in close proximity to the one being treated.

fulcrum line, *n* See line, fulcrum.

fulguration (ful′gyərā′shən), *n* the destruction of soft tissue by an electric spark that jumps the gap from an electrode to the tissue without the electrode touching the tissue. See also electrocoagulation.

function, *n/v* the normal or special action of a part. As a noun, *function* has the following synonyms: *role, capacity, task, use, purpose, service, activity,* and *direction.* As a verb, it has the following synonyms: *act, operate, work, perform, go, take effect,* and *serve.* Use of the term to express intended purpose may be misleading.

function, auxiliary, *n* a function that is supplementary or additional to the function for which the part or organ is primarily intended.

function, dental, normal, *n* the correct action of opposing teeth in the process of mastication; sometimes referred to as *normal occlusion.*

function, group, *n* the simultaneous contact of opposing teeth in a segment or group.

function, heavy (occlusal function), *n* an increase in functional activities of the tooth, which may result in compensatory changes in the attachment apparatus (e.g., a stronger periodontal ligament) with an increase in the number of fibers, a reinforcement of the supporting bone by formation of new bone, and the formation of cemental spikes, which are calcifications of the cemental fibers. Such changes take place so that the increased stress may be withstood without damage.

function, impaired, *n* a diminished, weakened, or less-than-optimal work or action.

function, insufficiency of, *n* the hypofunction of the tooth, which may lead to regressive changes in the attachment apparatus and supporting bone. The severity of lesions varies with the degree of hypofunction. See also atrophy of disuse.

function, muscle, *n* the action of muscle, which is principally contraction.

function, occlusal, *n* See function, heavy.

function, physiologic, *n* the degree of activity that stimulates the physical structures but that is so limited as not to irritate those tissues.

function, skeletal, *n* the role of the skeleton in relation to the maintenance of body functions. The bony skeleton welds together and protects the softer vital visceral organs, supports and maintains the body form, and accomplishes body movement for locomotion, respiration, manual skills, and the functions associated with mandibular motion.

function, subcortical, *n* the function controlled by all the structures of the brain except the outer cortical rim of the cerebrum; most of the nonconscious activities of a sensory and motor nature.

functional, *adj* **1.** pertaining to the movements and actions of a part. **2.** of or pertaining to the functions of an organ, part, or prosthesis.

functional jaw orthopedics, *n* the objectives of activator-type appliances.

functionally dependent elderly, *n.pl* persons who have experienced a deterioration of physical capacities due to advanced age and must rely on mechanical assistance or the assistance of others.

functionally independent elderly, *n.pl* persons who are physically well despite advanced age. Also called *well elderly.*

fundoplication (fun′dōpləkā′shən), *n* a surgical procedure involving making tucks in the fundus of the stomach around the inferior end of the esophagus. The operation is used in the treatment of gastric acid reflux into the esophagus.

fungal infection, *n* an infection caused by a fungus or yeast organism.

fungate (fung′gāt), *v* to produce funguslike growths; to grow rapidly like a fungus.

fungus (fung′gəs), *n* a class of vegetable organisms of a low order of development, including mushrooms, toadstools, and molds. Examples include *Candida albicans* and *Histoplasma, Trichophyton, Actinomyces,* and *Blastomyces* organisms. Oral and systemic moniliasis (thrush) is produced by overgrowth of *C. albicans,* which is a normal resident in the oral cavity. When the patient's health is compromised, the organism may assume a pathogenic role (opportunistic infection).

furca, *n* **1.** the bone that separates the distal and mesial roots of molars. *n* **2.** the area where a tooth root divides.

furcal concavity (fur′kəl konkav′itē), *n* a depression present in the furcation area of the root of a tooth.

furcation (furkā′shən), *n* the region of division of the root portion of a tooth.

furcation defects, *n.pl* the structural defects that occur in the region of the division of the root of a tooth into two, three, or four divisions. Generally, these constitute a communication channel between the pulp and the periodontal space.

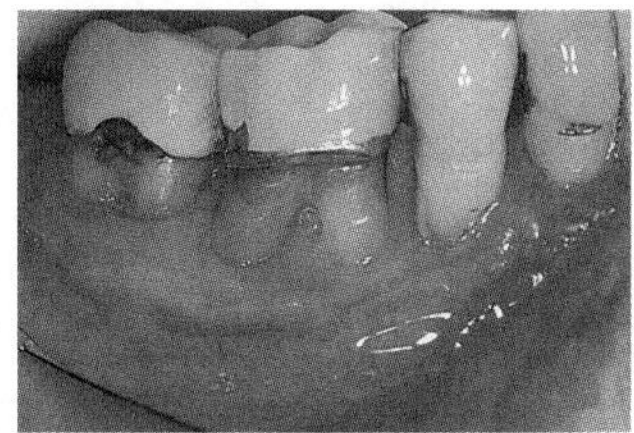

Furcation. (Daniel/Harfst/Wilder, 2008)

furcation crotches (furkā′shən krôch′ez), *n* the area between the roots of a tooth at the furcation.

furcation invasion, n the loss of bone at the point where the roots of a multirooted tooth divide.

furcation probe **(furkā′shən),** *n* See probe, furcation.

furcation, root, n the interradicular bone resorption in multirooted teeth caused by periodontal disease.

furnace, *n* an apparatus in which to generate heat.

furnace, inlay, n a furnace used for eliminating the wax from an inlay mold and establishing the proper condition and temperature of the investment to receive the molten casting gold.

furnace, porcelain, n a furnace used for fusing, firing, or fusion.

furosemide (fyŏŏrō′səmīd), *n brand names:* Lasix, Lasix Special; *drug class:* loop diuretic; *action:* acts on loop of Henle to decrease reabsorption of chloride and sodium and resultant diuresis; *uses:* pulmonary edema, edema in CHF, liver disease, ascites, hypertension.

fused teeth, *n.pl* the teeth that are joined together during tooth development by one or more of the hard tissues: enamel, dentin, or cementum.

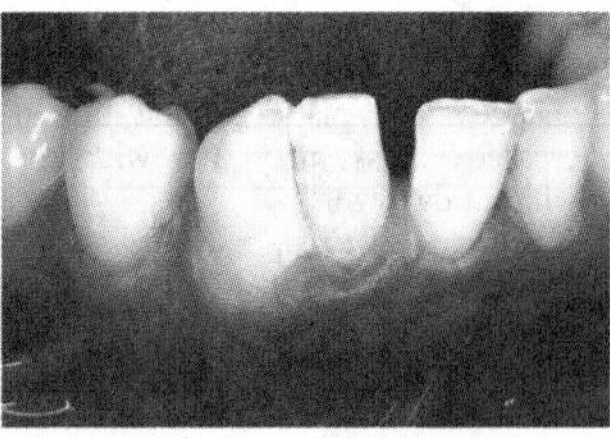

Fused teeth. (Neville/Damm/Allen/Bouquot, 2002)

fusiform bacilli, morphologic form of (fū′zifôrm), *n.pl* the fused strands of the narrow filaments of bacteria, tapered at both ends. See also *Fusobacterium fusiforme.*

fusion, *n* **1.** the uniting or joining together of two or more entities. The fusion temperature of an alloy lies just below the lower limit of its melting range, which is particularly important in soldering operations because temperatures near or above fusion temperature will decrease ductility. **2.** the process of producing fused teeth. **3.** during prenatal development, the joining of embryonic tissues of two separate surfaces or the elimination of a groove between two adjacent swellings. See also crescence and range, melting.

fusion, nuclear, n the union of atomic nuclei to form heavier nuclei, resulting in the release of enormous quantities of energy when certain light elements unite.

fusion of metal, n See metal, fusion of.

Fusobacterium **(fū′zōbaktir′ēəm),** *n* a genus of bacteria containing gram-negative, nonsporeforming, obligately anerobic rods that produce butyric acid as a major metabolic product. These organisms are normally in the oral flora; some species are pathogenic.

F. fusiforme **(fūzifôr′mā)** *(Vincent's bacillus), n* a microorganism that, along with *B. vincentii,* is implicated in the causation of necrotizing ulcerative gingivitis. Although *F. fusiforme* and *B. vincentii* are inhabitants of the oral cavity, they may become pathogenic when tissue resistance is impaired.

F. nucleatum, n a genus of schizomycetes bacterium often seen in necrotic tissue and implicated, but not conclusively, with other organisms in the causation and perpetuation of periodontal disease.

G

g, *n* See gram.

gabapentin (gab′əpen′tin), *n brand name:* Neurontin; *drug class:* anticonvulsant; *action:* anticonvulsant action is unclear; *use:* adjunctive therapy in adults with partial seizures.

gadolinium (Gd) (gadəlin′ēəm), *n* a rare-earth metallic element with an atomic number of 64 and an atomic weight of 157.25. It is used as a phosphor to intensify radiography screens.

gag, *n* a surgical device for holding the oral cavity open.

gag reflex, n a normal neural reflex

elicited by touching the soft palate or posterior pharynx; the response is a symmetric elevation of the palate, a retraction of the tongue, and a contraction of the pharyngeal muscles. It is used as a test of the integrity of the vagus and glossopharyngeal nerves.

gagging, *n* an involuntary retching reflex that may be stimulated by something touching the posterior palate or throat region.

gait (gāt), *n* a manner of walking; a cyclic loss and regaining of balance by a shift of the line of gravity in relationship to the center of gravity. A person's gait is as characteristic and as individual as a fingerprint.

gait, cerebellar, *n* an unsteady, irregular gait characterized by short steps and a lurching from one side to the other; most commonly seen in multiple sclerosis or other cerebellar diseases.

gait, festinating, *n* a gait characterized by rigidity, shuffling, and involuntary hastening. The upper part of the body advances ahead of the lower part. It is associated with paralysis agitans and postencephalitic Parkinson's syndrome.

gait, sensor ataxic, *n* an irregular, uncertain, stamping gait. The legs are kept far apart, and either the ground or the feet are watched, because there has been a loss of knowledge of the position of the lower limbs. This gait is caused by an interruption of the afferent nerve fibers and may be associated with tabes dorsalis and sometimes with multiple sclerosis and other lesions of the nervous system.

gait, spastic, *n* (creeping palsy) a slow, shuffling gait in which the patient appears to be wading in water. Knee and hip movements are restricted. This gait may be associated with multiple sclerosis, syphilis, combined systemic disease, or other diseases affecting the spinal pyramidal tracts.

gait, staggering, *n* a reeling, tottering, and tipping gait in which the individual appears as if he may fall backward or lose his balance. It is associated with alcohol and barbiturate intoxication.

gait, waddling, *n* an exaggerated alteration of lateral trunk movements, with an exaggerated elevation of the hip, suggesting the gait of a duck; characteristic of progressive muscular dystrophy.

galactin (gəlak′tin), *n* See hormone, lactogenic.

galactosamine, *n* a chondrosamine; a derivative of galactose, occurs in various mucopolysaccharides, notably of chondroitin sulfuric acid and B blood group substance.

galactose (gəlak′tōs), *n* a simple sugar found in the dextrorotatory form in lactose (milk sugar), nerve cell membranes, sugar beets, gums, seaweed, and, in the levorotatory form, in flaxseed mucilage. Galactose, a white crystalline substance, is less sweet and less soluble in water than glucose but is similar in other properties.

galactosemia (gəlak″tose′meə), *n* an inherited condition that prevents normal metabolism of galactose due to a lack of the galactose-*l*-phosphate uridyl transferase enzyme.

gallic acid (gal′ik), *n* an astringent used topically, made from tannic acid or nutgalls, and chemically known as 3,4,5-trihydroxybenzoic acid.

gallium (gal′ēəm), *n* a metallic element with an atomic number of 31 and an atomic weight of 69.72. It is used in high-temperature thermometers, and its radioisotopes are used in total-body scanning procedures.

galvanic current, *n* See current, galvanic.

galvanic skin response (GSR), *n* a reaction to certain stimuli as indicated by a change in the electric resistance of the skin. The GSR is used in some polygraph examinations.

galvanism, *n* See current, galvanic.

galvanotherapy, *n* See ionization.

gamma globulins, *n.pl* plasma proteins that are essential antibodies that circulate in the immune system. The most significant gamma globulins are antibodies or immunoglobulins. See also immunoglobulins.

gamma rays, *n* an electromagnetic radiation of short wavelength emitted by the nucleus of an atom during a nuclear reaction. Composed of high-energy photons, gamma rays lack mass and an electric charge and travel at the speed of light.

G

ganciclovir (gansī′klōvir), *n brand names:* Cytovene, DHPG; *drug class:* antiviral; *action:* inhibits replication of most herpes viruses in vitro; in vivo by selective inhibition of human cytomegalovirus (CMV) DNA polymerase and by direct incorporation into viral DNA; *uses:* CMV-retinitis in patients with AIDS.

ganglion(ia) (gang′glēon), *n/n.pl* an accumulation of neuron cell bodies outside the central nervous system.

ganglion, basal, *n* a group of forebrain nuclei that, with the related structures of the brain, play an important role in the regulation of muscle tone and motor control. The cell groups of these ganglia and their respective nerve tracts are classified as the *extrapyramidal motor system* to differentiate them from the *pyramidal motor system,* which goes directly from the cerebral cortex to the lower motor neuron. Disease associated with the basal ganglia is manifested by three principal motor abnormalities: disturbance of muscle tone, derangement of movement, and loss of associated or automatic movement.

ganglion, ciliary, *n* a parasympathetic nerve ganglion in the posterior part of the orbit. The ciliary ganglion receives preganglionic fibers from the region of the oculomotor nucleus and sends postganglionic fibers via short ciliary nerves to (1) the constrictor muscle of the iris (constriction of pupil) and (2) circular fibers of the ciliary muscle (accommodation for vision).

ganglion, otic, *n* a ganglion located medial to the mandibular nerve just below the foramen ovale in the infratemporal fossa. It supplies the sensory and secretory fibers for the parotid gland. Its sensory fibers arise from the facial and glossopharyngeal nerves.

ganglion, sphenopalatine **(sfē′nōpal′ətīn),** *n* a ganglia located deep in the pterygopalatine fossa that is intimately associated with the maxillary nerve. It lies distal and medial to the maxillary tuberosity. Its fibers supply the oral mucosa of the oropharynx, tonsils, soft and hard palates, and nasal cavity. The mucous and serous secretions of all the oral mucosa of the oropharynx are also mediated by this ganglion.

ganglion, submandibular, *n* a ganglion located on the medial side of the mandible between the lingual nerve and the submandibular duct. The submandibular ganglion is distributed to the sublingual and submandibular glands. The sensory fibers arise from the lingual branch of the trigeminal nerve; i.e., the chorda tympani of the facial nerve.

ganglion, trigeminal **(trī′jem′ənəl),** *n* a cluster of nervous tissue located on the root of the fifth cranial (trigeminal) nerve.

ganglionectomy (gang′lēōnek′təmē), *n* the excision of a ganglion.

ganglionitis, acute posterior (gang′glēənītis), *n* See herpes zoster.

gangrene (gang′grēn), *n* the death of tissue en masse, usually the result of loss of blood supply, bacterial invasion, and subsequent putrefaction. E.g., gangrene of the pulp is total death and necrosis of the pulp. All types require the removal of the necrotic tissue before healing can progress.

gangrene, dry, *n* a late complication of diabetes mellitus that is already complicated by arteriosclerosis in which the affected extremity becomes cold, dry, and shriveled and eventually turns black.

gangrene, gas, *n* the necrosis accompanied by gas bubbles in soft tissue after trauma or surgery. It is caused by anaerobic microorganisms such as various species of *Clostridium,* particularly *C. perfringens.* If untreated, it is rapidly fatal.

gangrene, moist, *n* a condition that may follow a crushing injury or an obstruction of blood flow by an embolism, tight bandages, or a tourniquet. This form of gangrene has an offensive odor, spreads rapidly, and may result in death in a few days.

Gantrisin, *n.pr* the brand name for sulfisoxazole, an antibacterial sulfonamide, which is effective in the treatment of acute, recurrent, or chronic urinary tract infections, meningococcal meningitis, and acute otitis media.

gap arthroplasty, *n* the surgical correction of ankylosis by creation of a space between the ankylosed part and the portion in which movement is desired.

gap, interocclusal, *n* See distance, interocclusal.

Gardner-Diamond syndrome, *n.pr* a condition resulting from autoerythrocyte sensitization, marked by large, painful, transient ecchymoses that appear without apparent cause but often accompany emotional upsets, various collagen disorders, and abnormalities of protein metabolism. Treatment includes topical and systemic corticosteroids. Also called *autoerythrocyte sensitization syndrome.*

gargoylism, *n* See syndrome, Hurler's.

GAS, *n* See syndrome, general adaptation.

gas, *n* a fluid with no definite volume or shape whose molecules are practically unrestricted by cohesive forces.

gas, laughing, *n* See nitrous oxide.

gas, noble, *n* a gas that will not oxidize; the inert gases (e.g., helium and neon).

gas, olefiant, *n* a machine that uses ethylene oxide gas to sterilize objects that cannot withstand high temperatures, such as soft plastic and cloth.

gasometer (gasäm′ətur), *n* a calibrated instrument or vessel for measuring the volume of gases. Used in clinical and physiologic investigation for measuring respiratory volume.

gastric acid, *n* the hydrochloric acid secreted by the gastric glands in the stomach; aids in the preparation of food for digestion.

gastric intrinsic factor (GIF), *n* a substance secreted by the gastric mucosa that is essential for the intestinal absorption of vitamin B_{12}; also known as *intrinsic factor.*

gastric juice, *n* the digestive secretions of the gastric glands in the stomach, consisting mainly of pepsin, hydrochloric acid, rennin, and mucin.

gastric mucosa, *n* the lining of the stomach.

gastrinoma, *n* a gastrin-secreting tumor associated with the Zollinger-Ellison syndrome.

gastritis (gastrī′tis), *n* an inflammation of the lining of the stomach that occurs in both acute and chronic forms. Acute gastritis may be caused by aspirin or other antiinflammatory agents, corticosteroids, drugs, foods, condiments, and alcohol and chemical toxins. The symptoms are anorexia, nausea, vomiting, and discomfort after eating. Chronic gastritis is usually a sign of underlying disease, such as peptic ulcer or pernicious anemia.

gastritis, atrophic, *n* a chronic form of gastritis with atrophy of the mucous membrane and destruction of the peptic glands, sometimes associated with pernicious anemia or gastric carcinoma.

gastroenteritis (gas′trōen′tərī′tis), *n* an inflammation of the stomach and intestines accompanying numerous gastrointestinal (GI) disorders. Symptoms are anorexia, nausea, vomiting, abdominal discomfort, and diarrhea.

gastroenterology, *n* the study of diseases affecting the GI tract, including the esophagus, stomach, intestines, rectum, gallbladder, and bile duct.

gastroesophageal reflux disease (GERD) (gas′trōisof′əjē′əl), *n* a backflow of the contents of the stomach into the esophagus that is often the result of incompetence of the lower esophageal sphincter. Gastric juices are acid and therefore produce burning pain in the esophagus and possibly demineralize the teeth.

gastrointestinal disease, *n* an abnormal state or function of the GI system.

gastrointestinal system, *n* the chain of organs of the GI tract, from the oral cavity to the anus.

gastroscopy, *n* the visual inspection of the interior of the stomach by means of a flexible fiberoptic tube inserted through the oral cavity and passing the length of the esophagus into the stomach.

gastrostomy, *n* the surgical creation of an artificial opening into the stomach through the abdominal wall, used to feed a patient who has cancer of the esophagus or other kind of barrier to oral feeding.

gate-keeper system, *n* a managed-care concept used by some alternative benefit plans, in which enrollees elect a primary care dental professional, usually a general practitioner or pediatric dental professional, who is responsible for providing nonspecialty care and managing referrals, as appropriate, for specialty and ancillary services.

gauge, *n* an instrument used to determine the dimensions or caliber of an object.

gauge, Boley, n.pr a vernier type of instrument used for measuring in the metric system. It is accurate to tenths of millimeters.

gauge, leaf, n a device for measuring the distance between two objects. A leaf gauge consists of a series of thin strips of plastic or metal, each calibrated and arranged in a sequential fashion in ascending or descending thicknesses, usually expressed in millimeters or fractions of millimeters. In dentistry, the leaf gauge is used to measure interocclusal space or the magnitude of an interocclusal interference.

gauge, undercut, n an attachment used in conjunction with a dental cast surveyor to measure the amount of infrabulge of a tooth in a horizontal plane.

gauze strip, for flossing, *n* a folded 6- to 8-inch pieces of sterile gauze used to clean abutment teeth, teeth located at the end of a row, the space underneath dental appliances that cannot be completely removed, and between teeth that are exceptionally far apart.

gel (jel), *n* a colloid in solid form, jellylike in character. Hydrocolloid impression materials are examples of gels.

gel, brush-on, fluoride, n a gelatinous preparation used to promote remineralization of teeth and discourage further demineralization, intended to augment daily brushing and flossing. Formulas contain either 1.1% sodium fluoride or 0.4% stannous fluoride in a glycerin base.

gel strength, n See strength, gel.

gel time, n See time, gel.

gelatin, *n* a protein formed from collagen by boiling in water. Medically, gelatin is used as a hemostat, a plasma substitute, and a protein food adjunct in severe cases of malnutrition. Gelatin is used in the manufacture of capsules and suppositories. It is also used in the production of radiographic films as the medium for suspending the crystal salts on the surface of the acetate film.

gelation time (jelā′shən), *n* See time, gel.

gemfibrozil (jemfī′brəzil′), *n brand name:* Lopid; *drug class:* antihyperlipidemic; *action:* reduces plasma triglycerides and very-low-density lipoproteins; *uses:* type IIb, IV, and V hyperlipidemia.

gemination (jem′ənā′shən), *n* the formation of two teeth from a single tooth germ.

gene, *n* See family practice.

gene, homeobox **(ho′meoboks″),** *n* a gene containing a DNA sequence called the homeobox, which is very similar between species and encodes a DNA-binding domain in the resulting protein molecule. Homeobox genes usually play a role in controlling development of the organism.

gene locus, n See locus, gene.

gene, sex-linked, n a gene located in a sex chromosome.

gene therapy, n a procedure that involves injection of "health genes" into the bloodstream of a patient to cure or treat a hereditary disease or similar illness.

general supervision, *n* a circumstance of treatment in which the dental professional must diagnose and authorize the work to be performed on the patient by the dental staff but is not required to be on the premises while the treatment is carried out.

generated path (chew-in), *n* See path, generated occlusal.

generator, *n* one who, or that which, begets, causes, or produces.

generator, electric, n a device that converts mechanical energy into electrical energy.

generator, radiographic, n a device that converts electrical energy into electromagnetic energy (photons).

genetic counseling, *n* the process of advising a patient with a genetic disease, or child-bearing parents of a patient with a genetic disease, about the probabilities and risks of future genetic accidents in conception, and counseling such persons about future family planning.

genetic disease, *n* a disease that is caused by a defect or anomaly in the genetic inheritance of the patient.

genetic effects of radiation (jənet′ik), *n.pl* the changes produced in the individual's genes and chromosomes of all nucleated body cells, both somatic and gonadal, due to exposure to radiation. The more common meaning relates to the effect produced in the reproductive cells. Radiation received by the gonads before the end of the reproductive period has the potential to add to the number of undesirable genes present in the population.

genetic marker, *n* a specific gene that produces a readily recognizable genetic trait that can be used in family and population studies or in linkage analysis.

genetic testing, *n* the analysis of a person's DNA, usually to determine predispositions for or diagnoses of certain inherited conditions. See also DNA.

genetics, *n* the science that deals with the origin of the characteristics of an individual.

genial tubercle, *n* See tubercle, genial.

genioplasty (jē′nēōplastē), *n* a surgical procedure, performed either intraorally or extraorally, to correct deformities of the mandibular symphysis.

genital wart (condyloma acuminatum), *n* a soft, wartlike growth found on the warm, moist skin and mucous membranes of the genitalia, caused by a virus and transmitted by sexual contact. Also called *acuminate wart.*

genome (jē′nōm), *n* the total gene complement of a set of chromosomes found in higher life forms.

genome, human, *n* the complete set of genes in the chromosomes of each cell.

genotype (jē′nōtīp), *n* the aggregate of ordered genes received by offspring from both parents; e.g., a person with blood group AB is of genotype AB.

gentamicin sulfate, *n* (ophthalmic), *brand names:* Garamycin Ophthalmic, Gentak; *drug class:* aminoglycoside antiinfective ophthalmic; *action:* inhibits bacterial protein synthesis; *use:* infection of external eye.

gentian violet (jen′shən), *n* See violet, gentian.

geographic tongue, *n* See tongue, geographic.

geometric unsharpness, *n* an impairment of image definition resulting from the geometric penumbra. See also penumbra, geometric and radiograph beam.

geometry of radiographic beam, *n* the effect of various factors on the spatial distribution of radiation emerging from a radiographic generator or source. See also law, inverse square; penumbra, geometric; and radiographic beam.

geriatric assessment, *n* the evaluation of the physical, mental, and emotional health of elderly patients.

geriatric dentistry, *n* a branch of dentistry that deals with the special and unique dental problems of the elderly. See also elderly.

geriatrics (jer′ēat′riks), *n* the department of medicine or dentistry that treats health problems peculiar to advanced age and the aging, including the clinical problems of senescence and senility.

germ cell, *n* a sexual reproductive cell in any stage of development; that is, an ovum or spermatozoon or any of their preceding forms.

germanium (Ge) (jərmā′nēəm), *n* a metallic element with some nonmetallic properties. Its atomic number is 32 and its atomic weight is 72.59.

germicide (jur′misīd), *n* a substance capable of killing a wide variety of microorganisms, more specifically, one capable of killing all microorganisms, except for spores, with which it is in contact for a standard period.

gerodontics (jer′ōdon′tiks), *n* (gerodontology) the branch of dentistry that deals with the diagnosis and treatment of the dental conditions of aging and aged persons.

gerodontology (jer′ōdontol′ōjē), *n* See gerodontics.

gerontology (jer″ontol′əje), *n* the comprehensive (physical, psychologic, and social) study of aging.

gestation, *n* the period of development between fertilization and birth.

gestational age, *n* the age of a fetus or newborn, usually expressed in weeks dating from the first day of the mother's last menstrual period.

giant cell, *n* an abnormally large tissue cell. It often contains more than one nucleus and may appear as a merger of several normal cells.

giantism, *n* (macrosomia), excessive growth resulting in a stature larger than the range that is normal for age and race.

giantism, infantile, n excessive growth occurring before adolescence.

giantism, primary, n excessive growth not attributable to a definite cause.

giantism, secondary, n excessive growth secondary to a disorder of the adrenal, pineal, gonadal, or pituitary gland.

Giardia **(jēär′dēə),** *n* a common genus of the flagellate protozoans. Many species normally inhabit the digestive tract and cause inflammation in association with other factors that produce rapid proliferation of the organism.

giardiasis (jēärdī′əsis), *n* an inflammatory intestinal condition caused by overgrowth of the protozoan *G. lamblia.* The source of infection is usually contaminated water. Also called *traveler's diarrhea.*

GIF, *n* See gastric intrinsic factor.

Gillies' operation, *n.pr* See operation, Gillies'.

Gillmore needle, *n.pr* See needle, Gillmore.

Gilson fixable-removable bar, *n.pr* See connector, cross arch bar splint.

gingiva(e) (jin′jivə), *n/n.pl* the fibrous tissue that immediately surrounds the teeth. Colloquial term is *gums.*

gingiva, adequate attached (AAG), n the amount of attached gingival tissues needed to prevent recession of the gingival tissues.

gingivae, attached, n the portion of the gingivae extending from the free gingival groove, which demarcates it from the marginal (free) gingivae, to the mucogingival junction, which separates it from the alveolar mucosa. This tissue is firm, dense, stippled, and tightly bound down to the underlying periosteum, tooth, and bone.

gingivae, attached, extension, n See extension, gingiva, attached.

gingiva, detached by calculus, n the recession and ultimate disconnection of gingival tissue from tooth surfaces that occurs as the result of the presence of large amounts of calculus.

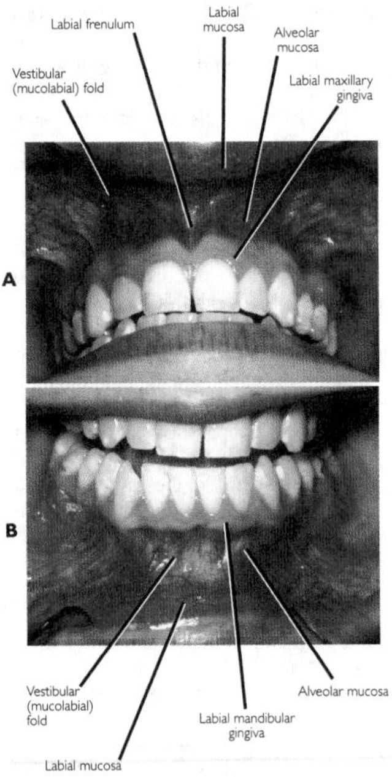

Vestibule and vestibular gingivae of oral cavity. A, Maxilla. B, Mandible. (Liebgott, 2001)

gingivae, erythemic **(erəthē′mik),** *n.pl* the unusually red gingival tissue that may be caused by either inflammation or excessive blood in the tissue. The condition may occur as a result of excess vitamin A.

gingivae, free, n.pl an older term for the unattached coronal portion of the gingiva that encircles the tooth to form the gingival sulcus. More commonly called *marginal gingiva.*

gingivae hyperplasia, n.pl See hyperplasia, gingival, Dilantin.

gingiva, inadequate attached (IAG), n a condition in which the amount of attached gingival tissues in a surveyed area is less than 1 mm, which may result in gingival recession and other periodontal conditions.

gingiva, interdental, n (interproximal gingiva[e]), the soft supporting gingival tissue, consisting of prominent horizontal collagen fibers, that normally fills the space between two contacting teeth.

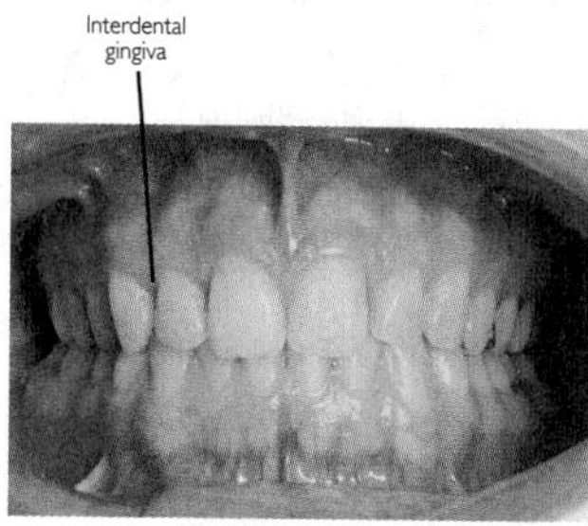

Interdental gingiva. (Bird/Robinson, 2005)

gingiva, interproximal, *n* See gingiva, interdental.

gingiva, lymphatic drainage of, *n* the lymphatic drainage that follows the course of the gingival blood supply; i.e., from the lymphatic vessels on the gingival side of the periosteum of the alveolar process to the lymphatic vessels in the periodontal membrane to vessels connecting into the alveolar bone.

gingiva, marginal, *n* the free gingiva at the labial, buccal, lingual, and palatal aspects of the teeth.

gingivae, microscopic appearance of, *n.pl* the stratified squamous epithelium that varies in degree of keratinization and overlies the lamina dura of connective tissue with interspersed blood vessels and nerves. Rete pegs of epithelium project downward into the connective tissue corium, except from the base of sulcular epithelium. The gingival fiber apparatus is also present.

gingival (jin′jəvəl), *adj* pertaining to or in relation to the gingiva.

gingival abrasion, *n* the attrition (scraping or wearing away) of the gingival tissue by harsh irritants such as coarse foods or faulty toothbrushing.

gingival anatomy, *n* the gingiva, which is a dense connective tissue covered by keratinized mucosa except in the sulcus, where it is nonkeratinized. The margin is curved buccolingually with the peaks (papillae) interdentally. The sulcus depth normally is the apical limit to the free (unattached) gingiva, the attached gingiva extending from the free gingiva to the oral mucosa.

gingival architecture, *n* the gingival form.

gingival blanching, *n* the lightening of gingival color resulting from stretching with diminution of blood supply; usually of a temporary nature. Can occur with the injection of a vasoconstrictor found in a local anesthetic agent.

gingival bleeding, *n* a prominent symptom of periodontal disease produced by ulceration of the sulcular epithelium and an inflammatory process. It can occur on probing or when the tissues are manipulated by instrumentation, oral hygiene, or eating. The blood comes from the lamina propria after ulceration of the epithelial lining.

gingival blood supply, *n* the vascular supply to the gingivae arises from the vessels that pass on the gingival side of the outer periosteum of bone and anastomoses with blood vessels of the periodontal ligament and intra-alveolar blood vessels.

gingival color, *n* the color of the gingival tissues in health and in disease. It varies with the thickness and degree of keratinization of the epithelium, blood supply, pigmentation, and alterations produced by diseased processes affecting the gingival tissues. In health often described as coral pink, with possible areas of pigmentation.

gingival consistency, *n* the visual and tactile characteristics of healthy gingival tissue. Visual consistency varies from a smooth velvet to that of an orange peel, either finely or coarsely grained. The tactile consistency of the gingival tissue should be firm and resilient.

gingival crater, *n* a concave depression in the gingival tissue. Especially seen in the area of the former apex of the interdental papilla as a result of gingival destruction associated with necrotizing periodontal disease or when food impaction occurs against the tissue subjacent to the contact points of adjacent teeth.

gingival crevicular fluid, *n* an older term for the serum transudate found in the gingival sulcus. Irritation and inflammation of the gingival tissue increase the flow and alter the constituents of crevicular fluid. More commonly called *gingival fluid.*

gingival cyanotic tissue, *n* gingival tissue that appears slightly bluish red due to a reduction in oxygenated hemoglobin; may occur in conjunction with vitamin C deficiency. See also cyanosis.

gingival cyst of the adult, *n* See cyst, gingival, of the adult.

gingival cyst of the newborn, *n* See cyst, gingival, of the newborn.

gingival discoloration, *n* a change from the normal coloration of the gingivae; associated with inflammation, diminution of blood supply, and abnormal pigmentation.

gingival enlargement, drug-influenced, *n* the growth of the gingival tissues, especially the interdental and papillae, resulting from the use of drugs such as those that block calcium channels or by Dilantin.

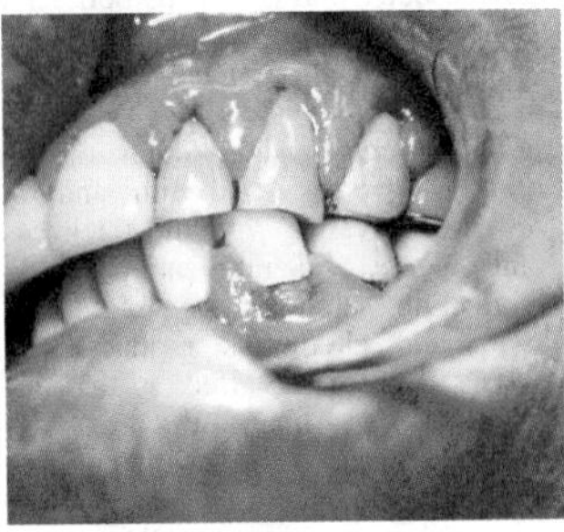

Gingival enlargement seen in a patient taking a calcium channel blocker. (Ibsen/Phelan, 2004)

gingival erythema, linear (LGE), *n* a characteristic of a necrotizing periodontal condition in an HIV-positive patient. A band of acute erythema located at the gingival margin.

gingival erythema, lingual, *n* a band of acute erythema located at the inside gingival margin (next to the tongue).

gingival fibroblast, *n* a formative cell that moderates wound healing and healing after treatment. See also fibroblast.

gingival fibromatosis, *n* See fibromatosis, gingival.

gingival graft, *n* See graft, gingival.

gingival hemorrhage, *n* the excessive bleeding of the gingival tissues; usually at the interpapillary crest, the gingival margin, or in the crevicular sulcus. It can be due to severe periodontal diseases or medical complications (e.g., leukemia).

gingival hormonal enlargement, *n* an enlargement of the gingivae associated with hormonal imbalance during pregnancy or puberty.

gingival mat, *n* the gingival connective tissue composed of coarse, broad collagen fibers that serve to attach the gingivae to the teeth and to hold the free gingivae in close approximation to the teeth.

gingival physiology, *n* the gingivae encircle the teeth and serve as a protective mucosal covering for the underlying tissues; the gingival fiber apparatus serves as a barrier to apical migration of the epithelial attachment and binds the gingival tissues to the teeth. The normal topography permits the free flow of food away from the occlusal surfaces and from the cervical and interproximal areas of the teeth.

gingival pigmentation, *n* the variations in gingival color may be correlated with the racial diversity of an individual or may be a reflection of pathologic influences, such as the melanin pigmentation associated with hypoadrenocorticism (Addison's disease), nevi, and depositions of heavy metals. See also melanin and melanosis.

gingival pocket, *n* a localized deepening of the gingival crevice of 2 mm or more.

gingival position, *n* the level of the gingival margin in relation to the tooth.

gingival recession, *n* the apical migration of the gingival crest.

gingival shrinkage, *n* the reduction in size of gingival tissue, principally by diminution of edema, usually as a result of therapeutic elimination of subgingival deposits and curettement of the soft tissue wall of the pocket.

gingival stippling, *n* a series of small depressions characterizing the surface of healthy gingivae, varying from a smooth velvet to that of an orange peel.

gingival sulcus, *n* the space between the free gingiva and the tooth.

gingival surface texture, *n* the texture of the attached gingivae, which normally is stippled; in inflammatory conditions, the edema, cellular infiltration, and concomitant swelling cause loss of the surface stippling, and the gingivae take on a smooth, shiny, edematous appearance.
gingival third, *n* the most apical one third of a given clinical crown or of an axial surface cavity or preparation.
gingival topography, *n* the form of the healthy gingival tissues. The marginal gingivae and the interdental papillae have a characteristic shape.

gingivectomy (jin′jivek′təmē), *n* the surgical excision of unsupported gingival tissue to the level where it is attached, creating a new gingival margin apical in position to the old.
gingivectomy in edentulous area, *n* the elimination of periodontal pockets surrounding abutment teeth; requires the removal of gingival tissue on the adjacent edentulous area.

gingivitis (jin′jivī′tis), *n* an inflammation of the gingival tissue. A major classification of periodontal disease.

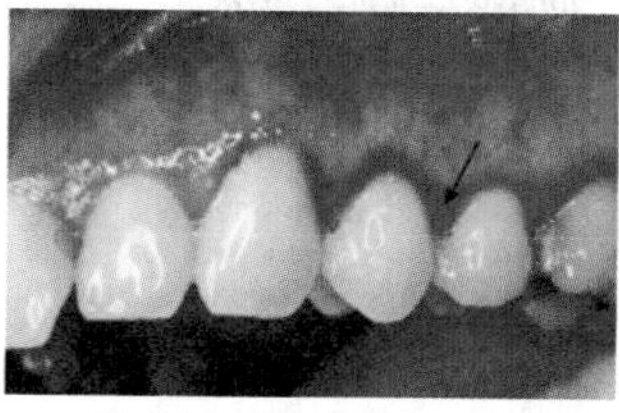

Gingivitis. (Bird/Robinson, 2005)

gingivitis and malposed teeth, *n* the malposition may predispose the gingivae to inflammation by permitting food impaction or impingement, by providing irregular spaces in which calculus may be deposited, and by making oral hygiene difficult.
gingivitis, bacteria in, *n* the causative organisms in gingival inflammation. The common chronic forms of gingivitis, from a bacterial standpoint, are nonspecific, with the exception of acute necrotizing ulcerative gingivitis, in which there is an apparent specificity of the bacterial flora: the fusospirochetal organisms.
gingivitis, bismuth, *n* a metallic poisoning caused by bismuth given for treatment of systemic disease; characterized by a dark, bluish line along the gingival margin.
gingivitis, chronic atrophic senile, *n* gingival inflammation characterized by atrophy and areas of hyperkeratosis; found primarily in elderly women.
gingivitis, desquamative **(des′kwəmā′tiv),** *n* an inflammation of the gingivae characterized by a tendency of the surface epithelium to desquamate. The disease is a clinical entity, not a pathologic entity. It is most frequently associated with menopause but may be associated with biologic stress. Older term: *gingivosis.*
gingivitis, eruptive **(ērup′tiv),** *n* the gingival inflammation occurring at the time of eruption of the primary or permanent teeth.
gingivitis, fusospirochetal, *n* See gingivitis, necrotizing ulcerative.
gingivitis gravidarum, *n* See gingivitis, pregnancy.
gingivitis, hemorrhagic, *n* the gingivitis characterized by profuse bleeding, especially that associated with ascorbic acid deficiency or leukemia.
gingivitis, herpetic, *n* an inflammation of the gingivae caused by herpesvirus. See also gingivostomatitis, herpetic.
gingivitis, hormonal, *n* the gingivitis associated with endocrine imbalance, the endocrinopathy being modified, in most instances, by the influence of local environmental factors.
gingivitis, hyperplastic, *n* the gingivitis characterized by proliferation of the various tissue elements. May be accompanied by dense infiltration of inflammatory cells.
gingivitis, idiopathic, *n* a gingival inflammation of unknown causation.
gingivitis, infectious, *n* a gingivitis not caused by plaque, but instead originating from bacteria, fungi, or viruses.
gingivitis, inflammatory cells in, *n* the inflammatory cells are, for the most part, lymphocytes, plasma cells, and some histiocytes, because the gingival inflammatory process is usually chronic and progressive in nature. With acute exacerbations, polymorphonuclear leukocytes are also present.

G

gingivitis, marginal, *n* an inflammation of the gingivae localized to the marginal gingivae and interdental papillae.

gingivitis, menstrual cycle–associated, *n* gingival inflammation that occurs during ovulation as a result of hormone-level changes.

gingivitis, necrotizing ulcerative, *n* (fusospirochetal gingivitis, NUG, trench oral cavity, ulcerative gingivitis, ulceromembranous gingivitis, Vincent's gingivitis, Vincent's infection) a form of necrotizing periodontal disease with an inflammation of the gingivae characterized by necrosis of the interdental papillae, ulceration of the gingival margins, the appearance of a pseudomembrane, pain, and a fetid odor.

gingivitis, nephritic, *n* (uremic gingivitis, uremic stomatitis), a membrane form of stomatitis and gingivitis associated with a failure of kidney function. It is accompanied by pain, ammonia-like odor, and increased salivation.

gingivitis, non–plaque-induced, *n* a gingivitis caused by factors other than plaque, such as allergic reaction, dermatologic disease, a genetic condition, infectious agents, response to a foreign body, or physical trauma.

gingivitis, plaque-induced, *n* a gingivitis caused by the accumulation of plaque.

gingivitis, pregnancy, *n* (gingivitis gravidarum, hormonal gingivitis), an enlargement of hyperplasia of the gingivae resulting from a hormonal imbalance during pregnancy.

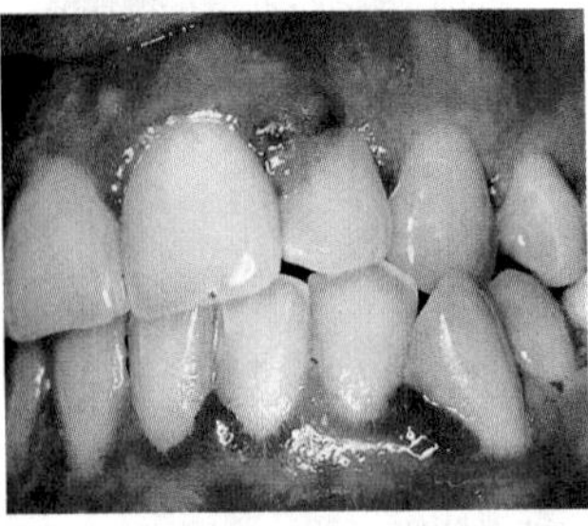

Pregnancy gingivitis. (Perry/Beemsterboer, 2007)

gingivitis, puberty, *n* an enlargement of the gingival tissues as a result of an exaggerated response to irritation resulting from hormonal changes.

gingivitis, scorbutic, *n* a gingivitis associated with vitamin C (ascorbic acid) deficiency.

gingivitis, systemic disease-induced, *n* a gingivitis occurring as a complication of a systemic disease, such as type 1 diabetes mellitus or acute leukemia.

gingivitis, uremic, *n* See gingivitis, nephritic.

gingivoplasty (jin′jivōplastē), *n* the surgical contouring of the gingival tissues to secure the physiologic architectural form necessary for the maintenance of tissue health and integrity.

gingivosis (jin′jivō′sis), *n* a noninflammatory degenerative condition of the gingivae. This older term is applied to desquamative gingivitis.

gingivostomatitis (jin′jivōstō′mətī′tis), *n* an inflammation that involves the gingivae and the oral mucosa.

gingivostomatitis, acute herpetic, *n* See stomatitis, herpetic, acute.

gingivostomatitis, herpetic, *n* an inflammation of the gingivae and oral mucosa caused by primary invasion of herpesvirus. Herpetic gingivostomatitis occurs mainly in childhood, one attack giving immunity to generalized stomatitis but not to isolated lesions (herpetic lesions), unless an adult has had an isolated upbringing. The symptoms are red and swollen gingivae; red mucosa, which soon shows vesicles and ulcers; painful oral cavity; and elevated temperature. The course is about 14 days.

gingivostomatitis, membranous, *n* a disease, or group of diseases, in which false membranes form on the gingivae and oral mucosa; the membranes are a grayish white color and are surrounded by a narrow red margin. Detachment of the membrane leaves a raw, bleeding surface. One cause is mixed pyogenic infection, in which *S. viridans* and *Staphylococcus* organisms predominate.

gingivostomatitis, white folded, *n* See nevus spongiosus albus mucosa.

ginglymus (hinge joint) (jing′gliməs), *n* a joint that allows motion around an axis.

glabella (gləbel′ə), *n* the smooth, elevated area on the frontal bone between the supraorbital ridges; the most anterior point on the frontal bone.

gland(s), *n/n.pl* an organ producing a specific product or secretion.

gland, parotid salivary, *n* the largest of the major salivary glands; its anterior position is situated between the ramus of the mandible, its posterior portion between the mastoid process and sternocleidomastoid muscle, and inferior to the zygomatic arch; irregularly wedge shaped, with the lateral surface flattened and the medial aspect more or less pointed toward the pharyngeal wall. Its secretion, which is serous, travels the parotid duct (Stenson's duct) to empty into the oral cavity at the ductal opening at the parotid papillae on the buccal mucosa opposite the maxillary molar teeth.

gland, pituitary, *n* (hypophysis), an endocrine gland located at the base of the brain in the sella turcica. The pituitary gland is composed of two parts: the pars nervosa, which is an extension of the anterior part of the hypothalamus, and the pars intermedia, which is an epithelial evagination of secretory tissue from the stomodeum of the embryo. By its structural and functional relationships with the nervous system and the endocrine glands, it acts as a mediator of both the nervous system and the endocrine system.

gland, sublingual salivary, *n* the smallest of the major salivary glands. It lies inferior to the floor of the oral cavity bilateral to the lingual frenum and is in contact with the sublingual depression on the inner side of the mandible. Its numerous ducts open directly into the oral cavity bilateral to the lingual frenum and join to form the sublingual duct (duct of Bartholin's), which enters into the submandibular duct (Wharton's duct). Its secretion is mucous in nature.

gland, submandibular salivary, *n* a major salivary gland that has an irregular form and is situated in the submandibular space, bordered anteriorly by the anterior belly of the digastric muscle and posteriorly by the stylomandibular ligament. Its mucoserous section is carried by the submandibular duct (Wharton's duct), whose openings lie at a small papilla (submandibular caruncle) bilateral to the lingual frenum.

gland, thymus, *n* See thymus.

glands, Blandin and Nuhn's, *n.pr* See spots, Fordyce's.

glands, endocrine, *n.pl* a gland of internal secretion; a hormone-secreting gland (e.g., the pituitary gland, thyroid gland, parathyroid glands, adrenal glands, ovaries, and testes).

glands, lacrimal, *n.pl* the ducted (exocrine) glands that produce lacrimal fluid, commonly called *tears.* See also lacrimal apparatus.

glands, minor salivary, *n.pl* the glands located at the posterior aspect of the dorsum of the tongue posterior to the circumvallate papillae (von Edner's) and along the lateral surface of the tongue; also located in the palate, floor of mouth, labial mucosa, and buccal mucosa. The secretion is mucous, and they do not have named ducts. Older term: *accessory salivary glands.* See also salivary glands, von Edner's.

glands, salivary, *n.pl* the glands in the oral cavity that secrete saliva. Three major salivary glands contribute their secretions to form the whole saliva; the minor mucous glands found within oral mucosa contribute a lesser amount. The major salivary glands are the parotid, submandibular, and sublingual.

glass, bioactive, *n* a form of glass that encourages bone growth. The compound consists of silica (glass) and other materials (often including calcium) in powder or molded form. In dental offices, bioactive glass is often used to repair bone structures during extractions or other procedures.

glass ionomer cement (īon′əmər), *n* a dental cement of low strength and toughness produced by mixing a powder prepared from a calcium aluminosilicate glass and a liquid prepared from an aqueous solution of prepared polyacrylic acid; used mainly for small restorations on the proximal surfaces of anterior teeth and for restoration of eroded areas at the gingival margin.

G

glass, lead, *n* the lead-impregnated glass used in windows of control booths and in protective shields to protect clinicians when taking radiographs.

glatiramer acetate (glahtear'a-meer as'ətāt), *n* a medication used to decrease or stop a relapse of multiple sclerosis. It is typically used to treat individuals resistant to the effects of interferon-β.

glaucoma (gloukō'mə), *n* an abnormal condition of elevated pressure within the eye because of obstruction of the outflow of aqueous humor.

G

glaucoma, acute, *n* (closed-angle) a condition that occurs if the pupil in an eye with a narrow angle between the iris and cornea dilates markedly, causing the folded iris to block the exit of aqueous humor from the anterior chamber.

glaucoma, chronic, *n* (open-angle) a condition that is much more common than closed-angle glaucoma and is often bilateral. Open-angle glaucoma develops slowly and is genetically determined and progressive with age. The obstruction is believed to occur within the canal of Schlemm.

glaze, *n* a critical stage in the final firing of dental porcelain when complete fusion takes place, with the formation of a thin, vitreous, glossy surface, or glaze.

glenoid (glē'noid), *n* the fossae in the temporal bone in which condyles of the mandible articulate with the skull.

gliadin (glī'ədin), *n* a protein substance that is obtained from wheat and rye. Its solubility in diluted alcohol distinguishes gliadin from glutenin.

glide(s), *n* **1.** the passage of one object over another as guided by their contacting surfaces. *n.pl* **2.** the sounds *w, wh,* and *y,* which are voiced as bilabial and palatal glides, respectively. The rapid movement of the lips or tongue from a set position toward a neutral vowel (*u,* as in up).

glide, mandibular, *n* the side-to-side, protrusive, intermediate movement of the mandible that occurs when the teeth or other occluding surfaces are in contact.

gliding occlusion, *n* See occlusion, gliding.

glimepiride (glimep'ərīd), *n brand name:* Amaryl; *drug class:* oral antidiabetic; *action:* a sulfonylurea type action; *use:* non–insulin-dependent diabetes, sometimes in combination with insulin support.

glioma (glē'ōmə), *n* the largest group of primary tumors of the brain, composed of malignant glial cells.

glipizide (glip'izīd), *n brand name:* Glucotrol; *drug class:* oral antidiabetic (second generation); *action:* causes functioning β cells in pancrease to release insulin, leading to a drop in blood glucose levels; *use:* stable adult-onset diabetes mellitus (type 2).

globin (glō'bin), *n* a group of four globulin protein molecules that become bound by the iron in heme molecules to form hemoglobin or myoglobin.

globulin (glob'yəlin), *n* a class of proteins.

globulin, antihemophilic, *n* See factor VIII.

globulin, antihemophilic A, *n* See factor VIII.

globulin, antihemophilic B, *n* See factor IX.

glomerular disease (glōmer'yələr), *n* a group of diseases in which the glomerulus of the kidney is affected.

glomerular filtration rate, *n* a kidney function test in which the results are determined from the amount of ultrafiltrate formed by plasma flowing through the glomeruli of the kidney. It may be calculated from insulin and creatinine clearance, serum creatinine, and blood urea nitrogen (BUN).

glomerulus (glōmer'yələs), *n* a cluster of blood vessels or nerve fibers, such as the cluster of blood vessels in the kidney that function as filters of the plasma portion of the blood.

glossalgia (glôsal'jēə), *n* painful sensations in the tongue.

glossectomy (glôsek'təmē), *n* the surgical removal of the tongue, a portion of the tongue, or a lesion of the tongue.

glossitis (glôsī'tis), *n* an inflammation of the tongue.

glossitis areata exfoliativa, *n* See tongue, geographic.

glossitis, atrophic, *n* (bald tongue,

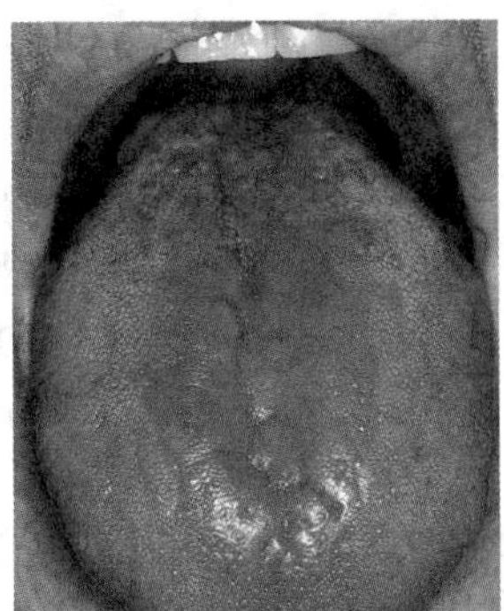

Glossitis. (Regezi/Sciubba/Pogrel, 2000)

smooth tongue) the atrophy of the glossal papillae, resulting in a smooth tongue. The tongue may be pallid or erythematous and may appear small or enlarged. It may be associated with anemias, pellagra, vitamin B complex deficiencies, sprue, or other systemic diseases or may be local in origin. Because atrophy may be one phase, and circumscribed, painful, glossal excoriations may be another phase of one or more of the same systemic disease(s), much confusion in terminology has arisen (e.g., Moeller's glossitis; Hunter's glossitis; slick, glazed, varnished, glossy, or bald tongue; chronic superficial erythematous glossitis; glossodynia exfoliativa; beefy tongue; and pellagrous glossitis).

glossitis, benign migratory, *n* See tongue, geographic.

glossitis exfoliativa, *n* See glossitis, Moeller's.

glossitis, interstitial sclerous, *n* (Clarke-Fournier glossitis), nodular, lobulated, indurated tongue associated with terminal syphilis.

glossitis, median rhomboid, *n* See atrophy, central papillary.

glossitis migrans, *n* See tongue, geographic.

glossodynia (glôs′ōdī′nēə), *n* painful sensations in the tongue; a sensation of burning in the tongue; a sore tongue.

glossopharyngeal air space (glos′ōfərin′jēəl er spās), *n* the empty area between the tongue and the pharynx at the back of the throat.

glossopharyngeal nerve (glos′ō-fərin′jēəl), *n* See nerve, glossopharyngeal (IX).

glossoplasty (glôs′ōplastē), *n* a surgical procedure performed on the tongue.

glossoplegia (glôs′ōplē′jēə), *n* a paralysis of the tongue; may be unilateral or bilateral.

glossoptosis, *n* a downward displacement of the tongue; a severe displacement may occlude the airway.

glossopyrosis (glôs′ōpīrō′sis), *n* a burning sensation of the tongue.

glossorrhaphy (glôsôr′əfē), *n* the suture of a wound of the tongue.

glossotomy (glôsot′əmē), *n* an excision or incision of the tongue.

glottal (glot′əl), *adj* pertaining to, or produced in or by, the glottis. The sound of *h* is a voiceless glottal fricative. The airstream on the exhalation phase moves unimpeded through the larynx, pharynx, and oral cavities.

glottis (glot′is), *n* the vocal apparatus of the larynx, consisting of the true vocal cords (vocal folds and the opening between them [rima glottidis]).

gloves or surgical gloves, *n.pl* the gloves used as an essential part of barrier protection in health care delivery.

glucagon (gloo′kəgon), *n* (hyperglycemic factor, hyperglycemic-glycogenolytic factor [HGF]) a hormone from the alpha cells of the pancreas that raises the blood sugar by increasing hepatic glycogenolysis.

glucans (gloo′kans), *n.pl* the polyglucose compounds such as cellulose, starch, amylose, glycogen amylose, and callose.

glucocorticoids (gloo′kōkôr′təkoidz), *n.pl* (antiinflammatory hormone, 11-oxycorticoids) the adrenocortical steroid hormones that affect glycogenesis in the liver. They are antiinflammatory, are active in protection against stress, and affect carbohydrate and protein metabolism. Typical of the group are cortisol and cortisone.

glucokinase, *n* a hexokinase or phosphotransferase that catalyzes the conversion of glucose to glucose-6-phosphate by ATP.

gluconeogenesis (gloo′kōnē′ōjen′əsis), *n* the formation of glycogen or glucose from noncarbohydrate sources (e.g., the glycogenic amino acids, glycerol, lactate, and pyruvate) by pathways mainly involving the citric acid cycle and glycolysis.

glucose (gloo′kōs), *n* a six-carbon (hexose) sugar that is the principal sugar in blood and serves as a major metabolic source of energy.

glucose, casual plasma, n the amount of glucose in the blood at any time, unrelated to eating.

glucose, fasting plasma (FPG), n a self-administered test of blood glucose levels for diabetes patients. The blood is tested after at least 8 hours of fasting. If results of the test are consistently at or above 126 mg/dL, the patient is commonly diagnosed with diabetes mellitus.

glucose meter, n an electronic device used to measure blood glucose levels that can be used by a patient at home. The device provides an accurate reading of blood glucose level with only a drop of blood from a pricked finger.

glucose oxidase, n an antibacterial flavoprotein enzyme obtained from *P. notatum* and other fungi. It is antibacterial in the presence of glucose and oxygen.

glucose, postprandial plasma, n the level of glucose in the blood plasma based on a sample of blood taken after ingesting a meal; used to diagnose diabetes.

glucose tolerance, impaired, n one category of oral glucose tolerance test results. The diagnosis is not necessarily indicative of diabetes, but the patient may be at risk of diabetes mellitus and heart disease.

glucose tolerance test, n a metabolic test that measures the ability of the body to metabolize carbohydrates. A patient is administered a standard dose of glucose, and blood and urine samples are measured for glucose levels at periodic intervals following administration. It is most often used to assist in the diagnosis of diabetes mellitus.

glucoside (gloo′kōsīd), *n* a glycoside in which the sugar component is glucose.

glucosuria (gloo″kosu′reə), *n* See glycosuria.

glucuronidase (gloo′kəron′idās), *n* an enzyme that acts as a catalyst in the hydrolysis of various glucuronides with the liberation of glucuronic acid.

glutamic acid, *n* a nonessential amino acid occurring widely in a number of proteins. Preparations of glutamic acid are used as aids for digestion.

glutaraldehyde (gloo′təral′dəhīd), *n* a germicidal agent used for the disinfection and sterilization of instruments or equipment that cannot be heat sterilized. An effective agent used in solution for "cold" sterilization.

glutathione (gloo′təthī′ōn), *n* an enzyme whose deficiency is commonly associated with hemolytic anemia.

gluten, *n* an insoluble protein constituent of wheat and other grains consisting of a mixture of gliadin, glutenin, and other proteins. Gluten provides the elastic qualities of bread dough.

glyburide (glī′byərīd), *n brand names:* Apo-Glyburide, DiaBeta, Micronase; *drug class:* oral antidiabetic (second generation); *action:* causes functioning cells in pancreas to release insulin, leading to a drop in blood glucose levels; *use:* stable adult-onset diabetes mellitus (type 2).

glycemia (glīsē′mēə), *n* the existence of glucose in the bloodstream. See also hypoglycemia, hyperglycemia.

glyceride (glis′ərīd), *n* an ester of glycerin with one or more aliphatic acids.

glycerin (glis′ərin), *n* a sweet, colorless, oily fluid that is a pharmaceutical grade of glycerol. Glycerin is used as a moistening agent for chapped skin, as an ingredient of suppositories for constipation, and as a sweetening agent and vehicle for drug preparation. It is also spelled glycerine.

glycerite (glis′ərīt), *n* a solution or suspension of a drug in glycerin.

glycerol, *n.pr* an alcohol that is a component of fats. See also glycerin.

glycine, *n* a nonessential amino acid occurring widely as a component of animal and plant proteins. Synthetically produced glycine is used in solutions for irrigation, in the treatment of various muscle diseases, and as an antacid and dietary supplement.

glycogen (glī'kōjen), *n* a branched, homopolysaccharide of glucose held by α 1-4 and α 1-6 glucosidic bonds. Liver glycogen provides a ready source of blood glucose through glycogenolysis.

glycogen storage disease, n a group of inherited disorders of glycogen metabolism. An enzyme deficiency causes glycogen to accumulate in abnormally large amounts in various parts of the body. The full taxonomy runs from Type I to Type VII.

glycogenesis (gli'kōjen'əsis), *n* the synthesis of glycogen from glucose.

glycogenolysis (gli'kōjēnol'isis), *n* the formation of blood glucose by hydrolysis of stored liver glycogen.

glycolipids (gli"kolip'ids), *n.pl* the fats found in the brain and nervous system that contain a carbohydrate constituent.

glycolysis (glīkol'isis), *n* **1.** the oxidation of glucose or glycogen by cytoplasmic enzymes of the Embden-Meyerhof pathway to pyruvate and lactate. **2.** a series of enzymatically catalyzed reactions occurring within cells, by which glucose and other sugars are broken down to yield lactic acid or pyruvic acid, releasing energy in the form of adenosine triphosphate.

glyconeogenesis (gli"kone"ojen'əsis), *n* the synthetic creation of blood sugar from mediating metabolites. See also gluconeogenesis and glycogenolysis.

glycoprotein, *n* a large group of conjugated proteins in which the nonprotein substance is a carbohydrate. These include the mucins, the mucoids, and the chondroproteins.

glycopyrrolate, *n brand names:* Robinul, Robinul Forte; *drug class:* anticholinergic; *action:* inhibits acetylcholine at receptor sites in autonomic nervous system, which controls secretions, free acids in stomach; *uses:* decreased secretions before surgery, reversal of neuromuscular blockade, peptic ulcer disease, irritable bowel syndrome.

glycosaminoglycan, *n* See mucopolysaccharide.

glycosated hemoglobin concentration (gli'kōsā'tid hēm'əglō'bin kon'sentrā'shən), *n* a measurement of the percentage of red blood cells that are glycosated hemoglobin (hemoglobin cells that have joined with glucose). This percentage is an indication of a person's average blood glucose level over the past several weeks. It is used by diabetics to manage their blood glucose levels.

glycoside (gli'kōsīd), *n* a compound that contains a sugar as part of the molecule.

glycosuria (gli'kōsŏŏr'ēə), *n* the presence of sugar in the urine. It most commonly results from diabetes mellitus but may occur from a lowered renal threshold (renal glycosuria) in pregnancy, inorganic renal disease, and in patients taking adrenocorticosteroids.

glycosylated hemoglobin assay, *n* a laboratory test to determine the amount of glucose in the blood that is permanently bound to a molecule of hemoglobin; helps prevent development of long-term complications by monitoring glycemic control over a longer period.

Gm, *n* See gram.

gnathion (nā'thēon), *n* the lowest point in the inferior border of the mandible at the median plane. It is a point on the bony border palpated from below and naturally lies posterior to the tegumental border of the chin.

gnathodynamometer (nath'ōdī'nəmom'ətur), *n* an instrument used for measuring biting pressure.

gnathodynamometer, bimeter, n a gnathodynamometer equipped with a central bearing point of adjustable height.

Gnathograph (nath'ōgraf), *n.pr* an articulator that resembles the Hanau instrument but differs mainly by having a provision for increasing the intercondylar distance, an important determinant of groove directions in the occlusal surfaces of teeth.

Gnatholator (nāth'əlā'tər), *n.pr* an articulator design that has since been succeeded by an improved instrument called the Simulator (or Gnathosimulator).

gnathologic instrument, *n* a term often used as a synonym for an articulator. Any dental instrument used for diagnosis and treatment, such as a probe for determining the depth of a periodontal pocket, is a gnathologic tool.

G

gnathology (nāthol′əjē), *n* the study of the functional and occlusal relationships of the teeth; sometimes also used to identify a specific philosophy of occlusal function.

gnathoschisis (nathos′kisis), *n* See jaw, cleft.

gnathostatics (nath′ōstat′iks), *n* a technique of orthodontic diagnosis based on relationships between the teeth and certain landmarks on the skull. See also cast, gnathostatic.

goal, *n* the purpose toward which an endeavor is directed, such as the outcome of diagnostic, therapeutic, and educational management of a patient's health problem.

goggles, *n* the protective eyewear worn by dental personnel and patients during dental procedures.

goiter (goi′tur), *n* an enlargement of the thyroid gland.

goiter, colloid, *n* (endemic goiter, iodine deficiency goiter, simple goiter) a visible enlargement of the thyroid gland without obvious signs of hypofunction or hyperfunction of the gland resulting from inadequate intake or from an increased demand for iodine.

goiter, endemic, *n* See goiter, colloid.

goiter, exophthalmic, *n* a disease of the thyroid gland consisting of hyperthyroidism, exophthalmos, and goiterous enlargement of the thyroid gland. A diffuse primary hyperplasia of the thyroid gland of obscure origin; may occur at any age. It produces nervousness, muscular weakness, heat intolerance, tremor, loss of weight, lid lag, and absence of winking and may lead to thyrotoxic heart disease and thyroid crisis.

goiter, iodine deficiency, *n* See goiter, colloid.

goiter, nodular, nontoxic, *n* the recurrent episodes of hyperplasia and involution of colloid goiter, which result in a multinodular goiter. Symptoms are related to pressure.

goiter, simple, *n* See goiter, colloid.

goitrogens (goi′trōjenz), *n.pl* the agents such as thiouracil and related antithyroid compounds that are capable of producing goiter.

gold, *n* a precious or noble metal; yellow, malleable, ductible, nonrusting; much used in dentistry in pure and alloyed forms.

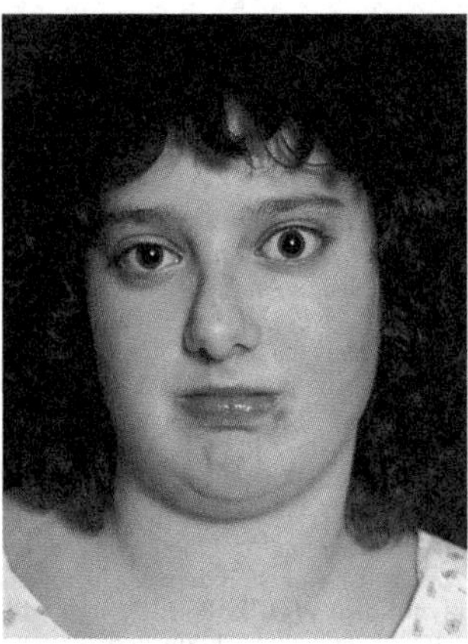

Exophthalmic goiter. (Zitelli/Davis, 2002)

gold alloys, *n.pl* an alloy that contains gold; usually alloyed with copper, silver, platinum, palladium, and zinc. The alloying of gold enhances certain properties such as hardness, or creates a lower melting point for gold solder.

gold, cohesive, *n* gold usually manufactured in thin sheets of foil, that has been treated to cause it to cohere, or stick together. This allows it to be easily formed into a variety of shapes.

gold compound, *n* a drug containing gold salts, usually administered with other drugs in the treatment of rheumatoid arthritis. Various radioisotopes of gold have been used in diagnostic radiology and in the radiologic treatment of certain malignant neoplastic diseases.

gold, crystal, *n* See gold, mat.

gold, fibrous, *n* See foil, gold.

gold file, *n* See file, gold.

gold foil, *n* See foil, gold.

gold foil cylinder, *n* See foil cylinder.

gold foil pellet, *n* See pellet, foil.

gold, inlay, *n* **1.** an alloy, principally gold, used for cast restorations. Desired physical properties may be obtained by selecting those with varying ingredients and/or proportions. Acceptable alloys are classified by the American Dental Association

(ADA) specifications according to Brinell hardness: Type A–soft, Brinell 40 to 75; Type B–medium, Brinell 70 to 100; Type C–hard, Brinell 90 to 140. *n* **2.** an intracoronal cast restoration of gold alloy fabricated outside the oral cavity and cemented into the prepared cavity.

gold knife, *n* See knife, gold.

gold, mat, *n* (crystal gold, sponge gold) a noncohesive form of pure gold prepared by electrodeposition. Sometimes used in the base of restorations and then veneered or overlaid with cohesive foil.

gold, powdered, *n* the fine granules of pure gold, formed by atomizing the molten metal or by chemical precipitation. For clinical use, powdered gold is available either as clusters of the granules or as pellets of the powder contained in an envelope of gold foil.

gold saw, *n* See saw, gold.

gold sodium thiosulfate, *n* an antirheumatic used in the treatment of rheumatoid arthritis.

gold, sponge, *n* See gold, mat.

gold, white, *n* a gold alloy with a high palladium content. It has a higher fusion range, lower ductility, and greater hardness than a yellow gold alloy.

Golden Proportions, *n* a mathematical proportion as a representation of aesthetic perfection.

Goldent, *n.pr* the brand name for a direct gold restorative material. It consists basically of varying amounts of powdered gold contained in a wrapping or envelope of gold foil.

Goldman-Fox knife, *n.pr* See knife, Goldman-Fox.

Golgi apparatus (gōl′jē), *n.pr* the small membranous structures found in most cells, composed of various elements associated with the formation of carbohydrate side chains of glycoproteins, mucopolysaccharides, and other substances. Also called *Golgi body* or *Golgi complex.*

Golgi's corpuscles (gol′jēz), *n.pr* See corpuscle, Golgi's.

gomphosis (gämfō′sis), *n* a form of joint in which a conical body is fastened into a socket, as a tooth is fastened into the jaw.

gonad (gō′nad), *n* an ovary or testis, the site of origin of eggs or spermatozoa.

gonadotrophin (gōnad′ōtrōf′in), *n* See gonadotropin.

gonadotropin (gōnad′ōtrōp′in), *n* (gonadotropic hormone) a gonad-stimulating hormone derived either from the pituitary gland (e.g., follicle-stimulating hormone [FSH] and luteinizing hormone [LH], which is also an interstitial cell-stimulating hormone [ICSH]) or from the chorion (e.g., chorionic gonadotropin, which is found in the urine of pregnant women).

gonadotropin, chorionic, *n* See hormone, pregnancy.

gonion (Go), *n* the most posteroinferior point of the angle of the mandible near the inferior border of the ramus.

gonorrhea (gon′ərē′ə), *n* a sexually transmitted disease of the genitourinary tract that is spread by direct contact with an infected person or fluids containing the infectious microorganism. It may also affect the conjunctiva, oral tissue, and other tissues and organ systems.

good faith, *n* honesty of intention. Generally, not a sufficient defense in a dental malpractice lawsuit.

good samaritan legislation, *n* the statutes enacted in some states protecting health care professionals from liability for aid rendered in emergency situations, unless there is a showing of willful wrong or gross negligence.

goodwill, *n* the intangible assets of a firm established by the excess of the price paid for the ongoing concern over its book value.

gothic arch tracer, *n* See tracer, needle point.

gothic arch tracing, *n* See tracing, needle point.

gout, *n* a disease associated with an inborn error of uric acid metabolism that increases production or interferes with the excretion of uric acid. Excess uric acid is converted to sodium urate crystals that precipitate from the blood and become deposited in joints and other tissues. The great toe is a common site for the accumulation of urate crystals. It can be exceedingly painful, with swelling of a joint and may be accompanied by chills and fever.

gown, *n* the protective garment worn by health care provider designed to prevent the spread of infection between the health care provider and the patient.

gr, *n* See grain.

grace period, *n* a specified time, after a plan's premium payment is due, in which the protection of the plan continues subject to actual receipt of the premium within that time.

G

graft, *n* a slip or portion of tissue used for implantation. See also donor site; recipient site.

graft, allo-, *n* a graft between genetically dissimilar members of the same species.

graft, allogenic, *n* a graft using tissue from the same species (i.e., person to person). See also allograft.

graft, alloplast **(al′əplast′),** *n* a graft of an inert metal or plastic material.

graft, auto-, *n* See graft, autogenous.

graft, autogenous **(ôtoj′ənəs),** *n* a graft taken from one portion of an individual's body and implanted into another portion of the individual's body.

graft, autogenous bone, *n* the bone that is removed from one area of a patient's body and transplanted into another area that requires additional bony material. Such bone grafts are advantageous because they contain live active cells that promote bone growth.

graft, bone, *n* the transplantation of healthy bone tissue to a defective bone cavity so that the new bone tissue meets the surrounding, unaffected surface and promotes healing and new growth.

graft, bone, allograft, *n* a bone graft using tissue obtained from an individual other than, but of the same species as, the host of the bone graft; sources include human cadavers, living relatives, and nonrelatives. Also called *allogeneic graft* and *homograft.*

graft, bone, autogenous, *n* See graft, autogenous.

graft, composite, *n* a transplant involving living tissue made of different materials, such as skin and cartilage.

graft donor site, *n* the site from which graft material is taken.

graft, filler, *n* the filling of defects, such as bone chips used to fill a cyst.

graft, free, *n* a graft of tissue completely detached from its original site and blood supply.

graft, full-thickness, *n* a skin graft consisting of the full thickness of the skin with none of the subcutaneous tissues.

graft, gingival, *n* a graft in which a thin piece of tissue is taken from the palate of the oral cavity, or moved over from adjacent areas, to provide a stable band of soft tissue around a tooth or implant.

graft, hetero-, *n* See graft, heterogenous.

graft, heterogenous **(het′əraj′ənəs),** *n* a graft implanted from one species to another.

graft, homo-, *n* See graft, homogenous.

graft, homogenous **(həmoj′ənəs),** *n* a graft taken from a member of a species and implanted into the body of a member of the same species.

graft, iliac, *n* a bone graft whose donor site is the crest of the ilium. Various locations of the iliac crest duplicate areas of the mandible and curvatures of the midfacial skeleton.

graft, iso-, *n* a graft between individuals with identical or histocompatible antigens.

graft, kiel, *n* a denatured calf bone used to fill defects or restore facial contour.

graft, mucosal, *n* a split-thickness graft involving the mucosa.

graft, onlay bone, *n* a graft in which the grafted bone is applied laterally to the cortical bone of the recipient site, frequently to improve the contours of the chin or the malar eminence of the zygomatic bone.

graft, particulate, *n* a surgical tissue implant or graft consisting of various particles, e.g., used in the stimulation of bone growth.

graft, pedicle **(ped′ikəl),** *n* a stem or tube of tissue that remains attached near the donor site to nourish the graft during advancement of a skin graft.

graft, ramus, *n* the surgically removed bone taken from the ascending ramus of the mandible for the purpose of transplantation.

graft, split-thickness, *n* a graft with varying thickness containing only mucosal elements and no subcutaneous tissue.

graft, swaging, *n* a procedure analogous to bone grafting. Also referred to as a *contiguous transplant,* which involves a greenstick fracture of bone bordering on an infrabony defect and the displacement of bone to eliminate the osseous defect.

graft, Thiersch's skin **(tērsh′əz),** *n.pr* a split-thickness skin graft containing cutaneous and some subcutaneous tissues, the line of cleavage through the rete peg layer.

graft-versus-host disease (GVHD), *n* See disease, graft-versus-host (GVHD).

grain (gr), *n* **1.** a unit of weight equal to 0.0648 g. *n* **2.** a crystal of an alloy.

grain boundary, *n* the junction of two grains growing from different nuclei, impinging and causing discontinuity of the lattice structure. Important in corrosion and brittleness of metals.

grain growth, *n* See growth, grain.

gram (Gm, g), *n* the basic unit of mass of the metric system. Equivalent to 15.432 gr.

gram-negative, *n* having the pink color of the counterstain used in Gram's method of staining microorganisms. Staining property is a common method of classifying bacteria. See also Gram's stain.

gram-positive, *n* retaining the violet color of the stain used in Gram's method of staining microorganisms. Staining property is a common method of classifying bacteria. See also Gram's stain.

gramicidin (gram′isī′din), *n* an antibacterial agent generally used in conjunction with nystatin, a specific anticandidal agent, and neomycin, a complementary antibacterial agent, in the treatment of angular cheilosis.

Gram's stain, *n.pr* a sequential process for staining microorganisms in which a violet stain is followed by a wash and then a counterstain of safranin. Gram-positive organisms appear violet or blue; gram-negative organisms appear rose pink.

granulation tissue, *n* a soft, pink, fleshy projections that form during the healing process in a wound not healing by first intent. It consists of many capillaries surrounded by fibrous collagen. Overgrowth is termed *proud flesh.* In dentistry, such tissue is evident at the opening to a fistulous tract or at the site of a recent tooth extraction.

granules, sulfur, *n.pl* See actinomycosis.

granulocyte (gran′yəlōsīt′), *n* a type of leukocyte (white blood cell) characterized by the presence of cytoplasmic granules.

granulocytopenia (gran′ūlōsī′tōpē′nēə), *n* a deficiency in the number of granulocytic cells in the bloodstream. See also agranulocytosis.

granuloma (gran′ūlō′mə), *n* a localized mass of granulation tissue characterized by an accumulation of macrophages, epithelioid macrophages, with or without lymphocytes, and giant cells into a discrete mass.

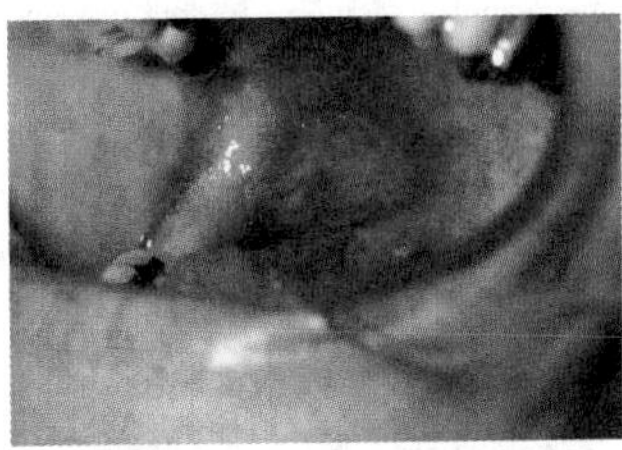

Granuloma. (Regezi/Sciubba/Jordan, 2002)

granuloma, central giant cell, *n* a painless, benign, expansile lesion on bone, usually on the anterior mandible, less frequently crossing the midline of the mandible. Usually contain a number of multinucleated giant cells.

granuloma, chronic, *n* (chronic apical periodontitis) a chronic inflammatory tissue surrounding the apical foramina as a result of irritation from within the root canal system.

granuloma, dental, *n* a mass of granulation tissue surrounded by a fibrous capsule attached at the apex of a pulp-involved tooth. It produces a radiolucency that is fairly well demarcated.

granuloma, eosinophilic **(ē′əsin′əfil′ik),** *n* a granulomatous inflammatory disease of unknown etiology, usually monofocal in bone but sometimes affecting soft tissues. Sheets of histiocytes and masses of eosinophils characterize the lesion histologically. See also disease, Langerhans cell.

granuloma, giant cell reparative, n an inflammatory lesion located near the gingival margin. It takes the shape of a mushroom, has a smooth, glossy surface, bleeds easily, and tends to reoccur after removal. It generally occurs in the third trimester of pregnancy. See also granuloma, pyogenic and granuloma, central giant cell.

granuloma inguinale **(ing′gwināl′),** *n* a sexually transmitted disease characterized by ulcers of the skin and subcutaneous tissues of the groin and genitalia. It is caused by infection with *C. granulomatis,* a small, gram-negative, rod-shaped bacillus.

granuloma, pyogenic, n a tumorlike mass of granulation tissue produced in response to minor trauma in some individuals. It is not suppuration producing, as the name suggests, but is highly vascular and bleeds readily. They are histologically identical to pregnancy granulomas, but they may be found in either gender in any location, and may occur at any age. Some prefer the term *lobular capillary hemangioma* to describe a pyogenic granuloma, as it more accurately describes the histologic findings.

granuloma, reticuloendothelial **(ritik′yəlōen′dōthē′lēəl),** *n* See disease, lipoid storage.

graph, *n* a diagram used to compare numerical relationships.

graphite, *n* a soft carbon substance with a metallic black or gray sheen and a greasy feel. It is used in pencils, as a constituent of lubricants, and for making refractories such as crucibles in which to melt gold and other metals.

grasp, *n* the manner in which an instrument is held.

grasp, finger, n a modification of the palm and thumb grasp; it is more useful with modern, smaller handled instruments. The handle is held by the four flexed fingers rather than allowed to rest in the palm, and the thumb is used to secure a rest. Used when working indirectly on the maxillary arch.

grasp, instrument, n a method of holding the instrument with the fingers in such a manner that freedom of action, control, tactile sensitivity, and maneuverability are secured. The most common grasp is the pen grasp.

grasp, modified pen, n a method for holding instruments that is designed to enhance control and sensitivity. The grasp consists of the tips of the thumb, index finger, and middle finger holding the instrument while the ring finger provides support. See also grasp, pen.

grasp, palm-and-thumb, n a grasp that is similar to the hold on a knife when one is whittling wood; the handle rests in the palm and is grasped by the four fingers, while the thumb rests on an adjoining object.

grasp, pen, n a grasp in which the instrument is held somewhat as a pen is held, with the handle in contact with the bulbous portion of the thumb and index finger and the shank in contact with the radial side of the bulbous portion of the middle finger (not crossing the nail), while the handle rests against the phalanx of the index finger.

grasp, pincer, n the grasping an object between the thumb and forefinger. The ability to perform this task is a milestone of fine motor development in infants, usually occurring from 9 to 12 months of age.

gratis, *adj* free, without reward or consideration.

Graves' disease, *n.pr* See goiter, exophthalmic.

gravity, specific, *n* a number indicating the ratio of the weight of a substance to that of an equal volume of water.

Gray (Gy), *n* a unit of measurement for an absorbed dose of radiation, from the French *Systéme International d'Unités;* converts to the traditional rad by the formula 100 rad = 1 Gy.

greater palatine foramen, *n* See foramen, greater palatine.

grid, *n* a device used to prevent as much scattered radiation as possible from reaching a radiographic film during the making of a radiograph. It consists essentially of a series of narrow lead strips closely spaced on their edges and separated by spacers of low-density material.

grid, crossed, *n* an arrangement of two parallel grids rotated in position at right angles to each other. See also grid, parallel.

grid, focused, *n* a grid in which the lead foils are placed at an angle so that they all point toward a focus at a specified distance.

grid, moving, *n* a grid that is moved continuously or oscillated throughout the making of a radiograph.

grid, parallel, *n* a grid in which the lead strips are oriented parallel to each other.

grid, Potter-Bucky, *n.pr* a grid using the principle of the moving grid, with an oscillating movement.

grid, stationary, *n* a nonoscillating or nonmoving grid; the image of its strips will be visible on the radiograph for which it is used.

grinding, selective, *n* a modification of the occlusal forms of teeth by grinding at selected places to improve function.

grinding-in, *n* the process of correcting errors in the centric and eccentric occlusions of natural or artificial teeth.

griseofulvin microsize/griseofulvin ultramicrosize (gris′ēōful′vin mī′-krōsīz′ ul′trəmī′krōsīz′), *n brand names:* Fulvicin U/F, Grifulvin V, Gris-PEG; *drug class:* antifungal; *action:* arrests fungal cell division at metaphase; binds to human keratin, making it resistant to disease; *uses:* mycotic infections: tinea corporis, tinea pedis, tinea cruris, tinea barbae, tinea capitis, tinea unguium if caused by *Epidermophyton, Microsporum, Trichophyton.*

grit, *n* the measurement of the abrasive particle size.

groin, *n* each of two areas where the abdomen joins the thighs.

groove, *n* a linear channel or sulcus.

groove, abutment, *n* a transverse groove that may be cut in the bone across the alveolar ridge to furnish positive seating for the implant framework and to prevent tension of the tissue.

groove, developmental, *n* a fine depressed line in the enamel of a tooth that marks the union of the lobes of the crown in its development.

groove, gingiva, free, *n* the shallow line or depression on the surface of the gingiva at the junction of the free and attached gingivae.

groove, interdental, *n* a linear, vertical depression on the surface of the interdental papillae; functions as a spillway for food from the interproximal areas.

groove, labiomental, *n* a natural indentation in the chin, just below the lips, that takes its form from the muscles and bones lying beneath the skin.

groove, linguogingival, *n* vertical groove on the lingual surface of certain anterior teeth that originates in the lingual pit and extends cervically and slightly distal onto the cingulum.

groove, marginal, *n* a developmental groove that forms across the marginal ridges of posterior teeth.

groove, nasolacrimal **(groov nā′zō-lak′rəməl),** *n* a linear depression that extends from the eye to the olfactory sac in an embryo and separates the lateral nasal process from the maxillary process.

groove, retention, *n* a groove formed by opposing vertical constrictions in the preparation of a tooth that provides improved retention of the restoration.

ground, electrical, *n* an electrical connection with the earth (or other ground).

ground state, *n* the state of a nucleus, an atom, or a molecule when it has its lowest energy. All other states are termed *excited.*

ground substance, *n* See matrix.

ground substance, of bone, *n* a major component of bone consisting of proteoglycans that contain chondroitin sulfate and hydroxyapatite. More recently called *intercellular substance.*

grounded, *adj* pertaining to an arrangement whereby an electrical circuit or equipment such as a radiographic generator is connected by an electrical conductor with the earth or some similarly conducting body.

group, blood, *n* See blood groups.

group function, *n* See function, group.

group practice, *n* the association of several health care providers to complement, facilitate, and extend their scope of health care delivery, not possible in a sole or single practice. See also practice, group.

group purchase, *n* the purchase of dental services, either by postpayment or prepayment, by a large group of people.

growth, *n* an increase in size.

growth and development, *n* the process of *growth* is defined as an increase in size; *development* is defined as a progression toward maturity. Thus the terms are used together to describe the complex physical, mental, and emotional processes associated with the "growing up" of children.

growth factor, *n* the chemical messengers that induce cell growth by tissue type (e.g., osteoinductive factor, epidermal growth factors).

growth failure, *n* a lack of normal physical and psychologic development as a result of genetic, nutritional, pathologic, or psychosocial factors. See also failure to thrive.

growth, grain, *n* a phenomenon resulting from heat treatment of alloys. In excessive amounts, this growth produces undesirable physical properties.

growth hormone (GH), *n* a single-chain peptide secreted by the anterior pituitary gland in response to growth hormone releasing factor (GHRF) from the hypothalamus. Growth hormone promotes protein synthesis in all cells, increased fat mobilization and use of fatty acids for energy, and decreased use of carbohydrates.

GTT, *n* See test, glucose tolerance.

guaiacol, *n* catecholomonomethyl ether, which is used as an expectorant and intestinal disinfectant.

guaifenesin (gwī'əfen'əsin), *n brand names:* Anti-Tuss, Robitussin; *drug class:* expectorant; *action:* acts as an expectorant by stimulating mucosal reflex to increase production of less viscous lung mucus; *use:* dry, nonproductive cough.

guanabenz acetate (gwän'əbenz), *n brand names:* Wytensin; *drug class:* centrally acting antihypertensive; *action:* stimulates central α_2-adrenergic receptors, resulting in decreased sympathetic outflow from the brain; *use:* hypertension.

guanadrel sulfate (gwän'ədrel), *n brand name:* Hylorel; *drug class:* antihypertensive; *action:* inhibits sympathetic vasoconstriction by inhibiting release of norephinephrine, depleting norepinephrine stores in adrenergic nerve endings; *use:* hypertension.

guanethidine sulfate (gwäneth'idēn), *n brand name:* Ismelin; *drug class:* antihypertensive; *action:* inhibits norepinephrine release, depleting norepinephrine stores in adrenergic nerve endings; *use:* moderate to severe hypertension.

guanfacine HCl (gwän'fəsēn), *n brand name:* Tenex; *drug class:* antihypertensive; *action:* stimulates central α-adrenergic receptors, resulting in decreased sympathetic outflow from the brain; *use:* hypertension in individuals using a thiazide diuretic.

guanosine (gwän'əsēn), *n* a compound derived from a nucleic acid, composed of guanine and a sugar, D-ribose. Guanosine is a major molecular component of the nucleotides guanosine monophosphate and guanosine triphosphate and of DNA and RNA.

guanosine triphosphate (GTP), *n* a high-energy nucleotide, similar to adenosine triphosphate, that functions in various metabolic reactions such as the activation of fatty acids and the formation of the peptide bond in protein synthesis.

guaranty (gar'əntē), *n* a contract that some certain and designated thing shall be done exactly as it is agreed to be done.

guard, bite, *n* an acrylic resin appliance designed to cover the occlusal and incisal surfaces of the teeth of a dental arch to stabilize the teeth and/or provide a flat platform for the unobstructed excursive glides of the mandible. See also plane, bite.

guard, night, *n* See guard, bite.

guard, oral cavity, *n* a resilient intraoral device worn during participation in contact sports to reduce the potential for injury to the teeth and associated tissue.

guardian, *n* a person appointed to take care of the person or property of another; one who legally has the care and management of the person or the property or both of a child until the child attains adulthood.

guardian ad litem, *n* a person appointed by the court to represent a child's or incapacitated person's best interests during legal proceedings.

Guérin's fracture (gāranz′), *n.pr* See fracture, Guérin's

guidance, *n* a mechanical or other means for controlling the direction of movement of an object.

guidance, angle, n See angle, incisal guidance.

guidance, condylar, n See guide, condylar.

guidance, condylar, inclination, n See guide, condylar, inclination.

guidance, developmental, n the comprehensive orofacial orthopedic control over the growth of the jaws and eruption of the teeth, with the objective of optimizing the achievement of the genetic potential of the individual. Requires a combination of carefully timed active appliance therapy and supervisory examinations, including radiography and other diagnostic records, at various stages of development. May be required throughout the entire period of growth and maturation of the face, beginning at the earliest detection of a developing malformation.

guidance, incisal, n the influence on mandibular movements of the contacting surfaces of the mandibular and maxillary anterior teeth.

guide, *n* a device for directing the motion of something.

guide, adjustable anterior, n an anterior guide, the superior surface of which may be varied to provide desired separation of the casts in various eccentric relationships.

guide, anterior, n the part of an articulator contacted by the incisal guide pin to maintain the selected separation of the upper and lower members of the articulator. The guide influences the changing relationships of mounted casts in eccentric movements. See also guide, incisal.

guide, condylar, n (condylar guidance) the mechanical device on an articulator; intended to produce guidance in articulator movement similar to that produced by the paths of the condyles in the temporomandibular joints.

guide, condylar, inclination, n (condylar guidance inclination) the angle of inclination of the condylar guide mechanism of an articulator in relation to the horizontal plane of the instrument.

guide, incisal, n (anterior guide) the part of an articulator that maintains the incisal guide angle.

guide, incisal, adjustment, n an occlusal adjustment that produces a minimum of overbite (vertical overlap) and a maximum of overjet (horizontal overlap), eliminates fremitus and racking effects on the anterior segment of teeth in the protrusive glide, and attains maximal incisive group function.

guide, incisal, angle, n See angle, incisal guide.

guide plane, n a fixed or removable orthodontic appliance designed to deflect the functional path of the mandible and alter the positions of specific teeth.

guidelines, *n.pl* a set of standards, criteria, or specifications to be used or followed in the performance of certain tasks.

gum(s), *n* the colloquial term for the fibrous and mucosal covering of the alveolar process or ridges or gingiva(e). See also gingiva.

gum pads, n edentulous segments of the maxillae and mandible that correspond to the underlying primary teeth.

gumboil, *n* an older term for an abscess of the gingiva and periosteum resulting from injury, infection, impacted food particles, or periapical infection. The gingival tissue is characteristically red, swollen, and tender. The abscess may rupture spontaneously, or it may require incision, as well as treatment of the underlying cause. See also abscess.

gumma (gum′ə), *n* a granulomatous, gummy lesion of tertiary syphilis. The palate and tongue are sites of predilection in the oral region. A similar lesion occurring with tuberculosis is designated a tuberculous gumma.

gummy smile, *n* condition in which gingival tissue is located more on the cervical third of the crowns than is normal, resulting in teeth that appear shorter and "gummy."

Gunn's syndrome, *n.pr* See splint, Gunning's.

gutta-percha (gut′ə-pur′chə), *n* the coagulated juice of various tropical trees that has certain rubberlike properties. Used for temporary sealing of dressings in cavities; also used in the form of cones for filling root canals and in the form of sticks for sealing cavities over treatment.

gutta-percha, baseplate, n the gutta-percha combined with fillers and coloring materials and rolled into sheets that are used as temporary bases for denture construction.

gutta-percha points, n.pl the fine, tapered cylinders of gutta-percha used, because of their radiopacity, for radiographic ascertainment of pocket depth and topography; used also as a root canal filling material.

gutta-percha, temporary stopping, n the gutta-percha mixed with zinc oxide and white wax. Used for temporary sealing of dressings in cavities.

gynecologist (gī′nikol′əjist), *n* a physician whose practice of medicine focuses on the care of women, including the treatment of conditions related to the female genitourinary tract, endocrine system, and reproductive organs.

gypsum (jip′sum), *n* the dihydrate of calcium sulfate ($CaSO_4$-$2H_2O$). α-Hemihydrate and β-hemihydrate are derived from gypsum. See also plaster of paris.

H

h II., *n* See hemophilia B.

h.s., *n* Latin phrase for "at bedtime"; used in writing prescriptions.

habilitation, *n* See rehabilitation.

habit, *n* the tendency toward an act that has become a repeated performance, relatively fixed, consistent, easy to perform, and almost automatic. Once learned, habits may occur without the intent of the person or may appear to be out of control and are difficult to change. In dentistry, habits such as bruxism, clenching, tongue thrusting, and lip and cheek biting may produce injury to the teeth, their attachment apparatus, oral mucosa, mandibular and temporomandibular musculature, and articulation.

habituation, *n* a state in which an individual involuntarily tends to continue the use of a drug. Generally refers to the state in which an individual continues self-administration of a drug because of psychologic dependence without physical dependence.

***Haemophilus* (hēmof′iləs),** *n* a genus of gram-negative pathogenic bacteria, frequently found in the respiratory tract of humans and other animals. *Haemophilus* are generally sensitive to cephalosporins, tetracyclines, and sulfonamides.

H. influenzae, n a small, gram-negative, nonmotile, parasitic bacterium that occurs in two forms, encapsulated and nonencapsulted, and in six types: A, B, C, D, E, and F. Almost all infections are caused by the encapsulated type B organisms. It is found in the throats of 30% of healthy, normal people. It may cause destructive inflammation of the larynx, trachea, and bronchi in children and debilitated older people.

Hageman trait (hä′gəmən), *n* See factor XII. (not current)

hair covering, *n* a part of an overall contamination-limiting strategy; hair should be pulled back from the shoulders and face. Longer hair may be completely concealed beneath a cap made from an approved material.

halazepam (halaz′əpam), *n brand name:* Paxipam; *drug class:* benzodiazepine (Controlled Substance Schedule IV); *action:* produces central nervous system depression by interaction with benzodiazepine receptor to facilitate action of inhibitory neurotransmitter γ-aminobutyric acid; *use:* anxiety.

halcinonide (halsin′ənīd), *n brand names:* Halog-E, Halog; *drug class:* corticosteroid, synthetic topical; *action:* interacts with steroid cytoplasmic receptors to induce antiinflammatory actions; *use:* inflammation of corticosteroid-responsive dermatoses.

half-life, *n* the time in which a radioactive substance will lose half of its activity through disintegration.

half-life, biologic, n the time in which a living tissue, organ, or individual eliminates, through biologic processes, half of a given amount of a substance that has been introduced into it.

half-life, effective, n the half-life of a radioactive isotope in a biologic organism, resulting from the combination of radioactive decay and biologic elimination.

half-life, physical, n the average time required for the decay of half the atoms in a given amount of a radioactive substance.

half-value layer (HVL), *n* the thickness of a specified material (usually aluminum, copper, or lead) required to decrease the dosage rate of a beam of radiograph at a point of interest to half its initial value. A determination of the half-value layer of a given radiographic beam is used to denote the quality of the radiographic beam. The half-value layer will vary depending on kilovolt peak and the amount of filtration at the source.

halisteresis (həlis′tərē′sis), *n* a theory of the method of bone resorption according to which bone salts can be removed by a humoral mechanism and returned to the tissue fluids, leaving behind a decalcified bone matrix; osteolysis. This is not considered to be the mechanism under which resorption occurs in periodontal disease.

halitophobia (hal′itōfō′bēə), *n* an abiding fear of having fetid breath, whether a valid concern or not. In some cases it may be symptomatic of mental illness.

halitosis (bad breath, bromopnea, fetor ex ore, offensive breath) (hal′itō′sis), *n* an offensive odor of the breath resulting from local and metabolic conditions (e.g., poor oral hygiene, periodontal disease, sinusitis, tonsilitis, suppurative bronchopulmonary disease, acidosis, uremia).

Haller's plexus, *n.pr* See plexus, Haller's.

hallucination (həloo′sinā′shən), *n* an artificial sensory experience without the presence of an external cause.

hallucinogens, abuse of (həloo′sinəjenz), *n* a regular use of mescaline or *d*-lysergic acid diethylamide (LSD) for reasons other than recognized medical applications. Street names include *cubes, acid, blue dragon, cupcake, big chief, sunshine, mesc,* and *buttons.*

halobetasol propionate (halōbā′-təsol prō′pēənāt′), *n brand name:* Ultravate; *drug class:* topical corticosteroid, group VI potency; *action:* interacts with steroid cytoplasmic receptors to induce antiinflammatory effects, possesses antipruritic/antiinflammatory actions; *uses:* psoriasis, eczema, contact dermatitis, pruritus.

halogen (hal′ōjen), *n* an element of a closely related group of elements consisting of fluorine, chlorine, bromine, and iodine.

halogenated hydrocarbons (hal′ō-jənātəd hī′drōkärbənz), *n.pl* the general anesthetic agents such as halothane and isoflurane, which work with a minimum of nausea and mucous membrane irritation. They produce drowsiness for several hours after the primary effects wear off.

haloperidol/haloperidol decanoate, *n brand name:* Haldol; *drug class:* antipsychotic/butyrophenone; *action:* blocks neurotransmission at dopaminergic synapses in the cerebral cortex, hypothalamus, and limbic system; *uses:* psychotic disorders, control of tics and vocal utterances in Gilles de la Tourette syndrome, short-term treatment of hyperactive children showing excessive motor activity.

halothane (hal′əthān), *n* a potent nonflammable and nonexplosive liquid anesthetic agent administered by inhalation. Common complications associated with other inhalation anesthetic agents are generally absent. Chemical name is 2-bromo-2-chloro-1,1,1-trifluoroethane.

hamartoma (ham′ärtō′mə), *n* a localized error in the composition of the tissue elements of an organ. May be automatically manifested in three ways, either singly or in combination: abnormal quantity, abnormal structure, or degree of maturation of the tissue components.

hamular notch, *n* See notch, pterygomaxillary.

hamular process, *n* See process, hamular.

hand condenser, *n* See condenser, hand.

hand pressure, *n* See pressure, hand.

Hand-Schüller-Christian disease (hand-shül′er-kris′chən), *n.pr* See disease, Hand-Schüller-Christian.

handicap, *n* a disability that hinders effective function; may involve any combination of physical, emotional, or social factors.

handpiece, *n* an instrument that is used to hold rotary instruments in the dental engine or condensing points in mechanical condensing units. It is connected by an arm, cable, belt, or tube to the source of power (e.g., motor, air, water).

handpiece, air-turbine, *n* a handpiece with a turbine powered by compressed air.

handpiece, contra-angle, *n* a binangled instrument for use with the dental engine; permits access to areas difficult or impossible to reach with a straight handpiece.

handpiece, high-speed, *n* a type of rotary or vibratory cutting tool that operates at speeds above 12,000 rpm. It is propelled by gears, a belt, or a turbine. Generally classified as an air turbine, a hydraulic turbine, or a high-speed handpiece on a conventional dental engine.

handpiece, high-speed, ultra, *n* a handpiece designed to permit rotational speeds of 100,000 to 300,000 rpm.

handpiece, right-angle, *n* a monangled instrument used with mechanical condensers to reach some operating areas.

handpiece, straight, *n* a handpiece whose axis is in line with the rotary instrument.

handpiece, water-turbine, *n* a handpiece with a turbine powered by water under pressure.

handwashing, *n* a fundamental part of standard precaution procedures and disease control for dental personnel; helps reduce or prevent infection and transmittal of microbes among people and objects; for regular dental procedures, liquid soap and water is sufficient but for surgical procedures, antimicrobial cleansers should be used.

Hansen's disease, *n.pr* See leprosy.

hapten (hap′tən), *n* a nonproteinaceous substance that acts as an antigen by combining with particular bonding sites on an antibody. Unlike a true antigen, it does not induce the formation of antibodies. A hapten bonded to a carrier protein may induce an immune response. Also called *haptene.*

hard disk drive, *n* the mechanism that controls the positioning, reading, and writing of the hard disk, which provides the largest amount of storage for the computer.

hard of hearing, *adj* a term applied to persons whose hearing is impaired but who have enough hearing left for practical use.

hard palate, See palate, hard.

hardener, *n* an ingredient (potassium alum) of the photographic and radiographic fixing solution that serves to harden the gelatin of the film to prevent softening and swelling of the gelatin.

hardening, *n* the process of setting or becoming firm.

hardening, age, *n* the precipitation of intermetallic compounds that alters certain physical properties in alloys; usually brought about through heat treatment.

hardening, precipitation, See tempering.

hardening solution, See solution, hardening.

hardening, strain, an increase in proportional limit resulting from distortion of the space lattice and fracture of grain boundaries through cold working. Ductility is markedly reduced.

hardening, work, *n* the hardening of a metal by cold work, such as repeated flexing.

hardness (of a substance), *n* the ability of a material to resist an indenting type of load.

hardness (of radiographs), *n* a term used to indicate in a general way the quality of x-radiation, with hardness being a function of the wavelength; the shorter the wavelength, the harder the x-radiation.

hardness, Mohs, *n* a relative scratch resistance of minerals based on an arbitrary scale: 10, diamond; 9, corundum; 8, topaz; 7, quartz; 6, orthoclase; 5, apatite; 4, fluorite; 3, calcite; 2, gypsum; and 1, talc.

hardness tests, See *tests, hardness.*

hardware, *n* the mechanical, magnetic, electronic, and electric devices or components of a computer.

harelip (cheiloschisis, cleft lip, congenital cleft lip) (her′lip), *n* an older term for a congenital nonunion or inadequacy of soft and hard tissues related to the lip. The deformity may be extensive enough to involve the nose, alveolar process, hard palate, and velum. The extent of the deformity varies among individuals. Various classifications have been established to identify the extent of a cleft. A rare midline cleft may occur in the lower lip at the embryonal junction of the two mandibular processes. See also lip, cleft and lip, congenital cleft.

harmony, functional occlusal, *n* an occlusal relationship of opposing teeth in all functional ranges and movements that will provide the greatest masticatory efficiency without causing undue strain or trauma on the supporting tissues.

harmony, occlusal, *n* the nondisruptive relationship of an occlusion to all its factors (e.g., the neuromuscular mechanism, temporomandibular joints, teeth and their supporting structures).

hashish, abuse of (hash′ish, həshēsh), *n* a regular use of the cannabis derivative hashish for reasons other than recognized medical applications. Street names are *hash* and *soles.*

Hatch clamp, See clamp, gingival, Hatch. (not current)

hatchet, *n* an angled cutting hand instrument in which the broad side of the blade is parallel with the angle(s) of the shank. Used to develop internal cavity form. May be bibeveled or single beveled like a chisel, in which case the instrument is paired with another.

haversian system, See osteon.

Hawley appliance, chart, retainer, (See under appropriate noun.)

Hawley retainer, See retainer, Hawley.

hay fever, *n* an acute seasonal allergic rhinitis, stimulated by tree, grass, or weed pollens. Also called *allergic rhinitis.*

hay rake, See appliance, hay rake.

hazard communication plan, *n* a set of written standards designed to reduce workplace illness and injury by ensuring that all employees are familiar with the names and potential hazards of the chemicals they handle and understand the precautions necessary for protecting themselves and others against any possible risks.

hazard, radiation, *n* the hazard that exists in any area in which a person is subject to radiation.

hazardous waste, *n* any material, gas, liquid, or solid substance that has the potential to cause injury or illness; that in an unprotected state poses a risk to the environment, including plant or animal life.

HDL, *n* the abbreviation or acronym for high-density lipoproteins. HDL molecules are considered a protective factor in coronary heart disease.

head covering, *n* a part of an overall contamination limiting strategy, a protective accessory that conceals most of the hair and head

head, steeple, See oxycephalia.

head tilt–chin lift maneuver, *n* a maneuver used to open the airway of an unconscious patient. The maneuver is performed by placing the palm of one hand on the patient's forehead and applying gentle backward pressure. The fingers of the other hand are placed on the bony part of the chin and the chin is lifted forward. This maneuver lifts the tongue from the back of the throat and reestablishes the airway.

headache, *n* a pain in the cranial vault resulting from intracranial, extracranial, or psychogenic causes: intracranial vascular dilation; space-occupying lesions; diseases of the eyes, ears, and sinuses; extracranial vascular dilation; sustained muscular contraction; hysteria; certain habit patterns (clenching); and reaction to stress.

headache, cluster, See neuralgia, facial, atypical.

headache, lower-half, See neuralgia, facial, atypical.

headache, migraine, *n* a vascular type of headache, typically unilateral in the temporal, frontal, and retroorbital area, but may occur midface. It is described as throbbing, burning, pulsating, exploding, or pressure and may become generalized and persist for hours or days. Onset of pain is usually preceded by prodromal symptoms that may include visual disturbances, scotomas, vomiting, and nausea. A migraine headache is usually considered to be a psychophysiologic (psychosomatic) disorder.

headcap, *n* the part of an extraoral orthodontic appliance that engages the back of the head, incorporating the skull as a source of resistance for tooth movement, and gives attachment to the intraoral element of the appliance.

headcap, plaster, *n* a cap that is constructed of plaster-of-paris gauze and embodies points for applying fixation and traction appliances in the treatment of mandibular and maxillofacial injuries.

headgear, *n* the apparatus encircling the head or neck and providing attachment for an intraoral appliance in use of extraoral anchorage.

headgear, radiologic, *n* a device that is used to protect the head from injury by radiation.

healing cap, *n* a device used during the second stage of dental implantation. It consists of a cylindrical head on the superior part and two downwardly projecting legs that are inserted into an anchor. It protects the area before the insertion of permanent prosthesis.

health, *n* a bodily state in which all parts are functioning properly. Also refers to the normal functioning of a part of the body. A state of normal functional equilibrium; homeostasis.

health, ASA classification, *n* a classification system for ranking the level of a patient's physical health, established by the American Society of Anesthesiologists (ASA). Patients are classified as ASA I, indicating a patient in a normal state of health, with no apparent disease. ASA II indicates a patient with a mild disease. ASA III indicates a patient with a serious disease, which may limit normal activity but does not cause incapacitation. ASA IV indicates a patient with a life-threatening and incapacitating disease. ASA V indicates a declining patient who is not expected to live beyond a day, regardless of medical attention. ASA E indicates emergency status when added to any of the normal status designations.

health assessment, *n* an evaluation of the health status of an individual by performing a physical examination after obtaining a health history. Various laboratory and functional tests may also be ordered to confirm a clinical impression or to screen for possible disease involvement.

health behavior, *n* an action taken by a person to maintain, attain, or regain good health and to prevent illness. Health behavior reflects a person's health beliefs.

health care clearing house, *n* an entity used to process or aid in the processing of information; may also be called a repricing company, billing service, community health information system, community health management information system, or "value-added" switch or network.

health care operations, *n.pl* the functions performed by a health care provider, health care plan, or health care clearing house to conduct administrative and business management activities.

health care professional, *n* a person who by education, training, certification, or licensure is qualified to and is engaged in providing health care.

health care provider, *n* an individual who provides health services to health care consumers (patients).

health education, *n* an educational

program directed to the general public that attempts to improve, maintain, and safeguard the health care of the community.

health hazard, *n* a danger to health resulting from exposure to environmental pollutants such as asbestos or ionizing radiation, or to a lifestyle influence such as cigarette smoking or chemical abuse.

health history, *n* previously diagnosed physical or mental condition of an individual. Also called *medical history.* See also health assessment and chart, history.

health information, *n* recorded information in any format (e.g., oral, written, or electronic) regarding the physical or mental condition of an individual, health care provision, or health care payment. See also *health assessment* and *health, patient.*

health information, individually identifiable, *n* recorded information in any format (e.g., oral, written, or electronic) regarding the physical or mental condition of an individual, health care provision, or health care payment. It contains demographic information able to specifically distinguish an individual. In some cases, this information may not be considered "protected." See also health information, protected.

health information, protected (PHI), *n* recorded information in any format (e.g., oral, written, or electronic) regarding the physical or mental condition of an individual, health care provision, or health care payment. It contains demographic information able to specifically distinguish an individual. See also health information, individually identifiable.

Health Insurance Portability and Accountability Act (HIPAA), *n* a public law enacted by Congress in 1996, consisting of two parts. Title I of the act protects workers and their families from the loss of health insurance coverage should they change or lose their jobs. Title II of the act calls for the establishment of national standards for electronic health care records, as well as national identities for health care providers, health insurance plans, and employers. In addition, Title II protects the privacy and security of an individual's health information.

health maintenance organization (HMO), *n* a legal entity that accepts responsibility and financial risk for providing specified services to a defined population during a defined period at a fixed price. An organized system of health care delivery that provides comprehensive care to enrollees through designated providers. Enrollees are generally assessed a monthly payment for health care services and may be required to remain in the program for a specified amount of time.

health, patient, *n* the state of bodily soundness of the patient; the patient's absolute or relative freedom from physical and mental disease.

health physics, *n* the study of the effects of ionizing radiation on the body and the methods for protecting people from the undesirable effects of radiation.

health policy, *n* **1.** a statement of a decision regarding a goal in health care and a plan for achieving that goal; e.g., to prevent an epidemic, a program for inoculating a population is developed and implemented. *n* **2.** a field of study and practice in which the priorities and values underlying health resource allocation are determined.

health promotion, *n* an educational program or effort directed at a targeted population to improve, maintain, and safeguard the health of that segment of society. See also health education.

health resources, *n* all materials, personnel, facilities, funds, and anything else that can be used for providing health care and services.

health risk, *n* a disease precursor associated with a higher than average morbidity or mortality. The disease precursors may include demographic variables, certain individual behaviors, familial and individual histories, and certain physiologic changes.

health risk appraisal, *n* a process of gathering, analyzing, and comparing an individual's prognostic characteristics of health with a standard age group, thereby predicting the likelihood that a person may develop prematurely a health problem associated with a high morbidity and mortality rate.

hearing, *n* the sense by which sound perception occurs; happens after sound waves are converted into impulses of the nerves and translated by the brain.

hearing aid, *n* an electronic device used to amplify and shape waves of sound entering the external auditory canal.

hearing aid, behind-the-ear, *n* an electronic device, situated over the ear, for amplifying and shaping sound waves entering the external auditory canal.

hearing aid, eyeglass model, *n* an electronic device, attached to the eyeglasses' thickened temple bar, for amplifying and shaping sound waves entering the external auditory canal.

hearing disorders, *n.pl* a structural or functional impairment of the ability to detect and recognize sound.

hearing disorders, indications of, *n.pl* symptoms such as an inability to pay attention or respond appropriately to spoken dialogue, heightened focus, increased use of a specific ear, frequent requests for repetition of spoken statements, and abnormal quality of speech.

hearing disorders, types of, *n.pl* classifications include a loss of central, mixed, sensorineural, or conductive hearing.

hearing loss, *n* a reduction in the acuity to detect and recognize sound.

hearing loss, conductive, *n* a hearing impairment of the outer or middle ear, which is due to abnormalities or damage within the conductive pathways leading to the inner ear.

hearing loss, mixed, *n* a hearing impairment that is the result of damage to both conductive pathways of the middle ear and to the nerves or sensory hair cells of the inner ear.

hearing loss, sensorineural **(sen′so-rēner′əl),** *n* a hearing impairment of the inner ear resulting from damage to the sensory hair cells or to the nerves that supply the inner ear.

hearsay, *n* **1.** the testimony given by a witness who relates not what is known personally but what others have stated. *n* **2.** the evidence that does not derive its value solely from the credit of the witness, but rests mainly on the veracity and competency of other persons and is admitted in court only in specified cases, from necessity.

heart, *n* the muscular pump that maintains and regulates the flow of blood through the body.

heart, artificial, *n* a mechanical device that acts to pump blood to and from the body tissues during repair of the heart.

heart attack, *n* See myocardial infarction; thrombosis, coronary; or occlusion, coronary.

heart block, *n* the condition in which the muscular interconnection between the auricle and ventricle is interrupted so that the auricle and ventricle beat independently of each other.

heart, compression of, *n* See massage, cardiac.

heart defect, *n* a fault in the structural integrity of the heart.

heart defect, congenital, *n* the structural errors in the heart formed during embryonic and fetal life.

heart disease, *n* a disorder in the normal functioning of the heart.

heart disease, dental concerns, *n.pl* the special considerations taken to eliminate oral disease by maintaining an elevated level of oral health and prevent infective endocarditis, an infection of the heart valves that may be caused by bacteremia created during dental treatments. Heart disease has also been linked with increased levels of periodontal disease.

heart disease, ischemic, *n* See disease, heart, ischemic.

heart disease risk factors, *n.pl* the hereditary, lifestyle, and environmental influences that increase one's chances of developing heart disease.

heart massage, *n* See massage, cardiac.

heart murmur, *n* the sound of blood flowing back through a defective heart valve. Two types are possible: organic or functional.

heart, normal, *n* a heart without anatomic defects that could cause an impairment in the function of the organ.

heart rate, *n* the rate or tempo of heart contractions recorded in beats per minute.

heart sounds, *n.pl* the normal noises produced within the heart during the cardiac cycle that can be heard over the precordium and may reveal abnormalities in cardiac structure or function. The use of the stethoscope over the left side of the chest is a common clinical technique to assess heart function. The typical sounds are a rythmic lub dup; abnormal sounds include clicks, murmurs, rubs, snaps, and gallops.

heart surgery, *n* a surgical procedure involving the heart, performed to correct acquired or congenital defects, to replace diseased valves, to open or bypass blocked vessels, or to graft a prosthesis or a transplant in place.

heart valves, *n.pl* one of the four structures within the heart that prevent backflow of blood by opening and closing with each heartbeat. They include two semilunar valves, the aortic and pulmonary; the mitral, or bicuspid, valve; and the tricuspid valve. They permit the flow of blood in only one direction, and any one of the valves may become defective, permitting the backflow associated with heart murmurs.

heart failure (härt′ fālyur), *n* a sudden, sometimes fatal, cessation of the heart's action.

heart failure, acute, *n* a rapid and marked impairment of the cardiac output.

heart failure, backward, *n* a type of congestive heart failure in which the initiating factor is increased venous pressure resulting from ventricular failure to empty the atria.

heart failure, congestive, *n* a clinical syndrome resulting from chronic cardiac decompensation associated with left-sided or right-sided heart failure. Left-sided failure may result from rheumatic mitral valvular disease, aortic valvular disease, systemic hypertension, or arteriosclerotic disease. Manifestations include orthopnea, paroxysmal dyspnea, pulmonary edema, cough, and cardiac asthma. Right-sided failure results most commonly from pulmonary congestion and hypertension associated with left-sided failure but may result from anemia, myocarditis, beriberi, or dysrhythmia. Manifestations include peripheral pitting edema, ascites, cyanosis, oliguria, and hydrothorax.

heart failure, forward, *n* a type of heart failure initiated by decreased cardiac output that leads to decreased blood supply to tissues, decreased excretion of salt (Na1) and salt retention, elevated venous pressure, and edema.

heartburn, *n* a painful burning sensation in the esophagus just below the sternum. It is usually caused by the reflux of gastric contents into the esophagus, but it may be caused by gastric hyperacidity or peptic ulcer.

heat, *n* the state of a body or of matter that is perceived as being opposite of cold and is characterized by elevation of temperature.

heat, applied, *n* the therapeutic application of wet or dry heat to increase circulation and produce hyperemia, accelerate the dissolution of infection and inflammation, increase absorption from tissue spaces, relieve pain, relieve muscle spasm and associated pain, and increase metabolism.

heat, applied, and cold, *n* the most commonly employed physical agents in dental practice; they modify the physiologic processes and have both a systemic and a local effect. The principal effect on the tissues is mediated by the alteration in the circulatory mechanisms. Properly used, they have a salutary therapeutic result; improperly used, they may produce serious pathologic consequences.

heat, applied, contraindications, *n.pl* the conditions that preclude the use of heat application: peripheral neuropathy, conditions in which maximum vasodilation and inflammation are already present, acute inflammatory conditions in which more swelling will cause acute pain and pulpitis, septicemia, and malignancies.

heat, applied, general physiologic effects, *n.pl* the physiologic effects of generally applied wet or dry heat; increase in body temperature, generalized vasodilation, rise in metabolism, decrease in blood pressure, increase in pulse rate and circulation, and increase in depth and rate of respiration.

heat, applied, local physiologic effects, n.pl the physiologic effects of locally applied wet or dry heat to the intraoral or extraoral tissues: increase in caliber and number of capillaries, increased absorption resulting from capillary dilation, increased lymph formation and flow, relief of pain, relief of spasm, increase of phagocytes, and a rise in local metabolism.

heat loss, metabolic causes, n.pl the biologic factors that influence heat loss: redistribution of blood vasodilation and vasoconstriction, variations in blood volume, tendency of fat to insulate the body, and evaporation.

heat loss, physical causes, n.pl the physical factors that influence heat loss: radiation, convection, and conduction; evaporation from the lungs, skin, and mucous membranes; the raising of inspired air to body temperatures; and the production of urine and feces.

heat production, metabolic causes, n.pl the chemical factors of the body that cause heat production: specific dynamic action of food, especially protein, that results in a rise of metabolism; a high environmental temperature that, by raising temperatures of the tissues, increases the velocity of reactions and thus increases heat production; and stimulation of the adrenal cortex and thyroid glands by the hormones of the pituitary glands.

heat treatment, See treatment, heat.

heat stabile, *adj* heat resistant. Also called *thermostabile.*

heavy function, *n* See function, heavy.

hebephrenia (hē′bəfrē′nēə), *n* a form of schizophrenia in which the individual behaves like a child (e.g., inappropriate laughter and silliness).

heel effect, *n* See effect, heel.

Heerfordt's syndrome, *n.pr* See fever, uveoparotid.

height of contour, *n* See contour, height of.

height, ramus, *n* the measurement of the expanse of a ramus. It is used to calculate the correct age of infants and toddlers with undetermined age statistics.

Heimlich maneuver (hīm′lik), *n.pr* an emergency procedure for dislodging food or other obstruction from the trachea to prevent asphyxiation. The choking person is grasped from behind by the rescuer, whose fist, thumb side in, is placed just below the victim's sternum and whose other hand is placed firmly over the fist. The rescuer then pulls the fist firmly and abruptly into the epigastrium, forcing the obstruction up the trachea.

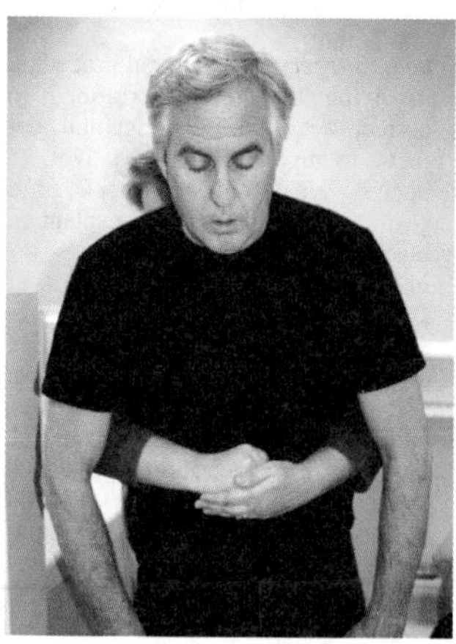

Heimlich maneuver. (Bird/Robinson, 2005)

Heimlich sign, *n.pr* a universal distress signal that a person is choking and unable to speak, made by grasping the throat with a thumb and index finger, thereby attracting the attention of others nearby.

***Helicobacter pylori* (hel′ikōbak′tər),** *n* a gram-negative, spiral-shaped bacteria that is active as a human gastric pathogen. It is associated with lesions or gastritis or peptic ulcers. See also ulcer, peptic.

helium (He) (hē′lēum), *n* a colorless, odorless, tasteless gas; one of the inert gaseous elements. Atomic number, 2; atomic weight, 4.003. Used in medicine as a diluent for other gases.

hellac base, See *base, shellac.* (not current)

helminths (hel′minths), *n.pl* the parasitic worms that cause disease and illness in humans such as tapeworm, pinworm, and trichinosis. They are usually transmitted via contaminated food, water, soil, or other objects. Adult worms live in the intestines and other organs. Minor infections may be asymptomatic, whereas stronger cases may cause dietary deficiencies or digestive, muscular, and nervous disorders.

Helsinki declaration (accords), *n.pr* a declaration signed by the representatives of member nations of the Conference on Security and Cooperation in Europe in Helsinki, Finland. The principle and practice of informed consent in health care grew from the Helsinki accords.

hemangioameloblastoma (hēman′jēōəmel′ōblastō′mə), *n* a neoplasm in the jaw that has characteristics of ameloblastoma and hemangioma.

hemangioendothelioma (hēman′jēōen′dōthē′lēō′mə), *n* a malignant tumor formed by proliferation of endothelium of the capillary vessels.

hemangiofibroma (hēman′jēōfī-brō′mə), *n* a benign neoplasm characterized by proliferation of blood channels in a dense mass of fibroblasts.

hemangioma (hēman′jēō′mə), *n* **1.** a benign neoplasm characterized by blood vascular channels. A cavernous form consists of large vascular spaces. A capillary form consists of many small blood vessels. *n* **2.** a benign tumor composed of newly formed blood vessels.

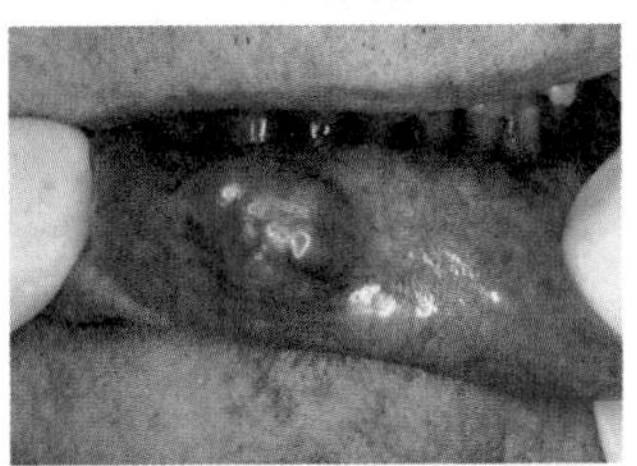

Hemangioma. (Ibsen/Phelan, 2004)

hemangiopericytoma (hēman′jēōper′isītō′mə), *n* a vascular tumor composed of pericytes.

hemarthrosis (he″mahrthro′sis), *n* the blood found in the cavity of a joint.

hemataerometer, *n* a device for determining the pressure of the gases in the blood. (not current)

hematemesis (hē′mətem′esis), *n* vomiting of blood.

hematocrit (hēmat′ōcrit), *n* (packed-cell volume), the percentage of the total blood volume composed of red blood cells (erythrocytes). Normal values average 42% to 45%. Specific groups averaging: children, 32% to 65%; adult men, 42% to 53%; adult women, 38% to 46%.

hematogenous (hemətoj′ĕnus), *adj* part of or originating in the blood, or distributed through the bloodstream.

hematogenous total joint replacement **(hemətoj′ĕnus),** *n* the replacement of a diseased or damaged joint with an artificial joint. The joint replacement is considered hematogenous if it comes into contact with the bloodstream.

hematologic disorders, *n.pl* the diseases of the blood and blood-forming tissues.

hematology (hē′mətol′əjē), *n* the scientific study of blood and blood-forming tissues.

hematology tests, *n.pl* the diagnostic tests of the blood and its constituent parts.

hematoma (hē′mətō′mə), *n* a mass of blood in the tissue as a result of trauma or other factors that cause the rupture of blood vessels.

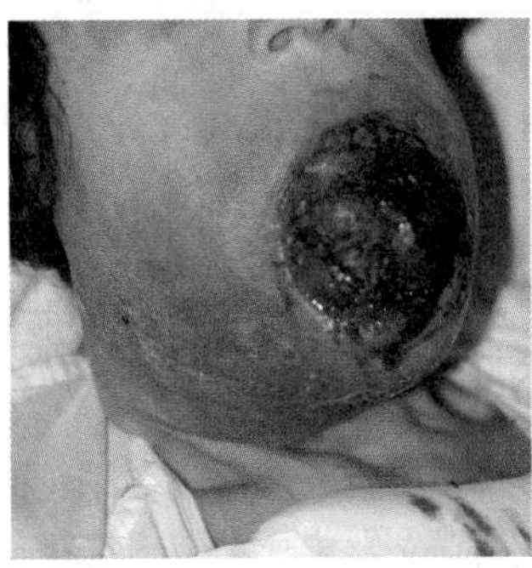

Hematoma. (Courtesy Dr. Charles Babbush)

hematoma, subdural, *n* a collection of extravasated blood trapped below the dural membranes of the brain causing pressure on the brain, resulting in pain and neural dysfunction. It may be life threatening.

hematopoiesis (hē′mətō′poiē′sis), *n* the normal formation and development of blood cells in the bone marrow.

hematosis (hē′mətō′sis), *n* the oxygenation or aeration of the venous blood in the lungs.

hematoxylin, *n* a dye or stain commonly used to treat tissue sections for microscopic examination, usually used in combination with eosin.

hematuria (hē′mətoo′rēə), *n* the presence of blood in the urine.

hematuria, gross, *n* the visible evidence of blood in the urine. It may occur from neoplasms of the kidney and bladder, hemorrhagic diathesis, hypertension with renal epistaxis, or acute glomerular nephritis.

hematuria, microscopic, *n* the demonstration of hematuria during the microscopic examination of centrifuged urine. It may result from the same causes as gross hematuria or from toxicity of drugs, embolic glomerulitis, vascular diseases, or chronic glomerular nephritis.

heme, *n* the pigmented, iron-containing, nonprotein portion of the hemoglobin molecule.

hemiachromatosia (hem′ēak′rōmətō′zhə), *n* a state of being color blind in only one half of the visual field.

hemianesthesia (hem′ēan′esthē′zhə), *n* the anesthesia or loss of tactile sensibility on one side of the body.

hemiatrophy (hem′ēat′rōfē), *n* an atrophy of one half of the body, an organ, or a part (e.g., facial hemiatrophy).

hemidesmosome (hem′ēdez′mōsōm), *n* **1.** one half of a cell junction (desmosome). **2.** the connection site between the surface of the tooth and the epithelium as a part of the epithelial attachment as well as the interface between the epithelium and connective tissues.

hemifacial microsomia (HFM) (hem′ifā′shəl mī′krəsō′mēə), *n* a condition in which one side of the lower face fails to develop properly. It is characterized by the malformation of the ear on the affected side and defects in the structure of the mandible. It is the second most common birth defect after clefts. Also called *brachial arch syndrome, oral-mandibular-auricular syndrome, lateral facial dysplasia,* or *otomandibular dysostosis.*

hemiglossectomy (hem′ēglôsek′təmē), *n* the surgical removal of half of the tongue.

hemihydrate, *n* a chemical compound in which the number of water molecules is half that of the other portion of the compound. In dentistry, hemihydrates are used in the manufacture of crowns, inlays, bridges, and dental molds.

hemihypertrophy (hem′ēhīpur′trəfē), *n* an excessive growth of half of the body, an organ, or a part (e.g., hemihyperplasia of the tongue).

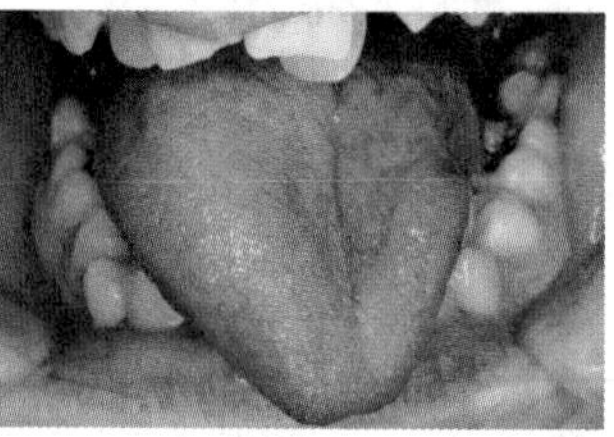

Hemihypertrophy. (Neville/Damm/Allen/Bouquot, 2002. Courtesy Dr. George Blozis)

hemiplegia (hem′ēplē′jēə), *n* the paralysis of one side of the body.

hemisection, *n* the complete sectioning through the crown of a tooth into the furcation region.

hemochromatosis (hē′mōkrō′mətō′sis), *n* an uncommon disorder, usually a complication of hemolytic anemia, that results in a surplus of iron deposits throughout the body. See also hemosiderosis; iron metabolism; siderosis; and thalassemia.

hemocyte, *n* a generic term referring to any cellular or formed element of the blood. Synonym: *hematocyte.*

hemodialysis (hē′mōdīal′isis), *n* a procedure in which impurities or wastes are removed from the blood. The patient's blood is shunted from the body through a machine for diffusion and ultrafiltration and returned to the patient's circulation. This procedure is used in treating renal failure and various toxic conditions. Without this, toxic wastes build up in the blood and tissues and cannot be filtered out by the ailing kidneys. This condition is known as uremia, which means "urine in the blood." Eventually, this waste buildup leads to death. Dental treatment should occur within 24 hours of hemodialysis. See also kidney failure.

hemodynamics, *n* the study of the physical aspects of blood circulation, including cardiac function and peripheral vascular physiology.

hemoglobin (hē'mōglōbin), *n* the oxygen-carrying red pigment of the red blood corpuscles. It is a reddish, crystallizable conjugated protein consisting of the protein globulin combined with the prosthetic group, heme.

hemoglobin A (HBA), *n* a normal hemoglobin. Also called *adult hemoglobin.*

hemoglobin estimation, *n* a determination of the hemoglobin content of the blood. By the Sahli method, 14 to 17 g/100 mL of blood is normal, and 15.1 Sahli units are taken as 100% for estimation of hemoglobin percentages.

hemoglobinopathy (hē'mōglō'binop'əthē), *n* a group of genetically determined diseases involving abnormal hemoglobin (e.g., sickle cell disease, in which hemoglobin S occurs, and hemoglobin C disease).

hemoglobinopathy, paroxysmal nocturnal, *n* an acquired hemolytic anemia of unknown cause characterized by increased hemolysis during sleep, resulting in the presence of hemoglobin in the urine on awakening.

hemogram, dental (hē'məgram'), *n* a simple blood test that measures the numbers, proportions, and morphologic characteristics of the blood cells. In dentistry, hemograms are used to determine the amount of bleeding in the dental pulp after the treatment of cavities.

hemohydremia, anhydremia, *n* a decrease in blood volume resulting from a decrease in the serum component of blood; occurs in shock or any condition in which blood fluid is passed into the tissue and results in hemoconcentration. (not current)

hemolysin (hēmol'isin), *n* an antibody that causes hemolysis of red blood cells in vitro.

hemolysis (himol'isis), *n* the breakdown of red blood cells and the release of hemoglobin that occurs normally at the end of the life span of a red blood cell.

hemophilia (bleeder's disease) (hē'mōfil'ēə), *n* a sex-linked genetic disease manifested in males and characterized by severe hemorrhage.

hemophilia A (classic hemophilia), *n* a hemorrhagic diathesis resulting from a deficiency of antihemophilic globulin (AHG); inherited as a recessive sex-linked characteristic and characterized by recurrent bouts of bleeding from even trivial injury. The coagulation time is prolonged, but the bleeding time is normal.

hemophilia B (Christmas disease, hemophilia II, hemophilioid state C), *n* a hemorrhagic diathesis resulting from a deficiency of plasma thromboplastin component (PTC); transmitted as a sex-linked recessive characteristic and characterized clinically by the same manifestations as classic hemophilia. There is a delay in the generation of thromboplastin. The platelet count, bleeding time, tourniquet test, and thrombin and prothrombin times are normal.

hemophilia C (plasma thromboplastin antecedent [PTA] deficiency, Rosenthal's syndrome), *n* a hemophilia-like condition believed to result from a deficiency of plasma thromboplastin antecedent (PTA), transmitted as a simple autosomal dominant trait and characterized by a moderate bleeding tendency after extraction of teeth or after tonsillectomy. Prothrombin consumption and thromboplastin generation are abnormal. See also factor XI.

hemophilia, classic, *n* See hemophilia A.

hemophilia, vascular, *n* a hereditary hemorrhagic disorder affecting both sexes and associated with a deficiency of antihemophilic globulin and vascular abnormalities characteristic of pseudohemophilia (von Willebrand disease). The bleeding time is prolonged, and severity of bleeding varies considerably among persons with this condition.

hemophilioid state C (hē'mōfil'ēoid), *n* See hemophilia B.

H

hemopoiesis (hē′mōpōē′sis), *n* See hematopoiesis.

hemoptysis (hēmop′tisis), *n* the expectoration of blood, by coughing, from the larynx or lower respiratory tract.

hemorrhage (hem′ərəj), *n* the escape of a large amount of blood from the blood vessels in a short period; excessive bleeding.

hemorrhage, pulpal **(hem′ərij pul′pəl),** *n* bleeding in the pulp of a tooth. Such bleeding may occur during dental extractions and restorations and are often controlled by the application of a hemostatic agent.

hemorrhagic bone cyst, *n* See cyst, hemorrhagic.

hemorrhagic diathesis, *n* an inherited predisposition to any one of a number of abnormalities characterized by excessive bleeding.

hemosiderin (hē′mōsid′ərin), *n* an intracellular storage form of iron; the granules consist of an ill-defined complex of ferric hydroxides, polysaccharides, and proteins having an iron content of approximately 33% by weight. It appears as a dark yellow-brown pigment.

hemosiderosis (hē′mōsid′ərō′sis), *n* a focal or general increase in tissue iron stores without associated tissue damage.

hemostasis (hē′mōstā′sis), *n* the arrest of an escape of blood.

hemostat (hē′mōstat), *n* a procedure or device that stops the flow of blood.

hemostatic (hē′mōstat′ik), *n* an agent used to reduce bleeding from small blood vessels by speeding up the clotting of blood or by the formation of an artificial clot.

***Hepadnaviridae* (hepad″nəvir′ĭdē),** *n* one of the major virus families, to which the hepatitis B virus belongs. Viruses in this family have a double-stranded incomplete circular molecular structure with icosahedral symmetry.

heparin/heparin calcium/heparin sodium, *n brand names:* Hep Lock, Liquaemin Sodium; *drug class:* anticoagulant; *action:* acts in combination with antithrombin III (heparin cofactor) to inhibit thrombosis; inactivates factor Xa and inhibits conversion of prothrombin to thrombin; affects both intrinsic and extrinsic clotting pathways; *uses:* anticoagulant in thrombosis, embolism, coagulopathies, deep vein thrombosis, dialysis, maintenance of patency of indwelling intravenous lines.

heparinized lock system, *n* an indwelling intravenous system by which multiple daily intravenous accesses can be accomplished and multiple penetrations of the veins can be avoided. The heparin chamber prevents the formation of a clot or thrombus at the needle site.

hepatitis (hep′ətī′tis), *n* an inflammation of the liver.

hepatitis C (Hep C, non-A, non-B hepatitis), n a type transmitted largely by blood transfusion or percutaneous inoculation, such as with intravenous drug users sharing needles. The disease progresses to chronic hepatitis in up to 50% of the patients acutely infected.

hepatitis, chronic active, n a hepatitis with chronic portal inflammation with regional necrosis and fibrosis, which may progress to nodular postnecrotic cirrhosis.

hepatitis, delta (Hep D), n a particularly virulent form caused by the delta hepatitis virus in conjunction with the hepatitis B virus (HBV), which is spread by contaminated needles or by direct exposure to blood or other body fluids from infected individuals. It occurs primarily in persons who have been repeatedly exposed to the HBV either through frequent blood transfusions or intravenous drug use. It may also be spread during the birthing process.

hepatitis delta virus (HDV), n the infectious agent that causes delta hepatitis, but only in the presence of the hepatitis B virus. The virus is usually superimposed on carriers of the hepatitis B surface antigen (HBsAg). It is also called the *delta agent.*

hepatitis E (Hep E, epidemic non-A, non-B hepatitis), n a self-limited type of hepatitis caused by the hepatitis E virus (HEV) that may occur after natural disasters because of fecal-contaminated water or food. There is currently no serologic test available.

hepatitis G, n a viral infection of the stomach and intestines, transmitted via blood and coinfection with the hepatitis C virus. The duration of the incubation period and range of symptoms are unknown, and no vaccine is available.

hepatitis, homologous serum (homologous serum jaundice, serum hepatitis, syringe jaundice, type B hepatitis), n a viral hepatitis clinically difficult to distinguish from epidemic infectious hepatitis. It is transmitted by human serum (that is, through parenteral injection, transfusions, lacerations). The incubation period is 40 to 90 days or longer. Principal manifestations are jaundice, gastrointestinal symptoms, anorexia, and malaise.

hepatitis, infectious (IH, type A hepatitis), n a viral hepatitis that is frequently epidemic in nature and has an incubation period of 1 to 4 or even 7 weeks. It is usually transmitted by the virus in fecal matter but may be transmitted by human (transfusions, lacerations, needle punctures).

hepatitis, non-ABCDE, n a viral infection of the stomach and intestines that is diagnosed by ruling out other forms of hepatitis. It may be transmitted orally, via injection, sexual contact, or fecal matter.

hepatitis, serum, n See *hepatitis, homologous serum.*

hepatitis, viral, n **1.** hepatitis caused by one of three immunologically unrelated viruses: hepatitis A virus; hepatitis B virus; and non-A, non-B virus. *n* **2.** hepatitis caused by a viral infection, including that by Epstein-Barr virus and cytomegalovirus.

hepatomegaly, abnormal (hep′ətōmeg′əlē), *n* an enlargement of the liver that is usually a sign of liver disease. It is usually discovered by percussion and palpation as part of a physical examination. It may be caused by hepatitis, fatty infiltration, alcoholism, biliary obstruction, or malignancy.

Herbst appliance, *n.pr* the only fixed, tooth-borne, functional orthodontic appliance in which jaw position is influenced by a pin-and-tube spring-loaded appliance that is cemented or bonded to the teeth.

hereditary benign intraepithelial dyskeratosis (həred′iter′ē bənīn′ in′trəep′əthē′lēəl dis′kerətō′sis), *n* a hereditary disease seen in triracial isolates (whites, Native Americans, blacks). It involves the oral mucosa and may cause periodic seasonal keratoconjunctivitis.

hereditary opalescent dentin (həred′iter′ē ō′pəles′ənt den′tin), *n* a developmental disturbance in the formation of dentin, better known as dentiogenesis imperfecta. The teeth range from gray to brownish violet and are translucent or opalescent. The crowns fracture easily because of an abnormal dentinoenamel junction.

heredity (hered′itē), *n* the inheritance of resemblance, physical qualities, or disease from a familial predecessor; the passage of characteristics from one generation to its progeny by genetic linkage.

Hering-Breuer reflex (her′ing-broi′ur), *n.pr* See reflex, Hering-Breuer.

hermetic seal, *n* See seal, hermetic.

hernia (hur′nēə), *n* the protrusion of an organ through an abnormal opening in the muscle wall of the cavity that surrounds it. It may be congenital, may result from the failure of certain structures to close after birth, or may be acquired later in life because of obesity, muscular weakness, surgery, or illness.

hernia, hiatal, n a protrusion of a portion of the stomach upward through the diaphragm. The condition occurs in approximately 40% of individuals and most people display few, if any, symptoms. The major difficulty is gastroesophageal reflux, which is the backflow of the acid contents of the stomach into the esophagus.

hernia, inguinal (direct), n a protrusion of the intestines into an opening between the deep epigastric artery and the edge of the rectus muscle; (indirect) involves the internal inguinal ring and passes into the inguinal canal.

heroin (her′ōin), *n* a highly addictive alkaloid prepared from morphine, previously used for cough relief. Use is prohibited by federal law because of its highly addictive properties and potential for abuse.

herpangina (hur′panjī′nə), *n* (Coxsackie A disease), a viral disease of children, usually occurring in summer, and characterized by sudden onset, fever (100° to 105° F; 38° to 40.5° C), sore throat, and oropharyngeal vesicles. Herpangina results from Coxsackie A viruses and is self-limiting.

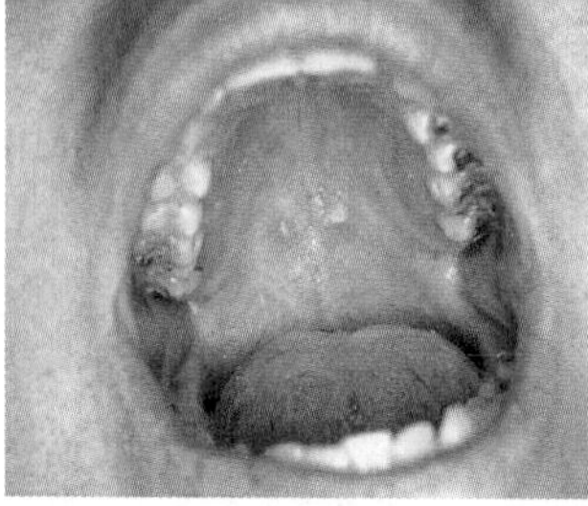

Herpangina. (Ibsen/Phelan, 2004)

herpangina aphthous ulcer, *n* See aphthous pharyngitis.

herpes labialis (hur′pēz lā′bēal′is), (cold sore), a disease of the lips caused by herpes simplex virus and characterized by vesicles that rupture, leaving ulcers. The local lesions are often called *fever blisters* or *cold sores.* Also called *herpes simplex of the lips.* See also herpes simplex.

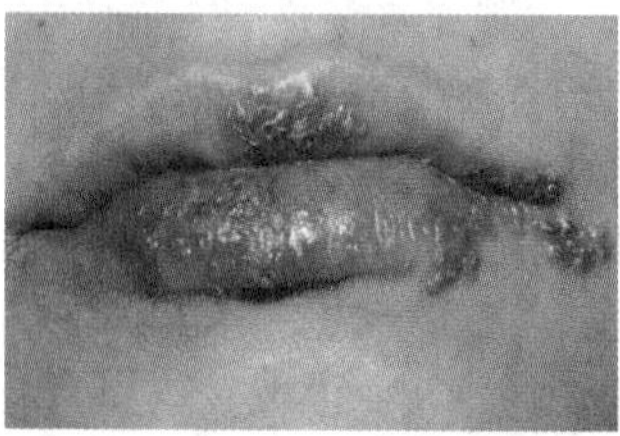

Herpes labialis. (Neville/Damm/Allen/Bouquot, 2002)

herpes simplex (hur′pēz sim′plex), *n* an infection caused by the herpes simplex virus. Primary infection, occurring most often in children between 2 and 5 years of age, may result in apparent clinical disease or such manifestations as acute herpetic gingivostomatitis, keratoconjunctivitis, vulvovaginitis, or encephalitis. Recurrent manifestations may include herpes labialis (fever blisters or cold sores), dendritic corneal ulcers, or genital herpes simplex. See also herpes labialis and gingivostomatitis, herpetic.

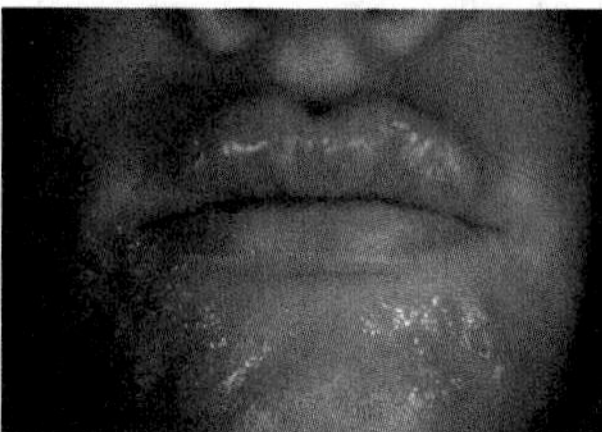

Herpes simplex. (Courtesy Dr. Donald Schermer)

herpes zoster (hur′pēz zos′tur), *n* an acute viral disease involving the dorsal spinal root or cranial nerve and producing unilateral vesicular eruption in areas of the skin corresponding to the involved sensory nerve. Pain is a prominent feature and may persist, although skin lesions subside in 1 to 2 weeks. It is caused by the varicella zoster virus, which is also responsible for childhood chickenpox. A vaccine against herpes zoster is now available. Colloquial term: *shingles.*

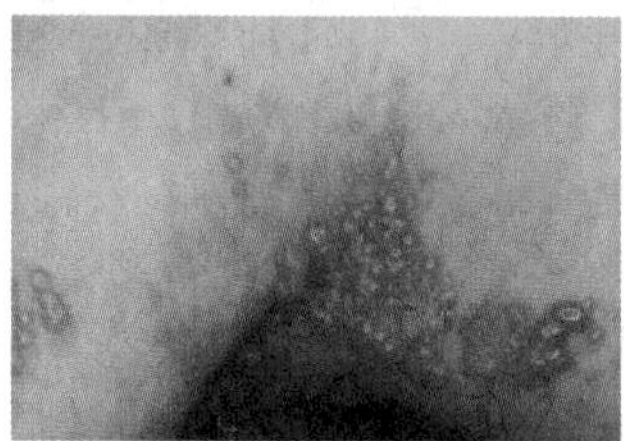

Herpes zoster. (Ibsen/Phelan, 2004)

Herpesviridae **(hər″pēzvi′rīde),** *n* one of the major virus families, to which the herpes simplex, varicella zoster, and Epstein-Barr viruses belong. Viruses in this family have a double-stranded linear molecular structure with icosahedral symmetry.

herpetic lesion, *n* See lesion, herpetic.

herpetic whitlow (hurpet′ik hwit′lō), *n* See whitlow, herpetic.

Hertwig's (epithelial) root sheath, *n* an elongation of the cervical loop, which helps determine the shape, size, and number of roots and which influences the formation of dentin in the root area during the developmental stages of a tooth.

heteresthesia (het′əresthē′zēə, -zhə), *n* a variation in the degree of cutaneous sensibility on adjoining areas of the body surface.

heterograft, *n* See graft, heterogenous.

heteropolysaccharides (het′ərō-pol′ēsak′ərīdz), *n.pl* the complex carbohydrates formed by combining carbohydrates with noncarbohydrates or carbohydrate derivatives; examples include pectin, lignin, glycoproteins, glycolipids, and mucopolysaccharides.

heterosexual, *n* a person with a sexual attraction to or preference for persons of the opposite gender; *adj* having erotic attraction to, predisposition to, or sexual activity with a person of the opposite gender.

heterotrophic (het′ərōtrof′ik), *adj* pertaining to an organism that must depend on others to provide sustenance. Parasitic.

heterozygous (het′ərōzī′gus), *adj* a term indicating that genes lying at equivalent loci on chromosome pairs are different.

hexamethonium (heksəmethō-nēəm), *n* a cholinergic blocking agent used to control bleeding and used in the treatment of peptic ulcers and hypertension. It produces ganglion blocking by occupying receptor sites.

hexosamine (heksō′səmēn), *n* the amine derivative (NH2 replacing OH) of a hexose such as glucosamine.

HGF, *n* See glucagon.

HIAA, *n.pr* the abbreviation for Health Insurance Association of America.

hiccup, *n* an involuntary spasmodic contraction of the diaphragm that causes a beginning inspiration that is suddenly checked by closure of the glottis, thus producing a characteristic sound.

hidradenoma, *n* a benign neoplasm derived from epithelial cells of sweat glands.

hidrocystoma (hī′drōsistō′mə), *n* a cystic form of sweat gland adenoma. A hidrocystoma is produced by the cystic proliferation of apocrine secretory glands. It is not uncommon, occurring in adult life in no particular age group, with males and females equally affected. The most common site is around the eye. Hidrocystomas are cured by surgical removal.

hierarchy (hī′ərär′kē), *n* **1.** system of persons or things ranked one above the other. *n* **2.** in psychology and psychiatry, an organization of habits or concepts in which simpler components are combined to form increasingly complex integrations.

hierarchy, Maslow's, See Maslow's hierarchy.

high blood pressure, *n* See hypertension.

high labial arch, *n* See arch, high labial.

high lip line, *n* See lip line, high.

high speed, *n* See speed, high.

high-pull headgear, *n* an apparatus designed to give an upward pull on the face-bow.

high-speed handpiece, *n* See handpiece, high-speed.

hilus (hī′lus), *n* an indentation appearing on an organ or other internal structure, such as a lymph node, at the point where nerves and vessels enter. Also called *hilum.*

hinchazon (hinch′əzon), *n* See beriberi.

hinge axis, *n* See axis, hinge.

hinge axis, determination, *n* See axis, condylar, determination.

hinge axis, orbital plane, *n* See axis, hinge, orbital plane.

hinge axis point, *n* See point, hinge axis.

hinge movement, *n* See movement, hinge.

hinge position, *n* See position, hinge.

hinge-bow, *n* the kinematic face-bow used to determine the location of the hinge axis. The hinge-bow is a three-piece instrument with independently adjustable arms controlled by micrometer screws that lengthen or shorten them. Other micrometer screws raise or lower the caliper points to find the spots in or on the skin near the tragi where only rotary movements occur when the jaw is opened and closed at the rearmost point. See also face-bow, kinematic.

HIPAA, *n.pr* See Health Insurance Portability and Accountability Act (HIPAA).

hippocampus (hip′ōkam′pəs), *n* a curved convoluted elevation of the floor of the inferior horn of the lateral ventricle of the brain. It is composed of gray substance covered by a layer of white fibers, or the alveus, and functions as an important component of the limbic system.

hippus, respiratory (hip′əs), *n* a dilation of the pupils occurring during inspiration and a contraction of the pupils occurring during expiration; often associated with pulsus paradoxus.

Hirschfeld-Dunlop file, *n.pr* See file, Hirschfeld-Dunlop.

Hirschfeld's method, *n.pr* See point, Hirschfeld's silver.

hirsutism (hir′sootizəm), *n* increased body or facial hair, which is especially noted in the female.

histamine (his′təmēn′), *n* a compound found in all cells that is produced by the breakdown of histidine. It is released in allergic, inflammatory reactions and causes dilation of capillaries, decreased blood pressure, increased secretion of gastric juice, and constriction of smooth muscles of the bronchi and uterus.

histamine blocker, *n* a drug used in the treatment of gastroesophageal reflux disease, including cimetidine, nizatidine, and ranitidine. The drug inhibits the release of stomach acid and reduces pain caused by introduction of stomach acids to esophagus.

histidine (his′tidēn), *n* an essential amino acids for infants and children. See also amino acid.

histiocyte (his′tēəsīt′), *n* a large phagocytic cell found in the interstices of the tissues; of reticuloendothelial origin.

histiocytosis, acute disseminated, X, *n* See disease, Letterer-Siwe.

histiocytosis, chronic disseminated X, *n* See disease, Hand-Schüller-Christian.

histiocytosis, Langerhans cell (histiocytosis X, Langerhans cell disease), *n* a group of diseases characterized by a proliferation of abnormal histiocytoid cells. Includes: **1.** Chronic disseminated histiocytosis (Hand-Schüller-Christian disease); **2.** Acute disseminated histiocytosis (Letterer-Siwe disease); and **3.** eosinophilic granulomas.

histiocytosis, nonlipid (his′tēōsītō′sis), *n* See disease, Letterer-Siwe.

histoclasia, implant (his′tōklā′zēə), *n* a condition of the tissues existing in the presence of an implant, in which the implant is not directly involved. It is a condition of the oral mucosal tissues, in which the pathologic condition results from some external cause (e.g., calculus, attached prosthetic appliances).

histocompatibility, *n* the compatibility of the antigens of donor and recipient of transplanted tissue.

histocompatibility testing, *n* the determination of the compatibility of the antigens of donor and recipient before tissue transplantation. Usually follows a blood typing protocol.

histocytoma (his′tōsītō′mə), *n* a tumor composed of histiocytes.

histodifferentiation (his′tōdif′ər-en′shēā′shən), *n* the process in which cells develop the distinctive characteristics of the tissues to which they are to belong.

histogenesis (his′tōjen′isis), *n* a series of integrated processes that occur during embryonic development wherein undifferentiated cells assume the characteristics of the various tissues contained in the human body. These undifferentiated cells comprise part of the three primary germ layers, the endoderm, mesoderm, and ectoderm.

histogram, *n* a bar graph; a graphic representation of a frequency distribution.

histology (histol′əjē), *n* microanatomy, which is the microscopic study of normal tissue and organs at the cellular level.

histology, oral, of soft tissues, *n* See epithelium, oral; lamina, propria; submucosa; and membrane, basement.

histomorphometry (his′tōmorfäm′ətrē), *n* a method used to accurately quantify the level of cellular activity and the amount of existing bone mass. Such methods include bone biopsies performed to determine the underlying cause for osteoporosis.

histopathology (his′tōpəthol′əjē), *n* the microscopic study of abnormal tissue and organs at the cellular level.

histoplasmosis (his′tōplazmō′sis), *n* a disease caused by the fungus *H. capsulatum* and affecting the reticuloendothelial system. Ulceration of the oral mucosa may occur.

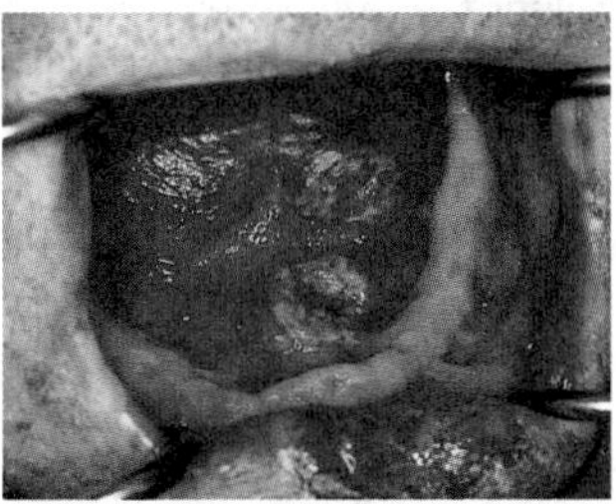

Histoplasmosis. (Regezi/Sciubba/Pogrel, 2000)

history, case, *n* a detailed and concise compilation of all physical, dental, social, and mental factors relative and necessary to diagnosis, prognosis, and treatment.

history, case, forms, *n.pl* questionnaires to aid the practitioner in taking medical history; should cover all aspects of patient's prior medical history; the American Dental Association distributes a basic health form that may provide a baseline.

history, case, hepatic disease, *n* as part of the process of taking a medical history, practitioner should ask patient for details of and occurrences of liver disease or drug metabolism problems.

history case, self-medication, *n* as part of the medical history process, practitioner should ask patient for descriptions of the type and frequency of self-administered medication as well as any history of substance abuse; this information can help eliminate complications in patient treatment schedules.

histotoxic (his′tōtăk′sik), *adj* relating to poisoning of the respiratory enzyme system of the tissues.

HIV, *n* See human immunodeficiency virus (HIV).

HIV gingivitis (HIV-G), *n* an aggressive form of periodontal disease presenting with a distinct type of gingivitis found in HIV-infected patients, characterized by an intensely red linear erythemic band (LGE) around the free gingiva that extends 2 to 3 mm apically into the attached gingiva. The involved gingiva tends to bleed spontaneously and may be present even in AIDS patients with good oral hygiene.

HIV periodontitis (HIV-P), *n* an aggressive form of periodontal disease with all the characteristics of HIV-G combined with those of periodontitis: soft tissue ulceration and necrosis and rapid destruction of the periodontium and bone. The condition is very painful. HIV-P may resemble acute necrotizing ulcerative gingivitis (ANUG). However, ANUG is limited to the soft tissue, whereas HIV-P disease extends into the crestal bone.

HIV-1, *n* the abbreviation for *human immunodeficiency virus type 1,* which is widely recognized as the causal agent of acquired immunodeficiency syndrome (AIDS). HIV-1 is characterized by its cytopathic effect and affinity for the T4-lymphocyte.

HIV-2, *n* the abbreviation *for human immunodeficiency virus type 2,* which is related to HIV-1 but carries different antigenic components with differing nucleic acid composition. It shares serologic reactivity and sequence homology with the simian lentivirus simian immunodeficiency virus (SIV) and infects only T4-lymphocytes expressing the CD4 phenotypic marker.

HIV-G, *n* See HIV gingivitis.

HIV-P, *n* See HIV periodontitis.

HIV-wasting syndrome, *n* a constitutional disease associated with AIDS, also known as the *slim disease.* Patients in this subgroup have a history of fever of more than 1 month, involuntary weight loss of more than 10%, or diarrhea persisting for more than 1 month.

hives, *n* See urticaria.

Hodgkin disease, *n.pr* See lymphoma, Hodgkin.

hoe, *n* an angled instrument with the broad dimension of its blade perpendicular to the axis of the shank of the shaft.

hold, *v* to possess by reason of a lawful title.

hold harmless clause, *n* a contract provision in which one party to the contract promises to be responsible for liability incurred by the other party. Hold harmless clauses frequently appear in the following contexts: (1) Contracts between dental benefits organizations and an individual dental professional often contain a promise by the dental professional to reimburse the dental benefits organization for any liability the organization incurs because of dental treatment provided to beneficiaries of the organization's dental benefits plan. This may include a promise to pay the dental benefits organization's attorney fees and related costs. (2) Contracts between dental benefits organizations and a group plan sponsor may include a promise by the dental benefits organization to assume responsibility for disputes between a beneficiary of the group plan and an individual dental professional when the dental professional's charge exceeds the amount the organization pays for the service on behalf of the beneficiary. If the dental professional takes action against the patient to recover the difference between the amount billed by the dental professional and the amount paid by the organization, the dental benefits organization will take over the defense of the claim and will pay any judgments and court costs.

H

holder, *n* an apparatus or instrument that is used to hold something.

film holder, precision, *n* a stainless steel device used to hold the film firmly in place during a dental radiographic procedure, which provides the rectangular collimation necessary for the paralleling technique.

film holder, Rinn X-C-P, *n* a name brand reusable film-positioning device with aiming capability made from a combination of plastic and stainless steel that is especially suited to the paralleling technique.

film holder, Stabe, *n.pr* a name brand disposable film-positioning device made from styrofoam that is especially suited to the paralleling or bisecting angle techniques.

holder, broach, *n* See broach holder.

holder, clamp, *n* See holder, rubber dam clamp.

holder, matrix, *n* See retainer, matrix.

holder, rubber dam, *n* an apparatus used to hold a rubber dam in place on the face and to secure the edges of the dam clear of the field of operation.

holder, rubber dam clamp (clamp holder), *n* See forceps, rubber dam clamp.

holistic health, *n* a concept in which concern for health requires a perspective of the individual as an integrated system rather than as a collection of parts and functions.

Hollenback condenser, *n.pr* See condenser, pneumatic.

hollow bulb, *n* a portion of a prosthesis made hollow to minimize weight.

holoprosencephaly (hō′lōpros′ən-sef′əlē), *n* a congenital defect caused by the failure of the prosencephalon to divide into hemispheres during embryonic development. It is characterized by multiple midline facial defects, including cyclopia in severe cases.

homatropine hydrobromide (optic) (hōmat′rōpēn′ hī′drōbrō′mīd), *n brand names:* AK-Homatropine, Isopto Homatropine; *drug class:* mydriatic (topical); *action:* blocks response of iris sphincter muscle and muscle of accommodation of ciliary body to cholinergic stimulation, resulting in dilation and paralysis of accommodation; *uses:* cycloplegic refraction, uveitis, mydriatic lens opacities.

home care, *n* the physiotherapeutic measures employed by the patient for the maintenance of dental and periodontal health. Includes proper cleaning with a toothbrush, floss, or other device. Older term: *oral hygiene.*

home health agency, *n* an organization that provides health care in the home. Medicare certification for a home health agency depends on the providing of skilled nursing services and of at least one additional therapeutic service, usually physical or occupational therapy.

homeostasis (hō′mēōstā′sis), *n* the term used to describe the tendency toward physiologic equilibration (e.g., acid-base balance, pH level of blood, blood sugar level).

homeostasis, cell, *n* the tendency of biologic tissues and processes to maintain a constancy of environment consistent with their vitality and well being. For cells to maintain their stability or equilibrium, the cell membranes must be in continuous interaction with both the internal (intracellular) environment and the external (extracellular) environment. When the equilibrium of any component is disturbed, the interaction permits automatic readjustment by giving rise to stimuli that result in restoration of the equilibrium.

homocystinuria (hō′mōsis′tinyoo′rēə), *n* a genetic disorder of amino acid metabolism in which the amino acid homocystine appears in the blood and urine; may respond to a low-protein diet and the administration of synthetic amino acids.

homograft, *n* See graft, homogenous.

homopolysaccharides (hō′mōpol′ēsak′ərēdz), *n.pl* the complex carbohydrates formed from at least six identical monosaccharides; examples include starch, glycogen, cellulose, and insulin.

homosexual, *n* a person with a sexual attraction to or preference for persons of the same gender; *adj* having erotic attraction to, predisposition to, or sexual activity with a person of the same gender.

homovanillic acid (hō′mōvənil′ik), *n* an acid that is produced by normal metabolism of dopamine and may be elevated in the urine in association with tumors of the adrenal gland.

homozygous (hō′mōzī′gus), *adj* a term indicating that genes lying at equivalent loci on chromosome pairs are the same.

hone, *v* to sharpen.

hook, skin, *n* a metallic instrument ending in a fine, sharp hook for handling soft tissues during surgery.

Hoover's sign, *n.pr* See sign, Hoover's.

HOP, *n* the abbreviation for high oxygen pressure.

horizontal bone loss, *n* a form of bone loss secondary to periodontal disease. This form of bone loss is more generalized than vertical bone loss and is characterized by the loss in height of the four walls surrounding the tooth roots. It may affect only the nearby teeth or may involve the entire dental arch.

horizontal overlap, *n* See overlap, horizontal.

horizontal plane, *n* See plane, horizontal.

horizontal position, *n* a posture in which the body lies flat and the feet and head remain on the same level. Also called *supine.*

horizontal scrub, *n* a form of tooth brushing in which the brush is held at a 45° angle to the neck of the tooth and is moved across the surface of the teeth in short horizontal movements.

hormone(s) (hôr′mōn[z]), *n.pl* the biochemical secretions of the endocrine glands that, in relatively small quantities, partially regulate the physiologic activity of the tissues, organs, organ systems, and other endocrine glands, and of the nervous system itself. Its secretions are conducted and distributed throughout the body by the circulation of the bloodstream and tissue fluids.

hormones, adenohypophyseal, *n.pl* the hormones secreted by the adenohypophysis. Includes seven distinct hormones: somatotropin (STH), thyrotropin (TSH), prolactin, follicle-stimulating hormone (FSH), luteinizing hormone (LH), melanocyte-stimulating hormone (MSH), and adrenocorticotropic hormone (ACTH).

hormones, adrenal medullary, *n.pl* the hormones secreted by adrenal medulla, including two catecholamines: epinephrine and norepinephrine.

hormones, adrenocortical, *n* the steroid hormones secreted by the adrenal cortex that are biologically active in one or more of the following states: stress, inflammation, metabolism of carbohydrates, proteins, electrolytes, and water.

hormones, adrenocorticotropic, *n* See ACTH.

hormones, adrenotropic, *n* See ACTH.

hormones, anabolic, *n.pl* the hormones that decrease blood glucose; an example is insulin. See also anabolic steroids.

hormones, androgenic, *n.pl* See hormones, sex, male.

hormones, anterior pituitary-like, *n* See hormone, pregnancy.

hormones, antidiabetic, *n* See insulin.

hormones, antidiuretic (ADH, vasopressin), *n* a hormone of the posterior pituitary gland that encourages resorption of water by acting on the epithelial cells of the distal portion of the renal tubule. It raises blood pressure by its effect on the peripheral blood vessels and exerts an antidiuretic effect (antifacultative resorption of water in the renal tubules). An absence of antidiuretic hormone causes diabetes insipidus.

hormones, antiinflammatory, *n.pl* See glucocorticoids.

hormones, catabolic, *n.pl* the hormones that increase blood glucose; examples include glucagon, epinephrine, steroid and growth hormones, and thyroxine.

hormones, chorionic gonadotropic, *n* a glycoprotein secreted by placental tissue early in normal pregnancy. This protein is also found in the urine or blood in association with chorioepitheliomas and some neoplastic diseases of the testes.

H

hormones, corticosteroid, *n* See steroid, adrenocortical.

hormones, corticotropic, *n* the ovarian or adrenal hormones (e.g., estradiol, estrone, estriol) that are capable of stimulating changes of a cyclic nature in the genital system. One of the ovarian or adrenal hormones capable of affecting the cyclic changes of the female genital system. See also ACTH.

hormones, female sex, *n.pl* the hormones secreted by the ovary. They include two main types: the follicular, or estrogenic, hormones produced by the graafian follicle, and the progestational hormones from the corpus luteum.

hormones, follicle-stimulating, a pituitary tropic hormone that promotes the growth and maturation of the ovarian follicle and, with other gonadotropins, induces secretion of estrogens and possibly spermatogenesis.

hormones, gastrointestinal, *n* the hormones that regulate motor and secretory activity of the digestive organs; that is, gastrin, secretin, and cholecystokinin.

hormones, gonadotropic, *n* See gonadotropin.

hormones, growth (somatotropic hormone, somatotropin), *n* a hormone that is secreted by the anterior lobe of the pituitary gland and that exerts an influence on skeletal growth. As long as the growth apparatus is functional, it is responsive to the effects of the hormone.

hormones, ketogenic, *n* the term used to describe a factor of the anterior pituitary hormone responsible for ketogenic effect. It is probably not an entity differing from known pituitary hormones.

hormones, lactogenic (galactin, mammotropin, prolactin), *n* a pituitary hormone that stimulates lactation.

hormones, luteal, *n* See hormones, progestational.

hormones, luteinizing, *n* a pituitary hormone that causes ovulation and development of the corpus luteum from the mature graafian follicle. It is called an *interstitial cell and stimulating hormone* because of its action on the testis in maintaining spermatogenesis and because of its role in the development of accessory sex organs.

hormones, male sex (androgenic hormone, C-19 steroids), *n.pl* the hormones found in the testes, urine, and blood. Included are testosterone found in the testes, andosterone excreted into the urine, and dehydro-3-epiandrosterone found in the blood.

hormones, melanocyte-stimulating (MSH, intermedin), *n* a hormone of the middle lobe of the pituitary gland that increases melanin deposition by the melanocytes of the skin.

hormones, N, *n* See hormone, nitrogen and steroid, C-19 cortico.

hormones, neurohypophyseal, *n.pl* the octapeptides of the neural lobe: oxytocin and vasopressin.

hormones, nitrogen (N hormone), *n.pl* the C-19 corticosteroids that have androgenic and protein anabolic effects.

hormones, parathyroid, *n* the secretory product of the parathyroid glands that promotes bone resorption and increases renal resorption of calcium and magnesium and diminishes that of phosphate. Excessive secretion produces generalized bone resorption, formation of fibrous marrow in the spongiosa, and, in young individuals, hypocalcification of the teeth.

hormones, pituitary, *n.pl* the hormones of the anterior lobe of the pituitary gland, including the growth hormones (somatotropin 1, lactogenic hormone, prolactin, galactin, mammotropin) and pituitary tropins (gonadotropins, thyrotropic hormone, and ACTH). Whether or not a true diabetogenic pituitary hormone exists is a question. The melanocyte-stimulating hormone is secreted by the middle lobe of the pituitary gland, and vasopressin and oxytocin are secreted by the posterior lobe of the pituitary gland.

hormones, pregnancy (anterior pituitary-like hormone, antuitrin S, chorionic gonadotropin), *n* a gonadotropic hormone found in the urine during pregnancy; it is a product of the very early placenta.

hormones, progestational (luteal hormone), *n.pl* the hormones produced during the phase of the menstrual cycle just preceding menstruation. Includes progesterone, pregnanediol, and pregneninolone.

hormones, proinflammatory, *n* See mineralocorticoids.

hormones, "S" (glucocorticoid factor, sugar hormone), *n* a factor in the secretions of the adrenal cortex related to the regulation of carbohydrate metabolism.

hormones, sex, *n.pl* the steroid hormones that are produced by the testes and ovaries and that control secondary sex characteristics, the reproductive cycle, development of the accessory reproductive cycle, and development of the accessory reproductive organs. Also included are the gonadotropins produced by the pituitary gland.

hormones, somatotropic, *n* See hormone, growth.

hormones, steroid, *n.pl* a group of biologically active organic compounds that are secreted by the adrenal cortex, testes, ovary, and placenta, and that have in common a cyclopentanoperhydrophenanthrene nucleus.

hormones, sugar, *n* See hormone, "S" and steroid, C-21 cortico-.

hormones, testicular, *n.pl* the hormones elaborated by the testes (mainly testosterone) that promote the growth and function of the male genitalia and secondary sex characteristics and that have potent protein anabolic effects.

hormones, thyroid, *n.pl* the hormonal variants, including thyroxin and triiodothyronine, derived from the thyroid gland. They act as a catalyst for oxidative processes of the body cell and thus regulate the rates of body metabolism and stimulate body growth and maturation.

hormones, thyroid, thyroid-stimulating, *n* See hormone, thyrotropic.

hormones, thyrotropic (thyroid-stimulating hormone [TSH]), *n* a pituitary hormone that regulates the growth and activity of the thyroid gland.

horn, pulp, *n* a small projection of vital pulp tissue directly under a cusp or developmental lobe.

hospice (hos′pis), *n* a program under medical direction and nurse coordination that provides a variety of inpatient and home care for individuals who are terminally ill and their family members; provides calming and accommodating care that meets the special needs arising from the variety of stresses experienced during the final phases of illness, death, and grieving (e.g., emotional, physical, social, economic, and spiritual).

hospital staff privileges, *n* the authority given to a clinician to practice at a hospital within the scope of privileges granted to him or her by that hospital.

host site, *n* an anatomic area surgically prepared to receive an implant or graft.

hostility, *n* the tendency of an organism to threaten harm to another or to itself.

Howard's method, *n.pr* See method, Howard's.

Howe's silver nitrate, *n.pr* See silver nitrate, ammoniacal.

Howe's silver precipitation method, *n.pr* See method, Howe's silver precipitation.

Howship's lacuna, *n.pr* See lacuna, absorption.

hub, *n* that part of a needle that connects to a syringe barrel. Usually made of plastic or metal.

huffing, *n* the inhalation of common household products such as glue, solvents, hair spray, or gasoline to obtain a temporary euphoria. Specifically, huffing refers to soaking a rag, toilet paper, or sock in the household substance and inhaling. Long-term huffing may result in weight loss, disorientation, muscle weakness, irritability, depression, and even death.

human genome project, *n* a federally sponsored research project to identify and map the entire gene pool.

human herpes virus-6 (HHV-6), *n* the herpes virus responsible for causing a skin rash similar to the type seen in persons infected with mononucleosis.

human immunodeficiency virus (HIV), *n* a type of retrovirus that causes AIDS. Retroviruses produce the enzyme reverse transcriptase, which allows transcription of the viral genome onto the DNA of the host cell. It is transmitted through contact with an infected individual's blood, semen, cervical secretions, cerebrospinal fluid, or synovial fluid. It infects T-helper cells of the immune system and results in infection with a long incubation period, averaging 10 years.

human leukocyte antigen (HLA), *n* a collection of human genes on chromosome 6 that encode proteins that function in cells to transport antigens from within the cell to the cell surface. These proteins are sometimes referred to as the MHC, or major histocompatibility complex.

human needs diagnostic model, *n* one of four approaches to patient care, employs an eight-point analysis of needs to gauge the status of the patient's oral cavity, teeth, and gingivae.

human parvovirus B19 (pär′vō-vī′rəs), *n* also called *Erythema infectiosum* or *fifth disease;* spread via the upper respiratory tract, this virus impacts on children more strongly than adults.

human rights, *n.pl* the legal and moral rights recognized by national and international laws.

humectant (hūmek′tənt), *n* **1.** a substance that prevents loss of moisture. *n.pl* **2.** a substance contained in toothpastes, gels, and powders that prevents their chemical or physical decomposition by maintaining moisture.

humidifier, *n* a device for adding moisture to dry air inside the home to help counteract the reduction in saliva that often occurs as a result of hyposalivation, radiation therapy, or other treatments that cause xerostomia.

humidity, *n* pertaining to the level of moisture in the atmosphere, the amount varying with the temperature. The percentage is usually represented in terms of relative humidity, with 100% being the point of air saturation or the level at which the air can absorb no additional water without an increase in temperature.

Hunt's syndrome, *n.pr* See syndrome, Ramsay Hunt.

Hunter's glossitis, *n.pr* See glossitis, Moeller's.

Huntington's chorea (hun′ting-tənz), *n.pr* a rare, abnormal hereditary condition characterized by chronic, progressive chorea and mental deterioration that terminates in dementia. The individual afflicted usually shows the first signs in the fourth decade of life and dies usually within 15 years. There is no known effective treatment but symptoms can be relieved with medications.

hurt, *v* **1.** to molest or restrain; not restricted to physical injuries; also includes mental pain, discomfort, or annoyance. *n* **2.** colloquial term for *traumatic injury.*

Hutchinson triad, *n.pr* See triad, Hutchinson.

Hutchinson's incisors, *n.pr* See incisors, Hutchinson's.

Hutchinson-Gilford syndrome, *n.pr* See syndrome, Hutchinson-Gilford.

HVL, *n* See half-value layer.

hyalinization (hī′əlin′izā′shən), *n* the appearance of an acellular, avascular, homogeneous area in the periodontal ligament, in which compression of the ligament between bone and tooth occurs as a result of orthodontic forces.

hyalinization of periodontal ligament, *n* a degenerative process resulting from long-continued occlusal trauma, in which the fibers become hyalinized into a homogeneous mass.

hyalinized (hī′ələnī′zd), *adj* refers to the transformation of a substance to a glasslike or transparent state. Hyalinized tissue is often found in the bronchial tubes of a person who has died of a viral respiratory infection.

hyaluronic acid (hīʹəlōōronʹik), *n* a mucopolysaccharide that forms the gelatinous substance in the tissue spaces. Hyaluronic acid is the intercellular cementing substance found throughout the tissues of the body.

hyaluronidase (hīʹəlyooronʹədās), *n* an enzyme that produces hydrolysis of hyaluronic acid, the cementing substance of the tissues. Produced by certain pathogenic bacteria and also formed by sperm.

hydralazine HCl, *n brand name:* Apreso-line; *drug class:* antihypertensive, direct-acting peripheral vasodilator; *action:* vasodilates arteriolar smooth muscle by direct relaxation; *uses:* essential hypertension.

hydraulic pressure, *n* See pressure, hydraulic.

hydremia (hīʹdrēʹmēə), *n* an increase in blood volume caused by an increase in serum volume. This may result from cardiac failure, renal insufficiency, pregnancy, or the intravenous administration of fluids.

hydroalcoholic (hīʹdrōalʹkōholʹik), *adj* containing both water and alcohol. See also *solution.*

Hydrocal (hīʹdrōkal), *n* the brand name for a gypsum product, a-hemihydrate, known as artificial stone. It is used for making casts.

hydrocele (hīʹdrōsēlʹ), *n* an accumulation of fluid in any saclike cavity or duct, specifically in the tunica vaginalis testis or along the spermatic cord.

hydrocephalus (hīʹdrōsefʹəlus), *n* an abnormal accumulation of cerebrospinal fluid in the cranial vault, resulting in a disproportionately large cranium.

hydrochloric acid, *n* a compound consisting of hydrogen and chlorine. Hydrochloric acid is secreted in the stomach and is a major component of gastric juice.

hydrochlorothiazide, *n brand names:* Esidrix, HydroDIURIL; *drug class:* thiazide diuretic; *action:* acts on distal tubule by increasing excretion of water, sodium, chloride, potassium; *uses:* edema, hypertension, diuresis, congestive heart failure.

hydrocodone (hīʹdrōkōʹdōn), *n* a semisynthetic narcotic analgesic and antitussive with multiple actions similar to those of codeine. Hydrocodone is an ingredient in prescription analgesics and cough medicines.

hydrocodone bitartrate, *n brand name:* Hycodan; *drug class:* narcotic analgesic, controlled substance schedule III; *action:* interacts with opioid receptor in the central nervous system to alter pain perception; acts directly on cough center in medulla to suppress cough; *uses:* hyperactive and nonproductive cough; mild to moderate pain.

hydrocolloid (hīʹdrōkolʹoid), *n.pl* **1.** the materials listed as colloid solids with water; used in dentistry as elastic impression materials. They can be reversible or irreversible. *n.pl* **2.** an agar-base impression material.

hydrocolloid, irreversible (alginate), *n* a type whose physical condition is changed by a chemical action that is not reversible. It is an impression material that is elastic when set. See also alginate.

hydrocolloid, reversible (agar-agar type), *n* a type whose physical condition is changed by temperature. The material is made fluid by heat and becomes an elastic solid on cooling.

hydrocortisone (hīʹdrōkôrʹtisōn), *n* (cortisol), a glucocorticosteroid secreted by the adrenal cortex in response to stimulation by ACTH. Hydrocortisone is antianabolic, stimulates gluconeogenesis, and probably acts on some cellular system in response to a need for adaptation to change (stress).

hydrocortisone acetate/hydrocortisone sodium phosphate/hydrocortisone sodium succinat, *n brand names:* Cortef, Cortifoam, Cortenema; *drug class:* corticosteroid; *action:* decreases inflammation by suppression of macrophage and leukocyte migration; reduces capillary permeability and inhibits lysosomal enzymes; *uses:* severe inflammation, shock, adrenal insufficiency, ulcerative colitis, collagen disorders.

hydrocortisone acetate/hydrocortisone valerate, *n brand names:* Acticort, Cortaid, Cort-Dome, Dermicort; *drug class:* topical corticosteroid; *action:* interacts with steroid cytoplasmic receptors to induce antiinflammatory effects; possesses antipruritic, antiinflammatory actions; *uses:* psoriasis, eczema, contact dermatitis, pruritus.

hydrodynamic theory, *n* the principles of physics relating to the study of fluidity and the movement of particles within fluids.

hydrofluoric acid, *n* a compound consisting of hydrogen and flourine. It is a very active, corrosive compound, used to etch glass and precious metals.

hydrogen (H), *n* a gaseous, univalent element. Its atomic number is 1 and its atomic weight is 1.008. It is the simplest and lightest of the elements and is normally a colorless, odorless, highly flammable diatonic gas.

hydrogen peroxide, *n* an unstable compound of hydrogen and oxygen that is easily broken down into water and oxygen. A 3% solution is used as a mild antiseptic for the skin and mucous membranes; more concentrated solutions may be used as a whitening (bleaching) agent. May be used to reduce gingival inflammation, but may not eliminate the responsible bacteria.

hydrogenation (hīdroj′ənā′shən), *n* the infusion of hydrogen into a compound. Also called *reduction.*

hydrokinetic activity (hī′drōkinet′ik), *n* refers to the movement or source of movement that causes fluid to be in motion.

hydrolysis (hīdrol′isis), *n* **1.** a reaction between the ions of salt and those of water to form an acid and a base, one or both of which is only slightly dissociated. A process whereby a large molecule is split by the addition of water. The end products divide the water, the hydroxyl group being attached to one and the hydrogen ion to the other. *n* **2.** the splitting of a compound into two parts with the addition of the elements of water.

hydromorphone HCl (hī′drōmor′fōn), *n brand names:* Dilaudid; *drug class:* synthetic narcotic analgesic (controlled substance schedule II); *action:* inhibits ascending pain pathways in the central nervous system, increases pain threshold, alters pain perception; *uses:* moderate to severe pain.

hydrophilic (hī′drōfil′ik), *adj* having an affinity for water. Opposite of lipophilic. See also ointment, hydrophilic.

hydrophobic, *adj* refers to the resistance of a substance to combine with water. Hydrophobic substances, such as oil, are composed of nonpolar molecules, which tend to clump together and repel water.

hydroquinone (hīdrōkwin′ōn), *n* **1.** a reducing agent used as an inhibitor in resin monomers to prevent polymerization during storage. *n* **2.** one of the two chemicals used as reducing agents in film-developing solutions. It is made from benzene (paradihydroxybenzene) and is sensitive to thermal changes. Above 70° F (21° C), the action of hydroquinone is rapid; below 60° F (15.5° C), hydroquinone becomes inactive. Its action is to control the contrast of the film.

hydrostatic pressure (hī′drōstat′ik), *n* See pressure, hydrostatic.

hydrotherapy (hī′drōther′əpē), *n* an empirical adjunct to oral physiotherapy where forced water irrigation is used to cleanse subgingival spaces, remove debris from interproximal spaces, and cleanse pockets.

hydroxide (hīdrok′sīd′), *n* an ionic compound that contains the OH_2 ion, usually consisting of metals or the metal equivalent of the ammonium cation (NH42) that inactivates an acid.

hydroxyapatite (hīdrok′sēap′ətīt), *n* a mineral compound of the general formula 3Ca3(PO4)2-Ca(OH)2, which is the principal inorganic component of bone, teeth, and dental calculus. It can also be used as bone graft material.

hydroxyapatite ceramic, *n* a synthetic substance composed of calcium and phosphate that is similar to a naturally occurring compound found in bones and teeth; used as the primary fabricating material or coating for dental implants.

hydroxychloroquine sulfate, *n brand name:* Plaquenil Sulfate; *drug class:* antimalarial; *action:* inhibits parasite replications, transcription of DNA to RNA by forming complexes with DNA of the parasite; *uses:* malaria, lupus erythematosus, rheumatoid arthritis.

hydroxyurea (hīdrok′sēyŏŏrē′ə), *n brand name:* Hydrea; *drug class:* antineoplastic; *action:* acts by inhibiting DNA synthesis without interfering with synthesis of RNA or protein; *uses:* melanoma, chronic myelocytic leukemia, recurrent or metastatic ovarian cancer.

hydroxyzine HCl/hydroxyzine pamoate, *n brand names:* Atarax, Quiess, Visaject, Hyzine; *drug class:* antianxiety antihistamine; *action:* depresses subcortical levels of the central nervous system, antagonist for histamine H1 receptors; *uses:* anxiety; preoperatively, postoperatively to prevent nausea, vomiting; to potentiate narcotic analgesics; sedation; pruritus.

hygiene (hī′jēn), *n* the science of health and its preservation.

hygiene, dental, continuing care, *n* a regular and continuing program of monitoring, evaluation, and therapy that strives to maintain a patient's optimal oral health by combining diligent self-care with periodic professional treatment.

hygiene, oral (oral cavity hygiene), *n* the practice of personal maintenance of oral cleanliness.

hygiene, oral, special needs persons, *n* the procedures using special skills and devices (e.g., suction or power-assisted toothbrushes) that are designed to promote the personal oral care of an individual who cannot participate in the cleaning process.

hygiene, radiation, *n* the art and science of protecting patients from injury by radiation. Because any amount of radiation is potentially harmful, the ideal objective is to prevent the exposure of any person without a definite medical purpose.

hygienist, dental, *n* a licensed dental professional who specializes in preventative care. Professional prophylaxis, radiographs, sealants, and nonsurgical periodontal therapy are among the procedures performed by a hygienist. Most are licensed to administer local anesthesia, depending on applicable regulations in their area. They usually work for a dentist in a dental office or clinic under a form of supervision. In some locations hygienists are allowed to practice without a dentist's supervision.

hygroma (hīgrō′mə), *n* a sac or cyst swollen with fluid.

hygroma colli cysticum (cystic hygroma, cystic lymphangioma), *n* a cavernous lymphangioma involving the neck. It may be large, thereby impairing breathing and swallowing.

hygroscopic (hī′grōskop′ik), *adj* having the property of absorbing moisture. When applied to gypsum products in contact with free water during their set, the resultant expansion is implied. See also expansion, hygroscopic.

hygroscopic investment, *n* See investment, hygroscopic.

hyoid bone (hī′oid), *n* a single U-shaped bone suspended from the styloid processes of the temporal bone behind and lower border of the mandible in front by muscle and ligament attachments.

hyoscyamine sulfate (hī′yəsī′əmēn′), *n brand names:* Anaspaz, Levsin, Levsinex, Gastrosed; *drug class:* anticholinergic; *action:* inhibits muscarinic actions of acetylcholine at postganglionic parasympathetic neuroeffector sites; *uses:* treatment of peptic ulcer disease in combination with other drugs; other gastrointestinal disorders; other spastic disorders such as parkinsonism; also preoperatively to reduce secretions.

hypalgesia (hī′paljē′zēə), *n* the diminished sensitivity to pain that results from a raised pain threshold.

hyper- (hī′pur), *pref* a prefix signifying above, beyond, or excessive.

hyperactivity, *n* the presence of abnormally heightened behaviors.

hyperadrenocorticism (hī′pərədrē′nōkôr′tisizəm), *n* an adrenocortical hyperfunction resulting from neoplasia of the cortex or hyperplasia of the cortex secondary to an increase in ACTH. Manifestations include hyperglycemia, edema, hypertension, glycosuria, negative nitrogen balance, acne, and hirsutism. See also syndrome, adrenogenital and syndrome, Cushing's.

hyperalgesia (hī′pəraljē′zēə), *n* a greater-than-normal sensitivity to pain that may result from a painful stimulus or a lowered pain threshold.

hyperalgia (hīpəral′jēə), *n* an abnormal sensitivity to pain.

hyperandrogenism (hī′pərandroj′əniz′əm), *n* a state characterized or caused by an excessive secretion of androgens by the adrenal cortex, ovaries, or testes. The clinical significance in males is negligible, so the term is used most commonly with reference to the female. The common manifestations in women are hirsutism and virilism. Hyperandrogenism is often caused by either ovarian or adrenal diseases.

H

hyperbaric oxygen (hī′purber′ik), *n* oxygen delivered to a patient in a pressurized (hyperbaric) chamber that delivers the oxygen in high concentrations for therapeutic benefits. It may be used prior to implant therapy for patients who underwent head and radiation therapy to reduce risks of osteoradionecrosis.

hyperbilirubinemia (hī′pərbil′ēroo′binē′mēə), *n* a greater than normal amounts of the bile pigment bilirubin in the blood, often characterized by jaundice, anorexia, and malaise. It is associated with liver disease and biliary obstruction, but it also occurs when there is excessive destruction of red blood cells, as in hemolytic anemia.

hypercalcemia (hī′pərkalsē′mēə), *n* (hypercalcinemia), **1.** an elevated blood calcium level. *n* **2.** an abnormal elevation of calcium in the blood. Causes include primary hyperparathyroidism, sarcoidosis, multiple myeloma, malignant neoplasms, prolonged androgen therapy, and massive doses of vitamin D. Symptoms suggestive of it are nausea, vomiting, constipation, polyuria, weight loss, muscular weakness, and polydipsia. The normal level of total serum calcium is 8.5 to 10.5 mg/100 ml.

hypercalcinuria, *n* See hypercalciuria.

hypercalciuria (hī′pərkal′sēoo′rēə), (hypercalcinuria), a condition in which there is an excessive increase in urinary calcium excretion. Major causes include primary hyperparathyroidism, hypervitaminosis D, excessive milk intake, metastatic malignancy, immobilization, and renal tubular acidosis. See also hypercalcemia.

hypercapnia (hī′pərkap′nēə), *n* the presence of more than the normal amount of carbon dioxide in the blood tissues resulting from an increase of carbon dioxide in the inspired air or a decrease in elimination.

hypercementosis (hī′purse′mentō′sis), *n* an excessive formation of cementum on the roots of one or more teeth.

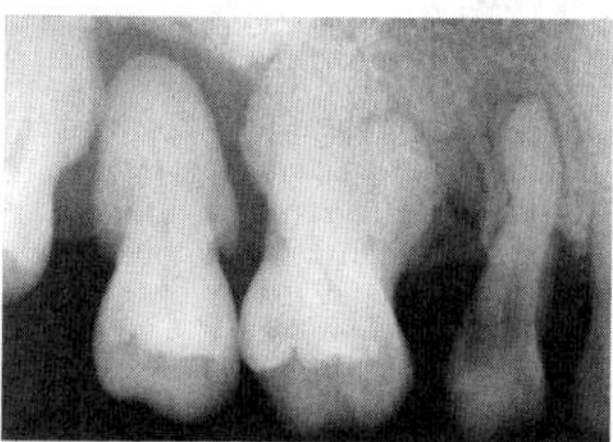

Hypercementosis. (Sapp/Eversole/Wysocki, 2004)

hypercenesthesia (hī′pursen′esthē′zhə), *n* a feeling of exaggerated well-being such as is seen in general paralysis and sometimes in mania.

hyperchloremia (hī′purklôrē′mēə), *n* an excessive concentration of chloride in the plasma. Normal range is 98 to 100 mEq/L. It may occur in water depletion, dehydration, decreased bicarbonate concentration, or metabolic acidosis.

hypercholesterolemia, *n* the presence of an abnormally large amount of cholesterol in the cells and plasma of the circulating blood.

hypercortisolism (Cushing syndrome), *n* a genetic or acquired condition resulting in elevated levels of glucocorticoids, often as a result of tumors in adrenal or pituitary glands. Leads to significant weight gain, particularly on the back (causing a "buffalo hump") and face. More commonly caused by steroid use/abuse, in which case it is called Cushing syndrome medicamentosus.

hyperdivergent, *adj* describes excessive vertical development of the posterior facial height or underdevelopment of the anterior facial height resulting in improper alignment of the bite. Also referred to as *long-face syndrome.*

hyperdontia (hī′pərdon′chēə), *n* a dental condition marked by the presence of excessive teeth in the oral cavity. See supernumerary teeth.

hyperemia (hī′pərē′mēə), *n* an increased and excessive amount of blood in a tissue. The hyperemia may be active or passive.

hyperemia, active, *n* a type caused by an increased flow of blood to an area by active dilation of both the arterioles and capillaries. It is associated with neurogenic, hormonal, and metabolic function.

hyperemia, passive, *n* a type caused by a decreased outflow of blood from an area. It may be generalized, resulting from cardiac, renal, or pulmonary disorders, or it may be localized, as in the oral cavity, and caused by pressure from mechanical or physical obstruction or by pressure from a tumor, denture, filling, or salivary calculus.

hyperemia, pulpal **(hī′pərē′mēə pul′pəl),** *n* a condition in which an injury, infection, or irritant causes the blood vessels around the tooth's pulp to dilate, resulting in painful pressure.

hyperesthesia (hī′pəresthē′zhə), *n* an excessive sensitivity of the skin or of a special sense.

hyperesthetic (hī′pəresthet′ik), *adj* pertaining to or affected with hyperesthesia.

hypergammaglobulinemia (hī′purgam′əglob′ūlinē′mēə), *n* an excess of gammaglobulin in the blood. It occurs in chronic granulomatous inflammations, chronic bacterial infections, liver disease, multiple myeloma, lymphomas, and dysproteinemias.

hyperglobulinemia (hī′purglob′ūlinē′mēə), *n* an abnormally high concentration of globulins in the blood.

hyperglycemia (hī′purglīsē′mēə), *n* an increase in the concentration of sugar in the blood. It is a feature of diabetes mellitus.

hypergonadism (hī′pərgō′nadizəm), *n* an excessive secretion of hormonal agents by the testes or ovaries. Gingival changes induced by the administration of estrogens and androgens include an increase in keratinization and hyperplasia of epithelial and connective tissue. (not current)

hyperhidrosis (hī′purhīdrō′sis), *n* the presence of excessive sweating, which may be generalized or localized.

hyperhidrosis, gustatory **(gus′tətor′ē),** *n* the presence of increased sweating in the preauricular region, forehead, or face associated with eating. See also syndrome, auriculotemporal.

hyperhidrosis, masticatory **(mas′tikətor′ē),** *n* excessive sweating associated with chewing. The cause is traumatic injury producing anastomosis of the facial nerve with a sympathetic branch.

hyperinsulinemia (hī′pərin′sələnē′mēə), *n* a state of elevated levels of insulin in the body due to an improper dose of synthetic insulin or a result of an insulin-secreting tumor. Symptoms include excessive hunger, shakiness, and hypoglycemia.

hyperkalemia (hi′purkəlē′mēə), *n* an abnormally elevated concentration of serum potassium. It may occur in renal failure, shock, and advanced dehydration, and in association with high intracellular potassium in Addison's disease. The normal adult range of serum potassium is 4.0 to 5.5 mEq/L.

hyperkeratosis (hī′purker′ətō′sis), *n* an excessive formation of keratin (e.g., as seen in leukoplakia).

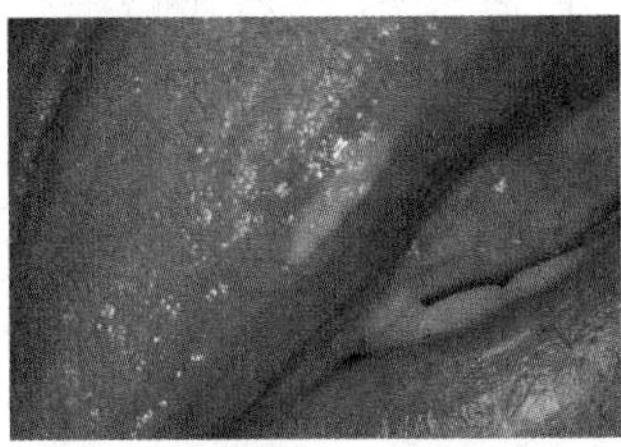

Hyperkeratosis. (Courtesy Dr. Charles Babbush)

hyperkeratosis, benign, *n* a nonmalignant form of a thickening condition that affects the keratin layer of the oral mucosa; generally appears as a white lesion.

H

hyperkinesis (hī′purkinē′sis), *n* the presence of excessive or frequent movement; fidgetiness.

hyperlipidemia, *n* an excess of lipids in the plasma, including the glycolipids, lipoproteins, and phospholipids.

hyperlipoproteinemia (hī′purlip′ōprō′tēnē′mēə), *n* a metabolic disorder in which large amounts of certain fatty substances accumulate in the blood along with small amounts of high-density lipoproteins (HDLs).

hypermagnesemia (hī′purmag′nəsē′mēə), *n* an excess of magnesium in the blood serum. Normal range is 1.5 to 2.5 mEq/L. It may result in respiratory failure and coma and may occur in untreated diabetic acidosis, renal failure, and severe dehydration.

H

hypernasality (hī′purnāzal′itē), *n* an excessive nasal resonance usually accompanied by emission of air through the nasal passageways.

hypernatremia (hī′purnətrē′mēə), *n* an abnormally elevated concentration of serum sodium. It may occur rarely in nephrosis, congestive heart failure, and Cushing's disease and after administration of adrenocorticotropic hormone (ACTH), cortisone, or deoxycorticosterone. Normal adult range of serum sodium is 135 to 145 mEq/L.

hyperocclusion (traumatic), *n* premature tooth contact during oral cavity closure.

hyperopia (hī′pərō′pēə), *n* a condition in which vision improves for far objects rather than near.

hyperosmotic diarrhea (hī′pərôsmôtik dī′ərē′ə), *n* describes diarrhea that produces abnormally rapid fluid loss. It is often a result of poor carbohydrate absorption and is most common in infants and toddlers.

hyperostosis (hī′pərostō′sis), *n* **1.** an excessive growth of bone, as in infantile cortical hyperostosis. *n* **2.** a hypertrophy of bone. See also exostosis.

hyperostosis, infantile cortical (Caffey's disease, Smyth's syndrome), *n* a disease of infants; of unknown cause and characterized by tender, soft tissue swelling that is followed by hyperostosis of the cortex of the underlying bone. The mandible, clavicle, and ulna are most frequently affected.

hyperoxaluria (hī′pərok′səlŏŏr′ēə), *n* an excessive level of oxalic acid or oxalates, primarily calcium oxalate, in the urine. The cause is usually an inherited deficiency of an enzyme needed to metabolize oxalic acid, which is present in many fruits and vegetables, or a disorder of fat absorption in the small intestine. An excess of oxalates may lead to the formation of renal calculi. Treatment may include pyridoxine, forced fluid, and a low-oxalate diet.

hyperoxaluria, primary, *n* an inherited deficiency of the enzyme that metabolizes oxalic acid, resulting in an excessive level of oxalic acid or oxalates in the urine.

hyperoxia (hī′pərok′sēə), *n* an excess of oxygen in the system.

hyperparathyroidism (hī′purper′ethī′roidizəm), *n* (generalized osteitis fibrosa cystica, von Recklinghausen's disease of bone), **1.** an increased parathyroid function resulting from primary hyperplasia, a functioning neoplasm of the parathyroid glands, or secondary hyperplasia related most often to chronic renal insufficiency. Manifestations are related to abnormalities of the bones, kidneys, and blood vessels. Skeletal changes are referred to as *generalized osteitis fibrosa cystica or von Recklinghausen's disease.* Brown tumors, which are essentially giant cell tumors, may develop generally, as well as in the jaws. Kidney changes include renal stones and nephrocalcinosis. Calcification of muscles in arteries occurs. Renal rickets is associated with secondary hyperparathyroidism in children with chronic renal disease. Laboratory findings include a high serum calcium level, low phosphorus level, and a normal or high alkaline phosphatase level. Renal impairment, such as occurs in secondary hyperparathyroidism, tends to nullify hypercalcemia because of an increased loss of calcium in the urine. *n* **2.** an abnormal increase in activity of the parathyroid glands, causing loss of calcium from the bones and resulting in tenderness in bones, spontaneous fractures, muscular weakness, and osteitis fibrosa. **3.** excessive production of parathormone by the parathyroid gland (as in parathyroid hyperplasia and/or adenoma), resulting in increased renal excretion of phosphorus by lowering of the renal threshold for this substance. The pathologic changes produced are osteoporotic or osteodystrophic in nature as a consequence of withdrawal of calcium and phosphorus from osseous tissues.

hyperparathyroidism, brown node of, *n* See node, brown, of hyperparathyroidism.

hyperphagia (hī′pərfā′jēə), *n* a disorder marked by an abnormal appetite and excessive ingestion of food, even to the point of gastric pain and vomiting. It is associated with the malfunction of the hypothalamus and is often linked to conditions such as Kleine-Levin syndrome and central nervous disorders.

hyperphosphatemia (hī′purfos′fətē′mēə), *n* an increased concentration of inorganic phosphates in the blood serum. Hyperphosphatemia may occur in childhood and also in acromegaly, renal failure, and vitamin D intoxication. Normal adult range of serum inorganic phosphorus is 2.5 to 4.2 mg/100 ml.

hyperphosphaturia (hī′purfos′fətoo′rēə), *n* an excessive excretion of phosphate in the urine.

hyperpigmentation, *n* an unusual darkening of the skin. Causes include heredity, drugs, exposure to the sun, and adrenal insufficiency.

hyperpituitarism (hī′purpitoo′iterizəm), *n* a condition caused by excessive production of the hormones secreted by the pituitary gland. An excess of the growth hormone results in giantism or acromegaly; an excess of ACTH produces Cushing syndrome.

hyperplasia (hī′purplā′zēə, -zhə), *n* the abnormal multiplication or increase in the number of normal cells in normal arrangement in a tissue or organ, resulting in a thickening or enlargement of the tissue or organ.

hyperplasia, denture (denture hypertrophy), *n* an enlargement of tissue beneath a denture that is traumatizing the soft tissue.

hyperplasia, drug-induced gingival, *n* the swelling of fibrous gingival tissue most often seen with sustained use of the drugs phenytoin (an antiseizural medication), cyclosporine (an immunosuppressant), and nifedipine (a calcium blocking agent).

hyperplasia, focal fibrous, *n* a small, firm nodule originating in the fibrous connective tissue, which forms on the tongue, lower lip, or oral mucosa lining of the oral cavity as the result of injury or chronic irritation.

hyperplasia, gingival, *n* **1.** an enlargement of the gingival tissue resulting from proliferation of its cellular elements. Hereditary or inflammatory causes may be involved. *n* **2.** the proliferation of gingival epithelium to form elongated rete pegs and proliferation of fibroblasts with increased collagen formation in the underlying connective tissue; leads to nodular enlargement of the gingiva in diphenylhydantoin sodium therapy. *n* **3.** gingival enlargement, primarily produced by proliferation of connective tissue elements; often accompanied by gingival inflammation as a result of trauma to the hyperplastic tissues and coincidental with or following the ingestion of diphenylhydantoin sodium and other medications.

hyperplasia, idiopathic gingival, *n* See fibromatosis gingivae.

hyperplasia, inflammatory fibrous, *n* See epulis fissurata.

hyperplasia, inflammatory papillary (inflammatory papillomatosis, multiple papillomatosis, papillary hyperplasia), *n* a condition of unknown cause but associated with the presence of maxillary dentures. Characterized by numerous red papillary projections on the hard palate.

hyperplasia, papillary, *n* a growth in the midline of the hard palate, usually in the relief area of a denture; characterized by a papillary, or raspberry, appearance.

hyperplasia, phenytoin-related gingival, *n* an enlargement of the gingivae caused by the use of phenytoin (Dilantin) in the management of epilepsy. Numerous other medications have also been associated with gingival hyperplasia.

hyperplastic tissue, *n* See tissue, hyperplastic.

hyperpnea (hī′purpnē′ə), *n* an abnormal increase in respiratory volume; an abnormal increase in the rate and depth of breathing.

hyperpotassemia (hī′purpot′əsē′mēə), *n* See hyperkalemia.

hyperproteinemia (hī′purprō′tēnē′mēə), *n* an abnormal increase in serum and plasma proteins.

hyperproteinuria (hī′purprō′tēnyoo′rēə), *n* See albuminuria.

hypersalivation, *n* See sialorrhea.

hypersensitive, *n* abnormally sensitive.

hypersensitiveness (hī′pursen′sitivnes), *n* a state of altered reactivity in which the body reacts more strongly than normal to a foreign agent.

H

hypersensitivity, *n* **1.** an adverse reaction to contact with specific substances in quantities that usually produce no reaction in normal individuals. *n* **2.** an allergic tendency. In general, a tendency to react with unusual violence to stimuli. *n* **3.** a common complaint after periodontal therapy in which dentin may be exposed, resulting in pain in the teeth or sensitivity to heat, cold, and sweet substances.

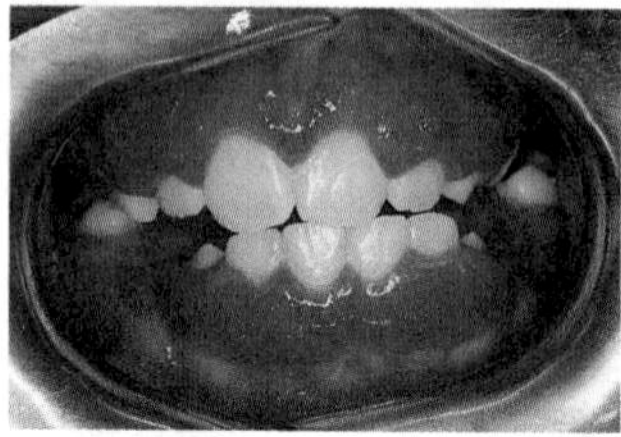

Contact hypersensitivity. (Regezi/Sciubba/Pogrel, 2000)

hypersensitivity, atopic, *n* See atopy.

hypersensitivity, bacterial, *n* delayed inflammatory reaction resulting from previous sensitization of the host by an antigen.

hypersensitivity, delayed, *n* a type involving a latent period between the antigen introduction and the reaction; cellular reactions mediated by the T lymphocytes (e.g., tuberculosis, and transplant reaction).

hypersensitivity, dentin, *n* refers to the pain caused by fractures, or gingival recession, which exposes the dentin of a tooth. This condition requires immediate treatment and can be corrected with topical agents or with periodontal or restorative procedures, such as gingival grafts or enamel bonding.

hypersensitivity, immediate, *n* a humoral reaction, mediated by the circulating B lymphocytes, which causes any of three immediate responses: anaphylactic hypersensitivity, cytotoxic hypersensitivity, and immune system hypersensitivity.

hypersensitivity reaction, cytotoxic, *n* a reaction in which the surface antigens of a cell join with an antibody, causing complement-mediated cell destruction, or other types of cell-membrane damage.

hypersensitivity reactions, immune complex, *n.pl* one of four types of hypersensitivity reactions to antigens in the body that acts as a barrier to disease. The reactions can cause tissue damage.

hypersensitization (hī′pərsen′sitizā′shən), *n* the process of rendering abnormally sensitive or the condition of being abnormally sensitive.

hypersplenism (hī′pərsplen′izəm), *n* a syndrome consisting of splenomegaly and a deficiency of one or more types of blood cells.

hypersthenuria (hī′pursthenyoo′rēə), *n* urine with an abnormally high specific gravity. It is seen in uncontrolled diabetes mellitus and in severe dehydration.

hypersusceptibility (hī′pursəsep′tibil′itē), *n* a condition of abnormal susceptibility to poisons, infective agents, or agents that are entirely innocuous in the normal individual.

hypersympathicotonus (hī′pursimpath′ikōtō′nus), *n* an increased tonicity of the sympathetic nervous system. See also sympathetic otonia.

hypertarachia (hī′purtərak′ēə), *n* extreme irritability of the nervous system.

hypertelorism (hī′purtel′ərizəm), *n* an excessive distance between paired organs. See also syndrome, Greig's.

hypertension (hī′purten′shən) (high blood pressure), *n* an abnormal elevation of systolic and/or diastolic arterial pressure. Systolic level is generally related to emotional stress, sclerosis of the aorta and large arteries, or aortic insufficiency. Diastolic level may result from obscure causes (essential), renal disease, or endocrine disorders. See also blood pressure.

hypertension, essential, *n* a type with an unknown cause.

hypertension, malignant, *n* an elevated blood pressure characterized by a progressive course uncontrollable by medication.

hypertension, orthostatic, *n* plummeting blood pressure that occurs upon standing up which may be accompanied by dizziness or fainting.

hypertension, portal, *n* a type originating in the portal system as occurring in cirrhosis of the liver and other conditions caused by an obstruction of the portal vein.

hypertension pulmonary, *n* a type resulting from pulmonary or cardiac disease such as fibrosis of the lung or mitral stenosis.

hypertensive agents, *n.pl* the agents that reduce or control blood pressure.

hyperthermia (hī′purthur′mēə), *n* an extremely high fever brought on by treatment.

hyperthermia, malignant **(məlig′nənt),** *n* an extremely high fever accompanied by muscle rigidity that occurs rapidly in susceptible individuals when they are exposed to certain types of anesthesia; may be fatal.

hyperthyroidism (hī′pərthī′roidiz′əm), *n* (Parry's disease), a condition with abnormalities of calorigenic mechanisms, body tissues, blood, and body fluids and of the circulatory, muscular, and nervous systems resulting from an excessive elaboration of thyroid hormone. Manifestations include increased sweating, increased appetite, intolerance to heat, weight loss, increased protein-bound iodine (PBI), early shedding of primary teeth and early eruption of permanent teeth, tachycardia, palpitation, tremors, nervousness, muscular weakness, diarrhea, increased excretion of calcium and phosphorus, hypocholesterolemia, creatinuria, and osteoporosis. May occur as the result of primary hyperplasia, hyperfunctioning nodular goiters, functional benign tumor, or adenoma of the thyroid gland. See also goiter, exophthalmic.

hypertonic (hī′purton′ik), *adj* having an osmotic pressure greater than that of the solution with which it is compared.

hypertrichosis (hī′purtrikō′sis), *n* an excessive growth of hair on the body, possibly as a result of endocrine dysfunction, as in the hirsutism accompanying excessive adrenocortical function.

hypertriglycerademia (hī′pərtrīglis′əridē′mēə), *n* an excess of triglycerides in the blood, which is often due to inherited conditions that affect the metabolism of lipoproteins.

hypertrophy (hīpur′trōfē), *n* an enlargement or overgrowth of an organ or part resulting from an increase in size of its constituent cells.

hypertrophy, denture, *n* See hyperplasia, denture.

hypertrophy, muscle, *n* a hypertrophy denotes an increase in the size or number of constituent fibers of a muscle. Any other condition such as inflammation, tumor, and fatty infiltration that increases the size of a muscle is called *pseudohypertrophy.* True or physiologic hypertrophy results from excessive activity of muscle. Genetic and hormonal factors play a role in determining the size of muscles; e.g., muscles in a man tend to be larger than in a woman in the temporal and facial regions. The histologic characteristics of hypertrophied muscle are normal. The fibrils are slightly wider in diameter than is normal, and the only change might be a slight increase in vascularity.

hyperventilation, *n* **1.** an abnormally prolonged, rapid, and deep breathing; also the condition produced by overbreathing of oxygen at high pressures. It is marked by confusion, dizziness, numbness, and muscular cramps brought on by such breathing. *n* **2.** rapid, deep, forced breathing frequently resulting from anxiety. It results in a transient loss of carbon dioxide and respiratory alkalosis. Symptoms include anxiety, circumoral numbness, tingling sensation, faintness, and occasionally, carpopedal spasms, tetany, and syncope.

hyperventilation, managing, *n* the steps that may be taken to assist a patient who experiences sudden, increased respiration that may be the result of anxiety or pain; may include verbal reassurances, repositioning, or deep breathing exercises.

hypervitaminosis A (hīpurvī′təminō′sis), *n* the effects of toxic doses of vitamin A. Manifestations include bone fragility, xeroderma, nausea, headache, and loss of hair.

hypervitaminosis D, *n* the toxic effects of ingesting large amounts of vitamin D. Manifestations include symptoms resulting from hypercalcemia, impairment of renal function, and metastatic calcification.

hypervolemia (hī′pərvolē′mēə), *n* increased blood volume.

H

hypesthesia (hī′pesthē′zhə), *n* a condition characterized by atypically decreased sensation.

hypnic (hip′nik), *adj* inducing or pertaining to sleep.

hypno- (hip′nō), *comb.* a combining form denoting a relationship to sleep.

hypnosis (hipnō′sis), *n* a condition of artificially induced sleep or of a trance resembling sleep induced by drugs, psychologic means, or both. Generally creating a condition of heightened suggestibility in the subject.

hypnotic (hipnot′ik), *n* **1.** a drug that induces sleep or depresses the central nervous system at a cortical level. *adj* **2.** causing sleep or a trance. See also sedative.

hypnotism (hip′nōtizəm), *n* **1.** the method or practice of inducing sleep. *n* **2.** in medical jurisprudence, a mental state rendering the patient susceptible to suggestion at the will and inducement of another.

hypnotize (hip′nōtīz), *v* to put into a state of hypnosis in which there is a condition of heightened suggestibility.

hypo (hī′pō), *n* an abbreviated form of the term hyposulfite, which is a synonym of sodium thiosulfate (Na2S2O3), a solution used in photography and radiography to fix and harden the manifest image. See also fixation.

hypo- (hī′pō), *pref* a prefix signifying beneath, under, or deficient.

hypoadrenocorticalism (hī′pōədrē′nōkôr′tikəlizəm), *n* an acute or chronic adrenocortical hypofunction, as in Waterhouse-Friderichsen syndrome or Addison's disease.

hypoadrenocorticism (hī′pōədrēnōkôr′tisizəm), *n* See hypoadrenocorticalism.

hypoalbuminemia (hī′pōalbū′mənē′mēə), *n* a condition marked by abnormally low amounts of the body's main serum-binding protein, albumin. Insufficient albumin can lead to edema and platelet malfunction.

hypoalgesia (hī′pōaljē′zēə), *n* a diminished sensation of pain resulting from a raised pain threshold.

hypoallergenic (hī′pōal′urjen′ik), *adj* descriptor of a substance ensuring a generally nonactivating property with regard to allergy-producing symptoms in individuals with certain chemical sensitivities.

hypobranchial eminence (hī′pōbrang′kəəl), *n* a small tissue structure formed from the second, third, and fourth pharyngeal arches during early embryonic development of the head and neck from which the tongue eventually takes shape.

hypocalcemia (hī′pōkalsē′mēə), *n* the presence of an abnormally low concentration of calcium in the blood; may be associated with hypoparathyroidism, rickets, osteomalacia, renal rickets, pancreatic disease, sprue, obstructive jaundice, or tetany.

hypocalcification (hī′pōkal′sifikā′shən), *n* a condition with a reduced amount of calcification, especially of enamel. It produces opaque white spots that may be discolored later. See also fluorosis.

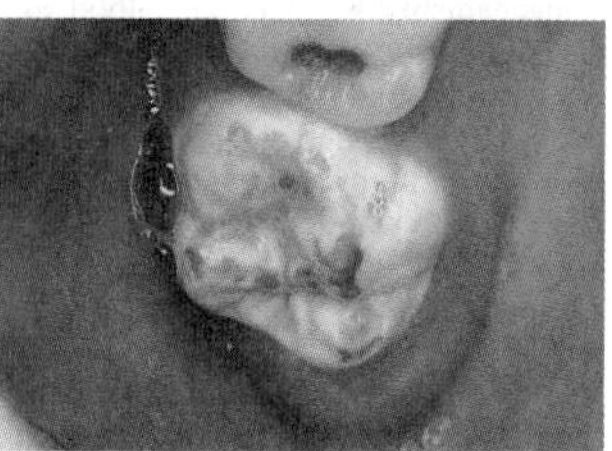

Hypocalcification. (Zitelli/Davis, 2002)

hypocalcification, hereditary enamel, *n* a hereditary anomaly of enamel formation affecting the primary and permanent dentition in which the enamel peels off after tooth eruption and exposes dentin, giving the teeth a yellow appearance.

hypocalciuria (hī′pōkal′sēoo′rēə), *n* a decrease in urinary calcium. Normal values vary considerably but are roughly related to calcium intake. Various values are given (e.g., 100 to 200 mg/day on a normal diet, or 350 to 400 mg/day for calcium intake of 10 mg/kg of body weight in children). Hypocalciuria may occur in hypoparathyroidism, rickets, osteomalacia, metastatic carcinoma of the prostate, and renal failure. See also test, Sulkowitch's.

hypocapnia (hī′pōkap′nēə), *n* a deficiency of carbon dioxide in the blood.

hypocarbia, *n* See hypocapnia.

hypochloremia (hī′pōklôrē′mēə), *n* a decrease below normal of chloride concentration in the plasma. The normal range is 98 to 100 mEq/L. It may occur in adrenal insufficiency, persistent vomiting, renal failure, acute infections, and dehydration with sodium depletion.

hypochlorous acid, *n* a greenish-yellow liquid derived from an aqueous solution of lime. An unstable compound that decomposes to hydrochloric acid and water; hypochlorous acid is used as a bleaching agent and disinfectant.

hypochondria (hī′pōkon′drēə), *n* anxiety about disease; a type of neurosis characterized by fear of disease or by simulated disease.

hypochondriasis (hī′pōkondrī′əsis), *n* See hypochondria.

hypochromia (hīpōkrō′mēə), *n* a reduced staining quality of cells, particularly pale staining red blood cells associated with hemoglobin deficiency.

hypodermoclysis (hī′pōdurmok′lisis), *n* a subcutaneous injection of fluid in large volume.

hypodontia (hī′pōdon′shēə), *n* a condition characterized by having fewer teeth than normal.

hypoesthesia (hī′pōesthē′zēə, -zhə), *n* a decreased sensitivity to touch or pressure.

hypoestrogenism (hī′pōes′trōjenizəm), *n* a diminished production of estrogenic substances by the ovaries, such as that which occurs during menopause. May produce desquamative lesions on the oral mucosa. See also gingivitis, desquamative.

hypofibrinogenemia (hī′pōfībrin′ōjənē′mēə), *n* a reduction of fibrinogen in the blood. Excessive bleeding may occur following trauma. The deficiency of fibrinogen may be congenital or may result from faulty synthesis associated with liver disease and defibrinogenation resulting from disorders of pregnancy involving the placenta and amniotic fluid. The normal range is 200 to 600 mg/100 ml of plasma. Clotting deficiencies do not occur until the concentration falls below 75 mg/100 ml.

hypogammaglobulinemia (hī′pōgam′əglob′ūlinē′mēə), *n* a deficiency of gammaglobulin, usually manifested by recurrent bacterial infections.

hypogeusia (hī′pōgoo′zēə), *n* a decreased sense of taste.

hypoglossal nerve, *n* see nerve, hypoglossal.

hypoglycemia (hī′pōglīsē′mēə), *n* a condition existing when the concentration of blood sugar (true blood sugar) is 40 mg/100 ml or less. Symptoms may not occur even when the concentration is considerably less. Symptoms include nervousness, hunger, weakness, vertigo, and faintness. Hypoglycemia may occur in the fasting state or following the injection of insulin.

hypoglycemia, fasting, *n* a type occurring in the postabsorptive state; occurs in renal glycosuria, lactation, hepatic disease, and in central nervous system lesions.

hypoglycemia, insulin, *n* a type resulting from improper administration of insulin. If hypoglycemia is severe, convulsions, coma, and death may occur. See also *shock, insulin.*

hypoglycemia, mixed, *n* a type occurring during the fasting state and after the ingestion of carbohydrates; occurs in idiopathic spontaneous hypoglycemia of infancy, in anterior pituitary and adrenocortical insufficiency, and with tumors of the islet cells of the pancreas.

hypoglycemia, reactive, *n* a type occurring after the ingestion of carbohydrates with an excessive release of insulin, as in functional hyperinsulinism.

hypoglycemia, spontaneous, n a type that is functional (such as in renal glycosuria, lactation, and severe muscular exertion) or is caused by organic disease such as in hepatic disease and adrenocortical insufficiency.

hypoglycemic agents (hī′pōglīsē′-mik), *n.pl* a large heterogeneous group of drugs prescribed to decrease or control the amount of glucose circulating in the blood; used in the prevention and treatment of diabetes.

hypogonadism (hī′pōgō′nad-izəm), *n* a gonadal deficiency resulting from abnormalities of the testes and ovaries or to pituitary insufficiency. Manifestations include eunuchism, eunuchoidism, Frohlich's syndrome, amenorrhea, and incomplete development or maintenance of secondary sex characteristics.

hypohidrotic ectodermal dysplasia (hī′pōhīdrot′ik ektōdur′məl dis-plā′zhə), *n* a syndrome consisting of hypodontia, hypotrichosis, hypohidrosis, and other defects related to the development of ectodermal structures.

hypokalemia (hī′pōkəlē′mēə), *n* an abnormally low serum potassium level. Hypokalemia may occur in metabolic alkalosis, chronic diarrhea, Cushing syndrome, primary aldosteronism, and excessive use of deoxycorticosterone, cortisone, or ACTH.

hypolarynx (hī′pōler′inks), *n* the infraglottic compartment of the larynx that extends from the true vocal cords to the first tracheal ring.

hypolethal (hī′pōlē′thəl), *adj* not quite lethal; said of dosage.

hypomagnesemia (hī′pōmag′nəs-ē′mēə), *n* a deficiency of magnesium in the blood serum (normal values range from 1.5 to 2.5 mEq/L). It may be associated with chronic alcoholism, starvation, and prolonged diuresis in congestive heart failure. Manifestations include muscular twitching, convulsions, and coma.

hyponasality (hī′pōnāzal′itē), *n* a lack of nasal resonance necessary to produce acceptable voice quality. The type of voice quality heard when the speaker's nose is occluded or when the speaker is suffering from a severe cold.

hyponatremia (hī′pōnətrē′mēə), *n* an abnormally low concentration of sodium in the blood serum. It may develop in adrenocortical insufficiency and chronic renal disease or with extreme sweating.

hypoparathyroidism (hī′pōper′ə-thī′roidizəm), *n* a decrease in parathyroid function, usually the result of surgical removal. Symptoms include tetany, irritability, and muscle weakness. The serum calcium is low, the blood phosphorus elevated, the blood magnesium reduced, and the alkaline phosphatase normal.

hypopharyngoscope (hī′pōfər-ing′gōskōp), *n* an apparatus devised for bringing the inferior portion of the pharynx or hypopharynx into view.

hypopharynx (hī′pōfer′inks), *n* the division of the pharynx that lies below the superior edge of the epiglottis and opens into the larynx and esophagus.

hypophosphatasia (hī′pōfos′fə-tā′zhə), *n* a familial disease in which the children may have very low serum alkaline phosphatase levels, total or partial aplasia of the cementum, and an abnormal periodontal ligament in the primary teeth; a decreased phosphatase level that has been linked to a premature loss of primary teeth in children. Examination reveals absence, hypoplasia, or dysplasia of cementum.

hypophosphatemia (hī′pōfos′fə-tē′mēə), *n* an abnormally low concentration of serum phosphates. Blood phosphorus levels are low in sprue, celiac disease, and hyperparathyroidism and in association with an elevated alkaline phosphatase in vitamin D-resistant rickets and other diseases involving a renal tubular defect in resorption of phosphate.

hypophyseal (hīpof′əsē′əl), *n* the structure of blood vessels responsible for transportation of hormones between the hypothalamus and anterior pituitary gland.

hypophysis, *n* See gland, pituitary.

hypopituitarism (hī′pōpitōō′it-erizəm), *n* a decrease in the hormonal secretions of the pituitary gland.

hypoplasia (hī′pōplā′zhə), *n* the defective or incomplete development of a tissue or structure.

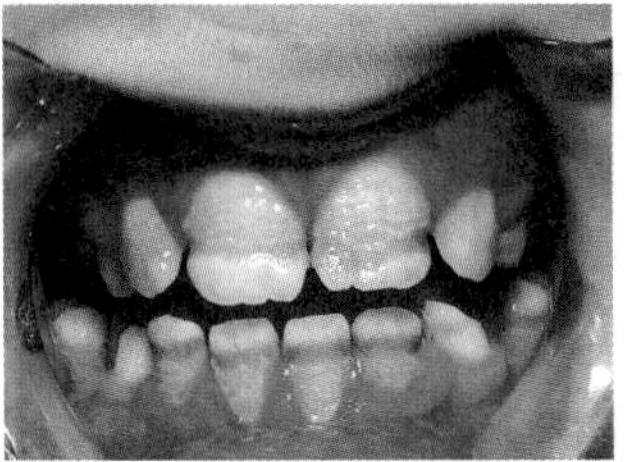

Hypoplasia. (Regezi/Sciubba/Pogrel, 2000)

hypoplasia, enamel, chronologic, *n* a prenatal or postnatal systemic type affecting amelogenesis occurring at the time of the systemic disorder.

hypoplasia, enamel, hereditary (hereditary brown tooth), *n* a hereditary anomaly of the enamel affecting the primary and permanent dentition in which a thin layer of hard enamel covering the yellow dentin gives the tooth a brown appearance.

hypoplasia, mandibular, *n* an abnormally small mandibular development (e.g., in micrognathia or brachygnathia).

hypoplastic, *adj* refers to an abnormality in dental enamel characterized by pits, fissures, and discoloration. Hypoplastic enamel may be genetically inherited or caused by conditions such as vitamin deficiency, disease, or trauma.

hypopnea (hīpop′nēə), *n* abnormally shallow and rapid respirations.

hypopotassemia (hī′pōpot′əsē′mēə), *n* See hypokalemia.

hypoproteinemia (hī′pōprō′tēnē′mēə), *n* a decrease in serum and plasma proteins.

hypoprothrombinemia (hī′pōprōthrom′binē′mēə), *n* a deficiency of prothrombin in the blood. It may be congenital or associated with vitamin K deficiency, large doses of salicylates, liver disease, or excessive anticoagulant. The normal level ranges from 70% to 120% plasma prothrombin concentration. There is little danger of hemorrhage if the prothrombin concentration is greater than 20% of normal.

hyposalivation (hī′pōsal′ivā′shən), *n* a decreased flow of saliva. It may be associated with dehydration, radiation therapy of the salivary gland regions, anxiety, the use of drugs such as atropine and antihistamines, vitamin deficiency, various forms of parotitis, and various syndromes (Sjögren's, Riley-Day, Plummer-Vinson, and Heerfordt's disease). See also asialorrhea.

hyposensitive (hī′pōsen′sitiv), *adj* less *sensitive.*

hyposthenuria (hī′pōsthen-yoo′rēə), *n* a condition in which the urine has an abnormally low specific gravity. Hyposthenuria may occur in cases in which renal damage impairs concentrating power or when the kidneys are normal but lack hormonal stimulus for concentrations, as in diabetes insipidus.

hypotension (hī′pōten′shən), *n* the presence of abnormally low blood pressure.

hypotension, orthostatic (postural) **(ôr′thōstat′ik),** *n* the plummeting of blood pressure that occurs when standing; dizziness and fainting may result.

hypothalamus (hī′pōthal′əmus), *n* a small extension of the brain that lies in the sella turcica in the cranium. It lies just at the superior level of the body of the sphenoid bone. It is intimately related structurally and functionally with the pituitary gland and is important in the central regulation of the endocrine glands, including the thyroid gland, pancreas, adrenal glands, and gonads. The most important visceral functions are under control of the hypothalamus because it functions in such close coordination with the endocrine glands. The control is mediated through its structural communication with the pituitary gland.

hypothermia (hī′pōther′mēə), *n* the presence of body temperature significantly below normal; 98.6°F, 37°C.

hypothetical question, *n* the assumed or proved facts and circumstances, stated to constitute a specific situation or state of facts, on which the opinion of an expert is asked, in producing evidence at a trial.

hypothyroidism (hī′pōthī′roidizəm), *n* a diminished activity of the thyroid gland with decreased secretion of thyroxin, resulting in lowered basal metabolic rate, lethargy, sleepiness, dysmenorrhea in females, and a tendency toward obesity. Occasionally there is accompanying gingival hyperplasia. The condition is called cretinism in children and myxedema in adults.

hypotonia (hī′pōtō′nēə), *n* an abnormality of the skeletal muscle tone, which is indicative of genetic disorders or nervous system dysfunction. Patients with hypoplastic tendencies display floppy limbs and an inability to sustain normal head position.

hypotonic (hī′pōton′ik), *adj* exhibiting less tension or firmness.

hypotrichosis (hī′pōtrikō′sis), *n* a less-than-normal amount of hair on the head or body.

hypoventilation, *n* an abnormal condition of the respiratory system, characterized by cyanosis, polycythemia, increased carbon dioxide arterial tension, and generalized decreased respiratory function. Hypoventilation occurs when the volume of air that enters the alveoli and takes part in gas exchanges is not adequate for the metabolic needs of the body.

hypoxanthine (hī′pōzan′thēn), *n* a purine present in the muscles and other tissues, formed during purine catabolism by deamination of adenine.

hypoxanthine phosphoribosyltransferase (hī′pōzan′thēn fos′fôrī′bōsil′transfərās′), *n* an enzyme present in human tissue that converts hypoxanthine and guanine to their respective 5 nucleotides, with 5-phosphoribose 1-diphosphate as the ribose-phosphate donor.

hypoxemia (hī′poksē′mēə), *n* a deficient oxygenation of the blood.

hypoxia (hīpok′sēə), *n* low oxygen content or tension.

hypoxia, anemic, n a type brought about by a reduction of the oxygen-carrying capacity of the blood because of a decrease in the complete blood counts or an alteration of the hemoglobin constituents.

hypoxia, anoxic, n a type resulting from inadequate oxygen in inspired air or interference with gaseous exchange in the lungs.

hypoxia, histotoxic, n a type resulting from the inability of the tissue cells to use the oxygen that may be present in normal amount and tension.

hypoxia, metabolic, n a type resulting from an increased tissue demand for oxygen.

hypoxia, stagnant, n a type resulting from decreased circulation in an area.

hyrax appliance, *n* a fixed orthodontic appliance used for the bilateral expansion of the maxillary posterior teeth or the bilateral expansion of the palate.

hysteresis (histerē′sis), *n* a physical phenomenon whereby a material such as a reversible hydrocolloid passes from a solid to a gel state at one temperature and a gel to a solid state at another.

hysteria (hister′ēə), *n* **1.** a disease or disorder of the nervous system, more common in females than males, not originating in lesions and resulting from psychic rather than physical causes. *n* **2.** a psychoneurosis characterized by lack of control over emotions or acts, exaggeration of sensory impression, and simulation of disease or pain associated with disease. In some patients, trismus, neuralgia, and temporomandibular joint disturbance may be hysterical in origin.

I

I and D (surgical fistulation), *n* the abbreviation for **incision and drainage,** which is the procedure of incising a fluctuant mucosal lesion to allow for the release of pressure and drainage of fluid exudate.

I cell disease, *n* a congenital disease, also known as *mucolipidosis II*. It is characterized by shortness of stature, psychomotor retardation, coarse facial features, and gingival enlargement. The progressive gingival enlargement may delay tooth eruption and may impair closure of the oral cavity.

iatrogenic (ī'atrōjen'ik), *adj* originating as a result of professional care; e.g., an iatrogenic pulpitis.

iatrosedation (īətrōsēdā'shən), *n* a relaxed state induced by actions rather than drugs; a method of anxiety reduction that is psychologically based.

ibuprofen (ī'būprō'fən), *n brand names:* Advil, Excedrin-IB, Midol-IB, Motrin IB; *drug class:* nonsteroidal antiinflammatory; *action:* inhibits prostaglandin synthesis by interfering with cyclooxgenase needed for biosynthesis; possesses analgesic, antiinflammatory, antipyretic properties; *uses:* rheumatoid arthritis, osteoarthritis, mild to moderate pain. Ibuprofen is useful for the temporary relief of minor aches and pains associated with the common cold, toothache, muscular aches, minor arthritic pain, and menstrual cramps and for fever reduction.

ichthyosis (ik'thēō'sis), *n* an inherited dermatologic condition in which the skin is dry, hyperkeratotic, and fissured, resembling fish scales. It usually appears at or shortly after birth and may be part of one of several rare syndromes. Some types respond temporarily to bath oils, topical retinoic acid, or propylene glycol. Also called *xeroderma.*

icterus (ik'terəs), *n* See jaundice.

icterus, acholuric, *n* See jaundice, hemolytic, congenital.

id (id), *n* the part of the psyche functioning in the unconscious that is the source of instinctive energy, impulses, and drives. It is based on the pleasure principle and has strong tendencies toward self-preservation. The full taxonomy includes the id, the ego, and the superego.

identity, *n* the fact that a subject, person, or thing before a court is the same as it is claimed to be.

idiopathic (id″eopath'ik), *adj* without apparent cause; of unknown origin.

idiopathic disease, *n* See disease, idiopathic.

idiopathic enlargement (id'ēōpath'ik), *n* See enlargement, idiopathic.

idiosyncrasy (id'ēōsing'krəsē), *n* **1.** the tendency to react atypically or with unusual violence to a food, drug, or cosmetic. **2.** a characteristic that is peculiar to an individual.

idoxuridine-IDU (ophthalmic), *n brand name:* Herplex; *drug class:* antiviral; *action:* inhibits viral replication by interfering with viral DNA synthesis; *uses:* herpes simplex keratitis, vaccinia virus keratitis, herpes simplex keratoconjunctivitis.

IgA, *n* the abbreviation for **immunoglobulin A.**

IgA deficiency, *n* a selective lack of immunoglobulin A, which constitutes the most common type of immunoglobulin deficiency, appearing in about 1 in 400 individuals. Immunoglobulin A is a major protein antibody in the saliva and the mucous membranes of the intestines and bronchi. It protects against bacterial and viral infections. IgA deficiency is common in patients with rheumatoid arthritis and in patients with systemic lupus erythematosus.

IgE, *n* the abbreviation for **immunoglobulin E.**

IgG, *n* the abbreviation for **immunoglobulin G.**

IgM, *n* the abbreviation for **immunoglobulin M.**

ignorance of law, *n* See law, ignorance of.

ilium (il'ēəm), *n* the most superior of the three bones that make up the innominate bone. The ilium forms part of the acetabulum. The iliac crest is a source of bone for mandibular and chin reconstruction and enhancement.

illegal, *adj* not authorized by law; illicit.

illuminator (light box), *n* a source of light with uniform intensity for viewing radiographs.

illusion, *n* a mistaken or erroneous perception of an object external to the individual. In some cases, the laws of physics explain the errors. In others, the explanation lies with the perceiver. Illusions should be distinguished from *hallucinations,* which are perceptions that lack external stimuli, and *delusions,* which are false beliefs. Illusions are seen in certain reactions to general anesthesia or intoxication.

illustration, *n* a drawing or photograph used to help clarify the patient's concept of proposed treatment and conditions present.

image enhancement, *n* the use of computer digital technology to improve the resolution of cathode ray images.

image, latent, *n* the invisible image produced on photographic or radiographic film by the action of light or radiation before development.

imaging, *n* the creation of digital, print, or film representations of anatomic structures for the purpose of diagnosis.

imbedded, *adj* See embedded.

imbibition (im′bibish′ən), *n* the absorption of liquid. Gel structures are particularly susceptible to imbibition.

imbrication lines (im″brĭka′shən līnz), *n.pl* **1.** the seams which are formed by overlapping layers of tissue in order to close a surgical wound. **2.** slight mesiodistal ridges in the cervical third of a tooth. They are associated with the lines of Retzius in the enamel.

imipramine HCl (imip′rəmēn), *n brand names:* Norfranil, Tipramine; *drug class:* tricyclic antidepressant; *action:* inhibits both norepinephrine and serotonin (5-HT) uptake in the brain; *uses:* depression, enuresis in children.

immediate denture, *n* See denture, immediate.

immediate functional loading, *n* a procedure for placement of an implant that involves the maxillary and mandibular teeth coming into contact with one another. The implant is placed upon removal of existing teeth. Also known as *immediate occlusal loading.*

immediate nonfunctional loading, *n* a procedure for placement of an implant that does not involve the maxillary and mandibular teeth coming into contact with one another. The implant is placed upon removal of existing teeth. Also known as *immediate nonocclusal loading.*

immediate temporization, *n* a procedure for placement of a temporary prosthesis (restoration) on an implant in which the maxillary and mandibular teeth may or may not come into contact with one another. The implant is placed upon removal of existing teeth. Also known as *immediate provisionalization.*

immersion, *n* the placing of a body or an object into water or other liquid so that it is completely covered by the liquid.

immobilization, *n* the act of securing in a fixed relationship to prevent damage and to promote healing, such as the use of a splint or cast to maintain the fractured pieces of bone in proper relationship to each other for healing to occur.

immune reaction, *n* See reaction, immune.

immune system, *n* a biochemical complex that protects the body against pathogenic organisms and other foreign bodies. It incorporates the humoral immune response, which produces antibodies to react with specific antigents, and the cell-mediated response, which uses T cells to mobilize tissue macrophages in the presence of a foreign body. It also protects the body from invasion by creating local barriers and inflammation. The principal organs include the bone marrow, the thymus, and the lymphoid tissues.

immune system, duality of, *n* the division of lymphocyte white blood cells into two classes of cells, types B and T. Type B cells help develop humoral immunities, while type T cells are active in cellular immunity.

immunity (imū′nitē), *n* **1.** an exemption from service or from duties that the law ordinarily requires most citizens to perform (e.g., jury duty). **2.** the condition of an organism whereby it successfully resists or is not susceptible to injury or infection. See also memory.

immunity, acquired, *n* **1.** the resistance to a particular disease (e.g., chickenpox) after recovering from that disease. **2.** the resistance to poisons or medications developed over a usually long period of gradually increasing exposure.

immunity, active, *n* the resistance to a disease or other biological or chemical agents acquired naturally as a result of exposure to the disease or agent; can also be acquired artificially by use of a vaccine containing a weakened or deadened form of the agent, stimulating the immune system to produce antibodies long after the initial exposure. See also passive immunity.

immunity, natural, *n* the inherited ability to remain resistant to or unaffected by a specific disease.

immunity, passive, *n* the short-term resistance to a specific disease that has been acquired either through the placenta from mother to fetus or as the result of receiving an injection of serum antibodies (gamma globulins) taken from an immune person or animal (inoculation). See also immunity, active and gamma globulins.

immunization (vaccination) (im′ūnəzā′shən), *n.pl* **1.** a process by which resistance to an infectious disease is induced or augmented. **2.** a fundamental element of preventative health care for dental workers, who should be fully immunized against influenza, hepatitis B, and all childhood diseases where a vaccine is available. See also immunity, active. HIV and hepatitis C vaccines are not available.

immunoassay (im′ūnōas′ā), *n* a competitive-binding assay in which the binding protein is an antibody.

immunoblotting, *n* the immunologic methods for isolating and quantitatively measuring immunoreactive substances. When used with immune reagents such as monoclonal antibodies, the process is known generically as *Western blot analysis.*

immunocompromised, *adj* having the quality of an immune response that has been weakened by a disease or immunosuppressive agent.

immunodeficiency (im′ūnōdəfish′ənsē), *n* a condition resulting from a defective immunologic mechanism. Primary form is caused by a defect in the immune system; secondary form is a result of another disease process such as HIV infection.

immunodiffusion (im′ūnōdifū′zhən), *n* a technique for the identification and quantification of an immunoglobulin.

immunoelectrophoresis (im′ūnōilek′trəfərē′sis), *n* a technique that combines eletrophoresis and immunodiffusion to separate and allow identification of complex proteins.

immunogens (antigens) (im′ūnojəns), *n.pl* agents that may be used to trigger the immune response, such as vaccines, or during disease, such as allergens. See also antigen.

immunoglobulins (Ig) (antibodies) (im′ūnōglob′ūlinz), *n.pl* serum proteins (γ globulins) synthesized by plasma cells that act as antibodies and are important in the body's defense mechanisms against infection. See also antibody and allergen.

immunoglobulin, IgA, *n* a type of immunoglobulin most commonly found in saliva, mucus, tears, urine, and other secretions.

immunoglobulin, IgD, *n* a type of immunoglobulin that operates as antibodies. Trace amounts of IgD proteins are found in the blood serum and the plasma membranes of B lymphocytes.

immunoglobulin, IgE, *n* a type of immunoglobulin that plays a role in regulating hypersensitivity reactions and reactions to parasitic infections.

immunoglobulin, IgG, *n* a type of immunoglobulin that plays a role in secondary immune responses. It is unique in that it can pass through the placental barrier.

immunoglobulin, IgM, *n* a type of immunoglobulin that reacts first to any given immune response.

immunohistochemistry, *n* the demonstration of specific antigens in tissues by the use of markers that are either fluorescent dyes or enzymes, especially horseradish peroxidase. See also peroxidase, horseradish.

immunology, *n* the study of the reaction of tissues of the immune system of the body to antigenic stimulation. See also immune system.

immunosuppressants, *n.pl* the agents that lower or reduce immune response; useful in organ transplant surgery to prevent organ rejection. Corticosteroid hormones given in large amounts; cytotoxic drugs, including antimetabolites and alkylating agents; antilymphocytic serum; and irradiation may result in immunosuppression.

immunosuppression, *n* **1.** the administration of agents that significantly interfere with the ability of the immune system to respond to antigenic stimulation by inhibiting cellular and humoral immunity. It may be deliberate, such as in preparation for bone marrow or other transplantation to prevent rejection by the host of the donor tissue. **2.** an abnormal condition of the immune system characterized by markedly inhibited ability to respond to antigenic stimuli.

immunotherapy (im′ūnōther′əpē), *n* a special treatment of allergic responses that administers increasingly large doses of the offending allergens to gradually develop immunity.

impact strength, *n* See strength, impact.

impacted tooth, *n* See tooth, impacted.

impaction, food, *n* the impaction of food generally interproximally because of open contact areas, uneven marginal ridge height, or "plunger" cusps.

impaction, tooth, *n* a situation in which an unerupted tooth is wedged against another tooth or teeth or otherwise located so that it cannot erupt normally.

impaired function, *n* See function, impaired.

impairment, *n* See function, impaired.

impeachment of witness, *n* the questioning of the veracity of a witness by means of evidence obtained for that purpose.

impetigo (im′pətī′gō), *n* an inflammatory disease of the skin mainly in children; characterized by pustules and yellow-colored crust. Caused by *Streptococcus* or *Staphylococcus.* Highly contagious.

impingement (impinj′mənt), *n* the striking or application of excessive pressure to a tissue by food or a prosthesis.

implant, *n* a device, usually alloplastic, that is surgically inserted into or onto the oral tissue. To be used as a prosthodontic abutment, it should remain quiescent and purely secondary to local tissue physiology.

implant, abutment of, n the portion of an implant that protrudes through the gingival tissues and is designed to support a prosthesis.

implant, anchor endosteal, n an implant with a narrow buccolingual wedge-shaped infrastructure that is designed to be placed deep into the bone. The outline of the implant appears similar to a nautical anchor, and there is a variety of sizes and shapes to satisfy many anatomic and prosthodontic needs. Endosteal anchor implants are cast of chromium-cobalt surgical alloy and annealed.

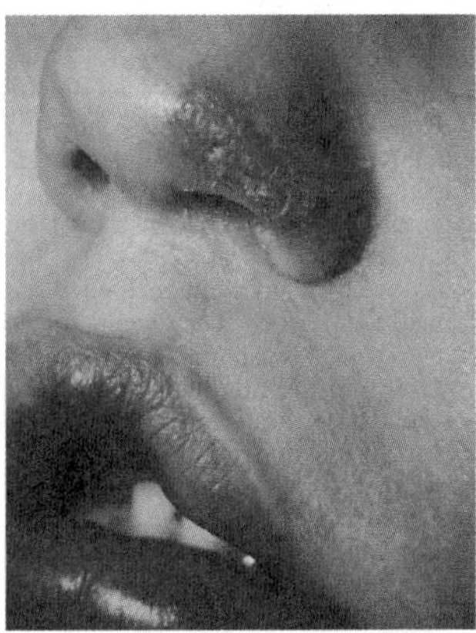

Impetigo. (Zitelli/Davis, 2002. Courtesy Dr. Michael Sherlock)

implant, anterior subperiosteal **(antē′rēər sub′perēos′tēəl),** *n* an implant placed in the anterior part of an edentulous mandible and designed to supply abutments in the two canine regions.

implant, arms of anchor endosteal, n the major portion of the implant infrastructure.

implant, arthroplastic **(ar′thrōplas′tik),** *n* a cast chrome-alloy glenoid fossa prosthesis available in right and left models.

implant, blade, n an implant with a bladelike shape used when a patient's jawbone is considered too narrow to receive a screw or a cylinder endosseous implant. Because of its shape, this implant can be inserted directly into a narrow jaw. These implants must be anchored to another blade implant, root form implants, or natural teeth to assist in handling lateral forces.

implant, blade endosteal, n an implant with a narrow (buccolingually) wedge-shaped infrastructure bearing openings or vents through which tissue grows to obtain retention.

implant, bone, *n* See graft, autogenous, bone; graft, iliac; graft,

implant, ceramic endosteal, *n* an endosteal implant of a variety of designs constructed of silicate or porcelain.

implant, cervix of, *n* that portion of an implant that connects the infrastructure with the abutment as it passes through the mucoperiosteum.

implant, CM (crête manche) spiral end-osteal, *n* a narrow-diameter screw implant designed for thin ridges.

implant, complete subperiosteal, *n* an implant used for an entire edentulous jaw.

implant, complete-arch blade endosteal, *n* a blade type of implant designed to be inserted into a completely edentulous ridge as a single appliance bearing multiple abutments.

implant, crown of anchor endosteal, *n* the abutment part of an anchor implant.

implant denture, *n* a prosthesis (denture) that is secured to the implants via the abutments or a connector bar.

implant, endodontic endosteal, *n* an implant with a threaded or nonthreaded pin that fits into a root canal and extends beyond the dental apex into the adjacent bone, thereby lengthening the clinical root.

implant, endosseous, *n* See implant, endosteal.

implant, endosteal, *n* an implant that is placed into the alveolar and/or basal bone and that protrudes through the mucoperiosteum.

implant, fabricated, *n* a custom-designed implant constructed for a specific operative site.

implant, fixation screw of subperiosteal, *n* the screws, 5 to 7 mm long, that are made of the same surgical alloy as the implant and are used to affix the implant to the underlying bone.

implant, flukes of anchor endosteal, *n* the end portions of the arms that rise to the most superficial portion within the bone.

implant, frame type of ramus endosteal, *n* a prefabricated mandibular full-arch implant consisting of two posterior ramus implants: an anterior (symphyseal) endosteal component and a conjunction bar.

implant, helicoid endosteal, *n* a two-piece end-osteal implant consisting of a helical steel spring that is inserted into bone as a female and a male that may be placed postoperatively and serves as the abutment.

implant, infrastructure of, *n* the part of an implant that is designed to give it retention.

implant, intraperiosteal, *n* an artificial appliance made to conform to the shape of a bone and placed beneath the outer, or fibrous, layer of the periosteum.

implant, mandrel of needle endosteal, *n* a hollow device available in full, half, and shallow depths into which needle implants fit. The mandrel, in turn, is used in the contraangle to drive the needle implant into place.

implant, mesostructure, *n* an intermediate superstructure. A series of splinted copings, each of which fits over an implant abutment or natural tooth and over which fits the completed prosthodontic appliance.

implant, needle endosteal, *n* (pin endosteal) a smooth, thin shaft (self-perforating) that serves as an implant usually in conjunction with two others, the three being placed in bone in tripodal conformity.

implant, nonsubmergible, *n* See implant, one-stage.

implant, one-stage, *n* an endosseous implant placed in the bone and immediately fitted with an abutment or an implant already having a transmucosal coronal portion as part of the implant design so that the implant is exposed to the oral cavity during the healing process. This eliminates the need for a second surgery. Also known as a *nonsubmergible implant* or a *single-stage implant.*

implant, oral, *n* See implant.

implant, polymer tooth replica, *n* an acrylic resin implant, shaped like the tooth recently extracted, that is placed into the tooth's alveolus.

***implant, prosthetic* (prosthet′ik),** *n* an apparatus such as an artificial limb or a crown, bridge, or denture that is affixed to an implant in order to compensate for a missing body part (teeth).

implant, pterygoid **(ter′igoid),** *n* an endosseous implant placed posterior to the maxillary first molar up into the pterygoid plate.

implant, ramus endosteal, *n* a blade type of implant designed for the anterior part of the ramus. See also implant, endosteal, blade.

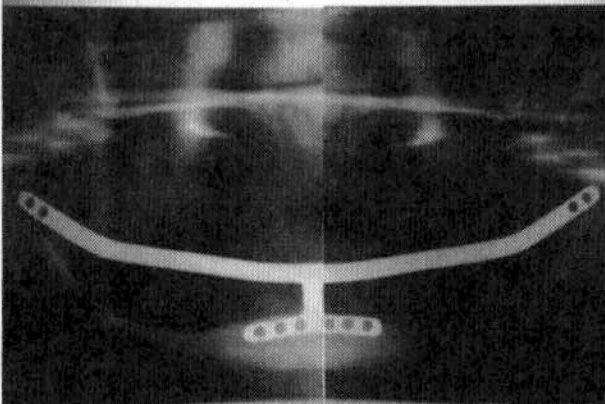

Ramus frame implant. (Courtesy Dr. Charles Babbush)

I

implant, ramus frame **(rā′məs),** *n* a full-arch endosseous implant set into both rami and the symphyseal area of the mandible with a horizontal connecting bar that sits along the gingival tissues, thus forming a design similar to a monorail with a tripodial effect.

implant, root form, *n* a cylindrical mechanism used to affix dental structures to the bone located under the soft tissue. These implants are classified under two forms: a threaded screw-type implant, and a smooth press fitted implant.

implant, seating instrument of anchor endosteal, arm type, *n* a bayonet-shaped device designed to assist in seating an anchor implant by straddling its arms over a specially designed *seating notch.*

implant, seating instrument of anchor endosteal, crown type, *n* a bayonet-shaped, double-ended device designed to assist in seating an anchor implant by cupping its crown or abutment.

implant, seating instrument of endosteal, *n* a device designed to be placed on a portion of an implant so that malleting on it will seat the implant into the bone. It usually has an angled or bayoneted shaft to enable it to protrude from the oral cavity in a more-or-less vertical direction.

implant, shaft of anchor endosteal, *n* the cervix of an anchor implant.

implant, shoulder of blade endosteal, *n* the unbroken surface of the wedge-shaped infrastructure that is widest and most superficial. This part is tapped during the seating of the implant.

implant, single-stage, *n* See implant, one-stage.

implant, single-tooth subperiosteal, *n* an implant designed to replace a single missing tooth; usually unsupported by adjacent natural teeth.

implant, spiral endosteal, *n* a screw type of implant, either hollow or solid, usually consisting of abutment, cervix, and infrastructure.

implant, staple, *n* a type of transosteal implant that allows the attachment of a lower denture to the abutments of two or four threaded posts that go transcortically from a curved plate, which has been inserted through a submental incision and fixed into place at the inferior border of the mandible, through to the canine areas of the alveolar crest of the mandible; retentive screws partially inserted into the inferior border affix the rest of the plate. Also known as *mandibular staple implant* and *transmandibular implant.*

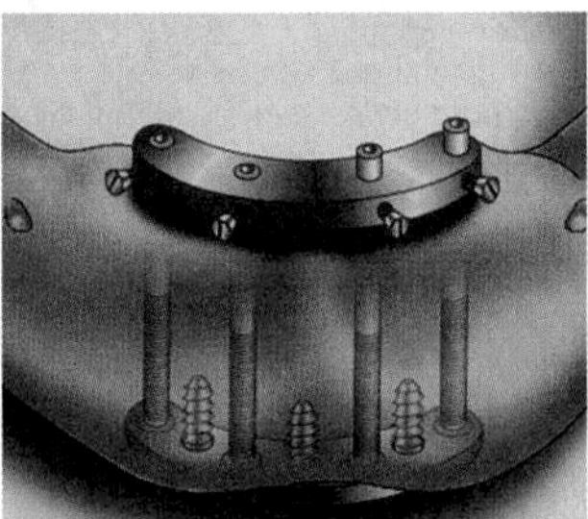

Mandible staple implant. (Courtesy Dr. Charles Babbush)

implant, stock, *n* an implant, usually endosteal, that is available in manufactured form in uniform sizes and shapes.

implant, strut of subperiosteal, *n* a thin, striplike component of an infrastructure.

implant, subperiosteal, *n* an appliance consisting of an open-mesh frame designed to fit over the surface of the bone beneath the periosteum.

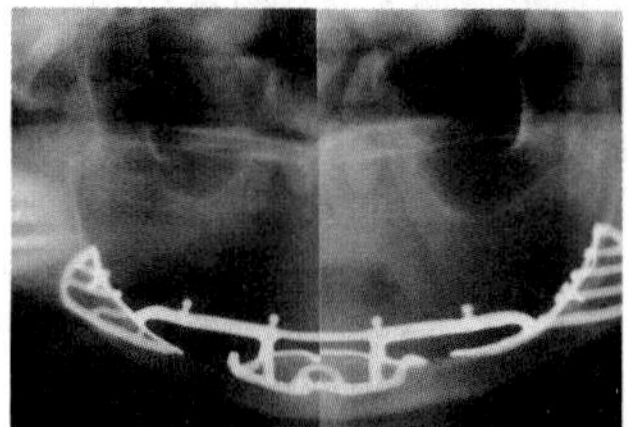

Subperiosteal implant. (Courtesy Dr. Charles Babbush)

implant, superstructure of, *n* a completed prosthesis that is supported entirely or in part by an implant. It may be a removable or fixed prosthesis but may be a single crown or a complete arch splint.

implant, threaded, *n* an endosseous implant with threads resembling a screw; also known as a *screw-type implant.*

implant, transosteal **(transos'tēəl),** *n* an implant that passes completely through the buccal and lingual aspects of a toothless ridge; also, an implant whose threaded posts pass completely through the mandible in the parasymphyseal region from the inferior border to the alveolar crest, allowing the attachment of a dental prosthesis. Also known as a *transosseous implant.* See also staple implant.

implant, two-piece, *n* an implant, either end-osteal or subperiosteal, having its infrastructure and abutment in separate parts. Generally, the abutment, which is threaded, is screwed to the infrastructure some weeks after its incision, so that healing has taken place.

implant, two-stage, *n* an endosseous implant placed in the bone, with the soft tissue over the implant being sutured closed in a stage-one surgery to allow osseointegration of the implant. A second surgery is performed later in which the soft tissue over the submerged implant is removed in order to thread an abutment into the implant so that a prosthesis can be attached; also known as a *submergible implant.*

implant, zygomatic **(zī'gəmat'ik),** *n* a long, screw-shaped endosseous implant placed in the area of the former first maxillary molar up into the zygomatic bone following an intrasinusal trajectory and used as an alternative to bone augmentation of a severely atrophic maxilla.

implantology, oral (im'plantol'əjē), *n* the art and science of dentistry concerned with the surgical insertion of materials and devices into, onto, and about the jaws and oral cavity for purposes of oral maxillofacial or oral occlusal rehabilitation or cosmetic correction.

implied, *adj* inferred; conceded.

implied consent, *n* assent to a clinical procedure that is recognized as an informed agreement by the patient, even if verbal or written consent is not explicitly given.

impression, *n* an imprint or negative likeness of an object from which a positive reproduction may be made.

impression, anatomic, *n* a type that records tissue shape without distortion.

impression, area, *n* See area, impression.

impression, boxing of an, *n* See boxing.

impression, bridge, *n* a type made for the purpose of constructing or assembling a fixed restoration, fixed partial denture, or bridge.

impression, cleft palate, *n* a type that records the upper jaw of a patient with a cleft (incomplete closure, or union) in the palate.

impression, closed oral cavity, *n* a type made while the oral cavity is closed and with the patient's muscular activity molding the borders.

impression, complete denture, *n* a type that records the edentulous arch made for the purpose of constructing a complete denture.

impression, composite, *n* a type consisting of two or more parts.

impression compound, *n* a hermoplastic material containing a mix of resin, filler, and lubricant components, which is useful in obtaining an imprint or impression of the teeth.

impression coping, *n* a medical device used to mark the placement of a dental implant in an impression of the teeth.

I

impression, correctable, *n* an impression with a surface that is capable of alteration by the removal from or addition to some area of its surface or border.

impression, dual, *n* See technique, impression, dual.

impression, duplicating, *n* See duplication.

impression, elastic, *n* a type made in a material that will permit registration of undercut areas by springing over projecting areas and then returning to its original position.

impression, final (secondary impression), *n* a type used for making the master cast.

impression, fluid wax, *n* an impression of the functional form of subjacent structures made with selected waxes that are applied (brushed on) to the impression surface in fluid form.

impression, functional, *n* a type that records the supporting structures in their functional form. See also structure, supporting, functional form of.

impression, hydrocolloid, *n* a type made of a hydrocolloid material.

impression, lower, *n* See impression, mandibular.

impression, mandibular (lower impression), *n* a type that records the mandibular arch and related tissues and dental structures.

impression, material, *n* See material, impression.

impression, maxillary (upper impression), *n* an impression of the maxillary jaw and related tissues and dental structures.

***impression, mercaptan* (mərkap′-tan),** *n* a type made of mercaptan (polysulfide), a rubber-base elastic material.

impression, partial denture, *n* a type that includes part or all of a partially edentulous arch made for the purpose of designing or constructing a partial denture.

impression, pickup, *n* a type made with the superstructure frame in place on the abutments in the oral cavity after the implant has been surgically inserted and the oral cavity has healed. The superstructure frame is included in the impression material, and an accurate impression of the oral mucosal tissue over the implant is obtained.

impression, preliminary, *n* (primary impression) a type made for the purpose of diagnosis or the construction of a tray for making a final impression.

impression, primary, *n* See impression, preliminary.

impression, secondary, *n* See impression, final.

impression, sectional, *n* an impression that is made in sections.

impression, silicone, *n* a rubber-base elastic type made using a material that contains a silicone. See also silicone.

impression, snap, *n* See impression, preliminary.

impression, surface, *n* See denture foundation area and surface, basal.

impression, surgical bone, *n* a type showing the likeness of the exposed bony surfaces necessary to support the implant substructure.

impression technique, *n* See technique, impression.

impression tray, *n* See tray, impression.

impression, upper, *n* See impression, maxillary.

impulse, *n* a surge of electric current for a short time span; e.g., in a 60-cycle AC current, there are 120 impulses per second. See also impression, maxillary.

impulse, muscle, *n* a wave of excitation along a muscle fiber initiated at the neuromuscular endplate; accompanied by chemical and electrical changes at the surface of the muscle fiber and by activation of the contractile elements of the muscle fiber; detectable electronically (electromyographically); and followed by a transient refractory period.

impulse, nerve, *n* a wave of excitation along a nerve fiber initiated by a stimulus; accompanied by chemical and electrical changes at the surface of the nerve fiber and followed by a transient refractory period during which further stimulation has no effect.

impulsive behavior, *n* action initiated without due consideration or thought as to the costs, results, or consequences.

in chief principal; directly obtained, *n* the evidence obtained from a witness on examination in court by the party producing the witness.

in pais (in pā′), *adj* a legal transaction that has been accomplished without legal proceedings.

in potestate parentis (in pōtestä′tā pəren′tis), *adj* under the authority of the parent.

in situ (in sē′too), *n* in the natural or original position. The phrase comes from the Latin for "in position." In dental and medical work, the phrase often describes work done on a dental or body structure in the patient (e.g., almost all dental fillings are done *in situ*).

in utero (in ūtərō), *adj/adv* pertaining to or occurring before birth, e.g., during the gestation period.

in vitro (in ve′tro), *adj/adv* occurring in a laboratory.

in vivo (in ve′vo), *adj/adv* occurring withing a living organism; alive.

in-house, *adj* a term that describes personal, mechanical, or electronic services that are located in the building where they are used, instead of being located remotely.

inactivate, *v* to render inactive; to destroy the activity of.

inactivator, *n* a substance added to a culture medium to prevent the activity of an inoculant. Penicillinase is added to the culture medium to prevent the activity of penicillin that might be carried over from a root canal treatment.

inadequacy, velopharyngeal (vel′ō-fərin′jēəl), *n* a lack of functional closure of the velum to the postpharyngeal wall.

inadmissible, *adj* that which cannot be admitted into evidence in a legal proceeding under the established rules of law.

inbreeding, *n* the production of offspring by the mating of closely related individuals, organisms, or plants; self-fertilization is the most extreme form, which normally occurs in certain plants and lower animals. The practice provides a greater chance for recessive genes for both desirable and undesirable traits to become homozygous and to be expressed phenotypically.

incentive plan, *n* a plan whereby the insurer pays an increasing share of the claim cost provided the covered individual visits the dental professional as stipulated during each incentive period (usually a year) and receives the prescribed treatment.

incentive program, *n* a dental benefits program that pays an increasing share of the treatment cost provided that the covered individual uses the benefits of the program during each incentive period (usually a year) and receives the treatment prescribed. E.g., a 70% to 30% copayment program in the first year of coverage may become an 80% to 20% program in the second year if the subscriber visits the dental professional in the first year as stipulated in the program. Most frequently, there is a corresponding percentage reduction in the program's copayment level if the covered individual fails to visit the dental professional in a given year (but never below the initial copayment level).

incidence (in′sidəns), *n* **1.** the number of times an event occurs. **2.** the number of new cases in a particular period. Incidence is often expressed as a ratio, in which the number of cases is the numerator and the population at risk is the denominator.

incipient (insip′ēent), *adj* beginning, initial, commencing.

incisal (insī′zəl), *adj* relating to the cutting edge of the anterior teeth, incisors, or canines.

incisal angle, n See angle, incisal.

incisal edge, n the cutting surface of the incisors.

incisal guidance angle, n See angle, incisal guidance.

incisal guide, n See guide, incisal.

incisal guide pin, n See pin, incisal guide.

incisal rest, n See rest, incisal.

incisal guidance, *n* See guidance, incisal.

incision (insizh′ən), *n* the act of cutting or biting.

incision and drainage, n See I and D.

incision of food, n the phase of the masticatory cycle, using the incisor teeth, that cuts or separates the bolus of food.

incision, preauricular, n the incision

of the soft tissue anterior to the external ear that permits access to the temporomandibular joint.

incision, relieving, *n* a cut into the soft tissues adjacent to a wound to permit a tension-free closure.

incision, Risdon's, *n* the incision of the soft tissues in the area of the mandibular angle that permits access to the lateral surface of the mandibular ramus, subcondylar neck, and condylar area.

incisive foramen, *n* See foramen, incisive.

incisive papilla, *n* See papilla, incisive.

incisor(s) (insī′zur), *n* a cutting tooth, one of the four anterior teeth of either jaw.

incisor, central, *n* the first incisor.

incisor, Hutchinson's, *n* the malformed teeth caused by the presence of congenital syphilis during tooth development. The incisors usually are shorter than normal, show a single permanent notch on each incisal edge, and are screwdriver shaped.

incisor, lateral, *n* the second incisor.

incisor point, *n* See point, incisor.

inclination (in′klinā′shən), *n* the angle of slope from a particular item of reference.

inclination, axial, *n* the alignment of a tooth in a vertical plane in relationship to its basal bone structure.

inclination, lateral condylar, *n* the direction of the lateral condyle path.

inclination of tooth, *n* See tooth, inclination of.

inclusion cyst, *n* an epidermal cyst formed of a mass of squamous epithelium cells with concentric layers of keratin.

income, *n* the return in money from one's business, practice, or capital invested; gains, profit.

income tax, *n* a tax upon an adjusted gross income (individual or corporate) imposed as a major source of governmental revenue at the state and federal levels.

incompatibility (in′kəmpat′ibil′itē), *n* a disharmonious relationship among the ingredients of prescriptions or other drug mixtures.

incompatibility, chemical, *n* a situation in which two or more of the ingredients of a drug interact chemically, with resulting deterioration of the mixture.

incontinentia pigmenti, *n* See syndrome, Bloch-Sulzberger.

incubation (in″kūbā′shən), *n* the maintenance of an ideal environment with regard to temperature, light, air, and humidity in order to foster development of an organism or culture.

incubation period, *n* the lapsed time between exposure to an infectious agent and the onset of symptoms of a disease.

incubator (in′kūbātur), *n* a laboratory container with controlled temperature for the cultivation of bacteria.

incurred claims, *n.pl* the outstanding obligations of the insurer for dental services rendered to the insured.

indapamide (indap′əmīd′), *n brand name:* Lozol; *drug class:* diuretic, thiazide-like; *action:* acts on distal tubule by increasing excretion of water, sodium, chloride, potassium; *uses:* edema, hypertension.

indemnification schedule, *n* See table of allowances.

indemnity benefit, *n* a contract benefit that is paid to the insured to meet the cost of dental services received.

indemnity plan, *n* **1.** a plan that provides payment to the insured for the cost of dental care but makes no arrangement for providing care itself. **2.** a dental plan in which a third-party payer provides payment of an amount for specific services regardless of the actual charges made by the provider. Payment may be made to enrollees or by assignment directly to dental professionals. Schedule of allowances, table of allowances, and reasonable and customary plans are examples of indemnity plans.

index, *n* **1.** the ratio of a measurable value to another. **2.** a core or mold used to record or maintain the relative position of a tooth or teeth to one another or to a cast. See also splint.

index, Broders's (Broders's classification), *n.pr* **1.** a system of grading of epidermoid carcinoma suggested by Broders. Tumors are graded from I to IV on the basis of cell differentiation. Grade I tumors are highly differentiated, with much keratin production; Grade IV tumors are poorly differentiated; the cells are highly

anaplastic, with almost no keratin formation. *n* **2.** the classification and grading of malignant neoplasms according to the proportion of malignant cells to normal cells in the lesion.
index, cardiac, *n* the minute volume of blood per square meter of body surface.
index, carpal, *n* the degree of ossification of the carpal bones noted in radiographs of the wrist; a method of determining the state of skeletal maturation.
index, cephalic, *n* head shape and size.
Index, Dean's Fluorosis **(flŏŏrō′-sis),** *n.pr* the most commonly used system for classifying dental fluorosis. Ratings are assigned based on the most severe fluorosis seen on two or more teeth.
index, DEF (decayed, extracted, filled), *n.pr* a dental caries index applied to the primary dentition in somewhat the same manner as the DMF index is used for classifying permanent teeth. Missing primary teeth are ignored in this index because of the uncertainty in determining whether they were extracted because of advanced caries or exfoliated normally.
index, DMF (decayed, missing, filled), *n.pr* a technique for managing statistically the number of decayed, missing, or filled teeth in the oral cavity. Analysis may be based on the average number of DMF teeth (sometimes called DMFT) per person or the average number of DMF tooth surfaces (DMFS).
index, facial height, *n* the ratio of posterior facial height to anterior facial height.
index, gingiva and bone count (Dunning-Leach index), *n* an index that permits differential recording of both gingival and bone conditions to determine gingivitis and bone loss.
index, gingival (GI), *n* an assessment tool used to evaluate a case of gingivitis based on visual inspection of the gingivae that takes into consideration the color and firmness of gingival tissue along with the presence of blood during probing.
index, gingival bleeding (GBI), *n* an assessment tool used to verify the presence of gingival inflammation based on any bleeding that occurs at the gingival margin during or immediately after flossing.
index, gnathic, *n* the relationship of jaw size to head size.
index, icterus, *n* See test, Meulengracht's.
index, malocclusion, *n* a measure of the severity of a malocclusion, obtained by assigning values to a series of defined observations.
index, measuring, *n* an expression of relationship of one measurable value to another, or a formula based on measurable values.
index, missing teeth, *n* See index, DMF.
index, oral hygiene, simplified (Greene-Vermillion index), *n* an index made up of two components, the debris index and the calculus index, which are based on numerical determination representing the amount of debris or calculus found on six preselected tooth surfaces.
index, periodontal (Ramfjord index), *n* a thorough clinical examination of the periodontal status of six teeth, with an evaluation of the gingival condition, pocket depth, calculus and plaque deposits, attrition, mobility, and lack of contact.
index, periodontal disease (Russell index), *n* an index that measures the condition of both the gingiva and the bone individually for each tooth and arrives at the average status for periodontal disease in a given oral cavity.
index, plaque, *n* an assessment tool used to evaluate the thickness of plaque at the gingival margin that may be applied to selected teeth or to the entire oral cavity.
index, PMA (Schour-Massler index), *n* an index used for recording the prevalence and severity of gingivitis in schoolchildren by noting and scoring three areas: the gingival papillae (P), the buccal or labial gingival margin (M), and the attached gingiva (A).
index, Pont's, *n* the relation of the width of the four incisors to the width between the first premolars and the width between the first molars.
index, Russell, *n.pr* See index, periodontal disease.

index, salivary **Lactobacillus (lak′-tōbəsil′əs),** *n* a count of the lactobacilli per milliliter of saliva; used as an indicator of present dental caries activity. The test is of questionable value in individual patients, although its use in large groups has led to valuable information on caries activity.

index, saturation, *n* a number indicating the hemoglobin content of a person's red blood cells as compared with the normal content.

index, sulcus bleeding, *n.pr* an assessment tool used to evaluate the existence of gingival bleeding in individual teeth and/or regions of the oral cavity upon gentle probing by assigning a score of 0-5, with 0 indicating a healthy appearance and no bleeding.

I

index, therapeutic, *n* the ratio of toxic dose to effective dose.

index, ventilation, *n* the index obtained by dividing the ventilation test by the vital capacity.

indication, *n* that which serves as a guide or warning.

indicator, *n* a mark or symptom specific to a condition or disease.

indicator, biologic, *n* a small quantity of harmless bacteria *(B. stearothermophilus)* placed into an object prior to sterilization, the subsequent death of which indicates that sterilization has taken place. See *B. stearothermophilus.*

indicator chemical, *n* a temperature-sensitive mark that changes color when a specific temperature has been reached. Used in the heat sterilization process but is by itself not proof that an object has been sterilized.

indicator diseases, *n* opportunistic infectious diseases or neoplastic diseases that are associated with primary immunodeficiency disease, such as caused by the retrovirus HIV-1.

indirect method, *n* See method, indirect restorative.

indirect pulp capping, *n* See capping, pulp, indirect.

indirect retention, *n* See retention, indirect.

indirect vision, *n* See vision, indirect.

indium (In) (in′dēəm), *n* a silvery metallic element with some nonmetallic chemical properties. Its atomic number is 49, and its atomic weight is 114.82. It is used in electronic semiconductors.

individual practice association (IPA), *n* **1.** an organization for the maintenance of the solo private practitioner as a lobbying force and vocal springboard. **2.** legal entity organized and operated on behalf of individual participating dental professionals for the primary purpose of collectively entering into contracts to provide dental services to enrolled populations. Dental professionals may practice in their own offices and may provide care to patients not covered by the contract as well as to IPA patients.

individual retirement account (IRA), *n* a savings certificate exempt from income tax until the time of withdrawal. There are limits to the amount that can be saved annually under this plan, and there are conditions of withdrawal for maximal interest and tax advantage.

individuality, *n* collective characteristics or traits that distinguish one person or thing from all others.

indomethacin/indomethacin sodium trihydrate (in′dōmeth′əsin sō′dēəm trīhī′drāt), *n brand names:* Indocin, Indocin SR, Indameth; *drug class:* nonsteroidal antiinflammatory; *action:* inhibits prostaglandin synthesis by interfering with cyclooxygenase needed for biosynthesis; possesses analgesic, antiinflamatory, antipyretic properties; *uses:* rheumatoid arthritis, osteoarthritis, ankylosing rheumatoid spondylitis, acute gouty arthritis.

induced, *adj* artificially caused to occur.

induction (induk′shən), *n* **1.** the act or process of inducing or causing to occur. **2.** the process by which the action of one group of cells on another leads to the establishment of the developmental pathway in the responding tissue.

inductive reasoning, *n* analyzing a problem by working from specific facts and discovering general principles. See also deductive reasoning.

indurated tissue (in′dərā′tid), *n* a soft tissue that is abnormally firm because of an influx of exudate or fibrous tissue elements.

induration, *n* **1.** the hardening of tissue, usually because of the accumulation of cells from an inflamed or infected site. Also called *sclerosis* when caused by inflammation. **2.** an accumulation of hard tissue.

industrial dentistry, *n* **1.** a type of dentistry that is concerned with the dental health of the worker as it affects the working environment. **2.** a dental service provided in the industrial plant, usually restricted to emergency care.

inert, *adj* inactive; without the ability to act, move, change, or resist.

inertia (inur′shə), *n* according to Newton's law of inertia, the tendency of a body that is at rest to remain at rest and a body that is in motion to continue in motion with constant speed in the same straight line unless acted on by an outside force.

infant, *n/adj* a child who is in the earliest stage of extrauterine life, a time extending from the first month after birth to approximately 12 months of age, when the baby is able to assume an erect posture; some extend the period to 24 months of age.

infant mortality, *n* the statistical rate of infant death during the first year after live birth, expressed as the number of such births per 1000 live births in a specific geographic area. Neonatal mortality accounts for 70% of infant mortality.

infantilism (infan′tilizəm), *n* a disturbance marked by mental retardation and retention of childhood characteristics into adult life. Teeth may be delayed in eruption or absent.

infarct (in′färkt), *n* the death of a tissue caused by partial occlusion of a vessel or vessels supplying the area.

infection (infek′shən), *n* an invasion of the tissues of the body by disease-producing microorganisms and the reaction of these tissues to the microorganisms and/or their toxins. The mere presence of microorganisms without reaction is not evidence of infection.

infection, adenovirus, *n* a proliferation of the adenovirus that may cause any number of illnesses, including "swimming pool conjunctivitis" and gastrointestinal or respiratory diseases, among others; it is possible to be infected without manifesting any symptoms.

infection, airborne, *n* an infection contracted by inhalation of microorganisms contained in air or water particles.

infection control, *n* procedures and protocols designed to prevent or limit cross-contamination in the health care delivery environment.

infection control, blood bank and blood transfusion, *n.pl* the precautions taken to ensure that blood-borne pathogens are not transmitted via donated blood; includes rejection of potential donors whose medical history shows evidence of viral hepatitis, drug addiction, or recent blood transfusions or tattoos, as well as laboratory testing of all donated blood for the presence of hepatitis B and C, syphilis, and the HIV-1 antibody.

infection control, surveillance, *n* the monitoring of the transmission of a disease in order to limit its occurrence.

infection, focal, *n* the process in which microorganisms located at a certain site, or focus, in the body are disseminated throughout the body to set up secondary sites, or foci, of infection in other tissues.

infection, hemolytic streptococcal, *n* **1.** an infection usually caused by Group A hemolytic streptococci. Such infections include scarlet fever, streptococcal sore throat, cellulitis, and osteomyelitis. **2.** an infection caused by streptococci that produce a toxic substance (hemolysin) that will lyse the erythrocytes and liberate hemoglobin from red blood cells.

infection, inflammatory, *n* an influx or accumulation of inflammatory elements (cellular and exudative) in the interstices of the tissues as a result of tissue injury by physical, chemical, microbiologic, and other irritants. Cellular elements include lymphocytes, plasma cells, polymorphonuclear leukocytes, and the macrophages of reticuloendothelial origin.

infection, latent, *n* a lingering infection that may lie dormant in the body for a time but may become active under certain conditions.

infection, local, n the prevention of excitation of the free nerve endings by literally flooding the immediate area with a local anesthetic solution.

infection, nosocomial, n an infection that first occurs during a patient's stay at a health care facility, regardless of whether it is detected during the stay or after.

infection, opportunistic, n an illness or condition that occurs when pathogens are able to exploit a vulnerable host. An infection that is able to take hold because resistance is low.

infection, primary, n the original outbreak of an illness against which the body has had no opportunity to build antibodies; the originating infection.

infection, recurrent, n a reoccurrence of the same illness from which an individual has previously recovered.

infection, Vincent's, n.pr See gingivitis, necrotizing ulcerative.

infection, waterborne, n an illness that occurs as the result of drinking contaminated water or of eating fish that has been taken from contaminated waters.

infection resistance, *n* the ability of an individual to fight off the detrimental effects of microorganisms and their toxic products. A complexity involving individual and interacting factors—e.g., antibody formation, adequate nutrition, tissue tone, circulation, and emotional stability.

infection susceptibility, *n* the degree of capability of being influenced by or involved in the pathologic processes produced by microorganisms and/or their toxins.

infectious, *adj* contagious; communicable; capable of causing infection.

infectious mononucleosis (mon′ō-noo′klēō′sis), *n* a benign lymphadenosis caused by the Epstein-Barr virus (EBV) and characterized by fever, sore throat, palatal petechiae, enlargement of lymph nodes and spleen, and prolonged weakness with a characteristic shift in the white blood cells during the course of the disease.

inferior, *n* a part of the body located below another; the opposite of *superior.* E.g., the legs are inferior to the hands when facing the body.

inferior alveolar nerve, *n* the nerve formed from the merger of the incisive and mental nerves that serves the tissues of the chin, lower lip, and labial mucosa of the mandibular anterior and premolar teeth and later joins the posterior trunk of the mandibular division of the trigeminal nerve.

infertile, *adj* unable to produce offspring.

infiltrate (infil′trāt), *n* **1.** the material deposited by infiltration. *v* **2.** to deposit material in a location.

infiltration (in′filtrā′shən), *n* **1.** an accumulation in a tissue of a substance not normal to it. **2.** the placement of a local anesthetic agent. See also anesthesia, infiltration.

inflammation (in′fləmā′shən), *n* the cellular and vascular response or reaction to injury. Inflammation is characterized by pain, redness, swelling, heat, and disturbance of function. It may be acute or chronic. The term is not synonymous with *infection,* which implies an inflammatory reaction initiated by invasion of living organisms.

inflammation, gingival, n See gingivitis.

inflammation, granulomatous, n a chronic inflammation in which there is formation of granulation tissue.

inflammation, periodontal, n See periodontitis and gingivitis.

inflation (inflā′shən), *n* the act of distending with air or a gas.

influences, local environmental, *n.pl* the factors or agents within the oral cavity that are responsible for the initiation, perpetuation, or modification of a pathologic state within the stomatognathic system.

influences, systemic environmental, *n.pl* the systemic factors that may initiate, perpetuate, or modify disease processes within the stomatognathic system. Generally, the oral manifestations of systemic disease are modified by the influence of local environmental factors.

influenza (in′flooen′zə), *n* a highly contagious infection of the respiratory tract caused by a myxovirus and transmitted by airborne droplet infection. Symptoms include sore throat, cough, fever, muscular pains, and weakness. Fever and constitutional symptoms distinguish influenza from the common cold. Three main strains of influenza virus have been recognized: Type A, Type B, and Type C. New strains of the virus emerge at regular intervals and are named according to geographic origin. Asian flu is a Type A influenza.

influenza-virus vaccine, *n* an active immunizing agent prescribed for immunization against influenza, generally recommended for at-risk populations, such as the elderly.

informed consent, *n* an agreement by a patient, verbal or written, after being told in sufficient detail of possible risks, to have a procedure performed.

infrabony pocket (in′frəbōnē), *n* See pocket, infrabony.

infrabulge (in′frəbulj), *n* the surface of the crown of a tooth cervical to the clasp guide line, survey line, or surveyed height of contour.

infraclusion (in′frəkloo′zhən), *n* (infraversion) the position occupied by a tooth when it has failed to erupt sufficiently to reach the occlusal plane.

infradentale (in′frədental′ē), *n* the most anterior point of the alveolar process of the mandible.

infrahyoid muscles (in′frəhī′oid), *n.pl* See muscle, suprahyoid and infrahyoid.

infraorbital foramen, *n* See foramen, infraorbital.

infraversion (in′frəvur′zhən), *n* See infraclusion.

infusion (infū′zhən), *n* **1.** the therapeutic introduction of a fluid, such as saline solution, into a vein. In contrast to injection, infusion suggests the introduction of a larger volume of a less concentrated solution over a more protracted period. **2.** a term used in pharmacy for a liquid extract prepared by steeping a plant substance in water.

ingate, *n* See sprue.

inhalant (inhā′lənt), *n* a medicine to be inhaled.

inhalation (inhəlā′shən), *n* the drawing of air or other gases into the lungs.

inhalation, endotracheal, *n* the inhalation of an anesthetic mixture into the lungs through an endotracheal catheter at low or atmospheric pressure.

inhaler, *n* **1.** a device that produces a vapor to ease breathing or is used to medicate by inhalation, especially a small nasal applicator containing a volatile medicament. Also called *nasal inhaler.* **2.** a device that is placed over the nose to permit inhalation of anesthetic agents.

inhibition (in′hibish′ən), *n* a neurologic phenomenon associated with the transmission of an impulse across a synapse. An impulse can be blocked from passing a synapse in a reflex situation by the firing of another, more dominant nerve. It can be achieved directly by preventing the passage of an impulse along an axon, or it can be achieved by liberation of a chemical substance at the nerve ending. This chemical inhibition is demonstrated by the sympathetic-parasympathetic control over smooth muscle activity in a blood vessel. Inhibition is the restraining of a function of a tissue or organ by some nervous or hormone control. It is the opposite of *excitation.*

inhibitor, *n* a substance that slows or stops a chemical reaction.

inhibitor of cholinesterase (inhib′itur əv kō′lines′terās), *n* a chemical that interferes with the activity of the enzyme cholinesterase.

inhibitor, proton pump, *n* a pharmacologic agent used to control heartburn by suppressing the production of stomach acid by blocking the action of the proton pump.

inion (in′ēon), *n* the most elevated point on the external occipital protuberance in the midsagittal plane.

initialize, *v* to set counters, switches, and addresses to 0 or other starting values at the beginning of, or at prescribed points in, a computer routine.

initiation stage, *n* the primary stage in the development of a tooth.

initiator (inish′ēātur), *n* a chemical agent added to a resin to initiate polymerization.

injection (injek′shən), *n* **1.** the injection of material into an area. **2.** the act of introducing a liquid into the body by means of a needle and syringe. Injections are designated according to the anatomic site involved.

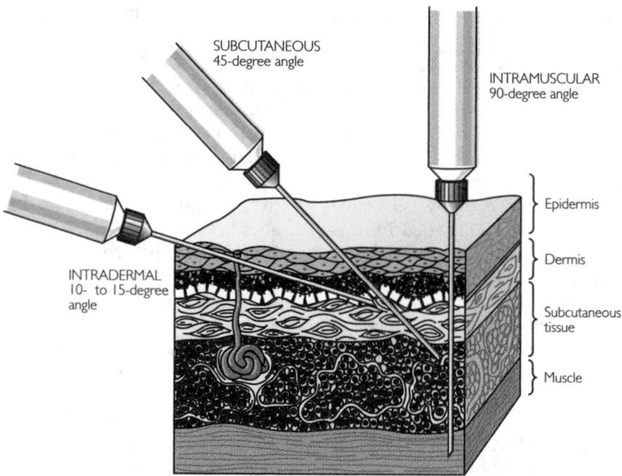

Injection into skin. (Chester, 1998)

The most common injections are intraarterial, intradermal, intramuscular, intravenous, and subcutaneous. The colloquial term is *shot.*

injection, Gow-Gates (GG), *n* See technique, Gow-Gates (GG) anesthetic.

injection, interseptal **(in′tersep′təl),** *n* an intraosseous injection of a local anesthetic agent in the interseptal bone between two teeth. Often used as a supplemental form of local anesthesia when more anesthesia is needed.

injection, intraosseous **(in′trəos′ēəs),** *n* an injection of a local anesthetic agent directly into the alveolar bone. Can include an interseptal injection and periodontal ligament injection.

injection molding, *n* See molding, injection.

injection, periodontal ligament (intraligamentary) **(per′ēōdon′təl lig′əmənt in′trəlig′əmen′tərē),** *n* an intraosseous injection of a local anesthetic agent directly to the alveolar bone surrounding the periodontal ligament. Often used as a supplemental form of local anesthesia when preliminary methods have proven ineffective.

injury, *n* the insult, harm, or hurt applied to tissues; may evoke dystrophic or inflammatory response from the affected part.

injury, root, *n* the damage to the root, especially to the cementum, when an excessive force is placed on the tooth.

injury, toothbrush, *n* the damage to the teeth and associated tissue produced by incorrect toothbrushing.

inlay, *n* **1.** a restoration of metal, fired porcelain, or plastic made to fit a tapered cavity preparation and fastened to or luted into it with a cementing medium. *v* **2.** to perform such a procedure.

inlay furnace, *n* See furnace, inlay.

inlay resin, *n* See resin, inlay.

inlay, setting, *n* the procedure of fitting a casting to a preparation; adjusting the occlusal function and contact areas; securing the proper, clean dry field; cementing the cleaned, polished casting in an aseptic, dry prepared cavity; and completing the final finishing and polishing of the restoration.

inlay wax, *n* See wax, inlay.

innervation (in′urvā′shən), *n* the distribution or supply of nerves to a part.

innervation, reciprocal, *n* the simultaneous excitation of one muscle with the inhibition of its antagonist. Rhythmic chewing is achieved efficiently when the masticatory muscles are reciprocally innervated, permitting alternate elevation and depression of the mandible in a smooth, coordinated sequence of actions.

inoculation (ĭnok″ula′shən), *n* a procedure in which a disease-causing substance is introduced into otherwise healthy tissue for the sole purpose of inducing immunity. See also immunization.

inorganic, *adj* having no derivation from living organisms; chemical compounds that generally do not contain carbon.

inositol (inō′sitol), *n* an essential growth factor in tissue culture with no known requirement. It has been used therapeutically in the management of diseases associated with the metabolism of fat.

input, computer, *n* the data to be processed.

input/output control (I/O control), *n* the portion of the central processor of some computer systems that contains software/firmware for supervising data flow between memory and the input/output devices connected to the CPU.

inquiry, *n* a request for information from storage in a computer.

insert, intramucosal (in′trəmūkō′səl), *n* (mucosal insert, implant button), a nonreactive metal appliance that is affixed to the tissue-bone surface of a denture and offers added retentive qualities to the denture. It consists of a base, cervix, and head.

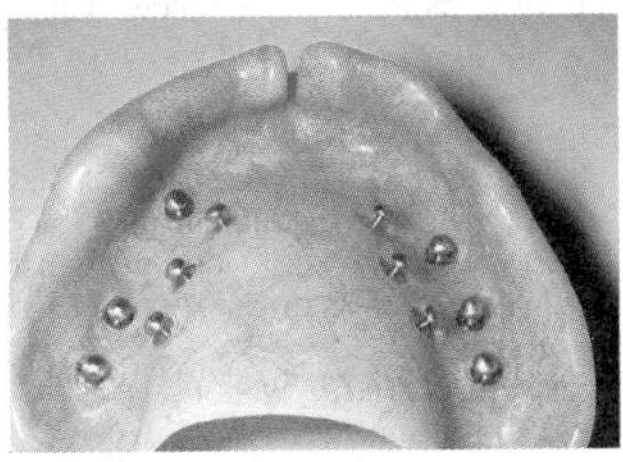

Mucosal inserts in a maxillary denture. (Courtesy Dr. Charles Babbush)

insert, mucosal, *n* See insert, intramucosal.

insertion (insur′shən), *n* the act of implanting or placing materials or introducing the needle into the tissues.

insertion, path of, n the direction in which a prosthesis is inserted and removed.

insidious disease (insid′ēus), *adj* a disease existing without marked symptoms but ready to become active upon some slight occasion; a disease not appearing to be as bad as it really is.

insoluble, *adj* not susceptible to being dissolved.

insomnia, *n* the chronic inability to sleep or remain asleep throughout the night.

inspection, *n* the visual examination of the body or portions thereof, which is an integral phase of the physical or dental examination procedure.

inspiration (in″spĭra′shən), *n* the act of drawing air into the lungs.

inspirometer (in′spirom′ətur), *n* an instrument for measuring the force, frequency, or volume of inspirations.

I

institutionalize, *v* to place a person in a health care or custodial facility for psychologic or physical treatment or for the protection of the person or society.

instruction, *n* a set of characters, together with one or more addresses, that defines a computer operation and, as a unit, causes the computer to operate accordingly on the indicated quantities; a term associated with software operation.

instruction of partial denture patient, n See denture, partial, instruction of patient.

instrument(s), *n* a tool or implement, especially one used for delicate or scientific work. See under the specific type of instrument (e.g., knife). See also instrumenting, instrumentarium.

instrument, air application, n a tool used to apply air in order to dry teeth, remove debris, and control saliva during treatment or in preparation for a specific procedure.

instrument, bibeveled cutting **(bī′bevəld),** *n* an instrument in which both sides of the end of the blade are beveled to form the cutting edge, as in a hatchet.

instrument blade, n the part bearing a cutting edge; it begins at the terminal angle of the shank and ends at the cutting edge.

instrument, blade face, n the innermost surface of a scaler or curet blade.

instrument, carving, *n* See carver.

instrument, classification of, names, *n* the classification of instruments by name to denote purpose (e.g., excavator), to denote position or manner of use (e.g., hand condenser), to describe the form of the point (e.g., hatchet), or to describe the angle of the blade in relation to the handle.

instrument, condensing, *n* a hand-held device used to adapt dental amalgams to a prepared cavity.

instrument, cutting, *n* an instrument used to cut, cleave, or plane the walls of a cavity preparation; the blade ends in a sharp, beveled edge. Unless otherwise specified, it refers to a hand instrument rather than to a rotary type.

instrument, diamond, *n* a rotary abrasive instrument, wheel, or mounted point. Made of fine diamond chips bonded into a desired form; used to reduce tooth structure.

instrument, double-ended, *n* a hand-held tool with two functional ends that are identical or complementary.

instrument, double-plane, *n* an instrument with the curve of the blade in a plane perpendicular to that of the angles of the shank.

instrument, formula name of, *n* a method of naming and describing dental hand instruments. Measurements are in the metric system. The working point is described first; then the formula is given, in three (or sometimes four) units. The first figure denotes the width of the blade, in tenths of millimeters; the second shows the length of the blade, in millimeters; and the third indicates the angle of the blade in relation to the shaft, in centigrades or hundredths of a circle. Whenever it is necessary to describe the angle of the cutting edge of a blade with its shaft, the number is entered in brackets as the second number of the formula. Paired instruments are also designated as right or left. In lateral cutting instruments the one used to cut from right to left is termed *right;* in direct cutting instruments with right and left bevels, the one having the bevel on the right side of the blade as it is held with the cutting edge down and pointing away from the observer is termed *right.*

instrument grasp, *n* See grasp, instrument.

instrument, hand, *n* an instrument used principally with hand force.

instrument, holding, *n* an instrument used to support gold foil while a foil restoration is inserted.

instrument, McCall's, *n.pr* a periodontal instrument used for gingival curettage and for removing deposits from the tooth surfaces.

instrument nib, *n* the counterpart of the blade in the condensing instrument; the end of the nib is the face.

instrument, parts, *n.pl* the handle or shaft, blade or nib, and shank.

instrument, plastic, *n* an instrument used to manipulate a plastic restorative material.

instrument, rotary cutting, *n* a power-activated instrument used in a dental handpiece, such as a bur, mounted diamond point, mounted carborundum point, wheel stone, or disk.

instrument, screwdriver, *n* an instrument made of surgical alloy; it may have at its tip a screw holder that is designed to drive screws into the bone.

instrument shaft/handle, *n* the part that is grasped by the clinician's hand while using the instrument.

instrument shank, *n* the part that connects the shaft and the blade or nib.

instrument sharpening, *n* See sharpening, instrument.

instrument, single-beveled cutting, *n* an instrument in which one side of the end of the blade is beveled to form the cutting edge, as in a wood chisel.

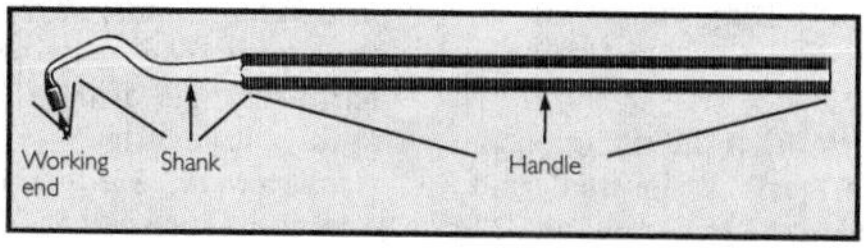

Parts of an instrument. (Bird/Robinson, 2005)

instrument, single-plane, n an instrument with all its angles and curves in one plane; when the instrument lies on a flat surface, the cutting edge and the blade will parallel the surface.

instrument, sonic, n a mechanical tool whose thin tip vibrates at high rates and is used to remove debris, deposits, or dead or damaged tissue.

instrument stop, n a device, usually metal, that can be placed on a reamer or file to mark the measurement of the root.

instrument, toe, n the tip or terminating end of the blade, may be rounded (blunt) or pointed (sharp).

instrument, universal, n a tool that may be used on all types of teeth surfaces.

instrumental values, n a person's innermost convictions concerning the means, as opposed to the ends, of a goal.

instrumentarium (in′strəmentar′ēəm), *n* the exact instruments required to perform a specific procedure.

instrumentation (in′strəmentā′shən), *n* the use of, or work done by, instruments in the treatment of a patient.

instrumentation, endpoint of, n the ultimate goal of instrument use in the periodontal process, which is to prepare the teeth and surrounding structures for healing and to maintain optimal oral health.

instrumentation zone, n the section of a tooth requiring the use of an instrument to remove deposits and debris.

instrumenting, *n* the colloquial term for the use of hand-activated tools to remove debris, plaque, and overhangs from the teeth.

insufficiency, adrenocortical (ədrē′nōkôr′tikəl), *n* See hypoadrenocorticalism.

insufficiency, functional, *n* the inadequacy of usage of stimulation to a part of the body, often resulting in atrophic tissue changes.

insufflation (in′səflā′shən), *n* the act of blowing a powder, vapor, gas, or air into a cavity such as the lungs.

insufflation, endotracheal, n the forcing of an anesthetic mixture into the lungs through an endotracheal catheter under pressure.

insufflation, mouth-to-mouth, n the oldest recorded procedure for artificially ventilating the lungs. The lungs are inflated by blowing into the oral cavity, and expiration either is passive or is assisted by compressing the thorax. Adequate ventilation is produced, and the procedure should be used when other techniques are not applicable; e.g., in thoracic injury. Auxiliary airway tubes are available for use when mouth-to-mouth insufflation is required. Such tubes maintain the airway and prevent the tongue from obstructing the glottis.

insufflator (in′sə-fla″tər), *n* an instrument used in insufflation.

insulator, thermal (in′səlātur), *n* a material having a low thermal conductivity.

insulin (antidiabetic hormone) (in′səlin′ an′tēdī′əbet′ik), *n* a hormone produced by the beta cells of the islets of Langerhans in the pancreas. It promotes a decrease in blood sugar. Its action may be influenced by the pituitary growth hormone, adrenocorticotropic hormone; hormones of the adrenal cortex; epinephrine; glucagon; and thyroid hormone.

insulin (obtained from beef or pork, or human recombinant technology), *n brand names:* Velosulin, Humulin R, Novolin R, Lente Insulin; *drug class:* exogenous insulin, antidiabetic; *action:* decreases blood glucose; important in regulation of fat and protein metabolism; *uses:* ketoacidosis; type 1 and type 2 diabetes mellitus; hyperkalemia; hyperalimentation.

insulin, exogenous **(eksoj′ənəs),** *n* a type that comes from a source external to a diabetic patient's body, taken to offset the patient's natural deficiency of insulin.

insulin, intermediate-acting, n a type that is a medium between rapid-acting and long-acting insulins; the onset is not as fast as rapid-acting insulin, but it reaches its peak action over a 4- to 12-hour period.

insulin, Lente **(len′te),** *n.pr* an intermediate-acting type that reaches its peak action over a 4- to 12-hour period.

I

insulin, Lispro, n.pr a rapid-acting type that reaches its peak action in 30 to 90 minutes.

insulin, long-acting, n a type that has a slow onset but reaches its peak action from 12 to 16 hours after administration.

insulin, NPH, n a synthetic type used to treat diabetes. Classified as intermediate acting; peak action occurs 4 to 10 hours after administering.

insulin, rapid-acting, n a synthetic type of insulin used to treat diabetes. Reaches peak action 30 to 90 minutes after administering.

insulin, regular, n a synthetic type used to treat diabetes. Classified as short acting; peak action occurs 2 to 3 hours after administering.

insulin resistance, n a complication of diabetes mellitus characterized by a need for more than 200 units of insulin per day to control hyperglycemia and ketosis. The cause is associated with insulin binding by high levels of antibody.

insulin shock, n See shock, insulin.

insulin, short-acting, n a synthetic type used to treat diabetes. Reaches peak action 2 to 3 hours after administering. Also called *regular insulin.*

insulin, ultralente **(ul′trəlen′te),** *n* a synthetic type used to treat diabetes. Classified as long acting, with peak action occurring 12 to 16 hours after administering.

insulin-like growth factors (IGF), *n* a group of polypeptides responsible for the activity of growth hormones, similar in chemical structure to insulin.

insurance, *n* a contract, or policy, whereby, for a stipulated consideration, or premium, one party (the insurer or underwriter) promises to compensate the other (the insured or assured) for loss on a specified subject (insurable interest) by specified perils or risks.

insurance benefits, n the contractual payout agreed to by the carrier for the policy holder.

insurance carriers, n.pl the organizations that for a contractual fee underwrite the payment of losses or costs incurred by the policy holder within the conditions of the policy.

insurance, group, n the type that covers a group of persons, usually employees of a single employer or members of a union local, under one contract for the benefit of the members of the group.

insurance, guaranteed renewable, n a policy that is renewable at the option of the insured until a stated time, such as the seventieth birthday of the insured. See also noncancellable insurance.

insurance, health, n the type that provides financial return when the dental professional is unable to practice because of prolonged illness.

insurance, liability, n insurance protecting the dental professional from financial loss resulting from liability suits.

insurance, life, n a protective contract providing for compensation to the beneficiaries of the insured.

insurance, malpractice, n in dentistry, insurance covering accidents or catastrophes that may occur during the performance of professional duties.

insurance, retirement, n a life insurance that carries, as an additional benefit, payments to the insured when he or she reaches a specific age.

insured, *n* a person covered by an insurance program. See also beneficiary.

insurer, *n* an organization that bears the financial risk for the cost of defined categories or services for a defined group of beneficiaries. See also third party.

intake, *n* the substance or quantities thereof taken in and used by the body.

intelligence, *n* mental potential or capacity; an individual's total repertoire of problem-solving and cognitive discrimination responses that are usual and expected at a given age level and in the large population unit; that which is measured by an intelligence test.

intelligence dental, quotient, n an estimated appraisal of a patient's knowledge and appreciation of dental services.

intelligence quotient (IQ), n an estimate of intelligence level; an index determined by dividing the mental age in months by the chronologic age in months and multiplying the result by 100. Thus the IQ of a child of 100 months with a mental age of 110 months would be 110.

intensifying screen, *n* See screen, intensifying.

intensity of a radiographic beam, *n* the amount of energy in a radiographic beam per unit volume or area.

intensity, radiation, *n* the energy flowing through a unit area perpendicular to the beam per unit of time. It is expressed in ergs per square centimeter or in watts per square centimeter.

intensive care, *n* the constant, complex, detailed health care as provided in various acute life-threatening conditions, such as multiple trauma, severe burns, and myocardial infarction, and after certain kinds of surgery.

interaction, *n* according to Newton's law of interaction, the phenomenon in which every force is accompanied by an equal and opposite force. For every force there are two bodies—one to exert the force and one to receive it. Furthermore, whenever there is one force, another force must also be involved. If there is force to the right on one body, there is force to the left on another. Because the one force acts as long as the other, the impulses are equal. The total momentum of the two interacting bodies cannot change. Continuous interaction is demonstrated between the food that is masticated and the force applied to the food.

interalveolar space (in'təralvē'ōlur), *n* See distance, interarch.

interarch distance, *n* See distance, interarch.

intercellular (in'tursel'ūlur), *adj* taking place between or among cells.

interceptive orthodontics, *n* an extension of preventive orthodontics that may include minor local tooth movement in an otherwise normally developing dentition.

intercondylar distance (in'turkon'dilur), *n* the distance between the vertical axes of a pair of condyles.

intercuspation (in'turkuspā'shən), *n* the cusp-to-fossa relationship of the maxillary and mandibular posterior teeth to each other.

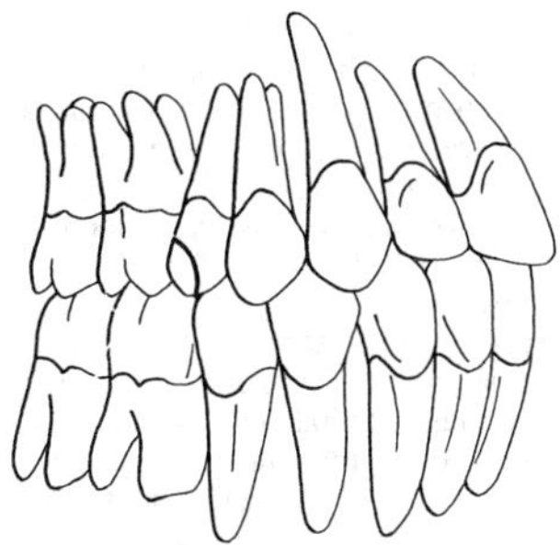

Intercuspation. (Roberson/Heymann/Swift, 2006)

interdental (in'turden'təl), *adj* situated between the proximal surfaces of adjacent teeth.

interdental canal, *n* See canal, interdental.

interdental embrasure, *n* See embrasure, interdental.

interdental gingiva, *n* See gingiva, interdental.

interdental septum, *n* See septum, interdental.

interdental splint, *n* See splint, interdental.

interdental tip, *n* an oral hygiene tool that features a rubber tip shaped like a small cone or pyramid; used to assist in the removal of plaque and other matter from between teeth. Also effective in and around the gingival area.

interdigitation (in'turdij'itā'shən), *n* See intercuspation.

interdisciplinary team, *n* a group that consists of specialists from several fields combining skills and resources to present guidance and information.

interface (in'turfās), *n* the surface, such as a plane surface, formed between the walls of a prepared cavity or extracoronal preparation and a restoration. It forms a common boundary between the tooth structure and the restorative material.

interface, computer, *n* a common boundary (connection) between automatic data processing systems or parts of a system.

interfacial surface tension, *n* See tension, interfacial surface.

interference, cuspal, *n* See contact, deflective occlusal.

interference marking, *n* the mark-

I

ing of the occlusive surfaces of the teeth while the jaw is at rest, usually performed by having the patient tap the teeth on a piece of special marking paper.

interference, occlusal, *n* tooth-to-tooth contact that interferes with jaw movement.

interferon (in′tərfir′on), *n* a small class of glycoproteins capable of exerting antiviral activity in homologous cells through metabolic processes involving synthesis of RNA.

interferon alpha, n a type formed by leukocytes in response to viral infection or by stimulation with double-stranded RNA. These protein products are used as antineoplastic agents. Specifically used as an antineoplastic agent for the treatment of Kaposi's sarcoma in AIDS patients. See also interferon alfa-2a.

interferon alfa-2a/interferon alfa-2b/interferon alfa-n1/interferon alfa-n3, n brand names: Roferon-A, Intron-A, Alferon N; *drug class:* biologic response modifier; *action:* antiviral action inhibits viral replication by reprogramming virus; antitumor action suppresses cell proliferation; immunomodulating action phagacytizes target cells; *uses:* hairy-cell leukemia in persons older than 18 years, metastatic melanoma, AIDS, Kaposi's sarcoma, bladder carcinoma, lymphomas, malignant myeloma, mycosis fungoides.

interferon beta, n a type formed by fibroblasts by stimulation similar to the alpha form.

interferon gamma, n a type formed by lymphocytes in response to mitogenic stimulation. See also interferon gamma-1b.

interferon gamma-1b, n brand name: Actimmune; *drug class:* biologic response modifier; *action:* species-specific protein synthesized in response to viruses, enhances antibody-dependent cellular cytotoxicity, enhances natural killer cell activity; *uses:* serious infections associated with chronic granulomatous disease.

interim denture, *n* See denture, interim.

interim prosthesis, *n* See prosthesis, temporary.

interincisal angle (in′tərinsī′zəl), *n* the A-P angle made by the intersection of the long axis of the maxillary central incisor with the mandibular central incisor. Statistically, a normal angle is about 130°. A more acute angle may indicate a proclined incisor, and a more obtuse angle may indicate a retracted incisor.

interleukin-1 (IL-1) (in′tərloo′kin), *n* a protein with numerous immune system functions, including activation of resting T cells, and endothelial and macrophage cells, mediation of inflammation, and stimulation of synthesis of lymphokines, collagen, and collagenases. It can also induce fever, sleep, and nonspecific resistance to infection. A number of interleukin proteins with varying immune-response properties exist. They are identified by numbers of 1 through 8.

interleukin-2, *n* a hormone produced by T helper and suppressor lymphocytes that functions to control the expansion and reactivity of T lymphocytes. Used to boost the immune system in HIV-positive patients.

intermaxillary (in′tərmak′səler′ē), *adj* between the maxillae and mandible.

intermaxillary anchorage, n See anchorage, intermaxillary.

intermaxillary elastic, n See elastic, maxillomandibular.

intermaxillary fixation, n See fixation, maxillomandibular.

intermaxillary relation, n See relation, maxillomandibular.

intermaxillary traction, n See traction, maxillomandibular.

intermediate chain linkage, *n* a chemical link between the aromatic portion and the amine used in local anesthetics. The intermediate chain link is either an ester or an amide, which influences how the anesthetic is metabolized and the allergic potential of the anesthetic.

intermedin (inturmē′din), *n* See hormone, melanocyte stimulating.

intern, *n* a dental or medical college graduate serving and residing for 12 months in a hospital, usually during the first year after receiving a D.D.S., D.M.D., D.O., or M.D. degree.

internal connection, *n* a prosthetic connection inside the implant, such as the internal hexagon and the Morse taper.

internal medicine, *n* the branch of medicine concerned with the study of the physiology and pathology of the internal organs and with the medical diagnosis and treatment of diseases and disorders of these organs.

International Classification of Diseases (ICD), *n.pr* the diagnostic codes designed for the classification of morbidity and mortality information for statistical purposes, for the indexing of hospital records by disease and operations, and for data storage and retrieval.

International Dental Hygienists' Federation (IDHF), *n.pr* an international organization of dental hygiene associations formed in Oslo, Norway, on June 28, 1986. The IDHF is a nonprofit organization that seeks to promote dental health across the world.

international numbering system, *n* a method of charting teeth in which each tooth is identified by a two-digit hyphenated number. The first number indicates quadrant and the second number indicates the particular tooth.

International Organization for Standardization (ISO), *n.pr* a nongovernmental, international organization that sets standards for industry, business, trades, and consumer products. These standards provide governments with a technical base for determining health, safety, and environmental legislation.

interneurons (in′tərner′ons), *n.pl* the combinations or groups of neurons between sensory and motor neurons, which govern coordinated activity.

internship, *n* the course work or practicum conducted in a professional dental clinic. The student-to-teacher ratio is low, allowing each student to receive personal attention from the instructor. During the internship, students perform patient procedures while sitting chairside with a dental professional. Students also perform radiographs and operate dental equipment. The goals are to prepare students for the successful completion of statewide exams and to provide them with practical experience so they can become dental professionals.

interocclusal (in′tərəkloo′səl), *adj* between the occlusal surfaces of the maxillary and mandibular teeth.

interocclusal clearance, *n* See clearance, interocclusal.

interocclusal contacts, *n* tooth contact between maxillary and mandibular teeth in closure.

interocclusal distance, *n* the distance between the maxillary and mandibular teeth when the mandible is in the rest position or other defined position of the mandible to maxillary. See also distance, interocclusal.

interocclusal gap, *n* See distance, interocclusal.

interocclusal record, *n* See record, interocclusal.

interocclusal rest space, *n* See distance, interocclusal.

interoceptors (inter′ōsepturz), *n.pl* the sensory nerve end receptors lining the mucous membrane of the respiratory and digestive tracts. They are similar to exteroceptors but differ from them essentially in their location in the viscera.

interphase, *n* the metabolic stage in the cell cycle during which the cell is not dividing.

interpolate (intur′pōlāt), *v* to insert intermediate terms in a series according to the trend of the series; to calculate intermediate values according to observed values.

interposition arthroplasty (är′thrōplastē), *n* the surgical correction of ankylosis by the separating of the immobile fragment from the mobilized fragment and the interpositioning of a substance, such as fascia, cartilage, metal, or plastic, between them. See also ankylosis.

interpretation, *n* the translation of radiographic changes seen by the clinician into real variations in the object radiographed for diagnostic purposes.

interpretation, radiographic (radiologic interpretation, roentgenographic interpretation), *n* an opinion formed from the study of a radiograph.

interpretation, radiographic, external oblique ridge, *n* radiopaque line formed by an elevated bony surface on the mandible.

interpretation, radiographic, genial tubercles, *n* the submandibular radiopaque structures that represent the attachment site for genohyoid and genioglossus muscles.

interpretation, radiographic, inferior border on mandible, *n* the radiopaque area that represents the cortical bone.

interpretation, radiographic, internal oblique ridge, *n* the radiopaque line that represents a bony ridge on the mandibular surface, the attachment site of the mylohyoid muscles.

interpretation, radiographic, lingual foramen, *n* the small area of radiolucency located centrally in the genial tubercles.

interpretation, radiologic, *n* See interpretation, radiographic.

interproximal (in′tərprôk′səməl), *adj* between the proximal surfaces of adjoining teeth.

interradicular (in′terrədik′yələr), *adj* referring to spaces between tooth roots and to furcations.

interradicular alveoloplasty (alvē′ōlōplastē), *n* (intraseptal alveoloplasty), the removal of the interradicular bone and the collapsing of the cortical plates to a more normal alveolar contour. See also alveolectomy.

interradicular osseous defect (os′ēəs), *n* the radiographic evidence of a discontinuity in the bony image in the area between the roots of a multirooted tooth.

interradicular septum, *n* a thin, bony divider within the tooth socket that separates the roots of a multirooted tooth.

interridge distance, *n* See distance, interarch.

interstitial (in′turstish′əl), *adj* pertaining to the tiny spaces between tissues.

intervention studies, *n.pl* the epidemiologic investigations designed to test a hypothesized cause and effect relation by modifying the supposed causal factor(s) in the study population.

interview, *n* **1.** a question-and-answer conference at which the parties concerned state the principles and facts regarding their relationship. In dental practice, this usually refers to the relationship between employer and employee, and between dental professional and patient. *v* **2.** to query a potential employee for employment.

intolerance, *n* inability to endure or withstand.

intraarterial (in′trəärtir′ēəl), *adj* situated within an artery or arteries.

intracellular (in′trəsel′ūlur), *adj* situated or occurring within a cell or cells.

intracoronal (in′trəkôrō′nəl), *adj* pertaining to the inside of the coronal portion of a natural tooth.

intracoronal attachment, *n* See attachment, intracoronal.

intracoronal retainer, *n* See retainer, intracoronal.

intracranial pressure (in′trəkrā′nēəl), *n* the pressure that occurs within the cranium. Trauma to the head, inflammation, or infection of the linings of the brain may cause an increase in pressure within the cranium, which is painful, dysfunctional, and may become life threatening.

intralabial gap (in′trəlā′bēəl), *n* the position of the upper and lower lips as measured from the midpoint of the lips when a patient is relaxed and smiling. When smiling, the gingival tissues should not be visible and only the cervical two thirds of the maxillary incisors are exposed. The acceptable upper limit of interlabial gap is 3 mm.

intraligamentary (in′trəligəmen′tərē), *adj* within a ligament.

intramaxillary anchorage, *n* See anchorage, intramaxillary.

intramaxillary elastic, *n* See elastic, intramaxillary.

intramucosal insert, *n* See insert, intramucosal.

intramuscular (in′trəmus′kūlur), *adj* situated in the substance of a muscle.

intraocular pressure (in′trəok′yələr), *n* the internal pressure of the eye, regulated by resistance to the flow of aqueous humor through the fine sieve of the trabecular meshwork. Obstruction within the trabecular meshwork will cause an increase in the intraocular pressure. High persistent levels may lead to blindness.

intraoral (in′trəôr′əl), *adj* within the oral cavity.

intraoral tracing, *n* See tracing, intraoral.

intraosseous (in′trəôs′ēəs), *adj* within the bone.

intraosseous fixation (in′trə-os′ēus), *n* See fixation, intraosseous.

intrapartum, *adj/adv* pertaining to or occurring during the delivery of offspring.

intrapulmonary (in′trəpul′mənerē), *adj* situated in the substance of a lung.

intrathecal (in′trəthē′kəl), *adj* pertaining to a structure or substance contained within a sheath; in drug delivery, the injection of a therapeutic agent into the sheath surrounding the spinal cord.

intravascular (in′trəvas′kūlur), *adj* within a blood vessel.

intravenous (in′trəvē′nus), *adj* in, into, or from within a vein or veins.

intraversion, *n* a term indicating teeth or other maxillary structures that are too near the medial plane.

intrinsic (intrin′zik), *adj* naturally occurring within; inherent; essential.

intrinsic coloring, *n* a coloring from within; the incorporation of pigment within the material of a prosthesis.

intrude, *v* to move a tooth apically.

intrusion, *n* a depression; an inward projection.

intrusion upon seclusion, *n* an offensive invasion of someone's personal affairs or property.

intubate (in′toobāt), *v* to treat by intubation.

intubation (in′toobā′shən), *n* the insertion of a tube; especially the introduction of a tube into the larynx through the glottis for the introduction of an anesthetic gas or oxygen.

intubator (in′toobātur), *n* an instrument used in intubation.

inulin (in′yəlin′), *n* a fructose-derived substance used as a diagnostic aid in tests of kidney function, specifically glomerular filtration. Inulin is not metabolized or absorbed by the body but is readily filtered through the kidney.

inunction (inungk′shən), *n* the local application of a drug in an oily or semisolid vehicle, such as an ointment, or the preparation that is thus applied.

invagination, epithelial (invaj′ənā′-shən epəthē′lēəl), *n* the downgrowth of epithelium along the cervical tract of an implant.

invasion of privacy, *n* a legal term defining a mistreatment of another's private life. See also false light, intrusion upon seclusion, and appropriation.

inventory, *n* an itemized compilation of materials on hand.

inventory, equipment, n a detailed listing of all the nonexpendable items owned and used in the practice of the profession.

inventory, materials, n a detailed listing of expendable supplies that are on hand in the practice. This is a constantly fluctuating list, depending on the quantity of the various materials presently on hand.

inverse-square law, *n* See law, inverse-square.

inversion, *n* the state of being upside down.

invest (invest′), *v* to surround, envelop, or embed in an investment material; e.g., a gypsum product.

investing (inves′ting), *n* the process of covering or enveloping an object wholly or in part.

investing, vacuum, n the investing of a pattern within a vacuum to form a mold.

investment (invest′ment), *n* the material used to enclose or surround a pattern of a dental restoration for casting or molding or to maintain the relations of metal parts during soldering.

investment, casting, n a type in which the casting mold is made in fabrication of gold or cobalt-chromium castings.

investment, gypsum-bonded casting, n a type that can be bonded by a-hemihydrate, a derivative of gypsum, because the fusion temperatures of the metal alloys to be cast in it are relatively low. All gold alloy investments and some low-fusing cobalt-chromium alloy investments are gypsum bonded.

investment, hygroscopic **(hī′grə-skop′ik),** *n* a type specially designed for use with the hygroscopic investing techniques.

investment, phosphate-bonded casting, n a type that is bonded by a phosphate and a metallic oxide that react to form a hard mass; generally used for high-fusing alloys.

investment, refractory, n a type in which the investing materials can withstand the high temperatures used in soldering or casting.

investment, sectional, n a type using a mold made in sections.

investment, silica-bonded casting, n a type that is bonded by a silica gel that reverts to cristobalite in heating and is generally used for high-fusing alloys.

investment, soldering, n a quartz type, preferably one with a very low thermal expansion, used for the investment of appliances during the soldering procedure.

Invisalign aligners, *pr.n* a clear, custom-fabricated device used for straightening teeth. These retainers are designed to gradually realign teeth and are meant to replace traditional braces. Cosmetically, invisible retainers are more appealing because they are difficult to notice, making them particularly popular among adults who wish to straighten their teeth without the use of traditional metal braces. Such retainers are easily removed during eating and tooth brushing.

involucrum (in′vəlookrum), *n* a covering of new bone around a sequestrum.

involuntary, *adj* performed independently of the will.

involute (in′vəloot), *v* to decrease normally, in size and functional activity, an organ whose role in the body economy is temporary or confined to certain periods of life. Involute should be distinguished from *atrophy,* which means to waste away from abnormal causes.

involvement, *n* the state of becoming involved.

involvement, bifurcation **(bīfurkā′-shən),** *n* the extension of pocket formation into the interradicular area of multirooted teeth in periodontitis.

involvement, pulp, n a condition wherein consideration of the vitality or health of the dental pulp is a factor.

involvement, trifurcation, n See involvement, bifurcation.

iodine (I) (ī′ədīn′), *n* a halogen element that is nonmetallic in nature; atomic weight is 126.91. As a nutritional element, iodine is vital to the production of thyroxin by the thyroid gland. In radioactive form, iodine is used as a diagnostic substance to determine the ability of the thyroid gland to take up iodine. In tincture form, iodine is used as a locally applied antiseptic, germicide, and disclosing solution.

iodine number, n the amount of iodine absorbable by 100 g of a fat or an oil; the lower the level of unsaturated fatty acids in the fat or oil, the higher the iodine number.

iodine, protein-bound (PBI), n the iodine bound to protein, mainly thyroxin in the plasma. The thyroid hormone is precipitated by protein-denaturing agents, and, in general, the amount of iodine in a protein precipitate indicates the amount of thyroid hormone present and is thus an index of thyroid activity. Various values are given for thyroid function: hypothyroidism, 0 to 3.5 μg/ml of protein-bound iodine; euthyroidism, 3.5 to 8 μg/ml; hyperthyroidism, values higher than 8 μg/ml.

iodism (iodine poisoning) (ī′ə-diz′əm), *n* an acute or chronic intoxication caused by the ingestion or absorption of iodides. Manifestations of acute poisoning include abdominal pain, nausea, vomiting, hypersalivation, conjunctivitis, and collapse. Chronic manifestations include hypersalivation, fever, acute rhinitis, swelling and tenderness of the salivary glands, and dermatitis and stomatitis in hypersensitive individuals. Iodism is a toxic condition that sometimes follows the use of preparations containing iodine.

iodophor (īō′dəfôr), *n* a loose chemical compound of iodine with certain organic compounds; e.g., polyvinylpyrrolidone.

iodoquinol (ī′ōdō′kwinôl), *n* an antimicrobial agent that acts against the parasite *Entamoeba histolytica.* It is used in the treatment of intestinal disease.

ion (ī′on), *n* an atomic particle, atom, or chemical radical bearing an electrical charge, either negative or positive.

ion exchange chromatography, n the process of separating and analyzing different substances according to their affinities for chemically stable but very reactive synthetic exchangers, which are composed largely of polystyrene and cellulose. The process uses an absorbent containing ionizing groups and accommodates the exchange of ions between a solution of substances to be analyzed and the absorbent. Ion exchange chromatography is often used to separate components of nucleic acids and proteins.

ion pair, *n* the two particles of opposite charge, usually the electron and the positive atomic residue resulting after the interaction of ionizing radiation with the orbital electrons of atoms. The average energy required to produce an ion pair is approximately 33 (or 34) electron volts.

ion-selective electrode, *n* a potentiometric electrode that develops a potential in the presence of one ion (or class of ions), but not in the presence of a similar concentration of other ions.

ionization (īʹänizāʹshən), *n* the process or the result of a process by which a neutral atom or molecule acquires either a positive or negative charge.

ionization chamber, *n* See chamber, ionization.

ionization, chamber, air-equivalent, *n* See chamber, ionization, air-equivalent.

ionization density, *n* the number of ion pairs per unit volume.

ionization path (ionization track), *n* the trail of ion pairs produced by ionizing radiation in its passage through matter.

ionization potential, *n* the potential necessary to separate one electron from an atom, resulting in the formation of an ion pair.

ionizer, *n* See electrolyzer.

ionomer (īonʹəmər), *n* a polymer containing ion. In dentistry, ionomers are a mixture of glass and an organic acid. They are clear but vary in the amount of translucency. For this reason, their aesthetic potential does not match that of composite resins. However, ionomers are not likely to shrink or be subject to the microleakage seen in composite resins because the bonding mechanism of ionomers is an acid-base reaction rather than a polymerization reaction.

iontophoresis (īonʹtōfôrēʹsis), *n* the application, by means of an appropriate electrode, of a galvanic current to an ionizable agent in contact with a surface to hasten the movement into the tissue of the ion of opposite charge to that of the electrode. See also ionization.

ipratropium bromide (ipʹrətrōʹpēəm brōʹmīd), *n brand name:* Atrovent; *drug class:* anticholinergic bronchodilator; *action:* inhibits interaction of acetylcholine at receptor sites on the bronchial smooth muscle, resulting in bronchodilation; *uses:* bronchodilation during bronchospasm in those with chronic obstructive pulmonary disease, bronchitis, emphysema, asthma; not for rapid bronchodilation; maintenance treatment only.

ipsilateral (ipʺsīlatʹərəl), *adj* originating or occurring on the same side of the body.

IQ, *n* See intelligence quotient.

iridium (Ir) (iridʹēəm), *n* a silvery-bluish metallic element. Its atomic number is 77 and its atomic weight is 192.2.

iris, *n* a circular, contractile disc suspended in aqueous humor between the cornea and the crystalline lens of the eye and perforated by a circular pupil. It regulates the amount of light passing into the chambers of the eye.

iron (Fe), *n* a common metallic element essential for the synthesis of hemoglobin. Its atomic number is 26 and its atomic weight is 55.85. Normal blood levels range between 60 and 190 micrograms.

iron oxide, *n* a compound of iron and oxygen which is often used for laboratory polishing of precious metals. See also jeweler's rouge.

irradiation (irāʹdēāʹshən), *n* **1.** the exposure of material to roentgen or other radiation. (One speaks of *radiation therapy* but not of *irradiation of the patient.*) **2.** the exposure to radiation.

irreversibility (irʹēvurʹsibilʹitē), *n* incapable of being returned to the original state.

irreversible (irʹēvurʹsebəl), *adj* incapable of being reversed or returned to the original state.

irreversible hydrocolloid, adj See hydrocolloid, irreversible.

irrigation (ir′igā′shən), *n* the technique of using a solution to wash or flush debris from the root canal or from a wound. See lavage.

irrigation, supragingival, n the flushing of liquid using a handheld device to remove bacterial plaque from dental surfaces above or even with the gingivae line. Can be performed by either the clinician or patient.

irrigator, *n* dental tool used to force liquid through a given area for irrigation; features a soft tube that draws liquid from a contained source. See also irrigation.

irritability, *n* the quality of being irritable or of responding to a stimulus.

irritant, *n* **1.** an agent that causes an irritation or stimulation. **2.** an agent that is toxic, bacterial, physical, or chemical and is capable of inducing functional derangements or organic lesions of the tissues.

irritant, chemical, n a chemical agent that causes irritation. The primary agents that have an etiologic relationship to periodontal disease are plaque and calculus. Other agents that serve as a medium for the growth of microorganisms include food debris, sloughed cells, and necrotic material.

irritation, *n* the act of stimulating. A condition of functional derangement and nervous irritability.

irritation from overstimulation, n See impingement.

irritation, mechanical, n the tissue damage, injury, or insult by physical forces directed against the tissue—e.g., tissue irritation produced by incorrect toothbrushing.

irritation of gingival tissues, n See impingement.

ischemia (iskē′mēə), *n* a focal deficiency of blood to a part of the body or simply a local anemia. It results from encroachment of the lumen of an artery or the capillaries supplying the affected area. The reduction in the lumen may be caused by allergic hypersensitivity, degeneration of the tunica intima (atherosclerosis), inflammation, physical pressure, pharmacologic and toxic agents, or neurogenic disorders.

isobar (ī′sōbär), *n* in radiochemistry, one of two or more different nuclides having the same mass number.

isoelectric focusing, *n* the ordering and concentration of substances according to their isoelectric points.

isoelectric point, *n* the pH at which a molecule containing two or more ionizable groups is electrically neutral.

isoetharine HCl/isoetharine mesylate (ī′sōeth′ərēn mes′ilāt′), *n brand names:* Bronkosol, Bronkometer, Dispos-a-Med; *drug class:* adrenergic β_2-agonist; *action:* causes bronchodilation by β_2 stimulation, resulting in increased levels of cAMP and causing relaxation of bronchial smooth muscle with very little effect on heart rate; *uses:* bronchospasm or asthma.

isogenic (ī′sōjen′ik), *adj* originating from a common source; possessing the same genetic composition.

isolation of a tooth, *n* a technique to protect a tooth against contamination from oral fluids during a surgical or restorative procedure, usually through the application of a rubber dam or the use of cotton rolls.

isoleucine (ī′səloo′sēn), *n* one of the essential amino acids occurring in most dietary proteins. Isoleucine is essential for proper growth in infants and for nitrogen balance in adults. See also amino acid.

isomers (ī′sōmurz), *n.pl* **1.** organic compounds having the same empirical formula—i.e., the same number of the same atoms but different structural formulas and therefore different physical and chemical properties. *n* **2.** one of several nuclides having the same number of neutrons and protons but capable of existing, for a measurable time, in different quantum states with different energies and radioactive properties. The isomer of higher energy commonly decays to one with lower energy by a process known as isomeric transition.

isomers, optical, n.pl two isomers whose structures, dextro- and levo-, differ only in a spatial arrangement that makes them mirror images. This occurs only when there is an asymmetric carbon atom—i.e., one attached to four different substituents. The pharmacologic activity often resides very largely in one of the two forms.

isomers, stereo-, *n.pl* molecules that differ only in the spatial arrangement of the atoms. This term includes optical isomers.

isometric muscle contraction (ī′sōmet′rik), *n* See contraction, muscle, isometric.

isoniazid (INH) (ī′sənī′əzid), *n brand names:* Laniazid, Nydrazid; *drug class:* antitubercular; *action:* bactericidal interference with lipid, nucleic acid biosynthesis; *uses:* treatment and prevention of tuberculosis.

isoproterenol HCl/isoproterenol sulfate (ī′sōprəter′ənol sul′fāt), *n brand names:* Isuprel, Vapo-Iso, Aerolone; *drug class:* adrenergic β_1- and β_2-agonist; *action:* relaxes bronchial smooth muscle and dilates trachea and main bronchi by increasing levels of cAMP, which relaxes smooth muscles; causes increased contractility and heart rate; *uses:* bronchospasm, asthma, heart block, bradycardia, or shock.

isosorbide dinitrate (ī′sōsor′bīd dīnī′trāt), *n brand names:* Iso-Bid, Isotrate, Dilatrate-SR, Isordil; *drug class:* nitrate antianginal; action: decreases preload/afterload, which is responsible for decreasing left ventricular end-diastolic pressure, systemic vascular resistance; *uses:* chronic stable angina pectoris, prophylaxis of angina pain.

isosorbide mononitrate (ī′sōsor′bīd mon′ōnī′trāt), *n brand name:* ISMO; *drug class:* antianginal, organic nitrate; *action:* decreases preload/afterload, which is responsible for decreasing left ventricular end-diastolic pressure, systemic vascular resistance; arterial and venous dilation; *use:* prevention of angina pectoris caused by coronary artery disease.

isosthenuria (ī′sōsthənyoo′rēə), *n* the excretion of urine with fixed specific gravity. It may occur in terminal renal disease when the specific gravity reaches that of the glomerular filtrate, 1.010.

isotone (ī′sōtōn), *n* one of several different nuclides having the same number of neutrons in their nuclei, but different mass numbers.

isotonic (ī′sōton′ik), *adj* equivalence in osmotic pressure. Specifically used in reference to a solution whose osmotic pressure is equal to that of a body fluid, such as blood plasma or tears, to which the solution is compared.

isotonic muscle contraction, *n* See contraction, muscle, isotonic.

isotope (ī′sōtōp), *n* one of several nuclides having the same number of protons in their nuclei, and hence having the same atomic number but differing in the number of neutrons, and therefore in the mass number. The isotopes of a particular element have virtually identical chemical properties.

isotope, stable, *n* a nonradioactive isotope of an element.

isotretinoin (ī′sōtret′inoin), *n brand name:* Accutane; *drug class:* retinoic acid isomer, vitamin A derivative; *action:* decreases sebum secretion, improves cystic acne; *uses:* severe recalcitrant cystic acne.

isoxsuprine HCl (īsok′səprēn′), *n brand name:* Vasodilan; *drug class:* peripheral vasodilator; *action:* β-adrenoreceptor antagonist with β-adrenoreceptor-stimulating properties; may also act directly on vascular smooth muscle; causes cardiac stimulation, uterine relaxation; *uses:* symptoms of cerebrovascular insufficiency, peripheral vascular disease including arteriosclerosis obliterans, or Raynoud's disease.

Isradipine (israd′ipēn), *n.pr brand name:* DynaCirc; *drug class:* calcium channel blocker; *action:* inhibits calcium ion influx across cell membrane during cardiac depolarization; produces relaxation of coronary vascular smooth muscle, peripheral vascular smooth muscle; increases myocardial oxygen delivery in patients with vasospastic angina; *use:* essential hypertension.

itraconazole (it′rəkon′əzol′), *n brand name:* Sporanox; *drug class:* antifungal, systemic; *action:* inhibits cytochrome P-450 enzyme's blocking synthesis of essential membrane sterols in fungal organism; *uses:* blastomycosis, histoplasmosis.

Ivalon sponge (ī′vəlon′), *n.pr* a polyvinyl alcohol sponge.

Ivy loop wiring, *n.pr* See wiring, Ivy loop.

Ivy's test, *n.pr* See test, Ivy's.

J

jacket, *n* See crown, complete, veneer, acrylic resin and crown, complete, veneer, porcelain.

jackscrew, *n* a threaded device used in appliances for separation or approximation of teeth or jaw segments.

Jackson's sign, *n.pr* See sign, Jackson's.

Janet's test, *n.pr* See test, Janet's.

jaundice (jändis), *n* a condition characterized by an abnormal accumulation of bilirubin (red bile pigment) in the blood and manifested by a yellowish discoloration of the skin, mucous membranes, and cornea. It presents with hemolytic anemias, biliary obstruction, hepatitis, cholangiolitis, and cirrhosis of the liver. Oral mucosa may be pigmented.

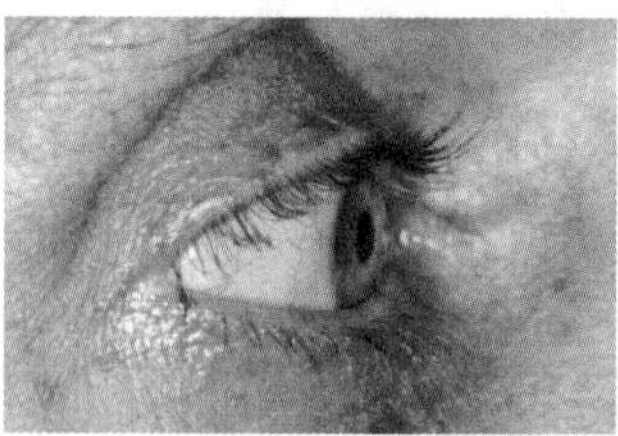

Jaundice. (Neville/Damm/Allen/Bouquot, 2002)

jaundice, acholuric **(ak′əlŏŏr′ik),** *n* a type without bile in the urine.

jaundice, congenital hemolytic **(kənjen′itəl hē′məlit′ik), (acholuric icterus, spherocytic anemia, hereditary spherocytosis) (sfer′ōsītō′sis),** *n* a familial hemolytic anemia transmitted as a Mendelian dominant trait. The intrinsic defects of the red blood cells include a spheroidal shape, which allows them to be trapped by the spleen, and increased mechanical fragility.

jaundice, epidemic, *n* See disease, Weil's.

jaundice, hemolytic (prehepatic jaundice), *n* excess bile pigments in the blood resulting from increased destruction of erythrocytes.

jaundice, hepatic, *n* See jaundice, hepatocellular.

jaundice, hepatocellular (hepatic jaundice, infective jaundice, medical jaundice, toxic jaundice), *n* a type resulting from disease of liver cells by infectious agents or toxins, decreasing the ability of the liver to handle the bile pigments that are continually produced by the destruction of red blood cells.

jaundice, homologous serum, *n* See hepatitis, homologous serum.

jaundice, infective, *n* See jaundice, hepatocellular.

jaundice, latent, *n* increased bilirubin in the blood without clinical signs of jaundice.

jaundice, medical, *n* See jaundice, hepatocellular.

jaundice, obstructive (posthepatic jaundice), *n* extrahepatic and intrahepatic obstruction of the biliary tract, resulting in retrograde retention of bile pigments and jaundice.

jaundice, posthepatic, *n* See jaundice, obstructive.

jaundice, prehepatic, *n* See jaundice, hemolytic.

jaundice, regurgitating, *n* jaundice resulting from reentry of conjugated bilirubin into the blood as a result of obstruction of the biliary tract or hepatocellular damage and failure to excrete conjugated bilirubin from liver cells.

jaundice, retention, *n* an increase in bilirubin in the blood from hemolysis; failure of the liver cells to conjugate bilirubin or remove free bilirubin.

jaundice, surgical, *n* extrahepatic obstruction of the biliary tract.

jaundice, syringe, *n* See hepatitis, homologous serum.

jaundice, toxic, *n* See jaundice, hepatocellular.

jaw, *n* a common name for either the maxillae or the mandible; the meaning is usually extended to include their soft tissue covering.

jaw, cleft (gnathouschisis), n See palate, cleft.

jaw cyst, n an abnormal bladderlike sac within the jaw. May occur in either the maxilla or mandible associated with or not associated with the dentition and its formation. See also cyst.

jaw, fibro-osseous, lesion, n See lesion, fibroosseous jaw.

jaw fracture, n a break in the continuity of the bone of the maxilla or mandible. See also fracture.

jaw, lumpy, n See actinomycosis.

jaw movement, n See movement, jaw.

jaw, phossy, n See poisoning, phosphorus.

jaw reflex, n See reflex, jaw.

jaw relation, n See relation, jaw.

jaw-to-jaw relationship, n See relation, jaw.

JCAHO/TJC, *n.pr* an acronym for the **Joint Commission on Accreditation of Healthcare Organizations.**

jealousy, *n* resentment against a rival or competitor. It may be a significant barrier to functional interpersonal relationships within any group.

jejunum (jəjoo′nəm), *n* the middle or intermediate of the three portions of the small intestine, connecting proximally with the duodenum and distally with the ileum. It has a slightly larger diameter, a deeper color, and a thicker wall than the ileum, and it contains heavy, circular folds that are absent in the inferior portion of the ileum.

jelly, petroleum, *n* See petrolatum.

jet injection, *n* a needleless system for delivering medications wherein a high-pressure stream of liquid is used to pierce the skin or oral mucosa and deposit medication into the subcutaneous tissues. The advantages of using jet injection are that patient discomfort is minimized and that the medication can be delivered in smaller doses with greater effect. See also syringe, jet injector.

jet tips, *n* the end of an oral irrigating device; engineered to deliver a directed flow of water into the subgingival area. Designs include monojet (single flow) and fractionated microjet (similar to a showerhead), and flow may be pulsating or nonpulsating. See also irrigator.

jeweler's rouge, *n* an iron oxide that has been pressed into a fine red powder, used to polish gold and metal alloys.

Johnston's method, *n.pr* See method, chloropercha.

Joint Commission on Accreditation of Healthcare Organizations (JCAHO/TJC), *n.pr* formerly the Joint Commission on Accreditation of Hospitals. The JCAHO conducts accreditation programs for most of the health care facilities in the United States. The American Dental Association is a corporate member of the JCAHO. Hospitals and clinics are surveyed on a regular basis for compliance with the standards and criteria for accreditation.

Joint Commission on Accreditation of Hospitals, *n.pr* See Joint Commission on Accreditation of Healthcare Organizations (JCAHO/TJC).

joint(s), *n* the junction of union between two or more bones or cartilages of the skeleton.

joint(s), Charcot's **(shärkōz′),** *n* a manifestation of late syphilis in which there is degeneration, hypertrophy, hypermobility, and loss of contour of a joint, usually a weight-bearing joint. It is most common in tabes dorsalis.

joint(s) diarthrosis **(dīärthrō′sis),** *n* a joint that moves freely in contact. The adjacent bone surfaces are typically covered by a film of cartilage and are bound by stout connective tissues, frequently enclosing a liquid-filled joint cavity.

joint(s) disease, n an inflammatory, infectious, or functional disorder within a joint.

joint(s), hinge, n See ginglymus.

joint(s) mice, n cartilaginous material present in the synovial spaces of a joint.

joint(s) prosthesis **(prosthē′sis),** *n* the addition to or replacement of a member(s) or of structural elements within a joint to improve and enhance the function of the joint. Principal joint prostheses include hip replacement and knee replacement. Less common is a joint prosthesis for the temporomandibular joint.

joint(s) synarthrosis **(sin′ärthrō′sis),** *n* (junctura fibrosa, fibrous joint) a joint in which the bony elements are connected by thin intervening layers of cartilage, connective tissue, or direct contact of bone to bone such as the rigid unions in the adult skull.

joint(s), temporomandibular, n See articulation, temporomandibular.

Jones protein, *n.pr* See protein, Bence Jones.

Jorgensen's drug administration principles (jor′gənsəns), *n.pr* the principles employed in the selection and administration of intravenous sedative agents that have a wide margin of safety and predictable effects and that, in combination, can elevate the pain threshold, produce euphoria, have an antisialogogue effect, and promote an amnesic response. The principles include the sequence and rate of administration while monitoring patient response signs.

J

judgment, *n* **1.** a legal finding. *n* **2.** the ability to discriminate between or among two or more states or conditions.

judicial process, *n* the rules that determine the role of judge and jury in the courtroom as well as the jurisdiction of the individual courts over specific areas of law.

junction (jungk′shən), *n* a place of coming together, or union.

junction, cementoenamel (CEJ) (cervical line), n the junction of the enamel of the crown and the cementum of the root of a tooth. The area above the junction corresponds to the anatomic crown of the tooth; the area apical to the junction constitutes the anatomic root of the tooth.

junction, dentinocemental (DCJ), n the line of union or apposition of the cementum and dentin of a tooth.

junction, dentinoenamel (DEJ) (dentoenamel junction), n the interface of enamel and dentin of the tooth crown, conforming in a general way to the shape of the crown. Older term is *dentoenamel junction.*

junction, dentoenamel, n See junction, dentinoenamel.

junction, dentogingival (DGJ), n the junction between the gingival attachment, a nonkeratinized epithelium, and the tooth surface.

junction, intercellular, n a special structure that exists between two or more cells with similar functionality. Most of these structures are anchored to the cytoskeleton and therefore provide mechanical stability to tissues. There are several types, including desmosomes that provide stability, tight junctions where the outer membranes of cells have become fused, and gap junctions where adjacent cells exchange cellular material.

junction, mucogingival, n the scalloped linear area denoting the separation of the gingivae and alveolar mucosa.

junctional epithelium (JE) (ep′əthē′lēəm), *n* a band of epithelial cells that surrounds the tooth and creates a seal at the gingival sulcus to hold it firmly in place.

jurisprudence (jŏŏr′isproo′dəns), *n* the philosophy of law.

jurisprudence, dental (forensic dentistry), n **1.** the science that teaches the application of every branch of dental knowledge to the purposes of the law; this also includes the elucidation of doubtful legal questions. *n* **2.** the state laws and codes covering the legal limitations of the practice of the profession of dentistry.

jurisprudence, medical n the science that applies the principles and practice of the different branches of medicine in the elucidation of doubtful questions in a court of justice. Also called *forensic medicine.*

jury, *n* a certain number of citizens selected according to law and sworn to inquire of certain matters of fact and to declare the truth on evidence submitted to them.

just, *adj* right; according to law and justice.

justice, *n* the constant and perpetual disposition to render every person his or her due. Also, the conformity of one's actions and will to the law.

juvenile periodontitis, *n* a distinct form of aggressive periodontitis that may present with symptoms such as localized or generalized inflammatory changes in the periodontium of prepubertal children. The disease is characterized by severe pocketing and rapid destruction of alveolar bone. Several subtypes of the disease are recognized such as localized or generalized (formerly called *periodontosis*).

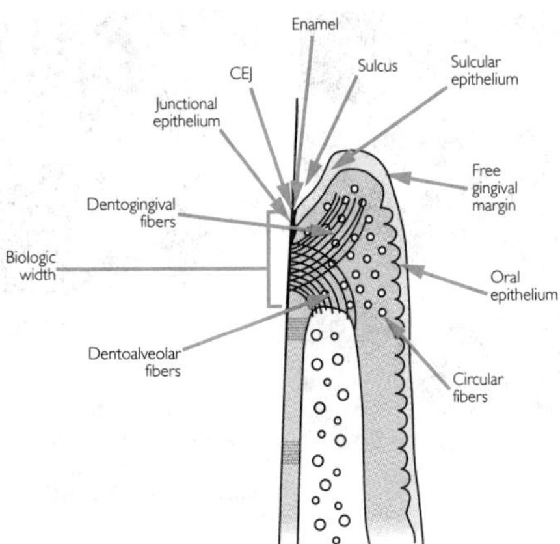

Junctional epithelium. (Daniel/Harfst/Wilder, 2008)

juxtaposition (juk′stəpəzish′ən), *n* adjacent situation; apposition or contact.

K

kakke (käk′kā), *n* See beriberi.

kallikrein (kal′ikrē′in), *n* a group of enzymes (plasma, tissue, pancreatic, urinary, submandibular kallikrein) that can convert kininogen to bradykinin or kallidin; trypsin and plasmin can also affect the conversion.

kallikrein-kinin system, *n* a proposed hormonal system that functions within the kidney, with the enzyme kallikrein in the renal cortex mediating production of bradykinin, which acts as a vasodilator peptide.

kanamycin (kānəmī′sin), *n* an aminoglycoside antibiotic that acts by inhibiting the synthesis of protein in susceptible organisms. Kanamycin requires close clinical supervision because of its potential toxicity and adverse side effects to the auditory and vestibular branches of the eighth cranial nerve and to the renal tubules.

kaolin (kā′əlin), *n* a fine, pure-white clay (hydrated aluminum silicate) used in porcelain teeth.

Kaposi's sarcoma, *n.pr* See sarcoma, Kaposi's.

karyotype (ker′ēōtīp) *n* the chromosomal arrangement of a single cell. The schematic representation of an individual's chromosomes, arranged in pairs according to number, form, and size.

Kazanjian's operation (kəzan′jēənz), *n.pr* See operation, Kazanjian's.

Kazanjian's procedure, *n.pr* See operation, Kazanjian's.

keloid (kē′loid), *n* a dense, proliferative growth on the skin (hypertrophy of scar tissue) that appears to be an abnormal reaction to trauma, especially burns. Keloids tend to recur after excision and occur more frequently in blacks than in whites.

keloplasty (kē′lōplastē), *n* the excision of scar tissue in the skin.

Kendall's compound B, *n.pr* See corticosterone.

Kendall's compound E, *n.pr* See cortisone.

Kennedy bar, *n.pr* See connector, minor, secondary lingual bar.

Kennedy classification, *n.pr* a method of classifying partially edentulous conditions and partial dentures; based on the location of the

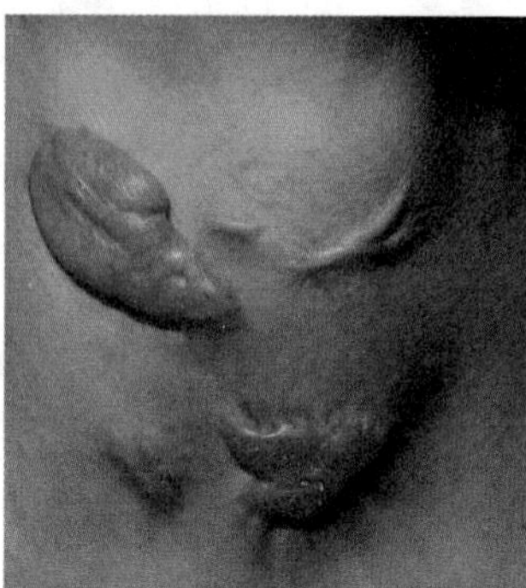

Keloids. (Zitelli/Davis, 2002)

edentulous spaces in relation to the remaining teeth.

keratin (ker′ətin), *n.* an insoluble sulfur-containing protein with a high content of the amino acids tyrosine and leucine; the main component of epidermis, hair, nails, keratinized epithelium. It contains a relatively large amount of sulfur, is insoluble in the gastric juices, and is sometimes used for coating enteric pills that are intended to be dissolved only in the intestine.

keratin layer, n the outer layer of cells of the epidermis, which contain a tough, fibrous protein (keratin). This layer acts as a protective barrier against outside elements.

keratinization (ker′ətin′izā′shən), *n* the process of becoming keratinized.

keratinocytes (kərat′inōsīts′), *n.pl* a cell of the living epidermis and certain oral epithelia that produces keratin in the process of differentiating into the dead and fully keratinized cells of the stratum corneum.

keratitis, *n* any inflammation of the cornea.

keratoacanthoma (ker′ətōak′anthō′mə), *n* ("self-healing carcinoma") a rapidly growing papular lesion with a superficial crater filled with keratin. Clinical and histopathologic features of this lesion are very similar to well-differentiated squamous cell carcinoma; however, most consider this growth to be benign. Treatment is conservative excision.

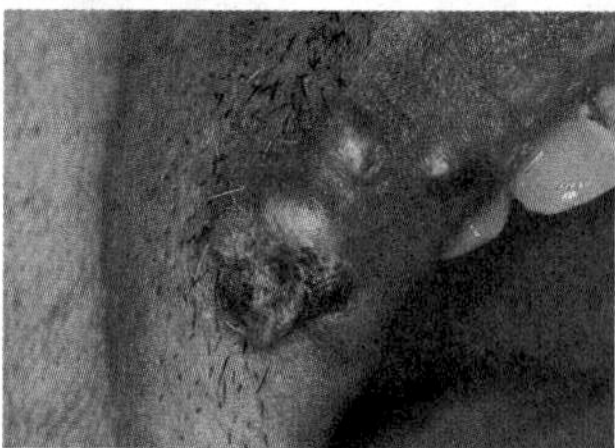

Keratoacanthoma. (Regezi/Sciubba/Pogrel, 2000)

keratoconjunctivitis sicca (ker′ətōkənjungk′tivī′tis sik′ə), *n* See syndrome, Sjögren's.

keratocyst (ker′ətōsist), *n* a homified cyst.

keratocystic odontogenic tumor (ker′ətōsist′ik ōdon′tōjen′ik), *n* a type of odontogenic cyst with a high rate of recurrence after surgery. Also distinguished by parakeratinized epithelial lining. Sometimes associated with nevoid basal cell carcinoma syndrome (Gorlin syndrome).

keratohyalin granules (ker′ətōhī′əlin), *n.pl* basophilic granules (0.2 to 4.5 micron) found in cells of the stratum granulosum that are presumed to play a role in keratinization.

keratolytic agents, *n.pl* agents that loosen or remove the horny outer layer of the skin.

keratoplasty, *n* corneal transplantation.

keratosis (ker′ətō′sis), *n* **1.** a horny or cornified growth (e.g., wart, callosity). *n* **2.** a condition characterized by cornification, or hyperkeratinization, of the tissues.

keratosis, actinic, n an overgrowth of the horny layer of the epidermis caused by excessive exposure to the sun.

keratosis blennorrhagia **(blen′ərā′jēə),** *n* a skin condition found in Reiter's syndrome characterized by pustules and crusting; once incorrectly associated with gonorrhea; more recently considered a genetic disorder occurring mostly in men between the ages of 20 and 25.

keratosis, chronic senile, n keratosis of the lips in elderly individuals. These lesions should be considered precancerous.

keratosis, focal, *n* localized areas of increased cornification (hyperkeratinization). Such lesions are seen particularly on the lips.

keratosis follicularis, *n* See disease, Darier's.

keratosis, seborrheic (basal cell papilloma, verruca senilis) **(seb'ərē'ik pap'əlōmə vəroo'kə sē'nilis),** *n* benign, pigmented, superficial epithelial tumors that clinically appear to be pasted on the skin of the trunk, arms, or face. Characterized histologically by marked hyperkeratosis, with keratin cyst formation, acanthosis of basal cells, and melanin pigmentation, all above the level of the adjacent epidermis.

keratosis, senile, *n* small, firm lesions occurring principally on the face and back of the hands in elderly people or those exposed to the sun. There is hyperkeratosis with irregular and atypical proliferation of the cells of the rete Malpighi. The condition is one of premalignancy with tendency toward epidermoid carcinoma. See also leukoplakia.

kernicterus (kurnik'tərəs), *n* a form of brain damage seen in newborns that is caused by an excessive level of red blood cells (polycythemia). As the body breaks down the red blood cells, bilirubin, a byproduct of cell destruction, becomes elevated and results in excessive jaundice. Typical symptoms include lethargy, high-pitched crying, and decreased muscle tone with intermittent periods of increased muscle tone. As the condition progresses, the newborn may exhibit a fever and may arch the head backward in a condition known as opisthotonus, or retrocollis.

ketamine, *n* a parenterally administered anesthetic that produces catatonia, profound analgesia, increased sympathetic activity, and little relaxation of skeletal muscles.

ketoacidosis (kē'tōas'idō'sis), *n* a form of acidosis characterized by an increased accumulation of ketone bodies (acetoacetic acid, β-hydroxybutyric acid, acetone) in the blood (e.g., the acidosis of uncontrolled diabetes mellitus).

ketoconazole (kē'tōkon'əzōl'), *n* a broad-spectrum synthetic antifungal agent applied to the skin to inhibit the growth of dermatophytes and yeasts, effective in *Candida* infections and in the treatment of seborrheic dermatitis; *brand name:* Nizoral; *drug class:* imidazole antifungal; *action:* alters cell membranes and inhibits several fungal enzymes; *uses:* systemic candidiasis, chronic mucocutaneous candidiasis, candiduria, coccidioidomycosis, histoplasmosis, chromomycosis, paracoccidioidomycosis, tinea pedis.

ketone (kē'tōn), *n* an organic chemical compound characterized by having in its structure a carbonyl or keto group attached to two alkyl groups. It is produced by oxidation of secondary alcohols.

ketone body, *n* See body, ketone.

ketonuria (kē'tōnyoo'rēə) *n* the indication of extra bodies of ketone within urine caused by decreased or unstable metabolism of carbohydrates; occurs more frequently in certain medical conditions (e.g., starvation acidosis and diabetes mellitus); may also be called *acetonuria.*

ketoprofen (kē'tōprō'fən), *n brand names:* Orudis, Oruvail, Actron; *drug class:* nonsteroidal antiinflammatory; *action:* inhibits prostaglandin synthesis by interfering with cyclooxygenase needed for biosynthesis; possesses analgesic, antiinflammatory, antipyretic properties; *uses:* osteoarthritis, rheumatoid arthritis, dysmenorrhea.

ketorolac/ketorolac tromethamine injection (kē'tōrō'lak trōmeth'əmēn'), *n brand name:* Toradol; *drug class:* nonsteroidal antiinflammatory; *action:* inhibits prostaglandin synthesis by interfering with cyclooxygenase needed for biosynthesis; possesses analgesic, antiinflammatory, antipyretic properties; *use:* acute mild to moderate pain; not for chronic pain use.

ketosis, *n* See ketoacidosis.

kev, *n* the abbreviation for 1000 electron volts.

keyway, *n* the slot into which the male portion of precision attachments fits.

kg, *n* See kilogram.

KHN, *n.pr* the abbreviation for Knoop hardness number. See also test, Knoop hardness.

kidney, *n* one of a pair of bean-shaped urinary organs in the dorsal part of the abdomen, one on each side of the vertebral column. The kidneys filter the blood and produce and eliminate urine. They use a complex filtration network and reabsorption system made up of nephrons, the functional unit of the organ. They also regulate the concentrations of hydrogen, sodium, potassium, phosphate, and other ions in the extracellular fluid. Diseases of the kidneys can lead to xerostomia, periodontal disease, and inflammation of the oral cavity and salivary glands. Medications may also need to be adjusted in these cases.

kidney dialysis, artificial, *n* a treatment used in patients with kidney failure. It performs the same function of normal kidneys, removing salts, waste products, and excess water. There are two types, peritoneal and hemodialysis.

kidney failure, *n* a disease in which the patient's kidney(s) fail to work properly, resulting in their inability to remove excess fluid and waste material from the blood. There are two types, acute and chronic.

kidney failure, acute, *n* a form of kidney disease that is more likely to occur in hospitalized patients whose health is already compromised by complicated surgery, injury to the kidney, or decreased blood flow to the kidney. Patients with acute kidney failure often can undergo intensive treatment and recover from the disease.

kidney failure, chronic, *n* a gradual, progressive form of kidney disease that often results from high blood pressure (hypertension) or diabetes.

killer cell, *n* a lymphocyte that develops in the bone marrow and lacks the characteristic surface markers of the B and T lymphocytes. Killer or null cells represent a small proportion of the lymphocyte population. Stimulated by the presence of an antibody, null cells can attach certain cellular targets directly and are known as *natural killer cells.*

kilo- (kil'ō), *pre* 1000.

kilocalorie, *n* 1000 calories, a unit of measure of the energy value in foodstuffs.

kilogram (kil'əgram), *n* 1000 g, or equivalent to approximately 2.2 pounds avoirdupois.

kilohertz (kil'ōhurts) *n* a frequency unit of 1000 cycles per second.

kilovolt (kil'əvōlt), *n* the unit of electrical potential equal to 1000 volts.

kilovolt peak (kvp), *n* the crest value of the potential wave in kilovolts in an alternating current cycle. When only half of the wave is used, the value refers to that of the useful half of the wave.

kilovolt potential, *n* refers to the intensitiy of the radiographic beam and the resulting image on the film. A higher kilovoltage radiograph increases the film density, whereas a lower kilovoltage radiograph increases contrast.

kilovoltage (kil'əvōl'təj), *n* the electrical potential difference between the anode and cathode of a radiographic tube.

kilovoltage, constant potential, *n* the potential of a constant voltage generator, in constant potential kilovolts (kvcp).

kilovoltage, equivalent (effective kilovoltage), *n* the kilovoltage of monoenergetic radiation having the same half-value layer (HVL) as the heterogeneous beam produced by the peak kilovoltage in question.

kinematic face-bow (kinəmat'ik), *n* See face-bow, kinematic.

kinesiology (kinē'sēol'əjē), *n* the study of motion that attempts to explain the manner in which movements of the body occur. The principles of kinesiology may be used to describe the laws of articulation and the several theories of mandibular movement.

kinetics (kənet'iks), *n* the study of the forces that produce, arrest, or modify the motions of the body. Kinetics is the application of Newton's first and third laws of inertia to body dynamics. The reaction forces of the muscles contribute to the equilibrium and motion of the body.

kinin (kī'nin), *n* a number of widely differing substances having pronounced and dramatic physiologic effects. Some are formed in blood by proteolysis secondary to some pathologic process. Kinins stimulate visceral smooth muscle but relax vascular smooth muscle, thus producing vasodilation. May be involved in periodontal disease.

kink, *n* a bend or twist.

Kirkland cement dressing, *n.pr* knife. See knife, Kirkland.

Kirschner wire, *n.pr* See wire, Kirschner.

Kirstein's method, *n.pr* See method, Kirstein's.

kissing disease, *n* a vernacular term for *infectious mononucleosis,* a viral infection frequently occurring in teenagers and young adults. See also infectious mononucleosis.

kleptomania (klep′tōmā′nēə) *n* an impulse control disorder distinguished by an uncontrollable urge to steal typically unnecessary objects.

Kline's test, *n.pr* See test, Kline's.

Klinefelter syndrome, *n.pr* a syndrome of gonadal defects, appearing in males with an extra X chromosome in at least one cell line. Characteristics are small, firm testes, long legs, gynecomastia, poor social adaptation, subnormal intelligence, chronic pulmonary disease, and varicose veins.

Kloehn headgear, *n.pr* an extraoral orthodontic appliance consisting of a facebow and a cervical strap used to retract maxillary teeth or to reinforce the anchorage during tooth retraction.

knee, *n* a joint complex that connects the thigh with the lower leg. It consists of 3 condyloid joints, 12 ligaments, 13 bursae, and the patella.

knife, *n* an instrument used for cutting that consists of a sharp-edged blade with a handle.

knife, amalgam, *n* a bladed metal instrument used in the margination process to remove excess amalgam and overhangs.

knife, buck, *n* a periodontal knife possessing spear-shaped cutting points; used for interdental incision during gingivectomy.

knife, electronic, *n* an electrosurgical scalpel used to incise or shave tissue.

knife, gold, *n* an instrument sometimes contraangled, with a blade or cutting edge; used to trim excess metal and develop contour in foil restorations.

knife, Goldman-Fox, *n.pr* a group of surgical instruments designed for the incision and contouring of gingival tissue.

knife, Kirkland, *n.pr* a heart-shaped knife, sharp on all edges, used for the primary gingivectomy incision.

knife, Merrifield's, *n.pr* a knife that has a long, narrow, triangular blade in a shank; used for gingivectomy incisions.

knitting yarn, *n* an alternative to floss, used to clean surfaces of teeth that are exceptionally far apart; also effective for cleaning isolated teeth, including those at the end of a row. Sometimes used with a floss threader to reach the difficult areas under pontics and around fixed and cantilevered dentures.

Knoop hardness test, *n.pr* See test, Knoop hardness.

Kobayashi ties (kō′bāäsh′ē), *n.pr.pl* the orthodontic ligature ties used to fix an orthodontic arch wire to the brackets attached to the teeth; also provides attachment for the use of inter- and intramaxillary elastic traction.

Koeber's saw, *n.pr* See saw, Koeber's.

koilocytosis (koil′əsītō′sis), *n* a histologic feature of the mucosal changes associated with the intraoral use of smokeless tobacco. The spinous cells of the squamous epithelium present with pyknotic, irregularly shaped nuclei surrounded by a perinuclear clear zone.

Koplik spots, *n.pr.pl* See spots, Koplik.

Korotkoff sounds (kôrot′kôf), *n.pr* the noises heard when taking a blood pressure reading, originated by blood passage causing vibrations in the walls of the blood vessel.

Kryptex, *n* See cement, silicophosphate.

krypton (Kr) (krip′ton), *n* an inert gas, present in small amounts in the atmosphere, with an atomic number of 36 and an atomic weight of 83.80.

KS, *n.pr* See sarcoma, Kaposi's.

Kurer anchor system, *n.pr* an endodontic post system with parallel sides, threaded and made of stainless material.

kV, *n* See kilovolt.

kVcp, *n* See kilovoltage, constant potential.

kVp, *n* See kilovolt peak.

kVp (kilovoltage peak) selector, *n* the control on a radiograph machine that selects the kilovoltage for a given radiographic film. See also radiograph, high kilovoltage radiograph, low kilovoltage.

kwashiorkor (kwä′shēôr′kôr), *n* a wasting disease of malnutrition that occurs in children after weaning as a result of severe protein deficiency. The word is Ghanan, meaning "the displaced child's visible condition."

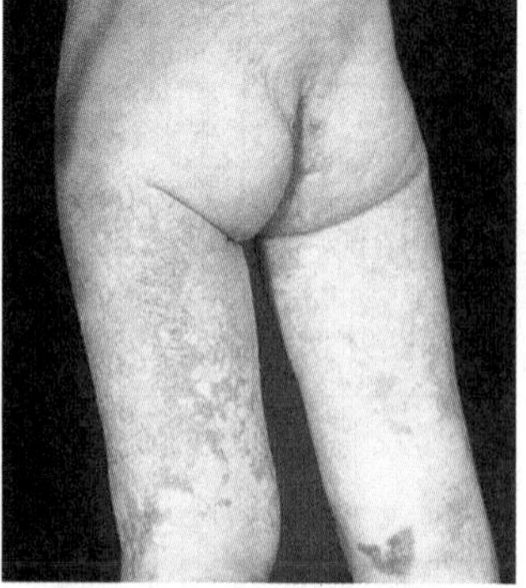

Kwashiorkor. (Zitelli/Davis, 2002)

kyphosis (kīfō′sis), *n* (Older term: humpback), an abnormal curvature of the spine with the convexity backward.

L

label (lā′bəl), *n* **1.** the portion of the prescription in which the directions for use are stated. **2.** one or more characters used to identify an item of data. Also called *key.* See also signa.

labetatol, *n brand names:* Normodyne, Trandate; *drug class:* nonselective adrenergic β-blocker and α-blocker; *action:* produces falls in BP without reflex tachycardia or significant reduction in heart rate through mixture of α-blocking and β-blocking effects; elevated plasma renins are reduced; *use:* mild to severe hypertension.

labial (lā′bēəl), *n* of or pertaining to a lip.

labial commissures, *n.pl* the lateral angles formed where the lips meet at the outer edges of the oral cavity; the corners of the oral cavity.

labial developmental depressions, *n.pl* the indentations extending from the cervix to the occusal surface on the crown of an anterior tooth in order to separate the tooth into labial developmental lobes.

labial mucosa, *n* tissue lining the inner lips within the oral cavity.

labial notch, *n* See notch, labial.

labial ridge, *n* See ridge, labial.

labile (lā′bīl), *adj* unstable, as labile fever.

labioversion (lā′bēōvur′zhən), *n* a deviation of a tooth toward the lips from the line of occlusion.

labium superius oris (lā′bēum soopir′ēus ō′ris), *n* the point of the upper lip lying in the midsagittal plane and a line drawn across the boundary of the mucous surface tangent to the curves.

laboratory, dental, *n* the area of the dental office where the dental professional performs nonpatient procedures.

laceration, *n* a wound produced by tearing; the process of tearing.

laches (lach′iz), *n* an inexcusable delay; a failure to claim or enforce a claim or right at a proper time; negligence.

lacquer, *n* a resin dissolved in a volatile solvent used to create a protective coating on the surface of an object.

lacrimal apparatus (lak′rəməl), *n* a network of structures of the eye that secrete tears and drain them from the surface of the eyeball. The parts include the lacrimal glands, the lacrimal ducts, the lacrimal sacs, and the nasolacrimal ducts.

lacrimal glands, *n.pl* See glands, lacrimal. See also lacrimal apparatus.

lacrimation, gustatory, *n* See syndrome, auriculotemporal.

lactalbumin (lak′talbū′min), *n* a simple, highly nutritious protein found in milk. Lactalbumin is similar to serum albumin.

lactate dehydrogenase (lak′tāt dē′hīdroj′ənās′), *n* an enzyme found in the cytoplasm of almost all body tissues, where its main function is to catalyze the oxidation of L-lactate to pyruvate.

***Lactobacilli*, cariogenic,** *n* a type of bacteria that may play an important role in tooth decay. It is usually found in small amounts in dental plaque. Its concentration increases with high sugar intake.

***Lactobacillius acidophilus* (lak'tōbəsil'ēəs as'idōfil'əs),** *n* a species of the genus *Lactobacillius* of the family Lactobacillaceae characterized by gram-positive rods found in cultured buttermilk and in the gastrointestinal tract of persons on a high milk-, lactose-, or dextrin-containing diet. *L. acidophilus* preparations may be effective in the treatment of some recurrent aphthous ulcers and for the prevention of candidiasis secondary to tetracycline and/or steroid therapy.

***L. casei* (kasā'ē),** *n* a species of *Lactobacillius* found in milk and cheese.

lactoferrin (lak'tōfer'in), *n* an iron-binding protein found in the specific granules of neutrophils where it apparently exerts an antimicrobial activity by withholding iron from ingested bacteria and fungi. It also occurs in many secretions and exudates such as milk, tears, mucus, saliva, and bile.

lactone, *n* an organic anhydride formed from a hyroxyacid by the loss of water between an 2OH and a 2COOH group.

lactoperoxidase (lak'tōpərok'sidās'), *n* a peroxidase enzyme obtained from milk.

lactose, *n* a disaccharide found in the milk of all mammals. Lactose is used as a component of formulas for infants; it is also used as a laxative and a diuretic.

lactose intolerance, *n* an inability to digest the lactose in milk and milk products.

lacuna (ləkoo'nə), *n* a term used in anatomic nomenclature to designate a small hollow cavity or pit.

lacuna, absorption (Howship's lacuna), *n* an area (pit) of bone resorption, usually irregular in outline, and often containing osteoclasts.

lacuna, osteocyte, *n* a hollow cavity within bone, containing osteocytes, from which canaliculi, containing protoplasmic processes of the osteocytes, radiate.

lambda (lam'də), *n* **1.** the eleventh letter of the Greek alphabet. **2.** the point in the skull at which the sagittal and lambdoid sutures meet. **3.** The strap of a rubber dam holder placed at this level will hold its position without slipping up or down.

lamellae (ləmel'ē), *n* the nearly parallel layers of bone tissue found in compact bone.

lamella, cemental **(ləmel'ə),** *n* the arrangement and deposition of cementum in incremental layers more or less parallel to the root configuration.

lamina (lam'inə), *n* a flat, thin plate.

lamina, dental, *n* a band of epithelial tissue that connects a developing tooth bud to the oral mucosa of the oral cavity.

lamina dura, *n* a radiographic term denoting the plate of compact bone (alveolar bone) that lies adjacent to the periodontal ligament.

lamina propria, *n* the zone of connective tissue subjacent to the epithelium of a mucous membrane such as the *oral mucosa.*

laminagraphy (lam'inäg'rəfē), *n* a body-section radiography.

laminate, *n* a thin slice of porcelain or plastic fabricated in a dental lab, which is cemented to the front of the teeth to cover gaps, whiten stained teeth, or reshape chipped or broken teeth. Laminates, or veneers, are generally natural in appearance and are long-lasting.

laminate veneer restoration, *n* a conservative esthetic restoration of anterior teeth to mask discoloration, restore malformed teeth, close diastemas, and correct minor tooth alignment. The materials of choice are acrylic veneers, processed composite resin veneers, and/or porcelain veneers that are bonded directly to a properly prepared tooth.

laminectomy, *n* the excision of a vertebral lamina, commonly used to denote the removal of the posterior arch.

laminin (lam'ənən), *n* a large polypeptide glycoprotein component of the basement membrane.

lamivudine (3TC), *n brand name:* Epivir; *drug class:* antiviral, nucleoside analog; *action:* inhibition of HIV reverse transcriptase; also inhibits RNA- and DNA-dependent DNA polymerase; *use:* in combination with zidovudine for the treatment of HIV infection.

lamotrigine (ləmōt′rijēn′), *n brand name:* Lamictal; *drug class:* antiepileptic; *action:* may be result of blockage of voltage-dependent sodium channels with inhibition of excitatory amino acids; *uses:* adjunctive treatment of refractive partial seizures in adults.

lamp, oral cavity, *n* a device to produce light or illumination directly in the oral cavity and transilluminate the dental tissues.

lance, *v* to cut open with a lancet; to incise.

lancinating, *adj* pertaining to a stabbing pain (e.g., the pain occurring in tic douloureux).

landmark, *n* an anatomic structure used as a guide for anatomic relationships.

***landmark, cephalometric* (sef′-əlōmet′rik),** *n* one of the points located on oriented-head radiographs from which lines, planes, and angles may be constructed to analyze the configuration and relationship of elements of the craniofacial skeleton.

Langerhans cells, *n.pl* the cells of the pancreas that produce insulin.

language, *n* a defined set of characters that is used to form symbols and words and the rules and connections for combining these into meaningful communications.

language, machine, *n* a language designed for interpretation and use by a computer system without translation. Also called *machine code.*

lansoprazole (lansō′prəzōl′), *n brand name:* Prevacid; *drug class:* antisecretory, proton pump inhibitor; *action:* suppresses gastric secretion by inhibiting hydrogen/potassium ATPase enzyme system in gastric parietal cell; *uses:* short-term treatment for healing and symptomatic relief of active duodenal ulcer and erosive esophagitis.

laparotomy (lap′ərot′əmē), *n* a surgical incision into the peritoneal cavity, usually performed under general or regional anesthesia, often on an exploratory basis.

large intestine, *n* the portion of the digestive tract comprising the cecum; the appendix; the ascending, transverse, and descending colons; and the rectum. The ileocecal valve separates the cecum from the ileum.

laryngectomy (lar′ənjek′təmē), *n* the surgical removal of the larynx, performed to treat cancer of the larynx.

laryngitis (lar′injī′tis), *n* an inflammation of the mucous membrane lining the larynx, accompanied by edema of the vocal cords with hoarseness (loss of voice).

laryngopharyngeal (ləring′gōfərin′jēəl), *adj* related jointly to the larynx and the pharynx.

laryngopharynx (ləring′gōfer′ingks), *n* the inferior portion of the pharynx, which extends from the corner of the hyoid bone or the vestibule of the larynx to the inferior border of the cricoid cartilage.

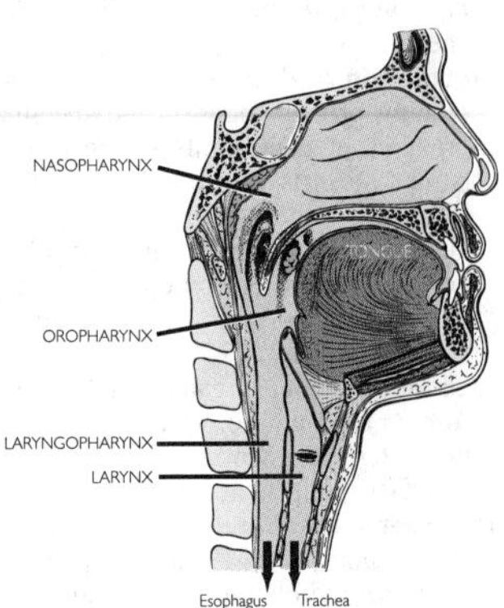

Laryngopharynx. (Liebgott, 2001)

laryngoscope (ləring′gōskōp), *n* a hollow tube equipped with electrical lighting, used to examine or operate upon the interior of the larynx through the oral cavity.

laryngoscopy, *n* the use of a laryngoscope to view the larynx.

laryngospasm (ləring′gōspazəm), *n* the spasmodic closure of the larynx, sometimes noted during the induction phase of general anesthesia or during the recovery period.

larynx (lar′ingks), *n* the organ of voice that is part of the air passage connecting the pharynx with the trachea.

laser, *n* a high-energy coordinated light source used in surgery, including the removal of the hard tissues and soft tissues of the periodontium.

laser whitening (bleaching), n a process for bleaching teeth whereby a bleaching powder or other agent is applied to the teeth and then activated by laser light.

last will and testament, *n* the legal document describing the desires of a person for the distribution of that person's worldly goods after death.

latent, *adj* hidden; beneath the surface; not obvious or active.

latent image, n See image, latent.

latent period, n See period, latent.

lateral (lat′ərəl), *adj* a position either to the right or the left of the midsagittal plane.

lateral abscess, n See abscess, periodontal.

lateral cervical cysts, n.pl a slowly growing cyst commonly developing on the oral cavity floor in children and teenagers, near the sternocleidomastoid muscle; removable by surgery. Also called *lymphoepithelial cyst* or *branchial cleft cyst.* See also lymphoepithelioma.

lateral checkbite, n See record, interocclusal.

lateral condylar inclination, n See inclination, lateral condylar.

lateral condyle path, n See path, lateral condyle.

lateral deviation, n **1.** a frontal asymmetry of the face in which one portion, usually the lower face, is lateral to the midsagittal plane. **2.** a condition of the temporomandibular joint, muscles of mastication, and the teeth that causes the mandible to move to one side on opening or forward thrust.

lateral excursion, n See excursion, lateral.

lateral fossa, n See fossa, lateral.

lateral jaw movement, n the movement of the jaw to one side.

lateral lingual swellings, n.pl the sections of tongue that appear along the midline during embryonic development of the tongue structure.

lateral movement, n See movement, lateral.

lateral nasal processes, n.pl protrusions of tissue that border the olfactory pits during early embryonic development of the face.

lateral periodontal cyst (botryoid odontogenic cyst), n See cyst, lateral periodontal (botryoid odontogenic cyst).

lateral pressure, n the minimum amount of pressure that must be exerted by an instrument against teeth or tissue to achieve the desired effect.

lateral protrusion, n See protrusion, lateral.

lateroretrusive (lat′ərōrētroo′siv), *n* pertaining to a movement direction in cusp or condyle thrusts that has both lateral and backward components of movement.

laterotrusion (lat′ərōtroo′zhən), *n* the outward thrust given by the muscles to the rotating condyle or the condyle on the bolus side.

laterotrusion, precurrent, n the laterotrusion in which the working side condyle is rotated as it is thrust laterally.

latex (lā′teks), *n* natural rubber.

latex allergy, n a hypersensitivity to natural rubber latex in which symptoms may range from minor skin irritations, hives, itchy eyes, and runny nose to asthma and life-threatening anaphylaxis. Because many items used during dental procedures contain rubber latex, patients should be routinely screened for this allergy.

latitude (lat′itood), *n* the range between the minimum and maximum film exposures to radiation that yields images of structures of which photographic density differences are discernible under normal viewing conditions. Latitude mainly varies directly with kilovoltage and inversely with contrast. See also contrast.

lattice, space (lat′is), *n* an arrangement of atoms in a definite relationship to each other, forming a lattice.

lavage (ləväzh′), *n* the irrigation, or washing out, as in oral lavage. See also irrigator or irrigation.

lavage, fluid, n spray washing of the periodontal pocket that occurs as the result of fluid flowing through the tip of a mechanized instrument.

law(s), *n* **1.** that which is laid down or established. An enforceable rule of conduct. *n.pl* **2.** that which must be obeyed and followed by citizens, subject to sanctions or legal consequences. The term is also used in opposition to fact. E.g., in a lawsuit, questions of law are to be decided by the court, whereas the jury decides questions in fact.

law, administrative, *n* a set of specific rules and regulations overseen by an administrative agency in order to enforce the law.

law, case, *n* the use of citations of previous court opinions in a court case, taken from the court decisions published by the state and federal government.

law, Charles's, *n* the principle that states that all gases expand equally upon heating and contract equally upon cooling.

law, constitutional, *n* the set of supreme laws set out in the U.S. Constitution. All other state and federal laws must be in accordance with the laws of the Constitution. The Constitution designates the roles of the three branches of government as well as setting forth which areas of law are in federal jurisdiction and which are left to the states.

law, Dalton's, *n* the principle that states that the pressure of a mixture of gases equals the sum of the partial pressures of the constituent gases.

law, ignorance of, *n* a want of knowledge or acquaintance with the laws of the land insofar as they apply to the act, relation, duty, or matter under consideration.

law, inverse-square, *n* principle stating that the strength of radiation from a point source varies inversely as the square of the distance.

law, judicial, *n* the interpretation of the written law by the courts. Decisions are often based on *stare decisis,* the doctrine that allows the court to follow the decision made in a previous case in the same jurisdiction. A departure from the legal precedents is known as a *landmark decision.*

law, moral, *n* the aggregate of rules and principles of ethics that relate to right and wrong conduct and prescribe the standards to which the actions of persons should conform in their dealings with each other.

law, neurologic, *n* See law of specific energy.

law of radiosensitivity, Bergonie-Tribondeau **(ber'gonē' trebondō'),** *n.pr* law stating that the resistance or sensitivity to radiation depends on the metabolic state of a cell, tissue, or an organ.

law of specific energy (neurologic law), *n* principle that states, in essence, that sensory quality is perceived according to the nerve that is excited, not according to the object that excites. If pressure placed on the eyeballs stimulates the retina, light is perceived, not pressure; similarly, electrical stimulation will produce sensations of smell, taste, touch, or pain in accordance with the nerve stimulated but not a sensation of electricity as such. The special as well as the general senses maintain this principle.

law, tort, *n* an area of law that deals with civil wrongs perpetrated against another person or private property. The primary concerns in dentistry are negligence and malpractice. A lapse in professional standards may be subject to proceedings for negligence or malpractice.

law, Wolff's, *n* principle that states that all changes in the function of bone are attended by definite alterations in its internal structure.

law(s), written, *n/n.pl* the law or laws created by express legislation or enactment, as distinguished from *unwritten* or *common law,* which includes all law or laws from any other legal source.

lay, *adj* nonprofessional.

layer, Beilby's (bil'bēz), *n.pr* an amorphous layer formed on the surface of metals by a disorientation of the crystalline structure during polishing.

LD50, *n* See dose, lethal, median.

LD_{50} time, *n* See time, median lethal.

LDL, *n.pl* See lipoproteins, low-density.

lead (Pb), *n* a common soft, blue-gray, metallic element. Its atomic number is 82, and its atomic weight is 207. In its metallic form, it is used as a protective shielding against radiographs. (In dentistry, lead acts as a protective shield against the radiographic beam and is found in the lead apron and walls of the surrounding operatory.) It is poisonous, a characteristic that has led to a reduction in the use of lead compound as pigments for paints and inks.

lead apron, n See apron, lead.

lead glass, n See glass, lead.

lead poisoning, n See plumbism.

lead-lined cylindrical position-indicating device, *n* a cylinder open at both ends that is lined with lead and used to aim a radiographic beam.

leaf gauge, *n* See gauge, leaf.

learning, *n* the process of acquiring knowledge or some skill by means of study, practice, and/or experience.

learning disability, n an inability to learn at a rate comparable to most members of a peer group. Some learning disorders have been traced to nutritional and behavioral causes, others stem from trauma or disease, and still others have genetic origins.

learning domains, n.pl the three spheres of learning—cognitive, affective, and psychomotor—that must be addressed by a teacher in order to influence behavioral change on the part of the learner. May be applied to the teaching of disease control.

learning-ladder continuum (kəntin′ūəm), *n* theory suggesting that learning takes place in sequential steps beginning with ignorance and culminating with habit. The process may be applied to the teaching of effective plaque control.

lease, *n* **1.** a conveyance of lands or tenements to a person for life, for a stated number of years, or at will, in consideration of rent or some other recompense. **2.** any agreement that gives rise to a landlord and tenant relationship.

least expensive alternative treatment (LEAT), *n* a limitation in a dental benefits plan that will only allow benefits for the least expensive treatment. Also referred to as *least expensive professionally acceptable alternative treatment (LEPAAT).*

lecithin (les′ithin), *n* a class of phosphatides containing glycerol, phosphate, choline, and fatty acids. They are widely distributed in cells and possess both metabolic and structural functions in membranes. Dipalmityl lecithin is an important surface-active agent in the lungs.

ledger sheet, *n* an accounting form for keeping track of debits, expenditures, credits, and charges.

leeway space, *n* the arch circumference difference between the primary canine, first primary and second primary molars, and the permanent canine and the first and second premolars. According to Black's means, the maxillary arch leeway space is 1.9 mm, and the mandibular arch leeway space is 3.4 mm.

LeFort fracture, *n.pr* See fracture, LeFort.

left justified, *n* data are left justified when the left-most digit or character occupies the left-most position of the space allotted for those data.

legal, *adj* **1.** in compliance with the law. **2.** not forbidden by law.

***Legionella* (lē′jənel′ə),** *n* a genus of areobic, motile, non–acid-fast, nonencapsulated, gram-negative bacilli that have a nonfermentative metabolism. They are water dwelling, airborne spread, and pathogenic for man.

L. pneumophila, n the causative agent of Legionnaires' disease.

Legionnaires' disease, *n.pr* an acute bacterial pneumonia caused by infection with *L. pneumophila* and characterized by an influenza-like illness followed within a week by high fever, chills, muscle aches, and headache. Contaminated air-conditioning cooling towers and stagnant water supplies, including water vaporizers and water sonicators, may be a source of organisms.

legislation, *n* the act of making or forming law, or the laws and/or statutes formed by the legislative process.

legumes (ləgyoomz′), *n* a plant belonging to the order Fabales and family Leguminosae. Examples of legumes are beans, peas, and lentils.

leiomyoma (lī′ōmīō′mə), *n* a benign tumor derived from smooth muscle.

leiomyosarcoma (lī′ōmī′ōsarkō′mə), *n* a malignant neoplasm of muscle that contains spindle cells of unstriated muscle.

leishmaniasis (lēsh′mənī′əsis), *n* an infection with a species of protozoan of the genus *Leishmania.*

length, *n* the longest measure of an object, or the measurement between the two ends.

length, muscle, n the variable end-to-end measurement of a muscle. The physical changes in muscle observed in the isotonic and isometric states of contraction are related to the alteration in the striated bands of muscle.

length of stay, n the expected length of time, usually a median, that institutionalized patients of similar age and diagnosis or condition in a hospital or other health care facility would be expected to remain.

length, tooth, n the distance along the long axis of the tooth from the apex of the root to the tip, or incisal edge, of the tooth.

lens, crystalline, *n* the lens of the eye.

lenses, curved, *n.pl* a transparent pieces of plastic or glass that are shaped, molded, or ground to refract light in a specific way, as in eyeglasses, microscopes, or cameras.

lentulo (lentoo′lə), *n* a flexible spiral-wire instrument used in a handpiece to apply paste filling materials in root canals.

leontiasis ossea (lē′əntī′əsis os′ēə), *n* an enlargement of the bones of the face, leading to a lionlike appearance. Osseous encroachment may cause obliteration of sinuses, blindness, and malocclusion.

leproma (leprō′mə), *n* a nodular lesion of leprosy seen on the skin, mucous membranes (including those of the eyes), upper respiratory tract, tongue, and palate.

leprosy (lep′rōsē), *n* a chronic granulomatous infection caused by *Mycobacterium leprae.* It may exist in lepromatous (contagious), tuberculoid (noncontagious), and intermediate forms.

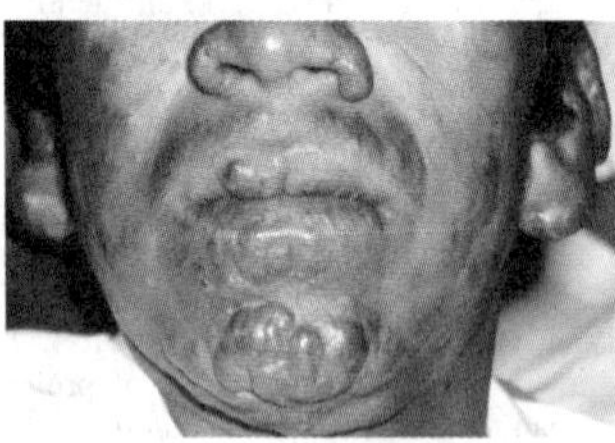

Leprosy. (Neville/Damm/Allen/Bouquot, 2002)

leptocytosis, hereditary (lep′tōsītō′sis), *n* See thalassemia.

***Leptothrix rocemosa* (lep′tōthriks),** *n* a filamentous microorganism, apparently not directly capable of pathogenicity, that may act as a nidus for the formation of dental calculus and its attachment to the tooth structure. May be associated with dental desease.

Lesch-Nyhan syndrome (lesh-nī′ən), *n.pr* a hereditary disorder of purine metabolism, characterized by mental retardation, self-mutilation of the fingers and lips by biting, impaired renal function, and abnormal physical development. It is transmitted as a recessive, sex-linked trait.

lesion (lē′zhən), *n* a pathologic disturbance of a tissue, with loss of continuity, enlargement, and/or function.

lesion, brown spot, n an area of demineralized tooth enamel that turns brown before progressing to an active caries.

lesion, carious, n also known as dental caries or tooth cavities. Typically caused by acid-producing bacteria, which lowers the pH of the oral cavity, causing demineralization. See caries.

lesion, coalescing **(ko′əles′ing),** *n* numerous raised nodules that often appear in groups on the skin surface of the knees, elbows, and lower extremities. The nodules coalesce to form a large patch that appears to be a single lesion.

lesion, of endodontic origin (LEO), n an abscess in the tooth root. Usually the result of caries, tooth fracture, or an invasive dental procedure.

lesion, extravasation, n See cyst, traumatic.

lesion, fibroosseous jaw, n an area in the jaw where normal alveolar bone has been replaced by a fibrous, mineral material.

lesion, flat oral, n a regularly or irregularly shaped laceration developing on the surface of the oral mucosa or normal skin.

lesion, herpetic, n a vesicle and/or ulceration of the mucosa caused by herpesvirus.

lesion, herpetiform, n a painful ulceration of the oral mucosa with a red center and yellow border; occurs as a solitary lesion or in groups and

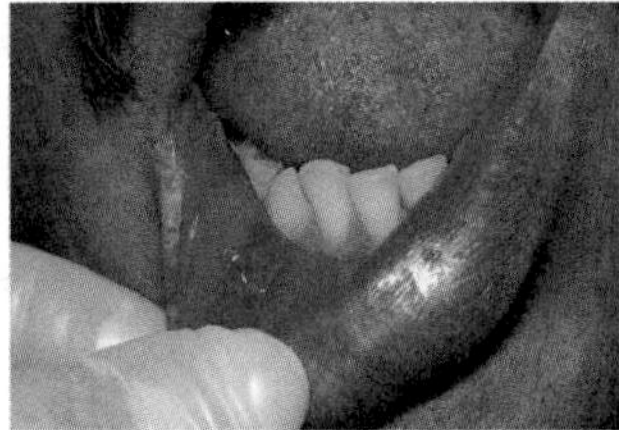

Flat oral lesions. (Regezi/Sciubba/Jordan, 2008)

appears similar to those lesions caused by herpesvirus. The term *herpetiform* is used as a clinical designation unless the viral cause has actually been demonstrated.

lesion, indefinite bone, *n* See cyst, extravasation.

lesion, mucous extravasation, *n.pl* See cyst, mucous.

lesion, noncarious dental, *n.pl* the abnormalities occurring on the surfaces of teeth that do not fall under the category of dental cavities. They may include enamel hypoplasia, attrition, erosion, abrasion, or tooth fractures.

lesion, precancerous, *n* a tissue abnormality or wound that although not yet malignant shows signs indicating the likely development of cancer in the future.

lesion, subsurface, *n* an area of softness below the tooth enamel that occurs as the result of acid retention. Can be corrected by fluoride administration.

lesion, traumatic bone, *n* See cyst, traumatic.

lesion, white spot, *n* a small, demineralized area of tooth enamel occurring under or near orthodontic brackets or bands.

LET, *n* See transfer, linear energy.

lethargy (leth′ärjē), *n* sluggishness or fatigue; a feeling of listlessness.

Letterer-Siwe disease, *n.pr* See disease, Letterer-Siwe.

leucine (loo′sēn), *n* one of the essential amino acids. See also amino acid.

leucovorin calcium (citrovorum factor/folinic acid), *n brand name:* Wellcovorin; *drug class:* folic acid antagonist antidote, antineoplastic adjunct; *action:* chemically reduced derivative of folic acid, converted to tetrahydrofolate; counteracts folic acid antagonists; *uses:* megaloblastic or macrocytic anemia caused by folic acid deficiency, overdose of folic acid antagonist, methotrexate toxicity caused by pyrimethamine or trimethoprim, or in colorectal cancer with fluorouracil.

leukemia (lookē′mēə), *n* a usually fatal disease of the blood-forming tissues characterized by the abnormal proliferation of leukocytes and their precursors and attended by fatigue, weakness, fever, lymphadenopathy, splenomegaly, and a tendency toward profuse tissue hemorrhage. Oral lesions include gingival enlargement, severe gingivitis, and necrosis. Lymphatic, monocytic, and myelogenous leukemias are the main types.

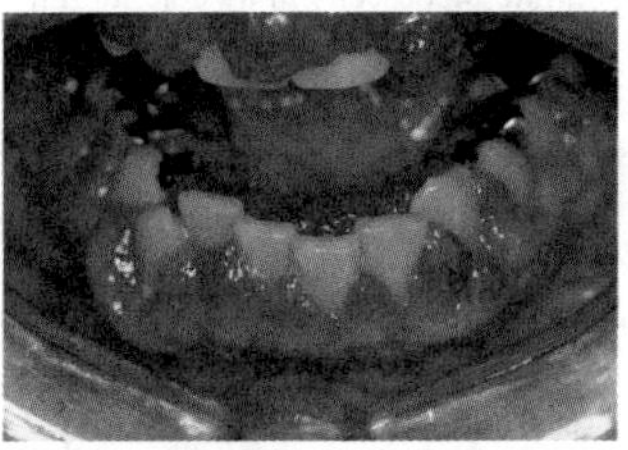

Leukemia. (Regezi/Sciubba/Jordan, 2008)

***leukemia, aleukemia* (ā′lookē′mēə),** *n* a phase of the leukemic state marked by proliferation of leukocytes within the blood-forming tissues but without an increase in the white blood cell count: relatively few precursor cells are found in the blood smear until the phase passes and the blood becomes flooded with white cells. Oral lesions, when present, are ulceronecrotic and hypertrophic.

leukemia, lymphatic (lymphoid leukemia), *n* a hyperplasia, of undetermined origin, affecting lymphoid tissue. Predominating cells are lymphocytes and lymphoblasts. Generally assumes a more chronic course than other forms of leukemia but may be acute. Oral lesions include swollen and hyperplastic gingivae, ulceronecrotic lesions, and marked tendency to gingival hemorrhage.

leukemia, monocytic, *n* a form characterized by an abnormal increase in the number of monocytes. Manifestations include progressive weakness, anorexia, lymphadenopathy, hepatomegaly, splenomegaly, and secondary anemia. Oral lesions may be ulceronecrotic or hemorrhagic.

leukemia, myelogenous, *n* a form in which the leukocytes are of bone marrow origin (e.g., polymorphonuclear leukocytes, myelocytes, myeloblasts). Oral manifestations may include gingival enlargement, hemorrhage, and necrosis.

leukocyte (lōō'kōsīt), *n* a white blood cell circulating in the blood. See also lymphocyte and monocyte.

leukocyte, basophilic (basophil), *n* a type that has coarse granules stainable with basic dyes and a bent lobed nucleus.

leukocyte count, *n* the number of white blood cells in a cubic millimeter of blood. Normal values range from 5000 to 10,000/mm^3.

leukocyte, eosinophilic (eosinophil), *n* a type that has coarse granules stainable with eosin and a bilobed nucleus.

leukocyte, immature, *n* a form of white blood cell usually found in disease (e.g., myelocytes, myeloblasts, lymphoblasts).

leukocyte, monocyte, *n* an agranulocyte white blood cell.

leukocyte, polymorphonuclear (PMN), (neutrophil), *n* **1.** a type with finely granular cytoplasm, an irregularly lobulated nucleus, and the appearance of a microphage. It is found in the tissues during acute inflammatory processes and in the superficial surface aspects of a lesion during subacute or chronic inflammation. It is the predominating leukocyte of the blood. Blood levels may be increased during acute inflammatory states and myelogenous leukemia, and decreased in agranulocytosis. See also neutropenia; polymorphonuclear leukocyte; neutrophilia.

leukocytosis (loo'kōsītō'sis), *n* an increase in the normal number of white blood cells; may be a defensive reaction, as in inflammation, or may result from a disturbance in white blood cell formation, as in leukemia. Various limits are given; e.g., leukocytosis in the adult is indicated when there are more than 10,000 white blood cells per cubic millimeter. See also eosinophilia; lymphocytosis; neutrophilia; monocytosis.

leukoedema (loo'kōədē'mə), *n* an innocuous oral condition characterized by a filmy, opalescent, white covering of the buccal mucosa consisting of a thickened layer of parakeratotic cells. It is most commonly associated with mechanical and chemical irritation.

leukopenia (loo'kōpē'nēə), *n* a decrease in the normal number of white blood cells in the circulating blood. Various lower limits are given; e.g., leukopenia signifies less than 4000 white blood cells per cubic millimeter. See also lymphocytopenia; neutropenia.

leukoplakia (loo'kōplā'kēə), *n* a white plaque formed on the oral mucosa from surface epithelial cells with an unknown etiology. It is leathery, opaque, and somewhat thickened. Excluded from this are the white lesions of lichen planus, white sponge nevus, burns, thrush, and other clinically recognizable entities. Histologically, hyperkeratosis, acanthosis, and subepithelial and perivascular infiltrate of round cells may be seen. Dyskeratosis may be present. These lesions may progress to malignancy, with cellular atypicism, dyskeratosis, epithelial pearl formation, and infiltration of malignant cells into connective tissue. See also dyskeratosis; hyperkeratosis.

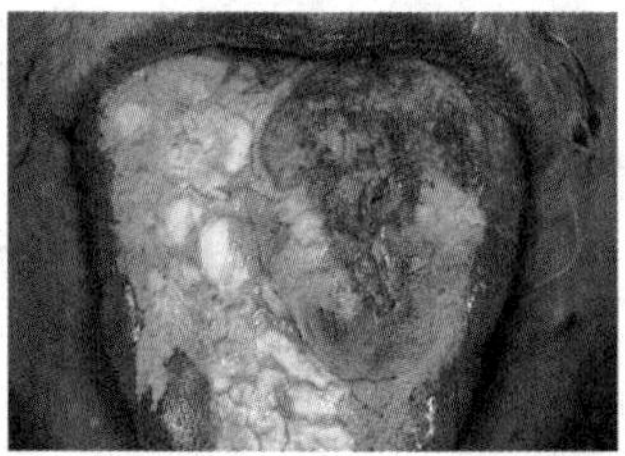

Leukoplakia. (Regezi/Sciubba/Pogrel, 2000)

leukoplakia, hairy, *n* a white lesion appearing on the lateral surface of the tongue and occasionally on the buccal mucosa of patients with AIDS. The lesion appears raised, with a corrugated or "hairy" surface as a result of keratin projections.

leukotaxine (loo'kōtak'sin), *n* a substance that appears when tissue is injured and can be removed from inflammatory exudates. Increases capillary permeability and the diapedesis of leukocytes.

lev-, *pref* See levo-.

levamisole HCl, *n brand name:* Ergamisol; *drug class:* immunomodulator; *action:* may increase the action of macrophages, monocytes, and T cells, which will restore immune function; *uses:* Dukes's stage C colon cancer, given with fluoruracil after surgical resection.

level (lev′əl), *v* to reduce the curve of Spee by intrusion and/or extrusion of the teeth in an arch.

leveling arch wire, *n* an arch wire used to align teeth in the same plane.

lever (lev′ur), *n* a bar or rigid body that is capable of turning about one joint or axis and in which are two or more other points where forces are applied. There are three classes of levers, and each has its own most effective use.

lever leverage **(lev′ərəj),** *n* the mechanical advantage gained by the use of a lever. A factor in the magnification of stresses generated by an extension-base partial denture.

lever, second-class, *n* a lever in which the force arm is longer than the work-producing arm; thus the work produced is always greater than the energy used, with a resultant high efficiency.

lever, third-class, *n* a lever in which the axis is at one end, the load at the other end, and the effort is exerted in between, as in a treadle.

levigated aluminum (lev′igā′təd), *n* the fine particles of aluminum oxide used to polish metals, but unsuitable for polishing teeth. See emery.

levo- (lev) (lē′vō), *pref* a prefix applied to the name of optical isomers that rotate the plane of polarized light to the left.

levobunolol hydrochloride (lev′ōbū′nōlol hī′drōklor′ād), *n brand name:* Akbeta, Betagan C Cap BID, Betagan C Cap QD, Betagan Standard; *drug class:* β-adrenergic blocker; *action:* reduces production of aqueous humor by unknown mechanisms; *uses:* chronic open-angle glaucoma, ocular hypertension.

levocabastine HCl (lev′ōkab′əstēn′), *n brand name:* Livostin; *drug class:* antihistamine, H_1-receptor antogonist; *action:* selective antagonist for histamine at H_1 receptors; little or no systemic absorption; intended for topical effect; *uses:* temporary relief of seasonal allergic conjunctivitis.

levodopa (lev′ōdō′pə), *n brand names:* Larodopa, Dopar; *class drug:* antiparkinson agent; *action:* levodopa is decarboxylated to dopamine, which can interact with dopamine receptors; *uses:* parkinsonism or parkinsonian symptoms.

levodopa-carbidopa (lev′ōdō′pə-kar′bidō′pə), *n brand names:* Sinemet, Sinemet CR; *drug class:* antiparkinson agent; *action:* decarboxylation of levodopa to periphery is inhibited by carbidopa; more levodopa is made available for transport to brain and conversion to dopamine in the brain; *uses:* treatment of idiopathic, symptomatic, or postencephalitic parkinsonism.

levomethadyl acetate HCl (lev′ōmeth′ədīl as′ətāt), *n brand name:* ORLAAM; *drug class:* synthetic opioid; *action:* mimics the action of opioid analgesics by interacting with CNS opioid receptors; *use:* management of opioid dependence.

levonordefrin (lē′vōnôrdef′rin), *n brand name:* Neo-Cobefrin; a vasoconstrictor added to a local anesthetic agent in a cartridge. It helps to contain the anesthetic in a specific area by reducing systemic absorption, decreasing blood flow, and prolonging effectiveness.

levonorgestrel implant (lēv′ənorjes′trəl), *n brand name:* Norplant System; *drug class:* contraceptive system; *action:* as a progestin, transforms proliferative endometrium into secretory endometrium; inhibits secretion of pituitary gonadotropins, which prevents follicular maturation and ovulation; *use:* prevention of pregnancy.

levothyroxine sodium (lē′vōthīrak′sēn), *n brand names:* Levo-T, Synthroid; *drug class:* thyroid hormone; *action:* increases metabolic rate, with increase in cardiac output, O_2 consumption, body temperature, blood volume, growth/development at cellular level; *uses:* hypothroidism, myxedema coma, thyroid hormone replacement, cretinism.

Leydig cells, *n.pr* the cells of the interstitial tissue of the testes that secrete testosterone.

liabilities, *n.pl* the claims against a corporation. They include accounts and wages and salaries payable, dividends declared payable, accrued taxes payable, and fixed or long-term liabilities, such as mortgage bonds, debentures, and bank loans.

liabilities, current, n.pl the short-term debts and obligations that must be paid within a period of 1 year.

liability (līəbil'itē), *n* the state of being bound by law or justice to do something or to make good something; legal responsibility.

libel (lī'bəl), *n* **1.** that which is written and published in order to injure the character of another by ridicule or contempt. **2.** a defamation expressed by print, writing, pictures, or signs.

license, *n* permission, accorded by a competent authority, granting the right to perform some act or acts that without such authorization would be contrary to law.

licensure (lī'sənshər), *n* the granting of permission by a competent authority (usually a government agency) to an organization or individual to engage in a practice or activity that would otherwise be illegal. Licensure is usually granted on the basis of education and examination rather than performance. It is usually permanent, but a periodic fee, demonstration of competence, or continuing education may be required. Licensure may be revoked by the granting agency for incompetence, criminal acts, or other reasons stipulated in the statutes or rules governing the specific area of licensure.

licensure, dental, n the permission to practice dentistry in a specific geopolitical area, granted by a government agency.

licensure, dental hygiene, n a form of regulation to protect the public from unqualified and unsafe practice. To be granted a license, an individual must state requirements by successfully completing a series of steps, such as graduating from an accredited dental program and passing national and regional exams.

lichen planus (lī'kən plā'nəs), *n* a dermatologic disease affecting the skin and oral mucosa; of unknown etiology but often associated with nervousness, fatigue, emotional depression, and allergy and considered to be a manifestation of quinacrine (Atabrine) therapy. Oral lesions often appear as white or blue-white striae forming an interweaving lacelike network of lines of epithelial thickening. Associated with the striated network; bullous or erosive lesions may be found. Histologically, varying degrees of hyperkeratosis and epithelial acanthosis may be found, with formation of sawtooth-shaped rete pegs of epithelium projecting into connective tissue. Subjacent to the epithelium is a bandlike infiltrate of round cells with perivascular accumulation of leukocytes. Treatment is symptomatic.

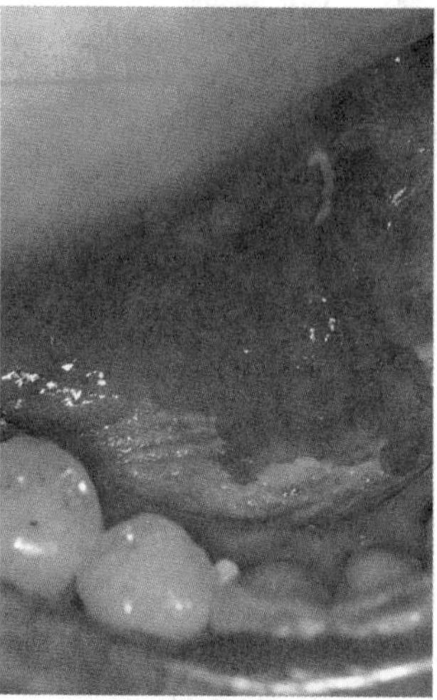

Lichen planus. (Courtesy Dr. Charles Babbush)

lichen planus, oral, n See lichen planus.

lidocaine HCl (cardiac) (lī'dōkān' kar'dēak), *n* *brand names:* Lidopen, Xylocaine, Xylocard; *drug class:* antidysrhythmic (Class IB); *action:* increases electrical stimulation threshold of ventricle and His-Purkinje system, which stabilizes cardiac membrane and decreases automaticity and excitability of ventricles; *uses:* ventricular tachycardia, ventricular dysrhythmias during cardiac surgery, cardiac catheterization.

lidocaine HCl (local), *n brand names:* Dalcaine, Dilocaine, Lidoject, Octocain, Xylocaine, Xylocaine-MPF; *drug class:* amide local anesthetic; *action:* inhibits ion fluxes across membranes, particularly sodium transport across cell membrane, decreases rise of depolarization phase of action potential, blocks nerve action potential; *uses:* local dental anesthesia, peripheral nerve block; caudal anesthesia; epidural, spinal, surgical anesthesia.

lidocaine HCl (topical), *n brand name:* Xylocaine Viscous; *drug class:* topically acting local anesthetic, amide; *action:* inhibits nerve impulses from sensory nerves, which produces anesthesia; *uses:* topical anesthesia of inflamed or irritated mucous membranes; to reduce gag reflex in dental radiologic examination or in dental impressions.

lien (lēn), *n* a qualified right of property that a creditor has in specific property of the debtor as security for the debt or for performance of some act.

life, effective half-, *n* See half-life, effective.

life expectancy, *n* the probable number of years a person will live after a given age, as determined by the mortality rate in a specific geographic area. This number may be individually qualified by the person's condition, race, sex, age, and other demographic factors.

life, radioactive, *n* See half-life.

ligament (lig′əment), *n* a tough, fibrous connective tissue band that connects bones or supports viscera. Some ligaments are distinct fibrous structures; others are folds of fascia or of indurated peritoneum; still others are the relics of unused fetal organs.

***ligament, alveolodental* (alvē′əlōden′təl),** *n* the principal fibers of periodontal ligament, made up of five groups: alveolar crest, horizontal, oblique, apical, and interradicular (if multirooted).

ligament, biologic width of periodontal, *n* the width of the periodontal ligament in normal, functioning teeth. It varies with the age of the individual and the functional demands made on the tooth. In health, the periodontal ligament is about 0.25 and 0.1 mm in width, narrowest at the center of the alveolus and widest at the margin and apex.

ligament, periodontal (PDL), *n* the method of attachment of the tooth to the alveolus. The ligament consists of numerous bundles of collagenous tissue (principal fibers) arranged in groups, between which is loose connective tissue, together with blood vessels, lymph vessels, and nerves. It functions as the investing and supportive mechanism for the tooth. Older term: *periodontal membrane.*

ligament, sphenomandibular, *n* a ligament extending from the spine of the sphenoid bone to the mandibular lingula.

ligament, stylohyoid, *n* a ligament attached superior to the styloid process of the sphenoid bone.

ligament, stylomandibular, *n* a ligament extending from the styloid process of the temporal bone and attached to the mandibular gonial angle.

ligament, temporomandibular, *n* a triangular-shaped ligament extending from the lateral aspects of the root of the zygomatic process of the temporal bone to the mandibular subcondylar neck.

ligand (līgənd), *n* **1.** a molecule, ion, or group bound to the central atom of a chemical compound, such as the oxygen molecule in hemoglobin, which is bound to the central iron atom. **2.** an organic molecule attached to a specific site on a surface or to a tracer element.

ligate (lī′gāt), *v* to tie or bind with a ligature or suture.

ligation (līgā′shən), *n* the binding together of tissue or teeth with wire, string, or thread for stabilization and immobilization.

ligation, surgical, *n* the exposure of an unerupted tooth with placement of a metal ligature around its cervix. The free ends of the ligature are fixed to a fine, precious-metal chain, which in turn is fixed to an orthodontic appliance for the purpose of placing traction on the unerupted tooth to cause its eruption.

ligature (lig′əchur), *n* **1.** a cord, thread, or fine wire tied around teeth for the purpose of holding a rubber dam in place on retained teeth with fractured roots or split crowns or on teeth that have been replanted. **2.** a wire or threadlike substance used to tie a tooth to an orthodontic appliance or to another tooth.

ligature, grass-line, *n* a type composed of the fibers of a grass-cloth plant (ramie); used for minor tooth movement. It depends for its activation in movement on the property of shrinkage of the ligature when it is wet by the saliva of the patient.

ligature, steel, *n* a type, available as steel filaments in several useful diameters.

light, *n* **1.** the electromagnetic radiation of the wavelength and frequency that stimulate visual receptor cells in the retina to produce nerve impulses that are perceived as vision. **2.** visible light ranges from 400 to 800 nm.

light box, *n* See illuminator.

light, chemiluminescent, *n* light produced by the conversion of chemical energy into light energy.

light fog, *n* See film fault, fogged.

light leaks, *n.pl* See film fault, dark.

light, operating, *n* a light with a strong beam that may be directed for concentrated illumination of a part being operated on.

light pen, *n* a pointerlike device available with some computer terminals. A light pen selects data displayed on the screen by being pointed at any desired item.

light touch, *n* See touch, light.

lighting, *n* the arrangement of a light source to create a certain effect. The lighting of a dental operatory is done to achieve a sufficient level of lighting to reduce eye strain in shifting from one field of vision to another and to achieve a light intensity across the spectrum to mimic natural light.

lignin (lig′nin), *n* the heteropolysaccharides contained in the cell walls of plants that provides dietary fiber for digestion.

limbic system (lim′bik), *n* a group of structures within the rhinencephalon of the brain that are associated with various emotions and feelings, such as anger, fear, sexual arousal, pleasure, and sadness. Unless it is modulated by other cortical areas, periodic attacks of uncontrollable rage may occur in some individuals. The function of the system is poorly understood.

limit, *n* restriction.

limit, elastic (proportional limit), *n* the greatest stress to which a material may be subjected and still be capable of returning to its original dimensions when the forces are released.

limit, proportional, *n* See limit, elastic.

limitations, *n* the restrictive conditions stated in a dental benefits contract, such as age, length of time covered, and waiting periods, which affect an individual's or group's coverage. The contract may also exclude certain benefits or services, or it may limit the extent or condition under which certain services are provided. See also exclusions.

limited treatment, *n* treatment directed at a limited objective; not involving the entire dentition. It may be directed at the only existing problem, or at only one aspect of a larger problem in which a decision is made to defer more comprehensive therapy.

lincomycin (ling′kəmī′sin), *n brand names:* Lincocin, Lincorex; *drug class:* antibacterial; *action:* binds to 50S subunit of bacterial ribosomes; suppresses protein synthesis; *uses:* infections caused by group A β-hemolytic streptococci, pneumococci, staphylococci (respiratory tract, skin, soft tissue, urinary tract infections; osteomyelitis; septicemia), and anaerobes. Lincomycin should be reserved for pencillin-allergic patients. Close clinical supervision is required because severe colitis has been associated with lincomycin therapy.

lindane (lin′dān), *n* γ-benzene hexachloride prescribed in the treatment of pediculosis and scabies.

line, *n* a boundary; demarcation.

line angle, *n* See angle, line.

line, basophilic, *n* a group of microscopic sections of bone that stains darkly with hematoxylin. Represents periods of bone inactivity.

line, Camper's, *n.pr* the line running from the inferior border of the ala of the nose to the superior border of the tragus of the ear.

line, cement, *n* the line of cement exposed at the margin of an inlay or crown.

line, cementing, *n* a basophilic line distinguishing adjacent lamellae of bone; represents periods of inactivity of bone formation and resorption.

line, cervical, *n* See junction, cementoenamel.

line, cross arch fulcrum, *n* See line, fulcrum, cross arch.

line, external oblique, *n* a ridge of osseous structure on the body of the mandible extending from the anterolateral border to the mandibular ramus, passing downward and forward, after covering the buccocervical portion of the mandibular third molar, and ending by blending into the molar teeth.

line, finish, *n* in cavity preparations, a minimal line of demarcation of the wall of the preparation at the cavosurface angle; usually results from a slice made by an abrasive disk.

line focus, *n* a principle employed in the design of radiographic tubes, by which the effective focal spot is sharply reduced relative to the actual (larger) focal spot desirable to deal with the heat generated. It involves focusing the cathode stream, in the pattern of a thin rectangle, onto an anode truncated at about 20° to the transverse axis of the tube. See also spot, focal, effective.

line, fulcrum, *n* an imaginary line around which a removable partial denture tends to rotate.

line, fulcrum, anteroposterior, *n* an imaginary line of rotation extending through the rest and other support areas along the same side of a removable partial denture.

line, fulcrum, cross arch, *n* an imaginary line through the tooth-supported rest areas nearest to soft tissue-supported areas and around which the partial denture will tend to rotate when forces are applied to the soft tissue-supported areas.

line, lead, *n* a bluish-black patch on the gingival tissues, usually about 1 mm from the gingival crest. Caused by the deposition of fine granules of lead sulfide in the tissues. A sign of lead absorption in lead poisoning (plumbism).

line, median, *n* the intersection of the midsagittal plane with the maxillary and mandibular dental arches. The center line divides the central body surface into right and left.

line, mercurial, *n* a linear area of abnormal pigmentation of the gingival tissues associated with mercury poisoning. Seen along the gingival margin, it has been variously described as bluish, brownish, dirty reddish, or purplish in coloration.

line, neonatal, *n* the microscopic imbrication line on a primary tooth marking the point at which prenatal growth stops and postnatal growth begins. See line, Owen contour.

line of credit, *n* an arrangement whereby a financial institution (bank or insurance company) commits itself to lend up to a specified maximum amount of funds during a specified period. The interest rate on the loan may be specified or not. Sometimes a commitment fee is imposed for obtaining the line of credit.

line of draw, *n* the direction or plane of withdrawal or seating of a removable or cemented restoration.

line of force, *n* See force, line of.

line of occlusion, *n* the alignment of the occluding surfaces of the teeth in the horizontal plane. See also plane, occlusal line.

line of Retzius, *n.pr* one of several microscopic incremental lines appearing in the mature enamel.

line, Owen contour, *n.pr* one of a series of adjoining microscopic imbrication lines in dentin that demonstrates a disturbance in body metabolism. See line, neonatal.

line, petrous **(pet′rəs),** *n* the line traced around the hard, dense portion of temporal bone that forms a case protecting the inner ear.

line printer, *n* a fast printing device. A line printer prints on paper each line of characters in one operation, rather than character by character.

line, protrusive, *n* one of the three tracings made on each of the six projection planes of a jaw motion data recorder.

line, survey, n a line produced on the various portions of a dental cast by a surveyor, scriber, or marker. It designates the greatest height of contour in relation to the orientation of the cast to the vertical scriber.

line, vibrating, n the imaginary line across the posterior part of the palate marking the division between the movable and relatively immovable tissues of the palate.

linea alba (lin′ēə al′bə), *n* a normal variation in the buccal mucosa that appears as a white line beginning at the corners of the oral cavity and extending posteriorly at the level of the occlusal plane. It is composed of keratinized oral mucosa.

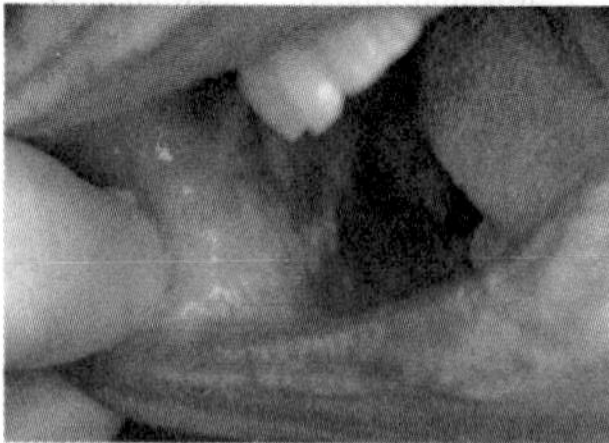

Linea alba. (Courtesy Dr. Charles Babbush)

linear energy transfer (LET), *n* the linear rate of loss of energy by an ionizing particle traversing a material medium.

linear models, *n.pl* statistical models in which the value of a parameter for a given value of a factor is assumed to be equal to $a + bx$, where a and b are constants. The models predict a linear regression.

linen strip, *n* See strip, abrasive.

liner, cavity, *n* See varnish, cavity.

liners, *n* the liquid material applied to teeth to protect them within a cavity preparation, to seal carious tissues, or to release beneficial chemicals such as fluoride.

lines, *n.pl* the elongated marks traced by a stylus on a gnathic projection plane, indicating direction of movement related variously to condyle movements.

lingual (ling′gwəl), *adj* pertaining to the tongue.

lingual appliances, n.pl orthodontic appliances that apply force from the lingual aspect of the anterior teeth. This mode of treatment is used to reduce the visibility of the appliance and thus improve the appearance of the smile during treatment.

lingual arch, n a space-holding arch or the basic arch for an active lingual orthodontic appliance. The arch usually spans around the inside of the dental arch from one first permanent molar to its antimere.

lingual bar, major connector, n See connector, major, lingual bar.

lingual button, n an attachment welded to the lingual side of the canine, premolar, or molar bands.

lingual cusps, n the bumps or projections on the tongue side of the chewing surface of teeth.

lingual foramen **(ling′gwəl fərā′mən),** *n* See foramen, lingual.

lingual fossa(e), n a depressed area that may appear on the lingual surface of selected anterior teeth.

lingual frenum, n a band of tissue that extends from the floor of the oral cavity to the inferior surface of the tongue.

lingual groove, n a furrow or channel that forms on the tongue side of selected anterior teeth.

lingual nerve, n See nerve, lingual.

lingual papillae, n the tiny, red protrusions covering the top surface of the tongue on which most of the taste buds can be found.

lingual peak, gingival, n a lingual peak that characterizes the normal interproximal tissue, which is composed of a lingual papilla and a buccal papilla connected interdentally in a triangular ridge depression termed a col.

lingual pit, n a pit that forms on the tongue side of the anterior teeth and certain maxillary posterior teeth.

lingual plate, n See connector, major, linguoplate.

lingual ridge, n a linear elevation that extends vertically from the chewing surface to the lingual developmental lobe on the tongue side of a canine tooth.

lingual tonsil, n See tonsil, lingual.

lingual veins, n the veins that run on the ventral surface of the tongue and terminate in the internal jugular vein.

lingula (ling′gūlə), *n* a small, tongue-like projection of bone forming the anterior border of the mandibular foramen.

linguoincisal edge (ling'gwōinsī'zəl), *n* the junction of the incisal or cutting edge of incisor teeth on the labial or lingual surface.

linguocclusion (linggwəkloo'zhən), *n* an occlusion in which the dental arch or group of teeth is lingual to normal.

linguoplate, *n* See connector, major, linguoplate.

linguoversion (ling'gwəver'zhən), *n* the state of being displaced toward the tongue.

lining mucosa, *n* See mucosa, lining.

linkage (ling'kəj), *n* the connection between two or more objects. In computer programming, coding that connects two separately coded routines.

linkage, cross, n See polymerization, cross.

linkage, sex, n the inheritance of certain characteristics that are determined by genes located in the sex chromosomes.

linoleic acid (lin'əlē'ik), *n* an unsaturated fatty acid essential to nutrition. Linoleic acid occurs in many plant glycerides.

liothyronine sodium (T_3) (lī'ōthī'rənēn'), *n brand names:* Cytomel, Triostat; *drug class:* thyroid hormone; *action:* increases metabolic rate with increase in cardiac output, O_2 consumption, body temperature, blood volume, growth/development at cellular level; *uses:* hypothyroidism, myxedema coma, thyroid hormone replacement, cretinism, nontoxic goiter.

liotrix (lī'ōtriks), *n brand names:* Euthroid, Thyrolar; *drug class:* thyroid hormone; *action:* increases metabolic rates, cardiac output, O_2 consumption, body temperature, blood volume, growth/development at cellular level; *uses:* hypothyroidism, thyroid hormone replacement.

lip, *n* **1.** either the upper or lower structure surrounding the opening of the oral cavity. **2.** a rimlike structure bordering a cavity or groove.

lip biting, n an oral habit in which either lip is placed between the teeth with more or less forcible application of the teeth to the lips.

lip, cleft, n See harelip.

lip, congenital cleft, n See harelip.

lip, double, n a redundant fold of tissue on the mucosal side of the upper lip that gives the appearance of a second lip and that may become accentuated by habitually being sucked between the teeth.

lip line, high, n the greatest height to which the lip is raised in normal function or during the act of smiling broadly.

lip line, low, n the lowest position of the lower lip during the act of smiling or voluntary retraction. The lowest position of the upper lip at rest.

lip pits (congenital lip fistulas), n.pl the congenital depressions, usually bilateral and symmetrically placed, on the vermilion portion of the lower lip. These pits may be circular or may be present as a transverse slit. The depression represents a blind fistula that penetrates downward into the lower lip to a depth of 0.5 to 2.5 cm. They often exude viscid saliva on pressure.

lip retractor, n a device to retract the lips when taking intraoral photographs.

lip, structures of, n.pl See vermilion border; vestibule, labial; frenum, labial.

lipase, *n* a fat-splitting or lipolytic enzyme.

lipid (lip'id), *n* a heterogeneous group of substances related actually or potentially to the fatty acids that are soluble in nonpolar solvents such as benzene, chloroform, and ether and are relatively insoluble in water. Included are the fatty acids, acylglycerols, phospholipids, cerebrosides, and steroids.

lipid, plasma, n the various plasma lipid classes include triacylglycerols, phospholipids, cholesterol, cholesterol esters, and unesterified fatty acids. Because of their hydrophobic nature, plasma lipids are carried in association with specific plasma proteins, the lipoproteins.

lipidosis (lip'idō'sis), *n* See disease, lipid storage.

Lipiodol (lipē'ōdəl), *n.pr* the brand name for an iodized oil used as an opaque contrast medium in radiography. When it is laced within periodontal pockets and radiographs are made, the depth and topography of

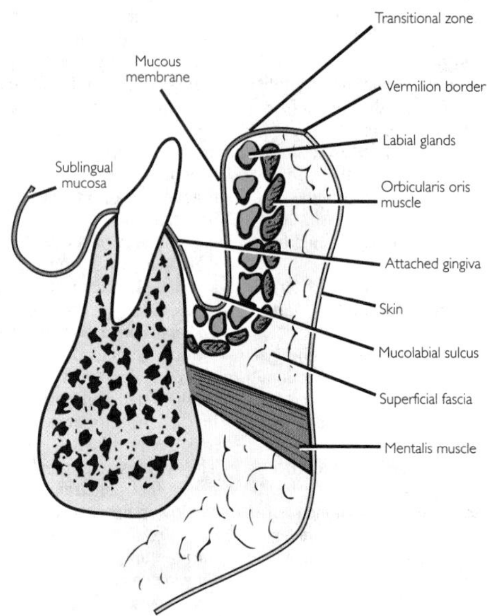

Lip structure. (Liebgott, 2001)

periodontal pockets may be ascertained.

lipodystrophy (lip′ōdis′trəfē), *n* an abnormality in the metabolism or deposition of fats.

lipogenesis (lip′ōjen′əsis), *n* the process that converts excess dietary carbohydrates into fat for storage as a source of long-term energy.

lipoids (lip′oidz), *n* a fatlike substance that may not actually be related to the fatty acids, although lipid and lipoid are occasionally used synonymously.

lipolysis (līpäl′əsis), *n* the process whereby fat stored in cells is broken down.

lipoma (lipō′mə), *n* a benign tumor characterized by fat cells.

lipophilic (lipōfil′ik), *adj* **1.** showing a marked attraction to, or solubility in, lipids. **2.** having an affinity for oil or fat.

lipopolysaccharides (lip′ōpol′ēsak′ərādz′), *n.pl* a compound or complex of lipid and carbohydrate.

lipoproteins (lip′ōprō′tēns), *n.pl* biochemical compounds that contain both lipid and protein. Most lipids in plasma are present in the form of lipoproteins. There are two main types: low density and high density.

lipoproteins, high-density (HDLs), *n.pl* the types containing approximately 50% protein that transport cholesterol to the liver for disposal. High HDL levels are associated with low body cholesterol and decreased risk of heart disease.

lipoproteins, low-density (LDLs), *n.pl* the types containing approximately 21% protein that deliver cholesterol from the liver to cells

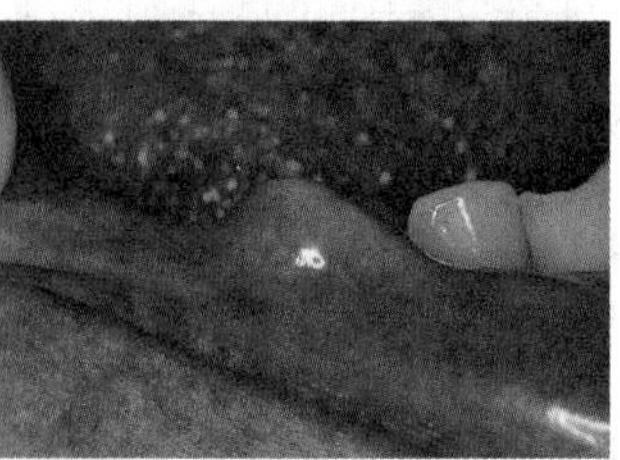

Lipoma of the lip. (Regezi/Sciubba/Pogrel, 2000)

throughout the body. High amounts of LDLs may raise cholesterol levels in the body and increase the risk of developing atherosclerosis.

liposomes (lip′əsōmz′), *n.pl* multi-layered spherical particles of a lipid in an aqueous medium within a cell.

lipoxygenase (lipok′səjənās′), *n* an enzyme that catalyzes the oxidation of unsaturated fatty acids with O_2 to form peroxides of the fatty acids.

lisinopril, *n brand name:* Zestril; *drug class:* angiotensin-converting enzyme (ACE) inhibitor; *action:* selectively suppresses renin-angiotensin-aldosterone system; inhibits ACE, which prevents conversion of angiotensin I to angiotensin II; *uses:* mild to moderate hypertension, post myocardial infarction if hemodynamically stable.

literature, *n* the entire body of writings on a given subject.

literature, dental, *n* the entire body of writing on dentistry. Most specifically, those writings published following a referee process to validate the scientific discipline in which the writings were produced.

lithium carbonate/lithium citrate, *n brand names:* Eskalith, Lithane, Lithobid, Lithotabs Cibalith-S; *drug class:* antimanic, inorganic salt; *action:* may alter sodium and potassium ion transport across cell membrane in nerve, muscle cells; may affect both norephinephrine and serotonin in CNS; *uses:* manic-depressive illness (manic phase), prevention of bipolar manic depressive psychosis.

litigation (lit′igā′shən), *n* the act or process of engaging in a lawsuit.

live birth, *n* the birth of an infant, irrespective of the duration of gestation, that exhibits any sign of life, such as respiration, heartbeat, umbilical pulsation, or movement of voluntary muscles. A live birth is not always a viable birth.

liver, *n* complex organ with many functions. Main functions include filtration of the blood, production of blood cells, and synthesis of blood-clotting components. It is divided into four lobes, with each containing thousands of lobules, and is served by two distinct blood supplies. The hepatic artery conveys oxygenated blood to the liver, and the hepatic portal vein conveys nutrient-filled blood from the stomach and the intestines.

liver cirrhosis **(sirō′sis),** *n* a degenerative disease of the liver in which hepatic tissue is replaced with connective tissue, commonly a result of chronic alcoholism. See jaundice.

liver failure, *n* a condition in which the liver fails to fulfill its function or is unable to meet the demand made on it. It may occur as a result of trauma, neoplastic invasion, prolonged biliary obstruction, viral infections (hepatitis C), or chronic alcoholism.

LJP, *n.pr* See localized juvenile periodontitis.

load, *n* an external force applied to an object.

load, occlusal, *n* the stresses generated by functional or habitual contacting of the occlusal surfaces of the upper and lower teeth. There are two components of such stress loads: the vertically directed components and those components that tend to move a tooth or denture laterally. See also force, occlusal.

loading, *n* the amount included in the premiums to meet liabilities beyond anticipated claims payments to provide administrative costs and contributions to reserve funds and to cover contingencies such as unexpected loss or adverse fluctuation.

lobbying, *n* the act of influencing, by argumentation, the course of action of a legislator.

lobectomy (lōbek′təmē), *n* the excision of a lobe of an organ, such as the submandibular gland or the lung.

Lobstein's disease (lōb′stīnz), *n.pr* See osteogenesis imperfecta.

local analgesia (an′əljē′zēə), *n* the loss of pain sensation over a specific area, caused by local administration of a drug that blocks nerve conduction.

localization, *n* a direct, exact site or restriction to a limited area, such as localization of abscess.

localization, radiographic, *n* determination, by means of radiographs, of the location of an object or structure in the body or head. Usually accomplished by obtaining radiographs made from different angulations to the part in question.

localization, tactile, *n* the property of localization associated with the sense of touch. Perception of the location of a stimulus is more precise in the regions of the lips and the fingertips than elsewhere. This more precise perception results from a greater density of special touch receptors in a given area.

localized juvenile periodontitis (LJP), *n* a type of aggressive periodontitis that presents as a localized periodontal tissue breakdown in prepubertal children in the primary or mixed dentition stage, apparently resulting from gingival pocket infection with *A. actinomycetemcomitans.* See also juvenile periodontitis.

location, practice, *n* place where equipment is set up to practice dentistry.

locking gate, *n* a portion of the peripheral frame of a maxillary subperiosteal implant; attached by a hinge. This device permits the implant to be placed into an area of undercut. After the implant is seated, the gate is closed and locked, and wire is wrapped around two locking buttons.

lockpin, *n* a soft metal pin used to attach an archwire to an orthodontic bracket.

locomotion, *n* the act or power to move from one place to another.

locomotor ataxia, *n* See tabes dorsalis.

locus, gene, *n* the position of a gene on the chromosome.

locus minoris resistentiae (lō′kus minôr′is rēsisten′chēā), *n* an area offering little resistance to invasion by microorganisms and/or their toxins. The junction between reduced enamel epithelium and oral epithelium within the epithelial wall of the gingival sulcus has been described as a weak link, providing a portal of entry for microorganisms and their toxins with initiation of pocket formation.

locus of control, *n* a psychologic concept that defines people as having either an internal or external locus of control, depending on whether they are more self-reliant and independent or more communally focused and dependent on others.

Lod score (lod), *n* the "Logarithm of the odds" score, which measures the likelihood of two genes being within measurable distance of each other.

lodoxamide tromethamine (lōdok′səmīd trōmeth′əmēn′), *n* *brand name:* Alomide; *drug class:* mast cell stabilizer; *action:* prevents release of mediators of inflammation from mast cells involved with Type 1 immediate hypersensitivity reactions; *uses:* vernal keratoconjunctivitis, vernal conjunctivits, keratitis.

logic, *n* a disciplined method of reasoning or argumentation that employs the principles governing correct or reliable inference.

logistic models, *n.pl* statistical models that describe the relationship between a qualitative dependent variable (that is, one that can take only certain discrete values, such as the presence or absence of a disease) and an independent variable. A common application is in epidemiology for estimating an individual's risk (probability of contracting a disease) as a function of a given risk factor.

logopedics (lôg′ōpē′diks), *n* the study and treatment of speech defects in children, involving habilitation or rehabilitation of speech.

lomefloxacin HCl (lō′meflok′səsin), *n* *brand name:* Maxaquin; *drug class:* fluoroquinolone antiinfective; *action:* a broad-spectrum bactericidal agent that inhibits the enzyme DNA gyrase needed for DNA synthesis; *uses:* lower respiratory tract infections (pneumonia, bronchitis); genitourinary infections (prostatitis); preoperatively to reduce UTIs in transurethral surgical procedures due to susceptible gram-negative organisms.

lomustine (lō′məstēn′), *n* *brand name:* CeeNU; *drug class:* antineoplastic alkylating agent; *action:* interferes with RNA and DNA strands, which leads to cell death; *uses:* Hodgkin disease; lymphomas; melanomas; multiple myeloma; brain, lung, bladder, kidney, colon cancer.

long face syndrome, *n* a malocclusion characterized by a long, narrow face; steep mandibular plane angle; and Class II Division 1 dental/skeletal relationship with anterior crowding and associated oral cavity breathing. The older term is *adenoid facies.*

long-term care (LTC), *n* the provision of medical, social, and personal care services on a recurring or continuing basis to persons with chronic physical or mental disorders.

longevity, *n* the length of life.

longitudinal studies, *n.pl* the epidemiologic studies that record data from a respresentative sample at repeated intervals over an extended span of time rather than at a single or limited number over a short period.

loop, vertical, *n* a U-shaped bend in the archwire that aids in the opening or closing of spaces in the arch.

loose premaxilla, *n* See premaxilla, loose.

loperamide HCl (lōper′əmīd′), *n brand names:* Diaraid, Imodium, Imodium AD, Kaopectate II, Maalox Antidiarrheal, Neo-Diaral, Pepto Diarrhea Control; *drug class:* antidiarrheal (opioid); *action:* direct action on intestinal muscles to decrease gastrointestinal peristalsis; *uses:* diarrhea (cause undetermined), chronic diarrhea, ileostomy discharge.

loracarbef (lor′əkär′bef), *n brand name:* Lorabid; *drug class:* antibiotic, 2nd-generation cephalosporin; *action:* inhibits bacterial cell wall synthesis, which renders cell wall osmotically unstable; *uses:* gram-negative *H. influenzae, E. coli, P. mirabilis, Klebsiella;* gram-positive *S. pneumoniae, S. pyogenes, S. aureus.*

loratadine (lərat′ədēn), *n brand name:* Claritin; *drug class:* antihistamine, H_1 histamine antagonist; *action:* acts on blood vessels, gastrointestinal system, respiratory system by competing with histamine for H_1-receptor site; decreases allergic response by blocking histamine; *uses:* seasonal rhinitis, allergy symptoms, idiopathic chronic urticaria.

lorazepam (lôraz′əpam), *n.pr brand name:* Ativan, Lorazepam Intensol; *drug class:* benzodiazepine antianxiety (Controlled Substance Schedule IV); *action:* depresses subcortical levels of the central nervous system, including limbic system and reticular formation; *uses:* anxiety, preoperative sedation, acute alcohol withdrawal symptoms, muscle spasm.

lordosis (lôrdō′sis), *n* an anteroposterior curvature of the spine with the convexity facing forward.

losartan potassium (lōsär′tan pətas′ēəm), *n brand name:* Cozaar; *drug class:* angiotensin II receptor antagonist; *action:* blocks the vasoconstrictor and aldosterone-secreting effects of angiotensin II; *use:* hypertension, as a single drug or in combination with other antihypertensives.

loss of attachment (LOA), *n* refers to the distance between the cementoenamel junction and the base of the sulcus. Typically measured with periodontal instruments. Includes both pocket depth and recession measurements, Also known as *attachment loss.*

loss of bone, *n* See resorption of bone.

loss ratio, *n* the relationship between the money paid out in benefits and the amount collected in premiums.

loupe, binocular (loop) (loop), *n* a magnifier that consists of lenses in an optical frame; it is worn like spectacles and is used with both eyes.

lovastatin (lō′vəstat′ən), *n brand name:* Mevacor; *drug class:* cholesterol-lowering agent; *action:* inhibits HMG-CoA reductase enzyme, which reduces cholesterol synthesis; *uses:* adjunct in primary hypercholesterolemia, mixed hyperlipidemia.

low lip line, *n* See lip line, low.

lower ridge slope, *n* See slope, lower ridge.

loxapine succinate/loxapine HCl (loksəpēn suk′sənāt′), *n brand name:* Loxitane; *drug class:* antipsychotic; *action:* depresses cerebral cortex, hypothalamus, limbic system, all of which control activity and aggression; blocks neurotransmission produced by dopamine at synapse; *uses:* psychotic disorders.

lozenge (läz′enj), *n* a medicated, disk-shaped tablet designed to dissolve slowly in the oral cavity.

lubrication, *n* **1.** the application of an agent, usually an oil or grease, to diminish friction. **2.** the natural secretions act as lubrication such as saliva in the oral cavity.

luciferase (loosif′ərās′), *n* an enzyme present in certain luminous organisms that act to bring about the

L

oxidation of luciferins; energy produced in the process is liberated as bioluminescence.

luciferin (loosif′ərin), *n* a chemical substance present in certain luminous organisms that, when acted upon by the enzyme luciferase, produces a glow called *bioluminescence.*

Ludwig's angina (lood′vigz), *n.pr* See angina, Ludwig's.

luetic (looet′ik), *adj* pertaining to or affected by syphilis.

lumbosacral region, *n* that area of the back that approximates level of the lumbar and sacral vertebrae. The lower third of the back.

lumen (loo′mən), *n* the space within a tube structure, such as a blood vessel, tube, or duct.

luminescence, *n* **1.** the emission of light by a material after excitation by some stimulus. **2.** the emission of light by intensifying screen phosphors after radiographic interaction.

lung, *n* the light, spongy organs in the thorax, constituting the main component of the respiratory system. They provide the tissue surface necessary for the exchange of gases between the environment and the blood. Oxygen is extracted from inspired air, and carbon dioxide is dispersed from the venous system back into the environment.

lung abscess, n a complication of an inflammation and infection of the lung, often caused by aspiration of infected material from the oral cavity.

lupus (loo′pus), *n* a disease of the skin and mucous membrane.

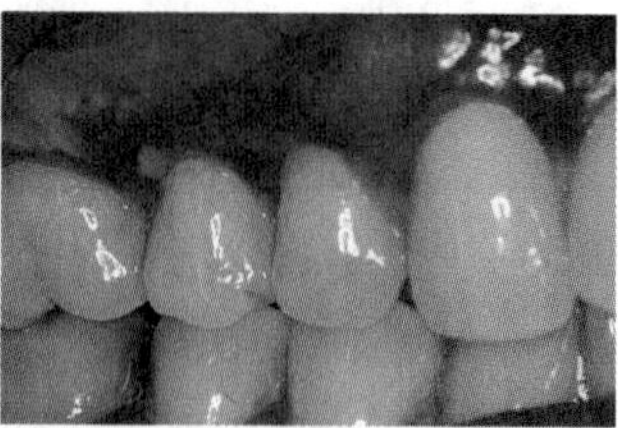

Lupus. (Newman/Takei/Klokkevold/Carranza, 2006)

lupus erythematosus (systemic lupus erythematosus, disseminated lupus erythematosus), n a chronic inflammatory disease of unknown etiology affecting skin, joints, kidneys, nervous system, serous membranes, and often other organs of the body. The classical facial "butterfly rash" facilitates diagnosis, although the rash need not be present. Other skin areas, particularly those exposed to the sun, may be involved by a scaly lesion that is referred to as *discoid lupus erythematosus.*

lupus erythematosus, discoid, n a form in which only cutaneous lesions are present. These commonly appear on the face as atrophic plaques with erythema, hyperheratosis, follicular plugging, and telangiectasia.

lupus vulgaris, n a cutaneous tuberculosis with characteristic nodular lesions on the face, particularly around the nose and ears.

luting agents (loo′ting), *n.pl* agents that bond, seal, or cement particles or objects together.

luxate (luk′sāt), *v* to be forced out of place or joint; to be displaced; to dislocate.

luxation (luk′sā′shən), *n* **1.** the act of luxating or state of being luxated, as in the dislocation or displacement of a tooth or of the temporomandibular joint. **2.** the dislocation or displacement of a tooth or of the temporomandibular articulation.

Lyme disease, *n.pr* an acute, recurrent inflammatory infection transmitted by a tick-borne spirochete, *B. burgdorferi.* Knees, other large joints, and temporomandibular joints are most commonly involved, with local inflammation and swelling. Chills, fever, headache, malaise, and erythema chronicum migrans (ECM), which is an expanding annular, erythematous skin eruption, often precede the joint manifestations.

lymph (limf), *n* a thin opalescent fluid originating in organs and tissues of the body that circulates through the lymphatic vessels and is filtered by the lymph nodes.

lymph node, n one of the many small oval structures that filter the lymph and fight infection, and in which are formed lymphocytes, monocytes, and plasma cells. See also each of the individual lymph nodes of the head and neck as they are listed.

lymph nodes, accessory, *n* the deep cervical lymph nodes situated near the accessory nerve.

lymph nodes, anterior jugular, *n* a type of superficial cervical lymph node located along the anterior jugular vein.

***lymph nodes, auricular* (ôrik′yələr),** *n* the superficial lymph nodes located surrounding the ear.

***lymph nodes, buccal* (buk′əl),** *n* the series of superficial lymph nodes in the face that lie above the buccinator muscle.

lymph nodes, deep cervical, *n* a group of lymph nodes situated around or near the internal jugular vein. Includes two groups, superior and inferior, based on the point where the omohyoid muscle crosses the vein.

***lymph nodes, deep parotid* (pərot′id),** *n* the lymph nodes located deep to the parotid salivary gland.

lymph nodes, external jugular, *n* a type of superficial cervical lymph node located along the external jugular vein.

lymph nodes, facial, *n* the superficial lymph nodes of the face, including the malar, nasolabial, buccal, and mandibular nodes.

***lymph nodes, jugulodigastric* (jug′yəlōdī′gas′trik),** *n* a type of the superior deep cervical lymph node located behind the mandible, inferior to the posterior belly of the digastric muscle. These nodes drain the tonsils and the posterior part of the tongue.

***lymph nodes, juguloomohyoid* (jug′yəlōō′mōhī′oid),** *n* a type of inferior deep cervical lymph node located in the angle between the internal jugular vein and the omohyoid muscle; these nodes drain the tongue.

lymph nodes, occipital, *n* the superficial nodes located on the posterior base of the head.

lymph nodes, superficial parotid, *n* the lymph nodes located just superficial to the parotid salivary gland.

lymphadenitis (limfad′ənī′tis), *n* **1.** an inflammation of a lymph node or nodes. **2.** an inflammation of the lymph glands, characterized mainly by swelling, pain, and redness.

lymphadenopathy (limfad′ənop′əthē), *n* a disease process that involves a lymph node or nodes.

lymphadenopathy, generalized, *n* the involvement of all or several regionally separated groups of lymph nodes by a systemic disorder.

lymphadenopathy, persistent generalized (PGL), *n* a swelling of the lymph nodes that is associated with HIV infection and AIDS. See acquired immunodeficiency syndrome (AIDS).

lymphadenopathy, regional, *n* the involvement of nodes draining a specific region (e.g., submental nodes draining the middle of the lower lip, floor of the oral cavity, skin of the chin).

lymphangioma (limfanjēō′mə), *n* a benign neoplasm of the lymph vessels characterized by lymph vessel proliferation.

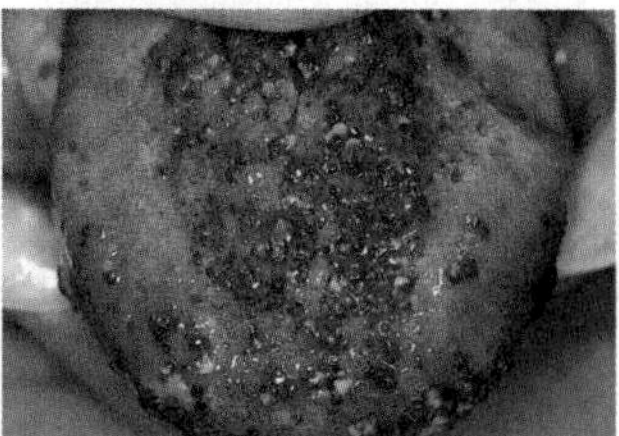

Lymphangioma. (Regezi/Sciubba/Pogrel, 2000)

lymphangioma, cystic, *n* See hygroma, cystic.

lymphatic system (limfat′ik), *n* a complex network of capillaries, thin vessels, valves, ducts, nodes, and organs that helps to protect and maintain the internal fluid environment of the entire body by producing, filtering, and conveying lymph and by producing various blood cells. See also vessels, afferent and vessels, efferent.

lymphatic vessels, *n.pl* See lymphatic system. See also vessels, afferent and vessels, efferent.

lymphocyte(s) (lim′fōsīt), *n* a form of white blood cell originating in lymphoid tissues; possesses a single spherical nucleus and a nongranular cytoplasm. It constitutes 25% of the white blood cells. Some, along with plasma cells and histiocytes, are found in clinically normal gingivae. Their numbers within the gingival connective tissue are increased in periodontal disease. With progress of gingival inflammation to the underlying bone, they are also found within the marrow spaces of the supporting bone.

lymphocytes-B, *n* short-lived, non–thymus-dependent lymphocytes that synthesize antibodies for insertion into their own cytoplasmic membranes. They are the precursor of the plasma cells.

lymphocytes, in pulp tissue, *n.pl* a subset of white blood cells that, when present, are located near the odontoblastic layer. An increase in lymphocyte count is indicative of inflammation.

lymphocytes-T, *n* long-lived lymphocytes that have circulated through the thymus gland and have differentiated to become thymocytes. When exposed to an antigen, they divide rapidly and produce large numbers of new T cells sensitized to that antigen. Some T cells are often called *killer cells,* because they secrete immunologically essential chemical compounds and assist B cells in destroying foreign protein. T cells also appear to play a significant role in the body's resistance to the proliferation of cancer cells.

lymphocytopenia (lim′fōsī′tōpē′nēə), *n* a decrease in the normal number of lymphocytes in the circulating blood. Various limits are given (e.g., a total number less than 600/mm^3). It may be associated with agranulocytosis, hyperadrenocorticism, leukemia, advanced Hodgkin disease, irradiation, and acute infections with neutrophilia.

lymphocytosis (lim′fōsītō′sis), *n* an absolute or relative increase in the normal number of lymphocytes in the circulating blood. Various limits are given; e.g., absolute form is said to be present if the total number of cells exceeds 4500/mm^3, whereas relative form is said to be present if the percentage of lymphocytes is greater than 45% and the total number of cells is less than 4500/mm^3. It may be associated with infancy, exophthalmic goiter, mumps, rubella, infectious mononucleosis, sunburn, lymphatic leukemia, pertussis, and pyogenic infections in childhood.

lymphoepithelial lesion, benign (lim′fōep′ithē′lēəl), *n* See disease, Mikulicz's.

lymphoepithelioma (lim′fōep′ithē′lēō′mə), *n* a malignant neoplasm arising from the epithelium and lymphoid tissue of the nasopharynx and characterized by cells of both tissues; may occur in the palate.

lymphokines (lim′fəkīnz′), *n.pl* the soluble substances, released by sensitized lymphocytes on contact with specific antigens, that help effect cellular immunity by stimulating activity of monocytes and macrophages. See also cytokine.

lymphoma (limfō′mə), *n* a neoplasm made up of lymphoid tissue.

lymphoma, B-cell, *n* a group of heterogenous lymphoid tumors generally expressing one or more B-cell antigens or representing malignant transformations of B lymphocytes.

lymphoma, Burkitt, *n* a type of B-cell lymphoma suspected to be related to infection by the Epstein-Barr virus (EBV). The classical (African) variation usually affects the bowels, whereas the endemic variation affects the jaws.

lymphoma, Hodgkin, *n* a group of malignant B-cell lymphomas suspected of being related to the Epstein-Barr virus. Characterized by the presence of Reed-Sternberg cells.

lymphoma, MALT, *n* a type of lymphoid tumor that can occur in any mucous tissue and in salivary glands. These tumors arise from benign lymphoepithelial lesions.

lymphoma, non-Hodgkin, *n* a group of malignant tumors of a lymphoid tissue that differ from Hodgkin disease, being more heterogeneous with respect to malignant cell lineage, clinical course, prognosis, and therapy. The only feature shared by these tumors is the absence of Reed-Sternberg cells, which are characteristic of Hodgkin disease.

lymphoma, T-cell, *n* an adult T-cell leukemia; an acute or chronic disease associated with a human T-cell virus, with lymphadenopathy, hepatosplenomegaly, skin lesions, peripheral blood involvement, and hypercalcemia.

L

lymphoreticulosis, benign inoculation (lim′fōretik′ūlō′sis), *n* See fever, cat-scratch.

lymphosarcoma (lim′fōsärkō′mə), *n* a malignant disease of the lymphoid tissues characterized by proliferation of atypical lymphocytes and their localization in various parts of the body. The jaws may be the sites of lymphosarcomas.

lypressin (līpres′in), *n brand name:* Diapid; *drug class:* pituitary hormone; *action:* promotes reabsorption of water by action on collecting ducts in kidney; decreases urine excretion; *uses:* nonnephrogenic diabetes insipidus.

lysin (lī′sin), *n* See plasmin.

lysine (lī′sēn), *n* one of the essential amino acids found in many proteins; needed for proper growth in infants and for maintenance of nitrogen balance in adults. See also amino acids.

lysis (lī′sis), *n* the gradual abatement of the symptoms of a disease. The disintegration or dissolution of cells by a lysin.

lysosomes (līsəsōmz), *n* the self-contained organelles found inside most cells, which contain hydrolytic enzymes that aid in intracellular digestion. If these enzymes are released into the cytoplasm, they cause the cell to self-digest.

lysozyme (lī′sōzīm), *n* an enzyme in major salivary secretions that may rupture bacterial cell walls and regulate the oral flora.

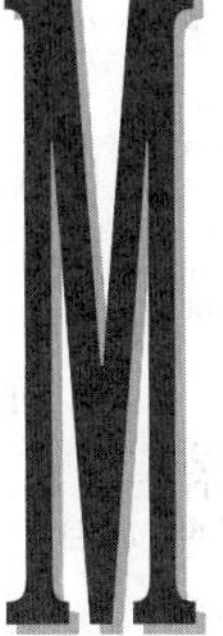

mA, *n* the abbreviation for milliampere.

macro, *pref* a prefix meaning excessively large or big.

macroalbuminuria (mak′rōalbū′mənur′ēə), *n* a type of albuminaria that is characterized by especially high levels of albumin in the urine (more than 300 mg in 1 day). This condition can be a symptom of many kidney diseases and disorders because its presence indicates that the kidney is leaking albumin (a protein found in blood). Also known as *proteinuria.*

macrocheilia (mak′rōkī′lēə), *n* an abnormally large lip.

macrocyte, *n* a red blood cell that is unusually large; usually seen in megaloblastic anemias (e.g., B_{12} deficiency).

macrodontia (makrōdon′shēə), *n* abnormally large teeth. It may be partial or complete.

macroglossia (mak′rōglôs′ēə), *n* an enlarged tongue resulting from muscle hypertrophy, vascular or neurogenic tumor, or endocrine disturbance.

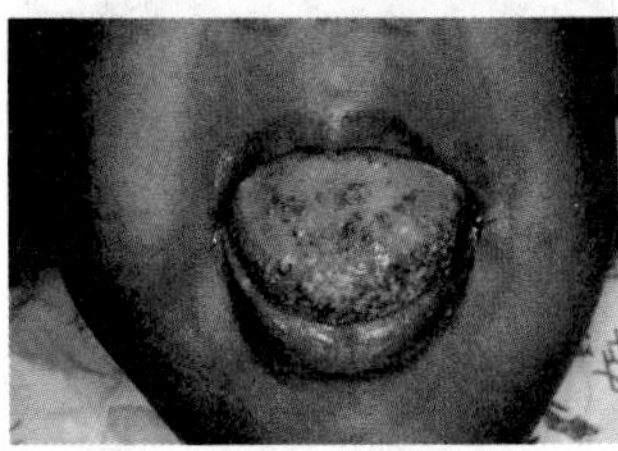

Macroglossia. (Sapp/Eversole/Wysocki, 2004)

macroglossia, amyloid, *n* See tongue, amyloid.

macrognathia (mak′rōnā′thēə), *n* a definite overgrowth of the maxillae and mandible.

macrolides (mak′rōlīdz), *n* a class of antibiotics discovered in *Streptomyces,* characterized by molecules made up of large-ring lactones. An example is erythromycin.

macromolecule, *n* a substance with molecules of colloidal size, notably proteins, nucleic acids, and polysaccharides.

macrophage (mak′rəfāj), *n* any phagocytic cell of the reticuloendothelial system including specialized Kupffer's cells in the liver and spleen, and histiocytes in loose connective tissue. See also histiocyte and monocyte.

macrophage, alveolar, *n* a dust cell, coniophage, a vigorously phagocytic macrophage on the epithelial surface of lung alveoli where it ingests inhaled particulate matter.

macroscopic (mak′rōskop′ik), *adj* relating to macroscopy, or the examination of areas such as surfaces of teeth without magnification.

macrosomia, *n* See giantism.

macrostomia (mak′rōstō′mēə), *n* an abnormally large opening of the oral cavity.

macule (mak′ūl), *n* a lesion that is not elevated above the surface.

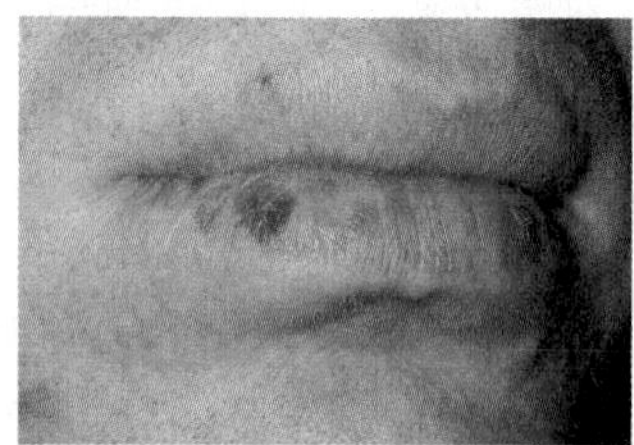

Oral melanotic macule. (Regezi/Sciubba/Jordan, 2008)

magaldrate (mag′əldrāt′), *n* (aluminum magnesium complex), *brand names:* Lowsium, Riopan, Riopan Plus; *drug class:* antacid/aluminum/magnesium hydroxide; *action:* neutralizes gastric acidity; *use:* antacid for hyperacidity.

magnesium (Mg), *n* an elemental metal with an atomic weight of 24.32. Magnesium is an essential nutritional substance. Deficiency produces irritability of the nervous system and trophic disturbances.

magnesium sulfate, *n* a salt of magnesium; also called Epsom salts, used as a therapeutic bath and as a purgative.

magnetic fields, *n.pl* the spaces in which magnetic forces are detectable; created by magnetostrictive ultrasonic scalers to cause the tips of instruments such as ultrasonic scalers to vibrate.

magnetic resonance imaging (MRI), *n* also known as nuclear magnetic resonance imaging. It is a diagnostic technique in which the phosphorus in cellular tissues is excited by magnetic force. The distribution and alignment of these cellular elements can be captured on phosphorus nuclear magnetic resonance instruments forming a high-resolution tissue image. A higher degree of resolution of soft tissues is possible using this technique than from radiographic techniques.

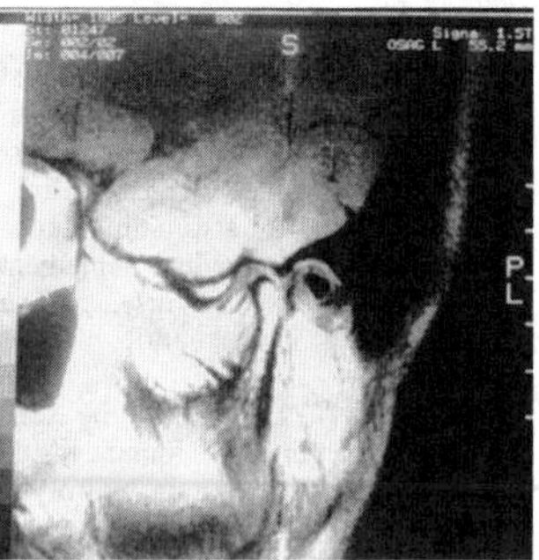

A magnetic resonance image. (Rosenstiel/Land/Fujimoto, 2006, courtesy Dr. J. Petrie)

magnetostrictive instruments (magne″tostrik′tiv), *n.pl* See ultrasonic scalers, magnetostrictive.

mainstream smoke, *n* a vaporous byproduct of burning tobacco products that is purposely taken into the lungs through the oral cavity.

maintenance, *n* to keep in a functional state or in the proper location.

maintenance, space, *n* See space maintainer.

maintenance phase, *n* the period following treatment for a specific condition during which the patient may undergo occasional examinations and treatments in order to regain optimal dental health.

major connector, *n* See connector, major.

major histocompatibility complex (his′tōkəmpat′əbil′itē), *n* the genetic region that contains the loci of genes that determine the structure of the serologically defined (SD) and lymphocyte-defined (LD) transplantation antigens, genes that control the structure of the immune response-associated (Ia) antigens, and the immune response (Ir) genes that control the ability of an animal to respond immunologically to antigenic stimuli.

making the turn, *n* the step in the procedure of inserting and condensing foil in a Class 3 cavity preparation, at which the line of force is changed from an incisogingival direction to a gingivoincisal direction.

mal-, *pref* a prefix denoting a bad or unfavorable condition.

malaise (məlāz'), *n* a general feeling of discomfort or uneasiness, often the first indication of an infection or other disease.

malar (mā'lur), *adj* pertaining to the cheek or the zygomatic bone.

malar bone, *n* See bone, malar.

malaria (məler'ēə), *n* a serious infectious illness caused by one or more of at least four species of the protozoan genus *Plasmodium,* characterized by chills, fever, anemia, an enlarged spleen, and a tendency to recur. The disease is transmitted from human to human by a bite from an infected *Anopheles* mosquito.

Malassez, epithelial rests of (mal'əsā'), *n.pr* See epithelial rests of Malassez.

maldevelopment, *n* an abnormal, imperfect, or deficient formation or development.

malfeasance (malfē'zəns), *n* an act that one should not do at all or the unjust performance of some act that one has no right to do.

malfunction, *n* a disorder in function or performance, which may or may not be related to a malformation of tissues, organs, or organ systems. See also dysfunction.

malice (mal'is), *n* a state of mind that disregards the law and legal rights of others but that does not necessarily involve personal hate or ill will.

malice, in the law of libel and slander, *n* an evil intent arising from spite or ill will; willful and wanton disregard of the rights of the person defamed.

malignant (məlig'nənt), *adj* **1.** resistant to treatment. **2.** able to metastasize and kill the host. **3.** describing a cancer.

malignant hypertension, *n* the most lethal form of high blood pressure. It is a fulminating condition, characterized by severely elevated blood pressure that commonly damages the intima of small vessels, the brain, retina, heart, and kidneys. It affects more persons with racial diversity and may be caused by a variety of factors such as stress, genetic predisposition, obesity, the use of tobacco, the use of oral contraceptives, high intake of sodium chloride, a sedentary lifestyle, and aging.

malignant hyperthermia, *n* an autosomal dominant trait characterized by often fatal hyperthermia with rigidity of muscles occurring in affected people exposed to certain anesthetic agents, particularly halothane and succinylcholine.

malingering, *n* the feigning of illness.

malleability (mal'ēəbil'itē), *n* the ability of a material to withstand permanent deformation under compressive forces without rupture.

mallet, *n* a hammering instrument.

mallet, hard, *n* a small hammer with a leather-, rubber-, fiber-, or metal-faced head; used to supply force or to supplement hand force for the compaction of foil or amalgam and to seat cast restorations.

malnutrition, *n* a disorder concerning nutrition. It may result from a poor diet or from impaired utilization of foods ingested.

malocclusion (mal'ōkloo'zhən), *n* (relationship of teeth in occlusion), a deviation in intramaxillary and/or intermaxillary relations of teeth that presents a hazard to the individual's oral health. Often associated with other orofacial deformities. Initial classification of cases is usually done by Angle's classification system. See also Angle's classification.

malocclusion, deflective, *n* a type of malocclusion occurring in persons who cannot close all their teeth while holding their condyles in the most posterior position. Instead, in closure they first contact one or two pairs of poorly coupled teeth. To gain occlusal contacts of the other teeth, they must move the jaw anteriorly, laterally, or anterolaterally, as the deflectors demand in their guidance.

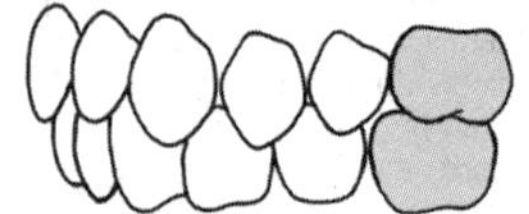

Normal occlusion

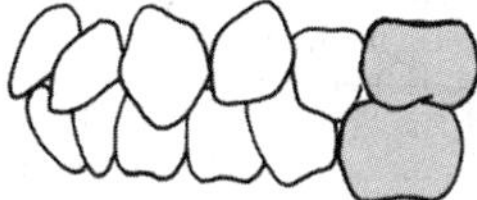

Class I malocclusion

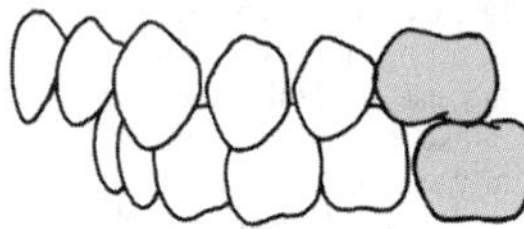

Class II malocclusion

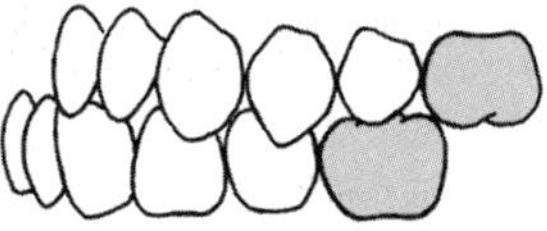

Class III malocclusion

Malocclusion classes as specified by Angle. (Proffit/Fields/Sarver, 2007)

malposed (malpōzd), *adj* in an abnormal position.

malposition, *n* a faulty or abnormal position of a part of the body.

malposition of jaw, *n* an abnormal position of the mandible.

malposition of teeth, *n* an improper position of teeth in relationship to the basal bone of the alveolar process, to adjacent teeth, or to opposing teeth.

M

malpractice, *n* in medicine and dentistry, a professional person's act or failure to act that was the proximate cause of an injury to a patient and that was below the standard of care required.

malrelation, *n* (of tooth, teeth, jaws, or facial structures), malalignment, malocclusion, and malposition are interrelated, so that one term frequently implies concurrent malrelationships of related teeth or structures.

maltose (môl'tōs), *n* malt sugar, a disaccharide formed in the hydrolysis of starch and consisting of two glucose residues bound by an α(1,4)-glycoside link.

mamelons (mam'ələns), *n* the three protrusions on the incisal edge of an incisor that has just erupted.

mammotropin (mam'ōtrō'pin), *n* See hormone, lactogenic.

manage, *v* to control and direct; to administer.

managed care, *n* **1.** a cost containment system that directs the utilization of health benefits by (a) restricting the type, level, and frequency of treatment; (b) limiting the access to care; and (c) controlling the level of reimbursement for services. *n* **2.** a health care system in which there is administrative control over primary health care services in a medical group practice. Patients may pay a flat fee for basic family care but may be charged additional fees for secondary care services of specialists.

management, *n* the planning, organizing, directing, and controlling of the enterprise's operation so that objectives can be achieved economically and efficiently through others.

management information system (MIS), *n* the specific type of data processing system that is designed to furnish management with information that may be of assistance in making decisions.

mandible, *n* the lower jawbone.

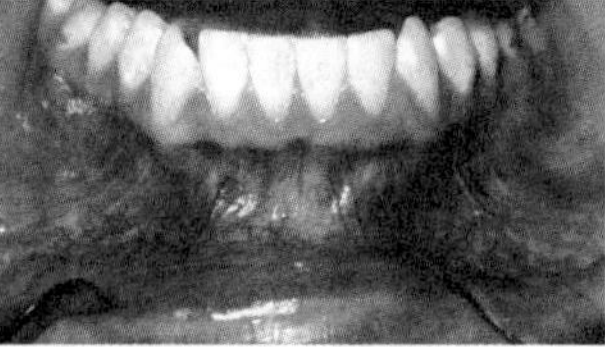

The mandible. (Liebgott, 2001)

mandible, inferior, *n* the border of the lower edge of the mandible. Begins anterior to the insertion of the masseter muscle at the inferior surface of the angles of the mandible and is continuous anteriorly with the incisor region.

mandible, movements of, *n.pl* See movement, mandibular.

mandible, posture of, *n* the physiologic rest position, or the rest vertical relation of the mandible.

mandibular (mandib′yələr), *adj* pertaining to the lower jaw.

mandibular angle, *n* See angle of the mandible.

mandibular axis, *n* See axis, mandibular.

mandibular border, *n* See border, mandibular.

mandibular canal, *n* See canal, mandibular.

mandibular centric relation, *n* the closing relation of the mandible with the fixed craniofacial complex as determined clinically by instruments that record jaw motion.

mandibular condyle, *n* See condyle, mandibular.

mandibular flexure, *n* See flexure, mandibular.

mandibular foramen, *n* See foramen, mandibular.

mandibular fracture, *n* a break in the continuity of the bone of the mandible. See also fracture.

mandibular glide, *n* See glide, mandibular.

mandibular guide prosthesis, *n* a prosthesis with an extension designed to direct a resected mandible into a functional relation with the maxillae.

mandibular hinge position, *n* See position, hinge, mandibular.

***mandibular labial frenum* (mandib′yələr lā′bēəl frē′nəm),** *n* a vertical band of oral mucosa located between the midlines of the mandibular central incisors, which connects the attached gingiva to the lower lip and safeguards against any excessive motions.

mandibular movement, *n* See movement, mandibular.

mandibular nerve, *n* See nerve, mandibular.

mandibular notch, *n* See notch, mandibular.

mandibular pain-dysfunction syndrome, *n* See temporomandibular joint pain-dysfunction syndrome.

***mandibular prognathism* (mandib′yələr prog′nəthiz′əm),** *n* a condition in which the mandible projects outward farther than the maxilla.

mandibular rest position, *n* See position, rest, mandibular.

mandibular retraction, *n* See retraction, mandibular.

mandibulofacial dysostosis (mandib′ūlōfā′shəl), *n* See syndrome, Treacher Collins.

mandrel (man′drəl), *n* a shaft that supports or holds any object to be rotated. An instrument, held in a handpiece, that holds a disk, stone, or cup used for grinding, smoothing, or polishing.

manganese (Mn) (mang′gənēz′), *n* a common metallic element found in trace amounts in tissues of the body, where it aids in the function of various enzymes. Its atomic number is 25 and its atomic weight is 54.9380.

mania, *n* the episode of intense euphoria found in people with bipolar disorder. Manic episodes may include rapid thought and speech, insomnia, setting unrealistic goals, or engaging in risky behaviors.

manifest anxiety scale, *n* a true-false questionnaire made up of items believed to indicate anxiety, in which the subject answers verbally the statement that describes him or her.

manifestation (man′ifestā′shən), *n* an obvious indication or specific evidence that a disease is present; a symptom.

manikin (man′ikin), *n* a replica of the complete body or its individual parts that is used for instructional purposes. Used interchangeably with mannequin. See typodont.

Mann-Whitney U test, *n.pr* See test, Mann-Whitney U.

mannitol (man′itol′), *n* a poorly metabolized sugar used as an osmotic diuretic and in kidney function tests.

mannose (man′ōs), *n* an aldohexose obtained from various plant sources.

manometer (mənom′itər), *n* a device for measuring the pressure of a fluid, consisting of a tube marked with a scale and containing a relatively incompressible fluid, such as mercury. The level of the fluid in the tube varies directly with the pressure of the fluid being measured. They are used to measure blood pressure.

manpower, *n* the number of persons required or needed to complete a task.

M

manual, *n* **1.** a book of instructions on performance of a task or the care of equipment. *adj* **2.** performed by the hand; used in the hand.

manual film processing, *n* See film processing.

manual scaling, *n* a procedure for removing bacterial plaque and calculus that utilizes a hand tool rather than a power-driven instrument.

map, *n* a drawing or diagram, to scale, of a surface object.

maprotiline HCl (məprō′təlēn′), *n* *brand name:* Ludiomil; *drug class:* tetracyclic antidepressant; *action:* blocks reuptake of norepinephrine and serotonin into nerve endings; *uses:* depression, depression with anxiety.

marasmus (məraz′mus), *n* a wasting disorder of malnutrition and partial starvation which occurs in infants and young children as a result of severe protein deficiency and insufficient caloric intake. See also kwashiorkor.

Marcaine, *n* a trade name for bupivacaine, a long-acting local anesthetic agent.

Marfan syndrome, *n.pr* a hereditary disorder of connective tissue characterized by tall stature, elongated extremities, subluxation of the lens, dilation of the ascending aorta, and "pigeon breast." It is inherited as an autosomal dominant trait.

margin, *n* **1.** the extreme edge of something. *n* **2.** the boundary of a surface. *n* **3.** in a cavity preparation for a restoration, the margin is the outside limit of the surgical preparation. See also cavosurface angle.

margin, bone, *n* the peripheral edge of a bone.

margin, cavosurface **(kā′vōsur′fəs),** *n* the point of contact between a tooth surface and the face of an associated cavity.

margin, enamel, *n* the part of the margin of a preparation that is laid in enamel.

margin, free gingival, *n* See margin, gingival.

margin, gingival, *n* **1.** the cavosurface angle of the wall of a cavity preparation closest to the apex of the root. *n* **2.** the crest or tip of the gingival tissues that forms the wall of the gingival sulcus. Also called *free gingival margin* or *gingival crest.*

margin of safety, *n* the margin between lethal and toxic doses.

margin, thickened bone, *n* See bone, thickened margin of.

marginal ridge, *n* See ridge, marginal.

margination (mär′jənā′shən), *n* the adhesion of leukocytes to the inner surface of blood vessel walls in the early stages of inflammation.

Marie's disease, *n.pr* See acromegaly.

marijuana, abuse of (mer′əwä′nə), *n* regular use of marijuana (e.g., Mary Jane, weed, pot, hemp, or grass), an example of a cannabinoid, for reasons other than recognized medical applications; may cause pupils to dilate and eyes to appear bloodshot, red, and inflamed as a result.

marital status, *n* the legal standing of a person in regard to his or her marriage state.

marketing, *n* the set of activities directed at facilitating and consummating exchanges. The following three elements must be present to define a marketing situation: two or more parties who are potentially interested in exchange; each party possessing things of value to others; and each party capable of communication and delivery.

marking medium, *n* See medium, marking.

marsupialization (märsoo′pēəlizā′shən), *n* the surgical formation of a pouch to treat a cyst when simple removal would not be effective. Under anesthesia, the cyst sac is opened and emptied. Its edges are sutured to adjacent tissues, and a drain is left in place. Over a period of several months, secretions will decrease and the sac space will be reduced until it is completely filled. See also operation, Partsch's.

MAS (MaS, mas, milliampere-second), *n* the product of the milliamperes and the exposure time in seconds (e.g., 10 ma × ½ sec = 5 MAS).

mask, *n* **1.** something that conceals from view. *n* **2.** a protective covering, especially for the face. *v* **3.** to cover up.

mask, nonbreather, *n* a plastic mask

worn over the oral cavity and nose in order to deliver additional oxygen to a patient who is able to breathe on his or her own. See also mask, oxygen.

mask, oxygen, *n* a device used during the delivery of oxygen that fits securely over the nose and oral cavity so that oxygen may be inhaled and carbon dioxide exhaled.

mask, rubber dam, *n* See pad, rubber dam.

mask, Wanscher's, *n* a mask for ether anesthesia.

mask, Yankauer's, *n* an open type of mask for administering ether.

masking, *n* an opaque covering used to camouflage the metal or other parts of a prosthesis.

Maslow's hierarchy of human needs, *n.pr* a term from sociology or social anthropology denoting the hierarchic hypothesis of Abraham Maslow of the basic needs of man. The first need is for air, food, and water; the second for safety, including protection and freedom from fear and anxiety. These are followed in order by the need to love and to be loved; the need for self-esteem; and ultimately, the need for self-actualization. The Maslow hypothesis states that the high needs, which are those at the end of the hierarchy, cannot be fully satisfied until the lower needs are met.

masoprocol (məsō′prəkol), *n brand name:* Actinex; *drug class:* antineoplastic (topical); *action:* inhibits lipoxygenase; *use:* actinic keratosis.

mass number (A), *n* the number of nucleons (protons and neutrons) in the nucleus of an atom.

mass screening, *n* the examination of large samples or populations to determine the presence or absence of some trait, condition, or behavior.

mass storage, *n* a storage medium in which data may be organized and maintained both sequentially and nonsequentially. Usually used for storage of files.

massage (məsäzh′), *n/v* the manipulation of tissues for remedial or hygiene purposes (as by rubbing, stroking, kneading, or tapping) with the hand or other instrument or device.

massage, cardiac, *n* a systematic, rhythmic application of pressure to the heart to cause significant blood flow in the treatment of a cardiac arrest; may be an open- or closed-chest procedure.

massage, gingival, *n* the massage of the gingival tissues.

mast cell, *n* a connective tissue cell whose specific physiologic function remains unknown; capable of elaborating basophilic, metachromatic, cytoplasmic granules that contain histamine.

mastalgia (mastal′jēə), *n* a pain, tenderness, or pressure in the breast. It is one of several physical symptoms of premenstrual syndrome.

master file, *n* a file of semipermanent information that is usually updated periodically.

masticate (mas′tikāt′), *v* **1.** to grind or crush food with the teeth to prepare it for swallowing and digestion. *v* **2.** to chew.

masticating apparatus, *n* See apparatus, masticating.

masticating cycle, *n* See cycle, masticating.

mastication (mas′tikā′shən), *n* **1.** the process of chewing food in preparation for swallowing and digestion. *n* **2.** the act of chewing accomplished by the coordinated activity of the tongue, mandible, mandibular musculature, and structural components of the temporomandibular joints, and controlled by the neuromuscular mechanism. See also chewing.

mastication, components of, *n.pl* the various jaw movements made during the act of mastication as determined by the neuromuscular system, temporomandibular articulations, teeth, and food being chewed. For purposes of analysis or description, the components of mastication may be categorized as opening, closing, left lateral, right lateral, or anteroposterior jaw movements.

mastication, forces of, *n.pl* See force, masticatory.

mastication, insufficiency of, *n* an inefficiency or inadequacy of the chewing act.

mastication, organ of, *n* See system, stomatognathic.

mastication, physiology of, *n* the movements of the mandible during the chewing cycle, which are controlled by neuromuscular action and are correlated with the structural attributes of the temporomandibular joints and the proprioceptive sense of the periodontal ligament. There are three phases in the physiology of mastication: the incision of food, the mastication of the bolus, and the act of swallowing. Accessory activity by the tongue and facial musculature facilitates the masticatory actions.

mastication, saliva in, *n* an increase in salivation, which serves to wet and lubricate the food to facilitate deglutition.

mastication, tongue in, *n* the muscular organ in the floor of the oral cavity whose function in the masticatory process consists of crushing some food by pressing it against the hard palate, forming it into a compact bolus, and assisting in placing it on the occlusal platform for tooth action.

masticatory force (mas′tikətôrē), *n* See force, masticatory.

masticatory movements, *n.pl* See movements, mandibular, masticatory.

masticatory muscles, *n.pl* See muscles, masticatory.

***Mastigophora* (mas′tigof′ôrə),** *n* a subphylum of sarcomastigophora consisting of parasitic protozoa, also called flagellates. Causes diseases such as enteritis, urethritis, vaginitis, and Chagas' disease by drinking contaminated water, contact with vaginal discharge, and through bug bite.

mastoid (mas′toid), *n* **1.** the protuberance of the temporal bone located directly behind the external ear that contains the air cells and on which the cervical muscles attach. *adj* **2.** breast-shaped.

mastoidale (mastoidālē), *n* the lowest point on the contour of the mastoid process.

materia alba (mətir′ēə al′bə), *n* a soft white deposit around the necks of the teeth, usually associated with poor oral hygiene; composed of food debris, dead tissue elements, and purulent matter; serves as a medium for bacterial growth.

materia medica, *n* the study of drugs and other substances used in medicine, their origins, preparation, uses, and effects.

material(s), *n* substance(s).

material, duplicating, *n.pl* the materials used to copy casts and models; usually hydrocolloids.

material, silicone rubber impression, *n* a dimethyl polysiloxane material whose polymerization is affected by an organ-metal compound and some type of alkyl silicate.

material testing, *n* the determination of the properties of a substance in comparison with a standard or specification.

materials, dental, *n.pl* the substances used to assist in rendering dental service.

materials, filling, *n* the substances (e.g., gutta-percha, silver cones, paste mixtures, or other substances) used to fill root canals.

materials, impression, *n* a substance or combination of substances used for making a negative reproduction or impression.

materials, impression, elastomer, *n* See elastomer.

materials, provisional, *n* the cements or resins used temporarily to protect soft, hard, or pulpal tissues, stabilize a tooth, allow the delivery of medications, provide the ability to chew, or encourage the comfort of the patient. See also filling, treatment.

materials, rigid impression, *n* inflexible substances (e.g., zinc oxide-eugenol, plaster, or compound) used to create casts and models for prosthodontic, orthodontic, and pedodontic appliances, or the construction of dentures.

maternal age, *n* the age of the mother at the period of conception.

matrix (mā′triks), *n* **1.** an intergranular substance that acts somewhat as a cementing material for other particles; e.g., zinc phosphate cement is made of undissolved zinc oxide particles, surrounded and held or cemented together by phosphate compounds. The phosphate compounds make up the matrix. *n* **2.** a mechanical or artificial wall that completes the mold into which plastic material is inserted. *n* **3.** a mold into which something is formed. See also bone; splint.

matrix, amalgam, *n* a metal form, usually of stainless steel, about 0.0015 to 0.002 inch thick, adapted to a prepared cavity to supply the missing wall so that the plastic amalgam will be confined when it is condensed into the cavity.

matrix, celluloid, *n* a strip of celluloid used to mold cement into the desired shape. See also strip, plastic.

matrix, custom, *n* a matrix made especially for a given location, tooth, or preparation.

matrix, fibrous, of alveolar bone, *n* collagen fibers in the alveolar bone, calcified by the accumulation of hydroxyapatite, a calcium salt.

matrix, fibrous, of bone, *n* a component of bone tissue consisting of collagen fibers.

matrix, fibrous, of periodontal ligament, *n* major component consisting of collagen and oxytalan fibers whose function is to provide support to the tooth.

matrix holder, *n* See retainer, matrix.

***matrix, intermicrobial* (in′turmīkrō′bēəl),** *n* an intercellular substance found in plaque, which is made from derivatives of saliva, gingival fluids, and microorganisms.

matrix, mechanical, *n* (proprietary matrix), a patented or manufactured type of matrix.

matrix, plastic, *n* a matrix of resin or plastic for use with cold-curing resin or cement.

matrix, platinum, *n* a matrix of wrought platinum foil, usually 0.001 inch or thinner, adapted to a die of a preparation for a fired porcelain restoration; serves as a vehicle to carry and maintain the applications of porcelain when they are placed in a furnace for firing.

matrix, proprietary, *n* See matrix, mechanical.

matrix retainer, *n* a mechanical device used to secure the ends of metal or plastic bands around a tooth to provide a form into which a restorative material can be condensed to replace a portion of tooth substance removed in cavity preparation. See also retainer, matrix.

matrix, T-band, *n* a matrix material cut with a T-shaped projection at one end; the lugs are bent over to engage the band as it encircles the tooth.

maturation (mach′ərā′shən), *n* the process through which an organism or body structure arrives at a state of complete development. In dentistry, this is the point at which an individual's periodontium or its parts have reached their full adult form, size, and function.

maxilla (maksil′ə), *n* the irregularly shaped bone forming half of the upper jaw or maxillary arch. It is composed of the two maxillae.

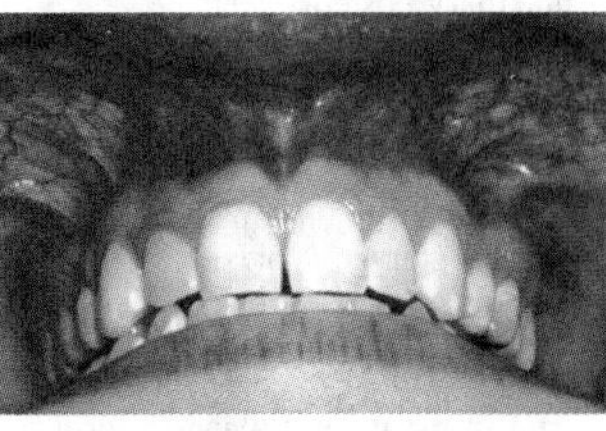

The maxilla. (Liebgott, 2001)

maxilla, frontal process of, *n* a projection of the maxilla that articulates with the nasal and frontal bones to form the nasal cavity.

maxillary (mak′siler′ē), *adj* pertaining to the superior jaw.

***maxillary antroplasty* (mak′siler′ē an′trōplas′tē),** *n* the addition of bone or other material to the antral floor of the sinus for the purpose of accommodating dental implants.

maxillary arch, *n* the upper dental arch and its supporting bone.

maxillary artery, *n* (internal maxillary artery), an artery that arises from the external carotid artery just below the level of the mandibular neck in the substance of the parotid gland. Its many branches include the middle meningeal, lower alveolar, temporal, pterygoid, masseteric, and buccal arteries, and the posterior superior alveolar and infraorbital arteries.

maxillary deficiency, *n* a maxilla whose structure is incomplete, such as in a cleft palate.

maxillary fracture, *n* a break in one or both of the maxillary bones; frequently sustained in automobile accidents and contact sports injuries.

maxillary labial frenum, *n* a vertical band of oral mucosa located between the midlines of the maxillary central incisors, which connects the attached gingiva to the upper lip and safeguards against any excessive motions.

maxillary nerve, *n* See nerve, maxillary.

maxillary retrusion, *n* See retrusion, maxillary.
maxillary sinus, *n* See sinus, maxillary.
maxillary sinusitis, *n* an inflammation of the mucosa lining the air sac in the maxillary bone. It can mimic in symptoms a pulpal infection of the maxillary posterior teeth.
maxillary torus **(mak′siler′ē tor′əs),** *n* See palatal torus.
maxillary tuberosity, *n* See tuberosity, maxillary.
maxillary vein, *n* a path of drainage for the pterygoid plexus of veins in the upper neck region. It is posterior to the mandibular condyle and merges with the superficial temporal vein in the parotid gland to form the retromandibular vein.

maxillofacial (maksil′ōfā′shəl), *adj* pertaining to the jaws and face.
maxillofacial injuries, *n.pl* the wounds to the midface area involving the premaxillary, maxillary, malar, lacrimal, nasal, and vomer bones and the tissues overlying these skeletal structures.
maxillofacial pain, *n* any pain in the region of the jaws or face. Usually coupled with oral pain; i.e., oral and maxillofacial pain may be present together. It frequently is associated with functional disorders of the temporomandibular joint and the muscles of mastication, which in turn may arise from structural problems in the occlusion of the teeth. Determining the cause may require comprehensive study of many possible factors or agents.
maxillofacial prosthetics, *n.pl* See prosthetics, maxillofacial.

maxillomandibular fixation (mak′silōmandib′yələr), *n* a temporary attachment of the maxilla to the mandible, usually with wires, to stabilize the bones of the jaw or face as fractures heal. Also known as *jaw wiring.*

maxillomandibular relation (maksil′ōmandib′ūlur), *n* See relation, maxillomandibular.

maxillotomy (mak′silot′əmē), *n* the surgical sectioning of the maxilla to allow movement of all or a part of the maxilla into the desired portion.

maximum allowance, *n* as specified in a fee schedule or table of allowances, the maximum dollar amount a dental plan will pay toward the cost of a dental service.

maximum benefit, *n* the maximum dollar amount a dental plan will pay toward the cost of dental care incurred by an individual or family in a specified policy year.

maximum fee schedule, *n* a compensation arrangement in which a participating dental professional agrees to accept a prescribed sum as the total fee for one or more covered services.

maximum recommended dose (MRD), *n* the highest amount of an anesthetic agent that can be given safely and without complication to a patient while maintaining its efficacy. It can also be adjusted to consider the patient's overall health and any extenuating factors that could hamper the patient's recovery.

mazindol (maz′indol′), *n brand names:* Mazanor, Sanorex; *drug class:* imidazoisoindole anorexiant (Controlled Substance Schedule IV); *action:* has amphetamine-like activity and may have an effect on satiety center of the hypothalamus; *use:* exogenous obesity.

Mazzini's test (məzē′nēz, mot-sē′nēz), *n.pr* See test, Mazzini's.

MCH, *n* See mean corpuscular hemoglobin.

MCHC, *n* See mean corpuscular hemoglobin concentration.

MCV, *n* See mean corpuscular volume.

MDR, *n* the abbreviation for minimum daily requirement, specifically the Minimum Daily Requirements for Specific Nutrients compiled by the United States Food and Drug Administration.

MDS, *n* See temporomandibular pain-dysfunction syndrome.

mean (x), *n* a measure of central tendency that is the calculated arithmetic average of a series of scores.
mean (x) corpuscular hemoglobin, *n* a measure of the weight of hemoglobin in a single red blood cell. The value is obtained by multiplying the hemoglobin value by 10 and dividing by the number of red blood cells. The normal range is between 27 and 31.

mean (x) corpuscular hemoglobin concentration (MCHC), *n* a measure of red blood cells useful in identifying the type of anemia. The MCHC is obtained by multiplying the value of hemoglobin by 100 and dividing by the value of the hematocrit. The normal range is between 31.5 and 35.5.

mean (x) corpuscular volume (MCV), *n* indicates the size of the red blood cells. The MCV is obtained by multiplying the hematocrit value by 10 and dividing by the number of red blood cells. The normal range is between 82 and 98.

mean (x) life, *n* See average life.

measles (mē′zəlz), *n* an infectious disease caused by a virus. There are two types: rubeola and rubella (German measles). Both have oral manifestations. See also spot, Koplik's.

measles, German, *n.pr* See rubella.

measles, three-day, *n* See rubella.

mebendazole (məben′dəzōl), *n* an anthelmintic agent that acts against pathogenic roundworms by inhibiting their glucose intake and secretory processes.

mecamylamine HCl (mek′əmil′əmēn′), *n brand name:* Inversine; *drug class:* antihypertensive, ganglionic blocker; *action:* occupies receptor site, prevents acetylcholine from attaching to postsynaptic nerve endings in autonomic ganglia; *uses:* moderate to severe hypertension, malignant hypertension.

mechanical toothbrush, *n* See automatic toothbrush.

mechanism, *n* a structure of working parts functioning together to produce an effect.

mechanism, cough, *n* a short inspiration, closure of the glottis, forcible expiratory effort, and then release of the glottis, with a rush of air at a flow rate of 3000 to 4000 cc/sec. It is essentially used or regarded as a process for removing foreign material from the lungs. It involves two phases. In the first, the combined action of the cilia and bronchiolar peristalsis moves the material up to the main bronchi and the bifurcation of the trachea. Further movement out of the respiratory system depends on the cough mechanism. In all medical conditions in which this mechanism is abolished or reduced, secretions and foreign material accumulate in the alveoli, with a resultant reduction in the aerating surface and a predisposition to infection. Because ventilation of the lungs depends on a patent airway, the cough mechanism should always be used by patients whose inadequate ventilation of lungs may be related to obstruction of the airway.

mechanism, inhibitory-excitatory **(inhib′itor′ē-eksī′tətor′ē),** *n* a mechanism that provides coordinated and continuous stimuli to the lower motor neuron for smooth, facile, and rapidly adjustable muscle contraction. This mechanism operates on every level of the central nervous system, from the final common pathway back up the spinal cord to the cerebrum. The excitatory phase of stimulation is transmitted directly to the nerve. Inhibition, however, is effected not by stimulating the motor output directly, as is done in the parasympathetic nerves, but rather by the interaction of inhibitory mechanisms on the excitatory impulses.

mechanism, respiratory control, *n* the mechanism by which the respiratory functions are controlled. Three major factors in the control of respiration concern the clinician: neurogenic control of respiration, chemical regulation of respiration, and mechanical events leading to pulmonary ventilation. These three factors are significant in practice procedures because the clinician influences each of these factors in routine dental care; e.g., the patency of the airways is always subject to alteration by instrumentation, dental prostheses, and the use of pharmacologic agents, and the physically induced responses modify the rate and magnitude of the respiratory mechanism.

mechanism, self-cleansing, *n* any of the structures within the oral cavity (e.g., teeth, saliva, oral mucosa, and tongue) that naturally allow the removal of substances entering the oral cavity that may affect the cleanliness of the cavity and promote the production of deposits.

mechanism, suspensory, *n* the hammocklike arrangement of the structures comprising the attachment apparatus.

mechanoreceptor, *n* a sensory nerve ending that responds to mechanical stimuli, such as touch, pressure, sound, and muscular contraction.

meclizine HCl (mek′lizēn′), *n brand names:* Antivert, Bonine, Dramamine II; *drug class:* antihistamine nonspecific antiemetic; *action:* a nonspecific central nervous system depressant with anticholinergic and antihistaminic activity; *uses:* dizziness, motion sickness.

meclofenamate (mek′lōfen′əmāt), *n brand name:* Meclofen, Meclomen; *drug class:* nonsteroidal antiinflammatory; *action:* inhibits prostaglandin synthesis by interfering with cyclooxygenase needed for biosynthesis; possesses analgesic, antiinflammatory, antipyretic properties; *uses:* mild to moderate pain, osteoarthritis, rheumatoid arthritis.

media (mē′dēə), *n.pl* the plural form of medium. See also medium.

M

medial (me′deəl), *adj* located in or directed toward the middle; closer to the body's midline.

median (mē′dēən), *adj* **1.** pertaining to the middle. *n* **2.** a measure of central tendency attained by a calculation or count that separates all cases in a ranked distribution into halves. The median may be used as an average score.

median lethal dose, *n* See dose, lethal, median.

median line, *n* See line, median.

median mandibular point, *n* See point, median mandibular.

median nerve, *n* one of the terminal branches of the brachial plexus that extends along the radial portions of the forearm and the hand and supplies various muscles and the skin of these parts.

median retruded relation, *n* See relation, centric.

median rhomboid glossitis, *n* See atrophy, central papillary.

median sagittal plane, *n* See plane, median sagittal.

mediastinitis (mē′dēas′tənī′tis), *n* an inflammation of the mediastinum.

mediastinum (mē′dēas′tənī′nəm), *n* a portion of the thoracic cavity in the middle of the thorax between the pleural sacs containing the two lungs. It extends from the sternum to the vertebral column and contains all the thoracic viscera except the lungs.

mediation intervention, *n* the act of a third person who interferes between two contending parties to reconcile them or to persuade them to adjust or settle their differences.

Medicaid, *n.pr* a federal assistance program established as Title XIX under the Social Security Amendments, which provides payment for medical care for certain low-income individuals and families. The program is funded jointly by the state and federal governments and administered by the states.

medical alert warning, *n* a coding of the patient's medical or dental record to indicate the presence of a serious medical condition that requires treatment planning consideration before treatment of any kind is initiated; possibly a pressure-sensitive red warning label containing a notation as to the exact nature of the compromising condition is placed on the record jacket or a note is made in the electronic record.

medical informatics, *n* the field of information science concerned with the analysis and dissemination of medical data through the application of computers to various aspects of health care and medicine.

medical record, *n* the portion of a patient's health record that is prepared by physicians and is a written or transcribed history of various illnesses or injuries requiring medical care, including inoculations, allergies, treatments, prognoses, and frequently health information about immediate family, occupation, and military service. Term can also be used by dental offices and clinics. See also health history.

medical staff, *n* physicians and dental professionals who are approved and given privileges to provide health care to patients in a hospital or other health care facility.

medical waste, *n* a discarded biologic product, such as blood or tissues, removed from operating rooms, morgues, laboratories, or other medical facilities. The term may also be applied to bedding, bandages, syringes, and similar materials that have been used in treating patients, as well as animal carcasses or body parts used in research. See also waste products, biohazard.

medical waste disposal, *n* the safe and proper handling of medical waste, prescribed by statute and institutional policy and designed to prevent cross contamination, reinfection, and transmission of disease.

medically necessary care, *n* the reasonable and appropriate diagnosis, treatment, and follow-up care (including supplies, appliances, and devices) as determined and prescribed by qualified appropriate health care providers in treating any condition, illness, disease, injury, or birth developmental malformation. Care is medically necessary for the purpose of controlling or eliminating infection, pain, and disease and restoring facial configuration or function necessary for speech, swallowing, or chewing.

Medicare, *n.pr* a federal insurance program enacted as Title XVIII of the Social Security Amendments that provides certain inpatient hospital services and physician services for all persons age 65 and older and eligible disabled individuals. The program is administered by the Health Care Financing Administration.

Medicare Part A, *n* provides hospital insurance to all qualified beneficiaries under the Medicare criteria.

Medicare Part B, *n* provides medical insurance coverage for services such as physician' s services, outpatient services, and home health care. Participation under Part B is voluntary, and beneficiaries pay monthly premiums. Part B is also called Supplementary Medical Insurance.

medication (med′ikā′shən), *n* **1.** a drug or other substance that is used as a medicine. *n* **2.** the administration of a medicine.

medication, antiretroviral, during pregnancy, *n.pl* substances used to treat RNA viruses (including HIV). The effects on fetal development are not known; however, antiretroviral medications are generally still administered to infected mothers.

medication, complete, *n* the combination of synergistic drugs used to sedate children undergoing prolonged or difficult dental procedures; the patient is in a state of sleep or light anesthesia.

medication, intracanal, *n* a drug used in the root canal system during the course of therapy.

medication, official, *n* See drug, official.

medication, officinal, *n* See drug, officinal.

medication, repository, *n* the slowly soluble drug mixtures intended for parenteral injection and gradual absorption into the blood and hence into other tissues of the body.

medication, sustained release, *n* an oral dosage form designed to be absorbed at various levels in the gastrointestinal tract, thus prolonging action.

medication, transdermal, *n* See transdermal delivery system.

medicine (med′isin), *n* **1.** a remedy. *n* **2.** the art of healing.

medicine, oral, *n* the discipline of dentistry that deals with the significance and relationship of oral and systemic disease.

medicine, practice of, *n* a pursuit that includes the application and use of medicines and drugs for the purpose of curing or alleviating bodily diseases; surgery is usually limited to manual operations generally performed by means of surgical instruments or appliances.

mediostrusive (mē′dēōstroo′siv), *n* nonfunctional side tooth contacts during lateral jaw movements.

mediotrusion (mē′dēōtroo′zhən), *n* a thrusting of the mandibular condyle inward (toward the median plane). When the right condyle is thrust outward (in laterotrusion) before it is rotated, the left condyle is thrust inward before it is orbited and is thus said to be in precurrent mediotrusion. If the left condyle is thrust outward before it is rotated, the right condyle is in precurrent mediotrusion.

Mediterranean anemia, *n* See thalassemia major.

medium (mē′dēum), *n* an interposed agent or material; a carrier; a material serving as an environment for the growth of microorganisms.

medium, computer, n the material on which data are recorded (e.g., CD-RWs, DVDs, external hard drives, magnetic tape).

medium, marking, n **1.** an agent, such as carbon paper or inked ribbon, used to indicate an occlusal interference. *n* **2.** an agent, such as stencil correction fluid, rouge and alcohol, or pressure indicator paste, used to determine areas of interference or pressure related to a removable prosthesis.

medium, radiopaque, n a substance that may be injected into a cavity or region to increase its density in radiographic examination and thereby aid in diagnosis. Lipiodol, Iodochloral, Parabodril, and Ioduron are examples of such materials.

medium, Sabouraud's, n.pr a nutrient agar used to grow fungi. It is especially useful for the growth and identification of *C. albicans,* the causative agent of thrush.

medium, separating, n a coating that is used on a surface and serves to prevent another surface or material from adhering to the first (e.g., tinfoil, cellophane, or alginate, all of which are used to protect an acrylic resin from the moisture in the gypsum mold).

MEDLARS, *n.pr* the abbreviation for Medical Literature Analysis and Retrieval System, which is a computerized literature retrieval service offered by the National Library of Medicine in Bethesda, Maryland.

MEDLINE, *n.pr* a National Library of Medicine computer data base of current references. The files duplicate the contents of the Unabridged Index Medicus. The references are available online.

medroxyprogesterone acetate (medrok′sēprōjes′tərōn as′ətāt), *n brand names:* Amen, Curretab, Cycrin; *drug class:* progestogen; *action:* inhibits secretion of pituitary gonadotropins, which prevents follicular maturation and ovulation; stimulates growth of mammary tissue; antineoplastic action against endometrial cancer; *uses:* abnormal uterine bleeding, secondary amenorrhea, endometrial cancer, metastatic renal cancer, contraceptive, with estrogens to reduce incidence of endometrial cancer.

medulla oblongata (mədul′ə oblôngä′tə), *n* the direct upward extension of the spinal cord that lies at the junction between the cerebrum and the spinal cord and is considered to be in a group with the pons and midbrain because the nuclei of all the cranial nerves except one are situated within this structural group. Its functions are associated with the nuclei of the glossopharyngeal, vagal, spinal accessory, and hypoglossal nerves. It controls the reflex actions of the pharynx, larynx, and tongue, which are related to deglutition, mastication, and speech, as well as the visceral reflexes of coughing, sneezing, sucking, vomiting, and salivating, and other secretory functions.

mefenamic acid (mef′ənam′ik), *n brand name:* Ponstel; *drug class:* nonsteroidal antiinflammatory; *action:* inhibits prostaglandin synthesis by interfering with cyclooxygenase needed for biosynthesis; possesses analgesic, antiinflammatory, antipyretic properties; *uses:* mild to moderate pain, dysmenorrhea, inflammatory disease.

megacolon (meg′əkō′lən), *n* an abnormal dilation of the colon that may be congenital, toxic, or acquired.

megacolon, acquired, n a result of a chronic refusal to defecate, usually occurring in children who are psychotic or mentally retarded.

megacolon, congenital, n caused by the absence of autonomic ganglia in the smooth muscle wall of the colon.

megacolon, toxic, n a serious complication of ulcerative colitis that may result in perforation of the colon, septicemia, and death.

megadontismus (megədontiz′mus), *n* See macrodontia.

megestrol acetate (məjes′trōl as′ətāt), *n brand name:* Megace; *drug class:* antineoplastic (progestin); *action:* affects endometrium by antiluteinizing effect; *uses:* breast, endometrial cancer, renal cell cancer.

meiosis (mio'sis), *n* a type of cell division of maturing sex cells that ensures that each daughter cell contains the necessary complement of chromosomes for future embryonic development.

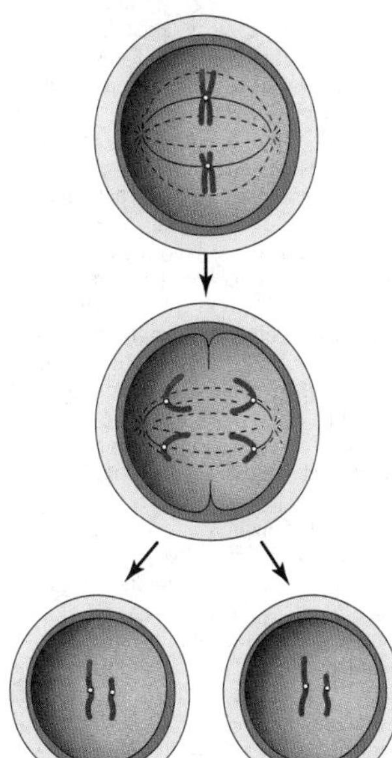

Second meiotic division. (Moore/Persaud, 2003)

Meissner's corpuscles (mīs'nurz), *n.pr* See corpuscle, Meissner's.

melanin (mel'ənin), *n* the dark amorphous pigment of melanotic tumors, skin, oral mucosa, hair, choroid coat of the eye, and substantia nigra of the brain.

melanocytes (mel'ənəsīts), *n.pl* the dendritic cells of the gingival epithelium that, when functional, cause pigmentation regardless of race.

melanoma (mel'ənō'mə), *n* a malignant epithelial neoplasm characterized by pigment-producing cells. It usually is dark in color but may be amelanotic, i.e., free of pigment. It can occur in skin as well as the oral cavity, where it usually would be a late finding. It can occur at the site of a mole (mainly) or another site.

melanosis (mel'ənō'sis), *n* the condition in which melanin pigments appear in the tissues. Melanosis is normal in the gingivae of most dark-skinned individuals and occasionally in those with light skin.

melatonin (mel'ətō'nin), *n* the only hormone secreted into the bloodstream by the pineal gland. It appears to inhibit numerous endocrine functions, including the gonadotropic hormones, and to decrease the pigmentation of the skin.

melena (melē'nə), *n* the passage of dark or black stools; the color is produced by altered blood and blood pigments.

melituria (mel'itoo'rēə), *n* the presence of any sugar in the urine (e.g., glucose, lactose, pentose, fructose, maltose, galactose, or sucrose).

melphalan (mel'fəlan'), *n brand name:* Alkeran; *drug class:* antineoplastic; *action:* responsible for cross-linking DNA strands, which leads to cell death; *uses:* palliative treatment of multiple myeloma and nonresectable epithelial carcinoma of the ovary.

melting range, *n* See range, melting.

member, *n* an individual enrolled in a dental benefits program. See also beneficiary.

membrane, *n* a thin layer of tissue that covers a surface or divides a space or organ.

membrane, barrier, *n* small pieces of meshlike material inserted between the gingival tissue flap and underlying bone, primarily during flap surgery. It is used to prevent grafted material from moving and to stop harmful cells from growing. It can be used alone or in combination with bone grafting.

membrane, basement, *n* the delicate, PAS-positive, noncellular membrane on which the epithelium is seated.

membrane bone, *n* See bone, membrane.

membrane, collagen, *n* a bioabsorbable, semipermeable membrane made of collagen. It is hemostatic, chemotactic, and well tolerated by adjacent tissue.

membrane, intramembranous **(in'trəmem'brənus),** *n* formed by differentiation of mesenchymal cells

M

into osteoblasts and bone matrix. See also bone, membrane and bone, membrane, formation.

membrane, mucous, *n* See mucosa.

membrane, Nasmyth's, *n.pr* See cuticle, primary.

membrane, occlusive, *n* See membrane, barrier.

***membrane, oropharyngeal* (ôr′ōfərin′jēəl),** *n* a layer of tissue on the cephalic end of the embryo in the region where the oral cavity will later be formed. Previously called *buccopharyngeal membrane.* See also oropharynx.

membrane, periodontal, *n* See ligament, periodontal.

membrane, subimplant, *n* the fibrous connective tissue that regenerates from the periosteum and that forms between the inner surface of the implant framework and the bone surface.

memory, *n* **1.** the ability to recall events, experiences, information, and skills. *n* **2.** a general term for a device that stores data in binary code on electronic or magnetic media in computers. *n* **3.** the ability of the immune system to greatly speed up the response to pathogens that have previously been encountered. See also immunity.

memory cycle, *n* the time it takes to access a character in memory.

memory location, *n* a place in the memory where a unit of data may be stored or retrieved.

memory, long-term, *n* the ability to recall events, experiences, information, or skills that occurred or were acquired in the distant past.

memory register, *n* a register in storage of a computer, in contrast with a register in one of the other units of the computer.

memory, short-term, *n* the ability to retain and recall recent events or experiences.

menadiol/menadiol sodium diphosphate (vitamin K_4) (men′ədī′ol sōdēəm dīfos′fāt), *n brand name:* Synkavite; *drug class:* synthetic vitamin K; *action:* needed for adequate blood clotting (factors II, VII, IX, X); *uses:* vitamin K malabsorption, hypoprothrombinemia, oral anticoagulant toxicity.

menarche (mənär′kē), the beginning of the menstrual function. See also menstruation.

Mendelian inheritance (mendē′lēən), *n.pr* (Mendel's laws, mendelian laws) two basic genetic principles were established: the law of segregation and the law of independent assortment. According to the law of segregation, the genetic characteristics of a species are represented in the somatic cells by a pair of units called genes that separate during meiosis so that each gamete receives only one gene for each trait. According to the law of independent assortment, the members of a gene pair on different chromosomes segregate independently from other pairs during meiosis, so that the gametes offer all possible combinations of factors.

Ménière's disease (menēerz′), *n.pr* a chronic disease of the inner ear characterized by recurrent episodes of vertigo, which is progressive sensorineural hearing loss. It may occur bilaterally and may include tinnitus.

meninges (mənin′jēz), *n.pl* the three membranes enclosing the brain and the spinal cord, comprising the dura mater, the pia mater, and the arachnoid.

meningioma (mənin′jēō′mə), *n* a mesenchymal fibroblastic tumor of the membranes enveloping the brain and spinal cord. They grow slowly, are usually vascular, and occur most commonly near the superior longitudinal, transverse, and cavernous sinuses of the dura mater of the brain.

meningism (mənin′jizəm), *n* an abnormal condition characterized by irritation of the brain and spinal cord and by symptoms that mimic those of meningitis. In meningism, however, there is no actual inflammation of the meninges.

meningitis (men′injī′tis), *n* an infection or inflammation of the membranes covering the brain and spinal cord. It usually is a purulent infection and involves the fluid of the subarachnoid space. The most common causes in adults are bacterial infection with *S. pneumoniae, N. meningitidis,* or *H. influenzae.* Aseptic meningitis may be caused by chemical irritation, neoplasms, or viruses.

Typical signs and symptoms include fever, headache, stiff neck, photophobia, or vomiting.

meningocele (məning'gəsēl'), *n* a saclike protrusion of either the cerebral or spinal meninges through a congenital defect in the skull or the vertebral column.

meningoencephalitis (məning'gōensef'əlī'tis), *n* an inflammation of both the brain and the meninges, usually caused by a bacterial infection.

meningomyelocele (məning'gəmī'ələsēl'), *n* a saclike cyst containing brain tissue, cerebrospinal fluid, and the meninges that protrudes through a congenital defect in the skull.

meniscectomy (men'isek'təmē), *n* the surgical removal of the meniscus or condylar disc, also referred to as *discectomy.* It is no longer a procedure of choice.

meniscus (mənis'kəs), *n* the cartilaginous intracapsular disc interposed between the mandibular condyle and the glenoid fossa of the temporal bone at the temporomandibular joint.

menopause (men'əpôz'), *n* the cessation of menstruation occurring variably from approximately 45 to 50 years of age. Menopause is accompanied by diminution of estrogen formation, often with atrophic changes occurring in the oral mucosa and gingivae. See also perimenopause.

menopause, hot flashes, *n* sudden surges of heat and perspiration encompassing the entire body that may occur day or night as the result of hormonal fluctuations during menopause.

menopause, oral symptoms of, *n* a burning sensation and dryness of the oral cavity; salty taste; edematous, reddened, atrophic-appearing, tender mucosa; glossitis; and often desquamative gingivitis.

menorrhagia (men'ərā'jēə), *n* an abnormally heavy or long menstrual period. Menorrhagia is a relatively common complication of benign uterine fibromyoma; it may be so severe or intractable as to require intervention such as hysterectomy. May occur during perimenopause.

menses (men'sēz), *n* See menstruation.

menstrual cycle, *n* a recurring cycle of change in the endometrium during which the decidual layer of the endometrium is shed, then regrows, proliferates, is maintained for several days, and is shed again at menstruation. The average length of the cycle is 28 days.

menstruation (men'strooā'shən), *n* the normal shedding of the necrotic mucosa of the endometrium and associated bleeding that occurs in the final phase of the menstrual cycle. The average duration of menstruation is 5 days, in which approximately 30 ml of blood is lost.

mental disorder, *n* any disturbance of emotional equilibrium as manifested in maladaptive behavior and impaired functioning, caused by genetic, physical, chemical, biologic, psychologic, or social and cultural factors. Also called *emotional illness, mental illness, psychiatric disorder.*

mental foramen, *n* See foramen, mental.

mental health, *n* a relative state of mind in which a person who is healthy is able to cope with and adjust to the recurrent stresses of everyday living in an acceptable way.

mental health service, *n* a group of government, professional, or lay organizations operating at a community, state, national, or international level to aid in the prevention and treatment of mental disorders.

mental protuberance, *n* a projection or eminence of the chin near the mesioanterior surface of the mandible. See also menton.

mental retardation, *n* a disorder characterized by certain limitations in a person's mental functioning and in skills such as communicating, taking care of him or herself, and social skills. It has many causes, including genetic conditions such as Down syndrome, fragile X syndrome, and phenylketonuria (PKU) as well as problems during pregnancy or at birth, or due to health problems such as diphtheria, measles, or meningitis. It can also be caused by extreme malnutrition, not getting enough medical care, or being exposed to poisons such as lead or mercury.

menthol, *n* a topical antipruritic with a cooling effect that relieves itching.

It is an ingredient in many topical creams and ointments.

menton, *n* the most inferior point on the chin in the lateral view; a cephalometric landmark.

mepenzolate bromide (məpenzōlāt brō′mīd), *n brand name:* Cantil; *drug class:* gastrointestinal (GI) anticholinergic; *action:* inhibits muscarinic actions of acetylcholine at postganglionic parasympathetic neuroeffector sites; *uses:* treatment of peptic ulcer disease, irritable bowel syndrome in combination with other drugs, other GI disorders.

meperidine HCl (məper′ədēn′), *n brand name:* Demerol; *drug class:* synthetic narcotic analgesic (Controlled Substance Schedule II); *action:* interacts with opioid receptors in the central nervous system to alter pain perception; *uses:* moderate to severe pain, preoperative administration in sedation techniques.

mephenesin (mefen′isin), *n* an antispasmodic drug, 3 ortho-toloxyl, 2 propanediol. Used for the preparation of apprehensive patients for dental and periodontal procedures because of its ability to produce muscular relaxation and euphoria. Usual dosage for an adult is 1 gm in either tablet or elixir form, 20 minutes before the dental procedure.

mephenytoin (məfen′ətō′ən), *n brand name:* Mesantoin; *drug class:* hydantoin anticonvulsant; *action:* reduces electrical discharges in motor cortex, reducing seizures; *uses:* generalized tonic-clonic seizures, single or complex-partial seizures.

mephobarbital (mef′ōbär′bital), *n brand name:* Mebaral; *drug class:* barbiturate anticonvulsant (Controlled Substance Schedule IV); *action:* a nonspecific depressant of the central nervous system; may enhance GABA activity in the brain; *uses:* generalized tonic-clonic (grand mal) or absence (petit mal) seizures.

mepivacaine HCl (local) (məpiv′əkān′), *n brand names:* Isocaine, Polocaine; *drug class:* amide local anesthetic; *action:* inhibits ion fluxes across membranes, particularly sodium transport across cell membranes; decreases rise of depolarization phase of action potential; blocks nerve action potential; *uses:* local dental anesthesia, nerve block, caudal anesthesia, epidural pain relief, paracervical block, transvaginal block or infiltration.

meprobamate (məprō′bamāt′), *n brand names:* Equanil, Miltown, Probate, Trancot; *drug class:* sedative-hypnotic, anxiolytic (Controlled Substance Schedule IV); *action:* nonspecific central nervous system depressant; acts in thalamus, limbic system, and spinal cord; *use:* anxiety disorders.

merbromin (murbrō′min), *n* a mercury-bromine compound used as a germicide for disinfection of the skin, mucous membrane, and wounds. Used in 10% alcoholic solution (Scott-Wilson reagent) in the treatment of moniliasis.

mercaptan (murkap′tən), *n* the basic ingredient of the polysulfide polymer employed in rubber base impression materials. See also Thiokol.

mercaptopurine (6-MP), *n brand name:* Purinethol; *drug class:* antineoplastic-antimetabolite; *action:* inhibits purine metabolism at multiple sites, which inhibits DNA and RNA synthesis; *uses:* chronic myelocytic leukemia, acute lymphoblastic leukemia in children, acute myelogenous leukemia.

mercurial (murkyoo′rēəl), *adj* a compound that owes its activity to the mercury it contains.

mercurial line, *n* See line, mercurial.

mercurialism (məkyŏŏr′ēəliz′əm), *n* (mercury poisoning), **1.** poisoning resulting from the ingestion of pure mercury, its salts, or its vapor. Manifestations of acute intoxication include nausea, vomiting, abdominal cramps, oral and pharyngeal pain, uremia, dehydration, diarrhea, and shock. Manifestations of chronic poisoning include hypersalivation, diarrhea, vertigo, depression, intention tremor, and stomatitis. See also acrodynia and stomatitis, mercurial. *n* **2.** poisoning by ingestion or absorption of mercury compounds. See also line, mercurial, and mercury poisoning.

mercuric chloride, *n* mercury bichloride or perchloride; a corrosive, highly toxic sublimate used as a topical antiseptic and disinfectant for inanimate objects.

Mercurochrome, *n* the brand name for merbromin.

mercury (Hg), a metallic element. Its atomic number is 80 and its atomic weight is 200.6. It is the only common metal that is liquid at room temperature, and it occurs in nature almost entirely in the form of its sulfide, cinnabar. It is used in dental amalgams, thermometers, barometers, and other measuring instruments. It forms many poisonous compounds. The major toxic forms are mercury vapor, mercuric salts, and organic mercurials. Elemental mercury is only mildly toxic when ingested because it is poorly absorbed.

mercury poisoning, n a toxic condition caused by the ingestion or inhalation of mercury or a mercury compound. The chronic form, resulting from inhalation of the vapors or dust of mercurial compounds, is characterized by irritability, excessive saliva, loosened teeth, gingival tissue disorders, slurred speech, tremors, and staggering. Symptoms of acute mercury poisoning usually appear no later than 30 minutes after exposure and include a metallic taste in the oral cavity, thirst, nausea, vomiting, severe abdominal pain, bloody diarrhea, and renal failure that may result in death. Its presence in the body is determined by a urine test.

merge, *v* to produce a single sequence of items, ordered according to some rule, from two or more sequences previously ordered according to the same rule. Merging does not change the items in size, structure, or total number.

Merrifield's knife, *n.pr* See knife, Merrifield's.

mes- (meso-), *pref* in the middle; intermediate as in position, size, type, and time degree.

mesalamine (məsal'əmēn'), *n brand names:* Asacol, Pentasa, Rowasa; *drug class:* antiinflammatory; *action:* unknown, may inhibit prostaglandin synthesis; *uses:* inflammatory bowel disease, ulcerative colitis.

mescaline, abuse of (mes'kəlēn, -lin), *n* the regular use of mescaline (e.g., mesc, big chief, or buttons), an example of a hallucinogen, for reasons other than recognized medical applications.

mesenchyme (mes'engkīm), *n* an embryonic connective tissue that migrates from the primitive epidermal and hypodermal layers and later produces the mesodermal layer. It is in this layer that embryonic tooth buds begin to form.

mesial (mē'zēəl), *adj* situated in the middle; median, toward the middle line of the body or toward the center line of each dental arch.

mesial migration, n the drifting of teeth toward the midline or forward in each dental arch to produce crowding in the permanent dentition of an older adult.

mesial, unilateral, adj mesiocclusion on one side.

mesiocclusion (mē'zēəkloo'zhən), *n* an occlusal relationship in which the mandibular teeth are positioned mesially, similar to the relationship in an Angle Class III malocclusion. See also distoclusion.

mesiodens (mē'zēədenz), *n* a supernumerary tooth appearing in an erupted or unerupted state between the two maxillary central incisors.

mesioversion (mēzēōvur'zhən), *n* when applied to a tooth, a term indicating that the tooth is closer than normal to the median plane or midline. When applied to the maxillae or mandible, it means that the jaw is anterior to its normal position.

meso-, *pref* See mes-.

mesocephalic (mes'ōsefal'ik), *adj* a descriptive term applied to a head size between dolichocephalic and brachycephalic (cephalic index 76 to 81).

mesoderm, *n* the middle of the three cell layers of the developing embryo. It lies between the ectoderm and the endoderm. Bone, connective tissue, muscle, blood, vascular and lymphatic tissue, and the pleurae of the pericardium and peritoneum are all derived from the mesoderm.

mesodontia (mes'ōdon'shēə), *n.pl* medium-size teeth.

mesognathic (mes'ōnāth'ik), *adj* having an average relationship of jaws to head. See also facial profile.

mesonephros (mez'ənef'rəs), *n* the second type of excretory organ to develop in the vertebrate embryo. The organ is the permanent kidney in lower animals, but in humans and various other mammals it is functional only during early embryonic development.

mesoridazine besylate (mez'ərid'əzēn bes'əlāt), *n brand name:* Serentil; *drug class:* phenothiazine antipsychotic; *action:* blocks neurotransmission at dopaminergic synapses in the cerebral cortex, hypothalamus, and limbic system; mechanism for antipsychotic effects is unclear; *uses:* psychotic disorders, schizophrenia, anxiety, alcoholism, behavioral problems in mental deficiency, chronic brain syndrome.

mesostomia (mes'ōstō'mēə), *n* an oral fissure of medium size.

mesostructure conjunction bar, *n* a connecting bar joining implant abutment copings together. Bar and copings together make up the mesostructure.

mesothelioma (mez'əthē'lēō'mə), *n* a rare malignant tumor of the mesothelium of the pleura or peritoneum associated with exposure to asbestos.

metaanalysis, *n* a quantitative method of combining the results of independent studies (usually drawn from the published literature) and synthesizing summaries and conclusions that may be used to evaluate therapeutic effectiveness and plan new studies, with application mainly in the areas of research and medicine and dentistry.

metabolic disease, *n* a disorder that causes dysfunction of the metabolic action of the body, resulting in loss of control of homeostasis.

metabolism (metab'ōlizəm), *n* the sum of chemical changes involved in the function of nutrition. There are two phases: anabolism (constructive or assimilative changes) and catabolism (destructive or retrograde changes).

metabolism, basal, *n* See basal metabolic rate.

metabolism, bone, *n* the continual complex of anabolism and catabolism taking place in bone when it is in physiologic equilibrium. Bone is a highly labile substance that reflects the adequacy of general body metabolism. See also bone, alveolar, metabolism.

metabolism, cell, *n* the complexity of anabolic and catabolic processes occurring within cellular structures.

metabolism, energy, *n* the transformation of energy in living tissues, consisting of anabolism (storage of energy) and catabolism (the dissipation of energy).

metabolism, substance, *n* the physical and chemical processes by which living organized tissues are produced and maintained.

metacarpus (met'əkär'pəs), *n* the five bones of the hand between the carpus (wrist) and the phalanges (fingers).

metal, *n* an element possessing luster, malleability, ductility, and conductivity of electricity and heat.

metal, base, *n* an older term referring to nonprecious metals or alloys such as iron, lead, copper, nickel, chromium, and zinc. In dentistry, the term usually refers to the stainless steel and chrome-cobalt-nickel alloys.

metal ceramic alloys, *n* the fusion of ceramics (porcelain) to an alloy of two or more metals for use in restorative and prosthodontic dentistry. Examples of metal alloys employed include cobalt-chromium, gold-palladium, gold-platinum-palladium, and nickel-based alloys.

metal, fusion of, *n* the blending of metals by melting together.

metal insert teeth, *n.pl* See tooth, metal insert.

metal, noble, *n* a precious metal, usually one that does not readily oxidize, such as gold or platinum.

metal, solidification of, *n* the change of metal from the molten to the solid state.

metal, wrought, *n* a cast metal that has been cold-worked in any manner.

metallic salts, *n.pl* the compounds such as potassium oxalate or strontium chloride used by dental professionals to help desensitize teeth. They work by forming a gritty film which blocks the dentin tubules.

metalloid (met'əloid), *n* a nonmetallic element that behaves as a metal under certain conditions. Carbon, silicon, and boron are three examples.

These elements may be alloyed with metals.

metalloprotein (mital'ōprō'tēn), *n* a protein with a tightly bound metal ion or ions, such as hemoglobin.

metallothioneins (MTs) (metal'ōthī'ōnēns), *n.pl* proteins and polypeptides containing very high levels of metal and sulfur. They are most common in the functional tissue of an organ and are considered useful in controlling the intracellular fixation and the free ion concentration of the trace elements zinc and copper, as well as defending the body against stress and toxic substances.

metallurgy, *n* the study of metals and their properties, including separating metals from their ores, the making and compounding of alloys, and the technology and science of working and heat-treating metals to alter their physical characteristics.

metanephrine (met'ənef'rin), *n* one of the two principal urinary metabolites of epinephrine and norepinephrine in the urine, the other being vanillylmandelic acid.

metaphen, tincture of (met'əfen), *n* the brand name for tincture of nitromersol.

metaphysis (mətaf'isis), *n* the line of junction of the epiphysis with the diaphysis of a long bone.

metaplasia (met'əplā'zhə), *n* a change in the type of adult cells in a tissue to a form that is not normal for that tissue.

metaproterenol sulfate (met'əprōter'ənol'), *n brand names:* Arm-A-Med, Metaprel, Prometa; *drug class:* selective β_2-agonist; *action:* relaxes bronchial smooth muscle by direct action on β_2-adrenergic receptors; *uses:* bronchial asthma, bronchospasm.

metastasis (mətas'təsis), *n* the transfer of a disease by blood vessels, lymph vessels, or the respiratory tract (through aspiration) from one organ or region to another not directly contiguous with it. Usually used in reference to malignant tumor cells, but bacteria can also metastasize (e.g., in focal infection).

meter, dose rate, *n* an instrument that measures radiation dose rate.

meter, integrating dose rate, *n* the ionization chamber and measuring system designed for determining the total accumulated radiation administered during an exposure.

meter, radiation, *n* an instrument for the measurement of exposure to radiation.

meter, radiation dosimeter (dōsim'itər), *n* an instrument used to detect and measure an accumulated exposure to radiation, commonly a pencil-size ionization chamber with built-in self-reading electrometer used in personnel radiation monitoring.

metformin HCl (metfor'min), *n brand name:* Glucophage; *drug class:* oral hypoglycemic, biguanide derivative; *action* exact mechanism unknown, requires insulin secretion to function properly; *use:* type II diabetes mellitus.

methacrylate (methak'rəlāt'), *n* an ester of methacrylic acid used as an enamel sealant. See also methyl methacrylate.

methadone HCl (meth'ədōn), *n brand names:* Dolophine, Methadone; *drug class:* synthetic narcotic analgesic (Controlled Substance Schedule II); *action:* interacts with opioid receptors in the central nervous system to alter pain perception; *uses:* severe pain, opioid withdrawal program.

methamphetamine HCl (meth'amfet'əmēn'), *n brand name:* Desoxyn Gradumet; *drug class:* amphetamine (Controlled Substance Schedule II); *action:* increases release of norepinephrine and dopamine in cerebral cortex to reticular activating system; *uses:* exogenous obesity, minimal brain dysfunction, attention deficit hyperactivity disorder (ADHD).

methantheline bromide (methan'thəlēn' brō'mīd), *n brand name:* Banthine; *drug class:* synthetic anticholinergic; *action:* inhibits muscarinic actions of acetylcholine at postganglionic parasympathetic neuroeffector sites; *uses:* treatment of peptic ulcer disease, irritable bowel syndrome, pancreatitis, gastritis, biliary dyskinesia, pylorospasm, reflex neurogenic bladder in children.

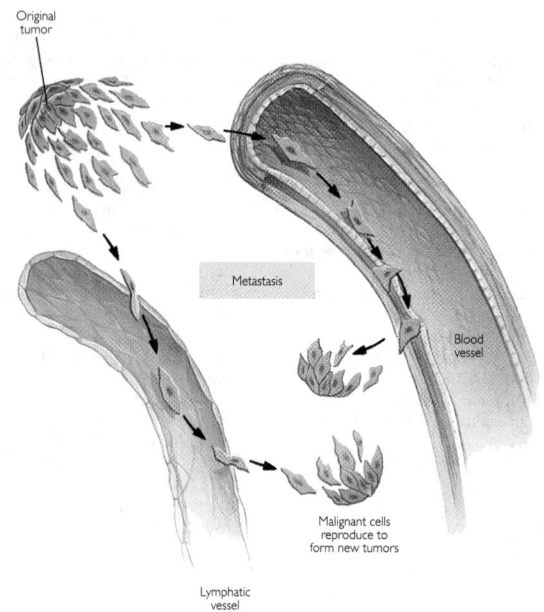

Metastasis. (Thibodeau/Patton, 2005)

methazolamide (meth′əzō′ləmīd′), *n brand name:* Neptazane; *drug class:* carbonic anhydrase inhibitor; *action:* decreases production of aqueous humor in the eye, which lowers intraocular pressure; *uses:* open-angle glaucoma or preoperatively in narrow-angle glaucoma.

methemoglobinemia (met′hēməglō′binē′mēə), *n* an abnormality of hemoglobin in which the iron is in the ferric state as a result of exposure to industrial substances or the ingestion of toxic agents such as phenacetin, sulfonamides, aniline nitrates, or nitrates. A rare congenital form is seen most commonly in persons with Greek heritage. Symptoms include generalized cyanosis, headache, drowsiness, and confusion. Methemoglobin does not carry oxygen. This condition has recently been associated with topical benzocaine spray when applied to the oropharynx.

methenamine salts (məthē′nəmēn′), *n brand names:* Hiprex, Urex; *drug class:* urinary antiinfective; *action:* in acid urine, it is hydrolyzed to ammonia and formaldehyde, which are bactericidal; *uses:* prophylaxis and treatment of uncomplicated urinary tract infections.

methicillin sodium, *n* a semisynthetic penicillin salt for parenteral administration. Restriction of its use to infections caused by penicillin G-resistant staphylococci is recommended.

methimazole (məthī′məzōl′), *n brand name:* Tapazole; *drug class:* thyroid hormone antagonist; *action:* inhibits synthesis of thyroid hormones by decreasing iodine use in manufacture of thyroglobulin and iodothyronine; *uses:* hyperthyroidism, preparation for thyroidectomy, thyrotoxic crisis, thyroid storm.

methionine (məthī′ənēn′), *n* one

of the essential amino acids. See also amino acid.

methocarbamol, *n brand name:* Carbacot, Delaxin, Robamol, Skelex; *drug class:* skeletal muscle relaxant; *action:* depresses multisynaptic pathways in the spinal cord; *uses:* adjunct for relief of spasm and pain in musculoskeletal conditions.

method, *n* a manner of performing an act or operation; a technique.

method, Callahan's, *n.pr* See method, chloropercha.

method, Charters', *n.pr* a method of toothbrushing in which the brush is held horizontally, with the bristles lying against the teeth and gingivae and pointed in a coronal direction at 45 degrees so that the bristles lie half on the teeth and half on the gingivae. A vibratory cycle of a very constricted diameter is negotiated so that the brush head moves in a circular movement but the brush bristles remain fairly stationary while being agitated. The circular vibration loosens debris and pumps the bristles into interproximal areas to massage the tissues.

method, chloropercha **(klō′rəpur′chə),** *n* (Callahan's method, Johnston's method), the method of filling root canals in which gutta-percha cones are dissolved in a chloroform-rosin solution in the root canal. The canal is flooded with the chloroform solution. A preselected gutta-percha cone is then pumped carefully into and out of the canal. As the cone dissolves, the material is forced into the apex as a plastic mass. Other cones and occasionally additional chloroform solution are added until the canal is sealed.

method, Collis, *n* a variation of toothbrushing that employs short, repetitive strokes with a Collis curved brush. Collis's brush design allows for brushing three surfaces of the tooth simultaneously. A 45° angle is used when brushing in and around the gingivae line. Favored by special needs patients, as well as parents and caretakers who perform the task of brushing for others. Also called *simultaneous sulcular.*

method, Fones', *n.pr* (Fones' technique), a toothbrushing technique in which, with the teeth occluded and with the brush at more or less right angles to the teeth, large sweeping, scrubbing circles are described. With the jaws parted, the palatal and lingual surfaces of the teeth are scrubbed using smaller circles. Occlusal surfaces are brushed in an anteroposterior direction.

method, Hirschfeld's, *n.pr* a toothbrushing method in which the bristles are placed against the axial surfaces of the teeth, with slight incisal or occlusal inclination from a right-angled application, in simultaneous contact with teeth and gingivae, and then rotated in a circle of exceedingly small diameter. Occlusal surfaces are brushed energetically.

method, Howard's, *n.pr* a method of artificial respiration. The patient is placed on the back, with the hands under the head, and a cushion is placed so that the head is lower than the abdomen. The physician applies rhythmic pressure upward and inward with the hands against the lower lateral parts of the patient's chest.

method, Howe's silver precipitation, *n.pr* a method of depositing silver in enamel and dentin by the application of ammoniacal silver nitrate solution and its reduction with formalin or eugenol.

method, indirect restorative, *n* the technique of fabrication of a restoration on a cast or model of the original (e.g., the indirect method of inlay construction, in which a die of amalgam or other material is made from an impression of the prepared tooth, a wax pattern is formed, and the cast inlay is fitted and finished on the die and then cemented to the tooth).

method, Johnston's, *n.pr* See method, chloropercha.

method, lateral condensation, *n* the method in which a preselected gutta-percha cone is sealed into the apex of the root. The balance of the space is filled with other gutta-percha cones forced laterally with a spreader.

method, Leonard, *n.pr* a method of teeth cleaning that advocates a vigorous drawing of the toothbrush up and down across the teeth. The teeth are held apart, so that each section is brushed separately. Also known as *vertical toothbrushing.*

method, modified Stillman, *n.pr* a toothbrushing technique characterized by the placement of the toothbrush head against the gingiva, vibrating it, then rolling the bristles over the rest of the tooth's surface. Each stroke is repeated five times for each section of the oral cavity.

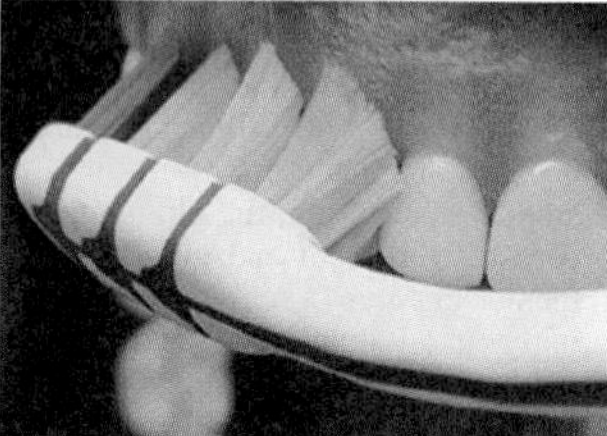

Modified Stillman method. (Daniel/Harfst/Wilder, 2008)

method, prebook, *n* a method of scheduling appointments in which the patient schedules the next appointment while checking out from the current one. A reminder postcard is filled out at this time, to be mailed later, or an e-mail reminder is stored.

method, rolling stroke, *n* a simple, introductory toothbrushing technique that does not include brushing of the gingival sulcus. Often taught to children as a precursor to the modified Stillman method, or as a preliminary framework for a more advanced technique incorporating vibration of the brush.

method, segmentation, *n* the method in which a preselected gutta-percha cone is cut into segments. The tip section is sealed into the apex of the root. The other segments are usually warmed and condensed against the first piece with a plugger. Additional pieces are then used until the space is obliterated.

method, silver cone, *n* the method in which a prefitted silver cone is sealed into the apex of the root canal. The space not sealed with the cone is obliterated with gutta-percha or sealer.

method, Smith's, *n.pr* a toothbrushing technique referred to as physiologic, in which the brush strokes mimic the path taken by food when it is chewed.

method, SOAP (subjective, objective, assessment, plan), *n* an acronym for the method for making notes to the problem-oriented record in which **S** stands for subjective data obtained from the patient or family; **O** refers to objective data acquired by observation, inspection, or testing; **A** relates to the assessment of the patient's current situation and progress made throughout the course of treatment; and **P** represents the actual patient care plan.

method, split cast, *n* **1.** a procedure for checking the ability of an articulator to receive or to be adjusted to a maxillomandibular relation record. *n* **2.** a procedure for indexing casts on an articulator to facilitate their removal and replacement on the instrument.

method, Stillman's, *n.pr* a toothbrushing technique that incorporates gingival stimulation and dental cleansing, in which the toothbrush is held against both the gingival and the dental surfaces and manually vibrated.

method, sulcal **(sul'kəl),** *n* a toothbrushing technique for controlling plaque involving placement of the bristles in the sulcus at an angle of 45° to the tooth's long axis and vibrating the bristles in a quick manner from side to side. Also called the *Bass method.*

methohexital sodium (meth'ō-hek'sitol), *n* an intravenous barbiturate prescribed for the induction of anesthesia in short surgical procedures as a supplement to other anesthetics.

methotrexate/methotrexate sodium (meth'ōtrek'sāt), *n brand names:* Folex, Mexate, Rheumatrex; *drug class:* folic acid antagonist, antineoplastic; *action:* inhibits an enzyme that reduces folic acid, which is needed for nucleic acid synthesis in all cells; *uses:* acute lymphocytic leukemia; in combination for breast, lung, head, neck cancer; lymphosarcoma, psoriasis; gestational choriocarcinoma, hydatid mole.

methoxamine HCl (methok'səmēn'), *n* an adrenergic that acts as a vasoconstrictor and is prescribed for use during anesthesia to maintain blood pressure and in the treatment of paroxysmal supraventricular tachycardia.

methsuximide (methsuk′simīd), *n* *brand name:* Celontin; *drug class:* anticonvulsant; *action:* inhibits spike wave formation in absence seizures (petit mal); decreases amplitude, frequency, duration, spread of discharge in minor motor seizures; *use:* refractory absence seizures (petit mal).

methyl methacrylate (meth′il methak′rilāt), *n* an acrylic resin, $CH_2 = C(CH_3)COOCH_3$, derived from methyl acrylic acid. Monomer is the single molecule and polymer is the polymerization product.

methylation (meth′əlā′shən), *n* **1.** the introduction of a methyl group, CH_3, to a chemical compound. *n* **2.** the addition of methyl alcohol and naphtha to ethanol to produce denatured alcohol.

methyldopa/methyldopate (meth′əldō′pə meth′əldō′pāt), *n* *brand name:* Aldomet; *drug class:* centrally acting antihypertensive; *action:* stimulates central inhibitory α-adrenergic receptors or acts as a false transmitter, resulting in reduction of arterial pressure; *use:* hypertension.

methylene blue (meth′əlēn′), *n* a bluish-green crystalline substance used as a histologic stain and as a laboratory indicator. It is also used in the treatment of cyanide poisoning and methemoglobinemia.

methylmalonicacidemia (meth′əlməlon′ikas′idē′mēə), *n* a genetic disorder of amino acid metabolism in which methylmalonic acid accumulates in the blood and urine at abnormally high levels. It may respond to a low-protein diet and the administration of synthetic amino acids. Also called *methylmalonicaciduria,* especially if the concentration is limited to or greatest in the urine.

methylphenidate HCl, *n* *brand names:* Methidate, Ritalin; *drug class:* central nervous system stimulant, related to amphetamines (Controlled Substance Schedule II); *action:* increases release of norepinephrine, dopamine in cerebral cortex to reticular activating system; exact mode of action not known; *uses:* attention deficit disorder with hyperactivity, narcolepsy.

methylprednisolone / methylprednisolone acetate/methylprednisolone sodium succinate (meth′əlprednis′əlōn′), *n* *brand names:* Medrol, Meprolone; *drug class:* immediate acting glucocorticoid; *action:* decreases inflammation by suppressing macrophage and leukocyte migration; reduces capillary permeability and inhibits lysosomal enzymes and phagocytosis; *uses:* severe inflammation, shock, adrenal insufficiency, collagen disorders.

methylxanthine (meth′ilzan′thēn), *n* diuretic agent (e.g., aminophylline, caffeine, or theophylline) that serves as a smooth muscle relaxant and cardiac muscle and CNS stimulant. Clinically, it is employed as a bronchodilator.

methysergide maleate (meth′isur′jī mā′lēāt), *n* *brand name:* Sansert; *drug class:* serotonin antagonist; *action:* competitively blocks serotonin HT receptors in central nervous system and periphery; *uses:* prophylaxis for migraine and other vascular headaches.

Meticorten, *n* the brand name for prednisone.

metoclopramide HCl (met′əklō′prəmīd′), *n* *brand name:* Clopra, Maxolon, Reglan; *drug class:* central dopamine receptor antagonist; *action:* enhances response to acetylcholine of tissue in upper GI tract, which causes contraction of gastric muscle, relaxes pyloric and duodenal segments, increases peristalsis without stimulating secretions; antiemetic action occurs centrally; *uses:* prevention of nausea, vomiting induced by chemotherapy, radiation, delayed gastric emptying, gastroesophageal reflux.

metolazone (metō′ləzōn′), *n* *brand names:* Diulo, Mykrox, Zaroxolyn; *drug class:* diuretic with thiazidelike effects; *action:* acts on distal tubule by increasing excretion of water, sodium, chloride, and potassium; *uses:* edema, hypertension, CHF.

metoprolol tartrate (met′ōprō′lol tar′trāt), *n* *brand name:* Nu Metop; *drug class:* antihypertensive selective β_1-blocker; *action:* produces fall in

M

blood pressure without reflex tachycardia or significant reduction in heart rate; *uses:* mild to moderate hypertension, acute myocardial infarction to reduce cardiovascular mortality, angina pectoris.

metric system, *n* See system, metric.

metronidazole (met′rənī′dəzōl′), *n* a generic synthetic antibacterial compound available for both oral and intravenous use. It is indicated in the treatment of serious infections caused by susceptible anaerobic bacteria. In dentistry, it is used in the treatment of HIV, periodontal disease, and aggressive periodontitis.

metronidazole HCl, *n brand name:* Flagyl, Metro IV, Protostat; *drug class:* trichomonacide, amebicide, antiinfective; *action:* direct-acting amebicide/trichomonacide binds, degrades DNA in organisms; *uses:* intestinal amebiasis, amebic abscess, trichomoniasis, refractory trichomoniasis, bacterial anaerobic infections.

MeV, *n* 1 million electron volts.

mexiletine HCl (mek′silətēn′), *n brand name:* Mexitil; *drug class:* antidysrhythmic (Class IB, lidocaine analog); *action:* blocks sodium channel in His-Purkinje system, which decreases the effective refractory period and shortens the duration of the action potential; *use:* documented life-threatening ventricular dysrhythmias.

micelle (mīsel′), *n* a space formed by the brush structure of fibrils in colloidal gels. The spaces are occupied by water in hydrocolloid impressions.

miconazole (mīkon′əzōl′), *n brand names:* Monistat, Monistat IV; *drug class:* antifungal; *action:* alters cell membranes and inhibits fungal enzymes; *uses:* coccidioidomycosis, candidiasis, cryptococcosis, paracoccidioidomycosis, fungal meningitis; IV used for severe infections only.

miconazole nitrate (topical), *n brand names:* Micatin, Monistat-7; *drug class:* antifungal; *action:* interferes with fungal cell membrane, which increases permeability, leaking of nutrients; *uses:* tinea pedis, tinea cruris, tinea corporis, tinea versicolor, vaginal or vulvar *C. albicans.*

microabrasion, *n* a procedure in which an abrasive compound is applied to the surface of teeth to remove a small amount of dental tissue.

microalbuminuria (mī′krōalbyoo′mənur′ēə), *n* a type of albuminaria that is characterized by relatively low levels of albumin in the urine (between 30 and 300 µg in 1 day). The increase in albumin secretion is generally too small to be detected by a conventional dipstick test but can indicate the beginnings of kidney disorders, especially those related to diabetes.

microangiopathy (mī′krōan′jēop′əthē), *n* a disease of the small blood vessels.

microbiology, *n* the branch of biology concerned with the study of microorganisms, including algae, bacteria, viruses, protozoa, fungi, and rickettsiae.

microbiota, *n* the microscopic organisms living within a particular region.

microcephalus (mī′krōsef′əlus), *n* an abnormally small head.

microchemistry, *n* the branch of chemistry concerned with the study of chemical processes at the cellular and subcellular levels.

microcirculation, *n* the flow of blood throughout the system of smaller vessels of the body, particularly the capillaries.

microcomputer, *n* a complete, multiuse, electronic, digital computer system consisting of a central processing unit, storage facilities, I/O ports, and a chip with megabytes of high-speed internal storage; it usually has only one user for personal, home, or office use.

microcurie, *n* one millionth of a curie.

microcyte, *n* an unusually small red blood cell associated with iron deficiency anemia.

microcytosis, hereditary (mī′krōsītō′sis), *n* See thalassemia; thalassemia major.

microdialysis, *n* a technique for measuring extracellular concentrations of substances in tissues, usually in vivo, by means of a small probe equipped with a semipermeable membrane. Substances may also be introduced into the extracellular space through the membrane.

microdontia (mī′krōdon′shēə), *n.pl* abnormally small teeth. The term may apply to one, several, or all the teeth.

M

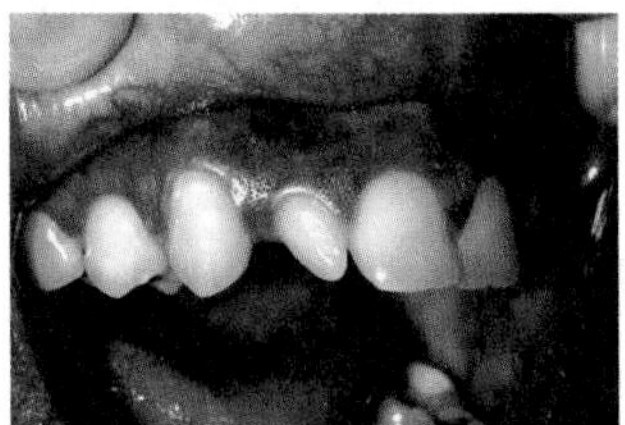

Microdontia. (Sapp/Eversole/Wysocki, 2004)

microelectrode, *n* an electrode of very fine caliber consisting usually of a fine wire or a glass tube of capillary diameter drawn to a fine point and filled with saline or a metal used in physiologic experiments to stimulate or record action currents of extracellular or intracellular origin.

microfilaments, *n.pl* any of the submicroscopic cellular filaments, such as the tonofibrils, found in the cytoplasm of most cells, that function primarily as a supportive system.

microflora, *n* a group or colony of microorganisms present in a specific, localized location.

microgenia (mī′krōjē′nēə), *n* an abnormal smallness of the chin.

microglossia (mī′krōglôs′ēə), *n* an abnormally small tongue.

micrognathia (mī′krōnāth′ēə), *n* an abnormally small jaw such as that seen in brachygnathia. See also brachygnathia; retrognathism.

microleakage, *n* the seepage of fluids, debris, and microorganisms along the interface between a restoration and the walls of a cavity preparation.

micrometer (mī′krōmēter), *n* a millionth of a meter (10^{-6} meter).

micron, *n* See micrometer.

micronutrient, *n* an organic compound such as a vitamin, or a chemical element such as zinc or iodine, that is essential only in small amounts for the normal physiologic processes of the body.

microorganism (mī′krō ōr′gənizəm), *n* a microscopic living organism, such as a bacterium, virus, rickettsia, yeast, or fungus. These may exist as part of the normal flora of the oral cavity without producing disease. With disturbance of the more or less balanced interrelationship among the organisms or between the organisms and host resistance, individual forms may overgrow and induce disease in the host's tissues. Those foreign to the individual may invade and produce pathologic processes.

microphthalmos, *n* a developmental anomaly characterized by abnormal smallness of one or both eyes.

micropore, *n* **1.** microscopic pores created by enamel etching in order to increase sealant adhesion. *n* **2.** an organelle in certain protozoa that develops at the site of a damaged membrane.

M

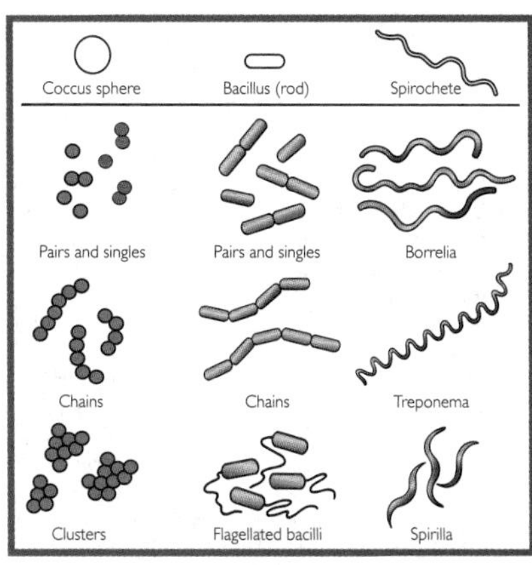

Three basic shapes. (Stepp/Woods, 1998)

microradiography (mī'krōrăd'ēog'rəfē), *n* a process by which a radiograph of a small or very thin object is produced on fine-grained photographic film under conditions that permit subsequent microscopic examination or enlargement of the radiograph within the resolution limits of the photographic emulsion, which approaches 1000 lines/mm.

microscope, *n* an instrument containing a powerful lens system for magnifying and viewing near objects.

Microscope, Confocal Laser Scanning (CLSM), *n.pr* a microscope equipped with a laser beam light source, electronic image detector, and computer for image storage and processing that is used in the laboratory to perform high-resolution, three-dimensional microscopy.

microscope, dark-field, *n* a microscope that has a special condenser and objective with a diaphragm or stop by which light is scattered from the object with the result that the object appears bright and the background dark.

microscope, electron, *n* a microsope in which electron beams with wavelengths shorter than those of visible light are used in place of visible light, allowing much greater resolution and magnification of the object.

microscope, electron, scanning (SEM), *n* an electron microscope capable of reflecting electrons from the specimen surface, resulting in a three-dimensional image of the surface that provides both high resolution and a great depth of focus view of the object.

microscope, interference, *n* a microscope designed to split entering light into two beams that pass through the specimen and are recombined in the image plane, allowing visualization of refractile object details that are not possible with a single beam.

microscope, phase-contrast, *n* a specially constructed microscope that has a special condenser and objective containing a phase-shifting mechanism whereby small differences in refraction can be made visible to intensity or contrast in the images. It is particularly helpful in examining living or unstained cells and tissues. This is an excellent aid in the education and motivation of patients in the understanding and control of dental plaque.

microscopy, *n* a technique for observing microscopic materials using a microscope.

microscopy, digital epiluminescence **(dij'itəl ep'iloo'mines'əns mīkros'kəpē),** *n* computer-aided technique that employs a binocular surface microscope to examine pigmented skin lesions.

Microsporum **(mī'krōspor'əm),** *n* a genus of dermatophytes of the family Monilaceae.

microstomia (mī'krōstō'mēə), *n* **1.** a small oral fissure. *n* **2.** the condition of having an abnormally small oral cavity.

microstrain, *n* a unit of measurement of strain. A microstrain equals the strain that produces a deformation of one part per million.

microsurgery, *n* surgery that involves microdissection and micromanipulation of tissues, usually accomplished with the aid of a binocular microscopic instrument.

microtia (mīkrō'shēə), *n* aplasia or hypoplasia of the pinna of the ear, with a closed or missing external auditory meatus.

microtubule (mī'krōtoo'būl), *n* a hollow cylindrical structure that occurs widely within plant and animal cells. Microtubules increase in number during cell division and are associated with the movement of DNA material.

microvilli (mī'krōvil'ē), *n.pl* tiny hairlike processes that extend from the surface of many cells. They are usually so small as to be visible only with an electron microscope.

midazolam HCl (midaz'əlam'), *n* *brand name:* Versed; *drug class:* benzodiazepine general anesthetic, anesthesia adjunct (Controlled Substance Schedule IV); *action:* depresses subcortical levels in central nervous system; may act on limbic system, reticular formation; may potentiate γ-aminobutyric acid (GABA) by binding to specific benzodiazepine receptors; *uses:* conscious sedation, general anesthesia induction, sedation for diagnostic endoscopic procedures, intubation, preoperative sedation.

midbrain (mid′brān), *n* the portion of the brain located superior to the pons and medulla and containing the motor nuclei of the ocular motor and trochlear nerves. It also contains the major pathways and decussations of fibers from the cerebrum and cerebellum.

middle age, *n* the period between young adult and elderly, usually 35 to 55 years of age; a period of great productivity. Also called *middle adult.*

midface, *n* the portion of the face comprising the nasal, maxillary, and zygomatic bones and the soft tissues covering these bones.

midline, *n* the line equidistant from bilateral features of the head.

midwife, *n* **1.** in traditional use, a (female) person who assists women in childbirth. **2.** a nurse practitioner trained and experienced in assisting women in childbirth.

migraine, *n* See headache, migraine.

migration, pathologic, *n* See tooth, migration of.

migration, tooth, *n* See tooth, drifting.

migratory glossitis (glosī′tis), *n* also known as *geographic tongue.* See also tongue, geographic.

migratory polyarthritis (pol′ēarthrī′tis), *n* a temporary form of arthritis caused by rheumatic fever.

milliammeter (mil′ēam′ētər), *n* a element on a radiograph machine used in dental procedures that controls the amount of current during a radiographic emission.

milliamperage control, *n* a crucial element in the operation of radiographic machinery used in dental procedures that regulates amperes and governs the current that flows toward the patient.

milliampere (mil′ēam′pir), *n* in radiography, milliamperage signifies the amount of current flowing in the tube circuit. With time (seconds), it is an indication of roentgen-ray quantity.

millicurie, *n* one thousandth of a curie.

milliliter (ml) (mil′ilē′tur), *n* the preferred unit of volume used in prescription writing. It is based on the fundamental unit, the liter. One liter equals 1000 milliliters. In prescriptions the abbreviations ml and cc are often used interchangeably because they are so nearly equal.

milling-in, *n* the procedure of refining or perfecting the occlusion of removable partial or complete dentures by placing abrasives between their occluding surfaces while the dentures make contact in various excursions on the articulator.

millirad (mil′irad′), (mr) *n* one-thousandth of a rad. Normal background radiation in this country varies from about 50 to 200 mr per year, depending on geographic location.

milliroentgen (mil′irent′gən), *n* a submultiple of the roentgen, equal to one thousandth of a roentgen.

Milwaukee brace, *n.pr* an orthotic device that helps immobilize the torso and the neck of a patient in the treatment or correction of scoliosis, lordosis, or kyphosis. Prolonged use may induce or complicate a malocclusion unless the teeth and jaws are supported with retaining appliances.

mineral oil, *n* See oil, mineral.

mineralization, *n* the bioprecipitation of an inorganic substance.

mineralized deposit, *n* calcified bacterial plaque, which may develop above or below the gingiva, on teeth, replacement teeth, or rehabilitative oral equipment.

mineralocorticoids (min′əral′ōkôr′tikoidz), *n.pl* (proinflammatory hormones), adrenal corticosteroids that are active in the retention of salt and in the maintenance of life of adrenalectomized animals. Typical are deoxycorticosterone and aldosterone. Aldosterone is a natural hormone for salt retention but also has some regulatory effect on carbohydrate metabolism.

minim (min′im), *n* a unit of volume in the traditional apothecary system. One minim equals 0.06 ml. A drop is sometimes used as a crude approximation of the minim.

minocycline HCl (min′ōsī′klēn), *n* *brand names:* Dyancin, Minocin; *drug class:* tetracycline antiinfective; *action:* inhibits protein synthesis, phosphorylation in microorganisms by binding 30S ribosomal subunits, reversibly binding to 50S ribosomal subunits; bacteriostatic; *uses:* syphilis, *Chlamydia trachomatis* infection, gonorrhea, lymphogranuloma venereum, rickettsial infections, inflammatory acne. Also used in the treatment of some periodontal infections, generally in conjunction with mechanical therapy.

minor, *n* **1.** a person of either gender under the age of majority, i.e., one who has not attained the age at which full civil rights are granted. *adj* **2.** describing a procedure or treatment that is non- or minimally invasive; describing an illness or condition that is temporary and minimally debilitating.

minor connector, *n* See connector, minor.

minoxidil (mənok′sədil′), *n brand names:* Loniten, Rogaine (topical); *drug class:* antihypertensive; *action:* directly relaxes arteriolar smooth muscle, reducing peripheral resistance; *uses:* severe hypertension not responsive to other therapy (used with a diuretic); topically to treat alopecia (mechanism unknown) and other forms of hair loss.

miosis (mīō′sis), *n* **1.** the contraction of the sphincter muscle of the iris, causing the pupil to become smaller. *n* **2.** an abnormal condition characterized by excessive constriction of the sphincter muscle of the iris, resulting in very small, pinpoint pupils.

miotic (mēot′ik), *n* a drug that constricts the pupil.

mirror, oral cavity, *n* a reflective device used to examine structures within the oral cavity and prevent the lips, cheeks, and tongue from obstructing the assessment.

misappropriation, *n* the act of benefitting financially by using someone's name or likeness without permission; e.g., using a dental patient's radiographs in an article without obtaining his or her permission.

miscible (mis′ĭbəl), *adj* may be blended or combined; mixable.

misconduct, *n* a deviation from duty by one employed in a professional capacity; a transgression of an established rule.

misfeasance (misfē′zens), *n* the improper performance of some act that one may lawfully do.

misoprostol (mī′sōprôs′til), *n brand name:* Cytotec; *drug class:* gastric mucosa protectant; *action:* a prostaglandin E_1 analog that inhibits gastric acid secretion; *uses:* prevention of nonsteroidal antiinflammatory drug-induced gastric ulcers.

misrepresentation, *n* an intentionally false statement regarding a matter of fact.

MIST, *n.pr* an acronym for Medical Information Service via Telephone. MIST is a consultation service offered by some state-operated university medical centers.

mistake, *n* an unintentional act, omission, or error resulting from ignorance, surprise, or misplaced confidence.

mitigation (mit′igā′shən), *n* alleviation; abatement or diminution of a penalty imposed by law.

mitigation of damages, *n* a reduction of damages based on facts showing that the plaintiff's course of action does not entitle the plaintiff to as large an amount as the evidence would otherwise justify the jury in allowing.

mitochondria (mī′tōkon′drēə), *n.pl* small, rodlike, threadlike, or granular organelles within the cytoplasm that function in cellular metabolism and respiration and occur in varying numbers in all living cells except bacteria, viruses, blue-green algae, and mature erythrocytes.

mitogen, *n* an agent that triggers mitosis.

mitosis, *n* a type of cell division that occurs in somatic cells and results in the formation of two genetically identical daughter cells containing the diploid number of chromosomes characteristic of the species.

mitotane (mī′tətān′), *n brand name:* Lysodren; *drug class:* antineoplastic; *action:* acts on adrenal cortex to suppress activity and adrenal steroid production; *use:* adrenocortical carcinoma.

mitotic index (mītot′ik), *n* the number of cells per unit undergoing mitosis during a given time. The ratio is used primarily as an estimation of the rate of tissue growth.

mitral valve, *n* a bicuspid valve situated between the left atrium and the left ventricle; the only valve with two, rather than three, cusps. It allows blood to flow from the left atrium into the left ventricle but prevents blood from flowing back into the atrium.

mitral valve prolapse (MVP), *n* the protrusion of one or both cusps of the mitral valve back into the left atrium during ventricular systole, resulting in incomplete closure of the valve. It may or may not be associated with mitral insufficiency (regurgitation) or a "leaky valve" and cause a heart murmur. Also called *"floppy" mitral valve.* In most cases, it is harmless and does not cause symptoms or need to be treated. Symptoms include sensation of feeling the heart beat (palpitations), chest pain (unrelated to coronary artery disease or a heart attack), difficulty breathing after exertion, fatigue, cough, shortness of breath when lying flat (orthopnea). Some forms seem to be hereditary. It has been associated with Marfan syndrome, Graves' disease, and other disorders.

mix, *v* to form by combining ingredients.

mixed dentition, *n* See dentition, mixed.

mixing, vacuum, *n* a method of mixing materials, such as gypsum products and water, in a vacuum.

MLD, *n* See dose, lethal, minimum.

MLT, *n* See time, median lethal.

MO cavity, *n* a cavity on the mesial and occlusal surfaces of a tooth. See also DO cavity, Class 2.

mobility, *n* the loosening of a tooth or teeth. It is an important diagnostic sign that may result not only from a decrease in root attachment or changes in the periodontal ligament but also from destruction of the gingival fibers and transseptal (interdental) fibers. Types are classified.

mobility of tooth, *n* See tooth mobility.

MOD cavity, *n* a cavity on the mesial, occlusal, and distal surfaces of a tooth. See also cavity, Class 2.

mode (mo), *n* a measure of central tendency that is the most frequently occurring score or value in a group of scores. The mode may be used as an average score.

model, *n* **1.** a replica, usually in miniature *n* **2.** a positive replica of the dentition and surrounding or adjoining structures used as a diagnostic aid and base for construction of orthodontic and prosthetic appliances. See also cast.

model, casting, *n* See cast, refractory.

model, implant, *n* See cast, implant.

model, of prepared cavity, *n* See die.

model, study, *n* See cast, diagnostic.

modeling compound, *n* See compound.

models, biologic, *n.pl* the use of the analog of a disease of man in some other animal species to study or compare the response or treatment of the disease before testing with humans.

models, statistical, *n.pl* statistical formulations or analyses that, when applied to data and found to fit the data, are used to verify the assumptions and parameters used in the analysis. Some examples of statistical models include the linear model, binomial model, polynomial model, and two-parameter model.

modem, *n* (modulator/demodulator), a device that converts data from a form compatible with computer manipulation to a form compatible with transmission equipment and vice versa.

moderator, *n* a chairman; one who presides over an assembly, group, or panel.

modiolus (mōdē′ōlus), *n* a point distal to the corner of the oral cavity where several muscles of facial expression converge.

modulins, microbial (moj′oolins mīkrō′bēəl), *n* the molecules that induce the synthesis of cytokine.

modulus (moj′ələs), *n* a constant that numerically indicates the amount in which a certain property is possessed by any object.

modulus of elasticity, *n* See elasticity, modulus of.

modulus of resilience, *n* See resilience, modulus of.

modulus of rigidity, *n* See rigidity.

modulus, Young's, *n.pr* See elasticity, modulus of.

moexipril hydrochloride (mōek′sipril′ hī′drōklor′īd), *n brand name:* Univasc; *drug class:* angiotensin-converting enzyme (ACE) inhibitor; *action:* selectively suppresses renin-angiotensin-aldosterone system; inhibits ACE;

M

prevents conversion of angiotensin I to angiotensin II; results in dilation of arterial, venous vessels; *use:* hypertension as a single drug or in combination with a thiazide diuretic.

Mohs scale, *n.pr* See hardness, Mohs.

Mohs surgery (mōz), *n.pr* a surgical technique used primarily in the treatment of skin neoplasms, especially basal cell or squamous cell carcinoma. This procedure is a microscopically controlled excision of cutaneous tumors either after fixation in vivo or after freezing the tissue. Serial examinations of fresh tissue specimens are most frequently done to ensure complete excision of the lesion.

molar, *n* **1.** a reference solution in which the concentration is stated with regard to the number of gram molecular weights per liter of solution. **2.** a tooth adapted for grinding by having a broad, somewhat ridged surface. It is one of the 12 teeth located in the posterior aspect of the maxillary and mandibular arches.

molar, mulberry, *n* a malformed first molar with a crown, suggesting the appearance of a mulberry. It may be a manifestation of congenital syphilis, although other diseases affecting the enamel organ during morphodifferentiation may produce a similar lesion.

molar sheath, *n* a rectangular metallic tube soldered or welded to the molar bands.

molars, second, *n* the molars posterior to the first molars and anterior to the third molars (wisdom teeth); also known as 12-year molars.

mold (mould), *n* a form in which an object is cast or shaped. The process of shaping a material into an object. The term is used to specify the shape of an artificial tooth or teeth.

molding, *n* shaping.

molding, border, *n* See border molding.

molding, compression, *n* the act of pressing or squeezing together to form a shape in a mold.

molding, injection, *n* the adaptation of a plastic material to the negative form of a closed mold by forcing the material into the mold through appropriate gateways. See also molding, compression.

molding, tissue, *n* See border molding.

mole, *n* a pigmented nevus; a benign lesion of melanin.

molecular biology, *n* the study of biology from the viewpoint of the physical and chemical interactions of molecules involved in life functions.

molecular weight, *n* See weight, molecular.

molecule, *n* a unit of matter that is the smallest particle of an element or chemical combination of atoms (as a compound) capable of retaining chemical identity with the substance in mass.

molimina, menstrual (molim′inə), *n* circulatory symptoms, psychic tension, irritable behavior, belligerence, and other personality alterations before or during menstruation. The cause is unknown.

molindone HCl (mō′lindōn′), *n* *brand name:* Moban, Moban Concentrate; *drug class:* antipsychotic; *action:* depresses cerebral cortex, hypothalamus, limbic system, which control activity, aggression; blocks neurotransmission produced by dopamine at synapse; mechanism for antipsychotic effects is unclear; *use:* psychotic disorders.

molluscum contagiosum (məlus′kəm kəntā′jēō′səm), *n* a disease of the skin and mucous membranes, caused by a poxvirus and found all over the world. It is characterized by scattered flesh-toned papules. The disease most frequently occurs in children and in adults with an impaired immune response. It is transmitted from person to person by direct or indirect contact and lasts up to 3 years.

molluscum fibrosum, *n* See neurofibromatosis.

Molt's mouth gag, *n.pr* See mouth prop, ratchet type.

molybdenum (Mo) (məlib′dənəm), *n* a grayish metallic element with an atomic number of 42 and an atomic weight of 95.94. Molybdenum is poisonous if ingested in large quantities.

momentum, *n* quantity of motion, expressed as the product of mass and velocity.

money, *n* the general term for the representation of value, currency, or cash.

moniliasis (mō′nilī′əsis), *n* infection by a fungus of the genus *Candida,* usually *C. albicans.* May involve the oral cavity (thrush), female genitalia, skin, hands, nails, and/or lungs. *Oral moniliasis* refers to thrush or to mycotic stomatitis. The latter term is sometimes applied to erythematous patches that are not typical of the usual white patches of thrush. See also thrush.

monitor, *n* to observe and evaluate a function of the body closely and constantly over time for diagnostic purposes.

monitoring, *n* the periodic or continuous determination of the dose rate in an occupied area by a person.

monitoring, ambulatory, *n* to observe and evaluate a patient while engaged in normal routine behaviors.

monitoring, area, *n* routine monitoring of the level of radiation of any particular area, building, room, equipment, or outdoor space.

monitoring, personal, *n* monitoring of a part of an individual (e.g., breath or excretions or any part of the clothing).

monitoring, personnel, *n* a systematic, periodic check of the radiation dose each person receives during working hours.

monitoring, physiologic, *n* the observation and evaluation of physiologic functions, usually with an electronic device with surface electrodes attached to specific areas of the body.

monoamine oxidase, *n* an enzyme that catalyzes the oxidation of amines.

monoamine oxidase inhibitor (MAOI), *n* an agent that blocks the oxidation and deamination of monoamines. The action of the inhibitor may increase the presence of catecholamines, which have antidepressant properties, but it is used for a range of disorders. It can include isocarboxazid (Marplan), phenelzine (Nardil), and tranylcypromine (Parnate). There are relative contraindications of the use of the drug with local anesthetic agents delivered in the dental office.

monobloc, *n* See activator.

monocyte (mon′osīt), *n* a large mononuclear leukocyte with an ovoid or kidney-shaped nucleus, containing chromatin material with a lacy pattern and abundant gray-blue cytoplasm filled with fine, reddish, and azurophilic granules. They are produced by the bone marrow from hematopoietic stem cell precursors called monoblasts and circulate in the bloodstream for about 1 to 3 days and then typically move into tissues throughout the body. They make up 3% to 8% of the leukocytes in the blood. In the tissues, monocytes mature into different types of macrophages at different anatomic locations. They are responsible for phagocytosis (ingestion) of foreign substances in the body. They can perform phagocytosis using intermediary (opsonising) proteins such as antibodies or complement that coat the pathogen, as well as by binding to the microbe directly via pattern-recognition receptors that recognize pathogens. They are also capable of killing infected host cells via antibody, termed *antibody-mediated cellular cytotoxicity.* They can increase in amount with certain disease. See also monocytosis.

monocytosis (mon′ōsītō′sis), *n* an increase in the number of monocytes in the peripheral bloodstream. Various limits are given (e.g., a total number in excess of 800/mm^3, regardless of the percentage, or a total greater than 8% with the total number less than 800). It may be associated with chronic pyogenic infections, bacterial endocarditis, infectious hepatitis, monocytic leukemia, rickettsial disease, and protozoan infections.

monofilament, *n* a single strand of untwisted synthetic material such as nylon; used to create surgical sutures.

monogenic (mon′əjen′ik), *adj* a trait controlled by a single gene or a single pair of genes. Monogenic traits often are associated with hereditary disorders.

monomer (mon′ōmur), *n* a single molecule. In commercial resin products, the term applies to the liquid, which is usually a mixture of monomers.

monomer, residual, *n* the unpolymerized monomer remaining in the appliance or restoration after processing.

mononucleosis, infectious (mon′ōnoo′klēō′sis), *n* (acute benign lymphadenosis, "kissing disease"), an acute infectious viral disease most commonly affecting young adults and older children. Manifestations include fever, sore throat, cervical lymphadenopathy, petechial hemorrhages of the soft palate, and, at times, purpura with thrombocytopenia. Early leukopenia and relative lymphocytosis occur, with later increases in the number of large leukocytoid lymphocytes. The heterophil (usually sheep cell) antibody titer is significantly increased in most instances.

monostotic, *n* affecting a single bone.

Monotremata **(mon′ōtrē′mətə),** *n* the lowest order of mammals, including animals that lay eggs similar to those of reptiles, and nourish their young by a mammary gland that has no nipple, in a shallow pouch developed during lactation. The only living representatives are the spiny anteater and the duck-billed platypus.

Monson curve, *n.pr* See curve, Monson.

moot (mŏŏt), *adj* **1.** subject to argument, undecided. *adj* **2.** in law, in a moot case one seeks to determine that an abstract question does not arise on existing facts or rights.

moral, *adj* relating to the conscience or moral sense or to the general principles of correct conduct.

morale, *n* the mental state or condition as related to cheerfulness, confidence, and zeal.

morbidity, *n* the state of being diseased. Can be used as an outcome measure such as number of decayed, missing, and filled teeth.

moricizine (moris′izēn′), *n brand name:* Ethmozine; *drug class:* antidysrhythmic, type I; *action:* decreased rate of rise of action potential, which prolongs the refractory period and shortens the action potential duration; *use:* documented life-threatening dysrhythmias.

morphine (môr′fēn), *n* an effective prescription analgesic narcotic. Street names include *M, white stuff, Miss Emma, hocus,* and *monkey.* Constricted pupils may be a sign of abuse.

morphine sulfate, *n brand names:* Duramorph PF, MS Contin, Roxanol; *drug class:* narcotic analgesic (Controlled Substance Schedule II); *action:* depresses pain impulse transmission at the central nervous system by interacting with opioid receptors; *use:* severe pain.

morphogenesis, *n* the development and differentiation of the structures and the form of an organism, specifically the changes that occur in the cells and tissue during embryonic development.

morphology (môrfol′əjē), *n* the branch of biology that deals with the form and structure of an organism or part, without regard to function.

morphology, determinants of occlusal, *n.pl* variable factors that determine the forms given to the crowns of teeth restored in metals, such as mandibular centricity; the intercondylar distance; the distance of teeth from the sagittal plane; the character of lateral and protrusive paths of the condylar axes; and the overlaps of the anterior teeth and wear.

mortality, *n* the death rate.

mortgage, *n* a right given to the creditor over the property of the debtor for the security of the debt; invests the creditor with the power to have the property seized and sold in default of payment.

motion, *n* envelope of the three-dimensional space circumscribed by border movements and by occlusal contacts of a given point of the mandible. Also called *movement space.* See also movement, border, posterior.

motivation, *n* the stimulus, incentive, or inducement to act or react in a certain way. Purposeful behavior is motivated behavior, which means that either physiologic or social stimuli activate or motivate a person to do something.

motivation, external, *n* incentive that accrues as a result of influence from outside sources; inducement to act or change based on the expectations and examples of other people.

motivation, internal, *n* incentive that accrues from within an individual;

inducement to act or change based on an inherent or intrinsic desire.

motor, *n* pertaining to a muscle, nerve, or center that produces or affects movement.

motor neuron, *n* one of the various efferent nerve cells that transmit nerve impulses from the brain or from the spinal cord to muscular or glandular tissue.

motor neuron disease, *n* a progressive disease that tends to affect middle-age men with degeneration of anterior horn cells, motor cranial nerve nuclei, and pyramidal tracts (e.g., amyotrophic lateral sclerosis).

motor output, *n* the activity that results from the integrative phenomena associated with brain activity. It is expressed in function as muscle contraction of the smooth and striated muscle and as secretion of the exocrine and endocrine glands and, in effect, represents the total behavioral activity. Whereas sensory phenomena have many avenues that feed into the brain, motor activity is expressed in terms of the simple, direct state of muscle contraction and glandular secretion. Thus muscle activity is expressed in terms of locomotion, hand-learned skills, speaking, mastication, and all forms of activity that involve motion.

motor pathway, *n* all reflex actions of muscle are achieved by the passage of nerve impulses through the final common pathway—the muscle fibers. The lower motor neuron (the motor route of the cranial nerve) is the final pathway for the structures that are innervated by the cranial nerves. Impulses traverse these nerves to their respective muscles from every level of the spinal cord, hindbrain, midbrain, and cerebral cortex. The cranial motor neurons collate these multiple stimuli and transmit sequences of stimuli to the motor end-plate, which in the normal muscle effects a smooth, continuous, controlled contraction.

motor skill, *n* the ability to make the purposeful movements that are necessary to complete or master a prescribed task.

motor unit, *n* the entity consisting of the lower motor neuron, motor end-plate, and muscle fibers supplied by the end-plate. The final motor activity resulting from a sequence of stimulations to the lower motor neuron is considered a function of the motor unit. The proportion of nerve fibers to the muscle fibers in motor units is designated as the innervation ratio. They may have ratios ranging from 1:4 to 1:150. The closer the ratio approximates unity, the greater the finesse of specificity of the muscular action. The eye muscles have the highest ratio of striated muscles, and the tongue, facial, masticatory, and pharyngeal muscles succeed in that order.

mottled enamel, *n* See fluorosis, chronic endemic dental.

moulage (moolazh′), *n* a model of a part or a lesion (e.g., a model of the face). It may be of wax or plaster and usually is colored by painting.

moulage, facial **(moolazh′fā′shəl),** *n* a facial model made using an impression. These models are used to construct facial prostheses or custom face masks.

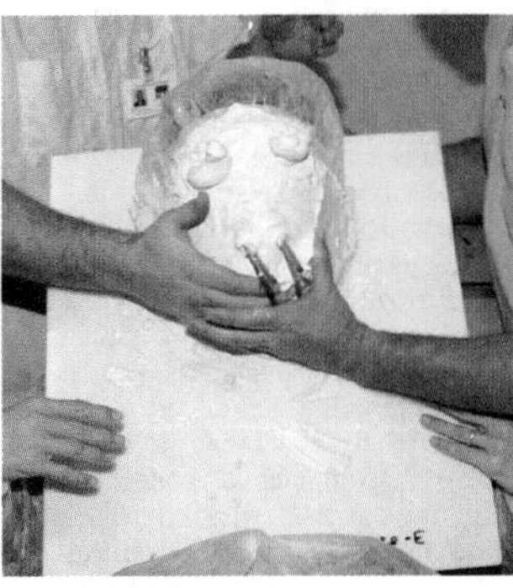

Facial moulage. (Courtesy Dr. David Nunez)

mould, *n* See mold.

mount, radiographic, *n* a windowed, stiff material on which non-digital radiographs are arranged in a specific order to correspond with the charts of the teeth.

mounting, *n* the laboratory procedure of attaching the maxillary or mandibular cast to an articulator or similar instrument.

mounting board, *n* a jig used in mounting the maxillary cast on the top articulator frame. The mounting board enables the dental professional to determine the patient's axis so that the maxillary cast can be positioned accurately.

mounting, split cast, *n* a cast with the margins of its base or capital beveled or grooved to permit accurate remounting on an articulator. Split remounting metal plates may be used instead of beveling or grooving in the casts.

mouth (mouth), *n* the oral cavity.

mouth breathing, *n* See breathing, mouth.

mouth, denture-sore, *n* traumatization and inflammation of the oral mucosa produced by ill-fitting dentures, hypersensitivity to the chemical components of the denture, or proliferation of *Candida albicans* with subsequent monilial infection.

mouth, floor of, *n* area within the oral cavity located beneath the ventral surface of the tongue.

mouth guard, *n* See guard, mouth.

mouth hygiene, *n* See hygiene, oral.

mouth preparation, *n* See preparation, mouth.

mouth rehabilitation, *n* See rehabilitation, mouth.

mouth, trench, *n* See gingivitis, necrotizing ulcerative.

mouthrinse, *n* See mouthwash.

mouthstick, *n* a device designed for use by quadriplegics and people with limited arm and hand mobility secondary to paralysis. The device fits into the oral cavity and enables the physically disabled to perform simple tasks such as dialing a telephone, using a computer keyboard, or turning the pages of a book.

mouthwash, *n* a mouth rinse possessing cleansing, germicidal, or palliative properties. Only some are approved by the ADA for treatment of gingivitis.

mouthwash, alcohol in, *n* a key ingredient in commercial oral rinses; helps oil-based ingredients blend into product. Typically constitutes from 15% to 30% of the solution. Serves to decrease surface tension while increasing the rinse's astringent properties. May be drying to the oral mucosa.

mouthwash, deodorants in, *n* a number of active ingredients including chlorophyll; added to oral rinses to decrease unpleasant smells that are the result of unbrushed teeth.

mouthwash, flavoring agents in, *n* an additive in oral rinses designed to enhance the product's taste. Agents are typically derived from aromatic waters and essential oils.

mouthwash, sodium benzoate, *n* a solution used prior to brushing teeth for the purpose of freshening the mouth. Long-term studies have not proved this to be effective in reducing gingivitis.

movement(s), *n* a change of place or of position of a body.

movement, Bennett, *n.pr* the bodily lateral movement or lateral shift of the mandible resulting from the movements of the condyles along the lateral inclines of the mandibular fossae during lateral jaw movement.

movement, bodily, *n* movement of a tooth so that the crown and root apex move the same amount in the same direction, thus maintaining the same axial inclination; opposed to tipping movement.

movement, border, *n* an extreme muscular movement limited by bone, ligaments, or other soft tissues.

movement, free mandibular, *n* mandibular movement made without tooth interference. An uninhibited movement of the mandible.

movement, hinge, *n* an opening or closing movement of the mandible on the hinge axis. A movement around a single axis.

movement, lateral, *n* a movement of a body to one side of its established position.

movement, mandibular, *n* any movement of the lower jaw.

movement, mandibular gliding, *n* side-to-side, protrusive, and intermediate movement of the mandible, occurring when the teeth or other occluding surfaces are in contact.

movement, nonfunctional mandibular, *n* movement of the mandible for other than the accepted range of functional movements; i.e., movements dictated by tension, emotion, or aggression. Also, mandibular movements may be misused to hold objects in either indulgent or work habits. These nonfunctional movements may result in a variety of pathologic manifestations.

movement, opening mandibular, n the movement of the mandible executed during jaw separation.

movement, posterior border, n a movement of the mandible occurring while the mandible is in its most posterior relation to the maxillae. This movement occurs in the vertical plane from the level of occlusal contact to the level of maximal opening of the jaws.

movement, tipping, n the movement of a tooth in any direction while its apex remains in almost the original position.

movement, tooth, n temporary or permanent deviation of a tooth from its normally fixed position in the dental arch. Also, mobility of teeth. When teeth exhibit mobility patterns, movement may be buccolingual, mesiodistal, occlusoapical, or rotational. Movement of teeth into different positions in the dental arch may be produced by repositioning them mesially, distally, buccally, lingually, or occlusally.

movement, translatory, n the motion of a body at any instant when all points within the body are moving at the same velocity and in the same direction.

movements, functional mandibular, n all natural, proper, or characteristic movements of the mandible made during speaking, chewing, yawning, swallowing, and other associated movements.

movements, intermediary (intermediate movement), n all mandibular movements between the extremes of mandibular excursions.

movements, jaw, n all changes in position of which the mandible is capable.

movements, masticatory mandibular, n the translatory and rotary movements of the mandible that are used in the course of chewing food.

moxibustion (mok′sibus′chən), *n* a method of producing analgesia or altering the function of a system of the body by igniting moxa, wormwood, or some other combustible, slow-burning substance and holding it as near the point on the skin as possible without causing pain or burning. It is also sometimes used in conjunction with acupuncture.

MPD, *n* See dose, maximum permissible.

MSH, *n* See hormone, melanocyte-stimulating.

mucin (mū′sin), *n* a mucopolysaccharide, the chief ingredient of mucus. It is present in most glands that secrete mucus and is the lubricant that protects body surfaces from friction or erosion.

mucobuccal fold, *n* See fold, mucobuccal.

mucocele (mū′kōsēl), *n* See mucous escape reaction.

mucoepidermoid tumor (mū′kōep′əder′moid), *n* a malignant neoplasm of glandular tissues, especially the ducts of the salivary glands. The tumor contains mucinous and epidermoid squamous cells.

mucogingival (mū′kōjin′jəvəl), *adj* **1.** of or pertaining to both the oral mucosa and the gingival tissues. **2.** of or pertaining to the line at which the oral mucosa and the gingival tissues join, such as in the mucogingival junction.

mucolabial fold, *n* See fold, mucolabial.

mucopolysaccharides (mū′kōpol′ēsak′ərīdz′), *n.pl* a generic term for a group of compounds composed of protein and complex sugars (polysaccharides), many of which are found in blood group substances.

mucopolysaccharidosis (MPS), *n* a genetic disorder involving mucopolysaccharide metabolism and leading to excess storage of the material in the tissues. Forms include MPS I, II, III, IV, V, and VI. Eponymic designations are Hurler, Hunter, Sanfilippo, Morquio, Scheie, and Maroteaux-Lamy syndromes.

mucosa (mūkō′sə), *n* (mucous membrane), a membrane, composed of epithelium and lamina propria.

mucosa, alveolar, n the covering on the alveolar process loosely attached to bone that extends from the mucogingival junction to the vestibular epithelium and from the mandible to the sublingual sulcus.

mucosa, lining, n a primary protective mucous membrane that lines the oral cavity. It covers the movable tissues of the soft palate, labial and buccal mucosa, ventral surface of the tongue, and the floor of the oral cavity. It comprises connective tissue and nonkeratinized stratified squamous epithelium.

mucosa, masticatory, n a mucosa comprising the connective tissue and keratinized, stratified squamous epithelium within the oral cavity that protects the areas frequently utilized for the chewing of food (e.g., hard palate and gingiva). See also mucosa, oral.

mucosa, nonkeratinized, n mucosa in which the cells of the stratified squamous epithelium maintain their cytoplasm and nuclei. It is associated with lining mucosa. See also mucosa, oral.

mucosa, oral, n the mucous membrane lining of the oral cavity, composed of stratified squamous epithelium and the underlying lamina propria.

mucosa, palatine, n the mucosa covering the palate.

M

mucoserous acinus (mu″kose′rəs as′ĭnəs), *n* a group of secretory cells of the salivary glands from which both mucous and serous salivary products are produced. See also acinus.

mucositis (mū′kōsī′tis), *n* an inflammation of the mucous membrane.

mucositis, chronic atrophic senile, n oral mucosal inflammation characterized by atrophy and found primarily in elderly women.

mucositis, fusospirochetal, n oral mucosal inflammation associated with fusiform and spirochetal microorganisms.

mucostatic, *adj* **1.** pertaining to the normal, relaxed condition of mucosal tissues covering the jaws. *adj* **2.** an agent that arrests the secretion of mucus.

mucous acinus (mū′kus as′ənəs), *n* a group of secretory cells of the salivary glands from which a type of mucous salivary product is produced.

mucous escape reaction (mucous extravasation phenomenon, mucocele), *n* nodular lesions (not cysts) on the oral mucosa caused by the escape of seromucous fluids from damaged minor salivary gland ducts. Such lesions fluctuate in size and can be treated by removing the affected minor salivary gland lobule.

mucous membrane, *n* See mucosa.

mucous membrane pemphigoid, *n* See pemphigoid, benign mucous membrane.

mucous patch, *n* See patch, mucous.

mucoviscidosis (mū′kōvis′idō′sis), *n* See disease, fibrocystic.

mucus (mū′kus), *n* the viscous, slippery secretions of mucous membranes and glands, containing mucin, white blood cells, water, inorganic salts, and exfoliated cells.

mulberry molars, *n.pl* the first permanent molars in which the occlusal surface is composed of an aggregate of enamel nodules. If all molars are involved, it is usually as the result of congenital syphilis.

mulling (mul′ing), *n* the final step of mixing dental amalgam; a kneading of the triturated mass to complete the amalgamation.

multiculturalism, *n* a philosophy that recognizes ethnic diversity within a society and that encourages others to be enlightened by worthwhile contributions to society by those of diverse ethnic backgrounds.

multifactorial, *adj* related to or produced by a number of elements or causes.

multilocular (mul″tĭlok′ulər), *adj* containing several cells, units, or spaces.

multiple sclerosis (sklərō′sis), *n* a progressive disease characterized by disseminated demyelination of nerve fibers of the brain and spinal cord. It begins slowly, usually in young adulthood, and continues throughout life with periods of exacerbation and remission. The first signs are paresthesias, or abnormal sensations in the extremities or on one side of the face. Other early signs are muscle weakness, vertigo, and visual disturbances.

multiple sclerosis, primary progressive, n form of multiple sclerosis in which the symptoms become progressively and steadily worse over time.

multiple sclerosis, progressive relapsing, n a very rare form of multiple sclerosis in which the symptoms become progressively worse over time, but in which the patient also experiences periods of accelerated deterioration.

multiple sclerosis, relapsing-remitting, *n* a form of multiple sclerosis in which the patient experiences periods of acute deterioration but is relatively stable between such periods.

multiple sclerosis, secondary progressive, *n* a form of multiple sclerosis in which the symptoms become progressively and steadily worse over time. May include periods of acute deterioration in patients with relapsing-remitting multiple sclerosis.

multiple trauma, *n* a number of injuries sustained during the same accident or assault.

multiprocessing, *n* the use of two or more processors in a system configuration. One processor controls the system, and the others are subordinate to it.

multiprogramming, *n* a technique for permitting more than one program to time-share machine components. This technique permits the concurrent handling of numerous programs by one computer.

multivariate analysis, *n* a set of techniques used when variation in several variables has to be studied simultaneously. In statistics, multivariate analysis is interpreted as any analytic method that allows simultaneous study of two or more dependent variables.

mumps, *n* (parotitis), a contagious parotitis caused by the mumps virus (paramyxovirus) and characterized by swelling of the parotid gland and sometimes swelling of the pancreas, ovaries, and testicles. The incubation period is 12 to 20 days; transmission is by droplet spread and direct contact; communicability begins about 2 days before the appearance of symptoms and lasts until swelling of the glands has abated. Vaccination is available in childhood. See also parotitis.

mumps, iodide, *n* (iodine mumps), an enlargement of the thyroid gland resulting from iodides.

mumps, iodine, *n* See mumps, iodide.

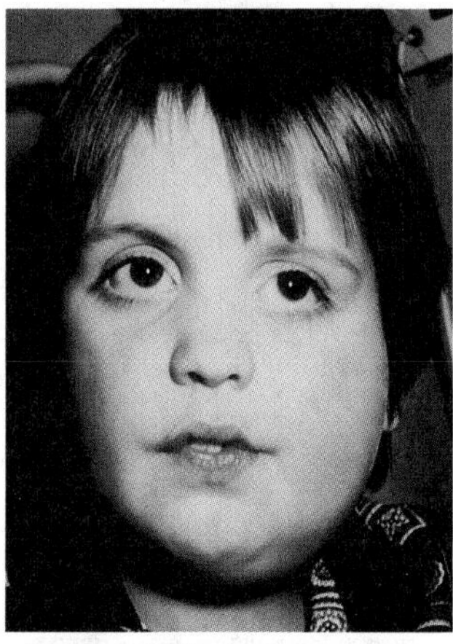

Mumps. (Zitelli/Davis, 2002. Courtesy GDW McKendrick)

mupirocin/mupirocin calcium (mūpir′ōsin), *n brand name:* Bactroban; *drug class:* topical antiinfective, pseudomonic acid A; *action:* inhibits bacterial protein synthesis; *uses:* impetigo caused by *Staphylococcus aureus,* β-hemolytic *Streptococcus, Staphylococcus pyogenes;* nasal membranes: *S. aureus.*

murmur, *n* a humming or blowing sound heard on auscultation.

murmur, aortic, a murmur resulting from insufficiency of the aortic valve secondary to involvement by rheumatic fever or tertiary syphilis.

murmur, apical diastolic, *n* a murmur heard over the apex of the heart and caused by mitral stenosis, relative mitral stenosis, or aortic insufficiency.

murmur, apical systolic, *n* a murmur heard at the apex of the heart in systole and caused by mitral insufficiency, which may result from rheumatic heart disease, or by relative mitral insufficiency, which may result from congestive heart failure associated with arteriosclerosis or hypertension. It may also have a functional basis.

murmur, basal diastolic, *n* a murmur heard over the base of the heart and caused by aortic insufficiency resulting from rheumatic heart disease or syphilis, relative aortic insufficiency associated with diastolic

M

hypertension, or a patent ductus arteriosus.

murmur, basal systolic, *n* a murmur heard over the base of the heart and caused by aortic stenosis resulting from rheumatic heart disease or by relative stenosis of the aortic valve resulting from aortic dilation secondary to arteriosclerosis or hypertension. It may also be functional or may result from congenital heart or vascular defects.

murmur, cardiac, *n* (heart murmur), an abnormal sound heard in the region of the heart at any time during the heart's cycle. They may be named according to the area of generation (mitral, aortic, pulmonary, or tricuspid) and according to the period of the cycle (diastolic or systolic).

murmur, functional, *n* (innocent murmur, inorganic murmur), a murmur resulting from the position of the body, severe anemia, or polycythemia. Not related to structural changes in the heart.

murmur, heart, *n* See murmur, cardiac.

murmur, innocent, *n* See murmur, functional.

murmur, inorganic, *n* See murmur, functional.

murmur, mitral, *n* a heart murmur produced by a defect in the mitral valve. It is the most common form of murmur in rheumatic heart disease.

murmur, organic, *n* a murmur resulting from structural changes in the heart or in the great vessels of the heart.

muscle(s), *n* an organ that, by cellular contraction, produces the movements of life. The two varieties of muscle structure are striated, which includes all the muscles in which contraction is voluntary and the heart muscle (in which contraction is involuntary), and unstriated, smooth, or organic, which includes all the involuntary muscles (except the heart), such as the muscular layer of the intestines, bladder, and blood vessels. See also each of the individual muscles of the head and neck as they are listed.

muscle, buccinator **(buk′sinātər),** *n* the muscle consisting of three bands and composing the wall of the cheek between the mandible and the maxilla; it causes the cheek to stay tight to the teeth and the lip corners to pull inward. It is often known as the "cheek muscle."

muscle, ciliary **(sil′ēer′ē),** *n* a tiny smooth muscle at the junction of the cornea and sclera, consisting of two groups of fibers: circular fibers, which exert parasympathetic control through the oculomotor nerve and the ciliary ganglion, and radial fibers, which exert sympathetic control. Ciliary muscles are responsible for accommodation for far vision through flattening of the lens.

muscle, concentric, contraction, *n* See contraction, muscle, concentric.

muscle contraction, *n* See contraction, muscle.

muscle, digastric **(dīgas′trik),** *n* suprahyoid muscle that helps activate the jaw for mastication and swallowing. It has both an anterior and a posterior belly. See also deglutition; mastication; muscle, hyoid.

muscle, eccentric, contraction, *n* See contraction, muscle, eccentric.

muscle, elasticity of, physical, *n* the physical quality of being elastic, of yielding to passive physical stretch.

muscle, elasticity of, physiologic, *n* the biologic quality, unique for muscle, of being able to change and resume size under neuromuscular control.

muscle fatigue, *n* the depletion of the metabolites necessary to sustain or repeat a muscle contraction.

muscle fiber, *n* the cell of muscle tissue. The three types of muscle fibers are striated (voluntary), cardiac, and smooth (involuntary).

muscle, functional changes of, *n.pl* asymmetric modifications in length, diameter, and bulk of muscle fibers as a result of variations in function. Muscle responds to normal function by maintenance of bulk. An increase in bulk is caused by an increase in the number of capillaries and in the mean diameter of individual muscle fibers. The response to function accounts for the asymmetry of the musculature, which is frequently found when the growth patterns have been influenced by a traumatogenic agent such as disease, injury, or surgery, and also by the functional processes of the body itself, such as posture and habit. Asymmetry is not necessarily pathologic; i.e., it may be the result of differences in habits of chewing, incision, speech sounds, and facial gestures.

muscle, genioglossus **(jē′nēōglô-s′us),** *n* an extrinsic tongue muscle that originates from the genial tubercles of the mandible and extends inside the tongue. It aids in tongue extension and prevents respiratory obstruction.

muscle, geniohyoid **(jē′nēōhī′oid),** *n* suprahyoid muscle attached to the superior surface of the hyoid bone. This muscle, which is used for mastication and swallowing, originates on the genial tubercles of the mandible and extends along the floor of the oral cavity. See also deglutition; mastication; muscle, hyoid.

muscle, hyoglossus **(hī′ōglôs′əs),** *n* an extrinsic tongue muscle that originates from the hyoid bone and extends on the lateral surface of the body of the tongue. It depresses the tongue during mastication and speech.

muscle, hypertenseness, *n* an increased muscular tension that is not easily released but that does not prevent normal lengthening of the muscle. Hypertenseness is found in patients with general nervousness.

muscle, innervation of, reciprocal, *n* a phenomenon of antagonistic muscles demonstrated during a concentric contraction such as that of the temporal muscle. Innervation of the antagonist, the external pterygoid muscle, is partially inhibited, so that freedom of action in flexing the temporomandibular joint is possible. This phenomenon demonstrates inhibition of antagonistic skeletal muscles in a reflex arc brought about automatically by a reduction of the motor discharges from the central nervous system. One of the two muscles in the reflex arc is activated, and the activity of the other is depressed.

muscle, isometric, contraction, *n* See contraction, muscle, isometric.

muscle, isotonic, contraction, *n* See contraction, muscle, isotonic.

muscle, lateral pterygoid **(lat′ərəl ter′igoid),** *n* the muscle whose superior head attaches to the sphenoid bone and whose inferior head attaches to the pterygoid plate. This muscle moves the jaw from side to side. Also known as the *external pterygoid muscle.*

muscle, masseter **(məsē′tər),** *n* one of the four muscles of mastication. The thick rectangular muscle in the cheek that functions to close the jaw. The masseter muscle arises from the zygomatic arch and inserts into the mandible at the corner of the jaw.

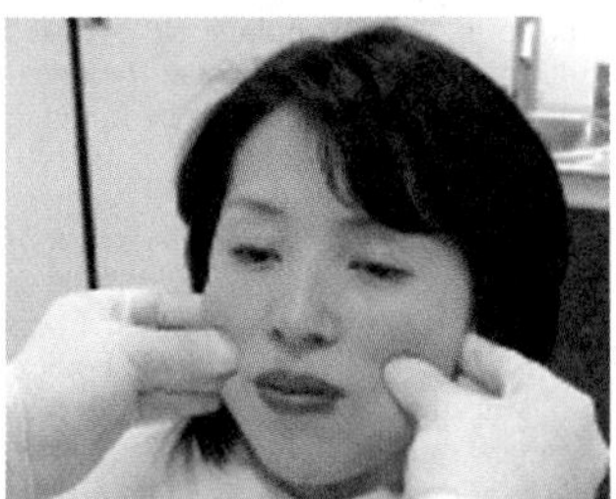

Palpation of the masseter muscle. (Rosenstiel/Land/Fujimoto, 2006)

muscle memory, *n* a kinesthetic phenomenon by which a muscle or set of muscles may involuntarily produce movement that follows a pattern that has become established by frequent repetition over a long period.

muscle, mentalis **(mental′əs),** *n* the muscle in the chin that originates in the incisive fossa and is inserted into the skin of the chin; it lifts the lower lip and wrinkles the skin of chin.

muscle, mylohyoid, *n* suprahyoid muscle originating from the mandible. It helps to raise the tongue and lower the mandible for mastication and swallowing and also forms the floor of the oral cavity. See also deglutition; mastication; muscles, hyoid.

muscle, omohyoid **(ō′mōhī′oid),** *n* infrahyoid muscle with both inferior and superior bellies. It is used for chewing and swallowing. See also muscles, hyoid.

muscle, orbicularis oris **(orbik′yəlar′əs or′is),** *n* the muscle that encircles the oral cavity; it encompasses both fibers proper to the lips as well as the adjacent facial muscles. Also known as the "kissing muscle" for its puckering role, it is intimately involved in the opening and closing of the oral cavity.

***muscle, palatoglossal* (pal′ətōglos′əl),** *n* the interior palate muscle that serves to raise and lower the posterior part of the tongue.

***muscle, palatopharyngeus* (pal′ətōferin′jēəs),** *n* the muscle that extends from the soft palate to the walls of the laryngopharynx and the thyroid cartilage to form the posterior facial pillars; it is used during swallowing to cover the opening of the nasopharynx by moving the palate and the posterior pharyngeal wall.

muscle, physical characteristics of primary, elasticity, *n.pl* a muscle is an elastic body. Its individual fibers follow Hooke's law of elastic bodies: that is, the amount of elongation is proportional to the stretching force. The muscle organs contain tissue other than muscle fibers and thus deviate slightly from this law. The human muscle fiber can contract to about half its total length.

M

***muscle, platysma* (plətiz′mə),** *n* the muscle that extends from the clavicle and shoulder, along the neck, to the mandible and the muscles surrounding the oral cavity; it allows the corners of the oral cavity to be pulled down in a grimace and the skin of the neck to be raised into ridges and depressions.

muscle, regeneration of reproduction or repair of muscle fiber, *n* a sequela to many types of muscle damage. Reparation is always associated with the proliferation of sarcolemmic nuclei. Connective tissue elements do not participate in this process except to bridge the gap and offer support for the regenerative fibers. The regenerative process takes place in two forms: regeneration by budding from the surviving parts of the muscle fibers, which occurs when segments of the muscle fiber and its sheath are destroyed, and regeneration by proliferation of cellular bands, which occurs when the sarcolemmic nuclei are spared and can form a sarcoplasmic band by linkage of the cytoplasmic processes.

muscle relaxation, *n* the resting state of a muscle fiber or a group of muscle fibers.

muscle reposition, *n* surgical replacement of a muscle attachment into a more acceptable functional position.

muscle, sequence of, development, *n* the pattern of embryologic muscular development. The muscles of the neck and trunk are the first to develop; they are followed by the lingual and facial musculature and then by the distal and proximal appendicular musculature.

muscle, smooth, *n* the simplest of the three types of muscle (smooth, striated, and cardiac). It is the muscle of the lining of the digestive tract, ducts of glands, and viscera associated with the gut. It also supplies the muscles for the genitourinary tract, structures of the blood vessels, connective tissues of the mucous membranes, and skin with its appendages. A typical fiber is a slender, spindle-shaped body averaging a few tenths of a millimeter in length. There is a single, centrally striated nucleus. The cytoplasm appears homogeneous. The cells are arranged in bands, or bundles, with interspersed connective tissue fibers uniting them into an effective common mass. They are innervated in part by nerve fibers and in part by the contraction of adjacent muscle tissues. The digestive tract, particularly, demonstrates waves of contraction that pass along a band of smooth muscle.

muscle, spasticity of, *n* increased muscular tension of antagonists that prevents normal movement; caused by an inability to relax (a loss of reciprocal inhibition) resulting from a lesion of the upper motor neuron.

muscle, sternocleidomastoid (SCM), *n* a muscle of the neck that is attached to the mastoid process and superior nuchal line and by separate heads to the sternum and clavicle. It functions with other muscles to turn the head from side to side and tilt the head to one side or the other. It separates the neck region into triangles.

muscle, sternothyroid (stur′nōthī′roid), *n* infrahyoid muscle that runs from the sternum to the thyroid cartilage and depresses the larynx and the thyroid cartilage for mastication and swallowing. See also deglutition; mastication; muscle, hyoid.

muscle, striated **(strī'ātəd),** *n* skeletal muscles forming the bulk of the body; the voluntary muscles derived from the myotomes of the embryo. Generally, they are organized as formed muscles that attach to and move the skeletal structures. The cells are large, elongated, and cylindric, with lengths ranging from 1 mm to several centimeters. The cells have multiple nuclei that are peripherally situated and scattered along the length of the fiber. The fiber contains a large number of elongated fibers that, under the microscope, appear as the alternating light and dark bands that give the characteristic striated appearance of striated muscle. The dimensional relationships between these light and dark bands are altered during contraction of the muscle fiber. The potential interaction between these bands permits the wide range of selective purposeful and rapid activity of the skeletal muscles.

muscle striations (strīā'shənz), *n.pl* the transverse alternating light and dark bands of skeletal muscles that result from differences in light absorption. The light bands contain actin and are called "I" bands because they are isotropic to polarized light. The dark areas contain myosin filaments and are called "A" bands because they are anisotropic to polarized light.

muscle, styloglossus **(stī'lōglôs'us),** *n* an extrinsic tongue muscle that originates from the styloid process and inserts on the lateral surface of the tongue. It is used to retract the tongue.

muscle, stylohyoid, *n* suprahyoid muscle that extends from the styloid process to the hyoid bone and is used for mastication and swallowing. See also deglutition; mastication; muscles, hyoid.

muscle, thyrohyoid, *n* infrahyoid muscle that extends from the thyroid cartilage to the hyoid bone and is used for mastication and swallowing. See also deglutition; mastication; muscles, hyoid.

muscle tonus, *n* the steady reflex contraction that resides in the muscles concerned in maintaining erect posture. Tonus has its basis in the positional interactions of the muscle and its accompanying nerve structure; e.g., a muscle holds the body (mandible) in a given position, and the awareness of this position is constantly being relayed by the sensory approaches to the cortex. A change in position or contractility of the muscle that affects its tonus is immediately relayed by the sensory apparatus for readjustment. Also called tone.

muscle tonus, facial **(tō'nus),** *n* the tone of the facial musculature, which is a major factor in providing the esthetic values of the face. The configurations of the face, which are maintained by good muscle tonus, are the modiolus, philtrum, nasolabial sulcus, and mentolabial sulcus. These functional contours are present when the nerve tissue is intact. They are altered by the loss of teeth or impaired nerve function. Their presence is an indication of a good state of health of the nerve and possibly of the dental arch.

muscle trimming, *n* See border molding and impression, correctable.

muscles, cervical, *n.pl* the large muscles used to turn or lower the head or to shrug the shoulders. This group includes the sternocleidomastoid and trapezius muscles.

muscles, elevator, *n* muscles of the body that serve to raise the body part with which they are associated. E.g., the mandibular elevator muscles raise the jaw.

muscles, facial, *n.pl* these muscles are quite variable in contour, are widely distributed over the scalp and face, and tend to be especially concentrated around the orbits, outer ear, and lips. It is the mobility of the lips that has extended the usefulness of these muscles in expressing emotion, speech, and intelligence. The muscles, as a group, have only one bony origin in the facial skeleton. The muscles form a circular rim around the perimeter of the facial bones and extend anteriorly as a tube of tissue in which the lumen narrows and terminates in the orbicularis oris. Their structure may be regarded as a truncated cone in which the base rests on the skeleton (origin) in a fixed position, whereas the truncated top of the cone (insertion in the orbicularis oris) is variable in diameter and height. The lips are thus extensible and retractable and can constrict like a purse string. The facial nerve provides neurologic control. Also called the *muscles of expression, mimetic muscles,* and *orofacial muscles.*

muscles, hyoid (hī′oid), *n.pl* a group of muscles used in mastication and swallowing. These muscles are attached to the hyoid bone, which is suspended in the neck and forms the base of the tongue and larynx. The muscles are divided into *suprahyoid* (superior) or *infrahyoid* (inferior) groups relative to the bone.

muscles, levator labii superioris alaeque nasi **(livā′tər lab′ēī soo′pērēor′is al′akū naz′ī),** *n* the muscle that elevates the upper lip and the alae of the nose, allowing the nostrils to dilate in a sneering expression.

muscles, levator veli palatini **(livā′tər vē′lī palatē′nē),** *n* the muscle located superior to the soft palate that extends from the inferior surface of the temporal bone to the median palatine raphe; it raises the soft palate, causing it to cover the opening of the nasopharynx during swallowing and speech.

muscles, masticatory **(mas′tikətôrē),** *n.pl* the powerful muscles that elevate and rotate the mandible so that the opposing teeth may occlude for mastication. Includes the temporal, masseter, lateral pterygoid, and medial pterygoid muscles. Also called the *muscles of mastication.*

muscles, mimetic **(mimet′ik),** *n.pl* See muscles, facial.

muscles, ocular, function of, *n.pl* the action of the eye muscles in moving the eyeballs. The eyes are in a position of rest (their primary position) when their direction is maintained simply by the tone of the ocular muscles. This condition prevails when the gaze is straight ahead into distance and not directed to any particular point in space. The visual axes are then parallel. When the eyes view some distant definite object, they are turned by contraction of the ocular muscles and converge so that the visual axes meet at the observed object, and an almost identical image of the object falls on a corresponding point on each fovea, the centralis of the retina. The adjustment of the eye movements for acute observation is called fixation, and the point where the visual axes meet is the fixation point. Thus the interplay of the ocular muscles permits rapid, reciprocally controlled movement of the eyeballs for fixation.

muscles, orofacial, *n.pl* See muscles, facial.

muscles, posterior suprahyoid **(sōō′prəhī′oid),** *n* the muscles situated superior to the hyoid bone and made up of the stylohyoid muscles and the posterior belly of digastric muscles; they are used during mastication.

muscles, suprahyoid and infrahyoid, *n.pl* the muscles grouped around the hyoid bone. They aid in depressing and fixing the mandible, hyoid bone, and larynx in the performance of their several respective functions.

muscle(s), tongue, extrinsic, *n.pl* the muscles of the tongue that provide a scaffolding by which the intrinsic muscles can be moved around in the oral cavity while the latter are continuously modifying their dimension and contour. The extrinsic muscles are paired and originate from both sides of the cranial skeleton, mandible, and hyoid bone to radiate medially and insert into the body of the tongue, which consists principally of the intrinsic muscles.

muscle(s), tongue, intrinsic, *n.pl* the muscles of the tongue that have no attachments in bone, terminating either within each other or in the extrinsic muscle group. The fibers of the intrinsic muscles also lie in all three planes of space and are called *longitudinal, vertical,* and *transverse fibers* to describe their distribution. They are capable of assuming an infinite variety of shapes. They depend, however, on the activity of the extrinsic muscles to be moved bodily through space.

muscular dystrophy (mus'kūlur dis'trōfē), *n* a group of genetically transmitted diseases characterized by progressive atrophy of symmetric groups of skeletal muscles without evidence of involvement or degeneration of neural tissue. In all forms of muscular dystrophy there is an insidious loss of strength with increasing disability and deformity. Serum creatine phosphokinase is increased in affected individuals and acts as a diagnostic aid. Diagnosis is confirmed by muscle biopsy, electromyography, and genetic pedigree.

muscular dystrophy, Duchenne **(dooshen'),** *n.pr* a genetic myopathic condition distinguished by the enlarged size of specific muscles (e.g., calves), noticeable indications of lordosis accompanied by a swelling of the abdominal region; diminished capacity to stand, walk, and maintain balance; a progressive deterioration of the muscles; and limited intellectual development.

muscular dystrophy, facioscapulohumeral **(fā'shēōskap'ūlōhyoo'mərəl),** *n* a genetic myopathic condition involving the facial muscles and distinguished by prominent scapula, weak muscles of the shoulders, and marked difficulty in lifting the arms and completely shutting the eyes.

musculature (mus'kūləchur), *n* a part of the muscular apparatus of the body; the source of power for the movement of the body or its parts.

musculature, cheek, *n* the muscles giving support, form, and function to the cheeks. Should disequilibrium exist between the functional forces exerted on the dentition by the tongue and cheek musculature, deviations in tooth alignment may occur.

musculature, lip, *n* the muscles that perform the physiologic or functional activities of the lips. The primary muscles include the orbicularis oris, quadratus labii superioris, risorius, and buccinators. If the tongue and the musculature of the lips do not exert equivalent forces against the teeth, movement of the teeth may occur.

musculoskeletal system (mus'kūlōskel'ətəl), *n* all the muscles, bones, joints, and related structures, such as the tendons and connective tissue, that function in the stability and movement of the parts and organs of the body. See also system, musculoskeletal.

mushbite, *n* a type of maxillomandibular record made by introducing a mass of soft wax into the patient's oral cavity and instructing the patient to bite into it to the desired degree. Not an accepted procedure. See also record, maxillomandibular.

mutagen (mū'təjiən), *n* a chemical or physical environmental agent that induces a genetic mutation or increases the mutation rate.

mutagenesis, *n* the induction or occurrence of a genetic mutation.

mutant, *n* an individual showing a mutation.

mutation (mūtā'shən), *n* a departure from the parent type, as when an organism differs from its parents in one or more heritable characteristics; caused by genetic change.

mutation, gene, *n* a sudden and permanent change in a gene. The term mutation is sometimes used in a broader sense to include chromosome aberrations.

mutation, lethal, *n* a mutation leading to death of the offspring at any stage.

mutism (mūtizəm), *n* a condition in which the patient is physically unable to speak or has emotional barriers to speaking. Sometimes accompanies deafness.

mutism, elective, *n* a continual refusal to speak in children who have a confirmed capacity to articulate.

mutual, *adj* interchangeable; reciprocal; joint.

myalgia (mīal'jēə), *n* pain in the muscles.

myasthenia gravis (mī'asthē'nēə grā'vis), *n* an autoimmune disease resulting in incomplete communication between the nerves, thereby causing fatigue and weakness of the muscles, with the facial muscles usually among the first affected.

myasthenic crisis, *n* a lack of acetylcholine, usually caused by insufficient medication, which results in an inability to speak, breathe, or swallow in patients with myasthenia gravis.

mycelium (mīsē'lēum), *n* the filamentous network of hyphae of a fungus.

Mycobacterium (mī'kōbakter'ēəm), *n* a genus of rod-shaped, acid-fast bacteria.

M. tuberculosis, *n* the bacterium responsible for tuberculosis, generally a respiratory infection in man; nonrespiratory tuberculosis is considered an indicator disease for AIDS. See also tuberculosis.

mycology, *n* that branch of microbiology that deals with yeasts and fungi.

mycophenolate mofetil (mī'kōfen'olāt mof'ətil'), *n brand name:* CellCept; *drug class:* immunosuppressant; *action:* selective inhibitor of inosine monophosphate dehydrogenase, thereby preventing the synthesis of guanosine nucleotide and resulting in cytostatic effect on T and B lymphocytes; *uses:* prophylaxis of organ rejection in patients receiving allogenic renal transplants (in combination with cyclosporine and corticosteroids).

Mycoplasma, *n* a genus of ultramicroscopic organisms lacking rigid cell walls and considered to be the smallest free-living organisms.

M. pneumoniae, *n* a species of *Mycoplasma* causing mycoplasma pneumonia, which is characterized by symptoms of an upper respiratory infection with a dry cough and fever.

mycosis (mīkō'sis), *n* a disease caused by a yeast or fungus.

mycosis fungoides, *n* a rare, chronic, lymphomatous skin malignancy resembling eczema or a cutaneous tumor that is followed by microabscesses in the epidermis and lesions simulating those of Hodgkin disease in lymph nodes and viscera.

mydriasis (midrī'əsis), *n* an abnormal condition of the eye characterized by contraction of the dilator muscle, resulting in widely dilated pupils.

mydriatic (mid'rēat'ik), *n* a drug that dilates the pupil.

myelin (mī'əlin), *n* a fatlike substance forming a sheath around certain nerve fibers. It is associated with volitional nervous system fibers and is believed to be related to the capacity of nerve structures for rapid transmission of nerve impulses. Various diseases, such as multiple sclerosis, can destroy these myelin wrappings.

myelocyte (mi'əlosīt), *n* a young white blood cell found in the bone marrow.

myeloma (mī'əlō'mə), *n* a neoplasm characterized by cells normally found in the bone marrow.

myeloma, multiple, *n* a primary malignant neoplasm of bone marrow characterized by proliferation of cells resembling plasma cells. Circumscribed radiolucencies are seen within the bones, and Bence Jones protein is usually found in the urine.

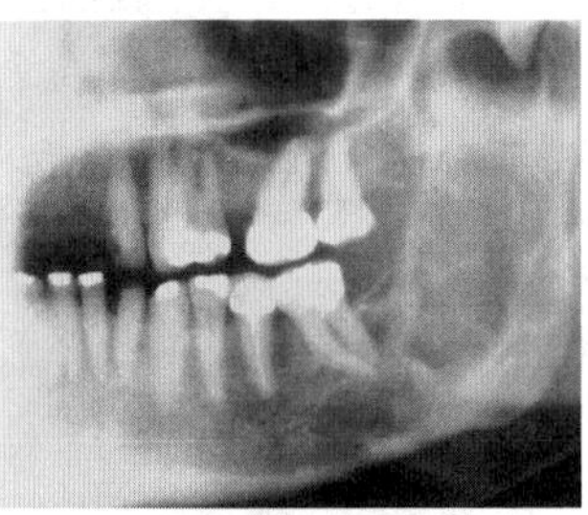

Multiple myeloma. (Regezi/Sciubba/Jordan, 2008)

myeloma, plasma cell, *n* a malignant neoplasm characterized by plasma cells. Solitary lesions may appear as radiolucencies in the bone and are sometimes considered benign, although most authorities believe that even these lesions become multiple and terminate fatally.

myeloma, solitary plasma cell, *n* an incompletely understood monostotic neoplasm of bone that is histologically identical with multiple myeloma. Laboratory findings, positive in multiple myeloma, are usually negative in solitary plasma cell myeloma. Although usually benign, solitary plasma cell myelomas may be malignant.

myelomeningocele (mī'əlōməning'gōsēl), *n* a condition in which part of the spinal cord protrudes from between the bones of the vertebrae. The condition can result in paralysis.

myelophthisis (mī'əlōfthī'sis), *n* a displacement of bone marrow by fibrous tissue, carcinoma, or leukemia.

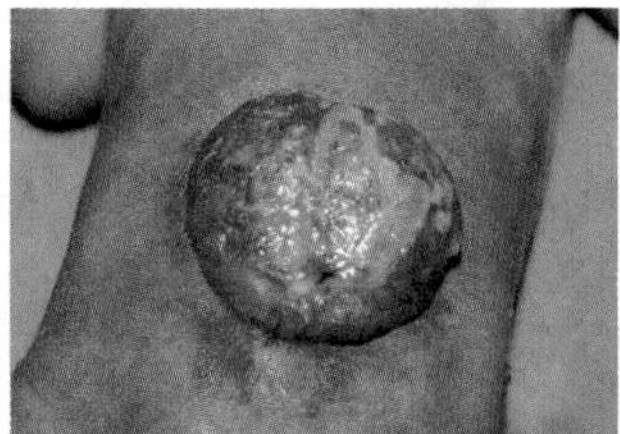

Myelomeningocele. (Moore/Persaud, 2003, Courtesy AE Chudley)

myelosuppression (mī′əlōsəpres′hən), *n* the suppression of blood cell and platelet production in the bone marrow.

mylohyoid ridge, cantilevered (mī′lōhī′oid kan′təlē′vərd), *n* a condition in which a major undercut occurs inferior to a broad mylohyoid ridge; creating a vertical groove into such an area often causes perforation of the medial cortical plate.

myoblastoma (mī′ōblastō′mə), *n* a benign neoplasm characterized by large polyhedral cells resembling young muscle cells. Occurs most frequently in the tongue.

myoblastoma, granular cell, *n* See tumor, granular cell.

myocardial infarction (heart attack), *n* an occlusion or blockage of arteries supplying the muscles of the heart, resulting in injury or necrosis of the heart muscle.

myocardial ischemia, *n* a loss of oxygen to the heart muscle caused by blockage of the coronary arteries or their branches.

myocardium (mī′ōkär′dēəm), *n* the thick, contractile middle layer of uniquely constructed and arranged muscle cells (cardiac muscle) that form the bulk of the heart wall.

myoclonus, *n* a spasm of muscle or group of muscles.

myoepithelial cell (mī″oep″ĭthē′-lēəl), *n* a contractile muscle cell found on the surface of some acini of the salivary glands, which is believed to facilitate the secretion of fluids from the gland.

myofascial pain, *n* pain associated with inflammation or irritation of muscle or of the fascia surrounding the muscle.

myofascial pain dysfunction syndrome (MPD), *n* a subset of the temporomandibular disorder (TMD) that presents with the triad of symptoms of unilateral pain in the muscles of mastication, clicking of the joint, and limitation of movement but without clinical or radiographic evidence of organic changes in the joint and a lack of tenderness in the joint when palpated from the external auditory meatus.

myolipoma (mī′ōlipō′mə), *n* a myxoma containing fatty tissue.

myoma (mīō′mə), *n* a neoplasm characterized by muscle cells.

myopathy (mīop′əthē), *n* weakness or degeneration of skeletal muscles associated with the many forms of muscular dystrophy. This should be distinguished from neuromuscular disorders.

myopia (mīō′pēə), *n* a form of defective vision resulting from excessive refractive power of the eye. In this condition, commonly called *nearsightedness,* or *shortsightedness,* light rays coming from an object beyond a certain distance are focused in front of the retina.

myosin (mī′əsin′), *n* a cardiac and skeletal muscle protein that makes up close to one half of the proteins that occur in muscle tissue. The interaction of myosin and actin is essential for muscle contraction.

myosin fibrils, *n.pl* strands of protein found in muscle tissue which are among the components necessary for muscle contraction.

myositis (mī′əsī′tis), *n* an inflammation of muscle tissue, usually of the voluntary muscles. Causes of myositis include infection, trauma, and infestation by parasites.

myotomy (mīot′əmē), *n* a cutting or resection of a muscle.

myotonia (mi″oto′neə), *n* a condition in which muscles remain tense or do not quickly relax after contraction.

myxedema (mĭksədē′mə), *n* See hypothyroidism.

myxofibroma (mik′sōfibrō′mə), *n* a benign neoplasm characterized by mucous and fibroblastic tissues.

myxoma (miksō′mə), *n* a benign tumor composed of fibroblastic cells that have reverted to embryonic growth and produce a mucoid matrix containing widely dispersed stellate cells that have multipolar processes.

myxoma, odontogenic, *n* a new growth of soft tissue, gelatinous in appearance, originating from the mesenchymal tissue of the tooth. The growth may invade tissues surrounding the region, and it does not metastasize or provide any bodily function.

myxosarcoma (mik′sōsärkō′mə), *n* a sarcoma containing myxomatous tissue.

N

N (n), *n* in statistics, the number of cases or observations.

N2, *n* a single-visit endodontic technique better known as the *Sargenti technique,* in which paraformaldehyde (a toxic chemical that can cause permanent tissue damage if not confined to the pulp chamber or root canal) is the principal ingredient in the endodontic paste. The technique is not approved by the Council on Dental Therapeutics, and it is not taught at any accredited dental school in the United States.

nabumetone (nəbū′mətōn′), *n brand name:* Relafen; *drug class:* nonsteroidal antiinflammatory; *action:* inhibits prostaglandin synthesis by interfering with cyclooxygenase needed for biosynthesis; possesses analgesic, antiinflammatory, and antipyretic properties; *uses:* osteoarthritis, rheumatoid arthritis.

nadolol (nadō′lol), *n brand name:* Corgard; *drug class:* nonselective β-adrenergic blocker; *action:* competitively blocks stimulation of β-adrenergic receptors within the heart; produces negative chronotropic and inotropic activity, slows conduction of AV node, decreases heart rate, which decreases oxygen consumption in myocardium; also decreases activity of the renin-aldosterone-angiotensin system; *uses:* chronic stable angina pectoris, mild to moderate hypertension.

nafcillin (nafsil′in), *n* a semisynthetic penicillin designed as an antistaphylococcal penicillin. Also effective in the treatment of infections caused by pneumococci and Group A β-hemolytic streptococci.

naftifine HCl (naf′tifēn), *n brand name:* Naftin; *drug class:* topical antifungal; *action:* interferes with cell membrane permeability in fungi; *uses:* tinea cruris, tinea corporis.

nalidixic acid, *n* an antibacterial prescribed in the treatment of urinary tract infections.

nalmefene HCl (nal′məfēn), *n brand name:* Revex; *drug class:* opioid antagonist; *action:* reverses the effects of opioids by competitive antagonism of opioid receptors; *uses:* management of opioid overdose and complete or partial reversal of opioid drug effects, including respiratory depression.

naloxone HCl (nalok′sōn), *n brand name:* Narcan; *drug class:* narcotic antagonist; *action:* competes with narcotics at narcotic receptor sites; *uses:* respiratory depression induced by narcotics, to reverse postoperative opioid depression.

naltrexone HCl, *n brand names:* ReVia, Trexan; *drug class:* narcotic antagonist; *action:* competes with opioids at opioid receptor sites; *uses:* treatment of opioid addiction following detoxification.

name, *n* a word or combination of words by which a person, object, or idea, or a group of persons, objects, or ideas is regularly known or designated.

name, generic, *n* a name that is usually descriptive of the substance. Strictly speaking, it is a name used to designate a class relationship. Often used synonymously with *nonproprietary name.*

name, nonproprietary, *n* a drug name that is not restricted by a trademark. Nonproprietary names are now selected in the United States by the United States Adopted Name (USAN) Council.

name, official, *n* the title under which a drug is listed in the *United States Pharmacopeia* (USP) or the *National Formulary* (NF).

name, proprietary, *n* a name assigned by the manufacturer that is restricted by trademark. A drug made by several companies may have more than one proprietary name.

Name, United States Adopted (USAN), *n* a name selected by the USAN Council (jointly sponsored by the American Medical Association, American Pharmaceutical Association, and United States Pharmacopeial Convention, Inc.) when a new drug is placed on the market. A nonproprietary or generic name.

Nance analysis of arch length, *n.pr* a method of determining whether there is sufficient arch length to accommodate the permanent dentition.

nandrolone deconate (nan′drəlōn dekō′nāt), *n* an androgen prescribed in the treatment of testosterone deficiency, osteoporosis, and female breast cancer and to stimulate growth, weight gain, and the production of red blood cells.

nanometer (nm) (nan′əmē′tər), *n* a billionth of a meter (10^{-9} meter). This term is now preferred over millimicron.

naphazoline HCl (nəfaz′əlēn), *n* *brand names:* AK-Con Ophthalmic, Allerest, Clear Eyes, VasoClear, Vasocon; *drug class:* ophthalmic vasoconstrictor; *action:* vasoconstriction of eye arterioles; decreases eye engorgement by stimulation of α-adrenergic receptors; *uses:* relieves hyperemia, irritation of superficial corneal vascularity.

naproxen/naproxen sodium (nəprok′sən), *n* *brand names:* Naprosyn, Anaprox, Aleve; *drug class:* nonsteroidal antiinflammatory; *action:* inhibits prostaglandin synthesis by interfering with cyclooxygenase needed for biosynthesis; possesses analgesic, antiinflammatory, antipyretic properties; *uses:* mild to moderate pain, osteoarthritis, rheumatoid, gouty arthritis, primary dysmenorrhea.

narcissism (när′səsizəm), *n* a personality disorder in which a person is so self-absorbed that the needs and feelings of others do not matter.

narcolepsy (när′kōlepsē), *n* a disease in which the patient is unable to stay awake.

narcoma, *n* a coma or stupor produced by narcotics.

narcosis (närkō′sis), *n* drug-induced unconsciousness.

narcotic (närkot′ik), *n/adj* a drug, usually with strong analgesic action and an addiction potential, that may be synthesized or derived from natural sources. Especially one of the opium alkaloids.

narcotism (när′kōtizəm), *n* a state of stupor induced by a narcotic.

narcotize (när′kōtīz), *v* to render unconscious by use of narcotics.

naris (nares), *n* one of two external openings into the nasal cavity; nostril.

nasal cavity, *n* See cavity, nasal.

nasal conchae, inferior (kong′kē), *n* the paired facial bones that project off the maxilla and form the lateral walls of the nasal cavity.

nasal lavage fluid, *n* a liquid, usually a saline-based water solution, used to cleanse the nasal passages.

nasal mucosa, *n* See mucosa.

nasal obstruction, *n* a narrowing of the nasal cavity, which reduces breathing capacity. Caused by an irregular septum, nasal polyps, foreign bodies, or enlarged turbinates.

nasal septum, *n* the partition dividing the nostrils. It is composed of bone and cartilage covered by mucous membrane.

nasality, *n* the quality of speech sounds when the nasal cavity is used as a resonator, especially when there is too much nasal resonance.

nascent (nas′ənt, nā′sənt), *adj* literal meaning: recently born. Also, just released from chemical combination.

nasion (nā′zēon), *n* the point at the root of the nose that is intersected by the median sagittal plane. The root of the nose corresponds to the nasofrontal suture, which is not necessarily the lowest point on its dorsum and which can usually be located with the finger.

Nasmyth's membrane (nas′miths), *n.pr* See cuticle, primary and stain, green dental.

nasoalveolar cyst (nā′zōalvē′ōlur), *n* an intraosseous cyst. A form of globulomaxillary cyst in which the epithelial inclusion is in the soft tissue fusion line.

nasolabial (nazōlā′bēəl), *adj* pertaining to the nose and the upper lip.

nasolabial angle, *n* the angle formed

by the labial surface of the upper lip at the midline and the inferior border of the nose. It is a measure of the relative protrusion of the upper lip.

nasolacrimal (nā′zōlak′rəməl), *adj* pertaining to the nose and the lacrimal apparatus.

nasolacrimal duct, *n* a tubular channel that drains lacrimal fluid (tears) from the lacrimal sac to the nasal cavity.

nasopharynx (nā′zōfar′ingks), *n* the most superior portion of the three regions of the throat, or pharynx, situated behind the nose and extending from the posterior nares to the level of the soft palate.

natal teeth, *n* the presence of teeth in the oral cavity at birth, usually caused by the premature eruption of primary teeth but may be an extra or supernumerary tooth. The presence may cause discomfort to the nursing mother.

National Board Dental Hygiene Examination, *n.pr* a written examination used to assist state boards in the licensure of dental hygienists; it is one of at least three requirements needed to obtain dental hygiene licensure. (An educational requirement and a clinical examination requirement make up the other two requirements.)

National Bureau of Standards (NBS), *n.pr* a federal agency in the Department of Commerce that sets accurate measurement standards for commerce, industry, and science in the United States.

National Dental Hygienists' Association (NDHA), *n.pr* an association established by African-American dental hygienists in order to focus on the professional needs of African-American dental hygienists; it is affiliated with the National Dental Association and offers limited scholarships to students of color.

National Formulary (NF), *n.pr* a publication containing the official standards for the preparation of various pharmaceuticals not listed in the *United States Pharmacopoeia.* It is revised every 5 years.

National Health Service Corps (NHSC), *n.pr* a program of the United States Public Health Service (USPHS) in which health care personnel are placed in areas that are underserved. Medical and dental professionals serve in rural and urban areas of need, usually as employees of local health care agencies. The USPHS pays most of the salary of each corps member.

National Institute for Occupational Safety and Health, *n.pr* an institute of the Centers for Disease Control and Prevention that is responsible for assuring safe and healthful working conditions and for developing standards of safety and health. Research activities are carried out pertinent to these goals.

National Institutes of Health (NIH), *n.pr* an agency within the United States Public Health Service comprising several institutes and constituent divisions, including the Bureau of Health Manpower Education, the National Library of Medicine, the National Cancer Institute, the National Institute for Dental Research, and a number of other research institutes and divisions.

natural bristles, *n* animal hair (usually from hogs) that can be used in toothbrushes. They are not as durable or effective as synthetic bristles because individual hair thickness and length is not uniform, the porous nature of the bristles makes contamination more probable, and their absorbency makes rapid wear and deterioration more likely.

nausea (nôz′ēə), *n* a sensation often leading to the urge to vomit. Common causes are motion sickness, early pregnancy, intense pain, emotional stress, gallbladder disease, food poisoning, and various enteroviruses. It is also the most common side effect of poorly administered nitrous oxide.

near-death experience, *n* the subjective observation of someone who has either been close to clinical death or who may have recovered after having been declared dead. Many claim to have witnessed similar episodes of passing through a tunnel toward a bright light and encountering people who have preceded them in death.

Necator americanus **(nikā′tər),** *n* the so-called New World hookworm. The adults of this species attach to villi in the small intestine and suck blood, causing abdominal discomfort, diarrhea and cramps, anorexia, loss of weight, and hypochromic microcytic anemia.

necatoriasis (nikā'tərī'əsis), *n* hookworm disease. See also *Necator americanus.*

necessary, *n/adj* anything indispensable or useful for the sustenance of life, such as food, shelter, and clothing.

necessary contracts of infants (minors), n things suitable to each child according to the child's circumstances.

necessary treatment, n a dental procedure or service determined by a dental professional to be necessary to establish or maintain a patient's oral health. Such determinations are based on the professional diagnostic judgment of the dental professional and the standards of care that prevail in the professional community.

neck of condyle, See process, neck of condyloid.

necrosis (nekrō'sis), *n* **1.** the death of a cell or group of cells in contact with living tissue. *n* **2.** the local death of cells resulting from, e.g., loss of blood supply, bacterial toxins, or physical or chemical agents.

necrosis, avascular **(nekrō'sis āvas'kylər),** *n* the consequence of temporary or permanent cessation of blood flow to the bones. The absence of blood causes the bone tissue to die, resulting in fracture or collapse of the entire bone.

necrosis, caseous **(kā'sēus),** *n* a change commonly associated with tuberculosis and characterized by dry, soft, and cheesy tissue.

necrosis, exanthematous **(eg'zanthē'mətəs),** *n* an acute necrotizing process involving the gingivae, jawbones, and contiguous soft tissues. It is of unknown cause, primarily affects children, and resembles noma. It differs from noma, however, in that it has a slight odor, tendency for self-limitation, low mortality rate, and normal leukocyte count. See also noma.

necrosis, gingival, n death and degeneration of the cells and other structural elements of the gingivae (e.g., necrotizing ulcerative gingivitis).

necrosis, interdental, n a progressive disease that destroys the tissue of the papillae and creates interdental craters. Advanced interdental necrosis leads to a loss of periodontal attachment.

necrosis, ischemic, n death and disintegration of a tissue resulting from interference with its blood supply, thus depriving the tissues of access to substances necessary for metabolic sustenance. It may occur in the periodontal ligament as a result of occlusal trauma.

necrosis of epithelial attachment, n the death of cells composing the epithelial attachment. In a specific periodontitis produced by organisms similar to *Actinomyces,* necrosis of the epithelial attachment may exist, permitting a rapid apical shift of the base of the pocket.

necrosis, periodontal ligament, n necrosis of a portion of the periodontal ligament, usually resulting from traumatic injury (e.g., in occlusal traumatism). Much of this necrotic change is the result of ischemia.

necrosis, radiation, n the death of tissue caused by radiation.

necrotic zone (nəkrot'ik), *n* one of the four microscopically identified layers of a necrotizing ulcerative gingivitis (NUG) lesion. The necrotic zone comprises decomposed tissue and bacteria, including many spirochetes.

necrotizing stomatitis, *n* an inflammatory disease of the oral cavity characterized by the destruction of epithelium, connective tissue, and papillae. The disease may cause a loss of periodontal attachment and the destruction of bone tissue. In advanced stages, it may lead to cancrum oris (noma) with exposed alveolar bone. It is associated with certain types of necrotizing periodontal disease such as occurs in people with HIV.

necrotizing ulcerative gingivitis, *n* See gingivitis, necrotizing ulcerative.

necrotizing ulcerative periodontitis (NUP), *n* an acute type of necrotizing periodontal disease characterized by erythema of the gingival and alveolar mucosa, ulcerated interdental papillae, interdental craters of the soft tissue and bone, and loss of periodontal attachment. May become chronic. See also gingivitis, necrotizing ulcerative (NUG).

nedocromil sodium (ned′ōk-rō′mil), *n brand name:* Tilade; *drug class:* antiasthmatic, mast cell stabilizer; *action:* stabilizes the membrane of the sensitized mast cell, preventing release of chemical mediators after an antigen-IgE interaction; *use:* prophylaxis only in reversible obstructive airway diseases such as asthma.

needle, *n* a sharp, metal shaft that is available in a variety of forms for penetrating tissue (e.g., in carrying sutures or injecting solutions).

needle, bevel, *n* the slanted part of a needle, which creates a sharp, pointed tip. The bevel of the needle allows for easy penetration of the oral mucosa in dentistry.

needle biopsy, *n* the removal of a segment of living tissue for microscopic examination by inserting a hollow needle through the skin or the external surface of an organ or tumor and rotating it within the underlying cellular layers to retrieve a tissue specimen for examination.

needle, gauge of, *n* the outside diameter of a needle.

needle, Gillmore, *n.pr* an instrument used in a penetration type of test for measuring the setting time of materials such as plaster or stone. A ¼-pound needle is used for determining the initial set, and a 1-pound needle is used for defining the final set.

needle holder, *n* a forceps used to hold and pass the needle through the tissue while suturing with a suture forceps.

needle, hub/syringe adaptor, *n* the proximal end of a needle, which attaches to the syringe barrel by means of a press-fit mechanism (Luer) or a twist-on mechanism (Luer-lock).

needle, lumen **(loo′mən),** *n* the interior diameter of a needle. The lumen, or bore, measurement is variable depending on the thickness of the catheter material. In general, the higher the needle gauge, the smaller the diameter of the lumen.

needle point tracer, See tracer, needle point.

needle, shank, *n* the length of a needle as measured from the hub (proximal end) to the bevel (distal end). In the United States, needle shanks are measured in inches and fractions of inches.

needle stick injuries, *n* accidental skin punctures resulting from contact with hypodermic syringe needles. Such injuries can be dangerous, particularly if the needle has been used in treatment of a patient with a severe blood-borne infection, such as hepatitis or AIDS. A strict federal protocol for the use and disposal of needles is required for all health care facilities and personnel engaged in direct patient care. The ADA has a policy for dental offices and clinics.

needle, suture, *n* a small, sterile, stainless steel implement used during and after surgery to sew stitches into various types of human tissue.

needle, swaged end of **(swājd),** *n* the opposite end of the sharp tip of a sterile, stainless steel implement, where the thread had been attached directly to it, so that threading is not necessary.

needle, tapered suture, *n* the pointed tip of a surgical mending tool.

needle, Vicat, *n.pr* an instrument used for measuring setting time by means of a penetration test.

nefazodone HCl (nəfā′zōdōn′), *brand name:* Serzone; *drug class:* antidepressant; *action:* inhibits neuronal uptake of serotonin and norepinephrine; *uses:* major depressive disorders.

neglect, *n/v* the failure to do something that one is bound to do; lack of due care. See also child neglect.

negligence (neg′lijəns), *n* the failure to observe, for the protection of another person, the degree of care and vigilance that the circumstances demand, whereby such other person suffers injury.

negligence, contributory, *n* negligence by an injured party that combines as a proximate cause with the negligence of the injurer in producing the injury. May bar recovery or mitigate damages.

negligence, imputed, *n* the principle that places the responsibility for negligence on a person other than the one that was directly negligent. This transfer of responsibility is based on some special relationship of the parties, such as parent and child or principal and agent (e.g., a dental professional may be responsible for the negligence of a dental assistant).

negotiate, *v* to deal or bargain with another or others to bring about an agreement or settlement.

Negri bodies, *n.pl* the intracytoplasmic inclusion bodies found in the brain and central nervous system cells of rabies victims.

***Neisseria* (nīsē′rēə),** *n* a genus of aerobic to facultatively anaerobic bacteria containing gram-negative cocci that occur in pairs with the adjacent sides flattened.

N. gonorrhoeae, *n* a species that causes gonorrhea.

N. meningitidis, *n* a species found in the nasopharynx of man. The causative agent of meningococcal meningitis.

Neivert whittler, *n.pr* an instrument used to sharpen the cutting edges of blades. The sharpening end consists of tungsten carbide steel, and the handle is stainless steel. It is particularly effective on curved scalers or curets.

nematodes (nē′mətōdz), *n* parasitic roundworms, such as hookworm and pinworm, that cause disease in humans.

Nembutal, *n.pr* the brand name for pentobarbital.

Neo-Synephrine, *n.pr* the brand name for phenylephrine, a vasoconstrictor and pressor drug chemically related to epinephrine and ephedrine. Commonly used as a decongestant. Contraindicated for prolonged use or in patients with severe hypertension.

neodymium (Nd) (nē′ōdim′ēəm), *n* a rare earth element with an atomic number of 60 and an atomic weight of 144.24.

neomycin (nē′ōmī′sin), *n* an antibiotic secured from cultures of *S. fradiae,* used for preoperative sterilization. It is a constituent of topically applied ointments, solutions, and troches because of its antibacterial action against gram-negative organisms.

neomycin sulfate (topical), *n brand name:* Myciguent; *drug class:* local antibacterial; *action:* interferes with bacterial protein synthesis; *use:* skin infections.

neonatal (nē′ōnā′təl), *adj* pertaining to a newborn child.

neonatal cytomegalovirus infection, *n* a disease caused by any of the viruses in the cytomegalovirus family (part of the herpesvirus family). It is transmitted to a newborn child through the birth process or contact with bodily fluids.

neonatal teeth, *n* the presence of teeth within 1 month of birth. See also natal teeth.

neoplasia (nē′ōplā′zhə), *n* the disease process responsible for neoplasm formation. See also neoplasm.

neoplasm, *n* (tumor), an abnormal mass of tissue, the growth of which exceeds and is uncoordinated with that of the normal tissues. It persists in the same excessive manner after cessation of the stimuli that evoked the change. Benign and malignant forms are recognized. See also neoplasia and tumor.

neoprene (nē′əprēn′), *n* an oil-resistant synthetic rubber.

neostigmine bromide/neostigmine methylsulfate (nē′ōstig′mēn brōmīd meth′əlsul′fāt), *n brand names:* Prostigmin Bromide/Prostigmin; *drug class:* cholinesterase inhibitor; *action:* inhibits destruction of acetylcholine, which facilitates transmission of impulses across myoneural junction; *uses:* myasthenia gravis, nondepolarizing neuromuscular blocker antagonist, bladder distention, postoperative ileus.

nephrocalcinosis (nef′rōkal′sənō′sis), *n* an abnormal condition of the kidneys in which deposits of calcium form in the parenchyma at the site of previous inflammation or degenerative change. Infection, hematuria, anal colic, and decreased function of the kidney may occur.

nephrology (nəfrol′əjē), *n* the study of the anatomy, physiology, and pathology of the kidney.

nephropathy (nəfrop′əthē), *n* kidney disease.

nerve, *n* a cordlike structure that conveys impulses between a part of the central nervous system and some part of the body and consists of an outer connective tissue sheath and bundles of nerve fibers. See also each of the individual nerves of the head and neck as they are listed.

nerve, abducent (VI), *n* the sixth cranial nerve; a small, completely motor nerve arising in the pons, supplying the lateral rectus muscle of the eye.

nerve, accessory, *n* See nerve, spinal accessory.

nerve, acoustic (VIII), *n* the eighth cranial nerve; the vestibulocochlear nerve; a sensory nerve consisting of a vestibular portion and an auditory (or cochlear) portion.

nerve(s), afferent, in pulp, *n* any nerve that originates as a terminal free nerve ending in the dental pulp tissue and travels to the second and third divisions (maxillary nerve and mandibular nerve) of the cranial trigeminal nerve (cranial nerve V).

nerve, alveolar, *n* afferent nerves that convey impulses from the pulp tissue and periodontium of the maxillary teeth to the maxillary division of the cranial trigeminal nerve.

nerve, anterior superior alveolar, *n* alveolar nerve that conveys impulses from the pulp tissue and periodontium of the maxillary anterior teeth to the infraorbital nerve.

N

nerve, auriculotemporal **(ôrik′yəlōtem′pərəl),** *n* a nerve that transmits feeling from the external ear, scalp, and parotid salivary gland to the mandibular division of the cranial trigeminal nerve.

nerve, branchial, *n* one of five cranial nerves that supply the derivatives of the branchial arches: trigeminal (V), facial (VII), glossopharyngeal (IX), vagus (X), and spinal accessory (XI). Each branchial nerve may have a variety of functions, including visceral motor and visceral and somatic sensory functions.

nerve, buccal (long), *n* afferent nerve that conveys impulses from the facial periodontium of the mandibular molars and gingiva to the mandibular division of the cranial trigeminal nerve.

nerve, chiasma, optic, *n* the decussation, or crossing, of optic nerve fibers from the medial side of the retina on one side to the opposite side of the brain.

nerve, chorda tympani **(kor′də tim′pənē),** *n* a parasympathetic and special sensory branch of the facial nerve supplying the submandibular and sublingual glands and the anterior two thirds of the tongue (taste).

nerve, cochlear **(kō′klēər),** *n* one of the two major branches of the eighth cranial nerve; a special sensory nerve for the sense of hearing that transmits impulses from the organ of Corti to the brain.

nerve, cranial, *n* any one of 12 paired nerves, classified in three sets, arising directly in the brain and supplying various tissues of the head and neck. The cranial nerves are the special somatic sensory nerves: olfactory (I), optic (II), and vestibulocochlear (acoustic) (VIII); the somatic motor nerves: oculomotor (III), trochlear (IV), abducent (VI), and hypoglossal (XII); and the branchial nerves: trigeminal (V), facial (VII), glossopharyngeal (IX), vagus (X), and spinal accessory (XI).

nerve, deep temporal, *n* an anterior and a posterior nerve that branch away from the mandibular nerve of the trigeminal nerve and extend deep into the temporalis muscle, which is used during mastication.

nerve degeneration, *n* the reversion to a less organized and functioning state, usually detected by the loss of ability to conduct or transmit nerve impulses. Advanced degeneration might show cellular decomposition.

nerve ending, *n* the terminal of a nerve fiber, usually in synapse with another fiber or in a sensory organ.

nerve, facial (VII), *n* the seventh cranial nerve; a mixed nerve supplying motor fibers to the facial muscles, the stapedius, and posterior body of the digastric; sensory fibers from the taste buds in the anterior two thirds of the tongue (via the chorda tympani); and general visceral autonomic fibers for the submandibular and sublingual salivary glands. It travels unilaterally over the face and at one point is located in the parotid salivary gland, which it does not serve. However, pain in the parotid gland indicates a glandular malignancy, and complications with an inferior nerve block can also result from its location there.

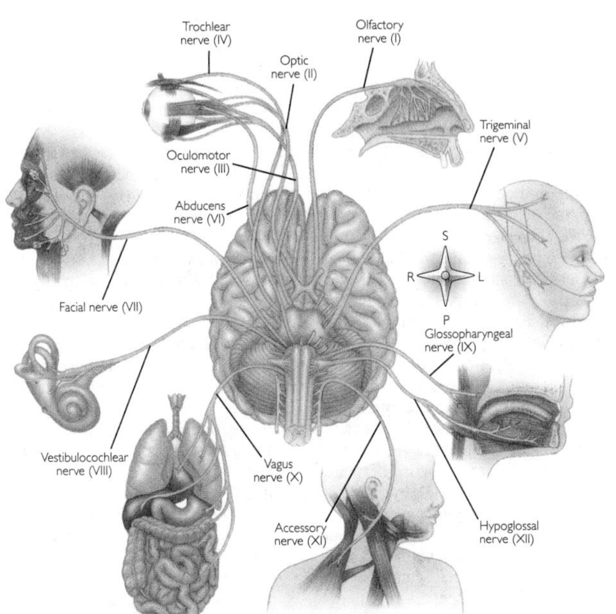

The cranial nerves. (Thibodeau/Patton, 2007)

N

nerve fiber, *n* a slender process of a neuron, usually the axon. Each fiber is classified as myelinated or unmyelinated.

nerve, frontal, *n* afferent nerve from the union of the superorbital and supratrochlear nerves that carries information from the forehead, scalp, nose, and upper eyelids to the ophthalmic division of the cranial trigeminal nerve.

nerve, glossopharyngeal (IX) **(glos′ōfərin′jēəl),** *n* the ninth cranial nerve; a mixed motor and sensory nerve arising in the medulla and supplying motor efferents to stylopharyngeal muscles and other pharyngeal muscles; visceral motor efferents via the otic ganglion for the parotid gland; special visceral afferents from the taste buds in the posterior third of the tongue; and general sensory afferents from the pharynx and posterior aspects of the oral cavity. It is essential to the sense of taste.

nerve, greater (anterior) palatine, *n* the nerve originating in the pterygopalatine ganglion that supplies the hard palate, part of the soft palate, and its associated lingual mucosa.

nerve, greater petrosal **(petrō′səl),** *n* one of the two nerves that branch off of the facial nerve and help control the muscles used in facial expression; this nerve also carries impulses to the lacrimal gland and the nasal cavity, and to and from the palate. The nerve has both afferent and efferent fibers.

nerve, hypoglossal (XII), *n* the twelfth cranial nerve; a motor nerve that arises in the medulla and supplies extrinsic and intrinsic muscles of the tongue. Each nerve has four major branches, communicates with the vagus nerve, and connects to the nucleus XII in the brain.

nerve, incisive, *n* afferent nerve that merges with the mental nerve to later create the inferior alveolar nerve in the mandibular canal. This nerve transmits feeling from the pulp tissue and facial periodontium of the mandibular anterior teeth and premolars to the mandibular division of the cranial trigeminal nerve.

nerve, inferior alveolar, *n* a motor and general sensory branch of the mandibular nerve, with mylohyoid, inferior dental, mental, and inferior gingival branches.

nerve, infraorbital, *n* afferent nerve that enters through the infraorbital foramen and canal to merge with the maxillary branch of the cranial trigeminal nerve.

nerve, intermediate, *n* the parasympathetic and special sensory division of the facial nerve with chorda tympani and greater petrosal branches.

nerve, lacrimal, *n* afferent nerve that is part of the ophthalmic division of the cranial trigeminal nerve and controls secretions in the upper eyelid, lacrimal gland, and the conjunctiva.

nerve, lingual, *n* a general sensory branch of the mandibular nerve having sublingual and lingual branches and connections with the hypoglossal nerve and chorda tympani.

nerve, mandibular, *n* the mandibular division of the trigeminal nerve, arising in the trigeminal ganglion and supplying general sensory and motor fibers via mesenteric, pterygoid, buccal, auriculotemporal, deep temporal, lingual, inferior alveolar, and meningeal branches.

N

nerve, maxillary, *n* the maxillary division of the trigeminal nerve arising in the trigeminal ganglion and supplying general sensory fibers via zygomatic, posterosuperior alveolar, infraorbital, pterygopalatine, and nasopalatine branches.

nerve, mental, *n* a nerve that branches off the inferior alveolar nerve, emerging from the mandible through the mental foramen and branching further to provide sensory innervation to the tissues of the chin and lower lip and the labial mucosa of the mandibular premolars and anterior teeth.

nerve, middle superior alveolar, *n* alveolar nerve that conveys impulses from the pulp tissue and periodontium of the gingiva and the maxillary premolar teeth to the infraorbital nerve. This nerve is not always present in all persons. If not present, the premolars are innervated by the posterior superior alveolar nerve.

nerve, mylohyoid, *n* a branch of the mandibular division of the cranial trigeminal nerve that serves the mylohyoid and digastric muscles of the oral cavity. It is thought to be a possible alternative innervation for the pulp tissues of the mandibular first molar in some cases.

nerve, nasociliary **(nā′zōsil′ēerē),** *n* one of three branches of the cranial trigeminal nerve that controls parts of the eyes, nasal cavity, and paranasal sinuses.

nerve, nasopalatine **(nā′zōpal′ətīn),** *n* afferent nerve that conveys impulses from the lingual periodontium of the maxillary anterior teeth bilaterally and the anterior hard palate to the maxillary division of the cranial trigeminal nerve.

nerve, oculomotor (III) **(ok′yəlōmō′tər),** *n* the third cranial nerve; primarily a motor nerve arising from the midbrain and supplying motor efferents to the superior rectus, medial rectus, inferior rectus, and inferior oblique eye muscles, as well as autonomic fibers via the ciliary ganglion to the ciliary body and the iris.

nerve, olfactory (I) **(olfak′tərē),** *n* the first cranial nerve; a special sensory nerve for the sense of smell.

nerve, ophthalmic **(ofthal′mik),** *n* the ophthalmic division of the trigeminal nerve, arising in the trigeminal ganglion and supplying general sensory fibers via the frontal, lacrimal, and nasociliary branches.

nerve, optic (II), *n* the second cranial nerve; a special sensory nerve for vision. It consists mainly of coarse, myelinated fibers that arise in the retinal ganglionic layer of the eye, traverse the thalamus, and connect with the visual cortex of the brain.

nerve, palatine, *n* the two afferent nerves of the maxillary division of the cranial trigeminal nerve. The greater palatine nerve innervates the posterior hard palate and lingual periodontium of the maxillary molar teeth, while the lesser palatine nerve innervates the soft palate and palatine tonsillar tissue.

nerve, posterior superior alveolar, *n* alveolar nerve that conveys impulses from the maxillary sinus, gingiva, pulp tissue, and periodontium of the maxillary molar teeth to the infraorbital nerve or to the maxillary nerve directly.

nerve regeneration, *n* the reconstruction and renewal of cell structure and function; generally restricted to myelinated nerve fibers.

nerve repositioning, *n* the surgical redirecting of the inferior alveolar and/or mental nerve to allow longer implants to be placed in a mandible that has extensive deterioration of the posterior ridge. Some temporary or long-term loss of sensation to the lip, tongue, chin and/or gingival tissue may result. Also known as *nerve lateralization* and *nerve transpositioning.*

nerve(s), somatic motor, *n* (cranial), the somatic motor nerves—oculomotor (III), trochlear (IV), abducent (VI), and hypoglossal (XII)—largely comparable to the ventral motor roots of the spinal nerves. They are composed almost entirely of somatic motor fibers that emerge ventrally from the brainstem. Their arrangement is closely correlated with the distribution of the myotomes in the head. The oculomotor, trochlear, and abducent nerves, which supply the eye musculature, have the same myotomic origin and arrangement as the somatic muscles of the trunk and extremities.

nerve(s), special somatic sensory, *n* the structural arrangements from typical sensory nerves by which the three main sense organs, nose, eyes, and ears, are innervated. The sensory nerves are the olfactory (I), optic (II), and vestibulocochlear (acoustic) nerves (VIII).

nerve(s), spinal, *n* any one of 31 pairs of mixed peripheral nerves (8 cervical, 12 thoracic, 5 lumbar, 5 sacral, and 1 coccygeal) that are connected segmentally with the spinal cord, dorsal sensory trunk, and ventral motor root.

nerve, spinal accessory (XI), *n* the eleventh cranial nerve; a motor nerve that derives its origin in part from the medulla and in part from the cervical spinal cord. Its internal ramus joins with the vagus nerve to supply some of the muscles of the larynx. Its external ramus joins with the spinal nerves to supply the sternocleidomastoid and trapezius muscles. The nerve and its relationship to head posture is important in maintaining stable occlusal relationships of vertical dimension and centric relation.

nerve, tensor tympani, *n* a small motor branch of the mandibular nerve.

nerve, trigeminal (V) **(trījem′ənəl),** *n* the fifth cranial nerve; a mixed motor and sensory nerve connected with the pons through three roots (motor, proprioceptive, and large sensory), the latter root expanding into the trigeminal ganglion, from which arise the ophthalmic, masseteric, and mandibular divisions. It serves the muscles of mastication and cranial muscles through its motor root and serves the teeth, tongue, and oral cavity and most of the facial skin through its sensory root.

nerve, trochlear (IV) **(trō′klēər),** *n* the fourth cranial nerve; a small motor nerve arising ventrally in the midbrain and supplying the inferior oblique muscle of the eye.

nerve trunk, *n* a particularly sizeable bundle of axons or nerve fibers.

nerve, vagus (X) **(vā′gəs),** *n* the tenth cranial nerve; a mixed parasympathetic, visceral, afferent, motor, and general sensory nerve with laryngeal, pharyngeal, bronchial, esophageal, gastric, and many other branches.

nerve, vestibular (VIII), *n* one of the two major branches of the eighth cranial nerve; a special sensory nerve for the sense of balance and the transmission of space-orientation impulses from the semicircular canals to the brain.

nerve, vestibulocochlear (VII), *n* the seventh cranial nerve; acoustic nerve; a sensory nerve consisting of a vestibular portion and an auditory, or cochlear, portion.

nerve, zygomatic **(zī′gōmat′ik),** *n* the afferent nerve of the maxillary division of the cranial trigeminal nerve that serves the skin of the cheek and temple. It also innervates the lacrimal gland.

nerve(s), dentinal, *n* any of the afferent or sensory neurons associated with the odontoblastic processes in the dentinal tubules and the attached cell body of the odontoblasts within the pulp tissue. These nerves may allow for an awareness of pain due to their monitoring of environmenal changes within the dentin. There is some controversy about their overall location in the dentin tubule (full length, partial, or not at all).

nerves, efferent, *n* motor nerves that carry impulses from the brain or spinal cord toward the periphery of the body to activate muscles, usually in response to impulses received from sensory nerves.

nerve(s), periodontal ligament, *n* the sympathetic fibers of the autonomic nervous system with enclosed nerve endings that control blood flow within the vessels and register pressure changes. Sensory or afferent fibers with free nerve endings cause an awareness of pain.

nerve(s), pulp, *n* the sympathetic fibers of the autonomic nervous system located within the tissue that control blood flow within the vessels. Sensory or afferent fibers with free nerve endings in close proximity to the odontoblasts may cause an awareness of pain.

N

nerve block, *n* **1.** the reversible interruption of conduction along a nerve trunk or its branches because of the absorption of a suitable agent. *n* **2.** a regional anesthesia secured by extraneural or paraneural injection in close proximity to the nerve whose conductivity is to be cut. See also anesthesia, block.

nerve block, anterior middle superior alveolar, *n* an injection delivered by digital syringe into the palate that is used to anesthetize the pulp, facial and lingual periodontal tissues of the ipsilateral maxillary anterior teeth and premolars. It does not cause lip or facial muscle anesthesia.

nerve block, anterior superior alveolar, *n* an injection delivered by traditional syringe that is used to anesthetize the pulp tissue and facial periodontium of the maxillary anterior teeth.

nerve block, buccal, *n* an injection using a traditional syringe that causes anesthesia of the facial periodontium of the ipsilateral mandibular molars.

nerve block, greater palatine **(pal′ətīn),** *n* an injection delivered into the palatal tissues that is used to anesthetize the lingual periodontium of the ipsilateral maxillary posterior teeth.

nerve block, incisive, *n* a local anesthetic agent injected near the incisive nerves at the mental foramen that serve the mandibular premolars and anterior teeth.

nerve block, infraorbital **(in′frə-ôr′bitəl),** *n* an injection anesthetizing the pulp tissue and periodontium of the ipsilateral maxillary anterior teeth and premolars, including the first molar and its mesiobuccal root in some cases. One side of the nose, the upper lip, and lower eyelid may also be anesthetized.

nerve block, mandibular (inferior alveolar), *n* an injection used to anesthetize the anterior two-thirds portion of the tongue, the pulp tissue of the mandibular teeth, the floor of the oral cavity, the facial periodontium of the mandibular first premolar and anterior teeth, the lingual periodontium of all mandibular teeth, the skin on the chin, and the lower portion of the lip.

nerve block, middle superior alveolar, *n* an injection used to anesthetize pulp tissue and facial periodontium of the maxillary premolars and the mesiobuccal root of the first molar in some cases.

nerve block, nasopalatine, *n* an injection used to bilaterally anesthetize the lingual periodontium of the maxillary anterior teeth.

nerve block, posterior superior alveolar, *n* an injection used to anesthetize pulp tissue and facial periodontium of the ipsilateral maxillary molars. It does not always anesthetize the mesiobuccal root of the first molar.

nervous system, *n* the extensive, intricate network of structures that activates, coordinates, and controls all the functions of the body. The nervous system is divided into the central nervous system, composed of the brain and spinal cord, and the peripheral nervous system, which includes the cranial nerves and the spinal nerves.

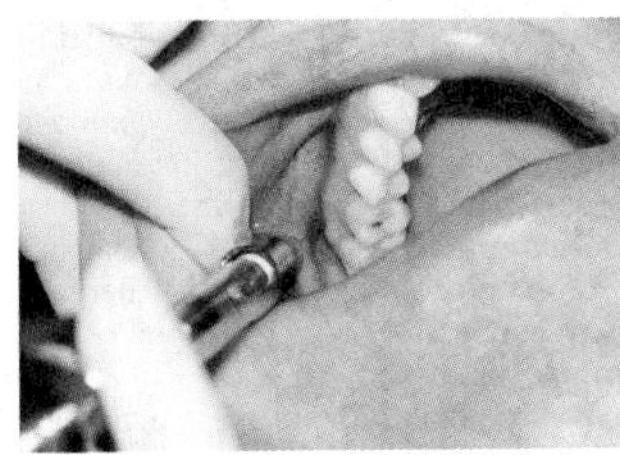

Posterior superior alveolar nerve block. (Fehrenbach/Herring, 2007)

net, *adj* devoid of anything extraneous; free from all deductions, such as charges, expenses, taxes; remaining after expenses.

net protein utilization (NPU), *n* a comparison between the amount of nitrogen taken into the body and the amount retained, which results in a percentage value; includes a determination of whether the protein containing the nitrogen is capable of being digested in the first place.

netilmicin sulfate (net′ilmī′sin sul′fāt), *n* a parenteral aminoglycoside antibiotic used for short-term treatment of serious or life-threatening bacterial infections.

neural crest cells (nŏŏr′əl), *n* the band of specialized cells from the neuroectoderm that lies along the outer surface of each side of the neural tube in the early stages of embryonic development. The cells migrate laterally throughout the embryo and give rise to certain spinal, cranial, and sympathetic ganglia. They also influence the ectomesenchyme to form dental tissues.

neuralgia (nyooral′jēə), *n* pain associated with a nerve or nerves (e.g., trigeminal and glossopharyngeal neuralgia).

neuralgia, atypical facial, *n* (cluster headache, lower-half headache, sphenopalatine neuralgia), severe unilateral pain behind the eye that spreads to the temple and behind the ear. It lasts 30 minutes to 3 hours and occurs once to several times a day and in cycles or clusters lasting several weeks. The clusters may be separated by several months or years. No trigger zones exist.

neuralgia, auriculotemporal, *n* (auriculotemporal causalgia neuralgia), sharp pain in the distribution of the auriculotemporal nerve.

neuralgia, buccal, *n* a throbbing, burning, and boring type of pain involving the cheeks, lips, gingivae, nose, and jaws. It may last a few minutes or several days. No trigger zones are present, although the pain may be initiated by chewing or thermal changes.

neuralgia, causalgia **(kozal′jēə),** *n* an intense, diffuse burning sensation in a limited area.

neuralgia, facial, *n* See neuralgia, trigeminal.

neuralgia, glossopharyngeal, *n* pain in the nerves of the tongue, pharynx, ear, and neck precipitated by swallowing, sneezing, coughing, talking, or blowing the nose.

neuralgia, Sluder's irritation of the sphenopalatine ganglion, *n.pr* diffuse pain may affect the eye, root of

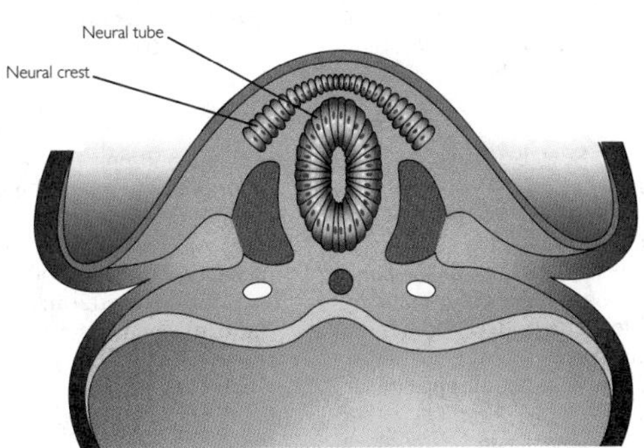

Neural crest. (Moore/Persaud, 2003)

the nose, teeth, and ear. Also, slight anesthesia and paralysis of the soft palate and palatine arch on the affected side may be present.

neuralgia, sphenopalatine, *n* See neuralgia, atypical, facial.

neuralgia, trifacial, *n* See neuralgia, trigeminal.

neuralgia, trigeminal, *n* (facial neuralgia, tic douloureux, trifacial neuralgia), an excruciating paroxysmal, stabbing, searing, or lancinating pain, usually occurring on the right side of the face and involving the distribution of the three divisions of the trigeminal nerve. It may last for a few seconds followed by additional episodes spontaneously or from stimulation of trigger zones. Intervals between attacks vary from a few hours to months or years.

neurasthenia (nyoo′rəsthē′nēə), *n* a neurotic reaction characterized by chronic physical fatigue, listlessness, mental sluggishness, and, often, phobias.

neurectomy (nyoorek′təmē), *n* the surgical excision of a nerve, or the more traumatic tearing away of nervous tissue from its anatomic position.

N

neurilemma (nyoo′rilem′ə), *n* the thin membranous outer covering surrounding the myelin sheath of a medullated nerve fiber or the axis cylinder of a nonmedullated nerve fiber. Neurilemma is associated with the booster mechanisms for the rapid transmission of impulses. Also called *sheath of Schwann.*

neurilemoma (nyoo′rilemō′mə), *n* (neurinoma, perineural fibroblastoma, schwannoma), a benign tumor of the neurilemma of disputed origin (Schwann cell vs. fibroblasts). May occur in soft tissue arid bone. Contains Verocay bodies. A malignant form occurs. See also body, Verocay and tissue.

neurinoma (nyoo′rinō′mə), *n* See neurilemoma.

neuritis (nyoorī′tis), *n* the inflammation of a nerve, accompanied by pain and tenderness over the nerves, anesthesia, disturbance of sensation, paralysis, wasting, and disappearance of reflexes.

neuritis, endemic multiple, *n* See beriberi.

neuroaminidase (nŏŏr′ōamin′idās), *n* an enzyme that is used in histochemistry to selectively remove sialomucins from bronchial mucous glands and the small intestine.

neuroanatomy, *n* the gross and microscopic structure of the nervous system.

neuroblastoma (nyoo′rōblastō′mə), *n* a malignant neoplasm characterized by proliferating nerve cells.

neuroectoderm (noor″oek′todərm), *n* specialized cells that differentiate from the ectoderm in the embryo from which the central and peripheral nervous systems develop.

neurofibroma (nyoo′rōfībrō′mə), *n* (neurogenic fibroma, perineural fibroblastoma), **1.** a benign neoplasm characterized by the various cells of a peripheral nerve (axon cylinders, Schwann cells, fibroblasts). *n* **2.** a connective tissue tumor of the nerve fiber fasciculi. Formed by the proliferation of the perineurium and endoneurium. See also neurilemoma.

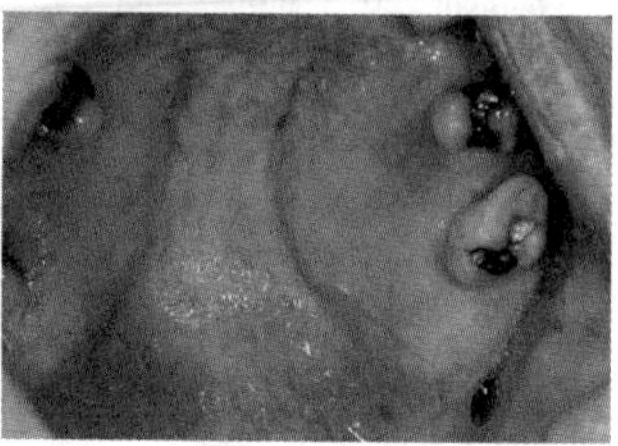

Neurofibroma. (Regezi/Sciubba/Jordan, 2008)

neurofibromatosis (nyoo′rōfī′brōmətō′sis), *n* (molluscum fibrosum, multiple neuroma, von Recklinghausen's disease of skin), a disease characterized by multiple neurofibromas. Most frequently affects the skin but possibly involves the oral mucosa.

neurokinin (A) (nŏŏ′ōkī′nin), *n* a mammalian deca-peptide tachykinin found in the central nervous system. The compound has bronchoconstrictor, smooth muscle constrictor, and hypotensive effects and also activates the micturition reflex.

neuroleptanalgesia (nŏŏr′ōlep′tanəljē′zēə), *n* a form of analgesia achieved by the concurrent administration of a neuroleptic and an analgesic. Anxiety, motor activity, and sensitivity to painful stimuli are reduced; the person is quiet and indifferent to the environment and surroundings. If nitrous oxide with oxygen is also administered, neuroleptanalgesia can be converted to neuroleptanesthesia.

neurology (nŏŏrol′əjē), *n* the field of medicine that deals with the nervous system and its disorders.

neuroma (nyoorō′mə), *n* technically, a benign neoplasm of nerve cells. As used in oral disease, the term usually refers to a traumatic neuroma, which is not a true tumor but an overgrowth of nerves associated with injury. The mental foramina and extraction scars are possible oral sites of this painful lesion.

neuroma, amputation, *n* See neuroma, traumatic.

neuroma, multiple, *n* See neurofibromatosis.

neuroma, traumatic, *n* (amputation neuroma), hyperplasia of nerve fibers and their supporting tissues in an exuberant attempt at repair after damage to, or the severing of, a nerve.

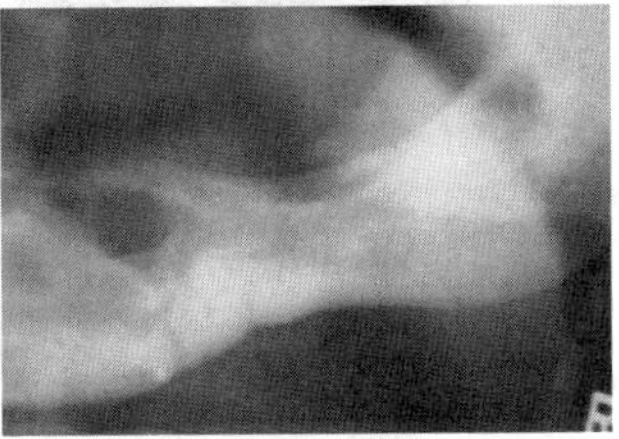

Traumatic neuroma. (Regezi/Sciubba/Jordan, 2008)

neuromuscular junction, *n* the area of contact between the ends of a large myelinated nerve fiber and a fiber of skeletal muscle. Also called *myoneural junction.*

neuron (nyoo′ron), *n* a nerve cell; the basic structural unit of the nervous system. There is a wide variation in the shape of nerve cells, but they all have the same basic structures: cell body, protoplasmic processes, axons, and dendrites. The neuron is the only body cell whose principal function is the conduction of impulses. It cannot regenerate when the cell body is destroyed; however, cell processes such as axons and dendrites can often regenerate.

neuron, sensory, *n* See neuron, afferent.

neuropathy, *n* an abnormal condition characterized by inflammation and degeneration of peripheral nerves.

neuropeptide, *n* any of a variety of peptides found in neural tissues, such as endorphins and enkephalins.

neurosis, *n* a diffusely defined term referring to a mental disorder for which professional help may be needed but that is milder than a psychosis; generally, a functional disorder in which there is no gross personality disorganization but there is an inability to cope effectively with some routine frustrations, anxieties, and daily problems. Somatic conditions may be factors in the cause and may be symptoms in a neurosis; however, the use of the term to describe a dysfunction of the nervous system is obsolete. Also called *psychoneurosis.*

N

neurostomatosis (nyoo′rōstō′mətō′sis), *n* an oral condition associated with psychosomatic or other psychologic factors; e.g., lichen planus and benign migratory glossitis may be considered types of neurostomatoses.

neurosurgery, *n* surgery involving the brain, spinal cord, or peripheral nerves.

neurosyphilis, paretic (nyoo′rōsi′filis), *n* See paresis.

neurotensin (nŏŏ′ōten′sin), *n* a 13-amino acid peptide neurotransmitter found in synapsomes in the hypothalamus, amygdala, basal ganglia, and dorsal gray matter of the spinal cord; it plays a role in pain perception. It also affects pituitary hormone release and gastrointestinal function.

neurotomy (nyoorot′əmē), *n* the severance of a nerve process.

neurotransmitter, *n* any one of numerous chemicals that modify or result in the transmission of nerve impulses between synapses. Neurotransmitters are released from syn-

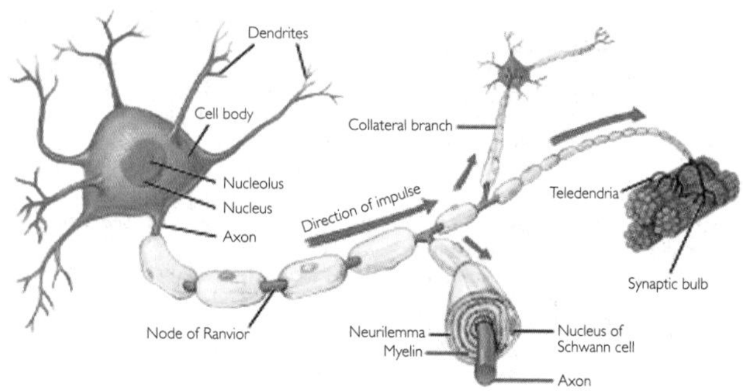

Neuron. (Applegate, 2006)

aptic knobs into synaptic clefts and bridge the gap between presynaptic and postsynaptic neurons.

neutral, *n* a solution that has a pH level of 7. Equal numbers of hydrogen and hydroxyl ions are formed on dissociation.

neutral zone, *n* See zone, neutral.

neutral position, *n* correct ergonomic positioning of the clinician's body in order to reduce stress and fatigue on muscles and joints during intraoral care of a patient, thereby reducing the possibility of neuromuscular disorders or repetitive strain injuries to the clinician.

N

neutralization, *n* the reaction of an acid with a base.

neutrocclusion, *n* normal mesiodistal occlusal relationships of the buccal teeth, similar to Angle class I.

neutron (noo′tron), *n* an elementary particle with approximately the mass of a hydrogen atom but without any electrical charge; one of the constituents of the atomic nucleus.

neutron activation analysis, *n* an activation analysis in which the specimen is bombarded with neutrons. Identification is made by measuring the resulting radioisotopes.

neutron ray, *n* See ray, neutron.

neutropenia (noo′trōpē′nēə), *n* a relative or absolute decrease in the normal number of neutrophils in the circulating blood. Various limits are given; e.g., absolute neutropenia may exist when the total is less than 1700 cells/mm^3 regardless of the percentage, whereas relative neutropenia may exist when the total percentage of neutrophils is less than 38% and the total number is not less than 1500/mm^3. It may be associated with viral infections, pernicious anemia, sprue, aplastic anemia, bone marrow, neoplasms, chronic intoxication with drugs or heavy metals, malnutrition, and nonpyogenic and overwhelming infections. See also neutrophil.

neutropenia, cyclic, *n* a condition in which there is a depression in the number of circulating white cells, especially the neutrophils, at intervals of about 21 days. It lasts for approximately 10 days; during this time, gingival inflammation and aphthous ulcer occur.

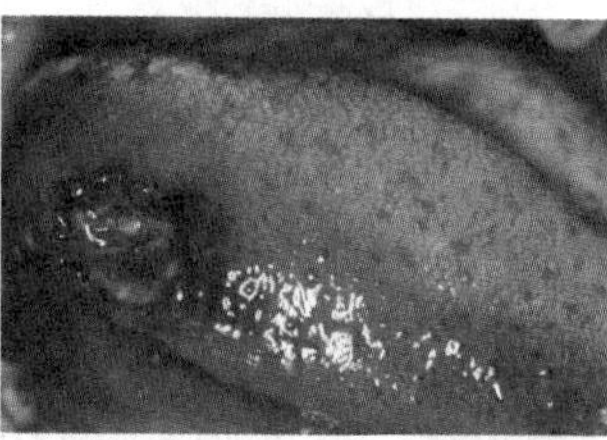

Cyclic neutropenia. (Sams/Lynch, 1996)

neutrophil, *n* a polymorphonuclear leukocyte (PMN). See also leukocyte, polymorphonuclear (PMN).

neutrophilia (noo′trōfil′ēə), *n* an absolute or relative increase in the normal number of neutrophils in the circulating blood. Various limits are given; e.g., an absolute neutrophilia may exist, regardless of percentage, if the total number of neutrophils exceeds 7000/mm^3, whereas a relative neutrophilia may exist if the percentage of neutrophils is greater than 70% and the total number of neutrophils is less than 7000/mm³. May be associated with acute infections, chronic granulocytic leukemia, erythemia, therapy with adrenocorticotropic hormone (ACTH) or cortisone, uremia, ketosis, hemolysis, drug or heavy metal intoxication, or malignancy, or it may follow severe hemorrhage.

nevus (nē′vus), *n* a circumscribed new growth of congenital origin that may be vascular (resulting from hypertrophy of blood or lymph vessels) or nonvascular (with epidermal and connective tissue predominating).

nevus, blue, *n* a benign neoplasm characterized by heavily pigmented spindle cells deep in the tissue; appears clinically as a dark mole.

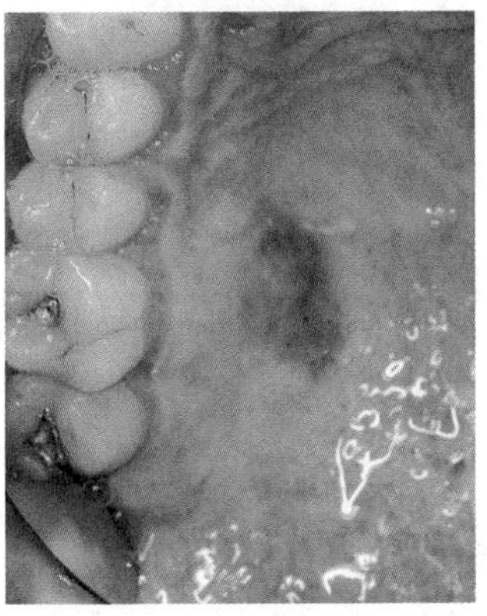

Blue nevus. (Sapp/Eversole/Wysocki, 2004)

nevus, cellular pigmented, *n* a nevus composed of melanin-producing "nevus" cells.

nevus, compound, *n* a nevus in which the melanin-producing nevus cells are found in the epidermis and dermis: the intradermal nevus plus the junctional nevus.

nevus, intradermal, *n* a nevus in which the melanin-producing nevus cells are found only in the dermis.

nevus, junctional, *n* a nevus in which the melanin-producing nevus cells are found within the epidermis at the junction with the dermis.

nevus, pigmented, *n* a dark-colored, benign neoplasm characterized by nevus cells. Junctional, intradermal, and compound types are recognized. Melanomas (malignant neoplasms) may develop from junctional or compound nevi.

nevus, white sponge (Cannon's disease; white folded gingivostomatitis), *n* an inherited disease of the oral mucosa characterized by generalized white mucosal surfaces with a spongelike appearance.

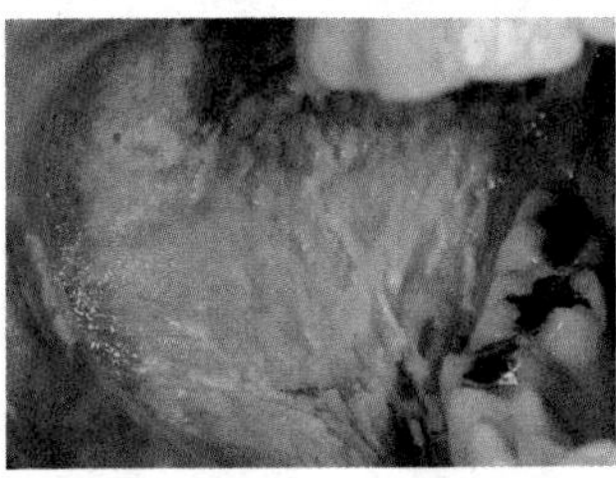

White sponge nevus. (Regezi/Sciubba/Pogrel, 2000)

new attachment, *n* a connection formed between epithelium or connective tissue and a root surface that has lost its original attachment; this new connection may involve new cementum, epithelial adhesion, and connective adaptation.

Ney surveyor, *n.pr* See surveyor, Ney.

NF, *n.pr* the National Formulary.

niacin (vitamin B_3) (nī′əsin), *n* *brand name:* generic niacin (nicotinic acid); *drug class:* vitamin B_3; *action:* needed for conversion of fats, protein, carbohydrates by oxidation-reduction; acts directly on vascular smooth muscle, causing vasodilation; *uses:* pellagra, hyperlipidemias, peripheral vascular disease.

nib, *n* the part of a condensing instrument corresponding to the blade of a cutting instrument. The end is called the *face* of the condenser.

nicardipine HCl (nīkär′dəpēn′), *n* *brand name:* Cardene; *drug class:* calcium channel blocker; *action:* inhibits calcium ion influx across cell membrane during cardiac depolarization; produces relaxation of coronary vascular smooth muscle, peripheral vascular smooth muscle; dilates coronary vascular arteries; decreases sinoatrial/atrioventricular (SA/AV) node conduction; *uses:* chronic stable angina pectoris, hypertension.

nickel, *n* a silvery-white metallic element. Its atomic number is 28 and its atomic weight is 58.69. Large numbers of people are allergic to nickel. Nickel causes more cases of allergic contact dermatitis than all other metals combined. Many cases of allergic contact dermatitis occur from exposure to the nickel content of jewelry, coins, buckles, and snaps, and from continued use of "carbonless" business forms.

nickel-chromium alloy, *n* See alloy, nickel-chromium.

niclosamide (niklō'səmīd), *n* an anthelmintic agent that acts against pinworms and most tapeworms by inhibiting oxidative phosphorylation in the mitochondria.

nicotine, *n* a poisonous alkaloid found in tobacco and responsible for many of the effects of tobacco. It is first a stimulant (small doses) and then a depressant (larger doses). It is highly addictive.

nicotine gum, *n brand name:* Nicorette (nicotine polacrilex); an over-the-counter chewable product containing the chemical nicotine. It is used for tobacco cessation.

nicotine inhaler, *n* a prescription inhalation device consisting of a mouthpiece into which a cartridge is inserted to deliver nicotine in gradually diminishing doses over time. It is used for tobacco cessation.

nicotine lozenge, *n* an over-the-counter dissoluble tablet that releases nicotine. It is used for tobacco cessation.

nicotine nasal spray, *n* a prescription nicotine-containing liquid that the user self-administers through the nose. It is used for tobacco cessation.

nicotine patch (nicotine transdermal system), *n brand names:* Habitrol, Nicoderm, Nicotrol, ProStep; an over-the-counter press-on patch that releases nicotine slowly into the body through the skin. It is used for tobacco cessation.

nicotine replacement therapy, *n* a tobacco cessation method intended to reduce nicotine cravings and ease the symptoms of withdrawal by substituting another source of nicotine, such as a specially formulated lozenge, gum, nasal spray, inhalant, or skin patch for tobacco products.

nicotinic stomatitis (nik'ətin'ik stō'mətī'tis), *n* See stomatitis, nicotinic.

nidus (nī'dus), *n* the focal point; an originating position or nucleus.

Niemann-Pick disease (nē'mon-pik'), *n.pr* See disease, Niemann-Pick.

nifedipine (nīfed'əpēn'), *n brand names:* Procardia, Procardia XL; *drug class:* calcium channel blocker; *action:* inhibits calcium ion influx across cell membrane during cardiac depolarization; produces relaxation of coronary vascular smooth muscle, dilates coronary arteries; increases myocardial oxygen delivery in patients with vasospastic angina; dilates peripheral arteries; *uses:* chronic stable angina pectoris, vasospastic angina, hypertension. Can cause gingival hyperplasia.

night guard, *n* See guard, night.

night-grinding, *n* See bruxism.

Nikolsky's sign (nikol'skēz), *n.pr* See sign, Nikolsky's.

niobium (Nb) (nīō'bēəm), *n* the chemical element with an atomic number of 41 and an atomic weight of 92.9064. It was formerly known as *columbium.*

nitric acid, *n* a colorless, highly corrosive liquid that may give off suffocating brown fumes of nitrogen dioxide on exposure to air. Commercially prepared nitric acid is a powerful oxidizing agent used in photoengraving and metallurgy.

nitrofurantoin/nitrofurantoin macrocrystals (nī'trōfyŏŏran'tōin), *n brand names:* Furadantin, Furalan, Macrobid, Macrodantin; *drug class:* urinary tract antiinfective; *action:* appears to inhibit bacterial enzymes; *uses:* urinary tract infections caused by *Escherichia coli, Klebsiella, Pseudomonas, Proteus vulgaris, Proteus morganii, Citrobacter,* and *Staphylococcus aureus.*

nitrogen (N), *n* a gaseous, nonmetallic element. Its atomic number is 7 and its atomic weight is 14.0067. It constitutes approximately 78% of the atmosphere and is a component of all proteins and a major component of most organic substances.

N

nitrogen monoxide, *n* See nitrous oxide.

nitrogen monoxidum, *n* See nitrous oxide.

nitrogen, nonprotein, *n* See nonprotein nitrogen.

nitrogen balance, *n* a determination made about the body's ability to meet its protein needs which is reached by comparing the amount of nitrogen taken in with the amount discharged via urine, hair, skin, or perspiration.

nitrogen balance, negative, *n* a condition in which nitrogen output exceeds nitrogen intake, resulting in the body's need to draw on its own stores of protein for energy; may be caused by dietary imbalances, illness, infection, anxiety, or stress.

nitrogen balance, positive, *n* a body condition in which nitrogen intake exceeds nitrogen output; a normal state for children, pregnant women, or individuals recovering from illness or surgery, whose bodies require extra protein in order to build tissue.

nitroglycerin (nī'trōglis'ərin), *n brand names:* Nitrogard, Nitro-Bid, Nitrostat; *drug class:* inorganic nitrate, vasodilator; *action:* decreases preload/afterload, which is responsible for decreasing left ventricular end-diastolic pressure, systemic vascular resistance; arterial and venous dilation; *uses:* chronic stable angina pectoris, prophylaxis of angina pain, congestive heart failure associated with acute myocardial infarction, controlled hypotension in surgical procedures. Metered spray has a longer shelf life than tablet form. Recommended for dental office or clinic emergency kits.

nitromersol, tincture (nītrōmur'sol), *n* a solution used in 1:200 strength as a topically applied antiseptic to temporarily minimize the bacterial count on an area of tissue.

nitrosamine (nītrō'səmēn), *n* compound present in tobacco that is linked to the development of cancer.

nitrous acid, HNO_2, a standard chemical reagent used in biologic and clinical laboratories.

nitrous oxide (N_2O) (nī'trəs ok'sīd), *n* (laughing gas, nitrogen monoxide, nitrogen monoxidum), a gas with a sweet odor and taste used with oxygen as an analgesic and sedative agent for the performance of minor operations. It is sometimes called *laughing gas* because it may excite a hilarious delirium preceding insensibility.

nizatidine (nīzat'ədēn'), *n brand name:* Axid; *drug class:* H_2-histamine receptor antagonist; *action:* inhibits histamine at H_2 receptor site in parietal cells, which inhibits gastric acid secretion; *uses:* duodenal ulcer, Zollinger-Ellison syndrome, gastric ulcers, hypersecretory conditions, gastroesophageal reflux disease, stress ulcers.

NMR (nuclear magnetic resonance), *n* See magnetic resonance imaging.

noble, *adj* an archaic term referring to inert gases and precious metals.

noble metal, *n* See metal, noble.

Nocardia, *n* a genus of aerobic nonmotile actinomycetes, which are transitional between bacteria and fungi. They are primarily saprophytic but may cause disease in man and other animals.

nocardiosis (nōkär'dēō'sis), *n* any of the pathologic entities that may follow infection with the bacterium *Nocardia.*

nociceptor (nō'sisep'tər), *n* somatic and visceral free nerve endings of thinly myelinated and unmyelinated fibers. They usually react to tissue injury but also may be excited by endogenous chemical substances.

node (nōd), *n* a swelling or protuberance.

node, brown, of hyperparathyroidism, *n* a central giant cell lesion of the bone seen in hyperparathyroidism. Its microscopic appearance is similar to giant cell reparative granuloma and giant cell tumor.

node of Ranvier gaps, *n.pl* nodes distributed at regularly spaced intervals along a myelinated nerve fiber. The intervals are 1 mm or more in length, and they function essentially as relay stations to facilitate the passage of an impulse.

nodule(s), *n* a small solid mass or knot that can be easily felt.

nodule, pulp **(nod'ūl),** *n* See denticle.

nodules, Bohn's, *n.pl* See also cyst, palatal, of the newborn.

noma (nō′mə), *n* a progressive necrotizing process originating in the cheek with secondary involvement of the gingiva and jawbone. Occurs primarily in debilitated children, and the mortality rate is high. There is a strong, foul odor; marked surrounding edema; absence of a specific erythematous halo; marked changes in the white blood cell count; and a high temperature. See also necrosis, exanthematous and stomatitis, gangrenous.

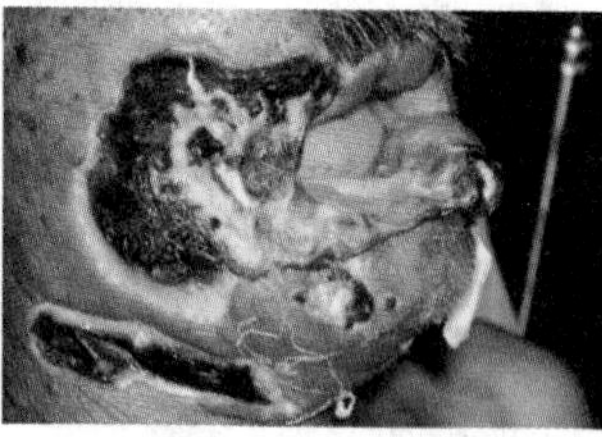

Noma. (Neville/Damm/Allen/Bouqout, 2002)

nomenclature (nō′menklā′chur), *n* the formally adopted terminology of a science, art, or discipline; the system of names or terms used in a particular branch of science.

nomenclature, anatomic, *n* a naming system used to identify and classify the structures and organs of the body.

non-Hodgkin lymphoma, *n* a form of lymphoma associated with AIDS. One of the indicator diseases of AIDS. See also lymphoma.

nonblisterform oral lesions, *n* solid wound with a firm texture located within the oral cavity that does not contain any fluid; may be a nodule, papule, plaque, or tumor.

noncohesive, *adj* lacking the property of sticking together, or cohesion.

noncontributory plan, *n* a method of payment for group insurance coverage in which the entire premium is paid by the employer or the union. Also referred to as *noncontributory program.*

nonduplication of benefits, *n* this term may apply if a subscriber is eligible for benefits under more than one plan. A dental benefits contract provision that relieves the third-party payer of liability for cost of services if the services are covered under another program. Distinct from a coordination of benefits provision because reimbursement would be limited to the greater level allowed by the two plans rather than a total of 100% of the charges. Also referred to as *less-benefit* or *carve-out.*

nonfeasance (nonfē′zəns), *n* the failure of a person to do some act that should be done.

nongonococcal urethritis (non′gon′ōkok′əl yoor′ithrī′tis), *n* an infection of the reproductive system caused by the bacterium *C. trachomatis.* Transmitted through sexual contact and can lead to infertility in women. See also *C. trachomatis.*

nonnutritive sucking, *n* a behavior of infants and toddlers that includes sucking on objects (fingers, pacifiers, etc.) out of habit or for psychologic comfort.

nonocclusion (non′əkloo′zhən), *n* a situation in which the tooth or teeth in one arch fail to make contact with the tooth or teeth of the other arch.

nonparticipating dental professional, *n* **1.** a dental professional with whom the underwriter (insurer) does not have an agreement to render dental care to members of the plan. *n* **2.** any dental professional who does not have a contractual agreement with a dental benefits organization to render dental care to members of a dental benefits program.

nonprofit insurers, *n.pl* service corporations organized under nonprofit laws for the purpose of providing dental care insurance.

nonprotein nitrogen (NPN), *n* the nitrogen of whole blood or serum exclusive of that of the proteins. The concentration of nonprotein nitrogen is a gross measure of renal function. The upper limit of normal is 35 mg/100 ml.

nonsuccedaneous (non″suk″səda′neəs), *adj* pertaining to those permanent teeth that are not preceded by a primary form (e.g., the molars).

nonsuit, *n* a failure on the part of a plaintiff to continue the prosecution of the suit; abandonment of a suit.

nor-, *comb* a prefix that indicates lack of a methyl group.

norepinephrine (nôr′epinef′rin), *n* the neurohormonal transmitter for neuroeffector junctions of adrenergic nerve fibers. Its official drug name in the United States is levarterenol. See also levarterenol.

norethindrone acetate (nôreth′in-drōn′ as′ətāt), *n brand names:* Aygestin, Micronor, Norlutate, Norlutin, Nor-QD; *drug class:* progesterone derivative; *action:* inhibits secretion of pituitary gonadotropins, which prevents follicular maturation, ovulation; *uses:* abnormal uterine bleeding, amenorrhea, endometriosis, contraceptive.

norfloxacin (nôrflok′səsēn), *n brand name:* Noroxin; *drug class:* fluoroquinolone antiinfective; *action:* a broad-spectrum bactericidal agent that inhibits the enzyme DNA gyrase needed for replication of DNA; *uses:* adult urinary tract infections.

norgestrel (nôrjes′trəl), *n brand name:* Ovrette; *drug class:* progesterone derivative; *action:* inhibits secretion of pituitary gonadotropins, which prevents follicular maturation, ovulation; *use:* oral contraception.

norm, *n* **1.** a statistical unit representative of the human species as a whole. *n* **2.** the numerical or statistical measures of the usual observed performance when related to health care provided to a given number of patients over time; often used in the building of profiles; can be the average or median or some other cutoff point in a series.

normal distribution, *n* a curve representing the frequency with which the values of a variable are obtained or observed when the number is infinite and variation is subject only to chance factors. The curve is a symmetrical, bell-shaped curve with the highest frequency occurring in the middle and gradually tapering toward the extremes. In a normal distribution, 68.2% of all scores cluster around the mean within approximately 1 standard deviation, 95.4% within approximately 2 standard deviations, and 99.7% within approximately 3 standard deviations. Also called *normal curve, Gauss' curve.*

normality, *n* a reference solution in which the concentration is stated with regard to the number of gram-equivalent weights present per liter of solution.

normalization, *n* the act of creating a lifestyle as similar as possible to that of a nonchallenged person for a person with disabilities.

normal-set powder, *n* an irreversible, hydrocolloid material used to make impressions of a patient's dentition; this alginate material has a working time of 2 minutes and a setting time of 4.5 minutes.

normoblast (nôr′mōblast), *n* a nucleated red blood cell found in the peripheral bloodstream in severe pernicious anemia and in some leukemias.

normotensive (nôr′mōten′siv), *adj* having or dealing with having normal blood pressure.

nortriptyline HCl (nôrtrip′təlēn′), *n brand names:* Aventyl, Pamelor; *drug class:* tricyclic antidepressant; *action:* blocks reuptake of norepinephrine, serotonin into nerve endings, which increases action of norepinephrine, serotonin in nerve cells; *use:* major depression.

Norwalk virus (nôr′wôlk), *n.pr* causative agent of acute gastrointestinal infection transmitted to humans through fecal-oral contact. Symptoms include cramping, fatigue, nausea, vomiting, and diarrhea.

nose, *n* the structure that protrudes from the anterior portion of the midface and serves as a passageway for air to and from the lungs. The nose filters, warms, and moistens the air on its passage into the lungs. The nose contains the end organs of smell.

nose, bones of, *n* paired facial bones that together shape the nasal bridge, the edges of which join with the frontal bone at the top and the upper cheek bones at the sides.

nosebleed, *n* See epistaxis.

nosocomial (nos′əkō′mēəl), *adj* related to a hospital; a condition described as nosocomial is one that occurs as a direct result of hospital treatment.

nostrum (nos′trəm), *n* a remedy not substantiated by scientific evidence or broadly accepted by the scientific community. Some herbal supplements may fall under this category.

not-for-profit third parties, *n.pl* service corporations or dental benefits organizations established under not-for-profit state statutes for the purpose of providing health care coverage (e.g., Delta Dental and Blue Cross, Blue Shield Plans).

notch, *n* an indentation.

notch, buccal, *n* the notch in the flange of a denture that accommodates the buccal frenum.

notch, coronoid **(kôr′ənoid),** *n* greatest concavity on the anterior border of the ramus of the mandible.

notch, hamular, *n* See notch, pterygomaxillary.

notch, labial, *n* the notch in the labial flange of a maxillary or mandibular denture that accommodates the labial frenum.

notch, mandibular, *n* a semicircular depression located on the mandible between the condyle and the coronoid process. Fibers arise from the anterior edge of the temporalis to form a distinct muscle, the temporalis minor, that inserts onto the mandibular notch.

notch, pterygomaxillary **(ter′igōmak′səlerē),** *n* (hamular notch), the notch or fissure formed at the junction of the maxilla and the hamular, or pterygoid, process of the sphenoid bone.

notch, sigmoid, *n* the concavity on the superior surface of the ramus of the mandible lying between the coronoid and condyloid processes.

note, promissory, *n* a written promise to pay to another, at a specified time, a stated amount of money or other articles of value.

notice, *n* **1.** knowledge; information; awareness of facts. *v* **2.** the knowledge of facts that would naturally lead an honest and prudent person to make inquiry constitutes "notice" of everything that such inquiry pursued in good faith would disclose. *v* **3.** to observe.

notochord (nō′təkôrd′), *n* an elongated strip of mesodermal tissue that originates from the primitive node and extends along the dorsal surface of the developing embryo beneath the neural tube, forming the primary longitudinal skeletal axis of the body of all chordates.

Novocain (nō′vəkān′), *n* the brand name for procaine hydrochloride, an ester, which is no longer used in the United States as an injectable. It is also the lay term for all types of dental local anesthesia.

noxious (nok′shus), *adj* hurtful; not wholesome.

NPN, *n* See nonprotein nitrogen.

NSAIDs, *n.pl* the acronym for nonsteroidal antiinflammatory drugs. See also naproxen.

nuclear family, *n* a family unit consisting of the biologic parents and their offspring. The nuclear family is less inclusive than the extended family. Although the nuclear family is a relatively recent product of Western society, it is threatened by the increasing dissolution of marriage.

nuclear magnetic resonance, *n* See magnetic resonance imaging.

nuclear medicine imaging, *n* the diagnostic imaging field that evaluates organ function by injecting isotopes into a structure and documenting the amount of radiation emanating from the tissues.

nucleic acid, *n* a family of macromolecules found in the chromosomes, nucleoli, mitochondria, and cytoplasm of all cells. In complexes with proteins, they are called *nucleoproteins.*

nucleic acid probes, *n* nucleic acid that complements a specific RNA or DNA molecule or fragment; used for hybridization studies to identify microorganisms and for genetic studies.

Nucleopolyhedrovirus **(noo′klēō′pol′ēhed′rōvī′rəs),** *n* (nuclear polyhedrosis virus), a genus of the family *Baculoviridae,* characterized by the formation of crystalline, polyhedral occlusion bodies in the host cell nucleus.

nucleoprotein (noo′klēōprō′tēn), *n* a special group of protein substances that are in combination with nucleic acid. The essential component is the phosphoric acid radical. The nucleoproteins are generally confined to the nucleus of the cell and are intimately associated with chromosome and gene function.

nucleoside (noo′klēəsīd′), *n* purine or pyrimidine bases attached to a ribose or deoxyribose.

nucleus (noo′klēus), *n* **1.** the small, central part of an atom in which the positive electric charge and most of the mass (protons and neutrons) are concentrated. *n* **2.** an easily recognized structural component of most cells, surrounded by a membrane and containing chromosomes and nucleolus.

Nuhn's gland (noonz), *n.pr* the anterior lingual gland embedded in the substance of the tongue near the apex and the midline on the inferior surface of the tongue. See also gland, Blandin and Nuhn's.

null cell, *n* a lymphocyte that develops in the bone marrow and lacks the characteristic surface markers of the B and T lymphocytes. Null cells stimulated by the presence of antibody can directly attack certain cellular targets and are known as "natural killers" or "killer cells."

null hypothesis, *n* a statistical hypothesis that predicts that no difference or relationship exists among the variables studied that could not have occurred by chance alone.

number, Brinell hardness (BHN), *n.pr* a numerical expression of the hardness of a material, determined by measuring the diameter of a dent made by forcing a hard steel or tungsten carbide ball of standard dimension into the material under specified load in a Brinell machine, which was devised by J.A. Brinell, a Swedish engineer. The larger the indentation, the smaller the Brinell hardness number. See also test, Brinell hardness.

number, Vickers hardness, *n.pr* hardness as measured by the Vickers hardness test. See also test, Vickers hardness.

nurse, *n* **1.** a person educated and licensed in the practice of nursing; one who is concerned with the diagnosis and treatment of human responses to actual or potential health problems. *v* **2.** to breastfeed an infant.

nurse anesthetist, *n* a registered nurse qualified by advanced training in an accredited program in the specialty of nurse anesthesia to manage the care of the patient during the administration of anesthesia in selected surgical situations.

nurse practitioner, *n* a nurse who, by advanced education and clinical experience in a specialized area of nursing practice, has acquired expert knowledge and skill in a special branch of practice. The nurse practitioner acts as a nurse clinician, functioning independently within standing orders or protocols and collaborating with associates to implement a plan of care.

nurse's aide, *n* a person who is employed to carry out basic nonspecialized tasks in the care of a patient, such as bathing and feeding, making beds, and transporting patients under the supervision and direction of a registered nurse.

nursing, *n* **1.** the performance of those activities that contribute to the health or recovery of a patient (or to a peaceful death). *n* **2.** the application of prescribed therapies and the management of the patient and environment to assist in healing.

nursing bottle caries, *n* dental caries of the maxillary primary teeth caused by the oral retention of milk or formula in the oral cavity.

nursing home, *n* a convalescent facility for the care of individuals who do not require hospitalization but who cannot be cared for at home. Preferred nomenclature: extended care facility.

nutrient, *n* the beneficial chemical in foods and beverages. Classified as carbohydrates, fats, proteins, water, vitamins, and minerals.

nutrient canal (noo′trēənt), *n* See canal, interdental.

nutrient dense, *adj* describes the ratio of beneficial chemicals to the number of calories in food when nutrient content is greater.

nutrient, essential, *n* See nutrient.

nutrition, *n* the process of assimilation and use of essential food elements from the diet (e.g., carbohydrates, fats, proteins, vitamins, mineral elements).

nutrition survey, *n* usually a questionnaire regarding dietary habits, but may include an objective evaluation of nutritional status through the administration of physical examinations and laboratory tests of metabolism of a target population.

nutritional requirements, *n* the food and liquids necessary for normal physiologic function.

nutritional status, *n* the assessment of the state of nourishment of a patient or subject.

nutritional support, *n* the supply of foods and liquids necessary to advance healing and support health.

nutriture (noo′trichur), *n* the nutritional status of a patient.

Nuva-lite, *n.pr* the brand name for an ultraviolet light used as a catalyst in the polymerization of Nuva-seal, a bonding agent used as an enamel sealant.

Nuva-seal, *n.pr* the brand name of a bonding agent used as an enamel sealant.

nylidrin HCl (nī′lidrən), *n brand name:* Arlidin; *drug class:* peripheral vasodilator, β-adrenergic agonist; *action:* acts on β-adrenergic receptors to dilate arterioles in skeletal muscles; increases cardiac output; may have direct vasodilatory effect on vascular smooth muscle; *uses:* arteriosclerosis obliterans, thromboangiitis obliterans, diabetic vascular disease, night leg cramps, Raynaud's disease, ischemic ulcer, frostbite, primary cochlear cell ischemia.

nystagmus (nīstag′mus), *n* the state of oscillatory movements of an organ or part, especially the eyeballs; irregular jerking movement of the eyes. Each movement of the cycle consists of a slow component in one direction and a rapid component in the opposite direction.

nystatin (nis′tətin), *n brand names:* Mycostatin, Nystex, O-V Statin; *drug class:* antifungal; *action:* interferes with fungal DNA replication; *uses:* *Candida* species causing oral, vaginal, and intestinal infections.

O

oath, *n* an affirmation of the truth of a statement that renders one who is willfully asserting untrue statements punishable for perjury.

obesity (ōbēs′itē), *n* a bodily condition marked by excessive generalized deposition and storage of fat.

obesity, adrenocortical, *n* one of the symptoms characteristic of Cushing's syndrome; an obesity that is confined mainly to the trunk, face, and neck. Also called *buffalo obesity.*

obesity, buffalo, *n* See obesity, adrenocortical.

object-film distance, *n* See distance, object-film.

obligation, *n* an assumed or assigned duty imposed by promise, law, contract, or society; the binding power of a vow, promise, oath, or contract.

observer variation, *n* the failure by the observer to measure or identify a phenomenon accurately, which results in an error. The observer may miss an abnormality or use faulty techniques, such as incorrect measurement or misinterpretation of the data. Two types are interobserver variation (the amount observers vary from one another when reporting on the same material) and intraobserver variation (the amount one observer varies between observations when reporting more than once on the same material).

obsessive-compulsive disorder (OCD), *n* the abnormal behavior of a person who tends to perform repetitive acts or rituals, usually as a means of releasing tension or relieving anxiety.

obstetrician (ob′stitrish′ən), *n* a physician whose practice of medicine focuses on the care of women during pregnancy, through childbirth, and immediately following delivery. Often informally known as *OB-gyn (obstetrician-gynecologist).*

obstetrics (obstet′riks), *n* the branch of medicine concerned with pregnancy and childbirth, including the study of the physiologic and pathologic function of the female reproductive tract and the care of the mother and fetus throughout pregnancy, childbirth, and the immediate postpartum period.

obtund (obtund′), *v* to diminish the ability to perceive pain and/or touch.

obtundent (obtun′dent), *n* an agent that has the property to diminish the perception of pain and/or touch.

obturation (ob′toorā′shən), *n* the act of closing or occluding.

obturation, retrograde, n See filling, retrograde.

obturation, root canal filling technique, n the procedure used for filling and sealing the root canal.

obturator (ob′toorātur), *n* a prosthesis used to close a congenital or acquired opening in the palate. See also aid, prosthetic speech.

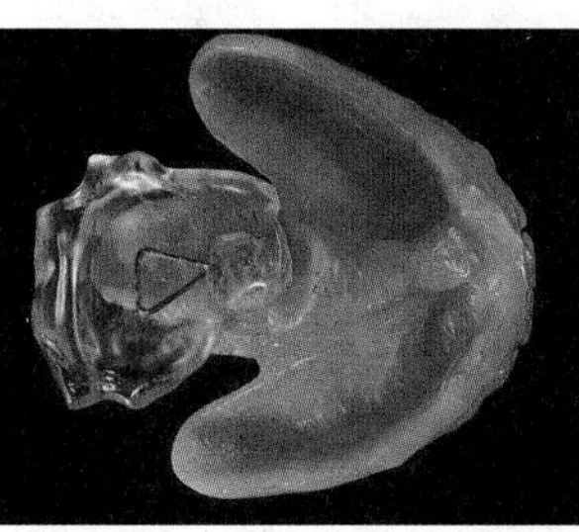

Cleft palate obturator. (Courtesy Dr. Charles Babbush)

obturator, hollow, n that portion of an obturator made hollow to minimize its weight.

occipital anchorage (oksip′itəl), *n* See anchorage, occipital.

occlude (ōklood′), *v* to close together. To bring together; to shut. To bring the mandibular teeth into contact with the maxillary teeth.

occluder, *n* a name given to some articulators. See also articulator.

occlusal, *adj* pertaining to the contacting surfaces of opposing occlusal units (teeth or occlusion rims). Pertaining to the masticating surfaces of the posterior teeth.

occlusal adjustment, n See adjustment, occlusal.

occlusal analysis, n See analysis, occlusal.

occlusal balance, n See balanced occlusion.

occlusal contacts, n.pl See contacts, deflective occusal and contact, interceptive occlusal.

occlusal contouring, n See contouring, occlusal.

occlusal correction, n See correction, occlusal.

occlusal curvature, n See curve of occlusion.

occlusal disharmony, n See disharmony, occlusal.

occlusal disturbances, n.pl See disturbances, occlusal.

occlusal embrasure, n See embrasure, occlusal.

occlusal equilibration, n See equilibration, occlusal.

occlusal force, n See force, occlusal.

occlusal form, n See form, occlusal.

occlusal function, n See function, heavy.

occlusal glide, See glide, occlusion.

occlusal guard, n See occlusal splint.

occlusal harmony, n See harmony, occlusal.

occlusal load, n See load, occlusal.

occlusal path, n See path, occlusal.

occlusal path registration, n See path, occlusal.

occlusal pattern, n See pattern, occlusal.

occlusal perception, See perception, occlusal.

occlusal pivot, n See pivot, occlusal.

occlusal plane, n See plane, occlusal.

occlusal position, See position, occlusal.

occlusal prematurities **(əkloo′zəl prē′məchoo′ritēz),** *n* premature contact of the occlusal surfaces of opposing teeth.

occlusal pressure, n See pressure, occlusal.

occlusal recontouring, n See contouring, occlusal.

occlusal rest, n See position, rest.

occlusal splint, n (occlusal guard) a bite plane designed and fabricated for patients with some types of functional temporomandibular joint disorders. Provides a stable occlusal platform from which to reconstruct a functional occlusion. See also splint.

occlusal stop, n See rest, occlusal.

occlusal surface, n See surface, occlusal.

occlusal system, n See system, occlusal.

occlusal table, *n* See table, occlusal.

occlusal template, *n* See template, occlusal.

occlusal therapy, *n* a treatment to establish and maintain a comfortable, stable, and functional occlusion for patients with one of several types of occlusal problems. Treatment may be limited to the teeth, the neuromuscular mechanisms of chewing, or a combination of both.

occlusal trauma, *n* See trauma, occlusal.

occlusal unit, *n* one of two kinds of cusps: (1) a stamp cusp coupled with a fossa, and (2) a shear cusp. The occlusal edges of the shear cusp are coupled with the edges of a stamp cusp, by which it passes closely without sliding contacts.

occlusal vertical dimension (OVD) **(əkloo′zəl),** *n* the distance between a point on a maxillary tooth and a point on the opposing mandibular tooth during occlusion; several methods are used to determine this measurement, including specific facial measurements that have been proven to be equal to the OVD.

occlusal wear, *n* See wear, occlusal.

occlusion, *n* **1.** the act of closure or state of being closed. *n* **2.** a contact between the incising or masticating surfaces of the maxillary and mandibular teeth.

occlusion, acentric, *n* See occlusion, eccentric.

occlusion, adjustment, *n* See adjustment occlusion.

occlusion, anatomic, *n* the ideal relation of the mandibular and maxillary teeth when closed.

occlusion, anterior determinants of cusp, *n.pl* the characteristics of the anterior teeth, i.e., occlusion, alignment, overlaps, and capacity to disclude conjointly with the trajectories given the condyles, that determine the cusp elevations and the fossa depressions of the postcanine teeth.

occlusion, attritional, *n* an occlusion in which each tooth of the dentition wears occlusally and proximally as it erupts.

occlusion, balanced, *n* **1.** an occlusion of the teeth that presents a harmonious relation of the occluding surfaces in centric and eccentric positions within the functional range of mandibular positions and tooth size. *n* **2.** the simultaneous contacting of the maxillary and mandibular teeth on both sides and in the anterior and posterior occlusal areas of the jaws. This occlusion is developed to prevent a tipping or rotating of the denture base in relation to the supporting structures. This term is used primarily in connection with the oral cavity, but it may be used in relation to teeth on an articulator.

occlusion, bilateral balanced, *n* the closure suitable for worn dentitions that are cuspless or have flat-sided cusps; it permits an increase of the amount of surface contact in centric closure and provides as much closure contact as possible for horizontal chewing. This kind of occlusion is a therapeutic form designed to keep dentures seated when fine-textured foods are chewed horizontally. It is not found in young, unworn natural dentitions.

occlusion, canine protected, *n* the lateral mandibular movements guided by the canine teeth.

occlusion, central, *n* See occlusion, centric.

occlusion, centric, *n* the relation of opposing occlusal surfaces that provides the maximum planned contact and/or intercuspation. It should exist when the mandible is in centric relation to the maxilla. Also called *central occlusion.*

occlusion, centrically balanced, *n* a centrically related centric occlusion in which the teeth close with even pressures on both sides of the oral cavity but have no occlusion of the postcanine teeth in attempted eccentric closures.

occlusion, components of, *n.pl* the various factors involved in occlusion (e.g., temporomandibular joint, associated neuromusculature, and teeth). In denture prosthetics, also the denture-supporting structures.

occlusion, convenience, *n* the assumed position of maximum intercuspation when there is occlusal interference in the centric path of closure. The convenience occlusion may be anterior, lateral, or anterolateral to the true centric occlusion. Also called *convenience jaw relation* and *convenience relationship of teeth.*

occlusion, coronary, *n* a coronary thrombosis resulting in closure of the coronary artery. See also thrombosis, coronary.

occlusion, cross-bite, *n* an occlusion in which the mandibular teeth overlap the maxillary teeth.

occlusion, determinants of, *n.pl* the classifiable factors in the gnathic organ that influence occlusion. These factors are divided into two groups: those that are fixed and those that can be modified by reshaping or repositioning the teeth. The fixed factors most mentioned are the intercondylar distance; anatomy, which influences the paths of the mandibular axes; mandibular centricity; and the mating of the jaws. The changeable factors most mentioned are tooth shape, tooth position, vertical dimension, height of cusps, and depth of fossae.

occlusion, eccentric, *n* any occlusion other than centric occlusion.

occlusion, edge-to-edge, *n* an occlusion in which the anterior teeth of both jaws meet along their incisal edges when the teeth are in centric occlusion.

occlusion, end-to-end, *n* See occlusion, edge-to-edge.

occlusion, faulty centric, *n* a condition in which centric occlusion does not correspond to a patient's centric jaw relationship, resulting in premature or interceptive or deflective tooth contacts in the centric path of closure.

occlusion, functional, *n* **1.** an occlusion in which attention is directed specifically to performance and is differentiated from structure and appearance. *n* **2.** any tooth contacts made within the functional range (according to the size) of the opposing tooth surfaces. An occlusion that occurs during function.

occlusion, gliding, *n* used in the sense of designating contacts of teeth in motion. A substitute for the term articulation.

occlusion, ideal, *n* **1.** the relationship existing when all the teeth are perfectly placed in the arches of jaws and have a normal anatomic relationship to each other. When the teeth are brought into contact, the cusp-fossa relationship is considered the most perfect anatomic relationship that can be attained. *n* **2.** the normal relationships of the inclines of the cusps of opposing teeth to each other in occlusion, when the alignment, proximal contacts, and axial positions of the teeth in both arches have resulted from normal growth and development in relation to all associated tissues and parts of the head.

occlusion, lateral, *n* right or left lateral movement of the mandible until the canines on the respective sides are in a cusp-to-cusp relationship. See also cross-bite.

occlusion, locked, *n* an occlusal relationship of such nature that lateral and protrusive mandibular movements are limited.

occlusion, malfunctional, *n* a disturbance in the normal or proper action of the masticatory apparatus produced by such factors as missing teeth or tilting and drifting of teeth.

occlusion, mechanically balanced, *n* an occlusion balanced without reference to physiologic considerations (e.g., on an articulator).

occlusion, normal, *n* See occlusion, ideal.

occlusion, pathogenic, *n* an occlusal relationship capable of producing pathologic changes in the teeth, supporting tissues, and/or other components of the stomatognathic system.

occlusion, physiologic, *n* an occlusion in harmony with functions of the masticatory system and presents no pathologic manifestation in the supporting structures of the teeth; the stresses placed on the teeth are dissipated normally, with a balance existing between the stresses and adaptive capacity of the supporting tissues.

occlusion, physiologically balanced, *n* a balanced occlusion in harmony with the temporomandibular joints and the neuromuscular system. See also occlusion, balanced.

occlusion, plane of, *n* See plane, occlusal.

occlusion, protrusive, *n* an occlusion of the teeth existing when the mandible is protruded forward from a centric position. See also position, rest, physiologic.

occlusion, rim, *n* See rim, occlusion.

occlusion, spherical form of, *n* an arrangement of teeth that places their occlusal surfaces on the surface of an imaginary sphere (usually 8 inches [20 cm] in diameter) with its center above the level of the teeth, as suggested by Monson.

occlusion, static, *n* See occlusion, ideal.

occlusion table, *n* See table, occlusal.

occlusion, terminal, *n* the relation of opposing occlusal surfaces that provides the maximum natural or planned contact and/or intercuspation.

occlusion, traumatic, *n* an occlusion that results in overstrain and injury to teeth, periodontal tissues, or the residual ridge or other oral structures.

occlusion, traumatogenic, *n* See occlusion, traumatic.

occlusion, working, *n* the occlusal contacts of teeth on the side toward which the mandible is moved. From the mesial or distal view, the buccal and lingual cusps of the maxillary teeth appear to be end-to-end with the buccal and lingual cusps of the lower teeth, respectively. Viewed from the lateral, each maxillary cusp is distal to the corresponding lower cusp. The mesial incline of each maxillary cusp makes contact with the distal incline of the opposing cusp in front of it, and the distal incline of each upper cusp makes contact with the mesial incline of the opposing cusp distal to it.

occupational disease, *n* a disease that results from a particular employment, usually from the effects of long-term exposure to specific substances or from the continuous or repetitive physical acts.

occupational exposure, *n* a person working in an environment with one or more risk factors present.

occupational hazard, *n* See occupational risk.

occupational health, *n* the ability of a worker to function at an optimum level of well-being at a worksite as reflected in terms of productivity, work attendance, disability compensation claims, and employment longevity.

occupational risk, *n* a hazard found or likely to occur in the workplace. The number and types of hazards a health care worker may encounter in the routine conduct of health care delivery.

Occupational Safety and Health Administration (OSHA), *n.pr* a federal agency charged with establishing guidelines and regulations regarding worker safety. These guidelines include storage and disposal of toxic chemicals and hazardous materials and the safety and proper use of clinical and office equipment.

OSHA coordinator, *n* the person within an organization, agency, or health care facility who is the designated "expert" on OSHA standards. As the person most knowledgeable about federal and state safety requirements, he or she should be consulted whenever operating procedures are developed or revised to ensure compliance with the law.

ocular herpes (ok′ūlur), *n* HSV-1 or HSV-2 infection of the eye, resulting in lesions on the eye. The infection can be transmitted by contaminated saliva contacting the eye.

odontalgia (ō′dontal′jə), *n* an older term for pain in a tooth; toothache.

odontalgia, phantom, *n* pain in the area from which a tooth has been removed. Also called *ghost pain.*

odontectomy (ō′dontek′təmē), *n* an older term for the removal of a tooth.

odontoblasts (ōdon′tōblasts), *n.pl* the cells that produce the dentin of the tooth and differentiate from the outer cells of the dental papilla.

odontoclasts (ōdon′tōklasts), *n.pl* the cells responsible for the resorption of cementum, dentin, and enamel. Active during exfoliation (shedding) of the primary dentition.

odontodysplasia, regional (ōdon′tōdisplā′zhə), *n* a developmental anomaly characterized by deficient tooth development. Deficiencies are noted in enamel and dentin formation. Also called *ghost teeth.* See also tooth, shell.

odontogenesis (ōdon′tōjen′əsis), *n* the process of tooth formation.

odontogenesis imperfecta, *n* a generic term that includes simultaneous defects in epithelial and mesenchymal tissue involved in tooth development.

O

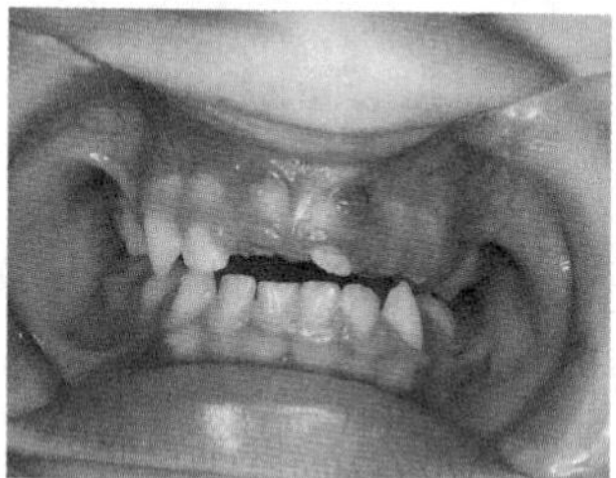

Odontodysplasia. (Regezi/Sciubba/Jordan, 2008)

odontogenic cysts, *n.pl* See cysts.

odontogenic keratocyst (OKC), *n* See tumor, keratocystic odontogenic.

odontogenic myxoma (ōdon′tōjen′ik miksō′mə), *n* a deep lesion in a maxillary or mandibular tooth germ's mesenchyme. It occurs equally in males and females between the ages of 10 and 30. The tumor may displace teeth and spread to other locations.

odontogenic tumors, *n.pl* See tumors.

odontoid process (ōdon′toid), *n* the toothlike projection that rises perpendicularly from the maxillary surface of the body of the second cervical vertebra or axis, which serves as a pivot point for the rotation of the atlas, or first cervical vertebra, enabling the head to turn in a horizontal plane.

odontolysis (odontol′isis), *n* See resorption, root.

odontoma (ō′dontō′mə), *n* a common hematoma made up of dentin, enamel, cementum, and pulp tissue. Two types exist: complex odontoma and compound odontoma.

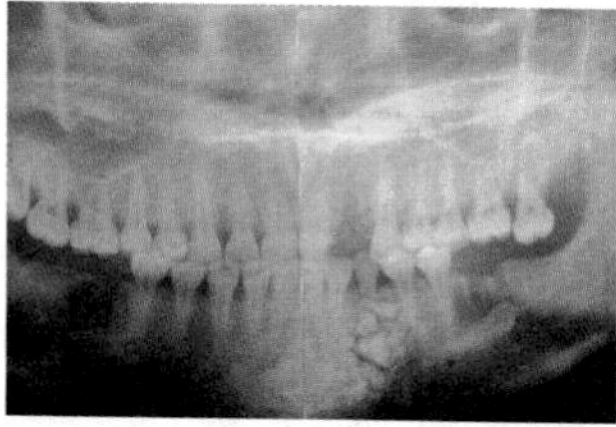

Odontoma. (Courtesy Dr. Charles Babbush)

***odontoma, ameloblastic* (əmel′ōblas′tik),** *n* a form characterized by the occurrence of an ameloblastoma within an odontoma. See also ameloblastoma; odontoma.

odontoma, complex, *n* an odontogenic tumor characterized by the formation of calcified enamel and dentin in an abnormal arrangement because of lack of morphodifferentiation.

odontoma, compound, *n* a tumor of enamel and dentin arranged in the form of anomalous miniature teeth. Several small abnormal teeth surrounded by a fibrous sac.

odontoma, cystic, *n* a form associated with a follicular cyst.

odontoma, gestant, *n* See dens in dente.

odor, *n* a scent or smell. The sense of smell is activated when airborne molecules stimulate receptors of the first cranial nerve.

office hours, *n.pl* See business hours.

office management, *n* the oversight of the business aspects of professional practice.

office planning, *n* the physical arrangement of the rooms available within the limitations of space designed to enable the dental staff to practice.

office routine, *n* See routine, office.

office visit, *n* a patient encounter with a health care provider in an office, clinic, or ambulatory care facility as an outpatient.

offline, *adj/adv* pertaining to the operation of input/output devices or auxiliary equipment not under direct control of the central processor.

offset, *n* a deduction; a counterclaim; a contrary claim or demand by which a given claim may be lessened or cancelled.

offset blade, *n* a blade that is set at an angle to the shank rather than perpendicular to it; in an area-specific curet, an offset blade is set at a 70° angle to the shank.

ofloxacin (ōflok′səsin), *n brand names:* Floxin, Floxin IV; *drug class:* fluoroquinolone antiinfective; *action:* broad-spectrum bactericidal agent that inhibits the enzyme DNA-gyrase needed for replication of DNA; *uses:* treatment of lower respiratory tract infections, genitourinary infections, skin and skin structure infections.

ofloxacin (optic), *n brand name:* Ocuflox; *drug class:* fluoroquinolone antiinfective, topical; *action:* broad-spectrum bactericidal agent that inhibits the enzyme DNA-gyrase needed for replication of DNA; *uses:* treatment of bacterial conjunctivitis caused by susceptible organisms.

oil, *n* an unctuous, combustible substance that is liquid, or easily liquefiable on warming, and soluble in ether but insoluble in water.

oil, essential, n a volatile, nonfatty liquid of vegetable origin having a distinct aroma and flavor, often pleasant. Also called *volatile oil.*

oil, fixed, n a nonvolatile oil consisting mainly of glycerides.

oil, mineral, n a grade of liquid petrolatum.

oil, volatile, n See oil, essential.

ointment (oint′ment), *n* a soft, bland, smooth, semisolid mixture that is used as a lubricant and as a vehicle for external medication.

ointment, hydrophilic, n an ointment that is miscible with water.

olfaction (olfak′shən), *n* the process of sensing certain odors during basic patient assessment, both intraoral and extraoral, in order to note changes in disease states; simply by detecting certain odors, the dental professional can suspect periodontitis, dental caries, necrotizing periodontal disease, diabetic acidosis, cigarette use, and alcohol abuse.

O

olfactory bulb (olfak′tərē), *n* the area of the forebrain where the olfactory nerves terminate and the olfactory tracts arise.

olfactory nerve, *n* first cranial nerve. See nerve, olfactory. See odor.

oligodendroglioma (ol′igōden′drōglēō′mə), *n* a relatively rare, moderately well-differentiated, relatively slow-growing glioma that occurs most frequently in the cerebrum of adults. It is grossly homogeneous, fairly well-circumscribed, moderately firm, and somewhat gritty in consistency, with interstitial calcification sufficiently dense to allow detection by radiographic imaging of the skull.

oligodontia (ol′igōdon′shēə), *n* a subcategory of hypodontia in which six or more teeth fail to develop.

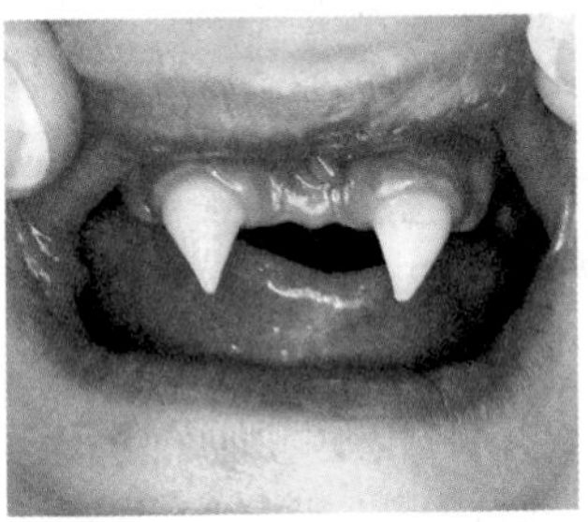

Oligodontia. (Sapp/Eversole/Wysocki, 2004)

oligodynamic (ol′igōdīnam′ik), *adj* effective in extremely small quantities.

oligomenorrhea (ol′igōmen′ərē′ə), *n* a condition in which a woman experiences fewer menstrual cycles than normal because each cycle lasts longer than 45 days.

oligomer (əlig′əmər), *n* an organic polymer consisting of two or more organic molecules; dimethacrylate (Bis-GMA) and urethane dimethacrylate (UDMA) oligomers are the basis of most common resins.

oligonucleotide, *n* a compound made up of the condensation of a small number of nucleotides.

oligosaccharides (ol′igōsak′ərīdz), *n.pl* carbohydrates that are formed by combining as few as two or as many as six monosaccharides.

oliguria (ol′igyoo′rēə), *n* a decreased output of urine (usually less than 500 ml/day), possibly associated with dehydration from diarrhea or excessive sweating, low fluid intake, lower nephron nephrosis resulting from burns, heavy metal poisoning, terminal renal disease, or an increase in extracellular fluid volume in untreated renal, cardiac, or hepatic disease.

olsalazine sodium (olsal′əzēn), *n brand name:* Dipentum; *drug class:* antiinflammatory, salicylate derivative; *action:* bioconverted to 5-amino-salicylic acid, which decreases inflammation in the colon; *uses:* maintenance of remission of ulcerative colitis in patients intolerant to sulfasalazine.

omeprazole (ōmep′rəzōl′), *n* *brand name:* Prilosec; *drug class:* antisecretory compound; *action:* suppresses gastric secretion by inhibiting hydrogen/potassium ATPase enzyme system in the gastric parietal cell; *uses:* gastroesophageal reflux disease (GERD), severe erosive esophagitis, pathologic hypersecretory conditions (Zollinger-Ellison syndrome, mastocytosis, multiple endocrine adenomas).

omission, *n* in speech, a phoneme left out at a place where it should occur.

on account, *adv* in partial payment; in partial satisfaction of an amount owed.

on or about, *adv* a phrase used in stating the date of an occurrence or conveyance to avoid being bound by the statement of an exact or certain date.

Onchocerca **(ong′kōsur′kə),** *n* a genus of elongated filariform nematodes that inhabit the connective tissue of their hosts, usually within firm nodules in which these parasites are coiled and entangled.

O. volvulus, *n* the blinding nodular nematode that causes dermatologic lesions and ocular complications that lead to blindness.

oncocytoma (ong′kōsītō′mə), *n* a rare, benign tumor usually occurring in the parotid glands in older patients. The lesion is encapsulated and composed of sheets and cords of large eosinophilic cells with small nuclei. Also called *acidophilic adenoma, oxyphilic adenoma.*

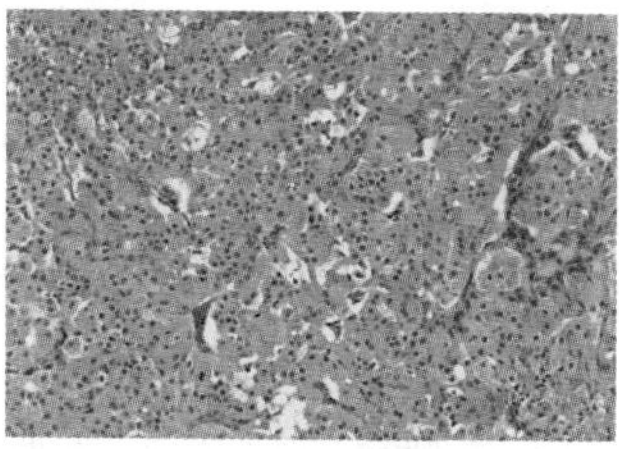

Oncocytoma. (Regezi/Sciubba/Jordan, 2008)

oncogene (ong′kəjēn), *n* a potentially cancer-inducing gene.

oncology (ongkol′əjē), *n* the scientific study that focuses on tumors and malignancy; the science of cancer.

ondansetron HCl (ondan′sətrōn), *n* *brand name:* Zofran; *drug class:* antiemetic; *action:* selective 5-HT3 antagonist; *uses:* prevention of nausea and vomiting associated with cancer chemotherapy.

ondontoplasty, *n* an older term for the cosmetic or rehabilitative rebuilding of a tooth.

onlay, *n* **1.** a cast type of restoration that is retained by frictional and mechanical factors in the preparation of the tooth and restores one or more cusps and adjoining occlusal surfaces of the tooth. *n* **2.** an occlusal rest portion of a removable partial denture that is extended to cover the entire occlusal surface of the tooth.

onlay bone, *n* See graft, onlay bone.

online, *adj/adv* a system of data processing under control of the central processing unit. Data reflecting current activity are introduced into the processing system as soon as they occur.

ontogeny (ontoj′ənē), *n* the natural life cycle of an individual as contrasted with the natural life cycle of the race (phylogeny). See also life expectancy.

opacification (ōpas′ifikā′shən), *n* **1.** the process of making something opaque. *n* **2.** the formation of opacities.

opalescent (ō′pəles′ent), *adj* resembling an opal in the display of various colors, as in opalescent dentin.

opalescent teeth, *n.pl* a translucent or opal-like appearance of teeth, usually associated with a genetic defect in odontogenesis.

opaque (ōpāk′), *adj* relatively impenetrable to light. See also opacity, optical.

open bite, *n* a malformation in which the anterior teeth do not occlude in any mandibular position.

open contact, *n* an increased area between adjacent teeth without interproximal contacts. It can be due to the abnormal position or absence of the teeth, oral disease, oral habits, or the overdevelopment of the frena. See also frenum and diastema.

open enrollment, *n* the annual period in which employees can select from a choice of benefits programs.

open panel, *n* a dental benefits plan characterized by three features: (1) any licensed dental professional may elect to participate, (2) the beneficiary may receive dental treatment from among all licensed dental professionals with the corresponding benefits payable to the beneficiary or the dental professional, and (3) the dental professional may accept or refuse any beneficiary. See also panel, open.

open scaling, *n* procedure for working on the subgingival surface that has been made accessible by the removal of or laying aside of the enclosing tissue. See also flap, periodontal.

open-end contract, *n* See contract, open-end.

opening click, *n* an audible or palpable click that may occur upon opening of the oral cavity, a measurement of which is noted while examining the range of mandibular motion.

opening movement, *n* See movement, mandibular, opening.

opening, vertical, *n* See dimension, vertical.

operate, *v* **1.** to work on the body with the hands or by means of cutting or other instruments to correct a deformity. **2.** to remove an anatomic part, or remove pathologic processes and/or tissues.

O

operating field, *n* See field, operating.

operating light, *n* See light, operating.

operating procedure, *n* See procedure, operating.

operation, *n* **1.** a surgical procedure. *n* **2.** the action of a drug or other remedy. *n* **3.** an act or series of acts performed on the body of a patient for relief or cure.

operation, Abbé-Estlander **(ab′ē-ēst′landər),** *n.pr* the transfer of a full-thickness section of one lip of the oral cavity to the other lip, using an arterial pedicle to ensure survival of the graft.

operation, blind, *n* a procedure in which the surgeon operates by using the sense of touch and knowledge of surgical anatomy without making a significant mucous membrane or cutaneous incision.

operation, computer, *n* the program step undertaken or executed by a computer (e.g., addition, multiplication, comparison, and data movement). The operation is usually specified by a functional command in the software used.

operation, exploratory, *n* a surgical procedure used to establish a diagnosis.

operation, Gillies', *n.pr* a technique for reducing fractures of the zygoma and the zygomatic arch through an incision in the temporal hairline.

operation, Kazanjian's **(kazan′jēənz),** *n.pr* a technique of surgical extension of the vestibular sulcus for improved prosthetic foundation of edentulous ridges. Also known as *Kazanjian's procedure.* See also extension, ridge.

operation, modified flap, *n* a variation of the flap procedure in oral and periodontal surgery. In this variation the vertical incisions of the flap procedure are not made, but the labial and/or lingual gingival walls are distended as far as possible to ensure sufficient access and an unobstructed view for instrumentation. See also flap, periodontal.

operation, open, *n* a procedure in which the surgeon operates with full view of the structures through mucous membrane or cutaneous incisions.

operation, Partsch's, *n.pr* the name applied to a technique of marsupialization.

operation, pedicle flap, *n* a procedure in mucogingival surgery designed to relocate or slide gingival tissue from a donor site in close proximity to an isolated defect, usually a tooth surface denuded of attached gingiva.

operation, Sorrin's, *n.pr* a type of flap approach in the treatment of a periodontal abscess; especially suitable when the marginal gingiva appears well adapted and gives no access to the abscess area. A semilunar incision is made below the involved area in the attached gingiva, leaving the gingival margin undisturbed; a flap is raised, allowing access to the abscessed area for curettage. Suturing follows.

operative dentistry, *n* the branch of dentistry that deals with the esthetic and functional restoration of the hard tissues of individual teeth.

operatory (op′ərətôrē), *n* the room or rooms in the dental office or clinic in which the dental staff performs professional dental services.

operculectomy (ōpur′kūlek′təmē), *n* the surgical removal of the operculum, a flap of tissue over a partially erupted tooth, particularly a third molar, in pericoronitis. See also operculum and pericoronitis.

operculitis (ōpur′kūlī′tis), *n* See pericoronitis.

operculum (ōpur′kūləm), *n* a flap of tissue over a partially erupted or unerupted tooth, particularly a third molar. It may result in pericoronitis with inflammation of the flap tissue. See also pericoronitis.

operon (op′əron′), *n* a segment of DNA consisting of an operator gene and one or more structural genes with related functions controlled by the operator gene in conjunction with a regulator gene.

ophthalmology (of′thəlmol′əjē), *n* the branch of medicine concerned with the study of the physiology, anatomy, and pathology of the eye and the diagnosis and treatment of disorders of the eye.

ophthalmoscope (ofthal′məskōp′), *n* a device for examining the interior of the eye. It includes a light, a mirror with a single hole through which the examiner may look, and a dial holding several lenses of varying strengths. The lenses are selected to allow clear visualization of the structures of the eye at any depth.

opiate (ō′pēət), *n* **1.** a remedy containing or derived from opium. *n* **2.** a drug that induces sleep.

opinion, *n* in the law of evidence, an inference or conclusion drawn by a witness from information known to him or her or assumed.

opioids, abuse of (ō′pēoidz), *n* a regular use of heroin, codeine, or morphine for reasons other than recognized medical applications.

opisthion (ōpis′thēôn), *n* the hindmost point on the posterior margin of the foramen magnum.

opisthocranion (ōpis′thōkrā′nēon), *n* the point in the midline of the cranium that projects farthest backward.

opium (ō′pēəm), *n* the actual juice of the poppy, *Papaver somniferum.* It contains morphine, codeine, nicotine, narceine, and many other alkaloids.

opportunistic infection, *n* an infection by a microbial organism to which the patient is usually resistant; however, because of reduced vitality or through suppression of the immune system, the patient has become infected.

opsin (op′sin), *n* a visual pigment protein found in the retinal rods.

optic chiasm (op′tik kī′azm), *n* a point near the thalamus and hypothalamus at which portions of each optic nerve cross over.

optic nerve, *n* See nerve, optic.

optics, *n* the science concerned with the properties of light, its refraction and absorption, and the properties of the media of the eye that refract and absorb light.

optimal (op′timəl), *adj* the best or most favorable.

optimism, *n* the tendency to look on the bright or happy side of everything, to believe that there is good in everything.

optometry (optom′itrē), *n* the professional discipline devoted to testing the eyes for visual acuity, prescribing corrective lenses, and recommending eye exercises and other health practices to preserve sight.

Orabase, *n* the brand name of a topical dental paste containing an adrenocorticoid. The base consists of gelatin, pectin, mineral oil, and sodium carboxymethylcellulose in a hydrocarbon gel. The adrenocorticoid is hydrocortisone acetate. It is used for temporary relief of symptoms associated with oral inflammation and ulcerative lesions.

oral, *adj* pertaining to the oral cavity.

oral biology, *n* the study of the health and disease of the oral cavity in the context of its proper biologic function.

oral cavity, *n* the mouth.

oral contraceptives, *n.pl brand names:* Demulen, Loestrin, Lo/Ovral, Nordett; *drug class:* estrogen/progestin combinations; *action:* prevents ovulation by suppressing follicle-stimulating and luteinizing

O

hormones; *uses:* pregnancy prevention, endometriosis, hypermenorrhea, hypogonadism. Also called *estrogens, mestranol androgens, ethinyl estradiol, levonorgestrel.*

oral environment, *n* See environment, oral.

oral evacuator, *n* a suction apparatus used to remove fluids and debris from an operating field. Also called *vacuum* or *suction.*

***oral hairy leukoplakia* (loo′kōplā′kēə),** *n* a filamentous, white plaque found on the lateral borders of the tongue that can spread across the entire dorsum of the tongue and onto the buccal mucosa. The Epstein-Barr virus (EBV) has been identified in biopsy specimens of these lesions. An indicator disease for AIDS. See also leukoplakia.

oral health diet score, *n* a motivational aid to good nutrition. Merit points are earned by an adequate intake of foods from the recommended food groups. Demerits are given for frequent intake of foods high in sugars. The difference is the oral health diet score. The technique is applicable to children with a high incidence of dental caries.

oral health index, *n* a statistical measure that quantifies one or more aspects of a person's or group's oral health status.

oral hygiene, *n* See hygiene, oral.

oral manifestation, *n* the presence of the signs, symptoms, and lesions of a systemic disease in and around the oral cavity.

oral medicine, *n* See medicine, oral.

oral mucosa, *n* See mucosa, oral.

oral physiology, *n* See physiology, oral.

oral self-examination, *n* the procedure shown to dental patients in order to look for indications of cancer. The patient monitors the tissues of his or her oral cavity, as well as those of the head and neck, reporting any changes to a dental professional.

oral surgery, *n* See surgery, oral.

oral warts, *n.pl* warts caused by human papillomavirus (HPV) that may be scattered throughout the oral cavity or localized in one area. They frequently recur. They are associated with AIDS infection.

orangewood, *n* the wood of choice for the working tips of porte polishers, due to its resistance to splitting and its ability to carry polishing agents. See porte polisher.

orbit, *n* **1.** in chemistry, refers to the movement of an electron around an atom's nucleus. **2.** the bony socket that contains the eyeball and all its supporting structures.

orbital (ôr′bitəl), *adj* pertaining to the orbit.

orbital exenteration, *n* the surgical removal of the entire contents of the orbit.

orbital marker, *n* a projecting part of a face-bow that marks the location of the orbitale. Used in the orientation of casts on an articulator in relation to cranial planes.

orbital plane, *n* See plane, orbital.

orbitale (ôr′bital′ē), *n* the lowest point in the margin of the orbit (directly below the pupil when the eye is open and the patient is looking straight ahead) that may readily be felt under the skin. The eye-ear plane passes through the orbitale and tragion.

orders, *n.pl* the written or verbal directions of a health care professional or dental staff member to a nurse or other assistant detailing the care to be given to a patient.

ordinal scale (or′dənəl), *n* the classification system by which objects are ordered in terms of their qualitative value, as opposed to a ranking performed strictly numerically or quantitatively.

organ, *n* a somewhat independent body part that performs a specific function or functions and that is formed from tissues.

organ transplantation, *n* the replacement of a diseased organ with a healthy organ from a donor with a compatible tissue type. Organs such as a kidney may be donated by living donors or harvested from brain-dead organ donors.

organelle(s) (ôr′gənel′), *n* the specialized structures within most cells that are permanent and metabolically active, which include the nucleus, mitochondria, the Golgi complex, the endoplasmic reticulum, the lysosomes, and the centrioles.

organism(s) (ôr′gənizəm), *n* any organized body of living economy.

organism(s), Vincent's, n.pr the fusospirochetal organisms associated with the initiation of necrotizing ulcerative gingivitis, necrotizing ulcerative stomatitis, or Vincent's angina.

organization, *n* an arrangement of distinct but mutually dependent parts, persons, or tasks to create, enhance, or improve a functioning unit.

organogenesis (ôr′gənōjen′əsis), *n* the formation of organs within an embryo. Organogenesis occurs within the first trimester.

orientation, *n* the ability to correctly place oneself in time, space, and relationship to others and one's work and environment.

orifice (ôr′ifis), *n* an older term for the opening, entrance, or outlet of any body cavity; any foramen or meatus.

O-ring, *n* a doughnut-shaped flexible gasket made of synthetic material. Used as an overdenture attachment.

Orlistat (ôr′listat), *n brand name:* Xenical; *drug class:* lipase inhibitors; *action:* interferes with the body's ability to digest fat but may cause gas and oily bowel movements; *uses:* reduction in fat absorption for weight loss.

ornithine (ôr′nəthēn′), *n* an amino acid, not a constituent of proteins, that is produced as an important intermediate substance in the urea cycle.

ornithine carbamoyltransferase, n an enzyme in the blood that increases in patients with liver and other diseases.

oroantral fistula (ôr′ōan′trəl), *n* an abnormal tract that connects the oral cavity with the maxillary sinus.

orodigitofacial dysostosis (OFD syndrome), *n* a syndrome characterized by abnormal development of the jaws and tongue, cleft lip and palate, hypoplasia of bones of the skull with ocular hypertelorism, nasal alar deformity, malformation of digits (frequently manifested as brachydactyly and syndactyly), mental retardation, granular skin, and alopecia of the scalp.

orofacial (ôr′ōfā′shəl), *adj* of or related to the face and oral cavity.

orofacial abnormality, *n* a structural and functional disorder of the oral cavity and face, usually arising from genetic or congenital defects.

orofacial pain, *n* pain within the structures of the oral cavity and face, usually of a diffuse pattern.

oronasal, *adj* pertaining to the oral cavity and nose.

oropharyngeal (ôr′ōfərin′jēəl), *adj* in anatomy, being part of or related to the oropharynx, the region of the pharynx that lies underneath the soft palate and posterior to the oral cavity.

oropharynx (ôr′ōfer′ingks), *n* the portion of the pharynx associated with the oral cavity; usually described as bounded superiorly by the uvula, inferiorly by the epiglottis, anteriorly by the tongue, and posteriorly by the posterior pharyngeal wall.

orosomucoid (ôr′əsōmū′koid), *n* a subgroup of the α_1-globulin fraction of the blood.

orphenadrine citrate (ôrfen′ədrēn sit′rāt), *n brand names:* Banflex, Flexoject, Norflex, Orflagen; *drug class:* skeletal muscle relaxant, central acting; *action:* acts centrally to depress polysynaptic pathways to relax skeletal muscle, inhibit muscle spasm; *uses:* pain in musculoskeletal conditions.

ortho-, *comb* straight or correct.

orthodentin (ôr′thōden′tin), *n* the tubular-shaped dentin situated between the enamel and pulp chamber of a tooth.

orthodontic (ôr′thədän′tik), *adj* pertaining to the orthopedic correction of abnormal dental relationships, including related abnormalities in facial structures.

orthodontic appliances, n.pl See appliance.

orthodontic appliances, functional, n.pl See appliances, removable.

orthodontic appliances, removable, n.pl See appliances, removable.

orthodontic bracket, n See bracket.

orthodontic retainer, n See appliance, retaining orthodontic.

orthodontic toothbrush, n See bilevel orthodontic toothbrush.

orthodontic wire, n See wire.

orthodontics (ôr′thədän′tiks), *n* the area of dentistry concerned with the supervision, guidance, and correction of the growing and mature orofa-

O

cial structures. This includes conditions that require movement of the teeth or correction of malrelationships and malformations of related structures by the adjustment of relationships between and among teeth and facial bones by the application of forces or the stimulation and redirection of functional forces within the craniofacial complex. Major responsibilities of the practice include (1) the diagnosis, prevention, interception, and treatment of all forms of malocclusion of the teeth and associated alterations in their surrounding structures; (2) design, application, and control of functional and corrective appliances; and (3) guidance of the dentition and its supporting structures to attain and maintain optimum occlusal relations in physiologic and esthetic harmony among facial and cranial structures. Also called *dentofacial orthopedics.*

orthodontist, *n* a dental specialist who has completed an approved, advanced course of at least 2 years in the special area of orthodontics.

orthognathic (ôr′thognā′thik), *adj* pertaining to the normal relationships of the jaws.

orthognathic surgery, *n* surgery to alter relationships of dental arches and/or supporting bones, usually accomplished with orthodontic therapy.

orthognathous (ôr′thognāth′us), *adj* pertaining to straight jaws; no projection of the lower part of the face. The facial angle is 85° to 90°.

orthokeratinized (ôr′thōker′ətinī′zd), *adj* of a specific type of epithelium; its four layers include a keratin component whose cells are nuclei-free. Most oral mucosa consists of parakeratinized epithelium, which contains nucleated keratinocytes.

Orthomyxoviridae **(ôr′thomik′sōvir′idā),** *n.pl* one of the major RNA virus families, to which the influenza virus belongs. Viruses in this family have a single-stranded, eight-segmented, linear molecular structure with helical symmetry.

orthopantograph (ôr′thōpan′tōgraf), *n* a panoramic radiographic device (Panorex) that permits visualization of the entire dentition, alveolar bone, and other contiguous structures on a single extraoral film.

orthopantomograph (ôr′thōpan′tōmōgraf), *n* a radiographic system (manufactured by Siemens) that uses three axes of rotation to obtain a panoramic radiograph of the dental arches and their associated structures.

orthopedic (ôr′thōpē′dik), *adj* pertaining to the correction of abnormal form or relationship of bone structures. May be accomplished surgically (orthopedic surgery) or by the application of appliances to stimulate changes in the bone structure by natural physiologic response (orthopedic therapy). Orthodontic therapy is orthopedic therapy applied through the teeth.

orthopnea (ôr′thopnē′ə), *n* an inability to breathe except in an upright position.

orthotic (ôr′thot′ik), *n* an orthopedic brace used to repair or support a joint or muscle in the body. Also called *orthosis.*

OSAP, *n.pr* an abbreviation for the Organization for Safety and Asepsis Procedures, a nonprofit organization that consists of dental and health care professionals and others interested in promoting infection control and effective health and safety practices. It also supports a research and development foundation.

Osler-Weber disease, *n.pr* See telangiectasia, hereditary hemorrhagic.

osmium (Os) (oz′mēəm), *n* a hard, grayish, pungent-smelling metallic element. Its atomic number is 76 and its atomic weight is 190.2. It is used to produce alloys of extreme hardness and is highly toxic.

osmosis (ozmō′sis), *n* the passage of pure solvent from the lesser to the greater concentration when two solutions are separated by a membrane that selectively prevents the passage of solute molecules but is permeable to the solvent. The principles of osmosis and the selective permeability of the cell membrane help to regulate the transfer of fluids and metabolites to and from the cells. Thus, they also maintain the stability of the salt/ion concentration in the extracellular and intracellular fluids.

O

osmotic, *adj* pertaining to osmosis.
osmotic pressure, n See pressure, osmotic.

osseointegration (os″eoin″təgra′-shən), *n* **1.** the growth action of bone tissue, as it assimilates surgically implanted devices or prostheses to be used as either replacement parts or anchors. *n* **2.** a specific endosseous dental implant technique involving very slow and precise bone drilling to minimize heat production; the procedure makes use of biocompatible metal and a defined healing environment. Also known as the *Branemark technique.*

osseous coagulum (osēəs kōag′yələm), *n* a blend of blood, bone, and saliva whose application in fostering bone regeneration has been the focus of scientific study.

ossification (os″ifikā′shən), *n* the development of forming bone.
ossification, endochondral (intracartilaginous), n the development of bone from cartilage rods, as in the development of arm or leg bones.
ossification, intramembranous, n the development of bone from tissue or membrane, as in the formation of the skull.

ossify (os′ifī), *v* to transform from soft tissue to hardened bone.

ostectomy (ostek′tōmē), *n* the excision of a bone or portion of a bone.
ostectomy, periodontal, n the removal of alveolar bone from around the tooth root to eliminate an adjacent pocket and secure physiologic osseous and gingival form.

osteitis (os′tēī′tis), *n* an inflammation of the bone; an inflammation of the haversian spaces, canals, and their branches but generally not of the medullary cavity. The disease is characterized by tenderness and a dull, aching pain. Enlargement of the bone may occur. Osteitis of the alveolar process after tooth extraction is commonly referred to as dry socket.
osteitis, alveolar localized, n See socket, dry.
osteitis, condensing, n a chronic inflammation associated with some nonvital teeth or located in the site of extraction of such teeth, resulting in abnormally dense bone.
osteitis deformans **(difôr′məns),** *n* See disease, Paget's, of bone.

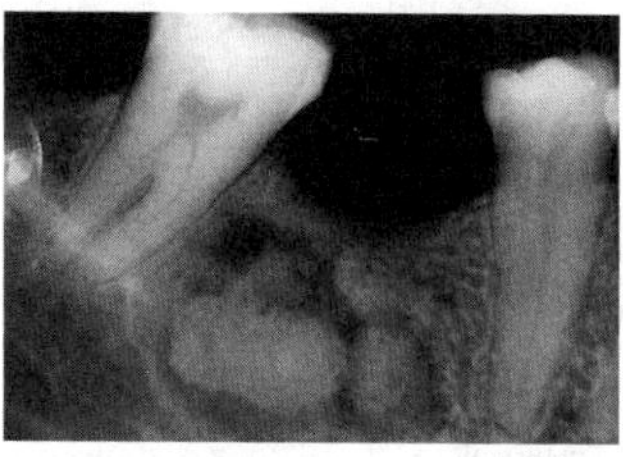

Osteitis. (Regezi/Sciubba/Jordan, 2008)

osteitis fibrosa cystica, generalized, (von Recklinghausen's disease of bone) **(fībrō′sə sis′tikə),** *n* **1.** a disease caused by parathyroid adenomas and characterized by cystlike radiolucencies in the bones (including the jaws), loosening of teeth, localized swellings, giant cell lesions, increased blood calcium and phosphatase levels, and lowered blood phosphorus levels. *n* **2.** increased resorption and destruction of bone caused by primary and secondary hyperparathyroidism.

osteoarthritis (ostēōärthrī′tis), *n* chronic degeneration and destruction of the articular cartilage leading to bony spurs, pain, stiffness, limitation of motion, and change in the size of joints. Considered to result from chronic traumatic injury and wear and tear. Heberden's nodes occur in a special form of the disease. Symptoms may be associated with hormonal, vascular, and/or nutritional disorders. The structural changes of advanced osteoarthritis may involve erosion of the articular cartilages or the subchondral bone. Also called *degenerative joint disease.*

osteoarthropathy, hypertrophic pulmonary (os′tēōärthrop′əthē), *n* a clubbing of the fingers and toes resulting from deposition of calcium in the subperiosteal tissues around the joint. Related to chronic pulmonary disease and occasionally to circulatory and digestive disease.

osteoblast (os′tēōblast), *n* the cell associated with the growth and development of bone; cuboidal in shape. In active growth, they form a continuous layer on mature bone like a sheet of epithelial cells; when the bone growth is arrested, the cells assume an elongated appearance like fibroblasts.

osteoblastoma (os′tēōblas′tōmə), *n* a bone tumor benign in nature but characterized by swelling and chronic dull pain. If left untreated, these tumors lead to such conditions as scoliosis.

osteocalcin (os′tēōkal′sin), *n* vitamin K–dependent calcium-binding protein synthesized by osteoblasts and found primarily in bone. Serum osteocalcin measurements provide a noninvasive specific marker of bone metabolism.

osteocementum (os′tēōsēmen′-tum), *n* a secondary cementum; the hard, bonelike cementum deposited after root formation is completed. See also atrophy of disuse.

osteochondritis (os′tēōkondrī′tis), *n* a disease of the epiphyses, or bone-forming centers of the skeleton, beginning with necrosis and fragmentation of the tissue and followed by repair and regeneration.

osteoclasia, traumatic (os′tēōklā′zhə), *n* See cementoma; fibroma, periapical.

osteoclast (os′tēōklast), *n* a large, multinucleated giant cell associated with the resorption of bone; the nuclei resemble the nuclei of the osteoblasts and osteocytes; the cytoplasm is often foamy, and the cell frequently has branching processes. They may arise from stromal cells of the bone marrow. They may represent fused osteoblasts or may include fused osteocytes liberated from resorbing bone. They are usually found in close relationship to the resorption of bone and frequently lie in areas of resorption (Howship's lacunae).

osteoclastoma, *n* See granuloma, giant cell reparative, peripheral.

osteocyte (os′tēōsīt), *n* an osteoblast that has been surrounded by a calcified interstitial substance; the cells are enclosed within lacunae, and the cytoplasmic processes extend through apertures of the lacunae into canaliculi in the bone. Like the osteoblast, the osteocyte may undergo transformations and assume the form of an osteoclast or reticular cell.

***osteocyte osteodystrophy* (os′tēōdis′trəfē),** *n* a condition marked by defective or deficient bone formation.

osteocyte, renal, *n* a form of dwarfism associated with osteoporosis produced by renal insufficiency during childhood. Periodontal changes include widening of the periodontal space and marked osteoporosis of the mandibular and maxillary bones. Similar to renal rickets. See also rickets, renal.

osteofibroma (os′tēōfībrō′mə), *n* See fibroma, ossifying.

osteogenesis, *n* the origin and development of bone tissue.

***osteogenesis imperfecta* (os′tēōjen′əsis),** *n* a congenital disease of unknown cause characterized by fragile, brittle, and easily fractured bones; presumed to stem from a failure in the formation of bone matrix. Variants are often hereditary or familial and include manifestations such as blue sclerae, dentinogenesis imperfecta, and otosclerosis. Also known as *brittle bone disease, fragilitas ossium, Lobstein's disease, osteopsathyrosis idiopathica.*

osteoid (os′tēoid), *n* the initial bony matrix laid down by the osteoblasts. It is later calcified, with inclusion of osteoblasts as osteocytes within lacunae, into bone.

osteoinduction (os′tēōinduk′shən), *n* the process by which undefined cells of loose makeup undergo mitosis and form osteoprogenitor cells.

osteointegration (os′tēōin′təgrā′shən), *n* the structural linkage made at the contact point where human bone and the surface of a synthetic, often titanium-based implant meet. Also called *osseointegration.*

osteology (os′tēol′əjē), *n* a subgroup of anatomic research concerning the scientific study of bones.

osteolysis (os′tēol′əsis), *n* a process of bone resorption whereby the bone salts can be withdrawn by a humoral mechanism and returned to the tissue fluids, leaving behind a decalcified bone matrix. Also called *halisteresis.*

osteoma (os′tēō′mə), *n* a benign neoplasm of bone or bone tissue.

osteomalacia (os′tēōməlā′shēə, -shə), *n* a systemic disorder of bone characterized by decreased mineralization of bone matrix possibly resulting from vitamin D deficiency, inadequate calcium in the diet, renal disease, and/or steatorrhea. Manifestations include incomplete fractures and gradual resorption of cortical and cancellous bone.

osteomyelitis (os′tēōmī′əlī′tis), *n* an inflammation of the bone marrow or of the bone, marrow, and endosteum.

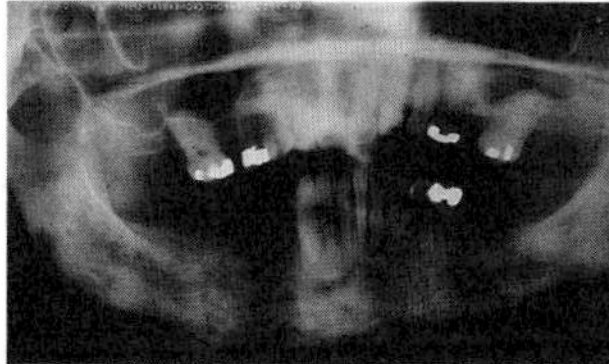

Osteomyelitis. (Regezi/Sciubba/Pogrel, 2000)

osteon (os′tēon), *n* the three-dimensional reconstruction of concentric lamellae arranged circumferentially about the course of a central blood vessel.

osteonecrosis (os′tēōnəkrō′sis), *n* the destruction and death of bone tissue. It may stem from ischemia, infection, malignant neoplastic disease, or trauma.

osteonecrosis, bisphosphonate-associated (BON) **(bisfos′fənāt′ əsō′shēā′təd),** *n* a condition that may develop in patients on bisphosphonate therapy in which pain, swelling and infection of soft tissue, drainage, loosening of teeth, and exposed bone may occur suddenly, usually at a previous tooth extraction site, as well as numbness and heaviness of the jaw.

osteonectin, *n* noncollagenous, calcium-binding glycoprotein of developing bone. It links collagen to mineral in the bone matrix.

osteopenia (os′tēōpē′nə), *n* the deterioration of bone density, decrease of calcification, or insufficient synthesis of uncalcified bone material.

osteopetrosis (ostēōpetrō′sis), *n* an osteosclerosis of unknown origin that obliterates the bone marrow regions, with resultant anemia. Delayed tooth eruption and severe osteomyelitis or necrosis after dental infection may be associated with the disease. Also known as *Albers-Schönberg disease, marble bone.*

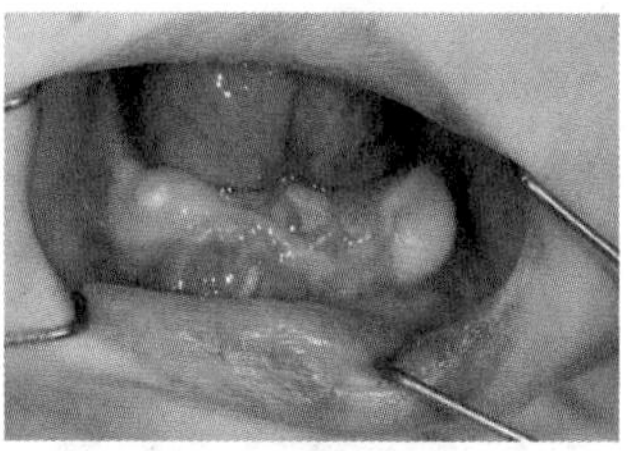

Osteopetrosis. (Regezi/Sciubba/Jordan, 2008)

osteoplasty (os′tēōplastē), *n* a surgical procedure to modify or change the configuration of a bone.

osteoporosis (os′tēōpôrō′sis), *n* an enlargement of the soft marrow and haversian spaces resulting from a decreased rate of formation of the hard bone matrix. With the exception of immobilized parts, it is a systemic disorder that occurs in advanced age (senile osteoporosis), during ACTH and cortisone therapy, during and after menopause, in limited physical activity, in Cushing syndrome, during malnutrition, and in other disorders of matrix formation such as hyperadrenalism, hyperthyroidism, vitamin C deficiencies, and deficiency of androgenic steroids. See also atrophy, bone and bone rarefaction.

osteoprogenitor (os′tēōprōjen′ətər), *n* a loosely organized cell that undergoes metamorphosis to become an osteoblast, a cell type with the capacity to form bone.

osteoradionecrosis (ORN) (os′tēōrā′dēōnekrō′sis), *n* bone necrosis secondary to irradiation and superimposed infection. It occurs because radiation inevitably destroys normal cells and blood vessels, as well as tumor cells. Damage to the small arteries reduces circulation to the area, depriving it of oxygen and other necessary nutrients. Sequestrum formation can be noted on the radiographs. Mainly treat with hyperbaric oxygen.

osteosarcoma (os′tēōsärkō′mə), *n* a malignant neoplasm of the bone-forming tissues.

osteosclerosis (os′tēōsklərō′sis), *n* an increased bone formation resulting in reduced marrow spaces and increased radiopacity.

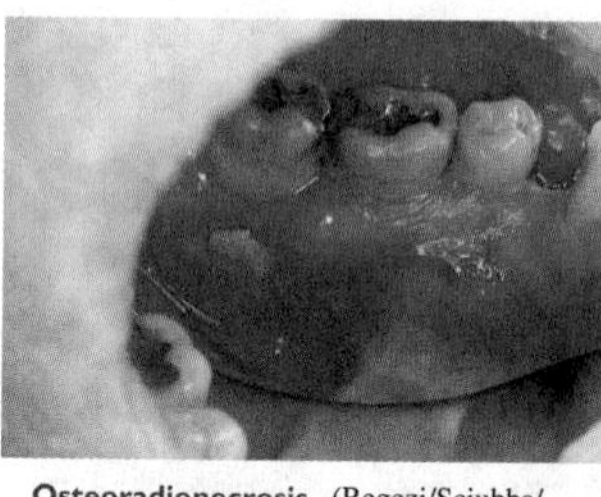

Osteoradionecrosis. (Regezi/Sciubba/Jordan, 2008)

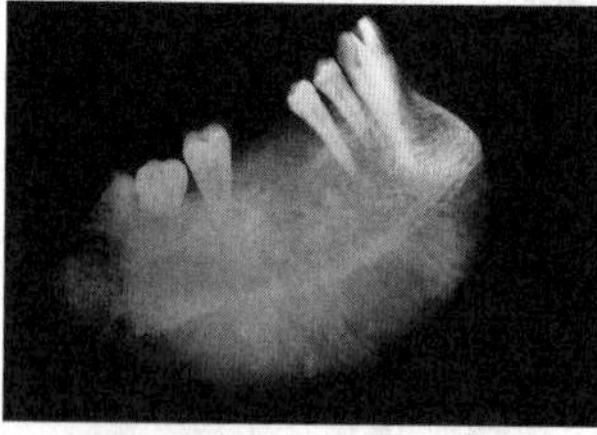

Osteosarcoma. (Regezi/Sciubba/Jordan, 2008)

osteosynthesis (os′tēōsin′thəsis), *n* See osseointegration.

osteosynthesis, miniplate, n an internal procedure for repairing fractures to the mandible by using titanium or stainless steel plates and screws to stabilize the bone fragments in proper alignment.

osteotome (os′tēətōm′), *n* a surgical tool used in procedures involving bone cutting or marking, including but not limited to tooth extraction.

osteotomy (os′tēot′əmē), *n* the surgical cutting or transection of a bone.

otalgia dentalis (ōtal′jēə), *n* a reflex pain in the ear resulting from dental disease; usually propagated along the auriculotemporal nerve.

OTC, *adj* See over-the-counter.

otic ganglion, *n* See ganglion, otic.

otitis, *n* an inflammation or infection of the ear.

otitis externa, n an inflammation or infection of the external canal or the auricle of the external ear. Major causes are allergy, bacteria, fungi, viruses, and trauma.

otitis media **(ōtī′tis mē′dēə),** *n* an inflammation of the middle ear that may be marked by pain, fever, abnormalities of hearing, deafness, tinnitus, and vertigo. It may originate in the pharynx and be transmitted by the eustachian tubes.

otolaryngologist (o″tolar″inggol′əjist), *n* a physician whose practice of medicine focuses on diagnosing and treating diseases of the ears, nose, and throat.

otolaryngology, *n* the branch or specialty of medicine that deals with diseases of the ear, nose, and throat.

otologist (ōtol′əjist), *n* a doctor who specializes in conditions and diseases of the ear.

otology (ōtol′əjē), *n* a division of medicine concerning diseases of the ear.

otosclerosis (ō′tōsklərō′sis), *n* a disorder of the middle ear that generally results in hardening and fusion of the ossicles of the ear, with resultant immobilization so that sound waves cannot be conducted along their paths.

otoscope, *n* an instrument used to examine the external ear, the eardrum, and, through the eardrum, the ossicles of the middle ear. It consists of a light, a magnifying lens, and a device for insufflation.

otoscopy, *n* viewing or inspecting the tympanic membrane and other parts of the outer ear with an otoscope.

outline form, *n* See form, outline.

outpatient, *n* a patient, not hospitalized or housed in an extended care facility, who is being treated in an office, clinic, or other ambulatory care facility.

output, *n* the transfer or exit of processed or in-process information from a computer to printers, video terminals, and other peripheral devices.

ovale foramen, *n* See foramen, ovale.

ovalocytosis (ō′vəlōsītō′sis), *n* See elliptocytosis.

ovaries (ō′vərēz), *n* the pair of female gonads found on each side of the inferior abdomen, beside the uterus, in a fold of the broad ligament.

overbilling, *n* a nondisclosure of waiver of patient copayment.

overbite, *n* a vertical overlapping of maxillary teeth over mandibular teeth, usually measured perpendicular to the occlusal plane. See also overjet and overlap, vertical.

overclosure, *n* the raising of the mandible too far before the teeth make contact; loss of occlusal vertical dimension is the cause. See also distance, large interarch.

overcoding, *n* reporting a more complex and/or higher cost procedure than was actually performed.

overcontour, *n* a process in which the normal anatomy of the restored tooth is altered by using too much restorative material. Overcontouring can destroy the natural cleaning processes present in the periodontium.

overdenture, *n* a complete or partial removable denture supported by retained roots that is intended to provide improved support, stability, and tactile and proprioceptive sensation and to reduce ridge resorption. See also root retention and root submersion.

overdose (OD), *n* an excessive use of a drug, resulting in adverse reactions ranging from mania or hysteria to coma or death.

overextended, *adj* **1.** the situation occurring when a prosthetic appliance is inadvertently constructed in such a way that part of the oral mucosa is injured by the appliance. *adj* **2.** pertaining to an extrusion beyond the apical opening into the periapical area. May be with instrumentation, medication, or root canal filling.

overfilled, *adj* See overextended.

overhang, *n* an excess filling material projecting beyond cavity margins.

overhead, *n* the production costs required to be expended by the dental professional to practice the profession (e.g., rent, utilities, salaries, laundry). Costs include any involved with management, supplies, equipment, salaries (taxes), and maintenance. Amounts deducted from the gross receipts of a dental practice before the dental professional's net income (take-home pay) is received.

overjet, *n* the horizontal projection of maxillary teeth beyond the mandibular teeth, usually measured parallel to the occlusal plane. When not otherwise specified, the term is generally assumed to refer to central incisors and is measured from the labial surface of the lower central incisors to the labial surface of the upper central incisors at the level of the upper incisor edge. Unique conditions may sometimes require other measuring techniques. See also overlap, horizontal.

overlap, deep vertical, *n* an excessive vertical overlap of the anterior teeth. Also called *closed bite, deep bite, deep overbite.*

overlap, horizontal, *n* a projection of the anterior or posterior teeth of one arch beyond their antagonists in a horizontal direction. Also called *overjet, overjut.*

overlap, vertical, *n* an extension of the maxillary teeth over the mandibular teeth in a vertical direction when the opposing posterior teeth are in contact in centric occlusion. It may also be used to describe the vertical relations of opposing cusps of posterior teeth. Also called *overbite.*

overlay, *n* See onlay.

overlay, computer, *n* a technique for bringing routines into memory from magnetic storage during processing so that several routines will occupy the same storage locations at different times. Overlay techniques are used when the total storage requirements for instructions exceed the available storage in memory.

overshooting accident, *n* the result of seating an endosteal implant beyond its normal host site (through the inferior mandibular border, into the mandibular canal or nasal or antral floor).

over-the-counter (OTC), *adj* describes medications that can be legally sold without a doctor's prescription. In the United States, such medications are strictly regulated by the Food and Drug Administration (FDA). These medications include sunscreens, antimicrobials or antifungals, analgesics such as aspirin and ibuprofen, and other miscellaneous topical products that have a therapeutic effect.

ovoid arch, *n* See arch, ovoid.

ovolacto vegetarian diet (ō′vōl-ak′tō), *n* a modified vegetarian diet that prohibits consumption of meat, poultry, and fish but that permits some animal products such as eggs, milk, and cheese. The diet provides important proteins, but care must be taken to ensure adequate iron intake.

ovum (ō′vəm), *n* (*pl* **ova**) a female reproductive or germ cell (egg) containing 23 chromosomes. The cell can be fertilized.

ownership, *n* the legal right of possession.

Owren's disease (ō′renz), *n.pr* See parahemophilia.

oxacillin sodium (ok′səsil′in), *n* *brand names:* Bactocill, Prostaphlin; *drug class:* penicillinase-resistant penicillin; *action:* interferes with cell wall replication of susceptible organisms; the cell wall, rendered osmotically unstable, swells and bursts from osmotic pressure; *uses:* effective for gram-positive cocci, infections caused by penicillinase-producing *Staphylococcus.*

oxalate, *n* a salt of oxalic acid.

oxandrolone (oksan′drəlōn′), *n* *brand name:* Oxandrin; *drug class:* androgenic anabolic steroid (Controlled Substance Schedule III); *action:* reverses catabolic tissue processes; promotes buildup of protein; increases erythropoietin production; *uses:* treating catabolic or tissue-wasting processes, such as extensive surgery, burns, infection, or trauma; HIV wasting syndrome; Turner's syndrome.

O

oxaprozin (ok′səprō′zin), *n* *brand name:* Daypro; *drug class:* nonsteroidal antiinflammatory; *action:* inhibits prostaglandin synthesis by interfering with cyclooxygenase needed for biosynthesis; possesses analgesic, antiinflammatory, antipyretic properties; *uses:* rheumatoid arthritis, osteoarthritis, and ankylosing spondylitis.

oxazepam (oksaz′əpam), *n* *brand name:* Serax; *drug class:* benzodiazepine (Controlled Substance Schedule IV); *action:* produces central nervous system depression by interacting with a benzodiazepine receptor to facilitate the action of the inhibitory neurotransmitter λ-aminobutyric acid (GABA); *uses:* anxiety, alcohol withdrawal.

oxidant (ok′sidənt), *n* the substance that is reduced in an oxidation/reduction reaction, thereby oxidizing the other component.

oxidation, *n* the combination of oxygen with other elements to form oxides. The process in which an element gains electrons.

oxidation, beta, *n* a metabolic process in which complex fatty acids are broken down into simple compounds.

oxidation, of metal, *n* the formation of a surface oxide during the casting or soldering of a metal or during subsequent use by the patient.

oxidative, *adj* having the ability or property to oxidize.

oxidative phosphorylation and electron transport (ok′sidā′tiv fos′fərəlā′shən), *n* the metabolic process that creates adenosine triphosphate (ATP), the compound needed to store energy in muscles.

oxide, *n* a compound of oxygen with another element or radical such as iron.

oxide divinyl, *n* See ether, divinyl.

oxidized cellulose, *n* *brand name:* Surgicel; *drug class:* cellulose hemostatic; *action:* mechanism unclear; may act physically to absorb blood and promote an artifical clot; *uses:* hemostasis in surgery, oral surgery, exodontia.

oximetry (oksim′itrē), *n* the measurement of the oxygen saturation of hemoglobin in a sample of blood with the use of an oximeter.

oxtriphylline (ok′strifil′ēn), *n* *brand names:* Choledyl, Choledyl SA; *drug class:* choline salt of theophylline, a bronchodilator; *action:* relaxes smooth muscle of respiratory system by blocking phosphodiesterase; *uses:* acute bronchial asthma, reversible bronchospasm in chronic bronchitis and COPD.

oxybutynin chloride (ok′sēbū′tinin klor′īd), *n* *brand name:* Ditropan; *drug class:* antispasmodic; *action:* relaxes smooth muscles in urinary tract; *use:* antispasmodic for neurogenic bladder.

oxycephaly (ok′sēsef′əlē), *n*, a high conical crown resulting from early closure of sutures and disturbed cranial development. Also called *steeple head.*

oxycodone (ok′sēkō′dōn), *n* *brand name:* Roxicodone; OxyIR; OxyContin; *drug class:* synthetic opioid analgesic (Controlled Substance Schedule II); *action:* attaches to opiate receptors in the central nervous system; *uses:* moderate to severe pain, normally used in combination with aspirin or acetaminophen, the opioid found in Percodan, Percocet, and Tylox. It is an easily abused substance. See also Percocet and Percodan.

oxygen (O), *n* a tasteless, odorless, colorless gas essential for respiration. Its atomic number is 8 and its atomic weight is 15.9994.

oxygen, E-cylinder tank, *n* the gas cylinder size most commonly used in the United States to store oxygen for individual patient delivery; the cylinder is color-coded green for quick recognition as oxygen.

oxygenate (ok′sijenāt), *v* to saturate with oxygen.

oxyhemoglobin (ok′sēhē′mōglō′bin), *n* a compound of hemoglobin with two atoms of oxygen.

oxymetazoline HCl (ok′sēmətaz′əlēn), *n brand names:* Afrin, Afrin Children's Nose Drops, Dristan Long-Lasting, Neo-Synephrine Nasal Decongestant, Sinarest 12-Hour, Vicks Sinex 12-Hour; *drug class:* nasal decongestant, sympathomimetic amine; *action:* produces vasoconstriction of arterioles, thereby decreasing fluid exudation and mucosal engorgement; *use:* nasal congestion.

oxymetholone (ok′sēmeth′əlōn′), *n brand name:* Anadrol-50; *drug class:* androgenic anabolic steroid (Controlled Substance Schedule III); *action:* reverses catabolic tissue processes; promotes buildup of protein, increased erythropoietin production; *uses:* anemia associated with bone marrow failure and red cell production deficiencies, aplastic anemia, myelofibrosis, and anemia caused by myelotoxic drugs.

oxytetracycline (ok′sētet′rəsī′klēn), *n* a tetracycline antibiotic prescribed in the treatment of bacterial and rickettsial infections.

oxytocin (ok′sētō′sin), *n* a hormone of the posterior pituitary gland that is the principal uterus-contracting hormone. Used in obstetrics to induce uterine contractions.

P

P point, *n* a measurement referring to the most posterior point relative to another feature.

PA skull, *n* See examination, radiographic; examination, extraoral; and examination, posteroanterior.

PAB, PABA, *n* an abbreviation for **paraaminobenzoic acid.**

PAC, *n* See aspirin, phenacetin, caffeine.

pacemaker, *n* an electrical device used to maintain a normal sinus rhythm in heart muscle contraction. Pacemakers can be permanent indwelling appliances. The use of electronic devices on patients with pacemakers is now considered permissible because of modern shields. The device may also have a defibrillator. Also called *cardiac pacemaker.*

pachymucosa alba (pak′imyookō′sə al′bə), *n* an appearance of the buccal mucosa that has a white surface and resembles elephant hide.

Pacini's corpuscle (pächē′nēz), *n.pr* See corpuscle, Pacini's.

pack, *n* a material used to protect tissue, fill space, or prevent hemorrhage.

pack, periodontal, *n* a surgical dressing applied to the necks of teeth and the adjacent tissue to cover and protect the surgical wound.

packing, *n* in dentistry, the act of filling a mold or a cavity preparation or placement of a cord into the suculus.

paclitaxel (pak′litak′səl), *n brand name:* Taxol; *drug class:* antineoplastic; *action:* obtained from Western Yew tree, unique action inhibits microtubule network reorganization essential for cell division; *use:* metastatic ovarian cancer.

pad, Passavant's (pas′əvänts), *n.pr* (Passavant's bar, Passavant's ridge), the bulging "transverse roll" of the posterior pharyngeal wall produced by the superior portion of the superior pharyngeal constrictor muscle during the act of swallowing or during vocal effort; an objectionable term. See also pharynx, activities of posterior and lateral pharyngeal wall.

pad, retromolar, *n* a mass of soft tissue, frequently pear shaped, which is located at the distal termination of the mandibular residual ridge. It is made up of fibers of the buccinator muscle, the pterygomandibular raphe, the superior constrictor muscle, the temporal tendon, and the mucous glands.

pad, rubber dam, (rubber dam mask), *n* an absorbent piece of flannelette, bird's-eye, or gauze of suitable shape to interpose between a rubber dam and the face to protect the face from contact with both the rubber and the clips of the dam holder.

Paget's disease (paj′əts), *n.pr* See disease, Paget's, of bone.

pain, *n* an unpleasant sensation created by a noxious stimulus mediated along specific nerve pathways to the central nervous system, where it is interpreted. The sensation of pain is a protective mechanism that warns of danger without giving too much information about the specific nature of the danger. It initiates nociceptive reflexes.

pain and suffering, *n* an element in a claim for damages in a liability lawsuit. It requests compensation to an individual for mental and physical pain and discomfort as a result of an injury.

pain, assessment, *n* an evaluation of the reported pain and the factors that alleviate or exacerbate a patient's pain; used as an aid in the diagnosis and the treatment of disease and trauma.

pain, chest, *n* pain that occurs in the chest region because of disorders of the heart (e.g., angina pectoris, myocardial infarction, or pericarditis), pulmonary artery (pulmonary embolism or hypertension), lungs (pleuritis), esophagus ("heartburn"), abdominal organs (aerophagia, biliary tract disease, splenic infarction, or gaseous distention in the splenic flexure), or the chest wall (neoplasia, costochondral strains, trauma, hyperventilation, or muscular tension).

pain clinic, *n* a multidisciplinary association of health care professionals devoted to the diagnosis and treatment of patients with acute and chronic pain.

pain, deep, *n* dull, aching, or boring pain originating in muscles, tendons, and joints. It is poorly localized and tends to radiate.

pain dysfunction syndrome, *n* in dentistry, a phrase used to describe a condition in patients who appear to have a psychophysiologic basis for stress overload on the temporomandibular joint. The preferred term is *mandibular stress syndrome*.

pain, ghost, *n* See odontalgia, phantom.

pain mechanism, *n* the network that communicates unpleasant sensations and the perceptions of noxious stimuli throughout the body in association with both physical disease and trauma involving tissue damage.

pain, nerve ending, *n* a receptor nerve ending that is relatively primitive and ends in an undifferentiated arborization. The nerve ending for the sensation of pain is a protective mechanism that warns of danger without giving too much information about the specific nature of the danger. The danger stimuli give rise to nociceptive reflexes, or defensive, protective, or withdrawal movements. The nociceptive reflexes supersede other, less urgent, reflexes that are thus inhibited.

pain, projected pathologic, *n* pain erroneously perceived to arise in a peripheral region because of a stimulus from end-organs supplying the region (e.g., sciatic pain). Actually the stimulus occurred somewhere along the pain pathway from the nerve to the cortex.

pain, reaction, *n* the individual's manifestation of the unpleasant sensation.

pain, referred, *n* pain caused by an agent in one area but manifested in another (e.g., pain caused by caries in the maxillary third molar may be referred to the mandible, so the source of pain appears to be in the mandible).

pain stimulus, *n* an agent that has the potential to induce pain, whether through chemical, mechanical, or thermal means.

pain, tactile stimuli, *n* any of a number of physical sources that may aggravate dentin hypersensitivity, such as dental instruments, toothbrush bristles, ill-fitting oral prostheses, and various personal oral habits a patient may have.

pain, thermal stimuli, *n* dentin hypersensitivity related to abrupt changes in temperature of teeth as a result of contact with very cold or very hot foods and liquids, rapid intake of air through the oral cavity, and during professional oral hygiene procedures requiring rapid drying of teeth.

pain threshold, *n* the point at which a stimulus causes pain. It varies widely among individuals.

pain, tolerance, *n* the maximum pain level an individual is able to withstand.

pair, ion, *n* See ion.

palatability (pal'ətəbil'itē), *n* the quality of a food that makes it acceptable or agreeable to one's personal taste.

palatal (pal'ətəl), *adj* **1.** relating to the palate. **2.** the lingual structures or tooth surfaces closest to the palate on the maxillary arch.

palatal bar, *n* See bar, palatal.

palatal cyst of the newborn, *n* See cyst, palatal, of the newborn.

palatal perforation, *n* See perforation, palatal.

palatal plate, *n* See connector, major.

palatal rugae, *n.pl* See rugae.

palatal seal, *n* See seal, posterior palatal.

palatal shelves, *n.pl* the outgrowths of the embryonic maxillae that come together during prenatal development to form the secondary palate.

palatal torus **(pal'ətəl tor'əs),** *n* a thick protrusion of bone arising from the hard palate's midline. Also called *torus palatinus.* See maxillary torus.

palate (pal'ət), *n* the bone and soft tissue that closes the space encompassed by the maxillary arch, extending posteriorly to the pharynx. The palate forms the "roof of the mouth" and connects to the nasal septum and floor of the nose in the midline.

palate, acquired cleft, *n* a noncongenital defect of soft or hard tissues of the hard and soft palate.

palate, cleft, *n* a cleft in the palate between the two palatal processes. It can vary in involvement and can be associated with cleft lip. If both hard and soft palates are involved, it is a *uranostaphyloschisis;* if only the soft palate is divided, it is a *uranoschisis.* The term *cleft palate* is often erroneously applied to clefts between the median nasal and maxillary processes through the alveolus. The proper term for this type of cleft is *cleft jaw,* or *gnathoschisis.*

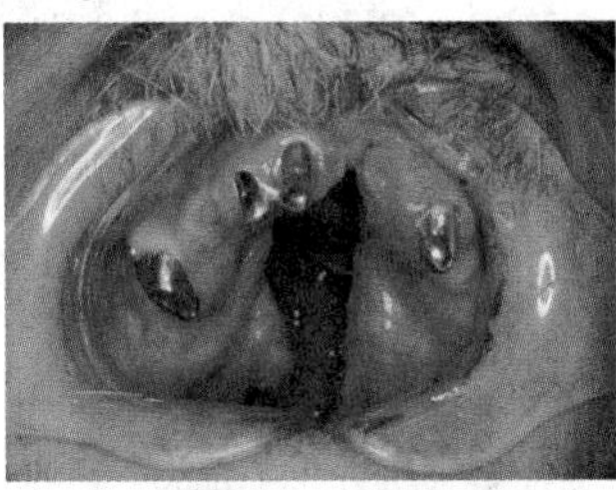

Cleft palate. (Courtesy Dr. Richard Streem)

palate, congenital cleft **(kənjen'itəl kleft),** *n* a congenital nonunion or inadequacy of soft and hard tissues related to the lip, nose, alveolar process, hard palate, and velum. The extent of these deformities varies among individuals. Varieties of classifications are available to identify the extent of the cleft.

palate, hard, *n* the anterior part of the palate, which is supported by and includes the palatal extensions of the maxillary and palatine bones.

palate, primary, *n* the shelf separating the oral and nasal cavities that is formed during early embryonic development from protrusions of tissue between the olfactory pits. It is also called *primitive palate.*

palate, secondary, *n* the final palate that is formed during embryonic development when projections from the nasal prominences come together to create portions of the maxillary arch.

palate, soft, *n* the part of the palate lying posterior to the hard palate, composed of only soft tissues without underlying bony support.

palate, soft, redivision, *n* the surgical incision or removal of a V-shaped area of tissue from the soft palate to facilitate the proper placement of the pharyngeal section of a prosthetic speech aid.

palate splitting appliance, *n* an orthodontic appliance cemented to buccal teeth on either side, incorporating a jackscrew that is progressively extended to accomplish forceful separation of the two lateral halves of the bony palate. Similar corrections also are accomplished with removable split-palate appliances.

palatine (pal′ətīn), *adj* associated with or being of the palate.

palatine arch (pal′ətin), *n* See arch, palatine.

palatine mucosa, *n* See mucosa, palatine.

palato- (pal′ətō), *comb* a prefix meaning "pertaining to the palate."

palatoglossal air space (pal′ətōglos′əl), *n* an opening between the tongue and the palate that occurs with contractions of the palatoglossus.

palatoplasty (pal′ətōplastē), *n* the surgical repair of palatal defects.

palatorrhaphy (pal′ətôr′əfē), *n* the surgical closure of a cleft palate using suturing.

palladium (Pd) (pəlā′dēəm), *n* a hard, silvery metallic element that is highly resistant to tarnish and corrosion. Its atomic number is 46 and its atomic weight is 106.42. Palladium is used in high-grade surgical instruments and in dental inlays, bridgework, and orthodontic appliances.

P

palliate (pal′ēāt), *v* to reduce the severity of.

palliative (pal′ēətiv), *n* an alleviating measure.

pallidotomy (pal′idot′əmē), *n* an operation in which the globus pallidus of the basal ganglia is removed to prevent the symptoms of parkinsonism.

pallor (pal′ər), *n* paleness; absence of skin coloration.

pallor, perioral, *n* paleness of soft tissues surrounding the oral cavity; an indication of impending syncope.

palm grasp, *n* See grasp, palm-and-thumb.

Palmer's method of tooth notation, *n.pr* a system for designating teeth by number and quadrant. The oral cavity is divided into quadrants and each tooth is designated by an Arabic numeral 1 to 8, starting with the central incisor in each quadrant and continuing posteriorly to the third molar. The quadrant is indicated by a right angle symbol oriented right or left and up or down. The system was popular in the 1950s but is no longer in general use except in orthodontic practices.

palpate (pal′pāt), *v* to examine the soft tissues with the fingers or hands.

palpation (palpā′shən), *n* **1.** the act of feeling with the hands or fingers. *n* **2.** a phase of the examination procedure in which the sense of touch is used to gather information essential for diagnosis.

palpation, bilateral, *n* a method of examination in which both hands are used to simultaneously examine and compare symmetrical body structures on opposite sides of the body.

palpitation (palpitā′shən), *n* an unduly rapid action of the heart that is perceptible to the patient.

palsy (pôl′zē), *n* a general term for *paralysis* but preferred by some to refer to certain types of paralysis.

palsy, Bell's, *n.pr* facial paralysis believed to result from inflammation in or around the facial nerve. One side of the face sags, the corner of the oral cavity droops, the eyelid does not close, and saliva dribbles from the corner of the oral cavity on the affected side. See also paralysis, facial.

palsy, cerebral, *n* **1.** a collective term for neurologic defects with associated disturbances of motor function. The disturbances vary in cause and anatomic type (e.g., acquired, hereditary, natal, postnatal, congenital palsy). *n* **2.** a nonspecific term representing a group of pathologic conditions having the following common, related characteristics: agenesis, or a lesion of nervous tissue within the cranium; interference with voluntary muscular movements; disabling disorders of a chronic nature, neither acute nor progressive; and occurrence of the original lesion at the date of birth of the patient or before the development of learned muscular function. **3.** a condition caused by damage to the motor centers of the brain, resulting in varying disturbances of motor function and often accompanied by mental subnormality.

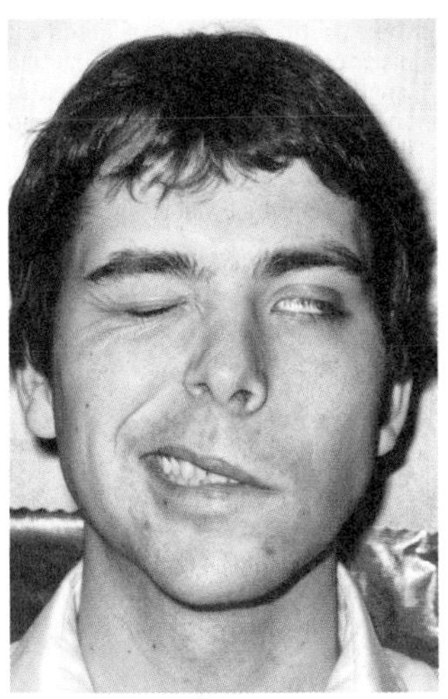

Bell's palsy. (Neville/Damm/Allen/Bouquot, 2002. Courtesy Dr. Bruce Brehm)

palsy, creeping, *n* See gait, spastic.

palsy, facial, *n* paralysis of the muscles supplied by the seventh cranial nerve. It may be associated with peripheral lesions, neoplasms invading the temporal bone, acoustic neuromas, pontine disease, and herpes zoster involving the geniculate ganglion. Bilateral paralysis may occur in uveoparotid fever and polyneuritis.

palsy, lead, *n* a weakness and paralysis of the hand, wrist, and fingers, associated with lead poisoning. See also lead (Pb).

pancreatin (pang′krēətin), *n* a concentrate of pancreatic enzymes from swine or beef cattle.

pancreatitis (pang′krēətī′tis), *n* inflammation of the pancreas that may be acute or chronic, characterized by severe abdominal pain radiating to the back, fever, anorexia, nausea, and vomiting.

pancrelipase (pang′krilip′ās), *n brand names:* Cotazym, Enzymase, Ilozyme, Protilase, Ultrase MT, Viokase, Zymase, others; *drug class:* digestant; *action:* pancreatic enzyme needed for proper pancreatic secretion insufficiency; *uses:* cystic fibrosis (digestive aid), steatorrhea, pancreatic enzyme deficiency.

pancuronium bromide (pang′kyərō′nēəm brō′mīd), *n* a skeletal muscle relaxant prescribed as an adjunct to anesthesia and mechanical ventilation.

pandemic (pandem′ik), *adj* describing an epidemic covering a widespread area such as a country or continent. It can describe a global epidemic.

panel, open, *n* a group dental plan characterized by three features: a licensed dental professional may elect to participate, the beneficiary may choose from among all licensed dental professionals, and the dental professional may accept or refuse any beneficiary.

pangamic acid (pang′gam′ik), *n* a substance that is a derivative of apricot pits and contains some potentially toxic substances. No evidence that this substance is a vitamin exists. Also called *vitamin* B_{15}.

panhypopituitarism (panhī′pōpitoo′itəriz′əm), *n* a deficiency involving all the hormonal functions of the pituitary gland. See also disease, Simmonds'.

panic attack, *n* an episode of acute anxiety that occurs unpredictably with feelings of intense apprehension or terror, accompanied by dyspnea, dizziness, sweating, trembling, and chest pain or palpitations. The attack may last several minutes and may occur again in certain conditions.

panic disorder, *n* See panic attack.

panneuritis endemica (pan′nyoorī′tis endem′ikə), *n* See beriberi.

panoral (panôr′əl), *adj* literally, "all of the oral region," a term used in diagnostic oral radiography to describe a technique that includes all the oral structures on one film.

panoramic radiograph, *n* See radiograph, panoramic.

Panoramix, *n.pr* a radiographic system in which the source of radiation is placed inside the oral cavity to expose a large film placed extraorally around the face.

pansinusitis (pan′sīnusī′tis), *n* inflammation of all the sinuses, as of the facial bones.

pantograph (pan′tōgraf), *n* a figurative term given to a pair of facebows fixed to both jaws and designed to inscribe centrically related points and then arcs leading to these points on segments of planes relatable to the three craniofacial planes of space. The maxillary planes are attached to the maxillary bow, and the inscribing styluses are attached to the mandibular bow.

pantomography (pantəmog′rəfē), *n* panoramic radiography for obtaining radiographs of the maxillary and mandibular dental arches and their associated structures.

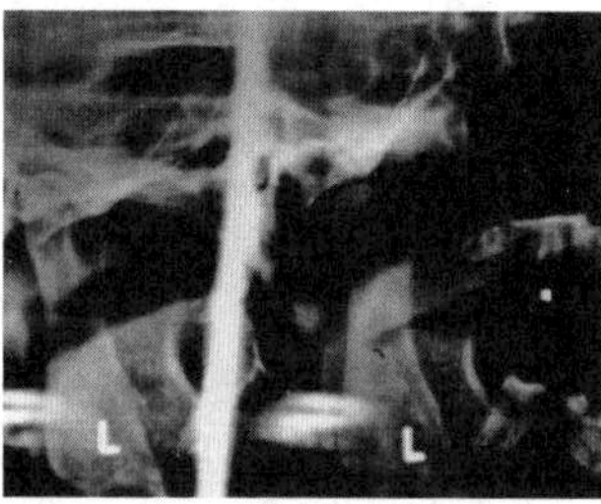

Pantomography of the temporomandibular joint. (Frommer/Stabulas-Savage, 2005)

pantothenic acid (pantəthēn′ik), *n* fatty acids. See also acid, pantothenic.

papain (pəpā′in), *n* an enzyme from papaya, a tropical fruit; used for enzymatic debridement of wounds and for promotion of healing.

papaverine HCl (pəpav′ərēn′), *n* *brand names:* Cerespan, Genabid, Pavabid, Pavacot, Pavagen, Pavased, others; *drug class:* peripheral vasodilator; *action:* relaxes all smooth muscle, inhibits cyclic nucleotide phosphodiesterase, which increases intracellular cAMP, causing vasodilation; *uses:* arterial spasm resulting in cerebral and peripheral ischemia; myocardial ischemia associated with vascular spasms or dysrhythmias, angina pectoris, peripheral and pulmonary embolism; visceral spasm, as in ureteral, biliary, gastrointestinal colic.

paper, articulating, *n* paper strips coated with ink or dye-containing wax, used for marking or locating occlusal interferences or deflecting occlusal contacts prior to making occlusal contacts. See also articulating paper.

paper point, *n* a cone of absorbent paper designed to be inserted into the length of the root canal and used to absorb fluid, carry medication into the canal, or inoculate cultures.

papilla(e) (pəpil′ə), *n* a small, nipple-shaped elevation.

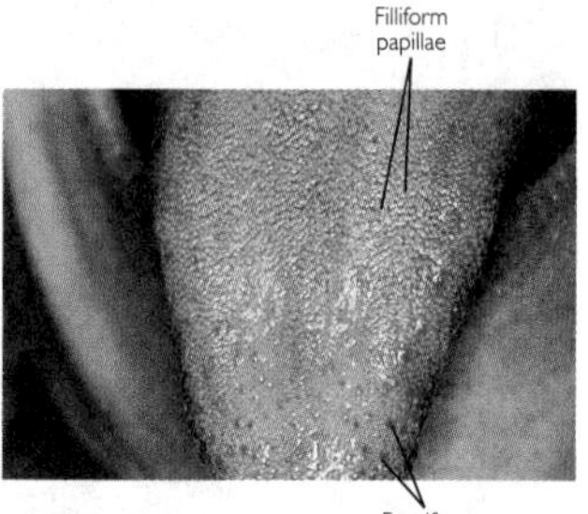

Papillae. (Bird/Robinson, 2005)

papilla, incisive, *n* the elevation of soft tissue covering the foramen of the incisive or nasopalatine canal.

papilla, retrocuspid, *n* benign nodules of the gingival tissues that occur lingual to the mandibular canines. These nodules are distinguished at a microscopic level by stellate fibroblasts within the fibrous connective tissue. Found in young adults and children, they are considered to be a normal variation of healthy tissue and should not be biopsied.

papilla(e), interproximal, *n* the cone-shaped projection of the gingiva filling the interdental spaces up to the contact areas when viewed from the labial, buccal, and lingual aspects. When viewed buccolingually or labiolingually, the crest of the interproximal papilla appears as a rounded concavity at an area below the contact point of the teeth. If recession has occurred, this concavity may become an area of pathology, and the entire papilla may require reshaping to restore health. Older term: *interdental papilla(e).*

papillae, central cell of the dental, *n* See cell, central of the dental papillae.

papillae, circumvallate lingual **(pəpil′ē surkəmval′āt ling′gwəl),** *n* the small projections located at the posterior of the tongue. These projections form a V-shaped pattern located just anterior to the sulcus terminalis of the tongue. The number of circumvallate papillae varies between three and fourteen. These papillae contain taste buds along their lateral walls.

papillae, lingual, *n* the small epithelial protuberances on the dorsal surface of the tongue. There are four types: circumvallate papillae, filiform papillae, foliate papillae, and fungiform papillae.

papillae, outer cell of the dental, *n* See cell, outer, of the dental papillae.

papillae, parotid **(pərot′id),** *n.pl* tiny tissue projections located on the inner portion of the buccal mucosa near the maxillary second molar that protect the parotid duct.

papillary, *adj* similar to a small, nipple-shaped elevation or projection.

papillary layer, *n* the most superior layer of the dermis. Characterized by papillae, fingerlike projections that interdigitate with the epidermis. Consists primarily of loose connective tissue.

papillary adenoma (pap′əlerē), *n* a benign epithelial tumor in which the membrane lining the glandular tissue forms papillary processes that project into the alveoli or grow out of the surface of a cavity.

papillary-marginal-attached, *n* See PMA.

papilledema (pap′ilədē′mə), *n* swelling of the optic disc caused by increased intracranial pressure.

papilloma (pap′ilō′mə), *n* an exophytic, pedunculated, cauliflower–like benign neoplasm of epithelium, often having a "warty appearance."

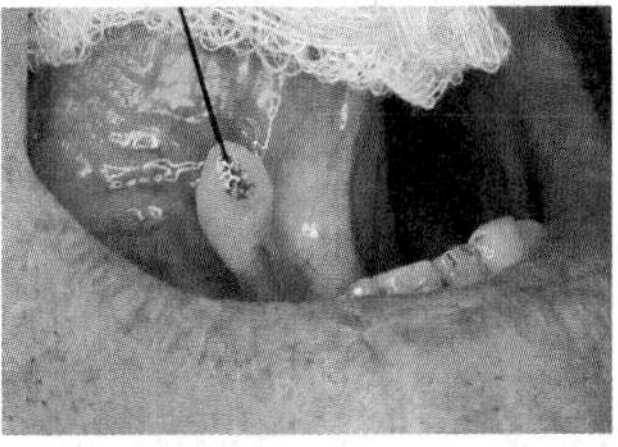

Oral papilloma. (Neville/Damm/Allen/Bouquot, 2002)

papilloma, basal cell, *n* See keratosis, seborrheic.

papilloma, squamous **(pap′əlō′mə skwäm′əs),** *n* a type of papilloma, or benign tumor of the skin or oral mucosa. Usually associated with infection by the human papilloma virus (HPV).

papillomatosis, inflammatory (pap′ilōmətō′sis), *n* See hyperplasia, papillary, inflammatory.

papillomatosis, multiple, *n* See hyperplasia, papillary, inflammatory.

papillomaviruses, *n. pl* viruses that cause infection of the hair, skin, and nails known as warts, including oral warts.

Papillon-Lefèvre syndrome (pap′iyōn-ləfev′), *n.pr* See syndrome, Papillon-Lefèvre.

papoose board (papoos′), *n* a board used to stabilize the position of a pediatric patient, or a patient with limited psychomotor control. It comes in various sizes and has soft flaps that surround and hold the patient.

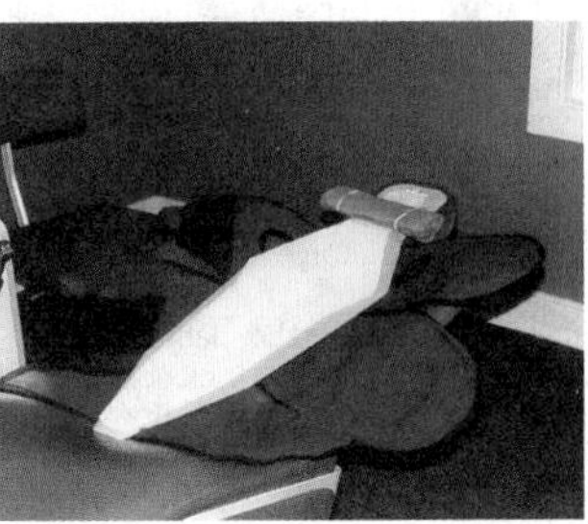

Papoose board. (Bird/Robinson, 2005)

Papovaviridae **(pap′əvəvir′idā),** *n.pl* a major deoxyribonucleic acid virus to which the papillomavirus and polyomavirus belong. Viruses in this family have a double-stranded, supercoiled, circular molecular structure with icosahedral symmetry.

papule (pap′ūl), *n* a small, circumscribed, solid elevated lesion.

papule, split, *n* a secondary lesion of syphilis seen at the angle of the lips, resulting from the formation of a papule that becomes fissured because of its position.

paradigm (par″ədīm), *n* a model or pattern. The set of values or concepts that represent an accepted way of doing things within an organization or community.

P

paradigm shift, *n* an adjustment in thinking that comes about as the result of new discoveries, inventions, or real-world experiences.

paradontosis (per′ədontō′sis), *n* See periodontosis.

paraffin (par′əfin), *n* a group of hydrocarbons or hydrocarbon mixtures of the paraffin series as indicated by the formula $C_{11}H_{(2n+2)}$. Examples include methane gas, kerosene, and paraffin wax.

paraffin bath, *n* the application of heat to a specific area of the body through the use of paraffin wax. The area is quickly immersed in heated liquid wax and then withdrawn so that the wax solidifies to form an insulating layer. The procedure is repeated until the layer is 5 to 10 mm thick, and then the entire area is wrapped in an insulating fabric. The technique is used primarily for patients with arthritis and rheumatism or any joint condition.

paraffin method, *n* a method used in preparing a selected portion of tissue for pathologic examination. The tissue is fixed, dehydrated, and infiltrated by and embedded in paraffin wax, forming a block that is cut with a microtome into slices 8 mm thick.

parafunction, *n* the habitual movements (e.g., bruxism, clenching, and rocking of teeth using teeth for tools) that are normal motions associated with mastication, speech, or respiratory movements and that result in worn facets and other problems associated with occlusal trauma. Also called *parafunctional habits* or *oral habits.*

parahemophilia (per′əhē′mōfil′ēə), *n* (Ac globulin deficiency, Owren's disease), a hemorrhagic disorder resulting from a deficiency of proaccelerin. Manifestations include mild to severe bleeding after extraction of teeth or other surgical procedures, epistaxis, easy bruising, monorrhagia, and hematomas. The one-stage prothrombin time is prolonged, but the bleeding time is ordinarily normal.

parainfluenza virus, *n* a myxovirus with four serotypes, causing respiratory infections in infants and young children and, less commonly, in adults.

parakeratosis (per′əkerətō′sis), *n* the persistence of nuclei in the stratum corneum keratin layer of stratified squamous epithelium. Associated with the masticatory mucosa of the attached gingiva; may be an immature form of orthokeratinized epithelium.

paralgesia (per′əljē′zēə), *n* **1.** a condition marked by abnormal and painful sensations. *n* **2.** a painful paresthesia.

parallax (per′əlaks), *n* the apparent change in position of an object when viewed from two different positions. The phenomenon is useful in determining the relative position of an object in a radiograph. Two or more radiographs are made from slightly different positions and the direction and amount of shift of the object is observed and measured.

parallel attachment, *n* See attachment, parallel.

parallelism (par′əleliz′əm), *n* the condition of two or more surfaces that, if extended to infinity, could never meet. In removable partial prosthodontics, such a condition is created on vertical tooth surfaces to act as guiding planes.

parallelometer (per′əlelom′ətur), *n* an apparatus used to determine parallelism or a lack of parallelism or to make a part or an object parallel with some other part or object. See also *surveyor.*

paralysis (pəral′isis), *n* **1.** the cessation of cell function. *n* **2.** the loss or impairment of the motor control or function of a part or region.

paralysis, diplegia **(dīplē′jēə),** *n* a loss of motor function in matching body parts (e.g., legs) on each side.

paralysis, facial, *n* paralysis of the muscles of facial expression resulting from supranuclear, nuclear, or peripheral nerve disease. With a mild case, when the face is at rest, the disorder is not readily observed. However, during muscular contraction (e.g., wrinkling the forehead, blinking the eyes, pursing the lips, speaking), the disorder is very noticeable. Only one lid may close, and the asymmetry of the oral cavity is pronounced because the normal buccinator muscle contracts and is unopposed by the weakness on the paralyzed side. This imbalance produces a significant asymmetry. The affected side remains smooth, and the normal side shows contraction. See also palsy, Bell's.

paralysis, infantile, *n* See poliomyelitis.

paralysis, motor, *n* a loss of the power of skeletal muscle contraction, resulting from interruption of some part of the pathway from the cerebrum to the muscle.

paralysis, transient, *n* the sudden loss of sensation or ability to move on one side or a single part of the body, which lasts briefly and may or may not recur and is often a symptom of cerebrovascular insufficiency or other underlying serious condition.

paralysis, transient facial, *n* a temporary unilateral loss of facial muscle function as a result of inadvertently injecting the parotid gland containing the facial nerve during the inferior nerve block.

parameter (pəram′ətur), *n* the values that refer to a population; characteristics of a population. Because a parameter is a value of a hypothetical, infinite, unknown population, it is always an estimate.

Paramyxoviridae **(per′əmik′sōvir′idā),** *n* one of the major ribonucleic acid virus families, to which the measles, mumps, parainfluenza, and respiratory syncytial viruses belong. Viruses in this family have a single-stranded, nonsegmented, linear molecular structure with helical symmetry.

paranasal sinuses (par′ənā′zəl), *n.pl* See sinus(es), paranasal.

paranesthesia (per′anesthē′zēə, -zhə), *n* anesthesia of the lower part of the body and limbs.

paranoia (per′ənoi′ə), *n* **1.** a psychosis characterized by delusions and hallucinations that are well systematized. **2.** the irrational belief that one is the object of special persecution by others or by fate.

parapharyngeal (par′əfərin′jēəl), *adj* refers to the parapharyngeal space, a cavity adjacent to the upper pharynx. Can also refer to tumors found in this cavity.

paraphilia (pər′əfil′ēə), *n* a condition in which a person derives pleasure from bizarre sexual fetishes.

paraplegia (par′əplē′jēə), *n* a paralysis characterized by motor or sensory loss in the lower limbs and trunk. Such events occur as a result of automobile and motorcycle accidents, sporting accidents, falls, and gunshot wounds.

parapsoriasis (par′əsərī′əsis), *n* a group of chronic skin diseases resembling psoriasis, characterized by maculopapular, erythematous, scaly eruptions without systemic symptoms. Parapsoriasis is resistant to all treatment.

parasite, *n* an organism living in or on and obtaining nourishment from another organism.

parasympathetic (par″əsim″pəthet′ik), *adj* pertaining to the part of the autonomic nervous system that controls craniosacral activity.

parasympatholytic (per′əsim′pathōlit′ik), *adj* See anticholinergic.

parasympathomimetic (per′əsim′pəthō′mimet′ik), *adj* See cholinergic.

Para-thor-mone (per′əthôr′mōn), *n.pr* a brand name for parathyroid hormone.

Parathyrin (per′əthī′rin), *n.pr* a brand name for parathyroid hormone.

parathyroidectomy, *n* the surgical removal of the parathyroid gland.

parenteral (pəren′tərəl), *adj* literally, "aside from the gastrointestinal tract"; not through the alimentary canal (i.e., by subcutaneous, intramuscular, intravenous, or other nongastrointestinal route of administration).

parenteral nutrition, *n* the administration of nutrients by a route other than the alimentary canal, such as subcutaneously, intravenously, intramuscularly, or intradermally. The parenteral fluid usually consists of physiologic saline with glucose, amino acids, electrolytes, vitamins, and medications, which are not nutritionally complete but maintain fluid and electrolyte balance.

paresis (pərē′sis), *n* a progressive psychosis associated with neurosyphilis.

paresthesia (per′esthē′zēə, -zhə), *n* an altered sensation reported by the patient in an area where the sensory nerve has been afflicted by a disease or an injury. The patient may report burning, prickling, formication, or other sensations.

paresthesia, oral, *n* a numbness or tingling that occurs in the mucosa or tissues of the oral cavity. It may be caused by a deficiency in vitamin B_{12} (cobalamine), trauma from surgery, or local anesthesia. It may be temporary, but in some cases it can be prolonged or permanent.

parietal bone (pərī′itəl), *n* the paired bones forming the sides of the cranium. Each articulates with five bones: the opposite parietal, occipital, frontal, temporal, and sphenoid.

parity (par′itē), *n* the use of a set of items, either even or odd in number, as a means for checking computer errors, such as in the transmission of information between various elements of the same computer.

parkinsonism, *n* an array of symptoms including stiffness, slow or restricted body movements, tremor, or postural problems. It has many causes, including Parkinson's disease.

parotid gland (pərot′id), *n* See gland, parotid salivary.

P

parotitis (per′ətī′tis), *n* inflammation of the parotid gland. See also mumps.

parotitis, endemic, *n* an acute viral infection characterized by unilateral or bilateral swelling of the salivary glands, especially the parotid.

parotitis, epidemic, *n* See parotitis, endemic.

parotitis, infectious, *n* See parotitis, endemic.

paroxetine, *n brand name:* Paxil; *drug class:* antidepressant; *action:* selectively inhibits the uptake of serotonin in the brain; *use:* depression.

paroxysm (per′əksizəm), *n* **1.** an abrupt increase or repeated occurrence of symptoms. *n* **2.** a sudden violent attack, contraction of muscles, or convulsion.

paroxysmal (per′əksiz′məl), *adj* recurring in paroxysms.

partial denture retention, *n* See retention, partial denture.

partial thromboplastin time (PTT), *n* a test for detecting coagulation defects of the intrinsic system by adding activated partial thromboplastin to a sample of test plasma and to a control sample of normal plasma. The time required for the formation of a clot is compared with the normal plasma. It is also used to monitor the activity of heparin in patients who are being treated for a variety of cardiovascular disorders.

participating dental provider, *n* a dental provider who has a contractual agreement with a dental benefits organization to render care to eligible persons.

particle, *n* a small amount of material.

particle, alpha, *n* (alpha ray, alpha radiation) a positively charged particulate ionizing radiation consisting of helium nuclei (two protons and two neutrons) traveling at high speeds. These rays are emitted from the nucleus of an unstable element.

particle, beta, *n* (beta ray, beta radiation) a particulate ionizing radiation consisting of either negative electrons (negatrons) or positive electrons (positrons) emitted from the nucleus of an unstable element. This phenomenon is called *beta decay.*

particulate bone grafts *n.pl* a type of autogenous bone graft that consists of small particles of cortical and cancellous bone and hematopoietic and mesenchymal marrow.

parties, *n.pl* the persons who take part in the performance of any act, who have a direct interest in a contract or conveyance, or who are actively involved in the prosecution and defense of a legal proceeding.

partnership, *n* **1.** the association of two or more persons for the purpose of carrying on business (or practice) together and dividing its profits. *n* **2.** a legal, binding contract defining the association of two or more persons in a business or professional relationship such as a dental practice.

partnership, notice of dissolution of intelligence, *n* by any of a variety of means, notice to creditors and the public that a partnership has been dissolved.

Partsch's operation, *n.pr* See operation, Partsch's.

parulis (pərū′lis), *n* an elevated nodule at the site of a fistula draining a chronic periapical abscess. These nodules occur most frequently in relation to pulpally involved primary teeth.

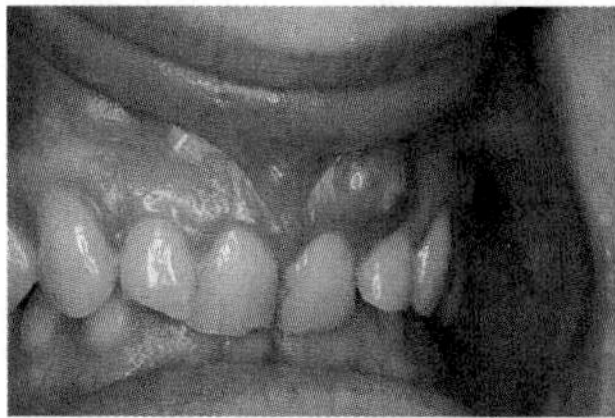

Parulis. (Neville/Damm/Allen/Bouquot, 2002)

Parvoviridae **(pär′vōvir′idā),** *n* one of the major deoxyribonucleic acid virus families to which the B_{19} virus belongs. These viruses have a single-stranded linear molecular structure with icosahedral symmetry.

Passavant's bar, *n.pr* See pad, Passavant's.

Passavant's pad, *n.pr* See pad, Passavant's.

Passavant's ridge, *n.pr* See pad, Passavant's.

passer, foil, *n* See foil passer.

passive, *n* in orthodontics, an orthodontic appliance that has been adjusted to apply no effective tooth-moving force to the teeth. Also called *self-ligation,* or *"frictionless."*

passive diffusion, n an absorption process that occurs in the body when carbohydrates are more highly concentrated in the intestine than in the blood.

passive immunity, n a form of acquired immunity resulting from antibodies that are transmitted naturally through the placenta to a fetus or through the colostrum to an infant or artificially by injection of antiserum for treatment or prophylaxis. Passive immunity is not permanent and does not last as long as active immunity.

passive reciprocation, n See reciprocation, passive.

passive smoking, n the inhalation by nonsmokers of the smoke from other people's cigarettes, pipes, and cigars. See also environmental tobacco smoke (ETS/passive smoke).

passive-aggressive behavior, *n* behavior that reflects hostility or resentment through indirect nonviolent means, such as procrastination, inefficiency, forgetfulness, and stubbornness.

passive-dependent personality, *n* a personality characterized by helplessness, indecisiveness, and a tendency to cling to and seek support from others.

passivity, *n* the quality or condition of inactivity or rest assumed by the teeth, tissues, and denture when a removable denture is in place but is not under masticatory pressure.

paste, *n* a soft, smooth, semifluid mixture, often medicated.

paste, filler, n a semisoft mixture of materials used to fill the root canal system, unlike solid filling material such as silver or gutta-percha cones.

paste, pressure-indicating, n a soft mixture used to disclose areas of contact or pressure in restorations.

paste, prophylactic, n a substance comprising several abrasive compounds and fluoride, which cleans and polishes the teeth.

Pasteurella **(pas′chərel′ə),** *n* a genus of gram-negative bacilli or coccobacilli, including species pathogenic to humans and domestic animals. *Pasteurella* infections may be transmitted to humans by animal bites.

patch (pach), *n* mucus, a large gray-white region overlying an area of ulceration and occurring on the oral mucosa as an expression of secondary syphilis; highly infectious. See also syphilis.

patch test, *n* a skin test for identifying allergens, especially those causing contact dermatitis.

patent (pat′ənt), *adj* open and unblocked, such as a *patent airway.*

patent ductus arteriosus (ahrtēr′ēōsis), *n* a congenital heart defect in which the passage between the aorta and the pulmonary artery is open, allowing blood to pool back into the lungs, causing the heart to work harder than necessary.

patent medicine, *n* a nonprescription drug available to the general public; usually referred to as an *over-the-counter medicine.*

paternity test, *n* a test based on genetic blood groups or other means and used mainly to exclude the possibility that a particular man could be the father of a specific child. Also called a *blood test.*

path, *n* a certain course that is usually followed.

path, condyle, *n* See condyle path.

path, generated occlusal, *n* a registration in the oral cavity of the paths of movement of the occlusal surfaces of teeth on a wax, plastic, or abrasive surface attached to the opposing dental arch.

path, idling, *n* the path that a stamp cusp travels when the bolus is being treated on the other side of the oral cavity.

path, lateral, *n* See condyle path, lateral.

path, occlusal, *n* **1.** a gliding occlusal contact. *n* **2.** the path of movement of an occlusal surface.

path of appliance insertion and removal, *n* See insertion, path of.

path of closure, *n* See closure, centric path of.

path of insertion, *n* See insertion, path of.

path of placement, *n* the direction in which a removable dental restoration is positioned in relation to the planned location on its supporting structures. The restoration is removed in the opposite direction. See also placement, choice of path of.

path, working, *n* the path that the stamp cusps make when working on the bolus. At first the bolus deflects the direction of these cusps, but after the fibers of the food have been reduced enough to be almost ready for swallowing, the travel coincides directionally with the working groove.

pathfinder, *n* See broach, smooth.

pathogen (path′ojən), *n* a microorganism responsible for causing disease.

pathogen, opportunistic, *n* an infectious agent that can only cause disease when the host's resistance is low.

pathogenesis (path″ojen′əsis), *n* the course of an illness or condition, from its origin to manifestation and outbreak.

pathogenic occlusion (path′ə-jen′ik), *n* See occlusion, pathogenic.

pathognomonic (pəthog′nəmon′ik), *adj* relating to a sign or symptom unique to a disease or one that distinguishes it from other diseases.

pathology (pəthol′əjē), *n* **1.** the branch of science that deals with disease in all its relations, especially with its nature and the functional and material changes it causes. *n* **2.** in medical jurisprudence, the science of disease; the part of medicine that deals with the nature of disease, its causes, and its symptoms.

pathology, experimental, *n* the study of disease processes induced, usually in animals; undertaken to ascertain the effect of local environmental changes or systemic disorders on particular tissues, parts, and organs of the body. This branch of medical science also attempts to correlate the interaction of local and systemic factors in the production, modification, and continuance of a disease.

pathology, oral, *n* the study of the characteristics, causes, and effects of diseases of the oral cavity and associated structures.

pathology, speech, *n* the study and treatment of the aspects of functional and organic speech defects and disorders.

pathology, surgical, *n* the study of the characteristics of diseased tissues and organs removed in the process of surgery.

pathophysiology (path′ōfiz′ēol′əjē), *n* the study of the disruption of normal bodily functions due to disease.

pathosis (pəthō′sis), *n* **1.** a disease entity. *n* **2.** a pathologic condition. More specifically a patient is said to have a *pathosis* rather than *pathology,* which is the study of disease.

pathway of inflammation, *n* in dentistry, the route of extension of chronic gingival inflammation into the subjacent structures, extending into the interdental septum from the gingivae, along the interdental vessels, or following the course of these blood vessels onto the periosteal side of the bone as well as into the bone marrow spaces.

patient, *n* a person under medical or dental care.

patient admission, *n* the formal acceptance of a patient for care into a clinic, hospital, or extended care facility.

patient, bedridden (homebound), n an individual from any age group confined to a private home, hospital, skilled nursing facility, hospice, nursing home, or institution.

patient compliance, n the degree or extent to which a patient follows or completes a prescribed diagnostic, treatment, or preventive procedure.

patient education, n the process of informing a patient about a health matter to secure informed consent, patient cooperation, and a high level of patient compliance.

patient load, n the number of patients treated by a dental professional or a group of dental professionals within a specified period.

patient satisfaction, n the perception of the patient(s) of one or more aspects of a dental care system; an outcome measure of quality.

patient transfer, n to convey the responsibility for the care of a patient from one entity to another. It may involve the discharge from one entity and the admission to another along with the patient's medical/dental records or copies.

Patient's Bill of Rights, *n.pr* a list of the patient's rights promulgated by the American Hospital Association (AHA). It offers some guidance and protection to patients by stating the responsibilities that a hospital and its staff have toward patients and their families during hospitalization, but it is not a legally binding document.

pattern, *n* a form used to make a mold, such as for a denture, an inlay, or a partial denture framework.

pattern, brachyfacial **(brak′ē-fā′shəl),** *n* a facial growth pattern in which the face appears short and wide, the mandible is considered strong and has a squared-off appearance, and the dental arches are broad. Deep anterior overbites, usually resulting from skeletal abnormalities, are present.

pattern, dolichofacial **(dō′likō-fā′shəl),** *n* a facial growth pattern in which the face is long and narrow, the dental arches often exhibit crowding of the teeth, and the musculature is weakened. Anterior open overbites are often present because of the vertical growth pattern of the mandible.

pattern, mesofacial **(mez′ōfā′shəl),** *n* a facial growth pattern in which there is a normal relationship between the mandible and maxilla and the face appears neither too long nor too wide. The jaw characteristics and dental arches are also harmonious.

pattern, occlusal, n the form or design of the occluding surfaces of a tooth or teeth. These forms may be based on natural or modified anatomic or nonanatomic concepts of teeth.

pattern, trabecular **(trəbek′yələr),** *n* the trabecular arrangement of alveolar bone in relation to marrow spaces; may be radiographically interpreted.

pattern, wax, n **1.** a wax model for making the mold in which the metal will be formed in casting. *n* **2.** a wax form of a denture that, when it is invested in a flask and the wax is eliminated, will form the mold in which the resin denture is formed.

pattern, wear, n the topographic attributes and distribution of areas of tooth wear (facets) resulting from attrition by food, tooth contacts during swallowing, terminal aspects of the masticatory cycle, and habits of occlusal neuroses. Wear patterns may be used to determine many of the functional and afunctional movements the mandible has been passing through in preceding years. Occlusal wear occurs with aging. The type of wear is termed the *wear pattern.*

Paul-Bunnell test, *n.pr* See test, Paul-Bunnell.

payable, *adj* pertaining to an obligation to pay at a future time. When used without restriction or modification, the term means that the debt is payable at once.

payback period, *n* the length of time required for the net revenues of an investment to return the cost of the investment.

payer, *n* in health care, generally refers to entities other than the patient that finance or reimburse the cost of health services. In most cases, this term refers to insurance carriers, other third-party payers, or health plan sponsors (employers or unions).

payment, *n* the performance of a duty or promise; the discharge of a

P

debt or liability by the delivery of money or something else of value.

payment, progress, *n* the interim payments by the purchaser of a dental plan contract to the carrier for use as an operating fund. A final accounting is always completed when actual costs are paid.

payroll record, *n* a printed form on which detailed records are kept of the amounts of money paid to auxiliaries. The record has columns for all the necessary tax deductions so that a detailed record is available for tax reporting and cost accounting.

PBI, *n* See iodine, protein-bound.

p.c. (post cibum), *n* a Latin phrase meaning "after meals"; the abbreviation may be used in prescription writing.

PCP, *n* an abbreviation for *Pneumocystis jiroveci pneumonia,* an opportunistic infection associated with acquired immune deficiency syndrome (AIDS) and used as an indicator of AIDS.

PDL, *n* See ligament, periodontal.

PDS, *n* See temporomandibular pain-dysfunction syndrome.

peak, *n* the buccal, outer high point of the normal interproximal tissue that rises to a peak; connected interdentally to a lingual peak by a triangular ridge, with a depression termed a *col.*

pearl, enamel (enameloma), *n* a small focal mass of enamel formed apical to the cementoenamel junction and resembling pearls. The bifurcation of molar roots is a favorite site for this. It appears as a radiopacity on radiographs.

pearls, Epstein's, *n.pr* See nodules, Bohn's.

pediatric dentistry, *n* See pedodontics.

pediatrics (pē′dēat′riks), *n* a branch of medicine concerned with the development and care of children. Its specialties are the particular diseases of children and their treatment and prevention.

pedicle flap, *n* See flap, pedicle.

Pediwrap, *n.pr* the brand name for a cloth bandage that is wrapped around a young patient from neck to ankles to stabilize the body or to minimize juvenile fidgeting. It comes in various sizes.

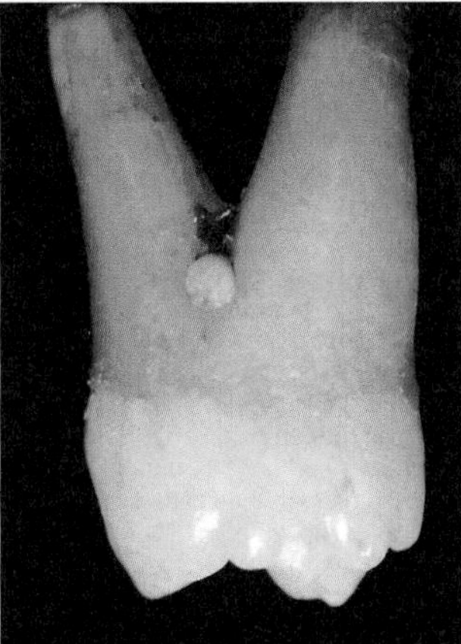

Enamel pearl. (Ibsen/Phelan, 2004. Courtesy Dr. Rudy Melfi)

pedodontics (pē′dədon′tiks), *n* the branch of dentistry that includes the following: training the child to accept dentistry; restoring and maintaining the primary, mixed, and permanent dentitions; applying preventive measures for dental caries and periodontal disease; and preventing, intercepting, and correcting various problems of occlusion.

pedunculated (pədung′kyəlā′tid), *adj* referring to a lesion attached with a narrow, stalklike base.

pedunculated lesion (pedung′kūlāted), *n* a raised lesion connected by a narrow stem.

peer review, *n* **1.** a retrospective consideration or an examination by one or more individuals of equal standing or rank. *n* **2.** a process established to provide for review by licensed dental professionals of the care by a dental professional for a single patient; disputes regarding fees; cases submitted by carriers and initiated by patients or dental professionals; and quality of care and appropriateness of treatment.

peer review organization (PRO), *n* an organization established by an amendment of the Tax Equity and Fiscal Responsibility Act of 1982 (TEFRA) to provide for the review of medical services furnished primarily in a hospital setting or in conjunction with care provided under the

Medicare and Medicaid programs. In addition to their review and monitoring functions, these entities can invoke sanctions, penalties, or other corrective actions for noncompliance in organization standards.

peer review system, *n* a professionally sponsored and operated system for the rendering of professional judgment on disagreements between or among dental professionals, patients, or fiscal intermediaries, respecting quality of care and related matters.

peg lateral, *n* a developmental anomaly of the maxillary lateral incisor that causes the tooth to resemble a small peg; developmental disturbance of partial microdontia.

peg third molar, *n* a developmental anomaly of the third molar (wisdom tooth) in which the crown fails to develop fully in any one of its four quadrants; developmental disturbance of partial microdontia.

pegs, epithelial, *n.pl* See rete ridges.

pellagra (pəlā′grə, pəlag′rə), *n* a nutritional deficiency resulting from faulty intake or metabolism of nicotinic acid, a vitamin B complex factor. It is characterized by glossitis, dermatitis of sun-exposed surfaces, stomatitis, diarrhea, and dementia. Thiamine, riboflavin, and tryptophan deficiencies may be associated.

pellet (pel′it), *n* a small, rounded mass of material.

pellet, cotton, *n* a rolled ball of cotton varying in diameter from approximately ⅜ inch to ⅛ inch. (The larger size is a cotton ball; the smaller size is a pledget.)

pellet, foil, *n* a loosely rolled piece of gold foil of various thicknesses; prepared from a portion—1/128, 1/96, 1/64, 1/48, 1/32, 1/16—cut from a 4-inch (10-cm) square of foil.

pellicle (pel′ikəl), *n* a film.

pellicle, brown, *n* a specific name for a brownish-gray to black film formed over time on the surfaces of the teeth as a result of not using an abrasive-containing dentifrice.

pellicle, salivary, *n* a thin, naturally occurring abacterial film from salivary proteins that regularly forms on teeth and other surfaces in the oral cavity, such as restorations or dentures. It may be brushed away, but it will reform within minutes. This serves as a base for plaque formation. Also called *acquired pellicle* or *organic dental pellicle.* See also plaque.

pelvis (pel′vis), *n* the lower portion of the trunk of the body, composed of four bones, the two innominate bones laterally and ventrally and the sacrum and coccyx posteriorly.

pemoline (pem′əlēn), *n brand name:* Cylert; *drug class:* central nervous system stimulant; Controlled Substance Schedule IV; *action:* exact mechanism unknown; may act through dopaminergic mechanisms; *use:* attention deficit disorder with hyperactivity.

pemphigoid, benign mucous membrane (pem′figoid), *n* a bullous disease that resembles pemphigus but is more chronic in nature. The oral mucosa, especially the gingiva where it resembles desquamative gingivitis, and conjunctiva are the sites of predilection. Skin is involved in approximately 20% of the cases.

pemphigus (pem′figus, pem-fī′gus), *n* a rare, serious skin disease of unknown cause characterized by the development of bullae on the skin and mucous membrane. See also bulla and sign, Nikolsky's.

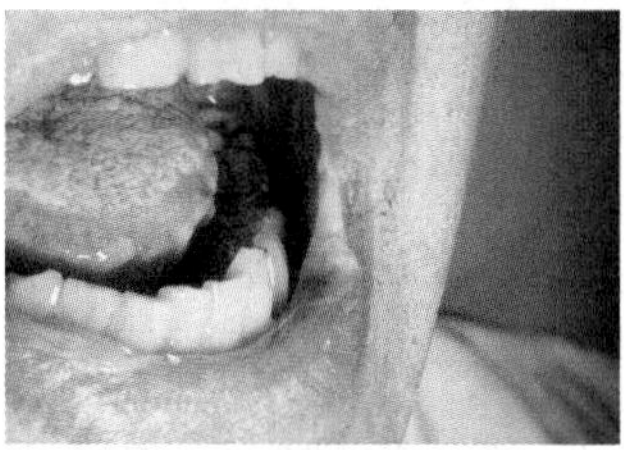

Pemphigus. (Courtesy Dr. Charles Babbush)

pemphigus, acute disseminated, *n* a serious disease of unknown cause, temporarily controlled by the administration of corticosteroids. Manifested by bullous formation on the skin and mucous membranes. Desquamation of the epithelium exposes a raw, burning, oozing submucosa. Adequate nutritional status is difficult to maintain; secondary infection is common; with progressive debility, pneumonia is common and is usually the cause of death.

pen grasp, *n* See grasp, pen.

penbutolol (penbū'təlôl), *n brand name:* Levatol; *drug class:* nonselective β-adrenergic blocker; *action:* competitively blocks stimulation of β-adrenergic receptors within the heart and decreases renin activity, all of which may play a role in reducing systolic and diastolic blood pressure; inhibits β_2 receptors in the bronchial system; *uses:* hypertension alone or with thiazide diuretics.

penetrability (pen'ətrəbil'itē), *n* the ability of an x-ray beam to pass through matter. The degree of penetrability is determined by kilovoltage and filtration.

penetration (pen'ətrā'shən), *n* the ability of radiation to extend down into and go through substances. The degree of penetration is determined by the kilovoltage.

penetrometer (pen'ətrom'ətur), *n* an aluminum step wedge or ladder exposed over a film to determine the quality or penetrating ability of a specific beam of x-radiation.

penicillin (pen'isil'in), *n* an antibiotic secured from cultures of *P. notatum,* being bactericidal for gram-positive cocci, some gram-negative cocci (gonococcus and meningococcus), and clostridial and spirochetal organisms. Its topical application to the oral mucusa membranes is discouraged because of the high risk of sensitization from local application of antibiotic substances.

penicillin G, *n* an acid-sensitive form of penicillin prepared as penicillin G benzathine and penicillin G procaine used for deep intramuscular administration. It is slowly released, resulting in prolonged effective blood levels. In past dentistry, it was used prophylactically for patients predisposed to bacterial endocarditis prior to any invasive dental procedure. Now it has been replaced by amoxicillin. It has a high allergy potential. See also penicillin G benzathine.

penicillin G benzathine, *n brand names:* Bicillin L-A, Permapen; *drug class:* benzathine salt of natural penicillin; *action:* interferes with cell wall replication of susceptible organisms; osmotically unstable cell wall swells and bursts from osmotic pressure; *uses:* respiratory infections, scarlet fever, erysipelas, otitis media, pneumonia, skin and soft tissue infections, and yaws.

penicillin V potassium/penicillin V, *n brand names:* Beepen-VK, Betapen-VK, V-Cillin K, Veetids, others; *drug class:* semisynthetic penicillin; *action:* interferes with cell wall replication of susceptible organisms; the cell wall, rendered osmotically unstable, swells and bursts from osmotic pressure; *uses:* effective for both gram-positive cocci and gram-negative bacilli.

pension plans, *n.pl* saving and investment programs designed to provide income at the time of retirement. These may be employer- or individual-based, in which portions of the funds may be protected from taxation at the time of earning but subject to taxation at the time of withdrawal.

pentaerythritol tetranitrate (pent'əerith'ritôl), *n brand names:* Duotrate, Pentylan, Peritrate, others; *drug class:* antianginal, organic nitrate; *action:* decreases preload, afterload, which is responsible for decreasing left ventricular end-diastolic pressure, systemic vascular resistance, arterial and venous dilation; *uses:* chronic stable angina pectoris, prophylaxis of angina pain.

pentamidine/pentamidine isethionate (pentam'idēn), *n brand names:* NebuPent, Pentam 300, others; *drug class:* antiprotozoal; *action:* interferes with deoxyribonucleic acid/ribonucleic acid synthesis in protozoa; *use: P. jiroveci* infections in immunocompromised patients.

pentazocine HCl/pentazocine lactate (pentaz'ōsēn), *n brand names:* Talwin, Talwin NX; *drug class:* synthetic opioid/mixed agonist/antagonist, Controlled Substance Schedule IV; *action:* interacts with opioid receptors in the central nervous system to alter pain perception; *uses:* moderate to severe pain alone or in combination with aspirin or acetaminophen.

pentobarbital/pentobarbital sodium, *n brand name:* Nembutal Sodium; *drug class:* sedative/hypnotic barbiturate, Controlled Substance

Schedule II; *action:* depresses activity in brain cells, primarily in reticular activating system of brain stem; *uses:* insomnia, sedation, preoperative medication. Useful as a preoperative sedative in dentistry.

pentoxifylline (pen′toksif′əlēn′), *n brand name:* Trental; *drug class:* hemorrheologic agent; *action:* decreased blood viscosity, stimulates prostacyclin formation, increases blood flow by increasing flexibility of red blood cells (RBCs), decreased RBC hyperaggregation, reduces platelet aggregation, decreases fibrinogen concentration; *uses:* intermittent claudication related to chronic occlusive vascular disease.

penumbra, geometric (pən-um′brə), *n* a partial or imperfect shadow about the umbra, or true shadow, of an object. In radiography, it is influenced by the size of the focal spot, focal-film distance, and object-film distance. See also geometric unsharpness.

peptic ulcer (pep′tik), *n* See ulcer, peptic.

peptide, *n* a compound of two or more amino acids in which the α-carboxyl group of one is united with the α-amino group of another, with the elimination of a molecule of water, creating a peptide bond —CO—NH—.

***Peptostreptococcus* (pep′tōstrep′tōko′kəs),** *n* a genus of nonmotile, anaerobic, chemoorganotrophic bacteria found in the oral cavity and intestinal tracts of normal humans. They may be pathogenic and may be found in pyogenic infections, putrefactive war wounds, and appendicitis.

percentile, *n* the number in a frequency distribution below which a certain percentage of fees will fall. E.g., the ninetieth percentile is the number that divides the distribution of fees into the lower 90% and the upper 10%, or that fee level at which 90% of dental professionals charge that amount or less and 10% charge more.

perception, occlusal, *n* the patient's cognizance of occlusal patterns and disharmonies, mediated by the proprioceptive sense of the nerve fibers of the periodontal ligament.

Percocet, *n.pr* the brand name for a narcotic analgesic containing a combination of acetaminophen and oxycodone. Prescribed for moderate to severe pain relief.

Percodan, *n.pr* a brand name for the combination of aspirin and oxycodone, a semisynthetic narcotic analgesic. It is a controlled substance.

percolation, *n* an extraction of the soluble parts of a drug by causing a liquid solvent to flow slowly through it.

percussion (perkush′ən), *n* the act of striking an area, a structure, or an organ as an aid in diagnosing a diseased condition by the sensations reported by the patient and by the sounds heard by the examiner.

percutaneous inoculation (pur′kūtā′nēus), *n* an inoculation accomplished by introducing microorganisms to a patient via a needle or through previously broken skin, such as a cut or burn.

percutaneous route (pur′kūtā′nē-us), *n* a path of entry via the skin.

perforation, palatal (pur′fôr-ā′shən), *n* a perforation that exists in the palatal area after the surgical repair of a cleft.

perforation, radicular, *n* an artificial opening made by boring or cutting through the lateral aspect of the root; also occurs as the result of internal or external resorption.

perforation, sublabial, *n* a perforation existing in the maxillary labial sulcus after surgical repair of the area. The perforation communicates between the oral and nasal cavities.

performance, *n* fulfillment of a promise, contract, or other obligation.

perfringens poisoning (perfrin′jəns), *n* an infection of the gastrointestinal tract caused by the bacterium *C. perfringens,* which is usually self-limiting. Symptoms include nausea, vomiting, and diarrhea.

perfusion (pərfūzhən), *n* a therapeutic measure whereby a drug intended for an isolated part of the body is introduced via the bloodstream.

periadenitis mucosa necrotica recurrens (PMNR) (per′ēad′ənī′tis), *n* involvement of the oral mucosa with deep-seated aphthouslike ulcers that tend to heal with scars. It may be impossible to differentiate the disease from Behçet's syndrome in the absence of a diagnosis of cyclic neutropenia. Also called *recurrent scarring aphtha, Sutton's disease, major aphthous.* See also disease, Miculicz'.

perialveolar wiring, See wiring, perialveolar.

periapex (per′ēā′peks), *n* the area of tissue that immediately surrounds the root apex.

periapical (per′ēā′pikəl), *adj* enclosing or surrounding the apical area of a tooth root.

periapical abscess, n an acute or chronic inflammation of the periapical tissues characterized by a localized accumulation of suppuration at the apex of a tooth. It is generally a sequela of pulp death of the tooth.

periapical granuloma, n an accumulation of mononuclear inflammatory cells with an encircling aggregation of fibroblasts and collagen at the apex of the root of a tooth caused by chronic inflammation. Also called *chronic apical periodontitis.*

periapical radiograph (PA), n a radiograph that includes the tooth apices and surrounding periodontium in a particular intraoral area.

periapical radiographic survey, n a complete series of intraoral radiographs that include the periapical portions of the tooth and its periodontium.

periapical tissue, n the tissue located at the root end of a tooth. Usually consists of the connective tissue forming an attachment between the root and the alveolar bone.

periauricular (per′ēôrik′ūlur), *adj* surrounding the external ear.

pericarditis (per′ikärdī′tis), *n* an inflammation of the pericardium associated with trauma, malignant neoplastic disease, infection, uremia, myocardial infarction, collagen disease, or idiopathic causes.

pericardium (per′ikärdēəm), *n* a fibroserous sac that surrounds the heart and the roots of the great vessels.

pericementitis (per′ēsē′mentī′tis), *n* See periodontitis.

pericoronitis (per′ēkôr′ənī′tis), *n* inflammation of the operculum or tissue flap over a partially erupted tooth, particularly a third molar. Inflammation around a crown, particularly the inflammation of a partially erupted tooth.

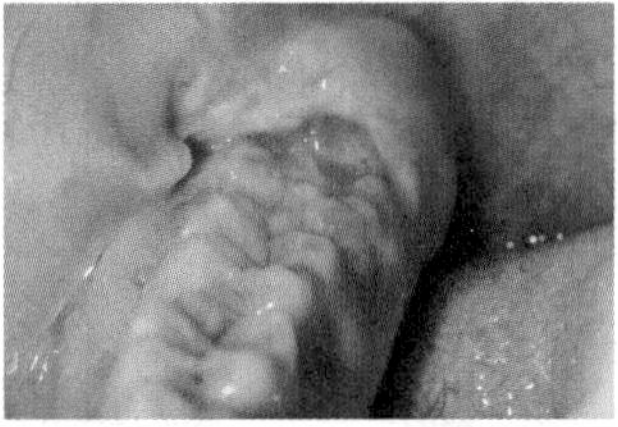

Pericoronitis. (Neville/Damm/Allen/Bouquot, 2002)

periimplant recession, *n* See recession, periimplant.

periimplant space, *n* the space between an implant and its investing tissues.

periimplantitis (per′ēim′plantī′tis), *n* an inflammation in and around the area of a dental implant that may also affect abutment areas.

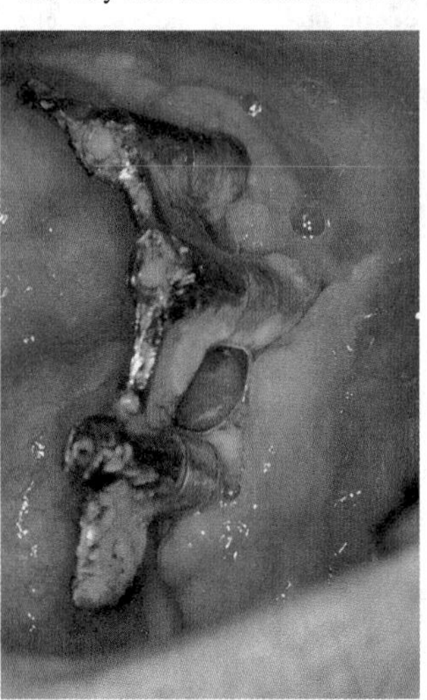

Periimplantitis. (Courtesy Dr. Charles Babbush)

perikymata (per″ĭki′mətə), *n* the wavy ridges on the surface of a permanent tooth, which signify overlaps in the enamel structure and that may disappear as the enamel wears over time.

perimenopause, *n* the premenopausal period of approximately 3 to 6 years during which menstrual cycles become erratic and estrogen levels fall, ending with the cessation of menstruation. See also menopause.

perimolysis (per′imol′isis), *n* erosion of tooth enamel by chemical means as a result of repeated vomiting; seen in those with eating disorders or chronic regurgitation.

perinatal, *adj* related to the time surrounding the birth process.

period, latent (lā′tənt), *n* the area of delay between the time of exposure of an organism to radiation and the manifestation of the changes produced by that radiation. This delay depends on many factors but particularly on the magnitude of the dose. The larger the dose, the earlier the appearance of the injury. In some instances the latent period for some effects may be as long as 25 years or more.

periodicity, *n* events that tend to repeat at predictable intervals.

periodontal (per′ēōdon′təl), *adj* relating to the periodontium.

periodontal abscess, n a localized area of acute or chronic inflammation found in the gingival tissues, infrabony pockets, or periodontal ligament. If it is located at the apex of the tooth, it is known as a *periapical abscess.* If located between the apex and the alveolar crest, it is known as a *lateral abscess.*

periodontal atrophy, n See atrophy, periodontal.

periodontal attachment loss, n a reduction in the connective tissue attaching the root of the tooth to the alveolar bone, usually caused by persistent inflammation of the gingival and periodontal tissues.

periodontal disease, n a group of inflammatory and infectious diseases affecting the periodontium of the teeth, with various classes noted.

periodontal disease, aggressive, n marked by the early onset of periodontal disease that affects the gingiva and periodontal tissues. If untreated, it may result in loss of teeth.

periodontal dressing, n a protective obtundent covering of the gingival and periodontal tissues used after periodontal surgery.

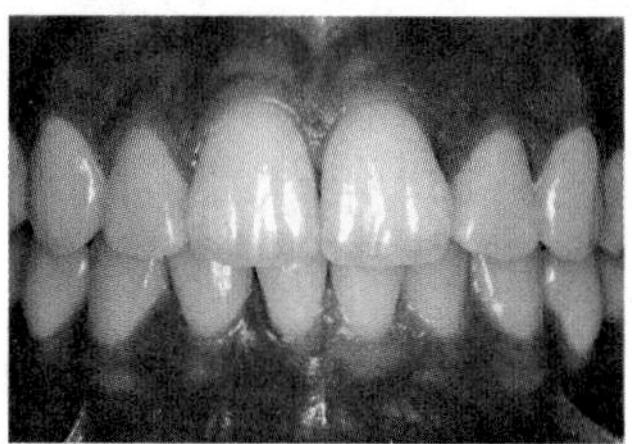

Aggressive periodontal disease. (Newman/Takei/Klokkevold/Carranza, 2006)

periodontal index, n a method for rating or ranking the severity of periodontal disease. An early index was the PMA, which ranked the number of *p*apillary, *m*arginal, and *a*ttached gingiva affected by gingivitis. A more contemporary index is the Russell Periodontal Index (PI), which is based on a 0-to-8 score system: from negative to advanced destruction.

periodontal ligament, n a system of collagenous connective tissue fibers that attaches the root of a tooth to its alveolus of bone by way of Sharpey's fibers. It contains blood vessels, lymph vessels, and nerves. The ligament consists of five groups of fibers: interdental, alveolar crestal, horizontal, oblique, and apical and possibly interradicular fibers if the tooth is multirooted.

periodontal pack, n See pack, periodontal.

periodontal pocket, n See pocket, periodontal.

periodontal probe, n See probe, periodontal.

periodontal prosthesis, n See prosthesis, periodontal.

Periodontal Screening and Recording (PSR), *n.pr* a proprietary method of briefly examining all of a patient's teeth, and recording the highest score in each of six regions of the oral cavity (mid-, mesio-, and distofacial and corresponding lingual areas). The process utilizes a blunt-tipped probe instrument and is intended to take only 2 to 3 minutes.

periodontal therapy, n See therapy, periodontal.

periodontal treatment planning, n the sequential arrangement of therapeutic procedures required to obtain a healthy periodontium.

periodontal surgery (per′ēōdon′təl), *n* an operative procedure used to treat disease or repair abnormalities in the periodontium and associated teeth. See also surgery.

periodontia (per′ēōdon′shēə), *n* See periodontics.

periodontics (per′ēōdon′tiks), *n* the art and science of examination, diagnosis, and treatment of diseases affecting the periodontium; a study of the supporting structures of the teeth, including not only the normal anatomy and physiology of these structures but also the deviations from normal.

periodontics, concept of cure in, *n* the idea that a successful result in periodontal therapy consists of restoring any tooth or collection of teeth to functional capability, regardless of whether they are able to function alone or require stabilization to survive.

periodontitis (per′ēōdontī′tis), *n* **1.** the alterations occurring in the periodontium with inflammation. Gingival changes are those of gingivitis, with the clinical signs associated with gingivitis. It has histologic characteristics, such as ulceration of the sulcular and junctional epithelium, epithelial hyperplasia, proliferation of epithelial rete pegs into the gingival tissues, apical migration of the epithelial attachment after lysis of the gingival fibers, increased cellular and exudative infiltrate, and vascularity of the lamina propria. Resorption of bone in an apical direction results in the loss of attachment of the periodontal fibers to the bone. A transseptal band of reconstituted periodontal fibers (interdental) walls off the gingival inflammation from the underlying bone. *n* **2.** a chronic, progressive disease of the periodontium. Considered under the classification of periodontal disease.

periodontitis, acute, *n* a sharply localized, acute inflammatory process involving the interproximal and marginal areas of two or more adjacent teeth, characterized by severe pain, purulent exudate from edematous inflamed gingivae, general malaise, fever, and sequestration of the crestal aspects of the alveolar process. It is now considered a stage of periodontal disease.

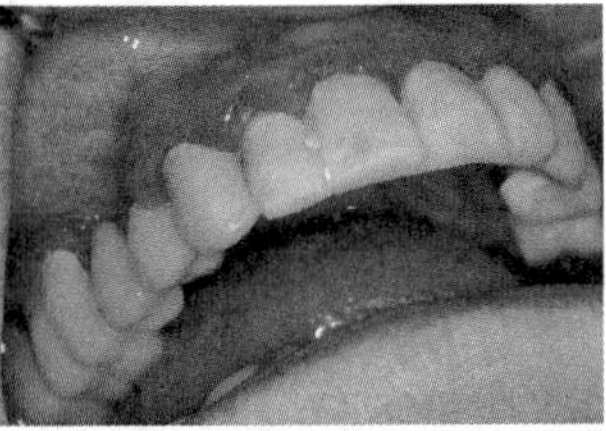

Periodontitis. (Courtesy Dr. Charles Babbush)

periodontitis, aggressive, *n* a periodontal disease that manifests before age 35. It causes rapid loss of the periodontium and does not respond easily to periodontal treatment. Now juvenile, early-onset, and refractory forms of periodontitis are considered under this classification of periodontal disease. See also periodontitis, juvenile and periodontitis, early-onset (EOP).

periodontitis, chronic periapical, *n* a periapical inflammation characterized by dental granuloma formation.

periodontitis, early-onset (EOP), *n* a periodontal disease affecting children which, if left untreated, may cause premature tooth loss. Used to be considered *prepubertal periodontitis* and is now considered under the classification of *aggressive periodontal disease.*

periodontitis in children, *n* See periodontitis, juvenile.

periodontitis, juvenile, *n* a periodontal disease present in children or adolescents, with radiographic and clinical findings similar to those observed in the adult, including gingivitis, periodontal pocket formation, and bone resorption but only in specific areas *(localized)* or throughout the oral cavity *(generalized).* Used to be called *periodontosis,* which is outdated, and now is considered under the classification of *aggressive periodontal disease.*

periodontitis, marginal, *n* the sequela to gingivitis in which the inflammatory process has spread apically to involve the alveolar process. It involves an inflammation of the marginal periodontium with resorption of the crest of alveolar bone. Apical migration of the epithelial attachment occurs with suprabony or infrabony pocket formation and cuplike resorptions and marginal translucence of the alveolar crest. In children the process may be more rapid and destructive than in adults. It is now considered a stage of periodontal disease.

***periodontitis, refractory* (per′ē-ōdontī′tis),** *n* a type of aggressive periodontal disease that persists despite proper treatment and oral hygiene. Previously classified as a separate form of periodontitis, it is now generally not considered to be a separate form of the disease but simply normal periodontitis that is exacerbated by numerous factors in the patient's history and physiology. See also periodontitis.

periodontium (per′ēōdon′shēum), *n* the tissues that support the teeth, which include the gingivae, cementum of the tooth, periodontal ligament, and alveolar bone).

periodontology, *n* See periodontics.

periodontometer (per′ēōdon-tom′ətur), *n* a device used to measure the amount of tooth movement.

periodontopathic (per″ēōdonto′path′ik), *n* a substance capable of starting diseases in the surrounding tissue and supporting structures of the teeth.

periodontosis (per′ēōdontō′sis), *n* See periodontitis, aggressive.

perioral structures (per′ēôr′əl), *n.pl* the anatomy around the oral cavity, generally the lips and muscles of facial expression within the lips.

periorbital (per′ēôr′bitəl), *adj* surrounding the eyes. The periorbital soft tissues are easily contused and produce marked inflammatory responses to trauma.

periosteal elevator (per′ē-os′tēəl), *n* See elevator, periosteal.

periosteum (per′ēos′tēum), *n* the layer of connective tissue that varies considerably in thickness in the different areas of bone. It consists of two layers: an outer layer, which is rich in blood vessels and nerves and shows a dense arrangement of collagenous fibers, and an inner layer, the cambium, in which the fibers are loosely arranged, the cells numerous, and the blood vessels relatively sparse. During active growth, this layer of osteoblasts covers the periosteal surface of the bone. In the quiescent state in the adult, the periosteum primarily provides support. However, the inner layer retains its osteogenetic potencies and in fractures is activated to form osteoblasts and new bone.

periostitis (per′ēostī′tis), *n* an inflammation of the periosteum in which it can become detached from the underlying bone, resulting from exudates produced by inflammation or infection.

Periotest (per′iōtest), *n* a commercial device designed to measure periodontal reaction to specific loads on the tooth crown.

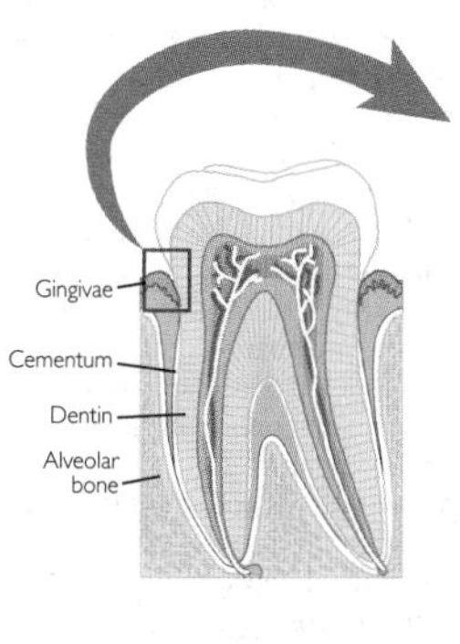

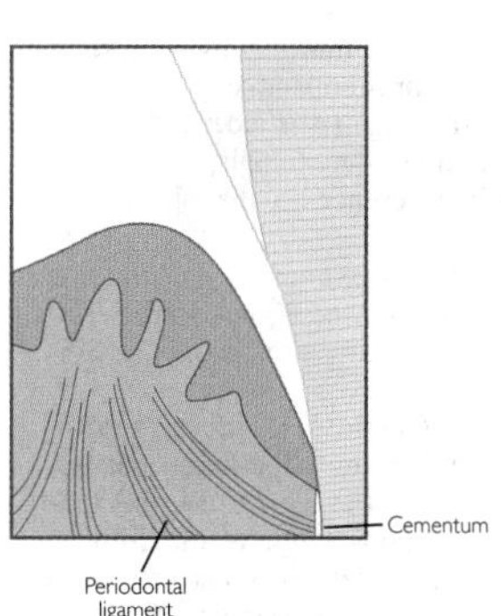

Structures of the periodontium. (Bird/Robinson, 2005)

P

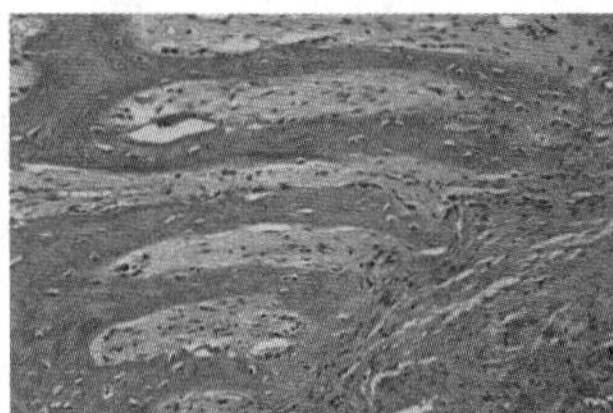

Periostitis. (Neville/Damm/Allen/Bouquot, 2002)

periotome (per′ēətōm′), *n* a dental tool utilized in tooth extraction, particularly in situations requiring the cutting of the periodontal ligament fibers.

peripheral circulation (pərif′ərəl), *n* See circulation, peripheral.

peripheral nervous system, *n* the motor and sensory nerves and ganglia outside the brain and spinal cord.

periphery (pərif′erē), *n* See border, denture.

periradicular (per″īrədik′ulər), *adj* pertaining to the area immediately outside or around the root of the tooth.

peritoneal cavity (per′itənē′əl), *p* the potential space between the parietal and the visceral layers of the peritoneum.

P

peritonitis (per′itənī′tis), *n* an inflammation of the peritoneum produced by bacteria or irritating substances introduced into the abdominal cavity by a penetrating wound or perforation of an organ in the gastrointestinal (GI) tract or the reproductive tract. Peritonitis is caused most commonly by rupture of the vermiform appendix.

peritonsillar (per′iton′silər), *adj* surrounding the tonsils. Generally used in reference to the pharyngeal tonsils.

peritonsillar abscess, *n* an infection of tissue between the tonsil and pharynx, usually after acute tonsillitis.

perlèche (perlesh′), *adj* a general term applied to superficial fissures occurring at the angles of the oral cavity. Lesions may result from a variety of causes but most often can be related to deep labial commissures, with associated drooling, licking of the lips, unhygienic conditions, and overgrowth of bacteria, yeast, or fungi. The term has also been applied to angular cheilosis resulting from riboflavin deficiency but not to the split papule of syphilis or to herpetic lesions.

permeability (pur′mēəbil′itē), *n* the degree to which one substance allows another substance to pass through it.

permissible dose, *n* See dose, maximum permissible.

permucosal extension (purmūkō′səl), *n* a dental implant that attaches to the body of the implant, which is anchored in the jaw, and rises above the marginal gingival tissues. These tissues are allowed to heal around the permucosal extension, which then provides access to the implant.

permucosal (biologic) seal, *n* permucosal tissue present between a dental implant and the soft tissue, the function of which is to prevent bacteria and inflammatory agents from entering the tissues.

permucosal route, *n* a path of entry via the mucous membranes.

peroral, *adj* through or about the oral cavity.

peroxidase horseradish, *n* an enzyme used in immunohistochemistry to label the antigen-antibody complex.

peroxidases, *n.pl* the hydrogen peroxide–reducing enzymes, occurring in animal and plant tissues, that catalyze the dehydrogenation (oxidation) of various substances in the presence of hydrogen peroxide.

peroxide, *n* See hydrogen peroxide.

perphenazine (pərfen′əzēn′), *n* *brand name:* Trilafon; *drug class:* phenothiazine antipsychotic; *action:* blocks neurotransmission at dopaminergic synapses in the cerebral cortex, hypothalamus, and limbic system; mechanism for antipsychotic effects unclear; *uses:* psychotic disorders, schizophrenia, alcoholism, nausea, vomiting.

personal, *adj* belonging to an individual; limited to the person; having the nature of the qualities of humans or of movable property.

personal representative, *n* a person designated to make health care decisions on another person's behalf. See also guardian.

personal supervision, *n* the supervision necessary for certain procedures in which the dental professional, while personally giving treatment to a patient, requires the dental staff to perform a supplementary or supportive procedure simultaneously.

personality, *n* **1.** the sum total of a patient's ideas, emotions, and behavior, including the rational and irrational, the conscious and unconscious, and the defensive and learned behavior patterns. It develops from both genetic factors and environmental factors. Thus the patient brings to a dental office an individual personality syndrome. It may be a well-adjusted, stable personality; a depressed, anxious, neurotic personality; or a manic, schizophrenic, psychotic personality. Patients have a broad spectrum of healthy and disordered personalities. *n* **2.** the characteristics of a person by which other people evaluate him or her.

personality assessment, *n* See personality test.

personality disorder, *n* a disruption in relatedness manifested in any of a large group of mental disorders characterized by rigid, inflexible, and maladaptive behavior patterns that impair a person's ability to function in society.

personality test, *n* a standardized test used in the evaluation of various facets of personality structure, emotional status, and behavioral traits.

personnel, *n* the persons employed in an enterprise. In dentistry, it refers to the staff employed.

personnel monitoring, *n* See monitoring, personnel.

pertussis (purtus′is), *n* a disease caused by *B. pertussis* in which the patient suffers from a cough that makes a "whooping" sound. Also called *whooping cough.*

pervasive, *adj* indicates that a condition permeates the entire development of the individual.

pesticide poisoning, *n* a toxic condition caused by the ingestion or inhalation of a substance used for the eradication of insects, fungi, and other pests.

petazocine (pet′əzō′sēn), *n* an analgesic approximately equivalent in analgesic effect to codeine; *brand name:* Talwin.

petechiae (pətē′kēā), *n.pl* a condition in which capillary hemorrhages produce small red or purplish pinpoint discolorations of the mucous membrane and skin. Petechiae are typical of blood dyscrasias, vitamin C deficiency, positive Rumpel-Leede test, liver disease, and bacterial endocarditis. Palatal lesions are noted in mononucleosis.

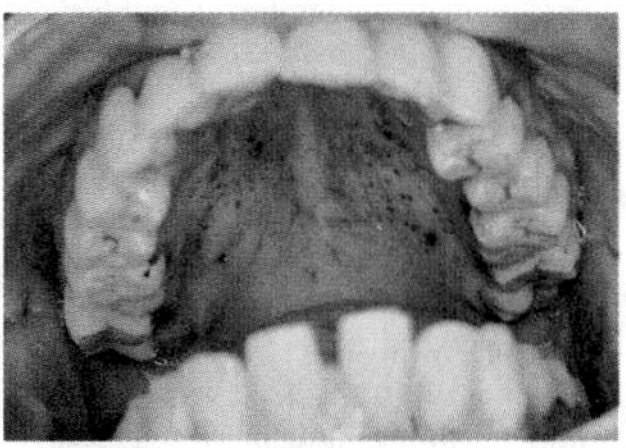

Petechiae. (Regezi/Sciubba/Jordan, 2008)

petri plate, *n* a shallow dish with a loose cover that is used in the laboratory for growing microorganisms.

petrolatum (pet′rəlā′tum), *n* a mixture of hydrocarbons obtained from petroleum. No longer used in the oral cavity because it does not work well with oral fluids and latex gloves.

Peutz-Jeghers syndrome (poits′-jeg′urz), *n.pr* See syndrome, Peutz-Jeghers.

pH, *n* the concentration of hydrogen ions expressed as the negative logarithm of base 10. A neutral solution (hydrogen ion activity equals hydroxide ion activity) has a pH of approximately 7. Aqueous solutions with pH values lower than 7 are considered acidic, whereas pH values higher than 7 are considered basic.

pH, critical, *n* the point at which the minerals in a substance begin to decrease. For enamel, critical pH is between 4.5 and 5.5 moles/L; radical (root) critical pH is 6.0 to 6.7 moles/L.

phagocyte (fag′əsīt), *n* a cell that ingests microorganisms, cells, or other substances.

phagocytosis (fag′əsītō′sis), *n* the engulfing of microorganisms, cells, and other substances by phagocytes. See also phagocyte.

phantom (fan′tum), *n* a device that absorbs and scatters x-radiation in approximately the same way as the tissues of the body.

pharmacist, *n* a person prepared to formulate and dispense drugs or medications through completion of an accredited university program in pharmacy. Licensure is required upon completion of the program and prior to serving the public as a pharmacist.

pharmacodynamics (fär′məkōdīnam′iks), *n* the science of drug action.

pharmacology (fär′məkol′əjē), *n* the total science of drugs, including their use in therapeutics.

pharmocokinetics (fâr′məkōkənet′iks), *n* a subdiscipline within pharmacology that studies how a body reacts to the presence of a drug, nutrient, or other foreign compound over the course of its introduction to its final elimination from the body.

pharmacotherapy (fär′məkōther′əpē), *n* treatment based on the use of drugs or pharmaceuticals.

pharmacy (fär′məsē), *n* **1.** the art and science of preparing and dispensing drugs. *n* **2.** place where drugs are dispensed.

pharyngeal (fərin′jēəl), *adj* related to or originating in the pharynx.

pharyngeal arch (fərin′jēəl), *n* See branchial arch.

pharyngeal flap, *n* a pedicle flap usually raised on the posterior pharyngeal wall and attached to the soft palate to reduce the size of the velopharyngeal gap.

pharyngeal pouches, *n.pl* the four pairs of evaginations from the lateral walls lining the pharynx between the branchial arches in a developing embryo.

pharyngitis (fer′injī′tis), *n* inflammation of the pharynx.

pharyngitis, gonococcal, n a throat infection caused by the same infectious microorganism that causes gonorrhea; spread by direct contact with an infected person or with fluids containing the infectious agent.

pharyngoplasty (fəring′gōplastē), *n* reconstructive operation to alter the size and shape of the nasopharyngeal opening.

pharyngospasm (fəring′gōspazəm), *n* spasm of the pharyngeal muscles.

pharyngotomy, *n* a cutting operation upon the pharynx, either from without or from within.

pharynx (fer′inks), *n* a funnel-shaped tube of muscle tissue between the oral cavity and nares and the esophagus, which is the common pathway for food and air. The nasopharynx lies above the level of the soft palate. The oropharynx lies between the superior edge of the epiglottis and the soft palate, whereas the laryngopharynx extends from the superior edge of the epiglottis to the superior end of the esophagus behind the larynx.

pharynx, activities of posterior and lateral pharyngeal wall, n.pl the bulging of the posterior and lateral pharyngeal wall produced by the superior pharyngeal constrictors and palatopharyngeus during the acts of swallowing and phonation; seen in individuals with a congenitally short soft palate, operated soft palate, or unoperated cleft of the soft palate. These activities are rarely present in the individual with the normal soft palate.

pharynx, implant surgical, n first stage: a major oral operation in which the mucoperiosteum is elevated, exposing the oral surface of the jawbone; the surgical jaw relations are established, and an impression is made of the exposed bone surfaces. Second stage: a major oral surgical operation in which the mucoperiosteum is reelevated, the prepared implant is placed on the bone surface, and the mucoperiosteum is coapted and sutured about the posts of the protruding implant abutments.

phase-contrast microscope, *n* a microscope with a special condenser and objective, which contains a phase-shifting ring by which small differences in the index of refraction become visible. The use of phase-contrast capabilities allows for direct viewing of transparent live cells and tissues. Phase-contrast microscopes are useful in educating patients about the oral flora associated with dental plaque and caries and periodontal disease.

phenacetin, caffeine, aspirin (fenas′ətin), *n* See aspirin, phenacetin, caffeine.

phenazopyridine HCl (fen′əzōpir′idēn), *n brand names:* Azo-Standard, Baridium, Eridium, Pyridiate, Urogesic, others; *drug class:* urinary tract analgesic; *action:* exerts analgesic anesthetic action on the urinary tract mucosa; exact mechanism of action is unknown; *use:* urinary tract irritation/infection.

phencyclidine (fensī′klidēn′), *n* an approved veterinary anesthetic. Illicitly, it is used as a hallucinogen. Also called *PCP, hog,* or *peace pill.*

phendimetrazine tartrate (fen′dīmet′rəzēn′ tar′trāt), *n brand names:* Adipost, Anorex SR, Appecon, Obalan, others; *drug class:* anorexiant, amphetamine-like Controlled Substance Schedule III; *action:* exact mechanism of action of appetite suppression is unknown but may have an effect on the satiety center of the hypothalamus; *use:* exogenous obesity.

phenelzine sulfate (fen′əlzēn′ sul′-fāt), *brand name:* Nardil; *drug class:* antidepressant, monoamine antioxidase inhibitor; *action:* increases concentrations of endogenuous epinephrine, norepinephrine, serotonin, dopamine in storage sites in central nervous system; *use:* depression when uncontrolled by other means.

phenobarbital/phenobarbital sodium (fē′nōbar′bitol′), *n brand names:* Ancalixor, Barbita, Luminal Sodium, Solfoton; *drug class:* barbiturate, anticonvulsant, Controlled Substance Schedule IV; *action:* a nonspecific depressant of the central nervous system; may enhance γ aminobutyric acid activity in the brain; *uses:* all forms of epilepsy, status epilepticus, febrile seizures in children, sedation, insomnia.

phenol (fē′nôl), *n* an organic compound in which one or more hydroxyl groups are attached to a carbon atom in an aromatic ring that contains conjugated double bonds.

phenol coefficient, *n* a basis of comparison in determining the relative effectiveness of antiseptics. Phenol is the standard for comparison with other agents for their ability to kill a well-dispersed suspension of *Salmonella* or *Staphylococcus.* It has little practical value.

phenolic, synthetic (sinthet′ik), *n* a form of a chemical agent used as a surface disinfectant that kills a wide range of microbes. It provides a residual level of treatment after initial application.

phenotype (fē′nōtīp), *n* term referring to the expression of genotypes that can be directly distinguished (e.g., by clinical observation of external appearance or serologic tests).

phenoxybenzamine HCl (fenok′sēben′zəmēn′), *n brand name:* Dibenzyline; *drug class:* antihypertensive; *action:* α-adrenergic blocker that binds to α-adrenergic receptors, dilating peripheral blood vessels; lowers peripheral resistance, lowers blood pressure; *use:* hypertensive episodes associated with pheochromocytoma.

phenprocoumon (fenprō′koomən), *n* a long-acting, orally effective anticoagulant.

phensuximide (fensuk′simīd′), *n brand name:* Milontin; *drug class:* anticonvulsant, succinimide; *action:* suppresses spike wave formation in absence seizures (petit mal); decreases amplitude, frequency, duration, spread of discharge in minor motor seizures; *use:* absence (petit mal) seizures.

phentermine HCl/phentermine resin (fen′tərmēn′ rez′in), *n brand name:* Adipex-P, Fastin, Ionamin, Obe-Mar, Panshape M, T-Diet, others; *drug class:* sympathomimetic, anorexiant, Controlled Substance Schedule IV; *action:* exact mechanism of action of appetite suppression unknown but may have an effect on satiety center of hypothalamus; *use:* exogenous obesity.

phentolamine mesylate (fentol′əmēn′ mes′ilāt′), *n brand name:* Regitine; *drug class:* antihypertensive; *action:* α-adrenergic blocker; binds to α-adrenergic receptors, dilating peripheral blood vessels, lowering peripheral resistance, lowering blood pressure; *uses:* hypertension, pheochromocytoma, prevention and treatment of dermal necrosis following extravasation of norepinephrine or dopamine.

phenylalanine (fen′ilal′ənēn), *n* one of the essential amino acids. See also amino acid.

phenylephrine HCl (fen′ilef′rin), *n brand names:* Neo-Synephrine, Vick's Sinex, others; *drug class:* nasal decongestant, sympathomimetic; *action:* produces rapid and long-acting vasoconstriction of arterioles; *use:* temporary relief of nasal congestion.

phenylketonuria (PKU) (fen′il-kē′tōnyoo′rēə), *n* a condition in which metabolism is severely compromised because of the absence of a phenylaline-processing enzyme resulting in mental retardation, although a prescribed diet can minimize its severity.

phenytoin sodium/phenytoin sodium extended/phenytoin sodium prompt (fen′itō′in sō′dēəm), *n brand names:* Dilantin, Diphenylan, Phenytex, others; *drug class:* hydantoin anticonvulsant; *action:* inhibits spread of seizure activity in motor cortex; *uses:* generalized tonic-clonic (grand mal) seizures, status epilepticus, nonepileptic seizures, trigeminal neuralgia, cardiac dysrhythmias caused by digitalis-type drugs.

P

pheochromocytoma (fē′ōkrō′mōsītō′mə), *n* a vascular tumor of chromaffin tissue of the adrenal medulla or sympathetic paraganglia, characterized by hypersecretion of epinephrine and norepinephrine, causing persistent or intermittent hypertension.

PHI, *n* See health information, protected.

philtrum (fil′trəm), *n* the vertical groove in the midline of the upper lip, extending downward from the nasal septum to the tubercle of the upper lip.

phlebectasia (fleb′ektā′zēə), *n* dilation of a vein.

phlebitis (fləbī′tis), *n* inflammation of a vein. See also thrombophlebitis.

phlebolith (fleb′ōlith), *n* a calcified thrombus in a vein.

phlegmon (fleg′mon), *n* **1.** an intense inflammation spreading through tissue spaces over a large area and without definite limits. *n* **2.** clinically, a hard, boardlike swelling without gross suppuration. See also cellulitis.

phobia (fō′bēə), *n* a specific hysterical fear.

phobia, social, *n* an anxiety disorder in which a person is afraid of social situations for fear of being judged unworthy by others.

phonation (fōnā′shən), *n* the production of voiced sound by means of vocal cord vibrations.

phonation, speech, *n* modification by the vocal folds of the airstream as it leaves the lungs and passes through the larynx, for the purpose of producing the various sounds that are the basis of speech. By opposing each other with different degrees of tension and space, the vocal folds create a slitlike aperture of varying size and contour; and by creating resistance to the stream of air, they set up a sequence of laryngeal sound waves with characteristic pitch and intensity.

phoneme (fō′nēm), *n* a group or family of closely related speech sounds, all of which have the same distinctive acoustic characteristics despite their differences; often used in place of the term *speech sound.*

phonetic values, *n.pl* See values, phonetic.

phonetics (fōnet′iks), *n* the study of the production and perception of speech sounds, including individual and group variations and their use in speech.

phosphatase(s) (fos′fətās), *n* a group of enzymes that are distributed throughout most cells and body fluids and are characterized by their ability to hydrolyze a wide variety of monophosphate esters to alcohols and inorganic phosphate.

phosphatase, acid, *n* a group of phosphatases (e.g., serum, liver, prostate) with optimal activity below a pH level of 7. Elevated serum levels have been observed in metastatic breast and prostatic cancer; Paget's, Gaucher's, and Niemann-Pick diseases and in myelocytic leukemia.

phosphatase, alkaline, *n* a group of phosphatases (e.g., serum, liver, bone) whose optimal activity ranges near a pH level of 9.8. Elevated blood levels occur in Paget's disease and pregnancy, whereas low levels are characteristic of dwarfism and a generalized nutritional protein deficiency.

phosphates (fos′fāts), *n.pl* the organic compounds of phosphorus. The blood phosphate level is normally 2.5 mg to 5 mg/100 ml. It is low in rickets and early hyperparathyroidism and high in tetany and nephritis.

phospholipase (fos′fōlip′ās), *n* an enzyme that catalyzes the hydrolysis of a phospholipid.

phospholipase C, n an enzyme removing choline phosphate from a phosphatidylcholine.

phospholipid, *n* a class of compounds, widely distributed in living cells, containing phosphoric acid, fatty acids, and a nitrogenous base.

phosphoprotein, *n* a protein containing phosphoric groups attached to the side chains of some of its amino acids, usually serine, casein, and vitellin.

phosphorescence (fos″fores′əns), *adj* the seeming ability to glow in the dark; occurs in substances that continue to emit light following exposure to and subsequent removal of a radiation source.

phosphoric acid (fosfôr′ik), *n* a clear, colorless, odorless liquid that is irritating to the skin and eyes and moderately toxic, if ingested. It is used in the production of fertilizers, soaps, detergents, animal feeds, and certain drugs.

phosphorus (P) (fos′fərus), *n* a nonmetallic element; atomic weight, 30.98. It is essential, as is the phosphate, for the mineralization of the organic matrix of teeth and bone. It is also essential in the intermediary metabolism of carbohydrates as a vital constituent of the various intermediary compounds (e.g., glucose 6-phosphate) and of the enzyme systems (e.g., adenosine triphosphate [ATP]).

phosphorylation (fos′fərəlā′shən), *n* the addition of phosphate to an organic compound.

phosphotungstic acid (PTA), *n* a mixture of phosphoric and tungstic acids used with hematoxylin for staining muscle tissue and cell nuclei. It is also used as a negative stain of collagen in electron microscopy.

phossy jaw (fos′sē), *n* See poisoning, phosphorus.

phosvitin (fosvī′tən), *n* a phosphated protein with anticoagulant properties that is found in the egg yolk.

photography, *n* the process of making images on a chemically sensitive plate or film, using the energy of light or other radiant source.

photometry, *n* the measurement of the intensity of light, usually in foot-candles.

photon (fō′ton), *n* a bullet or quantum of electromagnetic radiant energy emitted and propagated from various types of radiation sources. The term should not be used alone but should be qualified by terms that will clarify the type of energy (e.g., light photon, radiographic photon).

physical, *adj* relating to the body, as distinguished from the mind.

physical examination, n a diagnostic inspection of the body to determine its state of health, using palpation, auscultation, percussion, and smell.

physical fitness, n the ability to carry out daily tasks with alertness and vigor, without undue fatigue, and with enough energy reserve to meet emergencies or to enjoy leisure time.

physical medicine, n the use of physical therapy techniques to return physically diseased or injured patients to a useful life.

physical plant, n the entire architectural and decorated suite of offices in which the dental professional operates.

physical therapy, n the treatment of disorders with physical agents and methods, such as massage, manipulation, therapeutic exercises, cold, heat (including shortwave, microwave, and ultrasonic diathermy), hydrotherapy, electric stimulation, and light to assist in rehabilitating patients and in restoring normal function after an illness or injury. Also called *physiotherapy.*

physician, *n* a practitioner of medicine; one lawfully engaged in the practice of medicine.

Physicians' Desk Reference (PDR), *n* a comprehensive reference book detailing the composition and accepted applications of pharmaceuticals from major manufacturers. A supplemental edition, which covers the effective use of herbal and botanical products, is available, as well as online subscription and updated CD-ROM versions.

physics, *n* the study of material and energy, particularly as related to motion, force, heat, and light.

physiognomy (fiz'ēog'nəmē), facial features.

physiologic occlusion, *n* See occlusion, physiologic.

physiologic rest position, *n* See position, rest, physiologic.

physiology (fiz'ēol'əjē), *n* the study of tissue and organism behavior. The physiologic process is a dynamic state of tissue as compared with the static state of descriptive morphology (anatomy). Physiology is differentiated from descriptive morphology by the following qualifying properties: rate, direction, and magnitude. Physiologic processes are thus morphologic alterations in the three dimensions of space associated with a temporary (time) sequence. Physiologic processes relate to a wide spectrum of life activities on three levels: biochemical and biophysical activity of a subcellular nature, the activity of cells and tissues aggregated into organ systems, and multiorgan system activity as expressed in human behavior.

physiology, oral, *n* the physiology related to clinical manifestations in the normal and abnormal behavior of oral structures. The principal clinical functions in which the oral structures participate are deglutition, mastication, respiration, speech, and head posture.

P

physioprints (fiz'ēōprints), *n.pl* the photographs obtained by projecting a grid on the subject's face and superimposing two exposures. The resultant picture gives a three-dimensional approach for the diagnosis of facial contours and swelling.

physiotherapy, oral (fiz'ēōther'əpē), *n* older term for the collective procedures properly performed for the maintenance of personal hygiene of the oral cavity; those procedures necessary for cleanliness, tissue stimulation, tone, and preservation of the dentition. See also aid in physiotherapy.

physostigmine (fī'sōstig'mēn), *n* a cholinergic actylcholinesterase inhibitor prescribed in the treatment of some forms of glaucoma and to reverse effects of neuromuscular blocking agents.

phytic acid (fī'tik), *n* a component of some high-fiber foods, including many cereal grains that may, in excessive amounts, cause constipation or interfere with the body's ability to absorb minerals.

phytonadione (fī'tōnədī'ōn), *n* (vitamin K_1) *brand names:* AquaMEPHYTON, Konakion, Mephyton; *drug class:* vitamin K_1, fat-soluble vitamin; *action:* needed for adequate blood clotting (factors II, VII, IX, X); *uses:* vitamin K malabsorption, hypoprothrombinemia, prevention of hypoprothrombinemia caused by oral anticoagulants.

pica (pī'kə), *n* a persistent, pathologic desire to eat nonfood items such as paper or dirt.

Pick's disease, *n.pr* See disease, Niemann-Pick.

pickling, *n* the process of cleansing from metallic surfaces the products of oxidation and other impurities by immersion in acid.

pickup impression, *n* See impression, pickup.

PICO, *n* acronym for diagnostic questions based on these four areas of knowledge and action: **P**atient or problem; **I**ntervention, cause, or prognosis; **C**omparison or control; and **O**utcome. This evidence-based method is designed to make a valid, successful decision based on the skills and knowledge of the clinician, the values of the patient, and the best available evidence.

***Picornaviridae* (pīkôr'nəvir'idā),** *n* one of the major ribonucleic acid virus families, to which the polio-, rhino-, entero-, and hepatitis A viruses belong. Viruses in this family have a single-stranded, nonsegmented, linear molecular structure with icosahedral symmetry.

pier (pir), *n* an intermediate retaining or supporting abutment for a prosthesis. See also abutment.

Pierre Robin syndrome (pyer' rōban'), *n.pr* See retrognathism and syndrome, Pierre Robin.

piezoelectric instruments (pīē'zōəlek'trik), *n.pl* See ultrasonic scalers, magnetostrictive.

pigmentation, gingival, *n* See gingival pigmentation.

pigmentation, melanin (pig′məntā′shən mel′ənin), *n* the discoloration of tissues produced by the deposition of melanin. Seen normally in the oral mucous membranes (especially gingivae) of dark-complexioned individuals and abnormally in such conditions as adrenal hypofunction (Addison's disease).

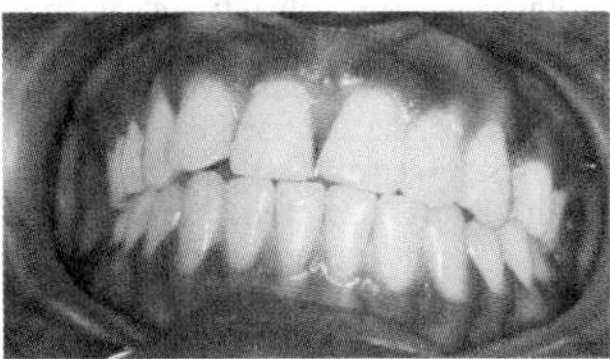

Melanin pigmentation. (Ibsen/Phelan, 2004)

pigtail explorer, *n* See explorer, cowhorn.

pilocarpine (pi″lokahr′pēn), *n* an alkaloid that causes parasympathetic effects (e.g., secretion of salivary, bronchial, and gastrointestinal glands). It stimulates the sweat glands and also causes vasodilation and cardiac inhibition.

pilocarpine HCl/pilocarpine nitrate (optic), *n brand names:* Adsorbocarpine, Akarpine, Isopto Carpine, Pilocar, Liquifilm, others *drug class:* miotic, cholinergicc agonist; *action:* acts directly on cholinergic receptor sites; induces miosis, spasm of accommodation, fall in intraocular pressure; *uses:* primary glaucoma, early stages of wide-angle glaucoma; also used to neutralize mydriatics used during eye examination. Also taken internally for non–drug-induced xerostomia such as Sjögren's syndrome and head and neck cancer patients.

pilot program, *n* an experimental program designed to test administrative and operational procedures and to collect information on service demands and costs that will serve as a basis for operating programs efficiently.

pimozide, *n brand name:* Orap; *drug class:* antipsychotic, antidyskinetic; *action:* blocks dopamine effects on central nervous system; *uses:* motor and phonic tics in Giles de la Tourette's syndrome.

pin, *n* a small cylindrical piece of metal.

pin, cemented, *n* a metal rod cemented into a hole drilled into dentin to enhance retention of a restoration.

pin, friction-retained, *n* a metal rod driven or forced into a hole to enhance retention. It is retained solely by elasticity of dentin.

pin, incisal guide, *n* a metal rod that is attached to the upper member of an articulator and that touches the incisal guide table. It maintains the established vertical separation of the upper and lower arms of the articulator.

pin, retention, *n* the frictional grip of small metal projections extending from a metal casting into the dentin of the tooth.

pin, self-threading, *n* a pin screwed into a hole prepared in dentin to enhance retention.

pin, sprue, *n* **1.** a solid or hollow length of metal used to attach a pattern to the crucible former. *n* **2.** a metal pin used to form the hole that provides the pathway through the refractory investment to permit the entry of metal into a mold.

pin, Steinmann, *n.pr* a firm metal pin that is sharpened on one end; used for the fixation of fractures. It is sometimes passed through the maxilla or mandible to provide external points for attachment of upward-supporting devices.

pinch, *n* a small amount of chewing tobacco (snuff) an individual takes to use the substance for its desired effect. A "pinch" is called a *quid* in Britain.

pindolol (pin′dəlol′), *n brand name:* Visken; *drug class:* nonselective β-adrenergic blocker; *action:* competitively blocks stimulation of β-adrenergic receptors within the heart and decreases renin activity, both of which may play a role in reducing systolic and diastolic blood pressure; *use:* mild to moderate hypertension.

pinna, *n* the external ear.

pinocytosis (pī′nōsītō′sis), *n* See phagocytosis.

pipe cleaner, *n* a small, brushlike device used to clean the spaces between the teeth (used also for other purposes). It should not be inserted all the way between the teeth, but rather just far enough to massage the tissue and remove any plaque.

pipe tobacco, *n* the dried tobacco leaves that come loosely packed in small, foldable bags for use in a handheld smoking implement that features a bowl on one end and a small cylinder for drawing in smoke on the other.

piperacillin sodium (pīper′əsil′in sō′dēəm), *n* a semisynthetic extended spectrum penicillin active against a wide variety of gram-positive and gram-negative bacteria.

piperazine (piper′əzēn), *n* an anthelmintic agent that acts against the roundworm *Ascaris lumbricoides* and the pinworm *Enterobius vermicularis* by interfering with their nerve transmissions, thereby causing paralysis.

pipette (pipet′), *n* a glass tube, usually graduated, which is used in the laboratory to measure and move liquids.

pirbuterol acetate (pirbū′tərol′ as′ətāt), *n brand name:* Maxair; *drug class:* bronchodilator; *action:* causes bronchodilation with little effect on heart rate by acting on β-receptors, causing increased cAMP and relaxation of smooth muscle; *uses:* reversible bronchospasms (prevention, treatment), including asthma, may be given with theophylline or steroids.

P

piroxicam (pīrok′sikam′), *n brand name:* Feldene; *drug class:* nonsteroidal antiinflammatory; *action:* inhibits prostaglandin synthesis by interfering with cyclooxygenase needed for biosynthesis; possesses analgesic, antiinflammatory, antipyretic properties; *uses:* osteoarthritis, rheumatoid arthritis.

pit, *n* **1.** a small depression in enamel, usually located in a developmental groove where two or more enamel lobes are joined. *n* **2.** a depression in a restoration resulting from nonuniform density.

pit, lingual, *n* See lingual pit.

pit and fissure cavity, *n* See cavity, pit and fissure.

pit and fissure sealant, *n* See sealant, enamel.

pituitary gland, *n* an endocrine gland suspended beneath the brain in the pituitary fossa of the sphenoid bone. It produces a number of hormones essential for growth, metabolism, reproduction, and vascular control.

pituitary hormones, *n.pl* the hormones of the anterior lobe of the pituitary gland controlled by hypothalamic releasing factors; they include growth hormone (somatotropin) prolactin, thyroid-luteinizing hormone, adrenocorticotropic hormone, and melanocyte-stimulating hormone. The posterior lobe is the source of vasopressin, which inhibits diuresis and raises blood pressure, and oxytocin, which stimulates the contraction of smooth muscle, especially in the uterus.

Pituitrin (pitoo′ətrin), *n.pr* brand name for an extract of the posterior lobe of the pituitary gland.

pityriasis rosea (pitərī′əsis rō′zēə), *n* a noncontagious skin disease with reddish, scaly patches and moderate fever.

pivot, adjustable occlusal, *n* an occlusal pivot that may be adjusted vertically by means of a screw or by other means.

pivot, occlusal, *n* an elevation artificially developed on the occlusal surface, usually in the molar region, and designed to induce sagittal mandibular rotation.

pK_a, *n* a mathematical function analogous to the calculation of pH. It is the negative log (p) of the constant of acid dissociation (K_a). When the pK_a of a buffering agent equals the pH of the solution to be buffered, the buffering system is most effective. According to the Henderson Hasselbach equation, pK_a = pH + log ([HOAc]/[OAc-]).

placebo (pləsēbō), *n* a substance that resembles medicine superficially and is believed by the patient to be medicine but that has no intrinsic drug activity.

placebo effect, *n* the real or imagined effect of a placebo, which may actually be the same effect ordinarily associated with the administration of a therapeutically active agent.

placement, *n* the act of placing an object (i.e., removable denture in its planned location on the dental arch).

placement, choice of path of, *n* determination of the direction of placement and removal of a removable partial denture on its supporting oral structures, which can be varied by altering the plane to which the guiding abutment surfaces are made parallel. The choice is a compromise to best fulfill five demands: to subject abutment teeth to a minimum or no torquing force, to encounter the least interference, to provide needed retention, to establish adequate guiding-plane surfaces, and to provide acceptable aesthetics.

placenta (pləsen′tə), *n* the organ of metabolic interchange between the fetus and the mother.

placenta abruptio **(əbrup′shēō),** *n* a condition in which a typically positioned placenta detaches from the uterine wall prior to delivery, which may threaten both the viability of baby and the life of the mother.

placenta previa **(pləsen′tə prē′vēə),** *n* atypical placental positioning and attachment within the inferior third of uterus, which may cover the cervix in part or fully.

placodes (plak′ōds), *n.pl* the thick, flat sections of embryonic ectoderm on the facial surface of the embryo from which the sense organs develop.

plagiarism (plā′jəriz′əm), *n* an appropriation of the work, ideas, or words of another without proper acknowledgment.

plagiocephaly (plā′jēōsef′əlē), *n* a condition characterized by an asymmetrical skull with flat spots. Temporomandibular joint disorder, as well as auditory and visual disturbances, may result if left untreated. If diagnosed during infancy, the condition can be treated with cranial orthotics.

plague (plāg′), *n* **1.** any disease of wide prevalence or of excessive mortality. *n* **2.** the vernacular term for bubonic plague, marked by inflammatory enlargement of the lymphatic glands, particularly in the axillae and groins.

plaintiff, *n* the party who sues in a personal legal action and who is so designated on the record.

plan, *n* program of action.

plan, bank, n See bank plan.

plan, preventive care, n a long-term strategy designed to preclude the development of a disease and promote overall health. See also preventive dentistry and preventive orthodontic treatment.

plan, provisional treatment, n a tentative treatment plan that may be modified or continued upon reevaluation of periodontal status after initial therapeutic procedures.

plan, treatment, n the intended sequence of procedures for the treatment of a patient.

plane, *n* an ideal flat surface that intersects solid bodies, extends uniformly in various directions (horizontally, vertically, laterally, or any relative combination thereof), and is determined by the position in space of three points.

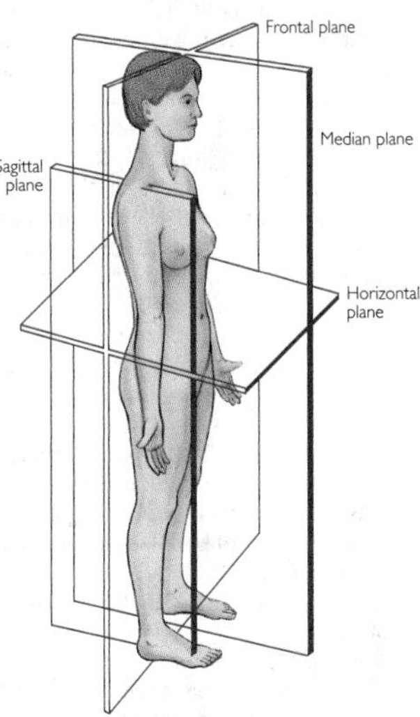

Body in anatomic position with median, sagittal, horizontal, and frontal planes noted. (Fehrenbach/Herring, 2007)

plane, axial, n a hypothetical plane parallel to the long axis of an object.

plane, axial, of teeth, n a term that applies to the mesiodistal or the buccolingual plane.

plane, axial wall, n an instrument used to plane and true the axial wall of a Class 3 preparation.

plane, axiobuccolingual, of teeth, n See plane of teeth, buccolingual.

plane, axiomesiodistal, of teeth, n See plane of teeth, mesiodistal.

plane, bite, n an appliance that covers the palate. It has an inclined or flat plane at its anterior border that offers resistance to the mandibular incisors when they come into contact with it. Also called *bite plate.*

plane, Bolton-nasion, *n.pr* imaginary surface passing through the nasion and the postcondylar notch, used in cephalometric analysis. See also point, Bolton.

plane, Broca's **(Brōkəz),** *n.pr* a plane extending from the tip of the interalveolar septum between the upper central incisors to the inferiormost point of the occipital condyle.

plane, brushing, *n* the top uniform edge of the bristles on the head of a toothbrush; forms the surface that comes in contact with teeth and gingival margin when brushing. The plane comes in a variety of designs that assist the user to remove plaque and clean the gingiva. Also called *trim.*

plane, buccolingual, of teeth, *n* a plane that passes through the tooth buccolingually parallel with its long axis. In incisors and canines, this is the labiolingual plane. Also called *axiobuccolingual plane.*

plane, Camper's, *n.pr* a plane extending from the inferior border of the ala of the nose to the superior border of the tragus of the ear.

plane, coronal, *n* the plane created by an imaginary line that divides the body at any level into anterior and posterior portions. Also called the *frontal plane.*

plane, eye-ear, *n* See plane, Frankfort horizontal.

plane, flush terminal, *n* a relationship between primary teeth in which the buccal surfaces of the opposing second molars are aligned when occlusion is centric.

plane, Frankfort horizontal, *n.pr* a craniometric plane determined by the inferior borders of the bony orbits and the upper margin of the auditory meatus. It passes through the two orbitales and the two tragions.

plane, frontal, *n* the frontal plane, in anatomy, is an imaginary plane that divides the body into anterior (ventral) and posterior (dorsal) halves along the longitudinal (left-right) axis.

plane, guide, *n* **1.** a mechanical device, part of an orthodontic appliance, having an established inclined plane that, when in use, causes a change in the occlusal relation of the maxillary and mandibular teeth and permits their movement to a normal position. *n* **2.** a plane developed in the occlusal surfaces of occlusion rims to position the mandible in centric relation. *n* **3.** two or more vertically parallel surfaces of abutment teeth shaped to direct the path of planement and removal of a remarkable partial denture. Also called *guiding plane.*

plane, guiding, *n* See plane, guide.

plane, Hamy's, *n.pr* a plane extending from the glabella to the lambda.

plane, His's, *n.pr* a plane extending from the anterior nasal spine to the opisthion.

plane, horizontal, *n* the plane created by an imaginary line that divides the body at any level into superior and inferior portions.

plane, horizontal, of teeth, *n* a plane that is perpendicular to the long axis of the tooth and may be supposed to cut through the crown at any point in its length.

plane, Huxley's, *n.pr* a plane extending from the nasion to the basion. Also called the *basicranial axis.*

plane, mandibular, *n* See border, mandibular.

plane, Martin's, *n.pr* a plane extending from the nasion to the inion.

plane, mean foundation, *n* the mean of the inclination of the denture-supporting (basal seat) tissues. The tissues constituting the denture foundation are irregular in form and consistency, and force may be applied from only one direction if it is to comply with the law of statics, which requires the exertion of force at a right angle to maintain support. Therefore the mean foundation plane forms a right angle with the most favorable direction of force. The ideal condition for denture stability exists when the mean foundation plane is almost at a right angle to the direction of force.

plane, mean occlusal, *n* the flat or horizontal plane or position and area between the cutting edge of the teeth.

plane, median, *n* See plane, midsagittal.

plane, median sagittal, *n* a plane passing through the median raphe of the palate at right angles to the Frankfort horizontal plane.

plane, median-raphe **(mē′dēən-rā′fē),** *n* the median plane of the head.

plane, mesiodistal, of teeth, *n* a plane that passes through the tooth mesiodistally parallel with its long axis. Also called *axiomesiodistal plane.*

plane, midsagittal **(midsaj′ətəl),** *n* the plane created by an imaginary line dividing the body into right and left halves. Also called the *median plane.*

plane, Montague's **(mon′təgūz),** *n.pr* the plane extending from the nasion to the porion.

plane, occlusal, *n* **1.** an imaginary surface that is related anatomically to the cranium and that theoretically touches the incisal edges of the incisors and tips of the occluding surfaces of the posterior teeth. It is not a plane in the true sense of the word but represents the mean of the curvature of the surface. *n* **2.** a line drawn between points representing one half of the incisal overbite (vertical overlap) in front and one half of the cusp height of the last molars in back. See also curve of occlusion.

plane of reference, *n* a plane that acts as a guide to the location of other planes.

plane of teeth, *n* for descriptive purposes, three planes are considered in the teeth proper: buccolingual, horizontal, and mesiodistal.

plane, orbital, *n* **1.** a plane perpendicular to the eye-ear plane and passing through the orbitale. *n* **2.** the plane that passes through the visual axis of each eye.

plane, sagittal, *n* a plane of the body created by an imaginary plane parallel to the median plane.

plane, Schwalbe's **(shväl′bez),** *n.pr* a plane that extends from the glabella to the inion.

plane, straight terminal, *n* See plane, flush terminal.

plane, vertical, of teeth, *n* an upright plane that is perpendicular to the horizon.

plane, von Ihring's **(ir′ingz),** *n.pr* a plane extending from the orbitale to the center of the bony external auditory meatus.

plaque (dental) (plak), *n* **1.** in dentistry, a biofilm noted in the oral cavity. It consists of salivary proteins, microorganisms, and other byproducts of the microorganism. A type of intercellular matrix is also present. It forms on the oral cavity surface after the formation of the salivary pellicle using selective attachment factors. It is a factor in initiation and continuation of dental caries and periodontal disease. Older terms: *mucin plaque, bacterial plaque.* **2.** deposits of cholesterol in the arteries, possibly causing disease.

plaque, cocci in **(kok′sī),** *n.pl* the gram-positive microorganisms occurring in early-developing plaque that are later replaced with filaments as the plaque matures.

plaque, epithelium-associated, *n* the loosely attached subgingival plaque found in the epithelium of the periodontal pocket that consists of gram-negative microorganisms and white blood cells.

plaque, fissure, *n* a plaque that develops in the pit and fissures of a tooth.

plaque, pigmented dental, *n* a colored plaque that is not related to the development of gingivitis and is often found in oral cavities that are almost plaque free. The plaque may be colonized by pigment-producing bacteria. The condition may be controlled by diligent plaque removal, but reoccurrence is possible. Also called *black line stain.*

plaque, subgingival, *n* a thick, noncalcified mass of plaque situated inferior to the gingival margin. It may or may not be attached to the epithelium or tooth and may cover subgingival calculus. It cannot be removed with flow of saliva or water. It can calcify with minerals from the lamina propria's blood vessels and become subgingival calculus.

plaque, supragingival **(soo′prəjinjī′vəl),** *n* a thick, noncalcified mass of plaque superior to the gingival margin. It cannot be removed with flow of saliva or water. It may or may not cover supragingival calculus. It may appear on any surface in the oral cavity. It can calcify from salivary minerals and become supragingival calculus. It can be stained with disclosing solutions. See also disclosing solution.

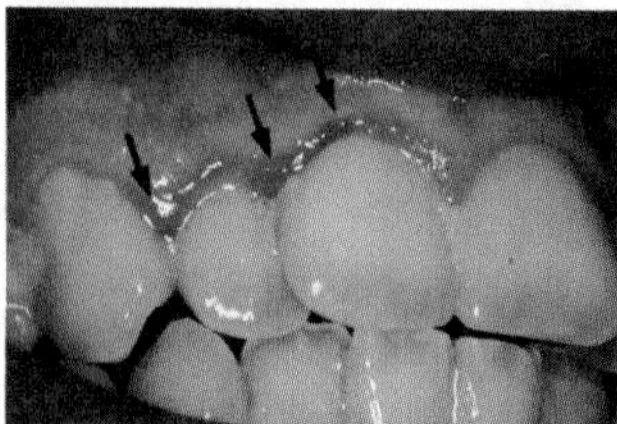

Supragingival plaque. (Newman/Takei/Klokkevold/Carranza, 2006)

plaque, tooth-surface-attached, *n* a type of subgingival plaque that uses selective attachment factors and is located in the subgingival area. This type of plaque is implicated in the formation of caries of the root and eventual breakdown of the root (resorption).

plasma (plaz′mə), *n* the fluid portion of the blood that, after centrifugation, contains all the stable components except the cells. It is obtained from centrifuged whole blood that has been prevented from clotting by the addition of anticoagulants such as citrate, oxalate, or heparin.

plasma accelerator globulin, *n* See proaccelerin and accelerator, prothrombin conversion, I.

plasma cell, *n* a lymphoid or lymphocyte-like cell found in the bone marrow, connective tissue, and sometimes the blood. Plasma cells are involved in the immunologic mechanism. See also cell, plasma.

plasma, normal human, *n* pooled sterile plasma from a number of persons to which a preservative has been added. It is stored under refrigeration or desiccated for later use as a substitute for whole blood.

plasma, platelet-rich (PRP), *n* a type of blood that contains high levels of platelets consisting of numerous growth factors. It can be used as one component assisting in the acceleration of tissue healing in bone regeneration.

plasma proteolytic enzyme, *n* See plasmin.

plasma spray, *n* the focused shooting of ceramic or metal powders on a hot plasma flame to initiate further heating and then rapid cooling, resulting in a thick coated surface on an implant.

plasma thromboplastin antecedent, *n* a factor required for the development of thromboplastic activity in plasma. Also called *antihemophilic factor C, factor XI, PTA,* and *plasma thromboplastin factor C.*

plasma thromboplastin component, *n* a clotting factor in normal blood necessary for the development of thromboplastic activity in plasma. A deficiency results in Christmas disease. Also called *antihemophilic factor B, autoprothrombin II, Christmas factor, factor IX, platelet cofactor II,* and *PTC.* See also factor IX.

plasmacytoma (plaz′məsītō′mə), *n* the primary soft tissue plasma cell tumors of the oral, pharyngeal, and nasal mucous membranes. The lesion consists of typical and atypical plasma cells, and its behavior is unpredictable. See also myeloma, solitary plasma cell and dyscrasia.

plasmacytoma, soft tissue, *n* a primary plasma cell tumor of the nasal, pharyngeal, and oral mucosa that has no apparent primary bone involvement. The lesions are sessile or polypoid sessile masses in the mucous membrane. The majority remain localized, but metastases have been reported.

plasmid, *n* a type of intracellular inclusion considered to have a genetic function.

plasmin (plaz′min), *n* collective term for one or more proteolytic enzymes found in the blood. The proteolytic enzymes are capable of digesting fibrin, fibrinogen, and proaccelerin. Plasminogen, the inactive form, may become active spontaneously in shed blood. An activator, fibrinokinase (fibrinolysokinase), is found in many animal tissues. Also called *fibrinolysin, lysin, plasma proteolytic enzyme,* and *tryptase.* See also plasminogen.

plasminogen (plazmin′ōjen), *n* the precursor of plasmin found in plasma. It is probably activated by a tissue factor or by a blood activator, which first must be activated by a blood or tissue fibrinolysokinase. Formerly called *profibrinolysin.* See also plasmin.

plaster (plas′tur), *n* colloquial term applied to dental plaster of paris.

P

plaster headcap, n See headcap, plaster.

plaster, impression, n plaster used for making impressions. Sets rapidly and is characterized by low-setting expansion and strength.

plaster, model, n plaster used for diagnostic casts and as an investing material.

plaster of paris, n the hemihydrate of calcium sulfate that, when mixed with water, forms a paste that subsequently sets into a hard mass. See also beta-hemihydrate.

plastic, *n* **1.** a restorative material (e.g., amalgam, cement, gutta-percha, resin) that is soft at the time of insertion and may then be shaped or molded, after which it will harden or set. *adj* **2.** malleable; capable of being molded.

plastic base, n See base, plastic.

plastic closure, n suturing of tissues that involves their displacement by sliding or rotation to create a surgical closure.

plastic strip, n a clear plastic strip of celluloid or acrylic resin used as a matrix when silicate cement or acrylic is inserted into proximal prepared cavities in anterior teeth.

plastic surgery, n branch of medicine that deals with the surgical alteration, replacement, restoration, or reconstruction of a visible part of the body to correct a structural or cosmetic defect.

plasticity (plastis′itē), *n* **1.** the quality of being moldable or workable. *n* **2.** the degree of permanent deformation resulting from stress application, usually associated with substances that are classed as solids or semirigid liquids.

plate, lingual, *n* See connector, linguoplate major.

plate, metal, *n* a titanium or stainless steel plate that is fastened to the bone by screws to bridge a fracture line and stabilizes bone fragments.

plate, palatal, See connector, major.

platelet (plāt′let), *n* a disc found in the blood of mammals that is involved in the coagulation and clotting of blood.

platelet ac-globulin, n See factor, platelet, 1.

platelet activating factor, n 1-0-alkyl-2-sn-glycero-3-phosphocholine. A phospholipid derivative formed by platelets, basophils, neutrophils, monocytes, and macrophages. It is a potent platelet-aggregating agent and inducer of systemic anaphylactic symptoms, including hypotension, thrombocytopenia, neutropenia, and bronchoconstriction.

platelet aggregation, n a clumping together of platelets in vitro, and likely in vivo, by a number of agents, such as adenosine diphosphate, thrombin, and collagen, as part of a sequential mechanism leading to the initiation and formation of a thrombus or hemostatic plug.

platelet aggregation inhibitors, n.pl the drugs or agents that antagonize or impair any mechanism leading to blood platelet aggregation.

platelet cofactor I, n See factor VIII.

platelet cofactor II, n See factor IX and plasma thromboplastin component.

platelet count, n the number of platelets found in 1 mm^3 of blood; the normal range is between 200,000 and 300,000 platelets.

platelet-derived growth factors (PDGF), n a type of protein released by platelets of the blood that aid in the repair and regeneration of connective tissue.

platelet disorder, n See disorder, platelet.

platelet-rich plasma (PRP), n See plasma, platelet-rich (PRP).

platelet transfusion, n **1.** the transfer of blood platelets from a donor to a recipient or reinfusion to the donor. *n* **2.** a treatment modality used in treating hemophilia and other conditions of impaired blood coagulation.

platinum (Pt) (plat′nəm), *n* a silvery-white, soft metallic element. Its atomic number is 78 and its atomic weight is 195.09. It is used in dentistry, jewelry, and the manufacture of chemical devices that must withstand high temperatures.

platinum matrix, n See matrix, platinum.

***Platyhelminthes* (plat′ēhelmin′thēz),** *n. pl* parasitic flatworms, such as tapeworms and flukes, that cause disease in humans.

pleadings, *n.pl* the written allegations of what is affirmed on the one side or denied on the other, disclosing the real matter to the court or jury having to try the case.

pledget (plej′ət), *n* a small pellet of absorbent cotton used for accurately controlled placement of medication or base. See also cotton, absorbent.

pleomorphic adenoma (plē′ōmôr′-fik ad′ənō′mə), *n* a benign tumor of the salivary gland containing varying proportions of epithelial and mesenchymal elements. The intermediate type of epithelial cells is in sheets, cords, and acini. The mesenchymal tissue varies from myxomatous to cartilaginous to densely hyalinized connective tissue. The marked variations in histologic pattern are responsible for the designation of pleomorphic. Also called *mixed salivary gland tumor.*

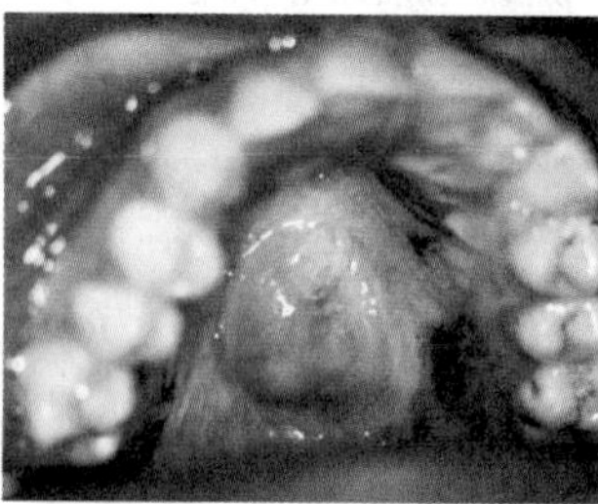

Pleomorphic adenoma. (Sapp/Eversole/Wysocki, 2004)

P

pleomorphism (plē′əmôr′fiz′əm), *n* the ability to change shape or form.

plethora (pleth′ərə), *n* a nonspecific increase in blood bulk. Clinically, the patient is flushed and has a feeling of tenseness in the head; the blood vessels are full, and the pulse is firm.

pleura (plŏŏr′ə), *n* a delicate serous membrane enclosing the lung, composed of a single layer of flattened mesothelial cells resting on a delicate membrane of connective tissue.

pleurisy (plur′əsē), *n* an inflammation of the pleura, with exudation into its cavity and on its surface.

plexus (plek′sus), *n* a network or tangle, especially of nerves, lymphatics, or veins.

plexus, Haller's, n.pr a nerve plexus of sympathetic filaments and branches of the external laryngeal nerve on the surface of the inferior constrictor muscle of the larynx.

plexus, intermediate, n a middle zone of the periodontal ligament situated between the cemental group of fibers attached to the root of the tooth and the alveolar group of fibers attached to the alveolar bone (Sharpey's fibers). The three groups of fibers are woven together by small, thick strands of collagen fibers. The interweaving of fiber bundles of the intermediate plexus allows for tooth eruption and tooth movement between the cemental and alveolar periodontal fibers.

plica fimbriata (plīkā fim′brēātā), *n* a fringed fold located on the ventral surface of the tongue near the location where it attaches to the floor of the oral cavity.

pliers, *n* a tool of pincer design with jaws of varying shapes; used for holding, bending, stretching, contouring, and cutting.

pliers, contouring, n a set of pliers with jaws curved to permit developing tooth contours in banding metal.

pliers, cotton, n a slender, tweezer-like instrument used to hold cotton pellets or pledgets, apply medicaments, and carry small objects to and from the oral cavity.

pliers, stretching, n pliers whose jaws are designed as a hammer and anvil, with the handles sufficiently long to develop a high leverage ratio. It is used to enlarge metal bands (gold, aluminum, copper) or to thin the contact area of matrix bands.

plosive (plō′siv), *n* any speech sound made by impounding the airstream for a moment until considerable pressure has been developed and then suddenly releasing it (e.g., *b, d,* and *g*). One of two types of stop consonants, the other being affricative (e.g., *ch*).

plug, *n* a peg or a mass filling a hole or closing an opening.

plugger, *n* an instrument used to compress the filling material in an apical and lateral direction when a root canal is being filled. See also condenser.

plumbism (plum′bizəm), *n* acute or chronic intoxication resulting from the ingestion, inhalation, or skin absorption of lead. Manifestations of acute poisoning include abdominal pain, paralysis, metallic taste, and collapse. Chronic manifestations include gastrointestinal disturbances, headache, peripheral neuropathy (foot drop and wrist drop), lead in the urine and blood, basophilic granular degeneration, coproporphyrinuria, and stomatitis. Also called *lead poisoning* and *saturnism.* See also stomatitis, lead.

Plummer-Vinson syndrome, *n.pr* See syndrome, Plummer-Vinson.

plunger cusp, *n* a stamp cusp, the tip of which is made to occlude in an embrasure; its shoulder has not been restored to occlude in a fossa.

PMA (papillary-marginal-attached), *n* a system of epidemiologic scoring of periodontal disease devised by Schour and Massler in which the symbols denote the areas involved in gingival inflammation.

pneumatic condenser (noomat′ik), *n* See condenser, pneumatic.

pneumococcal pneumonia (noo′məkok′əl nŏŏmōn′yə), *n* See *Streptococcus pneumoniae.*

pneumoconiosis (noo′mōkō′nēō′sis), any disease of the lung caused by chronic inhalation of dust, usually mineral dusts of occupational or environmental origin. The principal agents include coal, cotton, sand, and asbestos.

***Pneumocystis jiroveci* (noo′mōsis′tis),** *n* an opportunistic infection found in immunocompromised patients such as those with AIDS.

pneumocystis pneumonia, *n* See *Pneumocystis jiroveci.*

pneumonia (nŏŏmōn′yə), *n* an acute inflammation of the lungs, usually caused by inhaled microorganisms. The alveoli and bronchioles of the lungs become plugged with a fibrous exudate, seriously interfering with oxygen exchange.

pneumonitis (noo′mōnī′tis), *n* an inflammation of the lungs of an acute, localized nature.

pneumothorax (noo′mōthôr′aks), *n* an accumulation of air or gas in the pleural cavity. The air enters by way of an external wound, a lung perforation, a burrowing abscess, or rupture of a superficial lung cavity. It is accompanied by sudden, severe pain and rapidly increasing dyspnea.

pocket, *n* in dentistry, a deepened gingival sulcus. See also gingival sulcus.

pocket, bleeding, *n* an occurrence that denotes ulcerations of the pocket epithelium, with hemorrhaging through the broken surface from exposed connective tissue capillaries. May happen as a result of probing, oral hygiene, or other manipulation of the tissues such as dental procedures or eating.

pocket bottom, *n* the base of the pocket, marked or limited by the epithelial attachment to the cementum of the root (periodontal pocket) or the enamel of the crown (gingival pocket). The depth from the base of the pocket to the gingival crest is measured by the periodontal probe.

pocket, calculus, *n* the calcified deposits that usually occupy the pocket. It is attached to the tooth structure, with the gingival tissues tightly adapted to the surface of the calculus.

pocket, deepening, *n* an increase of the depth of the pocket, which depends on apical proliferation of the epithelial attachment alongside the cementum, with subsequent separation from the tooth, or on hyperplasia of the gingivae resulting from inflammation.

pocket, depth of, *n* the measurement, usually expressed in millimeters, of the distance between the gingival crest and the base of the pocket using a periodontal probe.

pocket, elimination, *n* the application of therapeutic measures to obtain a healthy gingival attachment and an intact, functioning epithelial attachment. The procedures employed include curettage (root and gingival), reattachment, or new attachment operations, gingivectomy and gingivoplasty, and osseous and mucogingival surgical procedures.

pocket, gingival, *n* a pseudopocket or false pocket formation; gingival inflammation with edema, hyperplasia, and ulceration of the sulcular epithelium but without apical proliferation of the epithelial attachment.

pocket in marginal periodontitis, *n* a condition in which the inflammatory process has progressed from the gingival tissues to the underlying alveolar process. The changes are those associated with gingivitis and, in addition, resorptive bone lesions. The base of the pocket is at the junction of the epithelial attachment to the cementum of the root.

pocket, infrabony, *n* a periodontal pocket, the base of which is apical to the crest of the alveolar bone. Consists basically of a vertical resorptive defect in alveolar and supporting bone, overlying which are a band of transseptal fibers connecting adjacent teeth, disintegrated fibers of gingival tissue, inflammatory cellular infiltrate, and hyperplastic pocket epithelium, accompanied by apical migration of the epithelial attachment. Clinical signs are those of periodontitis, associated with radiographic evidence of vertical bone resorption. It has been classified according to the number of remaining osseous walls supporting it for the purpose of therapeutic rationale. Also called *infracrestal pocket, intraalveolar pocket,* and *intrabony pocket.*

pocket, infracrestal, *n* See pocket, infrabony.

pocket, intraalveolar, *n* See pocket, infrabony.

pocket, intrabony, *n* See pocket, infrabony.

pocket ionization chamber, *n* See chamber, ionization.

pocket, marking, *n* the accurate determination and delineation of pocket depth and topography as an aid to diagnosis and prognosis or to provide a guide for the gingivectomy incision or other surgical procedures.

pocket, periodontal, *n* a pathologically deepened sulcus, with an ulcerated junctional epithelium and apical proliferation of the epithelial attachment. There is also a loss of bone and disorganization of the periodontal ligament.

pocket, suprabony, *n* an area of crestal alveolar bone loss that results in a deepened gingival sulcus.

pocket surgery, *n* a generic term referring to gingivectomy and gingivoplasty. See also gingivectomy and gingivoplasty.

podiatry (pədī′ətrē), *n* a health profession that deals with the diagnosis and treatment of diseases and other disorders of the feet.

pogonion (pōgō′nēon), *n* the most anterior point on the chin. A cephalometric landmark in the lateral view.

poikilocytosis (poi′kilōsītō′sis), *n* the presence in the blood of irregularly shaped red blood cells.

point, *n* **1.** a small spot or a small area. *n* **2.** a rotating instrument having a small cutting end or surface.

point A, *n* the deepest point in the bony concavity in the midline at the base of the anterior nasal spine, in the region of the incisor roots. A landmark on the lateral cephalometric view.

point, abrasive, rotary, *n* small abrasive instruments used in straight or contraangle handpieces. Also called *mounted carborundum, diamond.*

point angle, *n* See angle, point.

point B, *n* a mandibular point comparable to point A.

point, bleeding, *n* See bleeding points.

point, Bolton, *n* the highest point of the curvature between the occipital condyle and the basilar part of the occipital bone and located behind the occipital condyle. A substitute for the basion point when it cannot be ascertained on cephalometric headplates.

point, central-bearing, *n* the contact point of a central-bearing device. See also central-bearing device.

point, condenser, *n* the nib of a condensing instrument, which is a short instrument for condensing foil or amalgam that is inserted into a mechanical condenser or into a cone socket handle.

point, contact, *n* the area of contact of approximating surfaces of two adjacent teeth. The areas of contact are located at the line of junction between the occlusal and middle thirds of the posterior teeth and the incisal and middle thirds of the anterior teeth. Also called *contact area.* See also open contact.

point, convenience, *n* a small undercut in the cavity wall convenient for placing and retaining the first portion of a filling material. It is generally one of the retention points placed in a cavity preparation that provides the best access to the operator.

point D, *n* the center of the body of the symphysis.

point, faulty contact, *n* a defective contact between the proximal surfaces of adjacent teeth, produced by wearing of the contact areas, dental caries, improper restoration, or altered tooth position. See also open contact.

point, gutta-percha, *n* See gutta-percha points.

point, hinge axis, *n* a point placed on the skin corresponding with the opening axis of the mandible.

point, Hirschfeld's silver, *n.pr* a calibrated silver rod used to record the clinical depth of periodontal pockets radiographically for the purpose of diagnosis.

point, incisor, *n* the intersection of the mandibular occlusal and midsagittal planes. The point at the mesioincisal angles of the two mandibular central incisors.

point, loss of contact, *n* the failure of contact of convex proximal surfaces of adjacent teeth; produced by tooth migration, dental caries, or improper restoration.

point, median mandibular, *n* a point on the anteroposterior center of the mandibular ridge in the median sagittal plane.

point of centricity, *n* if the point of the buccal cusp of the mandibular right molar, put in lateral position, arcs around the upright axis of the right condyle, it will reach a station where further muscular efforts leftward will change the cusp's direction so that it will arc around the left condyle. The station where the right arc ends and the left arc begins is a point of mandibular centricity. While the right cusp point orbits (arcs) around the near vertical axis, all other points in the jaw join in orbiting (arcing). The left condyle arcs rearward until it reaches a cranial backstop; then the muscles start rotating it and carrying it leftward, and the right condyle begins arcing forward, downward, and medially. In the right and left swings of the jaw, a condyle reciprocally alternates between being a rotator and an orbiter. The point of centricity of the mandible is demonstrated usually on a horizontal plane, but it can be demonstrated on all three planes of projection. The point of centricity is rearmost, midmost (between the arcs of motion), and uppermost. See also face-bow and relation, centric.

point, paper, *n* See paper point.

point, registration, *n* a point considered as fixed for a particular pattern of analysis. Also, the midpoint of a perpendicular line from the sella turcica to the Bolton-nasion plane.

point, transition, *n* See Tg value.

point, treatment, *n* a piece of paper point, selected for the root canal being treated, that carries or holds the medication in place.

point, trial, *n* a cone of filling material placed in a canal and radiographed to check on the length and fit of the filling.

point, trigger, *n* the point from which referred pain initiates. In the myofascial pain syndrome, usually a localized, deep tenderness in a taut bundle of muscle fibers from which pain is referred to other sites.

point, yield, *n* **1.** the place on the stress-strain curve where marked permanent deformation occurs. It is just beyond the proportional limit. *n* **2.** the point where permanent deformation starts in a metal.

pointing, *n* a fluctuation pertaining to the area where the purulent exudate is eroding through tissues to an external surface. At this point an incision and drainage operation usually is performed.

poison, *n* a substance that, when ingested, inhaled, absorbed, injected into, or developed within the body, will cause damage to structures of the body and impair or destroy their function.

poisoning (poiz′əning), *n* the possibly fatal condition caused by exposure to poison.

poisoning, arsenic, *n* acute or chronic intoxication from the ingestion of insecticides or administration of organic arsenicals. Manifestations of acute poisoning include abdominal pain, nausea, vomiting, and collapse. Chronic manifestations include weakness, peripheral neuropathy, hyperkeratosis, skin rashes, and oral manifestations secondary to liver dysfunction and bone marrow depression. See also stomatitis, arsenical.

poisoning, bismuth, *n* See bismuthosis.

poisoning, chemical, n a form of poisoning caused by ingestion of a toxic chemical agent.

poisoning, iodine, n See iodism.

poisoning, lead, n See plumbism.

poisoning, mercury, n See mercurialism.

poisoning, metallic, n a toxic condition produced by excessive exposure to or intake of metals. In the oral cavity there may be definite signs of arsenic, bismuth, lead, phosphorus, radium, and other metals. Fluorides produce changes in developing teeth at levels far below those that are toxic.

poisoning, phosphorus, n the result of the ingestion of phosphorus, especially yellow phosphorus. Manifestations include burning of the oral cavity and throat, abdominal pain, vomiting, jaundice, liver damage, and death. In chronic poisoning, necrosis of the jaws (phossy jaw) occurs.

polacrilex (pol′əkril′eks), *n* See nicotine, polacrilex.

polarized, *adj* a state of concentration or alignment. E.g., polarized light is light that travels on a single plain as opposed to ordinary light, which is multidirectional.

policy, *n* the document embodying the insurance contract.

policy holder, n under a group purchase plan, the employer, labor union, or trustee to whom a group contract is issued. In a plan providing for individual or family enrollment, the person to whom the contract is issued.

policy period, n the time during which an insurance contract affords protection.

policy year, n the year commencing with the effective date of the insurance contract or with an anniversary of that date.

poliomyelitis (pō′lēōmī′əlī′tis), *n* a disease produced by a small viral organism that enters the body via the alimentary tract and produces upper pharyngeal, pharyngeal, and intestinal inflammation in its mentor form. In the more severe variety, a subsequent viremia is produced, with extension of the infection to the anterior pulp horn cells and ganglia of the spinal cord, producing a flaccid paralysis. In *bulbar poliomyelitis* the viral infection involves the medulla, resulting in impairment of swallowing, respiration, and circulation. It is now recognized that three types of viruses are responsible for the nonparalytic, paralytic, and bulbar varieties of poliomyelitis. The condition is rare in the United States due to vaccination by killed viruses (Salk) and attenuated mutant vaccines (Sabin).

polishing, *n* the process of making a surface smooth and glossy or giving luster to a surface, usually by friction.

polishing brush, n See brush, polishing.

polishing, coronal, n the removal of soft deposits such as materia alba, plaque, and stains from the clinical crowns of the teeth to provide cleaner-appearing dentition using a rubber cup or prophy jet. See also polishing, selective and polishing, air-powder.

polishing cup, n the working end of a powered rotary tooth-polishing tool. Attached in various ways including mounted, threaded, or slip-on and is made from synthetic or natural rubber. Can also be disposable type and attached to the prophy angle.

polishing disk, n See disk, polishing.

polishing, prophy jet, n See polishing, air-powder.

polishing, selective, n a method of coronal polishing in which selected teeth are targeted due to the presence of stains. This method helps minimize the loss of enamel on natural teeth due to the friction from the movement and polishing paste and also decreases the possibility of damage to restorations, such as porcelain crowns, or to exposed root surfaces.

politics, *n* **1.** the art and science of governance, particularly in a democracy or collegial body. **2.** the interpersonal relationships noted within group interactions such as can occur in a dental office or clinic.

pollakiuria (pol′əkēyoo′rēə), *n* an excessive frequent urination. It may result from partial obstruction, such as in prostatic enlargement, or it may be of nervous origin.

pollen (pol′ən), *n* a fertilizing element of plants that travels in the air and produces seasonal allergic responses (type I) such as hay fever or asthma in sensitive individuals. See hypersensitivity.

polyamines (pol′ēəmēnz′), *n.pl* many amines; polymers of amine, many of which normally occur in body constituents of wide distribution and are essential growth factors for microorganisms.

polyantibiotic (pol′ēan′tibīot′ik), *n* a combination of two or more antibiotics used to eliminate bacteria from a root canal.

polycarboxylate cement, *n* See cement.

polychlorinated biphenyls (pol′ēklôr′ənā′tid bīfē′nəlz), *n.pl* more than 30 isomers and compounds used in plastics, insulation, and flame retardants and varying in physical form from oily liquid to crystals and resins. All are potentially toxic and carcinogenic. Mild exposure may cause chloracne; severe exposure may result in hepatic damage.

polychromatophilia (pol′ēkrōmat′ōfil′ēə), *n* an irregular staining of cells, particularly red blood cells.

Polycillin (pol′ēsil′in), *n.pr* the brand name for ampicillin, an acid-stable semisynthetic penicillin effective against some gram-negative and gram-positive organisms.

polycythemia (pol′ēsīthē′mēə), *n* an increase in blood volume as a result of an increase in the number of red blood cells, the erythrocytes. It may result from a blood-forming disease that increases cell production, or it may be a physiologic response to an increased need for oxygenation in high altitudes, cardiac disease, or respiratory disorders.

polycythemia, phlebotomy for, *n* the drawing of blood to check for an overabundance of red blood cells.

polycythemia, primary, *n* See erythremia.

polycythemia, relative, *n* an overabundance of red blood cells due to plasma loss.

polycythemia rubra, *n* See erythremia.

polycythemia, secondary, *n* See erythrocytosis.

polycythemia vera, *n* See erythremia.

polydactyly (pol′ēdak′tilē), *n* a congenital anomaly characterized by the presence of more than the normal number of fingers or toes. It may be a part of a complex genetic syndrome. Early surgical treatment is generally used to correct the problem.

polydipsia (pol′ēdip′sēə), *n* an abnormally increased thirst.

polyglycolic acid, *n* a polymer of glycolic acid, used in absorbable surgical sutures.

polygon frequency (pol′ēgon), *n* a type of graph using lines to display uninterrupted data.

polymer (pol′emur), *n* a long-chain hydrocarbon. In dentistry, the polymer is supplied as a powder to be mixed with the monomer for fabrication of appliances and restorations.

polymerase chain reaction (PCR), *n* a process whereby a strand of deoxyribonucleic acid can be cloned millions of times within a few hours. The process can be used to make prenatal diagnoses of genetic diseases and to identify an individual by analysis of a single tissue cell.

polymerization (pol′imər′izā′shən), *n* the chaining together of similar molecules to form a compound of high molecular weight.

polymerization, addition, *n* a compound formed by a combination of simple molecules without the formation of any new products; e.g., methylmethacrylate.

polymerization, condensation, *n* the combination of simple, dissimilar molecules, with the formation of byproducts such as water or ammonia (e.g., vulcanite).

polymerization, cross, *n* (cross linkage, cross-linked polymerization), the formation of chemical bonds between linear molecules, resulting in a three-dimensional network. Used for artificial teeth and denture bases because of superior craze resistance.

polymerization, cross-linked, *n* See polymerization, cross.

polymerization, photo, *n* a process in which a light source is used for polymerization.

polymorphonuclear leukocytes (pol′ēmôr′fōnoo′klēər loo′kō-sīts), *n.pl* white blood cells with nuclei of varied forms. See also leukocyte polymorphonuclear (PMN) and neutrophil.

polymyxin (pol′ēmik′sin), *n* an antibiotic substance derived from cultures of *B. polymyxa.* Used topically, in troche form, in combination with bacitracin and neomycin in the treatment of various oral infections. Not used systemically; therefore sensitization is minimized. Systemic use may be attended by renal dysfunction and toxicity.

polymyxin B sulfate (sul′fāt), *n brand names:* Aerosporin; *drug class:* ophthalmic antiinfective; *action:* inhibits cell wall permeability in susceptible organism; *use:* superficial external ocular infections.

polyneuritis, endemic (pol′ē-nyoorī′tis), *n* See beriberi.

polyols (pol′ēôlz), *n.pl* substances made up of two or more alcohols. See also sugar alcohols.

polyostotic (pol′ēostot′ik), *adj* affecting more than one bone.

polyp (pol′ip), *n* a smooth, pedunculated growth from a mucous surface such as from the nose, bladder, or rectum.

polyp, pulp, n See pulpitis, hypertrophic.

P

polyphagia (pol′ēfā′jēə), *n* disproportionate appetite or eating.

polypharmacy, *n* the prescription or dispensation of unnecessarily numerous or complex medicines.

polypnea (pol′ipnē′ə), *n* a rapid or panting respiration.

polyposis, multiple (pol′ipō′sis), *n* See syndrome, Peutz-Jeghers.

polysaccharide, *n* a complex carbohydrate containing a large number of saccharide groups such as starch.

polystyrene (pol′ēstī′rēn), *n* a polymer of styrene, which is a derivative of ethylene; often one of the resins present in materials designed for denture construction by the injection molding technique.

polysulfide polymer (pol′ēsul′fīd pol′imur), *n* a rubber base impression material that makes use of a mercaptan bondage. It is prepared by mixing a base material (mercaptan) with either an inorganic catalyst (lead peroxide) or an organic catalyst (benzoyl peroxide).

polythiazide (pol′ēthī′əzīd′), *n brand name:* Renese; *drug class:* thiazide diuretic; *action:* acts on distal tubule by increasing excretion of water, sodium, chloride, potassium; *uses:* edema, hypertension, diuresis.

polyuria (pol′ēyoor′ēə), *n* the passage of an abnormally increased volume of urine. It may result from increased intake of fluids, inadequate renal function, uncontrolled diabetes mellitus or diabetes insipidus, diuresis of edema fluid, or ascites.

polyvinyl alcohol, *n* a complex alcohol that is soluble in water and is used as an emulsifier and adhesive.

polyvinyl chloride (pol′ēvī′nəl klor′īd), *n* a common synthetic thermoplastic material that releases hydrochloric acid when burned and that may contain carcinogenic vinyl chloride molecules as a contaminant.

pons (ponz), *n* a structure dorsal to the medulla and intimately related to the pathways to the cerebrum. The cranial nerves whose nuclei lie in the pons are the trigeminal, abducens, and facial nerves, and part of the acoustic nerve. It is intimately related to the medulla, has the same blood vessel supply, and is involved in many lesions that affect the medulla. It is especially involved with the cerebellar manifestations of disease and may cause serious muscular incoordination in motor function of the head, neck, and facial structures.

pontic (pon′tik), *n* the suspended member of a fixed partial denture; an artificial tooth on a fixed partial denture or an isolated tooth on a removable partial denture. It replaces a lost natural tooth, restores its function, and usually occupies the space previously occupied by the natural crown. See also abutment.

population, *n* the instances about which a statement is made; all events, organisms, and items of a stated kind occurring or in existence in a specified time. In statistics, a hypothetic infinite supply or universe of events or objects like those being studied and from which a sample was drawn.

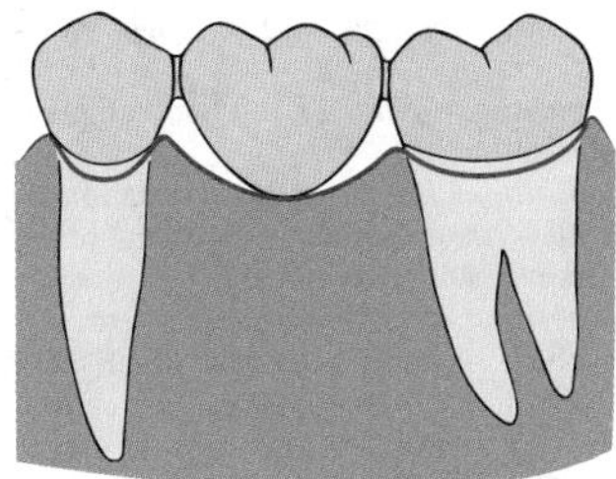

Pontic. (Rosenstiel/Land/Fujimoto, 2006)

population, at-risk, *n* the individuals belonging to a certain group or community who have the potential to contract a medical condition.

porcelain (pôr′səlin), *n* a material formed by the fusion of feldspar, silica, and other minor ingredients. Most dental porcelains are glasses and are used in the manufacture of artificial teeth, facings, jackets, and occasionally denture bases and inlays.

porcelain, baked, *n* See porcelain, dental.

porcelain, dental, *n* (baked porcelain, fired porcelain), a fused mixture that is glasslike and more or less transparent. Classification of the type of porcelain employed in inlays and crowns is based on the fusion temperature of the porcelain: high fusing, 2350°F to 2500°F (1287.5°C to 1371°C); medium fusing, 2000°F to 2300°F (1093.5°C to 1260°C); and low fusing, 1600°F to 2000°F (871°C to 1093.5°C).

porcelain, fired, *n* See porcelain, dental.

porcelain, synthetic, *n* See cement, silicate.

porion (pō′rēon), *n* the superior surface of the external auditory meatus. In craniometry, porion is identified as the margin of the bony canal on the skull. In cephalometrics it may be identified from the earpost of the cephalostat (machine porion) or from bony landmarks on the film (anatomic porion).

porosity (pōros′itē), *n* the presence of pores or voids within a structure.

porosity, back-pressure, *n* porosity produced in castings resulting from the inability of gases in the mold to escape through the investment.

porosity, occluded gas, *n* porosity produced by improper use of the blowpipe (i.e., heating the metal in the oxidizing portion of the flame).

porosity, shrink-spot, *n* an area of porosity in cast metal that is caused by shrinkage of a portion of the metal as it solidifies from the molten state without flow of additional molten metal from surrounding areas.

porosity, solidification, *n* porosity that may be produced by improper spruing or improper heating of the metal or the investment.

porotic dentin (pôrot′ik), *n* a condition in which the dentin of a tooth become porous. It may occur in conjunction with vitamin C deficiency.

porphyria, congenital (pôrfir′ēə), *n* See porphyria, erythropoietic.

porphyria, erythropoietic (ərith′rōpoiē′tik), *n* (congenital porphyria, photosensitive porphyria), an inborn error of metabolism (porphyrin synthesis) characterized clinically by skin photosensitivity, hypertrichosis, and reddish brown staining of the primary teeth.

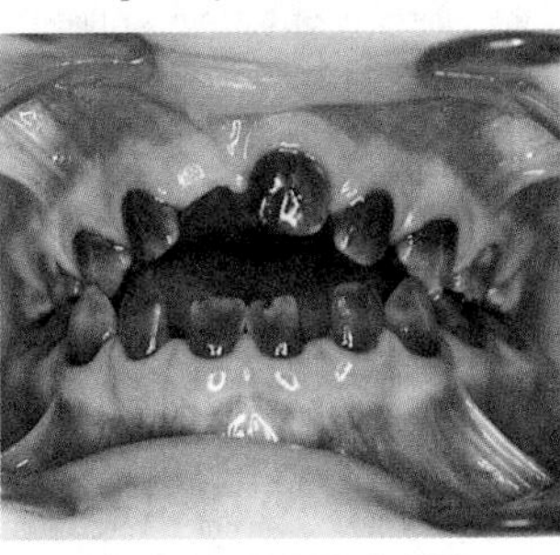

Porphyria. (Zitelli/Davis, 2002)

porphyria, photosensitive, *n* See porphyria, erythropoietic.

porphyrin (pôr′fərin), *n* any iron or magnesium-free pyrrole derivative occurring in many plant and animal tissues. Normal findings of porphyrins in urine are 60 mg to 200 mg/24-hour period.

Porphyromonas gingivalis **(pôr′firōmō′nas jin′jəval′is),** *n* a species of gram-negative, anaerobic, rod-shaped bacteria originally classified within the *Bacteroides* genus. This bacterium produces a cell-bound, oxygen-sensitive collagenase and is isolated from the oral cavity.

port, *n* in radiology, the opening through which radiographic photons or the useful beam of radiation exits from the head of a dental radiography machine.

portal of entry, *n* the area in which a microorganism enters the body. They may be cuts, lesions, injection sites, or natural body orifices.

porte polisher (port pol′ishur), *n* a manual dental polishing device featuring an orangewood tip attached at a contra-angle. Considered beneficial to gingival health, it is nonthreatening to patients wary of powered equipment.

position, *n* the placement or location of body parts to each other or the relationship of the body and its parts to other objects in space.

position, anatomic, *n* the upright, forward-facing stance used to reference the physical location of a body part. Arms are held down at the sides with palms, toes, and eyes all directed anteriorly.

position, axial, *n* the placement of the long axis of a tooth so that the tooth is positioned to withstand the occlusal forces exerted on it.

position, border, posterior, *n* the most posterior position of the mandible at any specific vertical relation of the maxillae.

position, centric, *n* **1.** the position of the mandible in its most retruded relation to the maxillae at the established vertical relation. *n* **2.** the constant position into which the patient will close the jaws; this relationship may be a convenience relationship or a true centric relationship.

position, condylar hinge, *n* **1.** mandibular joints at which a hinge movement of the mandible is possible. *n* **2.** the maxillomandibular relation from which a consciously stimulated true hinge movement can be executed.

position, eccentric, *n* (eccentric jaw position), any position of the mandible other than that in centric relation. See also relation, jaw, eccentric.

position, eccentric jaw, *n* See position, eccentric and relation, eccentric jaw.

position, finger, *n* See finger positions.

position, gingival, *n* See gingival position.

position, hinge, *n* the orientation of parts in a manner permitting hinge movements between them.

position, intercuspal, *n* the term applied to the cuspal contacts of teeth when the mandible is in centric relation. Also called *centric occlusion.*

position, mandibular hinge, *n* any position of the mandible that exists when the condyles are so situated in the temporomandibular joints that opening or closing movements can be made on the hinge axis. See also *axis, hinge.*

position, neutral, *n* a relaxed and level arrangement of specific parts of the body so as to minimize stress or strain on the joints, nerves, or spine. The neutral position is usually defined by the horizontal plane of the adjacent part(s).

position, physiologic rest, *n* the habitual postural position of the mandible when the patient is resting comfortably in the upright position and the condyles are in a neutral, unstrained position in the glenoid fossae. The mandibular musculature is in a state of minimum tonic contraction to maintain posture and to overcome its force of gravity. See also relation, rest jaw.

position, protrusive, *n* the occlusion of the teeth as the mandible and mandibular central incisors are moved straight forward toward the incisal edges of the upper central incisors; the normal anteroocclusal relationship; the forward end position, with the maxillary and mandibular incisors in edge-to-edge contact.

position, rest, *n* **1.** the position of the mandible when the jaws are in rest relation. See also position, physiologic rest, and relation, rest jaw. *n* **2.** the position that the mandible passively assumes when the mandibular musculature is relaxed.

position, semi-upright, *n* a way to position a patient suffering from respiratory or cardiovascular conditions.

position, terminal hinge, *n* the mandibular hinge position from which further opening of the mandible would produce translatory rather than hinge movement. See also position, hinge.

position, tooth, *n* the placement or location of the tooth in the dental arch in relation to the bone of the alveolar process, its adjacent teeth, and the opposing dentition.

position, Trendelenburg **(tren′delənbərg),** *n.pr* a position in which the patient is on his back with the head and chest lowered and the legs elevated.

positioner, *n* a removable elastic orthodontic appliance molded to fit the teeth in a "setup" made by repositioning the teeth from a plaster cast. The material may be rubber or elastomeric plastic. It is typically used to achieve fine adjustments and retain corrected positions in the finishing stages of treatment.

positioning, surgical, *n* the surgical repositioning or tilting of a tooth without injuring its blood supply.

positions at the chair, *n.pl* the posture and relative location of a clinician or chairside assistant in respect to the dental chair and patient. Classified as standing or sitting and as right side behind, right side in front, left side behind, left side in front, and directly behind. The position used should permit the most efficient performance of the current procedure and also keep paramount the health and comfort of the clinician and the patient. See also ergonomics.

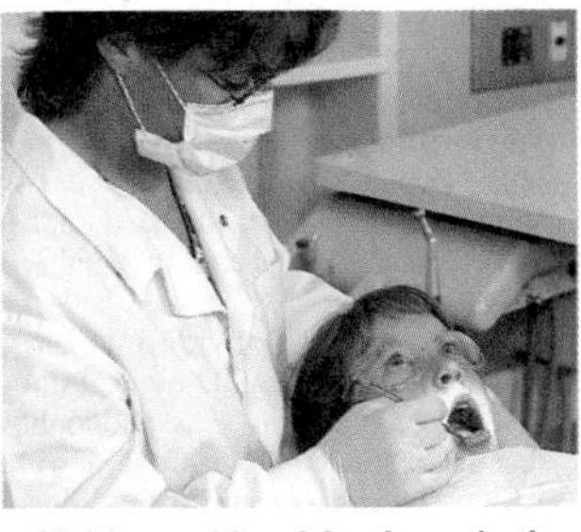

Clinician positioned by the patient's face. (Bird/Robinson, 2005)

positive reinforcement, *n* a technique used to encourage a desirable behavior. Also called *positive feedback,* in which the patient or subject receives encouraging and favorable communication from another person.

positron emission tomography (PET), *n* a computerized radiographic technique that employs radioactive substances to examine the metabolic activity of various body structures. Researchers and clinicians use PET to study blood flow and the metabolism of the heart and blood vessels.

possession, *n* the control or custody of anything that may be the subject of property as owner or as one who has a qualified right in it.

post cibum (pōst sī′bum), *adv* See p.c.

post-absorptive state, *n* the condition necessary for accurate measurement of the basal metabolic rate (BMR) in which the ambient temperature must be between 68° and 77° F (20° and 25° C) and the individual being tested must be fully awake, relaxed, and not ovulating.

postauricular (pōst′ôrik′yələr), *adj* describes the area behind the auricle, or external part of the ear.

postcondensation, *n* (aftercondensation), the procedure of completing the condensation of the surface of a gold-foil restoration after all the gold has been placed.

postdam area, *n* See area, posterior palatal seal.

posterior (postē′rēər), *adj* situated behind.

posterior nasal spine, *n* See spine, posterior nasal.

posterior palatal bar, *n* See connector, major, posterior palatal.

posterior palatal seal, *n* See seal, posterior palatal.

posterior palatal seal area, *n* See area, posterior palatal seal.

posteroanterior (pos′tərōantē′rēər), *adj* describes any back-to-front direction or motion.

posteroanterior extraoral radiographic examination, *n* See examination, posteroanterior extraoral radiographic.

postictal phase (pōstik′təl), *n* the period during which a patient recovers after an epileptic seizure. Also known as the *postconvulsion phase.*

postmortem changes, *n.pl* changes that occur after death.

postoperative care, *n* care after surgery or other invasive procedures, usually of a supportive nature.

postoperative complications, *n.pl* unexpected problems that arise following surgery. The most frequent are bleeding, infection, and protracted pain.

postoperative hemorrhage, *n* unexpected and abnormal (excessive) bleeding following surgery.

postpalatal seal, *n* See seal, posterior palatal.

postpalatal seal, area, *n* See area, posterior palatal seal.

postpartum, *adj* relating to or occurring during the period after birth.

postprandial (pōstpran′deəl), *adj* after having eaten.

posttreatment review, *n* See audit.

posture, normal, *n* the configuration of the body in the upright position, which varies considerably among individuals. However, normal posture can be described as follows: the shoulder, pelvis, and eyes are level; the sagittal plane is between the feet, and the line of gravity passes through the center of gravity at the lumbosacral joint. When observed from the following positions, the line of gravity intersects the following structures: lateral position—anterior border of the ear, and the shoulder, hip, knee, and ankle joints; anterior position—nose, symphysis pubis, and between the knees and feet; posterior position—occiput, spinous processes, gluteal crease, and between the knees and feet.

potassium (K) (pōtas′ēəm), *n* an alkali metal element, the seventh most abundant element in the earth's crust. Its atomic number is 19 and its atomic weight is 39.1. In the body, it constitutes the predominant intracellular cation, helping to regulate neuromuscular excitability and muscle contraction. The average adequate daily intake of potassium for most adults is 2 to 4 g.

potassium bicarbonate/potassium acetate/potassium chloride/potassium gluconate/potassium phosphate, *n brand name:* Effer-K, K-Lyte, Kapon-CL, K-Dur, Micro-K, K-G Elixir; *drug class:* potassium electrolyte; *action:* needed for adequate transmission of nerve impulses and cardiac contraction, renal function, intracellular ion maintenance; *uses:* prevention and treatment of hypokalemia.

potassium chloride, *n* a white crystalline salt used as a substitute for table salt in the diet of persons with cardiovascular disorders.

potassium dichromate **(dīkrō′māt),** *n* a compound of potassium used as an external astringent, antiseptic, and caustic.

potassium oxalate **(pōtas′ēəm ok′səlāt),** *n* a dentin desensitizing agent that occludes the openings of the dentinal tubules and blocks the hydrodynamics that initiate the pain response. *Brand name:* Protect.

potassium sulfate **(pōtas′ēəm sul′fāt),** *n* an accelerator used to speed the setting of gypsum products. Hydrocolloid impressions are fixed in a 2% solution of potassium sulfate.

potency (pō′tensē), *n* power.

potential, action, *n* See action potential.

potentiation (pōten′shēā′shən), *n* **1.** an increase in the action of a drug by the addition of another drug that does not necessarily possess similar properties. *n* **2.** the enhancement of action (e.g., of a drug).

Pott's disease, *n.pr* See disease, Pott's.

Potter-Bucky grid, *n.pr* See grid, Potter-Bucky.

pour hole, *n* an aperture in a refractory investment or another mold material leading to the pattern space into which prosthetic material is deposited.

povidone, *n* a polymerized form of vinylpyrolidone, which is a white hygroscopic powder that is easily soluble in water and used as a dispersing and suspending agent in drugs.

povidone iodine **(pōvidōn ī′ōdīn),** *n brand names:* ACU-dyne, Aerodine, Betadine; *drug class:* iodophor disinfectant; *action:* destroys a wide variety of microorganisms by local irritation and germicidal action; *uses:* cleansing wounds, disinfection, preoperative skin preparation; *dental use:* to irrigate periodontal pockets before debridement to control bleeding and pain.

powdered gold, *n* See gold, powdered.

power stroke, *n* See stroke, power.

***Poxviridae* (poksvir′idā),** *n* a major deoxyribonucleic acid virus family, to which the smallpox and vaccinia viruses belong. Viruses have a double-stranded, linear molecular structure with complex symmetry.

PPCF, *n* See factor V.

ppm (parts per million), *n* a standardized measurement used to describe the level of fluoride in products that contain it (e.g., toothpaste, mouthrinse, and water).

practice, *v* **1.** to follow or work at, as a profession, trade, or art. *n* **2.** the business operated by a medical professional.

practice administration, n the organization, operation, and supervision of the business and professional aspects of a dental practice.

practice building, n the process of increasing the number of patients and the number of services without sacrificing quality, by means of observing the principles of constantly improving professional care and maintaining effective relations with patients.

practice goal, n the planning of the objectives of a dental practice and the method of reaching those objectives. To be ascertained by the dental practitioner before or immediately on entering dental practice.

practice, group, n a large partnership formed for the purpose of practicing dentistry; may or may not include the services of the recognized specialties in dentistry.

practice guidelines, n a detailed description of a process of maintenance of health status or to slow the decline in health status in certain chronic clinical conditions. They are established to assist in the delivery of effective and efficient health care that preserves the resources of the provider, the patient, and the funding entity.

practice management, dental, n the administrative organization of a dental office, including but not limited to the supervision and control of patient flow, staff assignment and evaluation, record keeping, and financial overseeing.

practice, private, n the business and profession in which dental services are administered for a fee.

practicum (prak′tikəm), *n* See internship.

Prader-Willi syndrome, *n.pr* a metabolic condition characterized by congenital hypotonia, hyperphagia, obesity, and mental retardation. The syndrome is associated with a less-than-normal secretion of gonadotropic hormones by the pituitary gland.

pravastatin (prav′əstat′ən), *n brand name:* Pravachol; *drug class:* antihyperlipidemic; *action:* inhibits HMG-CoA reductase enzyme, which reduces cholesterol synthesis; *use:* as an adjunct in primary hypercholesterolemia (types IIa, IIb).

prazepam (prā′zəpam), *n brand name:* Centrax; *drug class:* benzodiazepine, antianxiety (Controlled Substance Schedule IV); *action:* produces central nervous system depression by interacting with a benzodiazepine receptor to facilitate the action of inhibitory neurotransmitter γ-aminobutyric acid (GABA); *use:* anxiety.

prazosin HCl (prā′zōsin), *n brand name:* Minipress; *drug class:* antihypertensive, α-adrenergic blocker; *action:* reduction in blood pressure results from blockage of α-adrenergic receptors and reduced peripheral resistance; *use:* hypertension.

preameloblast (pre″əmel′oblast″), *n* a cell within the enamel organ from which an ameloblast develops.

preanesthetic (prē′anesthet′ik), *n* a medicine for producing preliminary anesthesia (e.g., Avertin). See also premedication.

preauricular (prēôrik′yələr), *adj* describes the area in front of the ear between the ear's opening and the cheek.

preauricular lymph nodes, *n* the lymph nodes anterior to the auricle of the ear.

preauthorization, *n* **1.** the approval of or concurrence with the treatment plan proposed by a participating dental professional before the provision of service. Under some plans, preauthorization by the carrier is required before certain services

P

can be provided. *n* **2.** a statement by a third-party payer indicating that proposed treatment will be covered under the terms of the dental benefits contract. See also precertification and predetermination.

precancerous, *adj* a stage of abnormal tissue growth that is likely or predisposed to develop into a malignant tumor.

precautions, universal, *n* See universal precautions.

preceptorship, *n* the position of teacher or instructor to a new or recent graduate.

precertification, *n* confirmation by a third-party payer of a patient's eligibility for coverage under a dental benefits program. See also preauthorization and predetermination.

precipitate (prēsip′itāt), *n* an insoluble solid substance that forms from chemical reactions between solutions.

precipitating factor, *n* an element that causes or contributes to the occurrence of a disorder or problem.

precision attachment, *n* See attachment, intracoronal.

precision rest, *n* See rest, precision.

precordial, *adj* pertaining to the region over the heart or stomach: the epigastrium and inferior portion of the thorax.

precursor, fifth plasma thromboplastin, *n* See factor XII.

precursors (prēkur′sərz), *n.pl* particles or compounds that precede something. In biochemistry, carbohydrates may serve as precursors for structural and functional molecules. The -blast suffix indicates the precursor cell of a structure, such as in the term odontoblast.

predentin (preden′tin), *n* the dentin matrix produced by the odontoblasts that makes up the inner layer of the dentin and when matured becomes dentin.

predetermination, *n* an administrative procedure whereby a dental professional submits a treatment plan to the carrier before treatment is initiated. Then the carrier returns the treatment plan, indicating the patient's eligibility, covered service amounts payable, application of appropriate deductibles, copayment factors, and maximums. Under some programs, predetermination by the carrier is required when covered charges are expected to exceed a certain amount, commonly $100. Also known as *preauthorization, precertification, preestimate of cost,* and *pretreatment estimate.*

predisposition, *n* an increased vulnerability to a particular disease based on genetic factors or the existence of certain underlying conditions not yet active or revealed.

prednicarbate (pred′nəkär′bāt), *n brand name:* Dermatop Emollient Cream; *drug class:* topical corticosteroid, group III potency; *action:* possesses antipruritic, antiinflammatory actions; *uses:* relief of inflammatory and pruritic manifestations of corticosteroid-responsive dermatoses.

prednisolone/prednisolone acetate/prednisolone sodium phosphate/prednisolone tebutate (prednis′əlōn′ as′ətāt sō′dēəm fos′fāt teb′ōōtāt), *n brand names:* Delta-Cortef, Prelone, Pedaject-50, Hydeltra TBA; *drug class:* immediate-acting glucocorticoid; *action:* decreases inflammation by suppressing macrophage and leukocyte migration; reduces capillary permeability and inhibits lysosomal enzymes and phagocytosis; *uses:* severe inflammation, immunosuppression, neoplasms, adrenal insufficiency.

prednisone (pred′nisōn), *n brand names:* Deltasone, Sterapred; *drug class:* intermediate-acting glucocorticoid; *action:* decreases inflammation by suppressing macrophage and leukocyte migration, reduces capillary permeability and inhibits lysosomal enzymes and phagocytosis; *uses:* severe inflammation, immunosuppression, neoplasms, multiple sclerosis, collagen disorders, dermatologic disorders.

preeruptive (prē′ērup′tiv), *adj* refers to the development period that occurs while the tooth develops roots and before it erupts into the oral cavity through the gingival tissues.

preexisting condition, *n* in dentistry, the oral health condition of an enrollee that existed before his or her enrollment in a dental program.

preextraction cast, *n* See cast, diagnostic and cast, preextraction.

preextraction record, *n* See record, preoperative.

preferred provider organization (PPO), *n* a formal agreement between a purchaser of a dental benefits program and a defined group of dental professionals for the delivery of dental services to a specific patient population as an adjunct to a traditional plan, using discounted fees for cost savings.

prefiling of fees, *n* the submission of a participating dental professional's usual fees to a service corporation for the purpose of establishing, in advance, that dental professional's usual fees and the customary ranges of fees in a geographic area to determine benefits under a usual, customary, and reasonable dental benefits program.

pregnancy (preg′nəncē), *n* the gestational process, comprising the growth and development within a woman of a new individual from conception through the embryonic and fetal periods to birth. Pregnancy lasts approximately 266 days from the day of fertilization, but is clinically considered to last 280 days (40 weeks, or 10 lunar months) from the first day of the last menstrual period.

pregnancy gingivitis, *n* See gingivitis, pregnancy.

pregnancy tumor, *n* See granuloma, pregnancy; granuloma, pyogenic.

preicteric phase of hepatitis A (prē′ikter′ik), *n* the initial flulike symptoms a patient experiences when infected with hepatitis A.

prekallikrein, *n* a plasma protein that is the precursor of kallikrein. Plasma that is deficient in prekallikrein has been found to be abnormal in thromboplastin formation, kinin generation, evolution of a permeability globulin, and plasmin formation. Prekallikrein deficiency leads to Fletcher factor deficiency, a congenital disease.

preload, *n* the tensile force in the neck of a tightened screw that locks the screw in place without exceeding the screw material's elastic limit.

premature birth, *n* a birth in which the child is delivered before it has reached the full period of gestation (37 weeks).

prematurities, *n.pl* See contact, deflective occlusal and contact, interceptive occlusal.

premaxilla (prē′maksil′ə), *n* the embryonic structure that forms the anterior part of the maxillae.

premaxilla, floating, *n* See premaxilla, loose.

premaxilla, loose, *n* **1.** (floating premaxilla) the nonunion of the premaxillary process with the lateral maxillary segments, so that the premaxilla is loose, or floating. The position of the loose premaxilla in relation to the lateral maxillary segments varies among patients. *n* **2.** the administration of a tranquilizing drug, a drug that influences blood clotting time or any other drug that produces a preplanned set of conditions and is administered preceding any dental procedures.

premedication, *n* **1.** a sedative, tranquilizer, hypnotic, or anticholinergic medication administered before anesthesia. *n* **2.** the administration of medication before a stressful or invasive procedure.

premedication, antibiotic, *n* the administration of an antibiotic prior to an invasive procedure that prevents a dangerous infection, such as bacterial endocarditis, from occurring as a result of transient bacteria produced in the course of the procedure. See also endocarditis, bacterial.

premium, *n* the amount charged by a dental benefits organization for coverage of a level of benefits for a specified time.

premium, earned, *n* the portion of a policy's premium payment for which the protection of the policy has already been given.

premium rate, *n* the price per unit of insurance.

premium tax, *n* an assessment levied by a state government, usually on the net premium income collected in that state by insurance companies.

premium, unearned, *n* the part of the premium applicable to the unexpired part of the policy period.

premolar, *n* (bicuspid), one of the 8 teeth, 4 in each jaw, between the canines and first molars; usually has 2 cusps; replaces the molars of the primary dentition. Older term: *bicuspid.*

prenatal care, *n* the health care provided the mother and fetus before childbirth.

preoperative cast, *n* See cast, diagnostic.

preoperative record, *n* See record, preoperative.

prepaid dental plan, *n* a method of financing the cost of dental care for a defined population in advance of receipt of services.

prepaid group practice, *n* See closed panel.

preparation, *n* the selected form given to a natural tooth when it is reduced by instrumentation to receive a prosthesis or restoration (e.g., an artificial crown or a retainer for a fixed or removable prosthesis). The selection of the form is guided by clinical circumstances and physical properties of the materials that make up the prosthesis. See also preparation, oral cavity.

preparation, cavity, n a procedure in which carious material is removed from teeth and biomechanically correct forms are established in the teeth to receive and retain restorations. A constant requirement is provision for prevention of failure of the restoration through recurrence of decay or inadequate resistance to applied stresses. The colloquial term is *drilling.*

preparation, initial, n a procedure aimed at preparing the patient for final treatment. The objectives consist of eliminating or reducing all local causal factors and environmental influences before the operative procedures and establishing a sequence of therapy for the patient.

preparation, oral cavity, n a procedure applied to the oral cavity preparatory to the making of a final impression for a prosthesis.

preparation, slice, n a type of cavity preparation for Class 2 cast restorations. The proximal portion is formed by removing a sufficient slice of the proximal convexity of the tooth to achieve cleansable margins and a line of draw; a tapered keyway or two keyed grooves or channels in the proximal surface provide retention form.

preparation, surgical, n a surgical procedure that is required for preparing the oral cavity for prosthodontic treatment.

P

prepubertal (prēpū′burtəl), *adj* before the onset of puberty.

presbycusis (prez′bikū′sis), *n* the gradual loss of hearing that occurs naturally with age. The first sign is the diminished capacity to discern high-pitched tones.

presbyopia (prez′bīo′pēə), *n* a form of optical distortion affecting the vision of patients, particularly those of advancing age. It depends on diminution of the power of the accommodation of the lens as a result of loss of elasticity of the crystalline lens, causing the near point of distinct vision to be removed farther from the eye.

prescription (prēskrip′shən), *n* a written direction for the preparation and use of medicine or an appliance; a medical recipe; a prescribed remedy. Also used in dentistry to describe the treatment plan.

prescription, extemporaneous, n **1.** (magistral prescription) a prescription for a nonofficial drug. *n* **2.** a prescription that directs the pharmacist to compound the specified medication, as contrasted with a prescription that specifies medication available in precompounded form.

prescription, magistral, n See prescription, extemporaneous.

prescription, official, n a prescription for an official drug.

preservation, *n* a neurologic phenomenon such as the involuntary repetition of motor response or the continuation of a sensation after the adequate external stimulus has ceased.

preservative, *n* a substance added to prevent deterioration.

pressoreceptor, *n* a nerve ending that is sensitive to changes in blood pressure.

pressure, *n* a stress or strain that may occur by compression, pull, or thrust; an applied force.

pressure area, n See area, pressure.

pressure atrophy, n See atrophy, pressure.

pressure, biting, n the actual or potential power used in bringing the teeth into contact. See also pressure, occlusal.

pressure, blood, n See blood pressure.

pressure, deeper, n a pressure to the body—in excess of that which stimulates Meissner's corpuscles, Merkel's disks, or the hair receptors of light touch—that stimulates the deeper receptors such as Pacini's corpuscles. These latter deep-pressure perception organs lie in the inner layers of the dermis and in the muscle and tendon groups.

pressure, equalization of, n the act of distributing pressure evenly.

pressure, hand, n force applied by an instrument held in the hand.

pressure, hydraulic, n pressure transmitted by a liquid trapped between the tooth and a restoration being cemented.

pressure, hydrostatic, n the pressure in the circulatory system exerted by the volume of blood when it is confined in a blood vessel. The hydrostatic pressure, coupled with the osmotic pressure within a capillary is opposed by the hydrostatic and osmotic pressure of the surrounding tissues. Fluids flow from the higher pressure areas to the lower pressure areas.

pressure, intrapleural, n pressure within the pleura.

pressure, occlusal, n any force exerted on the occlusal surfaces of teeth. See also force, occlusal and load, occlusal.

pressure, osmotic, n the stress that develops when solutions containing different concentrations of solute in a common solvent are separated by a membrane that is permeable to the solvent but not the solute.

pressure, partial, n the pressure exerted by each of the constituents of a mixture of gases.

pressure, pulse, n the difference between systolic and diastolic pressure.

pressure sensibility, n the ability to detect light touch and deep pressure. See also corpuscle, Meissner's; corpuscle, Merkel's; and corpuscle, Pacini's.

pressure sore, n a decubitus ulcer caused when the bony protuberances of the body are subjected to chronic pressure from the weight of the body without breaks.

presumption, *n* an inference as to the existence of some fact, drawn from the existence of some other fact; an inference that common sense draws from circumstances usually occurring in such cases.

presurgical impression, *n* an overextended impression of the intact mandible before the first surgical stage. The cast made for this impression is altered so that the surgical tray may be fabricated on it.

preterm low birthweight, *n* a condition marked by a newborn weight of less than 5 pounds, 8 ounces, which may occur in an infant born before the end of the thirty-seventh week of pregnancy. Noted relationship with increased levels of periodontal disease.

pretreatment, *n* the protocols required before beginning therapy, usually of a diagnostic nature; before treatment.

pretreatment estimate, n See predetermination.

prevailing fee, *n* the term used by some dental benefits organizations to refer to the fee most commonly charged for a dental service in a given area.

prevalence (prevələns), *adj* in epidemiology, all the new and old cases of a disease or occurrence of an event during a particular period. It is expressed as a ratio in which the number of events is the numerator and the population at risk is the denominator.

prevent, *v* to keep from happening or existing, especially by precautionary measures.

preventive, *adj* avoiding occurrence.

preventive dentistry, n the procedures in dental practice and health programs that prevent the occurrence of oral diseases.

preventive maintenance, n a manner of avoiding future potential dental diseases or oral problems by practicing good oral hygiene on a regular basis.

preventive medicine, n the branch of medicine that is concerned with the prevention of disease and methods for increasing the power of the patient and community to resist disease and prolong life.

preventive orthodontic treatment, n the dental services intended to prevent the development of a malocclusion by maintaining the integrity of an otherwise normally developing dentition. Typical services include dental restorations, temporary prostheses (space maintainers) to replace prematurely lost primary teeth, and removal of primary teeth that fail to shed normally to allow the permanent successors to erupt satisfactorily.

***Prevotella* (prē′vōtel′ə),** *n* a genus of gram-negative, anaerobic, non–spore-forming, nonmotile rods. Organisms of this genus were originally classified as members of the *Bacteroides* genus but overwhelming biochemical and chemical findings indicated the need to separate them from other *Bacteroides* species; hence, this new genus was established.

***P. intermedia* (pre″votel′ə in″tər-me′deə),** *n* a bacilli found in gingival crevices that is believed to be responsible for gingivitis, chronic periodontitis, and other infections of the oral cavity.

prilocaine hydrochloride (local), *n brand name:* Citanest, Citanest Forte; *drug class:* amide local anesthetic; *action:* inhibits ion fluxes across membranes, particularly sodium transport across cell membrane; decreases rise of depolarization phase of action potential; blocks nerve action potential; *use:* local dental anesthesia.

P

prima facie (prī′mə fā′shē), *adv* a phrase that means "on the face of it"; so far as can be judged from the first appearance; presumably.

primaquine phosphate (prī′məkwēn′ fos′fāt), *n brand name:* generic; *drug class:* antiprotozoal; *action:* unknown; thought to destroy exoerythrocytic forms by gametocidal action; *use:* malaria caused by *P. vivax.*

primary, *n* a term indicating the first in time or the first in order in a series.

primary beam, *n* See radiation, primary.

primary care, *n* the first contact with a health care provider in a given episode of illness that leads to a decision regarding a course of action to resolve the health problem presented by the patient.

primary deficiency, *n* the insufficient intake of dietary nutrients that may be due to such factors as illness, ignorance, economic status, fad diets, food preferences, overuse of convenience foods, or poor oral health.

primary dentin, *n* the dentin produced after a tooth takes its position in the oral cavity but before the apical foramen is completed.

primary dentition, *n* See dentition, primary.

primary fixation, *n* the immediate postoperative fastening of an implant to bone by means of wires, screws, or a superstructure until, through natural healing and adhesion, final fixation occurs.

primary health care, *n* a basic level of health care that includes programs directed at the promotion of health, early diagnosis of disease or disability, and prevention of disease.

primary intention healing, *n* the healing of a wound directly at the incision site.

primary lymphoma of the brain, *n* a secondary neoplasm associated with acquired immunodeficiency syndrome (AIDS).

primary prevention, *n* an action performed to preclude the development of a disease. See also primary health care and secondary prevention.

primary radiation, *n* See radiation, primary.

primary cartilage, *n* See cartilage, primary.

primate (prī′māt), *n* a member of the biologic order of animals of the chordate class Mammalia. The primate order includes lemurs, monkeys, apes, and humans.

primate space, *n* the spacing between the primary canine and primary first molar that normally occurs in the anterior primary dentition in children.

primitive streak, *n* a furrowed, rod-shaped thickening in the middle embryonic disc that appears during the early formation of neural tissues and the mesoderm.

primodone (prī′mōdōn), *n brand name:* Myidone, Mysoline; *drug class:* anticonvulsant, barbiturate derivative; *action:* raises seizure threshold by unknown mechanism; may be related to facilitation of γ-aminobutyric acid; metabolized to phenobarbital; *uses:* tonic-clonic (grand mal), complex-partial psychomotor seizures.

primordium (primor′deəm), *n* the first evidence of an organ in a developing embryo.

principal, *adj* the leader; highest in rank; the source of authority.

principal in law of agency, *n* the employer; the person who gives authority to an agent to act for him.

prior authorization, *n* See predetermination.

privacy, *n* a culturally specific concept defining the degree of one's personal responsibility to others in regulating behavior that is regarded as intrusive.

private practice, *n* to engage in one's profession as an independent provider rather than as an employee.

privileges, *n* the authority granted to a physician or dental professional by a hospital governing board to provide patient care in the hospital. Clinical privileges are limited to the individual's license, experience, and competence.

p.r.n (pro re nata) (prō ray nahtah), *adv* a Latin phrase meaning "occasionally" or "according to circumstances"; the abbreviation is used in prescription writing.

pro forma (prō fôr′mə), *adj* pertaining to financial statement that shows the way that the actual statement will look if certain specified assumptions are realized. Pro forma statements are usually a future projection.

pro-SPCA, *n* See proconvertin.

proaccelerin (prō′aksel′ərin), *n* (factor V, labile factor, plasma accelerator globulin, plasma ac-globulin, proprothrombinase, prothrombin conversion accelerator I), an unstable protein found in the blood; the precursor of accelerin.

proandrogens (prōan′drōjenz), *n.pl* compounds that are not androgenic when applied locally but that have androgenic activity when metabolized in the organism. Included are cortisone and cortisol, which may be converted within the organism to androgens such as adrenosterone, 11-ketoandrosterone, and 11-hydroxyandrosterone.

probability, *n* **1.** an increased likelihood that something will occur. *n* **2.** a mathematic ratio of the number of times something will occur to the total number of possible occurrences.

probative (prō′bətiv), *adj* in the law of evidence, tending to prove or actually proving.

probe, *n* **1.** a slender, flexible instrument designed for introduction into a wound or cavity for purposes of exploration; in dentistry, it is mainly used for measuring and evaluating the sulcus or pocket region. *v* **2.** to use such an instrument.

probe, automated, *n* an automatically controlled instrument used to assess the severity of periodontal disease. It may provide more consistent readings than manual probes. Also called *controlled force probes.*

probe, automatic, *n* a device used to explore a cavity or a wound with minimal manual operation.

probe, depth, *n* the amount of space from the position of the tip of the periodontal probe to the gingival margin.

probe, furcation, *n* a hand-activated, blunt-tipped probing tool that is used to measure bone loss in teeth with multiple roots. See also probe, Nabers furcation.

probe, Hu-Friedy **(hū-frē′dē),** *n.pr* a thin, rounded and tapered handheld tool that is used to measure periodontal pocket depth. The millimeter marks are color coded for easier assessment.

probe, lacrimal **(lak′rəməl),** *n* an instrument useful in probing the lumen of duct structures, such as the nasolacrimal or salivary gland ducts.

probe, Marquis **(mar′kwis),** *n.pr* the probe is color coded by alternately colored or black and silver bands that mark 3, 6, 9, and 12 MM.

probe, Michigan O, *n.pr* a slender, round, conical-shaped device with a thin diameter used to assess the progression and extent of disease within the tissues of the oral cavity. The probe is marked at 3, 6, and 8 MM.

probe, Nabers furcation, *n.pr* an adapted device used to examine the layout and extent of an advanced furcation. See also furcation.

probe, periodontal, *n* a fine-calibrated instrument designed and used for measuring the depth and topography of gingival and periodon-

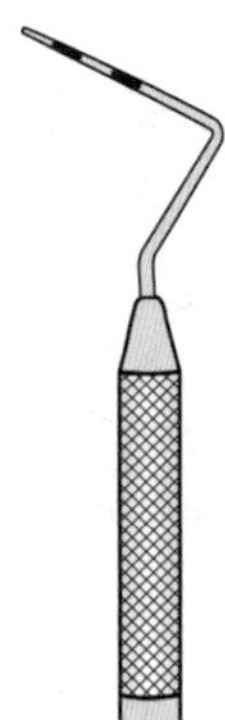

Marquis color-coded probe. (Daniel/Harfst/Wilder, 2008)

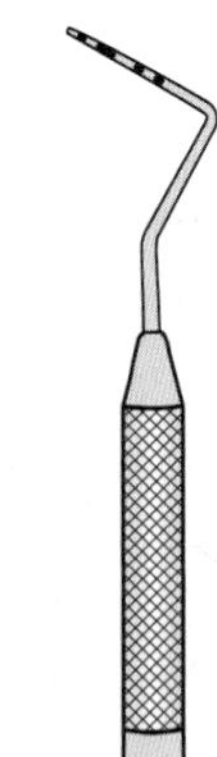

Williams probe. (Daniel/Harfst/Wilder, 2008)

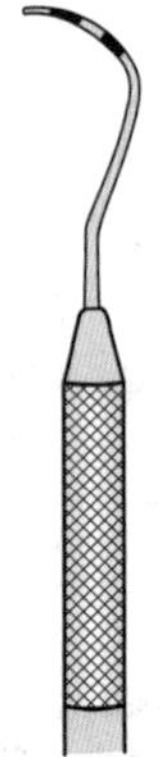

Nabers probe. (Daniel/Harfst/Wilder, 2008)

tal pockets. Also used to determine the degree of attachment and adaptation of the gingival tissues to the tooth. Automated devices are now available for dental offices and clinics.

probe, Williams, *n.pr* a round, conical-shaped device used to assess the progression and extent of disease within the tissues of the oral cavity. The probe has markings at 1, 2, 3, 5, 7, 8, 9, and 10 MM. The probe may be available with color coding.

probenecid (prōben′isīd), *n brand names:* Benemid, Probalan; *drug class:* uricosuric; *action:* inhibits tubular reabsorption of urates, with increased excretion of uric acids; *uses:* hyperuricemia in gout, gouty arthritis, adjunct to cephalosporin or penicillin treatment by reducing excretion and maintaining high blood levels of medication.

probucol (prōbyəkol′), *n brand names:* Bifenabid, Lesterol, Lorelco, Lurselle, Superlipid; *drug class:* antihyperlipidemic; *action:* increases bile acid excretion, catabolism of low-density lipoprotein (LDL) cholesterol; may block oxidation of LDL cholesterol; *use:* severe hypercholesterolemia when other treatment is unsuccessful.

procainamide HCl (prōkā′nəmīd), *n brand names:* Procan SR, Promine, Pronestyl; *drug class:* antidysrhythmic (Class IA); *action:* depresses excitability of cardiac muscle to electrical stimulation and slows conduction in atrium, bundle of His, and ventricle; *uses:* premature ventricular contraction, atrial fibrillation, paroxysmal atrial tachycardia, atrial dysrhythmias, ventricular tachycardia.

procaine hydrochloride (prōkān hī′drōklôr′īd), *n* an ester local anesthetic agent; 2-diethylaminoethyl 4-aminobenzoate hydrochloride, which is no longer available as an injectable due to its high allergenic potential. *Brand name:* Novocain.

procarbazine HCl (prōkarb′əzēn′), *n brand name:* Natulane; *drug class:* antineoplastic, miscellaneous; *action:* inhibits deoxyribonucleic acid, ribonucleic acid, protein synthesis; has multiple sites of action; a nonvesicant; also inhibits monoamine oxidase enzymes; *uses:* lymphoma, Hodgkin disease, cancers resistant to other therapy.

procedure (prōsē′jur), *n* a series of steps followed in a regular, orderly, definite way, by which a desired result is accomplished.

procedure, dental prosthetic laboratory, n the steps in the fabrication of a dental prosthesis that do not require the presence of the patient for their accomplishment.

procedure, invasive, n a series of steps that causes bleeding or the possibility of bleeding.

procedure, Kazanjian's **(kəzan′jēənz),** *n.pr* See operation, Kazanjian's.

procedure, operating, n the technique or method of conducting or performing an operation or form of treatment.

procedure, order of, n the sequence of steps made in performing an operation or following through a technique. In cavity preparation the sequence is as follows: (1) obtain the required outline form, (2) obtain the required resistance form, (3) obtain the required retention form, (4) retain the required convenience form, (5) remove any remaining carious dentin, (6) finish the enamel walls, and (7) make the debridement.

procedure, orthodontic, n the therapeutic measures employed to correct malalignment and malposition of the teeth and to immobilize and stabilize periodontally involved or previously moved teeth.

procedure, restorative, n a method or mode of action that reestablishes or reforms a tooth or teeth or portions thereof to anatomic or functional form and health.

process (pros′es, prō′ses), *n* **1.** in anatomy, a marked prominence or projection of a bone. **2.** in microanatomy, a protrusion of tissue. **3.** in dentistry, a series of operations that convert a wax pattern, such as that of a denture base, into a solid denture base of another material. See also denture curing.

process, alveolar, n the portion of the maxillae or mandible that forms the dental arch and serves as a bony investment for the teeth. Its cortical covering is continuous with the compact bone of the body of the maxillae or mandible, whereas its trabecular portion is continuous with the spongy bone of the body of the jaws. See also ridge, alveolar.

process, condyloid **(kon′diloid),** *n* a projection of the mandible arising on the posterosuperior aspect of the mandibular ramus. It consists of a neck and an elliptically shaped head or condyle that enters into the formation of the temporomandibular joint in conjunction with the articular disk and the glenoid fossa of the temporal bone.

process, coronoid, n the thin, triangular, rounded eminence originating from the anterosuperior surface of the ramus of the mandible. Provides insertion for the temporal muscle.

process, dehiscence of alveolar, n See dehiscence.

process, fenestration of alveolar **(fen′istrā′shən əv alvē′ələr),** *n* a circumscribed opening, located in the cortical plate over the root, that does not communicate with the crestal margin.

process, hamular **(ham′yələr),** *n* (pterygoid process) the pterygoid process of the sphenoid bone; appears as a vertical projection distal to the maxillary tuberosity.

process, horizontal resorptive, n the pattern of bone resorption, occurring with periodontal disease, in which the resultant level of bone is more or less flat or level in nature.

process, inferior articular, n the natural growth of bone that convexly projects in a forward lateral direction from the lumbar vertebrae.

process, lateral nasal, n the triangular cartilage that spans the bridge of the nose and is attached below the nasal bone and the front of the maxilla.

process, mandibular, n the stage of embryonic development during which two sections of the first branchial arch come together to create the mandibular arch.

process, maxillary, n the stage of embryonic development during which a prominence off of the first branchial arch unites with the corresponding median nasal prominence to form the upper jaw.

process, medial nasal, n a protrusion of tissue located midline to the olfactory pits during embryonic development from which the tip of the nose and philtrum of the lip develop.

process, neck of condyloid, n the part of the condyloid process that connects the condyle to the main part of the ramus.

process, odontoblastic **(ōdon′tōblas′tik),** *n* a structure of the tooth formed during dentogenesis. It becomes encased by predentin that eventually calcifies.

process, pterygoid **(ter′igoid′),** *n* See process, hamular.

process, Tomes', n a narrow extension of the ameloblast from which the enamel matrix is secreted.

process of care, *n* See plan, treatment.

processing (pros′esing), *n* in dentistry, the term that usually refers to the procedure of bringing about polymerization of appliances or working to the end product in denture or radiographic production.

processing, denture, n the conversion of a wax pattern of a denture or trial denture into a denture with a base made of another material, such as acrylic resin. See also process.

processing tank, n See tank, processing.

P

prochlorperazine edisylate/ prochlorperazine maleate (prōklorper′izēn′ ədis′əlāt′, mā′lēāt), *n brand name:* Compazine; *drug class:* phenothiazine antipsychotic; *action:* blocks neurotransmission at dopaminergic synapses in the cerebral cortex, hypothalamus, and limbic system; *uses:* antipsychotic; for nausea, vomiting.

proconvertin (prō′kənvur′tin), *n* (autoprothrombin I, cofactor V, cothromboplastin, factor VII, precursor of serum prothrombin conversion accelerator [pro-SPCA], stable factor), variously described as the inactive precursor of convertin. Recently proconvertin has been considered as a collective term for pro-SPCA and Stuart factor.

proconvertin-convertin, *n* See thromboplastin, extrinsic.

proctitis, *n* an inflammation of the rectum and anus caused by infection, trauma, drugs, allergy, or radiation injury.

procumbency (prōkum′bensē), *n* excessive labioaxial inclination of the incisor teeth.

procyclidine HCl (prōsik′lədēn), *n brand name:* Kemadrin; *drug class:* anticholinergic, antidyskinetic; *action:* blockage of central acetylcholine receptors; *uses:* Parkinson symptoms, extrapyramidal symptoms associated with neuroleptic drugs.

prodrome (prō′drōm), *n* a symptom, often noted prior to monitoring and diagnosis that may signal the beginning of a disease.

production, *n* the amount of work that can be accomplished in a specific length of time.

products, fission, *n.pl* See fission products.

profession, *n* a calling; vocation; a means of livelihood or gain.

professional autonomy, *n* the right and privilege provided by a governmental entity to a class of professionals, and to each qualified licensed caregiver within that profession, to provide services independent of supervision.

professional ethics, *n* the rules governing the conduct, transactions, and relationships within a profession and among its publics.

professional ethics liability, n **1.** the obligation of all professionals to their clients to do no harm. *n* **2.** the legal obligation of health care professionals, or their insurers, to compensate patients for injury or suffering caused by acts of omission or commission by the professionals.

Professional Ethics Standards Review Organization (PSRO), n a federal agency, established by Public Law 92-603, to determine the quality and appropriateness of health care services paid for, in whole or part, under the Social Security Act. Such determinations are to be made by local committees of providers.

profibrin (prōfī′brin), *n* See fibrinogen.

profile, *n* an outline or contour, especially one representing the lateral view of a head.

profile, extraoral radiographic examination, n See examination, profile extraoral radiographic.

profile, facial, *n* See facial profile.

profile, hematologic, *n* a thorough study of the blood and all its components that is used to diagnose diseases of the blood and to aid in the assessment of an individual's overall health condition. The results are compared with established normal blood values.

profile record, *n* See record, profile.

profit sharing, *n* a mechanism for funding a retirement plan for employees or members of a professional association. Members are eligible for a percentage of the net income based on predetermined formulae. Such plans, properly executed, are legal and ethical and are to be differentiated from fee splitting, which is illegal and unethical, in which a referring professional shares in the fee-for-service income of another professional.

progeria (prōjir′ēə), *n* See syndrome, Hutchinson-Gilford.

progesterone (prōjes′tərōn), *n* the ovarian hormone produced by the corpus luteum and responsible for preparing the endometrium for nidation and nourishment of the ovum. It also suppresses the production of the pituitary luteinizing hormone, estrus, and ovulation and stimulates the mammary glands.

progestin (prōjes′tin), *n* a hormone that suppresses the release of luteinizing hormone and thereby inhibits the onset of menstruation. Synthetically produced progestin and estrogen are used in combination as an effective contraception.

progestogen (prōjes′tōjen), *n* an agent capable of producing effects similar to progesterone; used to correct abnormalities of the menstrual cycle.

prognathic (prognath′ik), *adj* pertaining to a forward relationship of the jaws to the head (anterior to the skull); denoting a protrusive lower face.

prognathism (prog′nəthizəm), *n* a facial disharmony in which one or both jaws project forward. It may be real or false. Mandibular prognathism may exist when both the maxillae and the mandible increase in length or when the maxillae are of normal length but the mandible increases in length. It may be false when the maxillae are underdeveloped and short and the mandible is of normal length or when the maxillary and mandibular dental relationships are normal but there is an increase in the mental prominence of the mandible.

prognathous (prognath′əs), *n* the condition of having a marked projection of the mandible, usually resulting in a horizontal overlap of the mandibular anterior teeth in relation to the maxillary anterior teeth. See also prognathism.

prognosis (prognō′sis), *n* **1.** the foretelling of the probable course of a disease; a forecast of the outcome of a disease. *n* **2.** a forecast of the probable result of a regimen of treatment.

progressive loading, *n* the gradual increase of an external mechanical force on an artificial restoration and, consequently, the implant.

projection, *n* orthographic, a projection made on the assumption that the projection lines from the object to the plane of projection are at right angles to the plane.

projection, gnathic planes of orthographic, *n.pl* the three planes of projection to which gnathologically mounted casts are oriented: the horizontal, vertical, (frontal), and profile planes. The horizontal plane is the axis-orbital plane. The hinge axis is the line of intersection for both the horizontal and frontal planes. The profile plane is the mechanical midsagittal plane of the articulator.

prolactin, *n* See hormone, lactogenic.

prolapse (prōlaps′), *v* the falling, sinking, or sliding of an organ from its normal position or location in the body. See also mitral valve prolapse (MVP).

proliferation (prōlif′ərā′shən), *n* growth by reproduction of similar cells.

proliferation, epithelial, *n* a characteristic finding in inflammatory lesions affecting the gingival tissues; consists of hyperplasia of the pocket epithelium, with extension and elongation of epithelial rete pegs into the submucosa. Accompanying the hyperplastic changes in the crevicular epithelium, it is noticed that the epithelial attachment proliferates onto and alongside the cementum. Also, the multiplication of epithelial cells resulting either in increased thickness or new epithelial covering of a wound or an ulcer. See also pocket, periodontal.

proline (prō′lēn), *n* a nonessential amino acid found in many proteins of the body, particularly collagen.

promazine HCl (prō′məzēn), *n* *brand names:* Primazine, Prozine, Sparine; *drug class:* phenothiazine antipsychotic; *action:* blocks neurotransmission at dopaminergic synapses in the cerebral cortex, hypothalamus, and limbic system; mechanism for antipsychotic effects is unclear; *uses:* psychotic disorders, schizophrenia, nausea, vomiting, alcohol withdrawal.

promethazine HCl (prōmeth′əzēn), *n* *brand names:* Phenameth, Phenazine; *drug class:* antihistamine, H_1 receptor antagonist; *action:* acts on blood vessels, gastrointestinal and respiratory systems by competing with histamine for H_1 receptor site; decreases allergic response by blocking histamine; *uses:* motion sickness, rhinitis, allergy symptoms, sedation, nausea, preoperative or postoperative sedation.

promissory (prom′isôrē), *n* a promise; stipulation for a future act or course of conduct.

P

promotion, *n* **1.** the gaining and retaining of acceptance by others of the views, products, or services of the originator of the message. Components of promotion: personal selling, advertising, sales promotion, and publicity. **2.** achieving a higher-level position at a place of employment.

promotion, sales, *n* sales promotion includes those marketing activities, other than personal selling, advertising, and publicity, that stimulate consumer purchasing and dealer effectiveness. They include point-of-purchase displays, shows and exhibit demonstrations, and other nonrecurrent selling efforts.

pronasion (prōnā′zēon), *n* the most prominent point on the tip of the nose when the head is placed in the horizontal plane.

prone (prōn), *adj* lying flat with face down.

proof, *n* the establishment of a fact by evidence; to find the truth.

proof beyond a reasonable doubt, *n* in criminal law, such proof as precludes every reasonable hypothesis except that which it tends to support and is wholly consistent with the defendant's guilt and inconsistent with any other rational conclusions.

proof of loss, *n* the contractual right of the carrier or service corporation to request verification of services rendered (expenses incurred) by the submission of claim forms, radiographs, study models, or other diagnostic material.

prop, *n* a device inserted between the jaws to maintain an open position of the mandible.

prop, ratchet type, *n* a device placed in one side of the oral cavity that is used to keep the oral cavity of a patient open while work is performed on the other side. It can be set to various positions.

propafenone (prō′pəfē′nōn), *n* *brand name:* Rythmol; *drug class:* antidysrhythmic (Class IC); *action:* able to slow conduction velocity; reduces cardiac muscle membrane responsiveness; inhibits automaticity; increases ratio of effective refractory period to action potential duration; β-blocking activity; *use:* documented life-threatening dysrhythmias.

propagation (prop′əgā′shən), *n* the reproduction or continuance of an impulse along a nerve fiber in an afferent or efferent direction.

propantheline bromide (prōpan′thəlēn brō′mīd), *n* *brand name:* Pro-Banthine; *drug class:* anticholinergic; *action:* inhibits muscarinic actions of acetylcholine at postganglionic parasympathetic neuroeffector sites; *uses:* treatment of peptic ulcer disease, irritable bowel syndrome, duodenography, urinary incontinence.

proper equilibration, *n* the correct balance or stabilization between contrasting or opposing components.

property, *n* the rightful ownership; the exclusive right to a thing.

prophylactic (prō′filak′tik), *adj* preventing disease; relating to prophylaxis.

prophylaxis (prō′filak′sis), *n* the prevention of disease.

prophylaxis, oral (adult/child), *n* a series of procedures where plaque, calculus, and stain are removed from the teeth. This procedure is not the same as coronal polishing because the clinician can work subgingivally if needed. Only a licensed dental hygienist or dental professional is qualified to determine the need for oral prophylaxis and to perform the procedure. The colloquial term is *prophy.* See also coronal polishing.

propofol (prō′pōfol), *n brand name:* Diprivan; *drug class:* general anesthetic; *action:* produces dose-dependent central nervous system depression; mechanism of action is unknown; *use:* induction or maintenance of anesthesia as part of a balanced anesthetic technique.

proportional limit, *n* See limit, elastic.

propoxyphene napsylate/ propoxyphene HCl (prōpok′səfēn nap′səlāt), *n brand name:* Cotanal-65, Darvon, PP-Cap; *drug class:* synthetic opioid narcotic analgesic (Controlled Substance Schedule IV); *action:* depresses pain impulse transmission in the central nervous system by interacting with opioid receptors; *use:* mild to moderate pain.

propranolol HCl (prōpran′əlol′), *n brand name:* Inderal; *drug class:* nonselective β-adrenergic blocker; *action:* competitively blocks stimulation of β-adrenergic receptors within the heart and decreases renin activity, all of which may play a role in the reduction of systolic and diastolic blood pressure; *uses:* chronic stable angina pectoris, hypertension, supraventricular dysrhythmias, migraine, myocardial infarction prophylaxis, pheochromocytoma, essential tremor, hypertrophic cardiomyopathy, anxiety.

proprietary (prōprī′əterē), *adj* controlled by a private interest; protected by patent, trademark, or copyright.

proprietary name, *n* a brand name registered with the U.S. Patent Office under which the manufacturer markets his product. Also known as *brand name* or *trade name.*

proprioceptive (prō′preōsep′tiv), *adj* describes the body's ability to sense the movement and position of muscles without visual guides. It is essential for any activity requiring hand-eye coordination.

proprioceptive influence, *n* the influence of the muscle sense (kinesthetic sense) in guiding the jaw to close in such a way as not to be injurious to the teeth.

proprioceptors (prō′preōsep′-turz), *n.pl* the sensory nerve receptors situated in the muscles, tendons, and joints that furnish information to the central nervous system concerning the movements and positions of the limbs, trunk, head, and neck, and, more specifically for dentistry, the oral cavity and its associated structures.

proptosis (proptō′sis), *n* the forward displacement or protrusion of the eyeball. See also exophthalmos.

propylthiouracil (PTU) (prō′pəlthī′ōyŏŏr′əsil), *n brand name:* generic; *drug class:* thyroid hormone antagonist; *action:* blocks synthesis of thyroid hormones T_3 (triiodothyronine) and T_4 (thyroxine); *uses:* preparation for thyroidectomy, thyrotoxic crisis, hyperthyroidism, thyroid storm.

prorating (prōrā′ting), *n* a clause in a contract with participating dental professionals wherein they agree to accept a percentage reduction in their billings to offset the amount by which the total cost of services provided exceeds the total premium received. Prorating is a method of spreading a "loss" equitably among participating dental professionals.

prospective review, *n* the prior assessment by a payer or payer's agent that proposed services are appropriate for a particular patient, or the patient and the categories of service are covered by a benefits plan. See also preauthorization; precertification predetermination; and second-opinion program.

prospective study, *n* a study designed to determine the relationship between a condition and a characteristic shared by some members of a group. The population selected is healthy at the beginning of the study. Some of the members share a particular characteristic, such as cigarette smoking, whereas others do not. The study follows the population groups over a long period, noting the rate at which a condition, such as lung cancer, occurs in the smokers and in the nonsmokers.

prostaglandins (pros′təglan′dinz), *n.pl* a group of potent hormonelike substances that produce a wide range of body responses such as changing capillary permeability, smooth muscle tone, clumping of platelets, and endocrine and exocrine functions. They are involved in the pain process of inflammation.

prostate (pros′tāt), *n* a gland in men that surrounds the neck of the bladder and the urethra and produces a secretion that liquefies coagulated semen.

prostate cancer, *n* a slowly progressive adenocarcinoma of the prostate gland that affects an increasing proportion of males after the age of 50.

prostatitis, *n* an acute or chronic inflammation of the prostate gland, usually the result of infection.

prosthesis (prosthē′sis), *n* the replacement of an absent part of the body by an artificial part.

prosthesis, cleft palate, *n* a restoration to correct congenital or acquired defects in the palate and related structures if they are involved.

prosthesis, complete denture, *n* See denture, complete.

P

prosthesis, cranial, *n* an artificial material (alloplast) used to replace a portion of the skull.

prosthesis, definitive, *n* a permanent type that serves as a substitute for missing tissue.

prosthesis, dental, *n* a type that serves as an artificial replacement for one or more natural teeth or associated structures.

prosthesis, expansion, *n* a type used to expand the lateral segment of the maxilla in unilateral or bilateral cleft of the soft and hard palates and alveolar processes.

prosthesis, feeding, *n* a type worn by a young infant with a cleft palate to increase sucking power and to eliminate the escape of food through the nose.

prosthesis, fixed expansion, *n* a type that cannot be readily removed and stays in position for the required length of treatment.

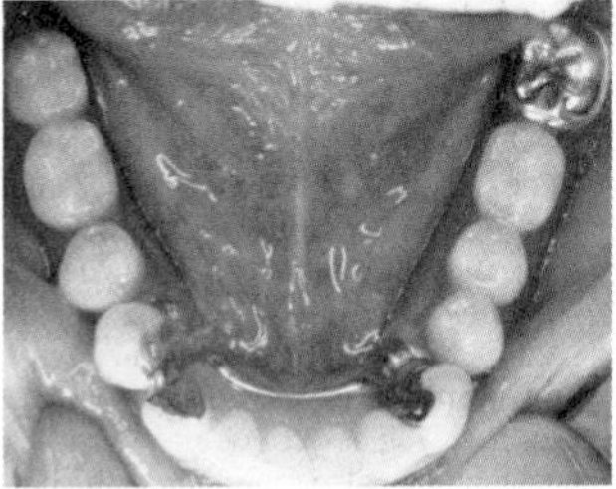

Dental prosthesis. (Rosenstiel/Land/Fujimoto, 2006)

prosthesis, hybrid, *n* a fixed denture that uses a combination of a metal framework and a complete denture. Also called a *high-water prosthesis.*

prosthesis, implant, *n* See implant prosthesis.

prosthesis, partial denture, *n* See denture, partial.

prosthesis, pediatric speech aid, *n* a type temporarily used to replace lost tissue in the palate of a child to remedy inarticulate speech. The device may be used to close an opening caused by a developmental defect or surgery.

prosthesis, periodontal, *n* a type that is used as a therapeutic adjunct in the treatment of periodontal disease.

prosthesis, postsurgical, *n* a type that serves as a replacement for a missing part or parts after surgical intervention.

prosthesis, removable expansion, *n* a type that can be removed from the oral cavity and replaced when indicated.

prosthesis, surgical, *n* a type that is used to assist in surgical procedures and placed at the time of surgery.

prosthesis, temporary, *n* a fixed or removable restoration for which a more permanent appliance is planned within a short period.

prosthetic appliance (prosthet′ik), *n* See appliance, prosthetic.

prosthetic restoration, *n* See prosthesis.

prosthetic speech aid, *n* See aid, speech therapy.

prosthetic valve endocarditis, *n* See endocarditis, infective.

prosthetics (prosthet′iks), *n* the art and science of supplying, fitting, and servicing artificial replacements for missing parts of the body.

prosthetics, complete denture, *n* **1.** the restoration of the natural teeth and their associated parts in the dental arch by artificial replacements. *n* **2.** the phase of dental prosthetics dealing with the restoration of function when one or both dental arches have been rendered edentulous.

prosthetics, dental, *n* See prosthodontics.

prosthetics, full denture, *n* See prosthetics, complete denture.

prosthetics, maxillofacial, *n* the branch of prosthodontics concerned with the restoration of stomatognathic and associated facial structures that have been affected by disease, injury, surgery, or congenital defect.

prosthetics, partial denture, *n* the dental service that, by replacing one or more but less than all the teeth of a dental arch, avoids the degenerative changes resulting from tooth movement and may thus achieve preventive measures of maximum benefit toward the maintenance of optimal oral health as well as reasonable restoration of dental functions.

prosthetist (pros′thətist), *n* the principal responsible individual involved in the construction of an artificial replacement for any part of the body.

prosthion (pros′thēon), *n* the point of the upper alveolar process that projects most anteriorly in the midline.

prosthodontia (pros′thōdon′shēə), *n* See prosthodontics.

prosthodontics (pros′thōdon′tiks), *n* the part of dentistry pertaining to the restoration and maintenance of oral function, comfort, appearance, and health of the patient by the replacement of missing teeth and contiguous tissues with artificial substitutes. It has three main branches: removable prosthodontics, fixed prosthodontics, and maxillofacial prosthetics.

prosthodontics, fixed, *n* the branch of prosthodontics concerned with the replacement or restoration of teeth by artificial substitutes that are not readily removable.

prosthodontist (pros′thōdon′tist), *n* a dental professional engaged in the practice of prosthodontics. A specialist in the practice of prosthodontics.

protective apron, *n* See apron, lead.

protective clothing, *n* clothing required to shield or guard the wearer from infectious, toxic, or harmful substances while engaged in employment. Federal and state statutes govern the use of such apparel.

protective devices, personal (PPD), *n.pl* articles designed to guard or shield an employee from harm, which include but are not limited to protective eye glasses and noise-dampening ear protectors. Federal and state statutes govern the use and placement of safety measures.

protective eyewear, *n* See eyewear, protective.

protein (prō′tēn), *n* a group of complex organic nitrogenous compounds; the principal constituent of cell protoplasm. Polymers of amino acids that are joined by peptide or amide bonds.

protein, anabolic, *n* See steroid, C-19 cortico.

protein, Bence Jones, *n.pr* a special protein found in the blood and urine of patients with multiple myeloma and occasionally other diseases involving bone marrow, such as sarcoma and leukemia.

protein, bone morphogenetic (BMP) **(môr′fogənet′ik),** *n* one of several genetically produced proteins that promotes the formation of bone and cartilage.

protein, C-reactive, *n* a mucoprotein whose presence in serum is always abnormal. It may be present in a variety of inflammatory or necrotic disease processes. It is almost always present in the serum in acute rheumatic fever.

protein chemical score (CS), *n* the result of a comparison between the amount of essential amino acid in a dietary protein and the amount in a reference protein.

protein, complementary, *n* a protein that is incomplete on its own but may become complete when combined with other proteins to provide all the amino acids necessary for normal metabolism.

protein, complete, *n* a protein that contains ample amounts of all the amino acids necessary for normal metabolism; animal proteins.

protein, deficiency, *n* See deficiency, protein.

protein efficiency ratio (PER), *n* a calculation designed to assess an individual protein's ability to sustain growth.

protein incomplete, *n* a protein that is missing one or more of the amino acids necessary for normal metabolism; vegetable protein.

protein kinase, *n* a protein that catalyzes the transfer of a phosphate group from adenosine triphosphate to produce a phosphoprotein.

protein, plasma, *n* blood serum contains 6.5 to 8 grams percent of a complex mixture of proteins, including albumin, globulin, and fibrinogen.

protein, reference, *n* a protein, usually egg, against which other proteins may be measured to evaluate their capability for supporting synthesis.

protein, spare, *n* one of several roles a carbohydrate food may play in a well-balanced diet. Many foods that are technically classified as carbohydrates, including some whole grains and beans, contain relatively significant amounts of protein that may, therefore, be referred to as spare.

protein specificity, *n* the arrangement of protein molecules in numerous spatial configurations to suit the special needs of the physical and chemical activities of the cell. The wide degree of variability of protein structures permits a high degree of specificity of tissue within one body. This characteristic of protein specificity is of great significance in blood transfusions, tissue grafts, and many allergic manifestations.

protein, thromboplastic, *n* See factor III.

proteinuria (prō′tēnyoo′rēə), *n* the presence of protein in the urine. It is an indication of kidney disease.

proteinuria, orthostatic, *n* (postural proteinuria) a type that occurs during daily activities but does not occur when the individual is recumbent.

proteinuria, physiologic, *n* See proteinuria, transient.

proteinuria, postural, *n* See proteinuria, orthostatic.

proteinuria, transient, *n* (physiologic proteinuria) a type that occurs in normal persons after a high-protein meal, violent exercise, severe emotional stress, or syncope. It may occur after an epileptic seizure or during pregnancy. It disappears after the cause subsides.

proteoglycans (prō′tēōglī′kans), *n.pl* the mucopolysaccharides bound to protein chains occurring in the extracellular matrix of connective tissue.

proteolytic (pro″teolit′ik), *adj* pertaining to substances that aid in the breakdown and assimilation of proteins.

Proteus **(prō′tēəs),** *n* a genus of motile, gram-negative bacilli often associated with nosocomial infections and normally found in feces, water, and soil. It may cause urinary tract infections, pyelonephritis, wound infections, diarrhea, bacteremia, and endotoxic shock.

prothrombase (prōthrom′bās), *n* See factor II and prothrombin.

prothrombin (prōthrom′bin), *n* a glycoprotein precursor of thrombin that is produced in the liver and is necessary for the coagulation of blood. A prothrombin deficiency is uncommon but may occur in liver disease. Vitamin K is essential for the synthesis of prothrombin.

prothrombin, B, *n* See factor II.

prothrombin, component A of, *n* See factor V.

prothrombin, component B of, *n* See factor VII.

prothrombin time, *n* a one-stage test for detecting certain plasma coagulation defects caused by a deficiency of factors V, VII, or X. Thromboplastin and calcium are added to a sample of the patient's plasma and, simultaneously, to a sample from a normal control. The amount of time required for clot formation in both samples is observed. A prolonged prothrombin time indicates deficiency in one of the factors. Normal findings are 11 to 12.5 seconds.

prothrombinase (prōthrom′binās), *n* (complete thromboplastin, direct activator of prothrombin, extrinsic prothrombin activator), an inferred direct activator of prothrombin common to tissue and plasma coagulation systems. See also factor V.

prothrombokinase (prōthrom′bōkin′ās), *n* See factor VIII.

prothromboplastin, beta (prōthrom′bōplas′tin), *n* See factor IX.

proton (prō′ton), *n* an elementary particle having a positive charge equivalent to the negative charge of the electron but possessing a mass approximately 1845 times as great; the proton is a nuclear particle, whereas the electron is extranuclear.

protoplasm (prō′tōplazəm), *n* a living substance; composed mainly of five basic materials: carbohydrates, electrolytes, lipids, proteins, and water and having the properties of both a complex solution and a heterogeneous colloid. The cell nucleus and cytoplasm are two major subdivisions of protoplasm.

protraction (prōtrak′shən), *n* a condition in which teeth or other maxillary or mandibular structures are situated anterior to their normal position.

protriptyline HCl, *n brand names:* Vivactil; *drug class:* tricyclic antidepressant; *action:* inhibits both norepinephrine and serotonin (5-HT) uptake in the brain; *use:* depression.

protrusion (prōtroo′zhən), *n* a situation in which the teeth or jaws protrude farther forward than normal.

protrusion, bimaxillary, *n* a relatively forward position, or prognathism, of the maxillary and mandibular teeth, alveolar processes, or jaws.

protrusion, double, *n* a definite labioversion of the maxillary and mandibular anterior teeth.

protrusion, forward, *n* a protrusion forward from the centric position.

protrusion, mandibular, *n* an abnormal protrusion of the mandible, as in a Class III malocclusion.

protrusion, maxillary, *n* an abnormal protrusion of the maxillae.

protrusive checkbite, *n* See record, interocclusal, protrusive.

protrusive occlusion, *n* See occlusion, protrusive.

protrusive position, *n* See position, protrusive.

protrusive record, *n* See record, protrusive.

protrusive relation, *n* See relation, jaw, protrusive.

Providencia **(prov′iden′sēə),** *n* a genus of gram-negative, rod-shaped, facultative anaerobic bacteria, associated with urinary tract and secondary tissue infections.

provider, *n* **1.** a governmental term used to denote health care institutions; sometimes used as a synonym for *practitioner.* **2.** used by insurance companies to denote the practitioner of the health care service(s).

provirus (prōvī′rus), *n* a type of virus incorporated into a host cell's genetic material that transmits from one generation of cells to the next via cell replication without triggering the separation or decomposition of the cell.

provisional prosthesis, *n* an interim prosthesis worn for varying periods.

provisional splint, *n* See splint, provisional.

provitamin (prōvī′təmin), *n* a substance in food that may be transformed into a vitamin within the body; a potential vitamin.

proximal (prok′səməl), *adj* describes an object location in reference to the nearest point to the center line of the body or the joint to which it is attached. The proximal surface of a tooth is the side that faces the centerline of the palate. The opposite of proximal is distal.

proximal surface (prok′səməl), *n* See surface, proximal.

proximate cause (prok′səmit), *n* one that directly produces an effect; that which in ordinary, natural sequence produces a specific result with no agencies intervening.

pruritus (proorī′tus), *n* itching.

Prussian blue, *n.pr* a chemical stain used on microscopic preparations. It demonstrates the presence of copper by developing a bright blue color.

pseudarthrosis (soo′därthrō′sis), *n* a false joint; sometimes seen after a fracture.

pseudo pocket (soo′dō), *n* a false pocket formed by gingival hyperplasia without apical migration of the epithelial attachment. See also pocket.

pseudoephedrine HCl/pseudoephedrine sulfate (soo′dōifed′rin), *n brand name:* Balminil, Benylin, Cenafed, Sudafed, Sufedrin; *drug class:* α-adrenergic

P

agonist; *action:* acts primarily on α-receptors, causing vasoconstriction in blood vessels; has more β activity and, to a lesser degree, central nervous system stimulant effects.

pseudoepitheliomatous hyperplasia (PEH) (soo′dōep′ithēlēōmətus hī′purplā′zēə, -zhə), *n* a type of epithelial hyperplasia associated with chronic inflammatory response; distinguished from squamous cell carcinoma by the lack of dysplastic cytologic characteristics.

pseudohemophilia (soo′dōhē′mōfil′ēə), *n* the term used to describe several hemorrhagic states: (1) von Willebrand disease, pseudohemophilia type B, vascular hemophilia; (2) a hereditary disease in which prolonged bleeding is the only consistent abnormality detected by currently available tests. See also purpura, thrombocytopenic.

pseudohypertrophic muscular dystrophy (soo′dōhī′purtrof′ik), *n* See muscular dystrophy.

pseudomembrane, *n* a loosely adherent, grayish false membrane typical of intracellular coagulation necrosis. It is formed by necrotic epithelium embedded in fibrin, leukocytes, and erythrocytes. It is seen in necrotizing ulcerative periodontal disease, apthous ulcers, and diphtheria. Removal leaves a raw, bleeding surface.

Pseudomonas **(soo′dōmō′nas),** *n* a genus of gram-negative bacteria that includes several free-living species of soil and water and some opportunistic pathogens isolated from wounds, burns, and infections of the urinary tract.

pseudopapillomatosis, *n* See hyperplasia, papillary.

pseudoprognathism (soo′dōprog′nəthiz′əm), *n* an acquired condition that results from malocclusions of the teeth, wherein the mandible is forced forward from its normal position in relation to the maxilla.

p.s.i., *n* pounds per square inch (lb/in^2); measurement describing the amount of pneumatic or hydraulic pressure in tanks and equipment used in pressurized dental procedures.

psoriasis (sôrī′əsis), *n* a papulosquamous inflammatory skin disease of unknown cause. Rare oral lesions consist of red patches with white, scaly surfaces.

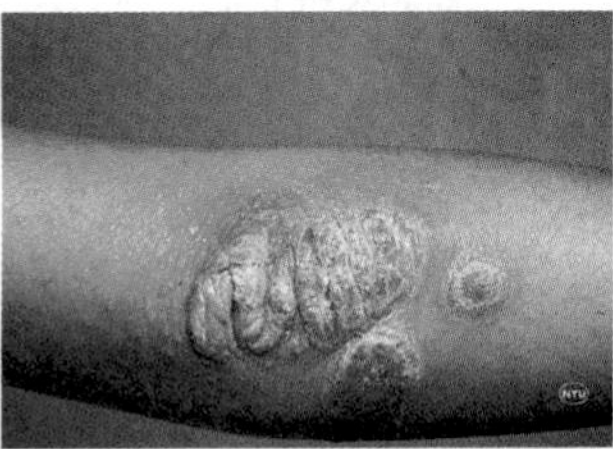

Psoriasis. (Courtesy Dr. Donald Schermer)

PSP test, *n* See test, phenolsulfonphthalein.

psychiatry, *n* the branch of medical science that deals with the causes, treatment, and prevention of mental, emotional, and behavioral disorders.

psychic, *adj* of or relating to the mind or the soul.

psychogenic (sī′kojen′ik), *adj* describes an illness or symptom of illness that originates in the mind rather than having physical causes.

psychologic age, *n* See age, psychological.

psychologic dependence, *n* mental state in which an individual considers a drug to be necessary for preserving health.

psychology (sīkol′əjē), *n* **1.** the study of behavior and the functions and processes of the mind, especially as related to the social and physical environment. *n* **2.** a profession that involves the practical applications of knowledge, skills, and techniques in the understanding of, prevention of, or solution to individual or social problems, especially in regard to the interaction between the individual and the physical and social environment.

psychomotor (sī′kōmō′tər), *adj* pertaining to or causing voluntary movements usually associated with neural activity.

psychomotor development, *n* the progressive attainment (by a child) of skills that involve both mental and muscular activity.

psychomotor domain, *n* the area of observable performance of skills that requires some degree of neuromuscular coordination.

psychoneurosis (sī′kōnyoorō′sis), *n* **1.** an abnormal reaction to the environment, including anxieties, phobias, hysteria, and hypochondria. *n* **2.** a term that includes neurasthenia, hysteria, psychasthenia, and mental disorders short of insanity.

psychopathology, *n* **1.** the study of the causes, processes, and manifestations of mental disorders. *n* **2.** the behavioral manifestation of any mental disorder.

psychopharmacology (sī′kōfär′məkol′əjē), *n* the scientific study of the effects of drugs on behavior and normal and abnormal mental functions.

psychosedative (sī′kōsed′ətiv), *n* a calming agent that reduces anxiety and tension without depressing mental or motor functions.

psychosis (sīkō′sis), *n* a functional or organic kind of mental derangement marked by a severe disturbance of personality involving autistic thinking, loss of contact with reality, delusions or hallucinations.

psychosis, manic-depressive, *n* (cyclothymia) a psychosis characterized by varying periods of depression and excitement. One state may predominate (e.g., manic-depressive reaction, manic type).

psychosomatic (sīkōsōmat′ik), *adj* **1.** pertaining to the expression of an emotional conflict through physical symptoms. *adj* **2.** pertaining to the mind-body relationship; having bodily symptoms of a psychic, emotional, or mental origin. See also disease, psychosomatic.

psychosomatic factors, *n* See factor, psychosomatic.

psychosomatic, medicine, *n* the branch of medicine concerned with the interrelationships between mental and emotional reactions and somatic processes, in particular the manner in which intrapsychic conflicts influence physical symptoms.

psychotherapy, *n* any of a large number of related methods of treating mental or emotional disorders by psychologic techniques rather than by physical means.

PTA, *n* See plasma thromboplastin antecedent.

PTC, *n* See plasma thromboplastic component.

pterygoid, lateral (lateralis), (ter′igoid), *n* one of the four muscles of mastication that functions to open the jaws, protrude the mandible, and move the mandible from side to side. Also called the *external pterygoid muscle.*

pterygoid, medial (medialis), *n* one of the four muscles of mastication. It lies medial to the ramus of the mandible and functions with the temporalis and masseter muscles to close the mandible. Also called the *internal pterygoid muscle.*

pterygoid plexus of veins, *n* the collection of veins that unite with the retromandibular and facial veins to carry blood from the face and brain back to the heart. It can play a role in spreading dental infection to the brain.

pterygoid process, *n* See process, hamular.

pterygomandibular fold (raphe) (ter″īgomandib′ulər, rafə), *n* a fibrous band of tissue posterior to the most distal mandibular tooth that spans the area between the mandible and the point at which the hard and soft palates meet, from the hamulus to the posterior end of the mylohyoid line.

pterygomandibular space (triangle), *n* the space between the medial area of the mandible and the medial pterygoid muscle, a target area for administering local anesthesia to the inferior alveolar nerve.

pterygomaxillary fissure (ter′igōmak′səlerē), *n* See fissure, pterygomaxillary.

pterygomaxillary notch, *n* See notch, pterygomaxillary.

PTF, *n* See factor, plasma thromboplastin.

PTF-A (plasma thromboplastin factor A), *n* See factor VIII.

PTF-B (plasma thromboplastin factor B), *n* See factor IX.

PTF-C (plasma thromboplastin factor C), *n* See factor XI.

ptosis, *n* a drooping of the upper eyelid.

PTT, *n* See partial prothrombin time.

ptyalectasis (tī′əlek′təsis), *n* See sialoangiectasis.

ptyalin (tī′əlin), *n* a salivary enzyme that changes starch into sugars.

ptyalism (tī′əlizəm), *n* See sialorrhea.

puberty (pū′burtē), *n* the age at which the reproductive system becomes functional, with concurrent development of secondary sex characteristics. Marked by increased estrogenic activity in the female and rise of androgenic activity in the male.

pubescence (pūbes′əns), *n* the age of sexual maturity.

public health, *n* a field of medicine that deals with the physical and mental health of the community, particularly in such areas as water supply, waste disposal, air pollution, and food safety.

public health authority, n a governmental agency responsible for matters of public health.

public health dentistry, n See community dentistry.

public opinion, *n* the pooled judgment or attitude of the public in regard to a specific issue. Public opinion is generally determined by polling a sample of the population, using statistical tools. Elections are formal public opinion polls by which registered voter citizens register their choice of candidates and referenda.

public relations, *n* the art and science of promoting good will within the public by a corporation or governmental agency.

puerperal (pūer′pərəl), *adj* relating to or occurring during childbirth or the period immediately following. See also postpartum.

pulmonary edema (pŏŏl′məner′ē edē′mə), *n* the accumulation of extravascular fluid in lung tissues and alveoli, caused most commonly by congestive heart failure.

pulmonary embolism (em′bəliz′əm), *n* the blockage of a pulmonary artery by foreign matter such as fat, air, tumor tissue, or a thrombus that usually arises from a peripheral vein. It is difficult to distinguish from myocardial infarction and pneumonia.

pulp (dental) (pulp), *n* the tissue in the central portion of the tooth, made up of blood vessels, nerves, and cellular elements, including odontoblasts, that forms dentin and is covered by it. Also called *tooth pulp.*

pulp amputation, n See pulpotomy.

pulp, anachoresis of **(an′əkorē′sis),** *n* the localization of microbes from the bloodstream in a damaged pulp.

pulp canal, n See canal, pulp.

pulp capping, n See capping, pulp.

pulp cavity, n See cavity, pulp.

pulp chamber, n See chamber, pulp.

pulp, dental, n See pulp.

pulp extirpation, n See pulpectomy.

pulp horn, n See horn, pulp.

pulp involvement, n See involvement, pulp.

pulp, mummification of, n a dry gangrene of the dental pulp in which the pulp dries and shrivels.

pulp removal, n See pulpectomy.

pulp stone, n See denticle.

pulp test, n the application of a physical stimulus (electrical, heat, or cold) to determine the degree of vitality of the pulp tissue.

pulp test, thermal, n a method of applying a hot or cold stimulus to any tooth to assess the amount and degree of vitality of the structure. The clinician may use heated water, cold drinks, ice sticks, or blasts of air.

pulp tester, n (vitalometer) an electric device of high or low frequency designed to determine the response of a pulp to an electrical stimulus.

pulp, tooth, n See pulp.

pulp vitality, n the health status of the pulp. When the pulp tissue of a tooth has undergone complete degeneration or has been removed, the tooth is termed pulpless or nonvital.

pulpal (pul′pəl), *adj* relating to the pulp or the pulp cavity.

pulpalgia (pulpal′jēə), *n* the sensitivity of the pulp to pain.

pulpectomy (pulpek′təmē), *n* (pulp extirpation, pulp removal), the complete removal of a pulp from the pulp chamber and root canal.

pulpectomy, complete, n the surgical removal of the pulp to the dentinocemental junction at the apex of the root.

pulpectomy, partial, n the surgical removal of only a part of the contents of the canal(s).

pulpitis (pulpī′tis), *n* an inflammation of the pulpal tissue of a tooth.

pulpitis, hypertrophic (pulp polyp), n the formation and proliferation of

P

granulation tissue from the surface of an exposed pulp.

pulpless (pulp′les), *adj* having a nonfunctioning pulp (untreated), or a pulp that has been replaced with an inert material (treated).

pulpless tooth, *n* See tooth, pulpless.

pulpotomy (pulpot′əmē), *n* (pulp amputation), the surgical amputation of the dental pulp coronal to the dentinocemental junction.

pulpotomy, partial, *n* the surgical removal of only a part of the tissue in the pulpal chamber.

pulpotomy, total or complete, *n* the surgical removal of the entire contents of the pulpal chamber at the entrance of the root canal(s).

pulse (pls) (puls), *n* the rhythmic expansion and contraction of arteries resulting from the surges of blood through the arteries. The pulse can be felt by the fingers in arteries that are close to the skin.

pulse, arterial, *n* the pulsation of an artery produced by the rise and fall in blood pressure as the heart goes into systole and diastole and observed clinically by palpation of the radial artery. The pulse rate at birth is approximately 130 beats/min and diminishes to approximately 70 beats/min in the healthy adult. The range of normalcy is around 60 to 80 beats/min.

pulse, brachial **(brā′kēəl),** *n* the rhythmic expansion and contraction of the artery located at the inside of the arm at the elbow.

pulse, carotid **(kərot′id),** *n* the rhythmic expansion and contraction of the carotid arteries. The carotid pulse can be measured from palpation of the carotid artery on either side of the neck.

pulse pressure, *n* See pressure, pulse.

pulse, venous, *n* pulsation of a vein, most easily felt in the right jugular vein.

pumice (pum′is), *n* a type of volcanic glass used as an abrasive. It is prepared in various grits and is used for finishing and polishing in dentistry. It is also used in the polishing of natural teeth during a coronal polish but is being replaced by less abrasive synthetic particles in some polishing pastes. See also polishing, coronal.

punch biopsy, *n* the removal of tissue for diagnostic purposes using a sharp, cylindrical, hollow instrument placed over the tissue to be excised and rotated with slight pressure until an incision of proper depth is achieved. The tissue within the incision is lifted, and the base is excised with a scissor or scalpel blade.

punch, rubber dam, *n* an instrument used to punch holes of varying sizes in a rubber dam so that it may be applied to the teeth.

punctate (pungk′tāt), *n* indicated with dots or points distinguished from the adjacent region by elevation, texture, or color.

pupil, Argyll Robertson, *n.pr* the pupillary abnormalities associated with tabes dorsalis (neurosyphilis), manifested by miosis, the absence of a ciliospinal reflex, and a reaction to accommodation but not to light.

purchaser, *n* a program sponsor, often an employer or union, that contracts with the dental benefits organization to provide dental benefits to an enrolled population.

purchasing cooperative, *n* a group of dental professionals pooling their financial resources to purchase large quantities of supplies and equipment for the purpose of obtaining a discount.

purging (purj′ing), *n* an effort to rid the body of food by vomiting or taking laxatives or diuretics.

purpura (pur′pyoorə), *n* an extravasation of blood into the tissues, resulting in blue to black lesions of the skin or mucosa (petechiae and ecchymoses).

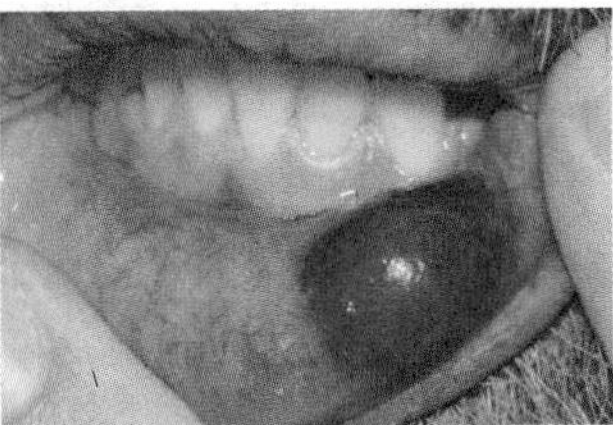

Purpura. (Neville/Damm/Allen/Bouquot, 2002)

purpura, allergic, *n* (anaphylactoid purpura) a thrombocytopenic or nonthrombocytopenic purpura related to an allergic reaction. Manifestations include the common symptoms of allergy.

***purpura, anaphylactoid* (an′əfəlak′toid),** *n* See purpura, allergic.

purpura, essential, *n* See purpura, thrombocytopenic, idiopathic.

***purpura hemorrhagica* (hem′əraj′ikə),** *n* See purpura, thrombocytopenic and purpura, thrombocytopenic, idiopathic.

purpura, idiopathic thrombocytopenic, *n* (essential purpura, land scurvy, primary purpura, purpura hemorrhagica) a type of unknown cause.

purpura, nonthrombocytopenic, *n* a type related to increased capillary permeability. Included are allergic purpuras and those resulting from vitamin C deficiency, bacterial toxins (scarlet fever, typhoid), drug intoxications, and metabolic toxins (nephritis, liver disease).

purpura, primary, *n* See purpura, thrombocytopenic, idiopathic.

purpura, secondary, *n* See purpura, thrombocytopenic, symptomatic.

purpura, symptomatic thrombocytopenic, *n* (secondary purpura) a type resulting from the effects of chemical, physical, vegetable, or animal agents or infections or related blood disorders.

***purpura, thrombocytopathic* (throm′bōsī′təpath′ik),** *n* a type associated with qualitative abnormalities of the platelets.

***purpura, thrombocytopenic* (throm′bōsī′təpē′nik),** *n* (essential thrombopenia, pseudohemophilia, hemorrhagica, Werlhof's disease) a type characterized by severe ecchymoses and petechiae associated with marked reduction in the numbers of blood platelets. There is prolonged bleeding time and poor clot retraction, but the coagulation and prothrombin times are normal. Hemorrhage may occur spontaneously from any area of the oral mucosa. This disease may be acute and fatal, whereas in other instances it may run a chronic course with intermittent attacks.

purpura, thrombotic thrombocytopenic, *n* a febrile disease of unknown cause characterized by hemolytic anemia, neurologic symptoms, hemorrhage into the skin and mucous membranes, icterus, hepatosplenomegaly, low platelet count, and platelet thrombi occluding capillaries and arterioles.

purulent discharge (pyoor′ūlent), *n* See pus.

pus (pus), *n* an inflammatory exudate formed within the tissues consisting of polymorphonuclear leukocytes, necrotic tissues, microorganisms, and tissue fluids. It may form within the tissues in periodontal disease and escape via the ulcerated pocket epithelium into the oral cavity. The material may be retained within the tissues when the opening of the periodontal pocket is blocked, thus creating a favorable circumstance for the formation of a periodontal abscess. It may also be involved in apical infections. Other term: *purulent discharge.* More current term: *suppuration.*

pustule (pus′chūl), *n* a vesicular lesion containing suppuration rather than clear fluid.

putrefaction (pū′trəfak′shən), *n* the rotting of matter through the use of enzymes, producing substances such as ammonia, mercaptans, and hydrogen sulfide.

putrescine (pūtres′ēn), *n* a foul-smelling toxic ptomaine produced by the decomposition of the amino acid ornithine during the decay of animal tissues, bacillus cultures, and fecal bacteria.

putty powder, *n* See tin oxide.

PVE, *n* an abbreviation for prosthetic valve endocarditis. See endocarditis, infective.

pyknic (pik′nik), *adj* characterized by a short, squat appearance especially of body structures.

pyknosis (piknō′sis), *n* increased basophilia and shrinkage of the nucleus of a dying cell.

pyogenic (pī′əjen′ik), *adj* suppuration-producing.

pyorrhea (pī′ərē′ə), *n* a term used to designate periodontal disease. Generally, it means "flow of pus," which previously was a feature of periodontal disease. Older term for *periodontal disease.*

P

pyramidal (pĭram′ĭdəl), *adj* having the shape that is peculiar to a pyramid (i.e., a solid with polygonal base and triangular faces that meet at a common point).

pyrazinamide (pir′əzin′əmīd′), *n brand name:* generic; *drug class:* antitubercular; *action:* bactericidal interference with lipid, nucleic acid biosynthesis; *use:* tuberculosis, as an adjunct with other drugs.

pyrexia (pīrek′sēə), *n* See fever.

pyridostigmine bromide (pir′ədōstig′mēn), *n brand names:* Mestinon, Regonol; *drug class:* cholinergic; *action:* inhibits destruction of acetylcholine, which increases concentration at sites where acetylcholine is released. This facilitates transmission of impulses across myoneural junction; *uses:* nondepolarizing muscle relaxant antagonist, myasthenia gravis.

pyridoxine deficiency (pir′idok′-sēn), *n* a lack of a required level of pyridoxine, which causes irritability and may lead to convulsions and peripheral neuritis.

pyridoxine HCl (pir′idok′sēn), *n* (vitamin B_6), *brand names:* Beesix, Nestrex; *drug class:* vitamin B_6, water soluble; *action:* needed for fat, protein, and carbohydrate metabolism as a coenzyme; *uses:* vitamin B_6 deficiency associated with inborn errors of metabolism, inadequate diet. See also vitamin B_6.

pyrimethamine (pir′imeth′əmēn), *n* a folic acid inhibitor that acts against *T. gondii* and *P. spp.*, which cause toxoplasmosis and malaria.

pyrolysis (pīrol′isis), *n* the breaking down of a substance through the application of heat.

pyromania (pī′rōmā′nēə), *n* an abnormal desire to start fires or an obsession with fire in general.

pyrometer (pīrom′ətur), *n* an instrument for measuring temperature by the change of electrical resistance within a thermocouple. It is a millivoltometer calibrated in degrees of temperature.

pyrophosphatase (pir′ōfos′fətās′), *n* an enzyme that cleaves an inorganic pyrophosphate from adenosyl triphosphate, leaving adenosine monophosphate.

pyrophosphate (pī′rōfos′fāt), *n* compound found in parotid saliva that helps delay calcification of bacteria plaque. It is also the active ingredient of commercial tarter-control oral hygiene products.

pyruvate kinase (pīroo′vāt kī′nās′), *n* an enzyme essential for anaerobic glycolysis in red blood cells.

pyuria (pīū′rēə), *n* abnormal numbers of white blood cells in the urine. Without proteinuria, it suggests infection of the urinary tract. With proteinuria, it suggests infection of the kidney (pyelonephritis).

Q

q.4.h. (quaque quarta hora), *adv* a Latin phrase meaning "every 4 hours"; used in prescription writing.

q.i.d. (quater in die), *adv* a Latin phrase meaning "four times a day"; used in prescription writing.

q.s. (quantum satis, quantum sufficit), *adv* a Latin phrase meaning "a sufficient quantity"; used in prescription writing.

quack, *n* one who professes to have medical or dental skill that is not possessed; one who practices medicine or dentistry without adequate preparation or proper qualification.

quad helix appliance, *n* a fixed, spring-loaded orthodontic appliance using four helix springs; used primarily to expand the maxillary dental arch.

quadrant, *n* one quarter of a circle; also used to describe one fourth of the combined dental arches. One half of the maxillary dental arch is one quadrant of the combined dental arches.

quadriplegia (kwod′rəplē′jēə), *n* an abnormal condition characterized by paralysis of both arms and legs and the trunk of the body below the level of the associated injury to the spinal cord.

qualified, *adj* having the required ability; fitted; entitled.

quality, *n* in reference to the voice, the acoustic characteristics of vowels resulting from their overtone structure or the relative intensities of their frequency component.

quality assessment, n **1.** the measurement of quality; generally includes the selection of an aspect of dental care or the dental care system to be evaluated; establishing criteria and standards for quality dental care and comparing treatment with these criteria and standards. *n* **2.** the measure of the quality of care provided in a particular setting.

quality assurance, n **1.** procedures for checking the quality of dental care provided by participating dental professionals and correcting any irregularities. Also called *quality control* or *quality evaluation. n* **2.** the assessment or measurement of the quality of care and the implementation of any necessary changes to maintain or improve the quality of care rendered.

quality assurance system, n a formally organized sequence of activities in dentistry that combines assessment of the existing situation, judgments about necessary changes, development of plans to effect such changes, implementation of these plans, and reassessment to determine that the desired changes have taken place.

quality of life, n a measure of the optimal energy or force that endows a person with the power to cope successfully with the full range of challenges encountered in the real world.

quality of radiation, n See radiation quality.

quality review committee, n a committee established by a professional organization or institution to assess and ensure quality. Unlike a peer review committee, it can function on its own initiative with regard to a broad range of topics.

quantum (kwon′təm), *n* a discrete unit of electromagnetic energy or of a roentgen. A quantity becomes quantized when its magnitude is restricted to a discrete set of values as opposed to a continuous set of values.

quantum theory, n See theory, quantum.

quarantine (kwôrantēn), *n* the isolation or confinement of a person or persons with a known or possible contagious disease.

quartz, *n* See silica.

quartz, fused, n a form of silica that is amorphous and exhibits no inversion at any temperature below its fusion point; of little use in dentistry.

quasi contract (kwäz′ē), *n* an obligation similar to a contract that arises not from an agreement of parties but from some relation between them or from a voluntary act of one of them.

quaternary (kwä′turnerē), *adj* having four elements. Widely used in medicine, quaternary ammonium salts are molecules containing four alkyl or aryl groups attached to a nitrogen atom.

quazepam (kwā′zəpam′), *n brand name:* Doral; *drug class:* benzodiazepine, sedative-hypnotic, Controlled Substance Schedule IV; *action:* produces central nervous system depression by interacting with a benzodiazepine receptor to facilitate the action of the inhibitory neurotransmitter γ-aminobutyric acid; *use:* insomnia.

quench, *v* to cool a hot object rapidly by plunging it into water or oil.

question, hypothetical, *n* a combination of assumed or proven facts and circumstances, stated so as to constitute a coherent and specific situation or state of facts, on which the opinion of an expert is asked by way of evidence at a trial.

questionnaire, *n* a form usually filled out by patients that provides data concerning their dental and general health.

questionnaire, health, n a list of key questions answered by the patient that permits the diagnostician to interpret the general and oral health of the patient.

quick-cure resin, *n* See resin, autopolymer.

quid, *n* See pinch.

quiescence (kwēes′ens), *n* a state of inactivity, quietness, or dormancy. In cell biology, it refers to that period when a cell is not dividing. E.g., if a neuron is not firing, or a muscle cell is not contracting, these cells are in a quiescent state.

quinacrine (kwin′əkrēn, -krin), *n* an anthelmintic and antiprotozoal agent used to treat giardiasis and tapeworm infections. It is not effective in treating malaria.

quinapril (kwin′əpril′), *n brand name:* Accupril; *drug class:* angiotensin-converting enzyme; *action:* selectively suppresses renin-angiotensin-aldosterone system; inhibits angiotensin-converting enzyme; prevents conversion of angiotensin I to angiotensin II; results in dilation of arterial and venous vessels; *use:* hypertension, alone or in combination with thiazide diuretics.

Quincke's disease (kwing′kēz), *n.pr* See edema, angioneurotic.

quinidine gluconate/quinidine polygalacturonate/quinidine sulfate (kwin′idēn, -din), *n brand names:* Cardioquin, CinQuin, Duraquin, Quinidex Extentabs, Quinora; *drug class:* antidysrhythmic (class IA); *action:* prolongs effective refractory period; decreases myocardial excitability, conduction velocity, and contractility; *uses:* premature ventricular contractions, atrial flutter and fibrillation, paroxysmal atrial tachycardia, ventricular tachycardia.

quinine (kwī′nīn), *n* an alkaloid derived from cinchona that is effective against malaria. It is also used as an antipyretic, analgesic, sclerosing agent, and stomachic and in the treatment of atrial fibrillation and myotonia congenita.

quinine sulfate, *n brand names:* Legatrin, M-Kya, Quinamm, Q-Vel; *drug class:* antimalarial; *action:* schizonticidal, but mechanism is unclear; increases refractory period in skeletal muscles; *uses: Plasmodium falciparum* malaria, nocturnal leg cramps.

quinolone (kwin′əlōn′), *n* a class of antibiotics that act by interrupting the replication of deoxyribonucleic acid molecules in bacteria.

quinsy, *n* a peritonsillar abscess.

quotient, *n* the number of times one amount is contained in another.

R

rabies (rā′bēz), *n* an acute, usually fatal viral disease of the central nervous system of animals. It is transmitted from animals to humans by infected blood, tissue, or most commonly, saliva.

racemic (rāsē′mik), *adj* referring to a mixture of equal quantities of the dextro- and levo-isomers of a compound.

rad (r), *n* a unit of absorbed dose of radiation: 1 r equals 100 ergs/Gm. See also rem.

radial keratotomy (ker′ətot′əmē), *n* a surgical procedure in which a series of tiny, shallow incisions are made on the cornea, causing it to bulge slightly to correct for nearsightedness. The operation is performed using local anesthesia and requires only a few minutes. Hospitalization is not necessary. Radial keratotomy usually corrects mild to moderate myopia.

radial pulse, *n* the pulse of the radial artery palpated at the wrist over the radius. The radial pulse is the one most often taken and recorded because of the ease with which it is located and palpated.

radiate (rā′dēāt), *v* **1.** to diverge or spread from a common point; to arrange in a radiating manner. *v* **2.** to expose to radiation, as x-radiation.

radiation (rā′dēā′shən), *n* **1.** the process of emitting radiant energy in the form of waves or particles. *n* **2.** the combined processes of emission, transmission, and absorption of radiant energy.

radiation, actinic, *n* radiation capable of producing chemical change (e.g., effect of light and roentgen rays on photographic emulsions).

radiation, background, *n* radiation arising from radioactive material other than the one directly under consideration. Background radiation resulting from cosmic rays and natural radioactivity is always present. Background radiation may also exist because of radioactive substances in other parts of a building (e.g., building material).

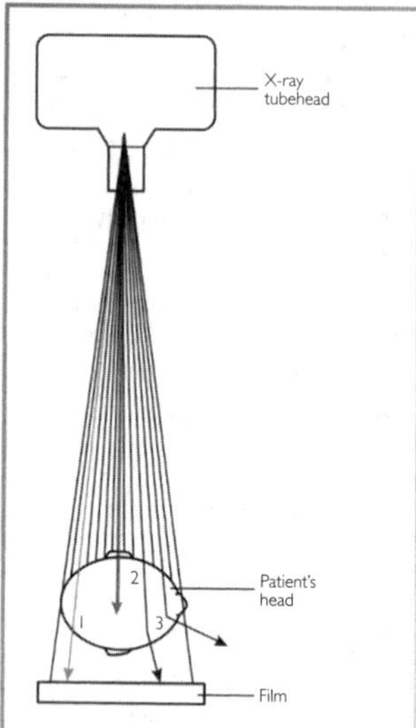

Radiation. (Bird/Robinson, 2005)

radiation, backscatter, *n* radiation that deflects off its target at an angle of deflection greater than 90°, possibly affecting those who may be off to the side of or behind the main beam. See also radiation, scattered.

radiation, biologic effectiveness of, *n* the ability of a particular type of ionizing radiation to produce biologic effects on an organism with small absorbed doses. See relative biologic effectiveness.

***radiation, bremsstrahlung* (brems-shträ′loong),** *n* (white), describes the distribution of roentgen rays from extremely low energy photons to roentgen rays originating from the highest kilovoltage applied to a radiographic tube. *Bremsstrahlung* translates to "braking radiation," referring to the sudden slowing of electrons that occurs when they encounter nuclei with a high positive charge.

radiation caries, *n* a type of tooth decay caused by the reduction in saliva that may result from the use of ionizing radiation in the treatment of oral and facial malignancies. Radiation caries is an unfortunate side effect of a necessary radical procedure to cure or prevent the spread of cancer.

radiation cataract, *n* a cataract that is caused by extended exposure of the eye to ionizing radiation in the course of treating facial cancers.

radiation, characteristic, *n* radiation that originates from an atom after removal of an electron or excitation of the nucleus. The wavelength of the emitted radiation is specific, depending only on the element concerned and on the particular energy levels involved. Also refers to the specific type of secondary radiation resulting when rays from a radio ray tube strike another substance, such as copper.

radiation, coherent scattering, *n* See coherent scattering.

radiation, Compton scatter, *n* See Compton scatter radiation.

***radiation, corpuscular* (kôrpus′kyə-lər),** *n* subatomic particles, such as electrons, protons, neutrons, or alpha particles, that travel in streams at various velocities. All the particles have definite masses and travel at various speeds. The properties are in opposition to electromagnetic radiations, which have no mass and travel in wave forms at the speed of light. See also radiation, electromagnetic.

radiation, cosmic, *n* See ray, cosmic.

***radiation, cumulative effect of* (kū′myələtiv),** *n* reactions vary depending on the dosage; if the radiation received is in several smaller doses, the reaction is not as severe as if the same amount of radiation is received all at once. Unless a tissue is completely destroyed by the radiation, some or all of it will be repaired, although cumulative damage may cause some irreparable conditions.

radiation, dermatitis, *n* See dermatitis, radiation.

radiation detector, *n* a device for converting radiant energy to a form more suitable for observation and recording. Examples include radiograph films and radiometers.

radiation, direct, *n* (primary radiation), radiation emanating from a tube aperture and comprising the useful beam, as compared with any stray radiation, such as that which comes from the tube container.

radiation, electromagnetic, *n* forms of energy propagated by wave motion, such as photons or discrete quanta. The radiations have no matter associated with them, as opposed to corpuscular radiations, which have definite masses. They differ widely in wavelength, frequency, and photon energy and have strikingly different properties. Covering an enormous range of wavelengths (from 10^{-6} to 10^{17} Å), they include radio waves, infrared waves, visible light, ultraviolet radiation, gamma rays, and cosmic radiation. See also radiation, corpuscular.

radiation exposure, *n* a measure of the ionization produced in air by roentgen rays or gamma rays. It is the sum of the electric charges on all ions of one sign that are produced when all electrons liberated by photons in a volume of air are completely stopped, divided by the mass of air in the volume element. The unit of exposure is the roentgen.

radiation field, *n* See radiographic beam, field size.

radiation, gamma, *n* See ray, gamma.

radiation, genetic effects of, *n* See genetic effects of radiation.

radiation, grenz, *n* See ray, grenz.

radiation, hard, radiation consisting of the short wavelengths (higher kilovolt peak equals greater penetration).

radiation hazard, *n* See hazard, radiation.

radiation, heterogeneous **(het′ərəj-ē′nēəs),** *n* a beam or "bundle" of radiation containing photons of many wavelengths.

radiation, homogeneous, *n* a beam of radiation consisting of photons that all have the same wavelength.

radiation hygiene, *n* See hygiene, radiation.

radiation intensity, *n* See intensity, radiation.

radiation, ionizing, *n* electomagnetic radiation such as roentgen rays and gamma rays; particulate radiation such as alpha particles, beta particles, protons, and neutrons; all other types of radiations that produce ionization directly or indirectly.

radiation leakage, *n* (stray radiation), the escape of radiation through the protective shielding of the radiography unit tube head. This radiation is detected at the sides, top, bottom, or back of the tube head; it does not include the useful beam.

radiation, monochromatic, *n* See radiation, homogeneous.

radiation necrosis, *n* See necrosis, radiation.

radiation, neutron, *n* See ray, neutron.

radiation oncology, *n* the study of the treatment of cancer using ionizing radiation

radiation osteomyelitis/osteonecrosis **(os′tēəmīəlītis os′tēōnəkrō′sis),** *n* an infection of the bone that occurs after exposure to radiation. Most commonly seen in cancer patients when radiation therapy damages healthy tissue surrounding the targeted tumor.

radiation, primary, *n* all radiation produced directly from the target in a radiographic tube. See also radiation, direct.

radiation protection, *n* provision designed to reduce exposure to radiation. For external radiation, this provision consists of using protective barriers of radiation-absorbing material, ensuring adequate distances from the radiation sources, reducing exposure time, and combinations of these measures. For internal radiation, it involves measures to restrict inhalation, ingestion, or other modes of entry of radioactive material into the body.

radiation quality, *n* the ability of a beam of radiographs to allow the production of diagnostically useful radiographs. Usually measured in half-value layers of aluminum and controlled by the kilovolt peak.

radiation quantity, *n* amount of radiation. The amount of exposure is expressed in roentgens (R), whereas quantity of dose is expressed in rads.

radiation, relative biologic effectiveness of (RBE), *n* a comparison between various types of ionizing radiation with respect to the ability to produce biologic effects with small doses.

radiation, remnant, *n* the radiation passing through an object or part being examined that is available either for recording on a radiographic film or for measurement.

radiation, scattered, *n* (backscatter radiation), radiation whose direction has been altered. It may include secondary and stray radiation.

radiation, secondary, *n* the new radiation created by primary radiation acting on or passing through matter.

radiation shield, *n* See shield, radiation.

radiation sickness, *n* a self-limited syndrome characterized by varying degrees of nausea, vomiting, diarrhea, and psychic depression after exposure to very large doses of ionizing radiation, particularly doses to the abdominal region. Its mechanism is not completely understood. It usually occurs a few hours after treatment and may subside within a day. It may be sufficiently severe to necessitate interrupting the treatment series, or it may incapacitate the patient.

radiation, soft, *n* radiation consisting of the long wavelengths (lower kilovolt peak results in less penetration).

radiation, speed of, *n* the speed of light, or approximately 186,000 miles per second.

radiation, stray, *n* See radiation leakage.

radiation survey, *n* See survey, radiation.

radiation therapy, *n* See therapy, radiation.

radiation, total body, *n* the exposure of the entire body to penetrating radiation. In theory, all cells in the body receive the same overall dose.

radiation treatment, *n* a cancer treatment method that uses roentgen rays to modify or destroy cancer cells; dental patients who are undergoing radiation therapy may exhibit an increased need for certain nutrients. See also therapy, radiation.

radiation, useful, *n* the part of the primary radiation that is permitted to pass from the tube housing through the tube head port, aperture, or collimating device. See beam, useful.

radical, *n* **1.** a group of atoms that acts together and forms a component of a compound. The group tends to remain bound together when a chemical reaction removes it from one compound and attaches it to another compound. A radical does not exist freely in nature. *adj* **2.** a drastic measure to cure or prevent the spread of a serious disease, such as the surgical removal of an organ, limb, or other body part.

radical neck dissection, *n* dissection and removal of all lymph nodes and removable tissues under the skin of the neck, performed to prevent the spread of malignant tumors of the head and neck that have a reasonable chance of being controlled by such aggressive treatment.

radicular (radik′ūlur), *adj* pertaining to the root. In restorative dentistry, the location at which the form of the preparation and restoration for the coronal portion of the natural tooth extends into the treated root canal of the pulpless tooth (e.g., radicular preparation, radicular restoration [dowel crown]).

radicular cyst, *n* See cyst, radicular.

radio-, *comb* denotes radiation from any source.

radioactive decay, *n* See decay, radioactive.

radioactive isotope, *n* See radioisotope.

radioactive tracer, *n* a molecule to which a radioactive atom has been attached so that it can be followed through a physiologic system with radiation detectors.

radioactivity (rā′dēōaktiv′itē), *n* spontaneous nuclear disintegration with emission of corpuscular or electromagnetic radiations. The principal types of radioactivity are alpha disintegration, beta decay (negatron emission, positron emission, and electron capture), and isometric transition. Double beta decay is another type of radioactivity that has been postulated, and spontaneous fission and the spontaneous transformations of mesons are sometimes considered to be types of radioactivity. To be considered radioactive, a process must have a measurable lifetime between approximately 1 and 10 seconds and 1017 years, according to present experimental techniques. Radiations emitted within a time too short for measurement are called *prompt;* however, prompt radiations, including gamma rays, characteristic roentgen rays, conversion and auger electrons, delayed neutrons, and annihilation radiation, are often associated with radioactive disintegrations because their emission may follow the primary radioactive process.

radioallergosorbent test (RAST) (rā′dēōəler′gōsor′bənt), *n* a test to determine whether an atopic allergy to a substance exists. A radioimmunoassay is used to identify and quantify IgE in serum that has been mixed with any of 45 known allergens. This is an in vitro method of demonstrating allergic reactions, as opposed to the patch test, which is the common in vivo method of determining allergens.

radiobiology, *n* the branch of the natural sciences dealing with the effects of radiation on biologic systems.

radiogram (rā′dēōgram), *n* See radiograph.

radiograph(s) (rā′dēōgraf), *n* an image or picture produced on a radiation-sensitive film emulsion by exposure to ionizing radiation directed through an area, region, or substance of interest, followed by chemical processing of the film. It basically depends on the differential absorption of radiation directed through heterogeneous media. See also x-ray.

radiograph, bite-wing (BWX), *n* a form of dental radiograph that reveals approximately the coronal halves of the maxillary and mandibular teeth and portions of the interdental alveolar septa on the same film. Bite-wings can be used at any point in the dental arch. Older term: *x-ray.*

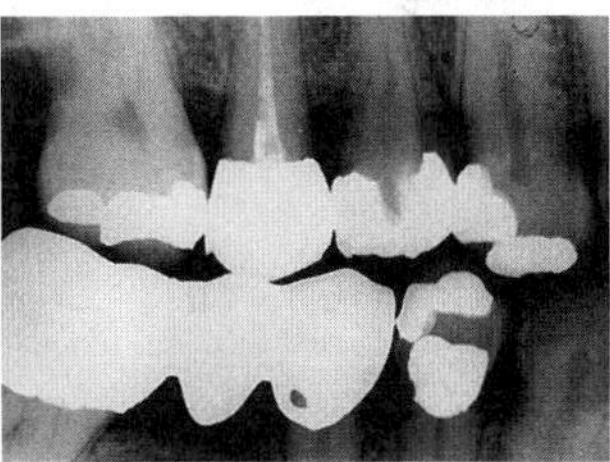

Bite-wing radiograph. (Frommer/Stabulas-Savage, 2005)

radiograph, body-section, *n* radiograph produced by rotation of the film and roentgen ray source around the region of interest in opposite directions during exposure, so as to blur interposed anatomic structures outside the region of interest.

radiograph, cephalometric **(sef′əlōmet′rik),** *n* a radiograph of the head made with precise reproducible relationships between radiograph source, subject, and film. The generally accepted distances between radiograph source and the center of the subject are 5 feet (152.4 cm) or 150 cm. The distance between subject and film is usually 12 cm but may be standardized at a different value or varied with patient size and recorded for each exposure. The two standard orientations are lateral (profile) and posteroanterior.

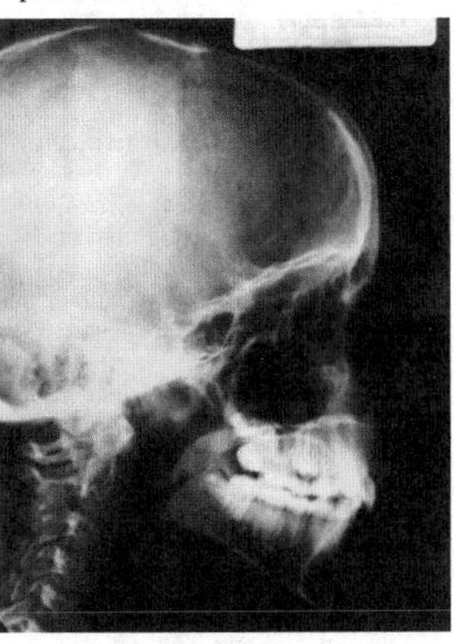

Cephalometric radiograph. (Bird/Robinson, 2005)

radiograph, composite, *n* radiograph made by superimposing a radiograph of osseous tissue whose exposed border has been cut away on a radiograph of soft tissue for the purpose of detecting radiographic information concerning both the soft tissues and the osseous tissues of the head and face from a single radiographic view.

radiograph, contrast media, *n* radiograph that records the shadow images of the secretory apparatus of any of the salivary glands, body cavities, or fistulous tracts after the injection of a liquid radiopaque solution.

radiograph, extraoral, *n* radiograph produced on a film placed extraorally.

radiograph, follow-up, *n* radiographs made during and after therapy to follow the progress or regress of a disease, determine the course of healing, or ascertain the results of treatment.

radiographs, full mouth (FMX), *n* a visual image of the entire oral cavity produced by radiography. They are repeated often in order to track a patient's oral history.

radiograph, high kilovoltage, *n* a radiograph taken using a higher kilovoltage than normal. This method provides a lower contrast film with more interpretive details and can be developed in a shorter time, but it subjects the surrounding areas to more radiation.

radiograph, intraoral, *n* radiograph produced by placing a radiographic film within the oral cavity. See also radiography, oral.

radiograph, microscopic examination, *n* See microradiography.

radiograph, occlusal, *n* a special type of intraoral radiograph made with the film held between the occluded teeth.

radiograph, oral, *n* the radiographic representation of shadow images of all the tissues, structures, and regions of the oral cavity and its adjacent areas and associated parts.

radiograph, panoramic, *n* a tomogram of the jaws, taken with a specialized machine designed to present a panoramic view of the full circumferential length of the jaws on a single film. Also known by several brand names of machines, most of which incorporate *pan* into the name.

radiograph, reference, *n* a training tool in which ideal dental radiographs are compared with recently taken radiographs to study, compare, and improve interpretation and investigative skills in dental office employees.

radiograph, salivary gland, *n* See sialography.

radiograph, stereoscopic **(ster′ēə-skop′ik),** *n* a pair of radiographs of a structure made by shifting the position of the radiographic tube a few centimeters between each of two exposures. Such pairs provide a three-dimensional, or stereoscopic, presentation of the recorded images.

radiograph, Towne's projection, *n.pr* the radiographic view of the mandibular condyles and the midfacial skeleton.

radiographer (rā′dēog′rəfur), *n* a specialist or technician in radiography.

radiographer anatomy, *n* See anatomy, radiographic.

radiographer contrast, *n* See contrast, radiographic.

radiographer density, *n* See density, radiographic.

radiographer diagnosis, *n* See diagnosis, radiographic.

radiographer examination, *n* See examination, radiographic.

radiographer grid, *n* a clear plastic device with the horizontal and vertical wires crossing each other at intervals of 1 mm; used in radiography techniques for the purpose of measurement.

radiographer interpretation, *n* See interpretation, radiographic.

radiographer localization, *n* See localization, radiographic.

radiographer, oral, *n* a specialist or technician in oral radiography.

radiographer survey, *n* See survey, radiographic.

radiographic (rā′dēōgraf′ik), *adj* relating to the process of radiography, the finished product, or its use.

radiographic beam, *n* the beam that emanates from a radiographic tube. X-ray photons produced at the target in the tube leave the tube as a divergent beam.

radiographic film, air bubbles on, *n* See film fault, white spots.

radiographic film sizes, *n* nonscreen films (e.g., No. 0, 22 × 35 mm; No. 1, 24 × 40 mm, No. 2, 31 × 41 mm; No. 3, 27 × 54 mm; and No. 4, 57 × 76 mm) or (e.g., 5 × 7 in, 5 × 12 in, and 8 × 10 in) used to produce radiographic images.

radiographic film storage methods, *n* an appropriate method of safekeeping to maintain the integrity of the materials (e.g., the placement of items in regions that will prevent exposure to radiation, heat, vapors from chemical substances, and moisture), as well as the creation of a filing system that ensures the oldest product is used first.

R

radiographic tube, *n* a vacuum tube containing electrodes that accelerate electrons and direct them to a metal anode where their impact produces a radiograph.

radiography (rā′dēog′rəfē), *n* the making of shadow images on photographic emulsion by the action of ionizing radiation. The image is the result of the differential attenuation of the radiation in its passage through the object being radiographed. *Roentgenography* refers to production of film by the use of roentgen rays only.

radiography, bone in, *n* radiography of bone and marrow tissue. Translucencies and opacities in bone in radiographs depend on the different densities that bone and marrow spaces present to the roentgen rays. The configuration of bone tissue represents the topography and arrangement of bone trabeculae, which register as opaque in contrast to the translucency of the marrow spaces.

radiography, computerized digital, *n* a radiography machine using computer technology to produce a digital image instead of using film; a digital sensor is placed in a disposable sheath inside the patient's oral cavity; then the sensor is exposed to radiation as in a traditional radiograph, except that the sensor produces an immediately accessible digital image that can be viewed on a computer screen.

radiography, digital subtraction, *n* a technique for eliminating unnecessary anatomic structures on a radiographic image by storing the pre- and postprocedure images in a computer and then combining them together digitally to display the final subtracted image, which emphasizes the differences between the two original films.

radiography, oral, *n* the specialized operative and technical procedures and practices for making successful radiographic surveys, with the understanding that it involves the selection of the dental radiography unit and its adjustments as well as the generation and application of roentgen rays to all phases of interest to the dental profession. It also takes into consideration all the processes necessary for the production of finished radiographs of the teeth and their supporting tissues, adjacent regions, and associated parts. See also radiograph(s).

radiography, subtraction, *n* the digital or photographic manipulation of a radiograph in which background images are eliminated to highlight areas for pre- and postoperative comparison.

radioisotope (rā′dēōī′sōtōp), *n* a chemical element that has been made radioactive through bombardment of neutrons in a cyclotron or atomic pile or found in a natural state.

radioisotope scan, *n* a two-dimensional representation of the gamma rays emitted by a radioisotope, showing its concentration in a body site such as the thyroid gland, brain, or kidney. Radioisotopes used in diagnostic scanning may be administered intravenously or orally.

radiologist (rā′dēol′əjist), *n* a person who has special experience in the science of radiant energy and radiant substances (including roentgen rays); especially a person engaged in the branch of medical science that deals with the use of radiant energy in the diagnosis and treatment of disease.

radiologist, oral, *n* a specialist in the art and science of oral radiology.

radiology (rā′dēol′əjē), *n* **1.** the branch of medicine dealing with the diagnostic and therapeutic applications of ionizing radiation. *n* **2.** the science of radiant energy, its use toward the extension of present knowledge, and its diverse beneficial applications.

radiology, oral, *n* all phases of the science and art of radiology that are of interest to the dental profession. Oral radiology involves the generation and application of roentgen rays for the purpose of recording shadow images of teeth and their supporting tissues, adjacent regions, and associated parts. It also includes the interpretation of the radiographic findings.

radiolucence (rā′dēōloo′sens), *n* relative term indicating the comparatively low attenuation of a radiographic beam produced by materials of relatively low atomic number. The image on a radiograph of such materials is relatively dark because of the greater amount of radiation that penetrates to reach the film.

radiolucency (rā′dēōloo′sensē), *n* a radiographic representation of decreased density of hard and soft tissue structures.

radiolucent (rā'dēōloo'sent), *adj* permitting the passage of radiant energy, with relatively little attenuation by absorption. The image of radiolucent materials on a radiograph ranges from shades of gray to black.

radiolysis of water (rādēōl'isis), *n* a separation of water via radioactive activity. The end result is the production of hydrogen peroxide.

radionuclide (rā'dēōnoo'klīd), *n* an unstable or radioactive type of atom characterized by the constitution of its nucleus and capable of existing for a measurable time. The nuclear constitution is specified by the number of protons *(A),* number of neutrons *(N),* and energy content, or alternatively by the atomic number *(Z),* mass number *(A – N + Z),* and atomic mass.

radiopacity (rā'dēōpas'itē), *n* relative term referring to the considerable attenuation of a radiographic beam produced by materials of relatively high atomic number. The image on a radiograph of such materials is relatively light because less radiation passes through, which prevents the exposure of the film in that area.

radiopaque (rā'dēōpāk'), *adj* permitting the passage of radiant energy, but only with considerable or extreme attenuation of the radiation by absorption. The image of radiopaque materials on a radiograph ranges from light gray to total white or clarity on the film. See also medium, radiopaque.

radioparent (rā'dēōper'ent), *adj* made visible by means of roentgen rays or other means of radiation. Permitting the passage of radiographs or other radiation.

radiopharmacy, *n* a facility for the preparation and dispensing of radioactive drugs and the storage of radioactive materials, inventory records, and prescriptions of radioactive substances. It is usually the correlation point for radioactive wastes, the unit responsible for waste disposal or storage and the center for clinical investigations using radioactive tracers.

radioresistance (rā'dēōrēzis'təns), *n* the relative resistance of cells, tissues, organs, or organisms to the injurious effects of ionizing radiation. See also radiosensitivity.

radiosensitivity (rā'dēōsen'sitiv'itē), *n* relative susceptibility of cells, tissues, organs, organisms, and other substances to the injurious action of radiation.

radiotherapy, *n* the treatment of neoplastic disease by using roentgen rays or gamma rays to prevent or slow the proliferation of malignant cells by decreasing the rate of mitosis or impairing deoxyribonucleic acid synthesis. See therapy, radiation.

radium (Ra) (rā'dēəm), *n* a radioactive metallic element of the alkaline earth groups. Its atomic number is 88. Four radium isotopes occur naturally and have different atomic weights: 223, 224, 226, and 228.

radium emanation, *n* radon. An element, used in radiotherapy, produced when radium disintegrates.

radon, *n* A byproduct of radium decomposition used in radiotherapy.

radon seed (rā'don), *n* a small sealed container or tube for carrying radon. It is made of gold or glass, is inserted into the tissues for the treatment of certain disease entities, and is visible radiographically.

rale (rāl), *n* **1.** abnormal sound that originates from the trachea, bronchi, or lungs. *v* **2.** to make such a sound.

Ramfjord teeth index (ram'fyurd), *n.pr* See index, periodontal.

ramify (ram'əfī), *v* to branch; to diverge in various directions; to traverse in branches.

ramipril (ram'əpril), *n brand name:* Altace; *drug class:* angiotensin-converting enzyme (ACE) inhibitor; *action:* selectively suppresses renin-angiotensin-aldosterone system; inhibits ACE; prevents conversion of angiotensin I to angiotensin II; results in dilation of arterial and venous vessels; *uses:* hypertension, alone or in combination with thiazide diuretics; congestive heart failure immediately after myocardial infarction.

ramus (rā'məs), *n* **1.** a branch of an artery, nerve, or vein. In the *Basle Nomina Anatomica* terminology, the term ramus is given to a primary division of a nerve or blood vessel. *n* **2.** any constant branch of a fissure, or sulcus, of the brain.

ramus, ascending **(rā′məs),** *n* the posterior, vertical portion of the mandible, which extends from the corpus to the condyle, and makes a joint at the temple. There are right and left ascending rami.

ramus graft, *n* See graft, ramus.

ramus, mandibular, *n* the upturned, angled bony process of the mandible that extends upward and backward from the horseshoe-shaped body and terminates in two processes: the articular condyloid process and the coronoid process.

random controlled trial, *n* a study plan for a proposed new treatment in which subjects are assigned on a random basis to participate in either an experimental group receiving the new treatment or a control group that does not.

random-access memory (RAM), *n* the part of a computer's memory available to execute programs and temporarily store data. The memory to which the operator has random access can usually be used for both reading and writing. Unless the file has been saved, RAM data are automatically erased when the computer is turned off.

range, *n* a crude measure of dispersion in a distribution; range is computed as the distance from the highest score to the lowest score plus one unit.

range, melting, *n* the temperature range from the time an alloy begins to melt until it is completely molten. It varies from 100°F to 200°F (38°C to 70°C), in gold-platinum-palladium alloys.

range of motion, *n* the maximum extent to which the parts of a joint can move in extension and flexion as measured in degrees of a circle.

ranitidine (rənit′ədēn′), *n brand name:* Zantac, Zantac EFFERdose, Zantac GELdose, Zantac 75; *drug class:* H_2-histamine receptor antagonist; *action:* inhibits histamine at H_2 receptor sites in parietal cells, which inhibit gastric acid secretion; *uses:* duodenal ulcers, gastric ulcers, hypersecretory conditions, gastroesophageal reflux disease.

Rankine scale (rang′kin), *n.pr* an absolute temperature scale calculated in degrees Fahrenheit. Absolute zero on the Rankine scale is –460°F, equivalent to –273°C.

ranula (ran′ūlə), *n* a large mucocele in the floor of the oral cavity. It usually results from obstruction of the ducts of the sublingual salivary glands. Less often, it results from obstruction of the ducts of the submandibular salivary glands.

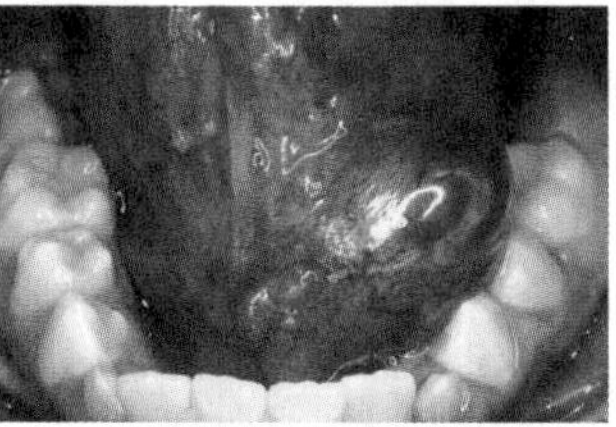

Ranula. (Neville/Damm/Allen/Bouquot, 2002)

Ranvier, nodes of (rän′vēā′), *n.pr* See node of Ranvier.

raphe (ra′fe), *n* (*pl* **raphae**) a crease or ridge that divides an organ in half.

raphe, median palatine (ra′fe), *n* the ridge of oral mucosa that marks the median line of the hard palate and the median palatine suture between the two palatal shelves to form the secondary palate embryonically.

rapport, *n* a sense of mutuality and understanding; harmony, accord, confidence, and respect underlying a relationship between two persons; an essential bond between a therapist and patient.

rare earth, *n* metallic elements used in intensifying screens. Also refers to fast-exposure roentgen-ray screen film.

rare earth screen, *n* a fluorescent material such as calcium tungstate used as the basis of roentgen-ray intensifying screens. In recent years, new materials, including the rare earths yttrium and gadolinium, have also found application in such devices. These rare earths enable lower radiation doses to be used while producing acceptable film densities.

rarefaction, bone, *n* See bone rarefaction.

rash, wandering, *n* See tongue, geographic.

rat, Sprague-Dawley, *n.pr* an inbred strain of albino rat commonly used in laboratory research. There are 12 strains of inbred rats listed under "Medical Subject Headings," a supplement to *Index Medicus.* The Wistar rat is an equally popular inbred strain of albino rat used in laboratory research.

ratchet wrench, *n* a wrench activated by its handle through a hinged catch (pawl) that causes the wrench to rotate in one direction only (may be adjusted for either direction).

rate, *n* measurement of a thing by its ratio or given in relation to some standard.

rate, basal metabolic, *n* See basal metabolic rate.

rate, DEF, *n* an expression of dental caries experience in primary teeth. The DEF rate is calculated by adding the number of decayed primary teeth requiring filling (D), decayed primary teeth requiring extraction (E), and primary teeth successfully filled (F). Missing primary teeth are not included in the count because whether they were extracted because of caries or exfoliated normally is often impossible to determine.

rate, DMF index, *n* a method of classifying the condition of the teeth based on the number of teeth in a given oral cavity that are decayed, missing, or indicated for removal and of those filled or bearing restorations.

rate, erythrocyte sedimentation **(ərith'rōsīt' sed'əməntā'shən),** *n* the rate of settling of erythrocytes by gravity under conditions in which all factors affecting the rate are corrected, standardized, or eliminated except for alterations in the physicochemical properties of the plasma proteins. These alterations are the basis for interpretation of the rate. There is an increase in the rate in most infections. Sedimentation velocity is useful in prognosis to determine recovery from infection. Normal values vary with the method used in the determination.

rate, heart, *n* the rate of the heartbeat, expressed as the number of beats per minute. The heart rate is reflected in the pulse rate. The cardiac rate of contraction is described as normal (70 beats/min), rapid (more than 100 beats/min), or slow (less than 55 beats/min). Disturbances in heart rate and rhythm may be paroxysmal or persistent. Descriptive terms are *tachycardia* (increased, shallow heart rate to compensate for inadequate cardiac output) and *bradycardia* (slow, firm heart rate caused by cardiac sinus mechanisms and the vagal effect over the sympathetic innervation of the heart).

rate, survival, *n* the percentage of survivals within a certain study; in dentistry, it refers to the percentage of implants that are functioning within acceptable standards.

ratification (rat'ifikā'shən), *n* confirmation of a previous act.

ratio, *n* proportion; comparison.

ratio, A:G, *n* the ratio of the protein albumin to globulin in the blood serum. On the basis of differential solubility with neutral salt solution, the normal values are 3.5 to 5 Gm% for albumin and 2.5 to 4 Gm% for globulin.

ratio, clinical crown: clinical root, *n* the proportion of the length of the portion of the tooth lying coronal to the epithelial attachment to the length of the portion of the root lying apical to the epithelial attachment. Radiographically the clinical crown is the portion of the tooth coronal to the alveolar crest; the clinical root is the part of the root apical to the alveolar crest. The radiographic crown: root ratio is useful in the evaluation and prognosis of periodontal disease.

ratio, crown-implant, *n* the proportional relationship between the height of the crown to the length of the implant that is surrounded by bone; the height of the crown is described as the length from the topmost point of the artificial crown to the point where the implant comes into contact with the bone.

ratio, grid, *n* the relation of the height of the lead strips to the width of the nonopaque material between them. Common grid ratios are 2:8, 2:12, and 2:16.

ratio, water:powder, *n* relative amounts of water and powder (usually gypsum products) in a mixture.

rationale (rash'ənal'), *n* the fundamental reasons used as the basis for a decision or action.

ray(s), *n* a line of light, heat, or other form of radiant energy. A ray is a more or less distinct or isolated portion of radiant energy, whereas the word *rays* is a very general term for any form of radiant energy, whether vibratory or particulate.

ray, alpha, *n* See particle, alpha.

ray, beta, *n* See particle, beta.

ray, cathode, *n* See electron stream.

ray, central, *n* the center of a radiographic beam.

ray, cosmic, *n* radiation that originates outside the earth's atmosphere. Cosmic rays have extremely short wavelengths. They are able to produce ionization as they pass through the air and other matter and are capable of penetrating many feet of material such as lead and rock. The primary cosmic rays probably consist of atomic nuclei (mainly protons), some of which may have energies of the order of 1010 to 1015 eV. Secondary cosmic rays are produced when the primary cosmic rays interact with nuclei and electrons (e.g., in the earth's atmosphere). Secondary cosmic rays consist mainly of mesons, protons, neutrons, electrons, and photons that have less energy than the primary rays. Practically all the primary cosmic rays are absorbed in the upper atmosphere. Almost all cosmic radiation observed at the earth's surface is of the secondary type.

ray, gamma, *n* photons with a shorter wavelength than those ordinarily used in diagnostic medical and dental radiography and that originate in the nuclei of atoms. A quantum of electromagnetic radiation emitted by a nucleus as a result of a quantum transition between two energy levels of the nucleus; e.g., as a radioisotope decays, it gives off energy, some of which may be in the form of gamma radiation.

ray, grenz **(grents),** *n* roentgen rays that are greater in length than 1 Å; used in radiography of soft tissues, insects, flowers, and microscopic sections of teeth and surrounding tissues. These rays are the result of using approximately 10 to 20 kV in a specially constructed radiation-generating device. They have a wavelength of about 2 Å.

ray, neutron, *n* particulate ionizing radiation consisting of neutrons. On impact with nuclei or atoms, neutrons possess enough kinetic energy to set the nuclei or atoms in motion with sufficient velocity to ionize matter or enter into nuclear reactions that result in the emission of ionizing radiation. The former variety is usually called the fast neutron, and the latter the thermoneutron, with gradations of epithermal and slow neutrons between them.

ray, roentgen (r) **(rent′gən),** *n* an international unit based on the ability of radiation to ionize air. The exposure to x- or gamma radiation such that the associated corpuscular emission per 0.001293 g of air produces, in air, ions carrying 1 esu of quantity of electricity of either sign (2.083 billion ion pairs).

Raynaud's phenomenon (rānōz′), *n* spasm of the digital arteries with blanching and numbness of the extremities, induced by chilling, emotional states, or other diseases.

RBC, *n* See red blood cell count.

RBE, *n* See radiation, biologic effectiveness of, relative.

RDA, *n.pr* an abbreviation for the **Recommended Dietary Allowances** of the Food and Nutrition Board of the National Research Council.

RDH, *n* an abbreviation for **registered dental hygienist.**

reaction (rēak′shən), *n* opposite action, or counteraction; the response of a part to stimulation; a chemical process in which one substance is transformed into another substance or substances.

reaction, acute dystonic **(diston′ik),** *n* extreme contraction of the jaw muscles, which can result in dislocation of the jaw bones and difficulty in opening the oral cavity. These symptoms may be caused by an adverse reaction to an antipsychotic drug.

reaction, alarm, *n* the first stage of the general adaptation syndrome of Hans Selye; occurs in response to severe physical and psychologic distress. Complete mobilization of body resources occurs in association with activity of the pituitary and adrenal glands and the sympathetic nervous system. See also syndrome, general adaptation.

reaction, anaphylactoid **(an′əfəlak′-toid),** *n* a reaction that resembles anaphylactic shock; probably caused by the liberation of histamine, serotonin, or other substances as a consequence of the injection of colloids or finely suspended material.

reaction, Arthus', *n.pr* See anaphylactic hypersensitivity.

reaction, heterophil **(het′ərōfil′),** *n* a heterophil agglutination test that measures the agglutination of the red blood cells of sheep by the serum of patients with infectious mononucleosis.

reaction, -id, secondary skin eruptions occurring at a distance from the primary lesion (e.g., tuberculid).

reaction, immune, *n* altered reactivity of the tissues to a foreign substance that was previously introduced into the body or in contact with it.

reaction, leukemoid **(lookē′moid′),** *n* an increase in normal or abnormal white blood cells in nonleukemic conditions; simulates myelogenous, lymphatic, and rarely, monocytic leukemia.

reaction, Shwartzman, *n.pr* an antigen AB local tissue response that occurs when an intravenous injection or challenge of a bacterial endotoxin that had previously been inoculated intradermally results in a hemorrhagic, often necrotic inflammatory lesion.

reaction, tissue, *n* the response of tissues to altered conditions.

reactor (rēak′tur), *n* an apparatus in which nuclear fission may be sustained in a self-supporting reaction at a controlled rate.

read-only memory (ROM), *n* the portion of a computer's memory in which information is permanently stored. The operator has random access to the memory but only for purposes of reading the contents. Special equipment is required to write or erase a read-only memory.

reading, lip, *n* a method of communication in which the motions of the oral cavity and face are "read" as a person is speaking. The British term is *speech reading.*

reagent (rēā′jənt), *n* a chemical substance known to react in a specific way.

reagin(s) (rē′ājin), *n* noncommittal term used for antibodies or antibody-like substances that differ in several respects from ordinary antibodies. It refers to the antibodies of allergic conditions (atopy) and to the antibody (reagin) concerned with the flocculation and complement fixation tests for syphilis.

real time, *n* an application of computerized equipment allowing data to be processed with relation to ongoing external events so that the operators can make immediate decisions based on the current data output. Ultrasound scanning uses real-time control systems, making results available almost simultaneously with the generation of the input data.

reamer (rē′mur), *n* an instrument with a tapered metal shaft, more loosely spiraled than a file; used to enlarge and clean root canals.

reasonable and customary (R&C) plan, *n* a dental benefits plan that determines benefits based only on "reasonable and customary" fee criteria. See also usual fee; customary fee; reasonable fee.

reasonable fee, *n* the fee charged by a dental professional for a specific dental procedure that has been modified by the nature and severity of the condition being treated and by any medical or dental complications or unusual circumstances; therefore may differ from the dental professional's "usual" fee or the benefit administrator's "customary" fee.

reasonably prudent person doctrine, *n* the concept that a person of ordinary sense will use ordinary care and skill in meeting the health care needs of a patient.

reattachment, *n* in dentistry the reattachment of the gingival epithelium to the surface of the tooth.

rebase, *v* a process of refitting a denture by replacing the denture base material without changing the occlusal relations of the teeth.

rebound (rē′bownd), *n/v* **1.** a recovery from illness. *n* **2.** an outbreak of fresh reflex activity after withdrawal of a stimulus

rebreathing, *n* breathing into a closed system. Exhaled gas mixes with the gas in the closed system, and some of this mixture is then reinhaled. Rebreathing is used as part of a general anesthesia technique in which a rebreathing bag functions as a reservoir for anesthetic gases and oxygen. The bag may be squeezed or pumped to assist in proper respiration while the patient is under deep anesthesia.

recall, *n* the procedure of advising or reminding a patient to have his oral health reviewed or reexamined; an important phase of preventive dentistry. Term is being replaced by *preventive maintenance appointment.*

receipt, *n* a written acknowledgment by one person of having received money or something of value from another.

receipt book, *n* the book in which one of the dental staff fills out forms verifying that a specific amount of money has been paid to the account.

reception room, *n* the area within the physical plant of the dental establishment through which patients enter the office. This is also the room in which patients await the attentions of the dental professional or receptionist. Older term: *waiting room.*

receptor(s) (rēsep′tur), *n* a site or location within a cell or its membrane that combines with a haptophore group of a toxin, drug, enzyme, hormone, or other substance and that may elicit a specific or general response; a sensory nerve terminal that responds to stimuli of various kinds.

receptor, sensory, *n* receptor system built on the theory that receptor organs are specialized and respond to the law of specific nerve energies; i.e., each type of end-organ, no matter what stimulus is applied, will respond (if it responds) with only a single appropriate type of sensation. Common experience shows this to be true; e.g., when a person receives a blow to the eye, light is experienced as a consequence of the blow. Another factor is that the impulse will travel in only one direction, from the receptor organ back to the central nervous system. The receptor system is thus the summation in the brain of all the sensory stimuli that come from the special senses, general senses, mucous membrane, skin, and deeper tissues and is the basis for instruction sent to the musculoskeletal system for action, as in the masticatory phenomenon.

receptors, adrenergic, *n* alpha and beta "units" associated with sympathetic neuroeffectors that react with sympathomimetic drugs to elicit the response of the effector cells.

receptors, beta, *n* sites on some cell membranes in the sympathetic nervous system that either activate or block the normal functions of the cell by binding with epinephrine (adrenaline). Cells with beta receptors normally control physiologic responses such as heart rate.

recession (rēsesh′ən), *n* a moving back or withdrawal.

recession, bone, *n* apical progression of the level of the alveolar crest associated with inflammatory and dystrophic periodontal disease; a bone resorption process that results in decreased osseous support for the tooth.

recession, gingival, *n* atrophy of the gingival margin associated with inflammation, apical migration (proliferation) of the epithelial attachment, and resorption of the alveolar crest.

recession, periimplant, *n* the loss of gingival tissues around a dental implant.

recidivism (rəsid′əviz′əm), *n* **1.** the tendency for an ill person to relapse or return to the hospital. *n* **2.** the return to a life of crime after a conviction and sentence.

recipient (rēsip′ēənt), *n* the person who receives a blood transfusion, tissue graft, or organ; also, a person who has received an honor, award, or grant.

recipient site, *n* the site into which a graft or transplant material is placed. See also donor site.

reciprocal arm (rēsip′rəkəl), *n* See arm, reciprocal.

reciprocal forces, *n.pl* the typical method of applying corrective orthodontic forces; each applied force is balanced by a reciprocal force elsewhere in the dentition or surrounding structures.

reciprocating action device, *n* a handheld, power-driven finishing tool with interchangeable tips that is used to shape, smooth, recontour, and polish restorations.

reciprocation (rēsip′rōkā′shən), *n* the means by which one part of a removable partial denture framework is made to counter the effect created by another part of the framework.

reciprocation, active, *n* reciprocation in a clasp unit achieved by the use of two opposing and balanced retentive clasp arms. Reciprocation cannot be achieved unless a similar and balanced arrangement on the opposite side of the dental arch occurs.

reciprocation, passive, *n* reciprocation in a clasp unit achieved by the use of a rigid part of the clasp, located on or above the height of contour line or on a guiding plane and opposite to the retentive arm. However, reciprocation cannot be achieved by a single clasp alone—a similar action must occur by another component of the removable partial denture located across the arch.

reciprocity (res′əpros′itē), *n* a mutual agreement to exchange privileges, dependence, or relationships, as in an agreement between two governing bodies to accept the credentials of a physician, dentist, licensed dental professional, or other health professional licensed in either jurisdiction.

Recklinghausen's disease (rek′linghowzenz), *n.pr* See neurofibromatosis; osteitis fibrosa cystica.

recombinant DNA hepatitis B vaccine, *n* a vaccine against hepatitis B that is cultured in yeast.

recombinant human bone morphogenetic protein (rhBMP) (rēkom′bənənt môr′fogənet′ik), *n* a protein created by recombinant DNA technology that induces bone formation.

R

reconstructive surgery, *n* surgery to rebuild a structure for functional or esthetic reasons.

recontour (rē′kon′tŏŏr), *n* a reshaping process that uses instruments, such as power-driven finishing tools, to remove excess restorative material and restore natural anatomic form.

recontouring, occlusal, *n* the reshaping of an occlusal surface of a natural or artificial tooth.

record, *n* information committed to and preserved in writing or electronically.

record base, *n* See baseplate.

record, centric interocclusal, *n* a record of the centric jaw position (relation).

***record, eccentric interocclusal* (in′terəkloo′səl),** *n* a record of a jaw relation other than the centric relation; a record of a lateral eccentric jaw position.

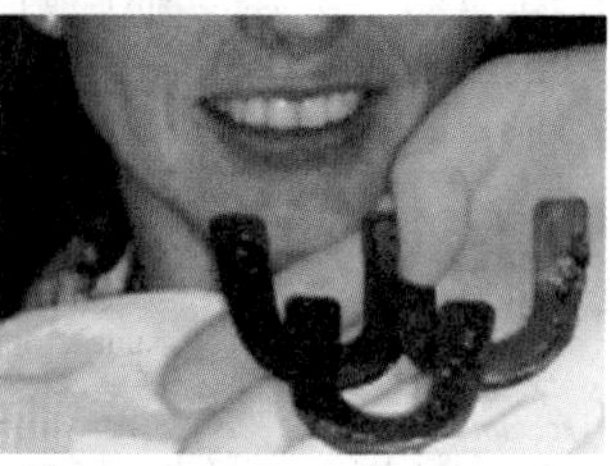

Eccentric interocclusal record. (Rosenstiel/Land/Fujimoto, 2006)

record, face-bow, *n* registration, by means of a face-bow, of the position of the mandibular axis or the condyles. The face-bow record is used to orient the maxillary cast to the opening and closing axis of the articulator.

record, functional chew-in, *n* **1.** a record of the natural chewing movement of the mandible made on an occlusion rim by teeth or scribing studs. *n* **2.** a record of the movements of the mandible made on the occluding surface of the opposing occlusion rim by teeth or scribing studs and produced by simulated chewing movements.

record, interocclusal, *n* a record of the positional relation of the teeth or jaws to each other; made on occlusal surfaces of occlusal rims or teeth in a plastic material that hardens, such as plaster of paris, wax, zinc oxide-eugenol paste, or acrylic resin.

record, jaw relation, *n* a registration of any positional relationship of the mandible in reference to the maxillae. The record may be of any of the many vertical, horizontal, or orientation relations.

record, maxillomandibular relationship, *n* See record, interocclusal.

record, occluding centric relation, *n* a registration of centric relation made at the vertical dimension at which the teeth make contact or are to make contact.

record, patient, legal aspects of, *n.pl* record must include proper identification of patient, signed consent forms, a complete medical and dental history, progress notes, and clinical observations from patient examinations. Improper record-keeping is grounds for malpractice. Records are also strictly confidential—unauthorized or inappropriate disclosure is an invasion of privacy and liable for legal action.

record, plaque control, *n* document used to measure and assist the progress of a patient undertaking a more purposeful approach to controlling bacterial plaque.

record, preoperative, *n* a record or records made for the purpose of study, diagnosis, or use in treatment planning or for comparison of treatment results with the pretreatment status of the patient.

record, profile, *n* a registration or record of the profile of a patient's face.

record, protrusive, *n* a registration of the relation of the mandible to the maxillae when the mandible is anterior to its centric relation with the maxillae.

record, protrusive interocclusal, *n* a record of a protruded eccentric jaw position.

record rim, *n* See rim, occlusion.

record, terminal jaw relation, *n* a record of the relationship of the mandible to the maxillae made at the vertical relation of the occlusion and at the centric position.

record, three-dimensional, *n* a maxillomandibular interocclusal record.

recording, *n* the act of making a written or electronic record of the data collected during examination.

recovery, *n* in a lawsuit, the obtaining or restoration of a right to something by a verdict, decree, or judgment of court.

recrystallization, *n* the return of a wrought metal to crystalline form because of excessive cold working or excessive application of heat.

rectification (rek′tifikā′shən), *n* conversion of electric current from alternating to direct (unidirectional).

rectifier (rek′tifīur), *n* a device used for converting an alternating current to a direct current; it also prevents or limits the flow of current in the opposite direction.

rectifier, full-wave, *n* an apparatus for rectifying the entire wave of an alternating current in a radiography machine by means of a mechanical rectifier or valve tube.

rectifier, half-wave, *n* an apparatus used in the rectifying of half of the sine wave in a radiography unit.

recumbent (rikum′bənt), *adj* to be lying down, leaning backward, or reclining.

recuperation, *n* the process of recovering health, strength, and mental and emotional vigor.

recurrence, *n* the reappearance of a sign or symptom of a disease after a period of remission.

red blood cell count, *n* the number of red blood cells (erthrocytes) in 1 mm^3 of blood; a useful diagnostic tool in the determination of several kinds of anemia. See also mean corpuscular hemoglobin.

red marrow, *n* the red vascular substance consisting of connective tissue and blood vessels, containing primitive blood cells, macrophages, megakaryocytes, and fat cells. Red marrow is found in the cavities of many bones. It manufactures and releases leukocytes and erythrocytes into the bloodstream.

redressment (rēdres′ment), *n* replacement of a part or correction of a deformity.

reduced fee plan, *n* a program in which the fees established for some or all services are lower than those usually charged by dental professionals in the community. In some industrial plans, employers make lower fees possible by partially subsidizing the cost of providing care (e.g., furnishing rent-free facilities and paying costs of utilities). In welfare plans with limited funds, dental professionals may in effect subsidize the programs by accepting lower fees than they usually charge.

reducer, *n* a solution used to remove some silver from the image on a radiograph and thereby produce a less intense image; an oxidizing agent used to remove excess density.

reduction in area, *n* a test to assess the ductility of a metal or an alloy, whereby the cross-sectional area of the fractured end of a wire or rod is compared with the original area. A tensile test is used to break the wire.

refereed journal, *n* a professional or literary journal or publication in which articles or papers are selected for publication by a panel of readers or referees who are experts in the field.

referral, *n* the recommendation of another health professional to a patient for a specified reason.

referred pain, *n* pain felt at a site different from that of an injured or diseased organ or part of the body. Angina pain is often felt at a site distant from the heart, such as arm or shoulder.

reflection, *n* the act of elevating and folding back the mucoperiosteum, thereby exposing the underlying bone.

reflection, mucobuccal, *n* See fold, mucobuccal.

reflex(es) (rē′fleks), *n* a reflected action or movement; the sum total of any specific involuntary activity.

reflex, arc, *n* See arc, reflex.

reflex, Breuer, *n.pr* See reflex, Hering-Breuer.

reflex, Cheyne-Stokes, *n.pr* See respiration, Cheyne-Stokes.

reflex emesis, *n* gagging or vomiting induced by touching the mucous membrane of the throat or as a result of other noxious stimuli. Also called *gag reflex.*

reflex, Hering-Breuer **(her′ing-broi′ər),** *n.pr* the nervous mechanism that tends to limit the respiratory excursions. Stimuli from the sensory endings in the lungs (and perhaps in other parts) pass up the vagi and tend to limit both inspiration and expiration during ordinary breathing.

reflex, jaw, *n* an extension-flexion reflex that is initiated by tapping the mandible downward. The masseter and other elevators of the mandible are the first stretched; then the reflex flexion-contraction elevates the mandible by flexion of elevator muscles while simultaneous stretching (extension) of the depressor muscles of the mandible occurs.

reflex, pharyngeal **(fərin′jēəl),** *n* contraction of the constrictor muscles of the pharynx, elicited by touching the back of the pharynx.

reflex, stretch, *n* one of the most important features of tonic contraction of muscle. It is the reflex contraction of a healthy muscle that results from a pull. It has been found that stretching a muscle by as little as 0.8% of its original length is sufficient to evoke a reflex response. A stretch of constant degree causes a maintained steady contraction, muscle spindles and stretch receptors in the tendons show very slow adaptation, and the reflex ceases immediately on withdrawal of the stretching force. The stretch reflex is obtained predominantly from those muscles maintaining body posture, among which are the masticating muscles that maintain the position of the mandible and the neck muscles holding the head erect. Together the masticating muscles and neck muscles are responsible for the maintenance of the air and food passages.

reflex, vagovagal **(vā′gōvā′gəl),** *n* a reflex in which the afferent and efferent impulses travel via the vagus nerve. The afferent impulses travel centrally via the sensory nucleus of the vagus. The efferent impulses travel via the motor fibers of the vagus nerve.

reflexes, allied, *n.pl* reflexes that join to effect a common purpose, such as mastication. They may arise from diverse stimuli, such as smell, taste of food, and texture, shape, and resistance of the food bolus. Collectively, they encourage salivation and a sequence of masticatory closures of the mandible, followed by deglutition.

reflexes, antagonistic, *n.pl* reflexes that cannot occupy the final pathway simultaneously. The weaker of these reflexes will give way to the stronger, especially if the latter is a protected reflex (e.g., a hot or nauseating food causes involuntary retching or even vomiting rather than the pleasurable gustatory experience associated with chewing and swallowing tasty food).

reflexes, flexion-extension, *n.pl* the reflexes based on the principle of reciprocal innervation. When a voluntary or reflex contraction of a muscle occurs, it is accompanied by the simultaneous relaxation of its antagonist. E.g., when the jaw reflex is initiated by tapping the mandible downward, the masseter and other elevators of the mandible are stretched. Then, reflex flexion-contraction of the elevators takes place, the mandible is elevated, and the depressor muscles of the mandible are stretched. Many combinations exist, not only between the agonists and the antagonists of a given joint but also between reflexes that cross over to muscle groups of contralateral extremities, joints, and muscles.

reflexes, pathologic, *n.pl* reflexes observed in the abnormal or inappropriate motor responses of controlled stimuli initiated in the sensory organ that is appropriate to the reflex arc. They may be initiated in the superficial reflexes of the skin and mucous membrane; in the deep myotatic reflexes of the joints, tendons, and muscles; and in the visceral reflexes of the viscera and other organs of the body. The pathologic reflexes are thus syndromes of abnormal responses to otherwise normal stimuli.

reflux, *n* the reverse flow of a liquid.

refractory (rēfrak′tərē), *adj* pertaining to the ability to withstand the high temperatures used in certain dental laboratory procedures. See also cast, refractory.

refractory periodontitis (per′ēōdontī′tis), *n* a progressive inflammatory destruction of the periodontal attachment that resists conventional mechanical treatment.

refusal, informed, *n* decision by the patient to forego a professional recommendation for dental care.

regeneration (rējen′ərā′shən), *n* the renewal or repair of lost tissue or parts.

regeneration, guided bone (GBR), *n* a technique in which a membrane is placed over a bone defect site to encourage new bone growth and direct its formation while preventing other tissues from interfering with osteogenesis.

regeneration, muscle, *n* repair of muscle tissue. When surgical intervention or inflammatory disease of dental structures injures the facial and masticatory muscles, two types of repair take place: repair by budding and repair by proliferation.

regeneration, muscle, by budding, *n* regeneration that takes place in destructive lesions of muscle, traumatic necrosis, hemorrhage, infarction, and suppurative myositis. The buds consist of undifferentiated plasmodial masses and certain sarcolemma nuclei. The rebuilt architecture is not classic and has bizarre and sometimes fibrous extensions that look like scarred defects.

regeneration, muscle, by proliferation, *n* regeneration in degenerating muscles by proliferation of bands of sarcoplasm in which the sarcolemma and its nuclei are preserved.

region, interprismatic (in′terprizmat′ik), *n* the area located between the parallel enamel rods.

region, mylohyoid (mī′lōhī′oid), *n* the region on the lingual surface of the mandible marked by the mylohyoid ridge and the attachment of the mylohyoid muscle; a part of the alveololingual sulcus.

regional, *adj* pertaining to a region or regions.

registered dietitian, *n* See dietitian, registered.

registered nurse (RN), *n* a professional nurse who has completed a course of study at an approved and accredited school of nursing and who has passed the National Council of Licensure Examination. RNs are licensed to practice by individual states.

registered record administrator (RRA), *n* a medical record administrator (health information manager) who has successfully completed the prescribed curriculum and the credentialing examination conducted by the American Medical Record Association.

registration, *n* the record of desired jaw relations that is made to transfer casts having these same relations to an articulator.

registration of functional form, *n* See impression, functional.

registration, tissue, *n* the accurate record of the shape of tissues under any condition by means of suitable material.

registration, wax-bite, *n* a wax impression used to record a patient's occlusion, which is then used to articulate diagnostic casts.

regression analysis, *n* a method of correlation for computing the most probable value of one variable, *y,* from the known value of another variable, *x;* a method for computing the amount of change in one variable for a unit change in another. It is spoken of as the regression of *x* on *y* and notated r_{xy}.

regulated waste, *n* refuse material made up of or contaminated by saliva, blood, or tissue (including teeth). Such waste includes contaminated sharp instruments as well as any solid waste materials that have been soaked or covered by the contaminants. Also called *infectious waste.*

regulator, *n* the mechanical part of a gas delivery system that controls gas pressure that allows a manageable flow of drug vapor to escape.

regurgitation (rēgur'jitā'shən), *n* a backward flowing (e.g., casting up of undigested food, backward flowing of blood into the heart or between the chambers of the heart).

regurgitation, heart valve, *n* blood flow in the wrong direction (from a ventricle to an atrium or into the heart from an artery) through a valve that has failed to close completely. See also heart valves.

rehabilitation (rē'həbil'itā'shən), *n* restoration of form and function.

rehabilitation, oral cavity, *n* (oral rehabilitation), restoration of the form and function of the masticatory apparatus condition to as near normal as possible.

rehalation, *n* rebreathing.

reimbursement, *n* payment made by a third party to a beneficiary or dental professional on behalf of the beneficiary toward repayment of expenses incurred for a service covered by the contractual arrangement.

reimplant, *v* to replace a lost or extracted tooth back into its alveolus.

reimplantation, *n* See replantation.

reinforcement, *n* the increasing of force or strength.

reinsertion, *n* the reimplantation and splinting of a tooth into the alveolus after dental trauma, such as avulsion, or following removal of the tooth. It is performed to prevent permanent tooth loss and to restore the dentition so the patient can speak and eat normally.

reinsurance, *n* insurance for third-party payers to spread their risk for losses (claims paid) over a specified dollar amount.

reintubation (rē'intoobā'shən), *n* intubation performed a second time.

Reiter's syndrome (rī'terz, -turz), *n.pr* See syndrome, Reiter's.

relapse, *v* to slip or fall back into a former state.

relation(s), *n* the designation of the position of one object as oriented to another (e.g., centric relation of the mandible to the maxillae).

relation, acentric, *n* See relation, jaw, eccentric.

relation, acquired centric, *n* See relation, jaw, eccentric, acquired.

relation, acquired eccentric jaw, *n* an eccentric relation that is assumed by habit to bring the teeth into a convenient occlusion.

relation, centric, *n* (centric jaw relation), the relation of the mandible to the maxillae when the condyles are in their most posterosuperior unstrained positions in the glenoid fossae, from which lateral movements can be made at the occluding vertical relation normal for the individual. Centric relation is a relation that can exist at any degree of jaw separation.

relation, centric jaw, *n* See relation, centric.

relation, cusp-fossa, *n* See cusp-fossa relations.

relation, dynamic, *n* relations of two objects involving the element of relative movement of one object to another (relationship of the mandible to the maxillae).

relation, eccentric, *n* See relation, jaw, eccentric.

relation, eccentric jaw, *n* (convenience relationship, eccentric relation, eccentric jaw position), any jaw relation other than centric relation.

relation, intermaxillary, *n* the relation between the right and left maxilla. See also relation, maxillomandibular.

relation, jaw, *n* a relationship of the mandible to the maxillae.

relation, lateral, *n* the relation of the mandible to the maxillae when the mandibular arch is in a position on either side of centric relation.

relation, maxillomandibular **(maksil'omandib'ūlur),** *n* any one of the many relations of the mandible to the maxillae, such as the centric

R

maxillomandibular relation or eccentric maxillomandibular relation.

relation, median, *n* See relation, centric.

relation, median jaw, *n* a jaw relationship existing when the mandible is in the median sagittal plane.

relation, median retruded, *n* See relation, centric.

relation, occluding, *n* the jaw relation at which the opposing teeth contact or occlude.

relation, posterior border jaw, *n* the most posterior relation of the mandible to the maxillae at any specific vertical dimension.

relation, protrusive **(prōtroo′siv),** *n* See relation, jaw, protrusive; position, rest, physiologic.

relation, protrusive jaw, *n* (protrusive relation), a jaw relation resulting from a protrusion of the mandible.

relation, rest, *n* See position, physiologic rest.

relation, rest jaw, *n* (rest), the postural relation of the mandible to the maxillae when the patient is resting comfortably in the upright position, the condyles are in a neutral unstrained position in the glenoid fossae, and the mandibular musculature is in a state of minimum tonic contraction to maintain posture.

relation, ridge, *n* the positional relation of the mandibular ridge to the maxillary ridges.

relation, static, *n* the relationship between two parts that are not in motion.

relation, unstrained jaw, *n* the relation of the mandible to the skull when a state of balanced tonus exists between all the muscles involved.

relation, vertical, *n* the relative position of the mandible in a vertical direction; one of the basic jaw relations.

relationship, *n* the condition of being associated or interconnected.

relationship, abnormal occlusal, *n* occlusal relationships that deviate from the regular and established type to produce esthetic disharmonies, interference with mastication, occlusal traumatism, and speech difficulties.

relationship, buccolingual **(buk′ō-ling′gwəl),** *n* the position of a space or tooth in relation to the tongue and cheek.

relationship, convenience, of teeth, *n* See occlusion, convenience.

relationship, normal, *n* a relationship in which structures conjoin as they should.

relationship, occlusal, *n* the individual and collective relationships of the mandibular teeth to the maxillary teeth and the relationship of the adjacent teeth in the same dental arch.

relationship, structure-activity (SAR), *n* the relationship between the chemical structure of a drug and its activity.

relationship, tissue-base, *n* the relationship of the base of a removable prosthesis to the structures subjacent to it. Three possibilities exist: the base may be entirely tissue-borne, it may be completely tooth-borne, or support may be shared by both the tissue subjacent to its base and the abutment that bounds the edentulous space at one terminus.

relative attachment level, *n* the physical measurement of the distance between the cementoenamel junction or gingival margin and the base of the periodontal pocket, as measured by a periodontal probe or stent. Such measurements are used to determine the loss of attachment at the periodontal ligament or the alveolar bone.

relative value system, *n* coded listing of professional services with unit values to indicate relative complexity as measured by time, skill, and overhead costs. Third-party payers typically assign a dollar value per unit to calculate provider reimbursement.

relaxant (rēlak′sənt), *n* an antispasmodic; a drug that relaxes spasms of smooth or skeletal muscle; a drug used to eliminate muscle spasms, thus facilitating the establishment of centric relation, centric occlusion, rest position, and so on. Also used in the treatment of painful muscle spasms associated with occlusal traumatism. Examples are mephenesin, the meprobamates, and methocarbamol (Robaxin).

relaxant, muscle, *n* a drug that specifically aids in lessening muscle tension.

relaxation training, *n* a stress-reduction technique that uses a sequence of progressive exercises under the direction of a therapist to lower the level of anxiety and its neuromotor manifestations.

release, *v* to give up as a legal claim; to discharge or relinquish a right.

release, sustained, adj See medication, sustained release.

reliability, *n* **1.** in research, the reproducibility of an experimental result; the extent to which an experiment, test, or measuring procedure yields the same result during independent, repeated trials. *n* **2.** the ability of two or more observers to examine the same data and arrive at a similar judgment within predefined bounds concerning the quality of care.

relicensure (rē′lī′sənshər), *n* being licensed to practice for a specific period with the license either being renewed at the end of that period or being forfeited. In some instances, evidence of continued competency must be submitted.

relief, *n* **1.** the mitigation or removal of pain or distress. *n* **2.** the reduction or elimination of pressure from a specific area under a denture base.

relief chamber, n See chamber, relief.

relief, gingival, n relief given to removable partial denture units at all gingival crossings to avoid impingement.

relief space, n See space, relief.

relieve, *v* **1.** to mitigate or remove pain or distress. *v* **2.** the procedure of placing hard wax in strategic areas.

reline, *v* to resurface the tissue side (basal surface) of a denture with new base material so that it will fit more accurately. See also rebase.

R

rem (roentgen-equivalent-man), *n* a unit of absorbed radiation dose adjusted for biologic effects equivalent to 1 rad of 250 kV roentgen rays (dental and cephalometric roentgen rays require less than 100 kV).

remedial (rəmē′dēəl), *adj* curative; acting as a remedy.

remineralization (rē′min′ərəlizā′-shən), *n* the reintroduction of complex mineral salts into bone, enamel, dentin, or cementum.

remineralize, *v* the replacement of depleted mineral content of bones and teeth. It is a naturally occurring process by the minerals contained in saliva. It may be promoted by certain dental treatments in the dental office and by the patient at home.

remission, *n* the partial or complete disappearance of the clinical and subjective characteristics of a chronic or malignant disease.

remit, *v* to send; to relinquish.

removable lingual arch, *n* See arch, removable lingual.

removable partial denture, *n* See denture, partial, removable.

removal, pulp, *n* See pulpectomy.

remuneration, *n* pay; recompense; salary.

renal (rē′nəl), *adj* pertaining to the kidneys.

Rendu-Osler-Weber disease, *n.pr* See telangiectasia, hereditary hemorrhagic.

rent, *n* a payment made by a tenant to an owner for the use of land or a building.

rental, *n/adj* the fee paid by the dental professional for the use of space in a building owned by someone else. Equipment may also be obtained under a rental or lease agreement.

reovirus (rē′ōvī′rəs), *n* any one of three ubiquitous, double-stranded ribonucleic acid viruses found in the respiratory and alimentary tracts in healthy and sick people. Reoviruses have been implicated in some cases of upper respiratory tract disease and infantile gastroenteritis.

reoxidation (rēok′sidā′shən), *n* the act of taking up oxygen again, as the hemoglobin of the blood.

repair, *n* **1.** the process of reuniting or replacing broken parts of a denture; a means for extending the usefulness of a denture. *v* **2.** to make sound; to mend; restoration to former condition. *n* **3.** formation of new tissues by processes such as fibroplasia, osteogenesis, and endothelioplasia to replace tissues damaged by disease or injury.

repair, cemental, n repair of areas of cemental resorption and cemental tears by apposition of cementum. Repair may be by formation of either cellular or acellular cementum.

repetitive strain injury (RSI), *n* a loose group of injuries that occur to muscles, nerves, and tendons as a result of repetitive movements of particular body parts. It is caused or aggravated by frequently repeated movements, such as computer strokes or the use of vibrating equipment. Symptoms include pain, tingling, or swelling of the affected body part. Also known as *overuse syndrome* or *cumulative trauma disorder.*

replacement, prosthetic, *n* See prosthesis.

replantation, *n* (reimplantation), replacement of a tooth (or teeth) that has been removed from the alveolus either intentionally or unintentionally, as in an accident.

replenisher, *n* a concentrated developing solution designed to maintain the active strength of developer through periodic addition to maintain original volume.

report generator, *n* a computer program for producing complete data processing reports giving only a description of the desired content and format of the output reports, as well as certain information concerning the input file.

reportable diseases, *n.pl* contagious diseases that must be reported by the physician to public health authorities. They include but are not limited to malaria, influenza, poliomyelitis, relapsing fever, typhus, yellow fever, cholera, and bubonic plague.

repositioning, jaw, *n* the changing of any relative position of the mandible to the maxillae, usually by altering the occlusion of the natural or artificial teeth.

repository, *n* long-acting drugs, usually administered intramuscularly. See also medication, repository.

repository, rapid, *n* mixtures of rapid-acting and slow-acting drugs, usually administered intramuscularly.

representative group, *n* a group whose members represent all the various sectors of a community or population under study.

reputation, *n* a person's credit, honor, and character; esteem in which one is held.

request for proposal (RFP), *n* a solicitation by a funding agency for proposals to accomplish a particular goal. The RFP lists the requirements a project must meet to receive funding.

require arch length, *n* the circumference of the dental arch sufficient to accommodate the sum of the mesiodistal widths of all the natural teeth in the dental arch.

res ipsa loquitur (rās′ ip′sə lō′kwitoor), *adj* a Latin phrase meaning "the thing speaks for itself." Used in actions for injury by negligence in which the happening itself is accepted as proof.

res judicata (rās′ joo′dikä′tə), *adj* decided or determined by judicial power; a thing judicially decided.

research, *v/n* the diligent inquiry or examination of data, reports, and observations in a search for facts or principles. Generally a disciplined protocol is followed to ensure objectivity and reproducibility. Most research employs the scientific method or a similar model.

research, analytical epidemiologic, *n* a method of investigation used to establish a disease origin or the existence of an contributory relationship between a cause and a disease.

research, convenience sample, *n* a method of investigation used when measuring an entire population is not possible. Participants are numbered as they enroll, then they are randomly assigned to either the control or experimental group.

research, epidemiologic **(ep′ədē′mēəloj′ik),** *n* a method of investigation (e.g., descriptive, analytical, and experimental) used to study the rate of occurrence, method of transmission, and control of a disease within a population.

research, epidemiologic survey, *n* a method of data collection from target population samples to establish factors causing or contributing to a disease and to develop potential methods for prevention.

research, experimental, *n* See controlled clinical trial.

research, experimental epidemiologic, *n* a method of investigation used after the establishment of a disease origin to determine the result of altering at least one cause.

resection, *n* excision of a considerable portion of an organ.

resection, root, *n* See amputation, root.

reserpine (res′ərpēn), *n brand names:* Serpalan, Serpasil; *drug class:* antiadrenergic agent, antihypertensive; *action:* depletes catecholamine stores in central nervous system and adrenergic nerve endings; *use:* hypertension.

reserve, *n* something kept in store for future use.

reserve, alkali, *n* See reserve, alkaline.

reserve, alkaline, *n* (alkali reserve), **1.** the amount of buffer compounds (e.g., sodium bicarbonate, dipotassium phosphate, proteins) in the blood capable of neutralizing acids; one of the buffer systems of the blood that can neutralize the acid valences formed in the body. It is made up of the base of weak acid salts and is usually measured by determining the bicarbonate concentration of the plasma. *n* **2.** the concentration of bicarbonate ions (HCO_3^-) in the blood. These ions serve as a reserve in that they may be displaced by anions (e.g., Cl^-, SO_4^{-2}, PO_4^{-3}). Displacement of bicarbonate ions occurs mainly by means of the chloride shift. The role of the buffer system is such that a large influx of acid or base ions from either metabolic function or ingestion can be neutralized by the alkaline reserves from the mineral and protein salts in the blood and tissue fluids. A strong acid is transformed into a weak base. Consequently, the pH level of the blood fluctuates very little, and the tissue cells are constantly bathed in a continuously buffered solution.

reserve, cardiac, *n* the reserve strength or pumping ability of the heart, which may be called on in an emergency.

reservoir bag, *n* a repository for excess gas that is attached to an anesthesia machine. It may be used as a source of gas during manual ventilation or to gauge the patient's respiratory rate and depth while under anesthesia.

resident, *n* a graduate and licensed dental professional or physician who has completed an internship and is serving in the hospital while pursuing advanced didactic and clinical studies in special disciplines of knowledge.

residual, *adj* pertaining to the portion of something that remains after an activity that removes the bulk of the substance; usually refers to the amount of air remaining in the lungs at the end of a maximum expiration.

residual ridge, *n* See ridge, residual.

residue, *n* remainder; that which remains after the removal of other substances.

resilience (rēzil′yəns), *n* **1.** an act of springing back. *n* **2.** capability of a strained body to recover its size and shape after deformation. *n* **3.** the recoverable potential energy of an elastic solid body or stricture resulting from its having been subjected to stress not exceeding the elastic limit.

resilience, modulus of, *n* the amount of energy stored up by a body when one unit volume is stressed to its proportional limit.

resin (rez′in), *n* broad term used to indicate organic substances that are usually translucent or transparent and are soluble in ether, acetone, and similar substances but not in water. They are named according to their chemical composition, physical structure, and means for activation or curing. Examples are acrylic resin, autopolymer resin (cold-curing resin), synthetic resin, styrene resin, and vinyl resin. See also methyl methacrylate; varnish, cavity.

resin, acrylic, *n* **1.** general term applied to a resinous material of the various esters of acrylic acid. It is used as a denture base material and also for trays and other dental restorations. *n* **2.** An ethylene derivative that contains a vinyl group (e.g., polymethacrylate [methyl methacrylate], the principal ingredient of many plastics used in dentistry).

resin, activated, *n* See resin, autopolymer.

resin, autopolymer, *n* (activated resin, autopolymerizing resin, cold-curing resin, direct restorative acrylic resin, self-curing resin), any resin that can be polymerized by an activator and a catalyst without the use of external heat.

resin cement, *n* resin-based materials used as alternatives to common cement base materials, such as zinc phosphate. They are used with nonmetallic fillings such as ceramic, which will not bond to zinc phosphate, and when used with enamel and dentin bonding agents produce a much stronger bond than zinc phosphate.

resin, composite, *n* a resin used for restorative purposes and usually formed by a reaction of an ether of bisphenol-A (an epoxy molecule) with acrylic resin monomers, initiated by a benzoyl peroxideamine system, to which is added as much as 75% inorganic filler (glass beads and rods, lithium aluminum silicate, quartz, and tricalcium phosphate).

resin, copolymer **(kōpol′əmər),** *n* a synthetic resin that is the product of the concurrent and joint polymerization of two or more different monomers of polymers.

resin, direct restorative, *n* See resin, autopolymer.

resin, epoxy, *n* a resin molecule characterized by reactive epoxy, or ethoxyline, groups that serve as terminal polymerization points. Used in dentistry for denture bases.

resin, heat-curing, *n* a resin that requires heat to activate its polymerization.

resin, inlay, *n* an applied dental filling contained within the tooth and made up of natural or synthetic resin-based materials.

resin, quick cure, *n* See resin, autopolymer.

resin, self-curing, *n* See resin, autopolymer.

resin, thermoplastic, *n* a synthetic resin that may be softened by heat and hardened by cooling.

resin, vinyl, *n* an ethylene-derivative copolymer of vinyl chloride and vinyl acetate; used at one time for denture bases.

resin-filled, *adj* pertaining to a resin, usually poly (methylmethacrylate), to which has been added an inert material such as glass beads or glass rods.

resistance, *n* ability of an individual to ward off the damaging effects of physical, chemical, or microbiologic injury; an immeasurable factor controlled and qualified by numerous local, systemic, and metabolic processes such as blood supply to tissues, nutritional status, age, and antibody formative ability.

resistance, abrasion, *n* an object's capacity to oppose the type of movement that results in physical weathering. A greater degree of abrasion resistance is beneficial in the long-term preservation of the teeth's appearance and structure.

resistance, cross-, *n* a state in which an organism is insensitive to several drugs of similar chemical nature.

resistance form, *n* See form, resistance.

resolution, *n* the discernible separation of closely adjacent radiographic image details.

resonance (rez′ənəns), *n* the vibratory response of a body or air-filled cavity to a frequency imposed on it.

resonance, speech, *n* the resonance of the body cavities and surfaces involved in the production of speech. The sound waves produced at the vocal folds are still far from the finished product heard in speech. The resonators give the characteristic quality to the voice. The resonating structures are the air sinuses; organ surfaces; cavities such as the pharynx, oral cavity, and nasal cavity; and chest wall. The resonating structures contribute no energy to the stream of air; they act to conserve and concentrate the energy already present in the laryngeal tone rather than to let it dissipate into the tissues. However, the resonated laryngeal tone still is not speech.

resorbable (rēsor′bəbəl), *adj* that which can be broken down and assimilated back into the body.

resorcinol (rizôr′sənôl′), *n* an antiseptic substance used as a keratolytic agent in dermatoses.

resorption (rēzôrp′shən), *n* **1.** loss of substance (bone) by physiologic or pathologic means; the reduction of the volume and size of the residual alveolar portion of the mandible or maxillae. *n* **2.** the cementoclastic and dentinoclastic action that often takes place on the root of a replanted tooth.

resorption, apical root, *n* dissolution of the apex of a tooth, resulting in a shortened, blunted root.

resorption, bone, *n* **1.** destruction or solution of the elements of bone. *n* **2.** loss of bone resulting from the activity of multinucleated giant cells, the osteoclasts, which are noted in irregular concavities on the periphery of the bone (Howship's lacunae).

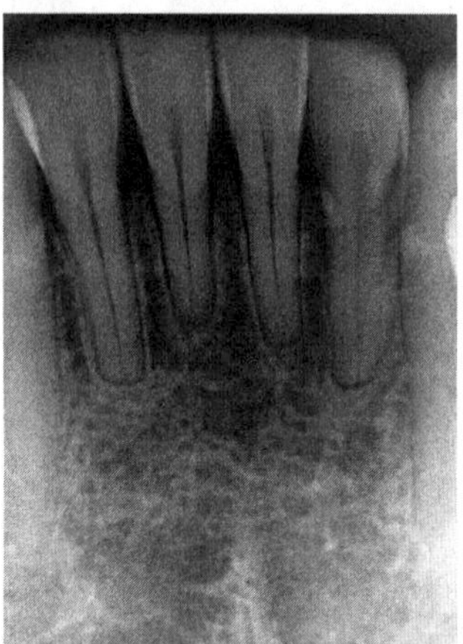

Apical root resorption. (Rosenstiel/Land/Fujimoto, 2006)

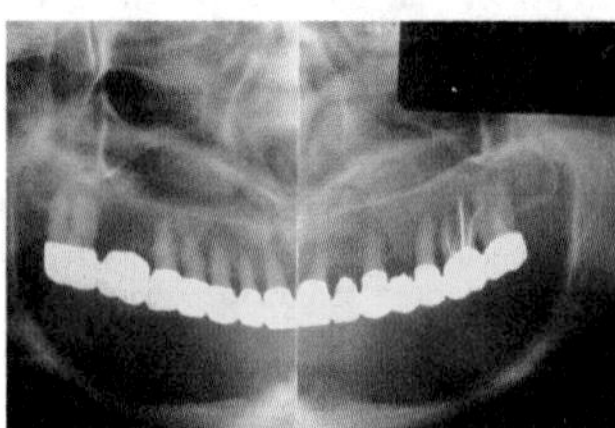

Severe bone resorption in the mandible. (Courtesy Dr. Charles Babbush)

R

resorption, cemental, *n* destruction of cementum by cementoclastic action. Noted as the presence of irregular concavities in the cemental surfaces.

resorption, frontal, *n* osteoclastic resorption of alveolar bone (lamina dura) by multinucleated cells on the osseous margin adjacent to the periodontal ligament.

resorption, horizontal, *n* a pattern of bone resorption in marginal periodontitis in which the marginal crest of the alveolar bone between adjacent teeth remains level; in these instances the bases of the periodontal pockets are supracrestal; a pattern of bone loss in which the crestal margins of the alveolar bone are resorbed. A horizontal pattern, rather than vertical loss along the root, is the typical type of bone loss in periodontitis.

resorption, idiopathic **(id′ēōpath′ik),** *n* resorption that is not attributable to any known disease or is without an apparent cause.

resorption, internal, *n* (idiopathic internal resorption, pink tooth), a special form of idiopathic root resorption from within the pulp cavity; granulation tissue is present within the tooth, apparently with the resportion of the dentin occurring from the inside outward. The cause is unknown.

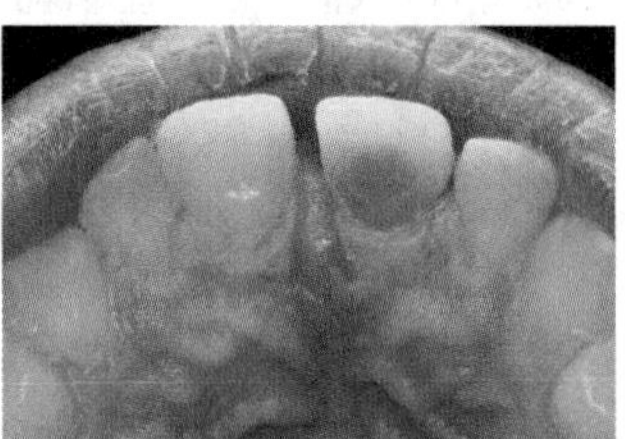

Internal resorption. (Neville/Damm/Allen/Bouquot, 2002)

resorption, lacunar, *n* See osteoclast.

resorption, osteoclastic **(os′tēōklas′-tik),** *n* loss of bone by cellular activity; osteoclasts are large, multinucleated cells seen in irregular concavities in the margin of the bone (Howship's lacunae) and currently believed to be directly responsible for the active destruction of bone.

resorption, pressure, of bone, *n* osteoclastic destruction of bone resulting from the application of sustained, excessive force. Remodeling of bone may occur to better adapt to these forces, or destruction may continue if the stresses are repeated and excessive.

resorption, rear, *n* See resorption, undermining.

resorption, root, *n* destruction of the cementum or dentin by cementoclastic or osteoclastic activity.

resorption, surface root, *n* localized resorptive areas on the cemental surface of the tooth root.

resorption, undermining, *n* indirect, as opposed to frontal, removal of alveolar bone where pressure applied to a tooth has resulted in loss of vitality of localized areas of the periodontal ligament.

resorption, vertical, *n* a pattern of bone loss seen in occlusal traumatism, marginal periodontitis, periodontosis, and other conditions; a pattern of bone loss in which the alveolar bone adjacent to a tooth is destroyed without simultaneous crestal loss, so that a vertical rather than a horizontal pattern of loss is observed.

respect, *n/v* to hold in high regard; to show consideration for another. Mutual respect is the basis for a good doctor-patient relationship.

respiration (res′pirā′shən), *n* the gaseous exchange between cells of the body and the environment. Four stages exist: pulmonary ventilation, diffusion of gases in the alveoli, transport of gases in the blood to and from cells, and regulation of the process.

respiration, artificial, *n* maintenance of respiratory movements by artificial means. When respiration has been arrested and no mechanical device is available, resuscitation by means of artificial respiration is the only practical means of ventilating the lungs.

respiration, Cheyne-Stokes **(chān′-stōks′),** *n.pr* (Cheyne-Stokes reflex), a type of breathing characterized by rhythmic variations in intensity that occur in cycles: rhythmic acceleration, deepening, and stopping of breathing movements.

respiration, controlled, *n* maintenance of adequate pulmonary ventilation in apneic patients.

respiration, external, *n* ventilation of the lungs and oxygenation of the blood.

respiration in speech, *n* in normal speech, the action of the respiratory apparatus during exhalation, which provides a continuous stream of air with sufficient volume and pressure (under adequate voluntary control) to initiate phonation. The stream of air is modified in its course from the lungs by the facial and oral structures, giving rise to the sound symbols that are recognized as speech.

respiration, internal, *n* the mechanism of gaseous exchange between blood and tissues.

respirator (res′pirātur), *n* an apparatus that qualifies the air breathed through it; a device for giving artificial respiration.

respiratory distress syndrome (RDS) of the newborn (res′pərətôr′ē), *n* an acute lung disease of the newborn, characterized by airless alveoli, inelastic lungs, more than 60 respirations per minute, nasal flaring, intercostal and subcostal retractions, grunting on expiration, and peripheral edema. The condition occurs most often in premature babies. It is caused by a deficiency of pulmonary surfactant. The disease is self-limited; the infant either dies in 3 to 5 days or completely recovers with no aftereffects. Treatment includes measures to correct shock, acidosis, and hypoxemia and the use of continuous positive airway pressure to prevent alveolar collapse.

respiratory failure, *n* a condition in which the level of oxygen in the blood is too low and the level of carbon dioxide is too high. This condition may be life threatening.

respiratory rate, *n* the normal rate of breathing at rest, about 12 to 20 inspirations per minute.

respiratory rhythm, *n* a regular, oscillating cycle of inspiration and expiration, controlled by neuronal impulses transmitted between the muscles of inspiration in the chest and the respiratory centers in the brain. The respiratory rate is influenced by metabolic rate, emotional state, neurologic disorders, and obstructive disease.

respiratory therapy, *n* a treatment that maintains or improves the ventilatory function of the respiratory tract.

respiratory tract, *n* the complex of organs and structures performing the pulmonary ventilation of the body and the exchange of oxygen and carbon dioxide between the ambient air and the blood circulating through the lungs. It includes all the structures from the external nares to the alveoli of the lungs.

respirometer (res′pirom′ətur), *n* an instrument for studying and determining the character and extent of respiration.

respondeat superior, *n* a legal doctrine that passes the legal responsibility for acts or omissions of an employee to the employer.

response, *n* action or movement resulting from the application of a stimulus.

response diagnosis, *n* the evaluation of previous treatment at the follow-up appointment. A method of assessing the previous treatment.

response time, *n* the period between the application of a stimulus and the response of a cell or tissue.

rest, *n* **1.** passive support. *n* **2.** an extension from a prosthesis that affords vertical support for a restoration.

rest area, *n* See area, rest.

rest, auxiliary, *n* the rest other than the one used as a component part of a primary direct retainer.

rest, finger, *n* See finger rest.

rest, incisal, *n* a metallic extension onto the incisal angle of an anterior tooth to supply support or indirect retention for a removable partial denture.

rest, lingual, *n* a metallic extension onto the lingual surface of an anterior tooth to provide support or indirect retention for a removable partial denture.

rest, occlusal, *n* (occlusal lug), a rest placed on the occlusal surface of a posterior tooth.

rest occlusion, *n* See position, rest, physiologic.

rest position, *n* See position, rest.

rest, precision, *n* a unit consisting of two closely fitted parts, the insert of which rests firmly against the gingival portion of the tubelike receptacle.

rest relation, *n* See relation, jaw, rest.

rest seat, *n* See area, rest.

resting potential, *n* the electrical potential across a nerve cell membrane before it is stimulated to release the charge. The resting potential for a neuron is between 50 and 100 mV.

restless legs syndrome, *n* a benign condition of unknown origin characterized by an irritating sensation of uneasiness, tiredness, and itching deep within the muscles of the legs, accompanied by twitching and sometimes pain. The only relief is walking or moving the legs.

R

restoration, *n* (prosthetic restoration), broad term applied to any filling, inlay, crown, bridge, partial denture, or complete denture that restores or replaces lost tooth structure, teeth, or oral tissues; a prosthesis.

restoration, amalgam, *n* a direct restoration made from an alloy consisting of mercury and other metals (e.g., silver, copper, or tin), which is carved and contoured after placement in the tooth; allow a minimum of 24 hours between placement and polishing.

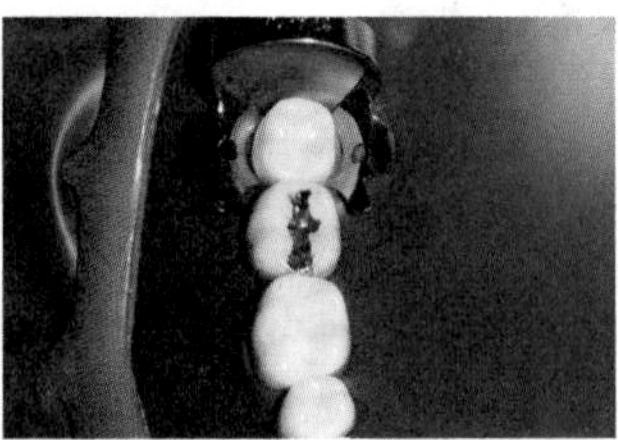

Amalgam restoration. (Bird/Robinson, 2005)

restoration, ceramic, *n* an indirect restoration made from metal and nonmetal compounds, which is carved and contoured before placement in the tooth; closely resembles natural teeth in strength, hardness, chemical inertness, and esthetic appearance.

restoration, dental prosthetic, *n* See prosthesis, dental.

restoration, direct, *n* a restoration prepared for immediate application to the tooth or cavity, as opposed to one prepared on a diagnostic cast and applied later.

restoration, faulty, *n* restoration in which there are imperfections or incorrect attributes (e.g., overhanging or deficient fillings, incorrect anatomy of occlusal and marginal ridge areas, faulty clasps). Such faults may be present in individual tooth restorations, fixed bridges, and removable partial dentures and are conducive to the initiation and perpetuation of inflammatory and dystrophic diseases of the teeth and periodontium.

restoration groove, *n* an opening between the restoration and the tooth structure, which results from either a broken flash or a material contraction; may also be called *ditch.*

restoration, implant, *n* the single-tooth implant crown or multiple-tooth implant, crown, or bridge that replaces a missing tooth or teeth.

restoration of cusps, *n* (preferred to tipping, capping, or shoeing cusps), reduction and inclusion of cusps within a cavity preparation and their restoration to functional occlusion with restorative material.

restoration, overcontoured, *n* a restoration containing so much excess restorative material that normal anatomic structure is altered; may cause plaque retention and open or deficient gingival margin.

restoration, PFM, *n* also called a *porcelain-fused-to-metal restoration.* A restoration made up of a metal substructure covered by an esthetic ceramic coating.

restoration, porcelain, *n* an indirect restoration made from a ceramic material that is cast in a laboratory prior to insertion in the oral cavity and finished during placement. See also ceramic restoration.

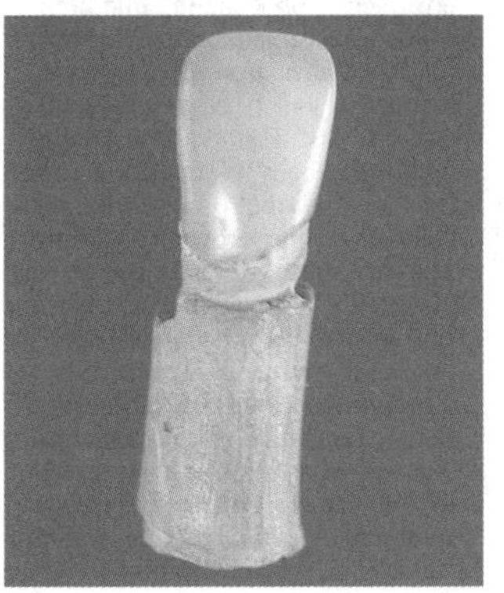

Porcelain restoration. (Bird/Robinson, 2005)

restoration, prosthetic, *n* See prosthesis.

restoration, temporary, *n* an artificial prosthesis used for a limited period to provide protective function and esthetics until a definitive prosthesis can be fixed into place.

restoration, undercontoured, *n* a restoration containing too little restorative material so that a space occurs between the margin and the cavity wall; may result when either the matrix band or wedge is improperly placed.

restorative (ristôr'ətiv), *adj* **1.** promoting a return to health or consciousness; a remedy that aids in restoring health, vigor, or consciousness. *adj* **2.** pertaining to rebuilding, repairing, or reforming.

restorative dentistry, *n* the branch of dentistry that deals with the reconstruction of the hard tissues of a tooth or group of teeth injured or destroyed by trauma or disease.

restorative materials, *n* materials used to reconstruct the hard tissues of teeth lost through trauma or disease.

restrainer, *n* a chemical ingredient (potassium bromide) of photographic developing solution. Its function is to inhibit the fogging tendency of the solution. Like the activator, the restrainer also controls the rate of development.

restraint, *n* any one of a number of devices used in aiding the immobilization of patients, especially children in traction.

restraint of trade, *n* an illegal act that interferes with free competition in a commercial or business transaction so as to restrict the production of a product or the provision of a service, affect the cost of a product or service, or control the market in any way to the detriment of consumers or purchasers of the service or product.

restrictive covenant (ristrik'tiv kuv'ənənt), *n* common clause found in a contract for the sale of a dental practice. The seller contracts that he or she will not practice dentistry within a certain time and area. A junior partner may be asked to sign such a covenant to guarantee that he or she will not compete with the partnership for a period after leaving the partnership. Also used in an employment situation.

resuscitation (rēsus'itā'shən), *n* restoration of life or consciousness to one who appears to be dead.

resuscitator (rēsus'itātur), *n* an apparatus for initiating respiration in asphyxia.

retail dentistry, *n* fee-for-service dentistry practiced in an exclusively retail environment (e.g., shopping center, department store) and directed to the clientele of that retail center, using the marketing technique of the parent retailer.

retail store dentistry, *n* dental services offered within a retail, department, or drug store operation. Typically, space is leased from the store by a separate administrative group that in turn subleases to a dental professional or dental group providing the actual dental services. The dental operation generally maintains the same hours of operation as the store, and appointments often are not necessary. It is considered to be a type of practice, not a dental benefits plan model.

retainer, *n* (retaining appliance), **1.** The part of a dental prosthesis that unites the abutment tooth with the suspended portion of the bridge. It may be an inlay, partial crown, or complete crown. *n* **2.** an appliance for maintaining the positions of the teeth and jaws gained by orthodontic procedures. *n* **3.** the portion of a fixed prosthesis attaching a pontic(s) to the abutment teeth (e.g., inlay, three-quarter crown). *n* **4.** a form of clasp, attachment, or device used for the fixation or stabilization of a prosthetic appliance. *n* **5.** an orthodontic appliance, fixed or removable, used to maintain teeth in corrected positions during the period of functional adaptation following corrective treatment.

retainer, continuous bar, *n* a metal bar that is attached to a major connector and contacts lingual surfaces of anterior teeth, on or incisal to the cingula; it aids in the stabilization of a distal extension removable partial denture.

retainer, direct, *n* a clasp, attachment, or assembly applied to an abutment tooth for the purpose of maintaining a removable restoration in its planned position in relation to oral structures.

retainer, extracoronal, *n* **1.** a type of retainer in which the preparation and its cast restoration lie largely external to the body of the coronal portion of the tooth and complement the contour of the crown. The retention or resistance to displacement is developed between the inner surfaces of the casting and the external walls of the prepared tooth. The extracoronal retainer may be a partial crown or a complete crown. *n* **2.** a direct retainer of the clasp type that engages an abutment tooth on its external surface in such a way as to afford retention and stabilization to a removable partial denture; a direct retainer of the manufactured type, the male portion of which is attached to the external surface of a cast crown on an abutment tooth (e.g., Dalbo and Crismani attachments).

retainer, Hawley, *n.pr* a wire and acrylic resin removable appliance designed to stabilize teeth after tooth movement; serves as a basis for tooth movement by providing an anchorage for the wires and rubber dam elastics used in orthodontic tooth movement.

retainer, indirect, *n* that part of a removable partial denture that resists movement of a free end denture base away from its tissue support through lever action opposite the fulcrum line of the direct retention.

retainer, intracoronal, *n* **1.** a type of retainer in which the prepared cavity and its cast restoration lie largely within the body of the coronal portion of the tooth and within the contour of the crown (e.g., inlay). The retention or resistance to displacement is developed between the casting and the internal walls of the prepared cavity. *n* **2.** the type of direct retainer used in the construction of removable partial dentures; it consists of a female portion within the coronal portion of the crown of an abutment and a fitted male portion attached to the denture proper. These retainers may be fabricated in the dental office or obtained through commercial sources.

retainer, matrix, *n* (matrix holder), a mechanical device designed to engage the ends of a matrix around the tooth.

retainer, radicular, *n* a type of retainer that lies within the body of the tooth and is usually confined to the root portion of the tooth (e.g., dowel crown). The retention or resistance to displacement and shear is developed by extending an attached dowel into the root canal of the tooth.

retainer, resin-bonded, *n* a prostheses fixed into an empty space created by a lost or congenitally missing tooth using bonding resin with intact or minimally restored abutment teeth in order to prevent abutment teeth from tilting or rotating.

retardation, *n* See mental retardation.

retarder, *n* a chemical added to a substance to slow a chemical reaction, prolong the set of the material, and provide more working time.

rete (epithelial) (rē′tē) ridges, *n.pl* extensions of the epithelium into the connective tissue. They occur to an excess where epithelium-lined tissues are irritated and inflamed such as the junctional epithelium during periodontal disease. Outdated term is *rete pegs.*

rete pegs, See rete ridges.

retention (rēten′shən), *n* **1.** power to retain; capacity for retaining; the inherent property of a restoration to maintain its position without displacement under stress; results from close adaptation of the restoration to the prepared form of the tooth, usually aided by cement. *n* **2.** term relating to the provision in cavity preparation for preventing displacement of a restoration. Retention supplements resistance form and is specifically created to resist any lateral or tipping force that may be brought against the restoration during and after its insertion. *n* **3.** resistance of a denture to removal in a direction opposite that of its insertion; the quality inherent in the denture that resists the force of gravity, adhesiveness of foods, and forces associated with the opening of the jaws. *n* **4.** the period of treatment during which the individual wears an appliance to maintain the teeth in the desired position.

retention arm, *n* See arm, retention.

retention, circumferential, *n* frictional resistance to displacement derived from completely veneering the exposed tooth surface.

retention, denture, *n* **1.** the means by which dentures are held in position in the oral cavity; the maintenance of a denture in its position in the oral cavity; the resistance to the movement of a denture from its basal seat in a direction opposite to that in which it was inserted. *n* **2.** the resistance of a denture to vertical movement in the occlusal direction from its basal seat.

retention, direct, *n* retention obtained in a removable partial denture by the use of attachments or clasps that resist removal from abutment teeth.

retention form, *n* See form, retention.

retention, indirect, *n* retention obtained in a removable partial denture through the use of indirect retainers.

retention, partial denture, *n* the fixation of a fixed partial denture by means of crowns, inlays, or other retainers.

retention, pin, *n* See pin, retention.

retention, pinhole, *n* one or more small holes, 2 to 3 mm in depth, placed in suitable areas of a cavity preparation parallel with the general line of draft to provide or supplement resistance and retention form.

retention, radicular, *n* retention derived from projections of metal into the root canals of pulpless teeth.

retention, removable partial denture, *n* the resistance to movement of a removable partial denture from its supporting structures, gained by the use of direct and indirect retainers or other attachments.

retention terminal, *n* See clasp, circumferential arm; clasp, circumferential, arm retentive.

reticular fibers, connective tissue, *n* fibers that come together to form a net of tissue in the lymph and bone marrow. These fibers may also be found in some glands and skin layers.

reticulocyte (ritik′yəlōsīt′), *n* an immature erythrocyte. Reticulocytes normally account for less than 2% of the circulating erythrocytes.

reticulocytosis (rētik′ūlōsītō′sis), *n* an increase in the normal number of reticulocytes in the circulating blood. Normal values range from 0.5% to 1.5% of the red blood cells.

reticuloendotheliosis, nonlipid (rētik′ūlōen′dōthē′lēō′sis), *n* abnormal increase of normal cells of reticuloendothelial tissue.

retina (ret'ənə), *n* a 10-layered, delicate nervous-tissue membrane of the eye, continuous with the optic nerve, that receives images of external objects and transmits visual impulses through the optic nerve to the brain.

retinal detachment, *n* a separation of the retina from the choroid in the back of the eye, usually resulting from a hole in the retina that allows the vitreous humor to leak between the choroid and retina. Severe trauma to the eye may be the proximate cause, but in the great majority of cases, retinal detachment is the result of internal changes in the vitreous chamber associated with aging or with inflammation of the interior of the eye.

retinitis (ret'inī'tis), *n* a condition in which the retina becomes inflamed.

retinoblastoma (ret'ənōblas'tōmə), *n* a congenital, hereditary neoplasm developing from retinal germ cells.

retinol equivalent (RE) (ret'inôl), *n* a unit of measurement used to determine the value of vitamin A in sources of vitamin A. Retinol equivalent is 3.3 IU of vitamin A. 1 retinol equivalent = 6 μg β-carotene or 1 μg retinol.

retinopathy (ret'ənôp'əthē), *n* a disease of the retina, excluding retinitis. Often named for the underlying condition which causes it, such as diabetic retinopathy.

retraction, *n* **1.** a drawing or shrinking back; the laying back of tissues to expose a given part. *n* **2.** distal movement of teeth; a distal or retrusive position of the teeth, dental arch, or jaw.

retraction, gingival, *n* laying back of the free gingival tissue to expose the gingival margin area of a preparation by mechanical, chemical, or electrical means.

retractor, *n* an instrument for retracting tissues to assist in gaining access to an area of operation or observation.

retractor, beaver-tail, *n* a broad-bladed periosteal elevator.

retractor, rake, *n* a metallic instrument with prongs set transversely for engaging and retracting soft tissues.

retractor, vein hook, *n* a metallic instrument ending in a rounded flange set transversely for engaging and retracting soft tissues.

retroclination, *n* posterior angulation (inclination) of anterior teeth.

retrofill, *v* obturation of the apex of a tooth root by the direct surgical approach.

retrognathic (ret'rōnath'ik), *adj* **1.** the condition of a mandible that is posterior to its normal relationship with other facial structures; may be a result of small mandibular size or posteriorly positioned temporomandibular fossae. *adj* **2.** mandibular retrusion. **3.** a facial profile with a protruding upper lip or the appearance of a recessive mandible and chin, or convex profile.

retrognathism (ret'rōnath'izm), *n* facial disharmony in which one or both jaws (usually the mandible) are posterior to normal facial relationships. This condition may be real or imaginary.

retrognathism, bird-face, *n* typical facial profile associated with an underdeveloped mandible; a retrognathia and small mandible usually associated with interference of condylar growth because of trauma or infection affecting the condyles. Surgical intervention is necessary for improvement.

retrognathism, Pierre Robin, *n.pr* See syndrome, Pierre Robin.

retrograde, *v* to move backward, degenerate, or return to an earlier state or worse condition.

retromolar pad, *n* See pad, retromolar.

retromylohyoid eminence, *n* See eminence, retromylohyoid.

retrospective review, a posttreatment assessment of services on a case-by-case or aggregate basis after the services have been performed.

retrospective study, a study in which a search is made for a relationship between one phenomenon or condition and another that occurred in the past (e.g., the exposure to toxic agents and the rate of occurrence of disease in the exposed group compared with a control group not exposed).

retrosternal pain (ret'rōster'nəl), *n* a pain behind the sternum that usually occurs on swallowing. If retrosternal pain is associated with oral or pharyngeal candidiasis, it may indicate candidiasis of the esophagus, which is an opportunistic infection indicative of acquired immunodeficiency syndrome.

retroversion (ret′rōvur′zhən), *n* a condition in which teeth or other maxillary and mandibular structures are located posterior to the normal or generally accepted standard.

Retrovir, *n.pr* brand name for zidovudine, a dideoxynucleoside used in the treatment of HIV-positive patients.

retrovirus (ret′rōvīrus), *n* a virus containing ribonucleic acid rather than deoxyribonucleic acid.

retruded contact position, *n* A tooth-to-tooth position at centric relation, sometimes referred to as centric relation occlusion.

retrusion (rētroo′zhən), *n* teeth or jaws posterior to their normal positions.

retrusion, mandibular, *n* abnormal retrusion of the mandible, as in a Class II malocclusion.

retrusion, maxillary, *n* abnormal retrusion of the maxillae.

reversal lines, *n.pl* stained scalloped microscopic lines caused by the resorption in bone and cementum.

reverse curve, *n* See curve, reverse.

reverse transcriptase (transkrip′tās), *n* an enzyme within a retrovirus that converts its ribonucleic acid into deoxyribonucleic acid (DNA), which then penetrates the cell nucleus and joins the host's DNA.

reverse Trendelenburg, *n.pr* a position in which the lower extremities are lower than the body and head, which are elevated on an inclined plane.

reverse-cut suture needle, *n* small, curved, handheld tool used to secure surgical stitches; characterized by three cutting surfaces; one on the outside edge of the curve of the needle, with the other two on opposite sides near the tip.

reversible, *adj* capable of going through a series of changes in either direction, forward or backward (e.g., reversible chemical reaction).

reversible hydrocolloid, *n* See hydrocolloid, reversible.

rewards, *n.pl* a motivation technique to improve patient compliance with oral hygiene protocols, generally used with young patients.

Rh factor, *n* an antigenic substance present in the erthrocytes of 85% of humans. A person having the factor is Rh positive, and a person lacking the factor is Rh negative.

Rh incompatibility, *n* a condition in which two groups of blood cells are antigentically different because of the presence of Rh factor in one group and the absence of the Rh factor in the other. See also Rh factor.

rhabdomyosarcoma (rab′dōmīōsärkō′mə), *n* a malignant tumor of striated, or voluntary, muscle.

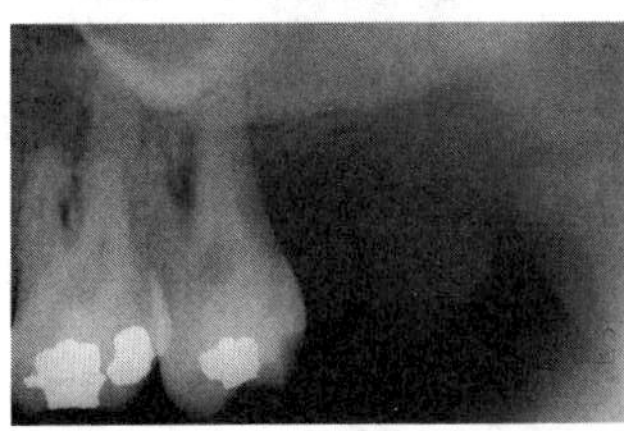

Rhabdomyosarcoma. (Regezi/Sciubba/Jordan, 2008)

Rhabdoviridae **(rab′dōvir′idā),** *n* one of the major ribonucleic acid virus families, to which the rabies virus belongs. Viruses have a single-stranded, nonsegmented, linear molecular structure with helical symmetry.

rhagades (rag′ədēz), *n.pl* fissures or cracks in the skin seen around body orifices and in regions subjected to frequent movement.

rheology (rēol′əjē), *n* the study of blood flow, pressure, and velocity through the vascular system.

rheostat (rē′ōstat), *n* a resistor for regulating a current by means of variable resistances.

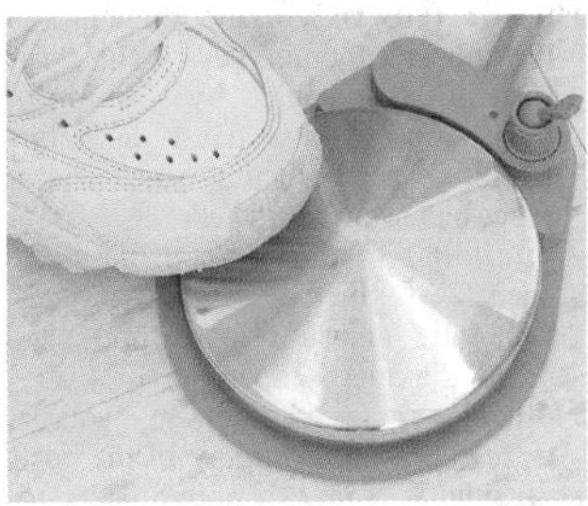

Rheostat pedal. (Bird/Robinson, 2005)

rheostat pedal, n foot pedal that controls the speed on rotary powered, variable speed dental polishing equipment.

rheumatic carditis (roomat′ik), *n* See rheumatic heart disease.

rheumatic fever, *n* See fever, rheumatic.

rheumatic heart disease, *n* damage to heart muscle and heart valves caused by episodes of rheumatic fever. Rheumatic heart disease may result when a susceptible person acquires a group A β-hemolytic streptococcal infection; an autoimmune reaction may occur in heart tissue, resulting in permanent deformities of heart valves or chordae tendineae.

rheumatism (roo′mətiz′əm), *n* (rheumatic disease), a nonspecific term indicating any painful disorder related to joints, muscles, bone, or nerves; acute rheumatic fever; or, as used by lay persons, rheumatoid arthritis, bursitis, myositis, or degenerative joint disease.

rheumatoid arthritis, *n* a chronic, destructive, sometimes deforming collagen disease that has an autoimmune component. Rheumatoid arthritis usually first appears in early middle age, between 36 and 50 years of age, and most commonly in women.

rheumatoid arthritis, juvenile, n a chronic disease affecting the immune system that occurs in children younger than age 16. Symptoms include joint inflammation in the spine, knees, and wrists and a limited ability to open the oral cavity.

rheumatoid factor (RF), *n* antiglobulin antibodies often found in the serum of patients with a clinical diagnosis of rheumatoid arthritis.

rhinitis (rīnī′tis), *n* inflammation of the mucous membranes of the nose, usually accompanied by swelling of the mucosa and a nasal discharge. Rhinitis may be acute, allegic, atrophic, or vasomotor.

rhinolalia (rī′nōlā′lēə), *n* nasalized speech, of which there are two types: rhinolalia clausa (closed port) and rhinolalia aperta (open port).

rhinoplasty (ri′nōplastē), *n* plastic or reconstructive surgery of the nose.

rhinovirus, *n* any of about 100 serologically distinct, small ribonucleic acid viruses that cause about 40% of acute respiratory illnesses. Infection is characterized by dry, scratchy throat, nasal congestion, malaise, and headache. Fever is minimal. Nasal discharge lasts 2 or 3 days.

rhizotomy, retrogasserian (rīzot′əmē, ret′rōgasser′ēən), *n* intracranial sectioning of the sensory root of the trigeminal nerve posterior to the semilunar ganglion; used in the treatment of severe trigeminal neuralgia.

rhodium (Rh) (rō′dēəm), *n* a grayish-white metallic element. Its atomic number is 45 and its atomic weight is 102.9055. Rhodium is used for providing a hard, lustrous coating on other metals and in the making of mirrors.

Rhodococcus **(rōdōkok′us),** *n* a genus of gram-positive, rod-shaped, aerobic bacteria, some of which are pathogenic in humans.

rhodopsin (rōdop′sin), *n* a purple light-receptive pigment found in the retina and consisting of opsin and retinal. Rhodopsin helps the eye adjust to drastic changes in environmental lighting.

rhythm (rith′əm), *n* a measured movement; the recurrence of an action or function at regular intervals.

rhythm, heart, n the rhythm pattern in the sequence of heart beats, which may be altered in the presence of cardiac disease.

rhytidoplasty (ritāidōplas′tē), *n* a procedure in reconstructive plastic surgery in which the skin of the face is tightened, wrinkles are removed, and the skin is made to appear firm and smooth.

ribavirin (rī′bəvir′in), *n* an antiviral agent that acts against many ribonucleic acid and deoxyribonucleic acid viruses by inhibiting protein synthesis and replication. Used in the United States only for aerosol therapy for infants to treat acute lower respiratory infections resulting from respiratory syncitial virus.

riboflavin (rī′bōflā′vin), *n* (vitamin B_2), *brand names:* many generic sources; *drug class:* vitamin B_2 water soluble; *action:* needed for normal tissue respiratory reactions; functions as a coenzyme; *uses:* vitamin B_2 deficiency.

ribonuclease (rī'bōnoo'klēās), *n* an enzyme that acts as a catalyst for ribonucleic acid hydrolysis. It may also be called *RNase.*

ribonucleic acid (RNA), *n* a nucleic acid, found in both the nucleus and cytoplasm of cells, that transmits genetic instructions from the nucleus to the cytoplasm. RNA functions in the assembly of proteins.

ribose, *n* a 5-carbon sugar that occurs as a component of ribonucleic acid.

ribosomal RNA (rī'bōsō'məl), *n* a type of protein-containing ribonucleic acid produced by the nucleolus and found connected to the endoplasmic reticulum or moving freely within the cytoplasm.

rickets (rik'əts), *n* a condition caused by deficiency of vitamin D or calcium in infants and children, with disturbance in the mineralization of osseous and dental tissues. Marked by bending and bowing of bones, nodular enlargements at the ends of bones, myalgia, delay in closure of fontanels, and other problems. See also osteomalacia.

rickets, adult, *n* See osteomalacia.

rickets, refractory, *n* See rickets, resistant.

rickets, renal, *n* a disturbance marked by excessive excretion of phosphorus and calcium resulting from a lowered renal threshold of excretion of these mineral elements. See also osteodystrophy, renal.

rickets, resistant, *n* (late rickets, refractory rickets), rickets that responds only to extremely large amounts of vitamin D.

***Rickettsia* (riket'sēə),** *n* a genus of microorganisms that combine aspects of both bacteria and viruses. Examples of rickettsial diseases are Rocky Mountain spotted fever and typhus.

ridge, *n* **1.** the remainder of the alveolar process after the teeth are removed. **2.** the linear elevations on the masticatory surface of both anterior and posterior teeth.

ridge, alveolar, *n* the bony ridge of the maxillae or mandible that contains the alveoli (sockets of the teeth). See also process, alveolar.

ridge, alveolar, remodeling, *n* an eroding of the residual ridge that occurs as the result of wearing dentures. It may cause changes to the bone structure of the face so that dentures must be repaired or replaced to obtain a secure, comfortable fit.

ridge augmentation, *n* the process of increasing the size of the alveolar ridge.

ridge, center of, *n* the buccolingual midline of the residual ridge.

ridge, central labial, *n* a groove appearing on the buccal midline of a canine tooth that is caused by a larger than usual middle labial developmental lobe.

ridge, cervical, *n* the height of the curve in the cervical third of a tooth's buccal surface.

ridge, crest of, *n* the highest continuous surface of the ridge, but not necessarily the center of the ridge; the top of a residual or alveolar ridge.

ridge expansion, *n* the surgical process of using chisels or osteotomes to widen the residual ridge laterally in order to allow an implant or bone graft to be inserted.

ridge extension, *n* See extension, ridge.

ridge, internal oblique, *n* the mylohyoid line located along each medial surface of the body of the mandible that extends posteriorly and superiorly, becoming more prominent as it ascends each body. It is the point of attachment of the mylohyoid muscle that forms the floor of the mouth.

ridge, key, *n* (zygomaxillare), the lowest point of the zygomaticomaxillary ridge.

ridge, labial, *n* a linear elevation or ridge located on the surfaces of the incisors that face the lips.

ridge lap, *n* the part of an artificial tooth that is adjacent to the residual ridge; the part of the artificial tooth that laps the ridge.

ridge mapping, *n* the act of using a graduated probe or caliper to pierce the anesthetized soft tissue along the residual ridge in order to determine the measurements needed to reproduce the shape of the ridge using a diagnostic cast.

ridge, marginal, *n* a ridge or elevation of enamel that forms the boundary of the occlusal surface of a tooth.

ridge, mental, *n* a dense ridge extending from the symphysis to the premolar area on the anterolateral aspect of the body of the mandible.

ridge, mylohyoid, *n* a dense line or ridge of bone on the medial surface of the body of the mandible that extends obliquely upward and posteriorly from the symphysis, covers the cervical portion of the third molar, and then goes upward and backward onto the vertical ramus. The mylohyoid muscle is inserted into this ridge of bone.

ridge, oblique, *n* See ridge, internal oblique.

ridge, Passavant's, *n.pr* See pad, Passavant's.

ridge relation, *n* See relation, ridge.

ridge, residual, *n* the portion of the alveolar ridge that remains after the alveoli have disappeared from the alveolar process after extraction of the teeth.

ridge support, *n* See area, supporting.

ridge, transverse, *n* an elevation that connects the buccal and lingual cusps and extends crosswise over the occlusal table of mandibular and maxillary posterior teeth.

ridge, triangular, *n* an elevation on a posterior tooth that extends from the tip of the cusp to the center of the occlusal table.

rifabutin (rif'əbūt'ən), *n brand name:* Mycobutin; *drug class:* antimycobacterial agent; *action:* inhibits deoxyribonucleic acid–dependent ribonucleic acid (RNA) polymerase synthesis of bacterial RNA; *uses:* prevention of disseminated *Mycobacterium avium* complex (MAC) disease with advanced HIV infection.

rifampin (rifam'pin), *n brand names:* Rifadin IV, Rimactane; *drug class:* antitubercular antiinfective; *action:* inhibits deoxyribonucleic acid–dependent ribonucleic acid (RNA) polymerase synthesis of bacterial RNA; *uses:* pulmonary tuberculosis, prevention of meningococcal caries.

right of action, *n* the right to sue; a legal right to maintain an action, based on a happening or state of fact.

right-to-know laws, *n.pl* laws that require employers to inform workers regarding health effects of materials they must handle, including toxic chemicals and radioactive substances. Right-to-know statutes are administered under the authority of the U.S. Occupational Safety and Health Administration (OSHA).

rigidity, *n* the characteristic of being nonflexible, which is essential in a connector, a reciprocal arm, or an indirect retaining unit of a removable partial denture.

rigor mortis, *n* the stiffening of skeletal and cardiac muscle shortly after death.

Riley-Day syndrome, *n.pr* See syndrome, Riley-Day.

riluzole (ril'əzōl'), *n brand name:* Rilutek; *drug class:* glutamate antagonist; *action:* inhibits presynaptic release of glutamic acid in central nervous system; *use:* treatment of amyotrophic lateral sclerosis (Lou Gehrig disease).

rim, *n* the outer edge; often curved or circular.

rim, occlusion, *n* (record rim), an occluding surface built on temporary or permanent denture bases for the purpose of making maxillomandibular relation records and arranging teeth.

rim, record, *n* See rim, occlusion.

rim, surgical occlusion, *n* a conventional occlusion rim, the base of which has been reduced until it is smaller than the surgical impression tray with which the surgical jaw relations are recorded.

rimantadine HCl (riman'tədēn), *n brand name:* Flumadine; *drug class:* antiviral; *action:* may inhibit viral uncoating; *uses:* adults, prophylaxis and treatment of illnesses caused by strains of influenza A virus; in children, prophylaxis against influenza A virus.

rimexolone (rimek'səlōn), *n brand name:* Vexol; *drug class:* corticosteroid; *action:* interacts with steroid cytoplasmic receptors to induce antiinflammatory effects; *uses:* inflammation of the eye associated with ocular surgery and uveitis.

ringworm, *n* a fungal infection of the skin, nails, and hair caused primarily by dermatophytes, symptoms of which include inflammation, patching, and scaling of lesions.

rinse bath, *n* a tank or container of water used in film processing to wash residual developer from the film before placement in the fixer.

Risdon wire, *n.pr* See wire, Risdon.

Risdon's incision, *n.pr* See incision, Risdon's.

risk factors, *n.pl* the elements that may contribute to or increase the risk to one's health, economic stability, or personal and professional liability.

risk management, *n* a program designed to identify, contain, reduce, or eliminate the potential for harm to patients, visitors, and employees and the potential financial loss to the facility if a compensable event occurs; usually concerned with the delivery system and site rather than practitioner performance.

risk pool, *n* a portion of provider fees or capitation payments withheld as financial reserves to cover unanticipated utilization of services in an alternative benefits plan.

risk-benefit analysis, *n* the consideration as to whether a medical or surgical procedure, particuarly a radical approach, is worth the risk to the patient compared with the possible benefits if the procedure is successful.

risorius (risō'rēəs), *n* a muscle of facial expression in the orofacial region that is used when smiling widely.

risperidone (risper'ədōn), *n brand name:* Risperdal; *drug class:* antipsychotic; *action:* may be related to antagonism for dopamine and serotonin receptors; also has affinity for alpha receptors and histamine (H_1) receptors; *use:* psychotic disorders.

RNA splicing, *n* the process by which base pairs that interrupt the continuity of genetic information in deoxyribonucleic acid are removed from the precursors of messenger ribonucleic acid.

RNA viruses, *n* See viruses.

Roach clasp, *n* See clasp, bar.

Rockwell test, *n.pr* See test, Rockwell.

Rocky Mountain spotted fever (RMSF), *n* a serious tick-borne infectious disease occurring throughout the temperate zones of North and South America, caused by *R. rickettsii,* and characterized by chills, fever, severe headache, myalgia, mental confusion, and rash.

rod, *n* a straight, slim, cylindric form of material, usually metal.

rod, analyzing, *n* the vertical part of a dental cast surveyor that is brought into contact with the surface contour of a tooth as a tangent related to a curve. It is used to determine the relative parallelism of one surface of a cast to other surfaces of the same cast. It is also used to estimate the cervical convergence of an infrabulge area of a tooth as it slopes from the contacting point of the surveying rod toward the cervical line, permitting evaluation of the retentiveness of the surface.

rod, condyle, *n* the adjustable pointers of a face-bow, which are placed over the condyles or at points on the face to mark the opening axis of the mandible.

rod, enamel, *n* a calcified column or prism, with an average diameter of 4 microns; extends in a wavy pattern through the entire thickness of the enamel and is generally perpendicular to the surface of the tooth.

rodent ulcer, *n* See basal cell carcinoma.

roentgen, equivalent man (rem) (rent'gən), the dose of any ionizing radiation that produces the same biologic effect as that produced by 1 roentgen of high-voltage x-radiation.

roentgen, equivalent physical (rep), *n* an unofficial unit of dose used with ionizing radiation other than roentgen rays or gamma rays. It is defined as the dose that produces an energy absorption of 93 ergs per gram of tissue. For most purposes the rep can be considered equal to the rad; the latter is gradually replacing the use of rep.

R

roentgeno- (rent'gənō), *pref* denotes radiation originating only from a radiographic tube.

roentgenogram (rent'gənōgram'), *n* See radiograph.

roentgenograph (rent'gənōgraf'), *n* See radiograph.

roentgenographer (rent'gənog'rəfur), *n* See radiographer.

roentgenographic detail, *n* See detail, radiographic.

roentgenography (rent'gənog'rəfē), *n* See radiography.

roentgenologist (rent'gənol'ōjist), *n* See radiologist.

roentgenologist, oral, *n* See radiologist, oral.

roentgenolucent (rent′gənōloo′-sent), *n* See radiolucent.

roentgenopaque (rent′gənōpāk′), *n* See radiopaque.

roentgenoparent (rent′gənōper′-ent), *n* See radioparent.

roentgenotherapy (rent′gənō-ther′əpē), *n* See therapy, radiation.

Romberg sign, *n.pr* an indication of loss of the sense of position in which the patient loses balance when standing erect, with feet together and eyes closed. Also called *Romberg test.*

rongeur forceps (rōnzhur′), *n* a strong and heavy cutting or biting forceps that is used for cutting bone.

root, *n* **1.** the part of a human tooth covered by cementum. *n* **2.** a nerve root; the part of a nerve adjacent to the center with which it is connected; in spinal and cranial nerves the part of the nerve between the cells of origin or termination and the ganglion.

root amputation, *n* See amputation, root.

root angulation, *n* the angle formed by the intersection of the tooth root and the long axes of the crown. Where roots are sufficiently angulated, adequate bone formation occurs between the adjacent roots, which is important if the patient is particularly susceptible to periodontal bone loss.

root apex, *n* the root tip.

root, apical **(ā′pikəl),** *n* the most inferior part or tip of the root of a tooth.

R

root axis line (RAL), *n* a hypothetical vertical line that could be drawn from the crown of a tooth to the root apex.

root, bifurcated, *n* the root structure of a tooth divided into two segments.

root canal, *n* **1.** the soft, hollow, canal-like tissues of a tooth that adjoin the pulp chamber. The root canals help secure the teeth in the jaw, provide nutrition to the teeth through their blood vessels, and help sense oral cavity activity through their nerves. Infected root canals can be extremely painful. **2.** the informal term for the endodontic procedure to remove infected root canal tissue and replace removed tissue with restorative material.

root canal, accessory, *n* a nonprimary passage typically located near the root's apex that extends from the cementum to the pulp. It may be located at a higher point on the tooth and connect to a periodontal pocket.

root canal instrument stop, *n* a device placed on a root canal instrument to mark the measured depth of instrument penetration.

root, clinical, *n* the portion of the tooth that is below the attached periodontal tissues and not exposed to the oral cavity.

root concavity, *n* a longitudinal depression located on the surface of a root.

root curettage, *n* See curettage, root.

root, dwarfed, *n* an abnormally short root with a normal-sized crown.

root, fused, *n* a tooth root that is joined with another.

root, intraalveolar **(in′trəalvē′ələr),** *n* the portion of a tooth root enclosed in and supported by alveolar bone.

root, mesiobuccal **(mezēəbuk′əl),** *n* the root of a tooth that is found near the mesial portion of the tooth and the buccal side of the alveolar ridge.

root morphology **(môrfol′əjē),** *n* the study of the topographic surfaces of the roots that allow for successful periodontal treatment.

root planing, *n* a procedure that smooths the surface of a root by removing abnormal toxic cementum or dentin that is rough, contaminated, or permeated with calculus.

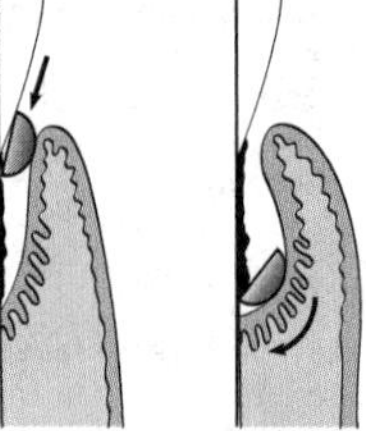
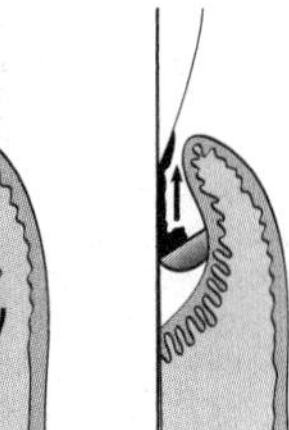

Root planing. (Newman/Takei/Klokkevold/Carranza, 2006)

root resection, *n* See apicoectomy.

root resorption of teeth, *n* the destruction of the cementum or dentin by cementoclastic or osteoclastic activity. It may result in a shortening or blunting of the root. Lateral root resorption may also occur, resulting in a loss of root substance along the side or length of the root. Severe lateral resorption may result in penetration of the pulp canal. Root resorption may be caused by inflammation resulting from trauma or infection, or it may be unknown or idiopathic. See also resorption.

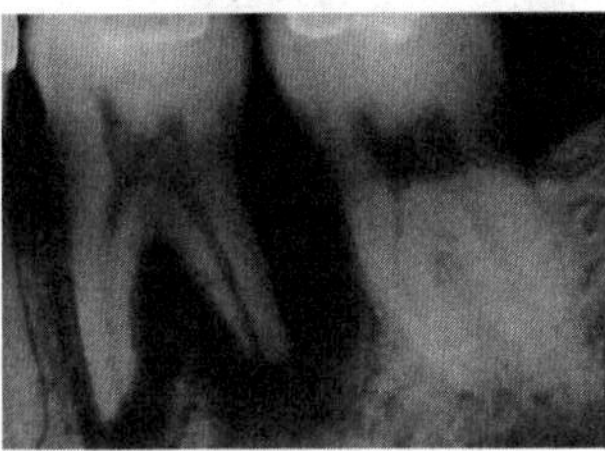

Root resorption of the teeth. (Ibsen/Phelan, 2004)

root retention, *n* removal of the crown of a root-canal–treated tooth, whose periodontium is not adequate to support a prosthesis but with enough retention of the root and gingival attachment to support a removable prosthesis. See also overdenture.

root submersion, *n* root retention in which the tooth structure is reduced below the level of the alveolar crest and the soft tissue is allowed to heal over it. It is believed that residual ridge resorption can be minimized by this approach. See also root retention.

root, trifurcated, *n* the root structure of a tooth divided into three segments.

root trunk, *n* the section of root nearest the crown from which multiple roots emerge.

Rorschach test (ror′shak), *n.pr* better known as the inkblot test, this test consists of 10 pictures of inkblots, five in black and white, three in black and red, and two multicolored, to which the subject responds by telling, in as many interpretations as is desired, what images and emotions each design evokes.

rosary, rachitic (rəkit′ik), *n* a beading of the ribs at the costochondral junction such as occurs in rickets.

rose fever, *n* a common misnomer for seasonal allergic rhinitis caused by pollen, most frequently of grasses, that is airborne when roses are in bloom.

rotary cutting instrument, *n* See instrument, cutting, rotary.

rotating anode, *n* See anode, rotating.

rotating condyle, *n* See condyle, rotating.

rotating spring, *n* an auxiliary wire used in conjunction with arch wire to rotate a tooth into proper position.

rotation, *n* **1.** the act of turning about an axis or a center. *n* **2.** movement of a tooth around its longitudinal axis.

rotation center, *n* See center, rotation.

rotavirus (rō′təvī′rəs), *n* a double-stranded ribonucleic acid molecule that appears as a tiny wheel, with a clearly defined outer layer or rim and an inner layer of spokes. It is a cause of acute gastroenteritis with diarrhea, particularly in infants.

rotundum foramen, *n* See foramen, rotundum.

rouge, *n* See jeweler's rouge.

rounds, *n* a teaching conference or meeting in which the clinical problems encountered in the practice of medicine, dentistry, nursing, or other service are discussed.

roundworm, *n* a worm of the class Nematoda, including *A. duodenale, A. lumbricoides, E. vermicularis,* and *S. stercoralis,* that may infect the gastrointestinal tract of humans.

routine, *n* **1.** a fixed pattern of procedures used in any phase of treatment. *n* **2.** a set of instructions arranged in proper sequence to direct the computer to perform a desired operation or series of operations.

routine, office, *n* a series of steps, to be followed in a carefully planned sequence, that provide a means of dealing with situations commonly encountered in dental practice.

rpm (revolutions per minute), *n* the speed of rotary dental surface polishing equipment. High speed is classified as 100,000 to 800,000 r.p.m. and low speed as 6000 to 10,000 r.p.m.

rubber dam, *n* See dam, rubber.

rubber dam clamp, *n* See clamp, rubber dam.

rubber dam clamp forceps, *n* an instrument used to place a clamp on a tooth, adjust a clamp, or remove it from a tooth. It engages the holes or notches of the flanges of the clamp.

rubber dam holder, *n* in endodontics, a rubber dam frame holder; in operative dentistry, a rubber dam frame.

rubber polishing cup, *n* See polishing cup.

rubefacient, *n* a substance or agent that increases the reddish coloration of the skin.

rubella (roobel′ə), *n* (German measles, 3-day measles), a highly contagious viral disease spread mainly by direct contact that has an incubation period of about 18 days. Manifestations include pharyngitis, regional lymphadenopathy, mild constitutional symptoms, and a maculopapular rash that becomes scarlatiniform. Oral lesions are red macules. When it occurs in pregnant women, it may cause congenital rubella syndrome with serious malformations of the developing fetus. Children infected with rubella before birth (a condition known as *congenital rubella*) are at risk for the following: growth retardation; malformations of the heart, eyes, or brain; deafness; and liver, spleen, and bone marrow problems.

rubeola (roobēō′lə), *n* See measles.

rudimentary, *adj* pertaining to something either vestigial or embryonic.

Ruffini's corpuscles (roofē′nēz), *n.pr* See corpuscle, Ruffini's.

rugae (roo′gē, roo′jē), *n.pl* the irregular ridges in the mucous membrane covering the anterior part of the hard palate.

rugae area, *n* See area, rugae.

rule, Clark's, *n.pr* a formula used to estimate the dosage of a drug for individuals whose weight varies significantly from the arbitrarily selected official standard of 150 pounds (67.5 kg). The dose is calculated by dividing the weight of the patient by 150 and multiplying by the dose to determine the current dose for a patient weighing more or less than 150 pounds.

rule of confidentiality, *n* a principle that personal information about others, particularly patients, should not be revealed to anyone not authorized to receive such information.

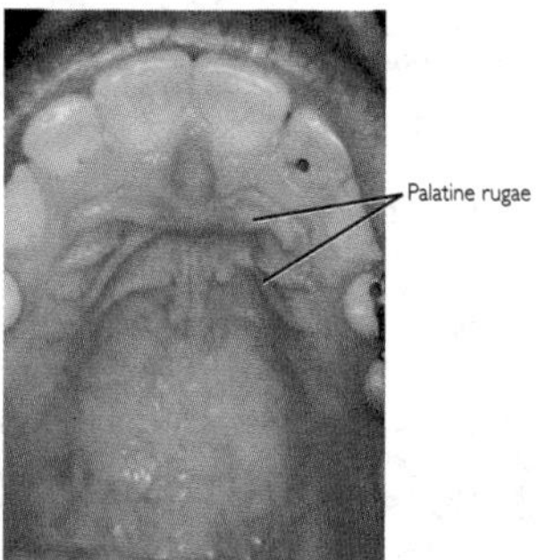

Rugae. (Fehrenbach/Herring, 2006)

rule, Young's, *n.pr* a mathematics expression used to determine a drug dosage for children. The correct dosage is calculated by dividing the child's age by an amount equal to the child's age plus 12 and then multiplying by the usual adult dose.

Rumpel-Leede test, *n.pr* See test, capillary resistance.

rupture, *n* a tear or break in the continuity or configuration of an organ or body tissue, including those instances when other tissue protrudes through the opening.

S

Sabouraud's medium (säbooröz′), *n* See medium, Sabouraud's.

saccharin, *n* the chemical sweetener benzosulfimide, which is 300 to 500 times as sweet as sucrose. Tests have demonstrated that large amounts may cause cancers in experimental animals. It is no longer in general use as a low-calorie sweetener.

Saccharomyces **(sak′ərōmī′sēz),** *n* a genus of yeast fungi, including brewer's and baker's yeast, as well as some pathogenic fungi, that cause such diseases as bronchitis, moniliasis, and pharyngitis.

sacroiliac joint (sak′rōil′ēak′), *n* an irregular synovial joint between the sacrum and ilium on either side of the pelvis.

saddle, *n* See base, denture.

saddle connector, *n* See connector, major.

saddle, metal, *n* See base, metal.

saddle, nose, *n* a sunken nasal bridge caused by injury or disease and resulting in damage to the nasal septum.

safelight, *n* a source of light in a darkroom of a color and intensity that does not fog radiographic film.

safelighting test, *n* a procedure used to determine whether darkroom lights are too bright. It involves bringing unprocessed film into the darkroom and placing a coin on the film. The safelight is then turned on for a short period of time, and the film is processed normally. Evidence of the coin's shape on the film will disqualify the safelight.

safety measures, *n.pl* actions (e.g., use of glasses, face masks) taken to protect patients and office personnel from such known hazards as particles and aerosols from high-speed rotary instruments, mercury vapor, radiation exposure, anesthetic and sedative gases, falls, inadequate sterilization, cuts, puncture wounds, and laboratory accidents.

sagittal (saj′ətəl), *adj* shaped like or resembling an arrow; straight; situated in the direction of the sagittal suture. Said of an anteroposterior plane or section parallel to the long axis of the body.

sagittal axis, *n* a hypothetical line through the mandibular condyle that serves as an axis for rotation movements of the mandible.

sagittal plane, *n* See plane, sagittal.

sagittal splitting of mandible, *n* an intraoral osteotomy of the ascending ramus and posterior body of the mandible in the sagittal plane for the correction of prognathism, retrognathism, or apertognathia. An alternative procedure confines the split to the body of the mandible.

Saint Vitus's dance, *n.pr* See chorea.

Sainton's disease, *n.pr* See dysostosis, cleidocranial.

salary arrangements, *n.pl* the clear understanding between the dental professional and auxiliaries concerning the amount of money they will be paid, the increase in pay they may expect, and the time interval between pay increases.

salicylamide (sal′isilam′īd), *n* an analgesic, antipyretic, and antiarthritic similar in action to aspirin.

salicylanilide (sal′isilan′ilīd), *n* an antifungal agent useful in the treatment of tinea capitis caused by *Microsporum audouinii.*

salicylates (səlis′əlāts), *n.pl* the salts or esters of salicylic acid; salicylates are used as preservatives, antiseptics, fungicides, and keratolytic agents.

salicylism (sal′isil′izəm), *n* a toxic state resulting from excess ingestion of salicylates.

saline (sā′lēn), *adj* salty; of the nature of a salt; containing a salt or salts.

saliva (səlī′və), *n* the clear mucoserous secretion formed mainly in the major glands of the parotid, submandibular, and sublingual, as well as minor glands. It has lubricative, cleansing, microbial, excretory, and digestive functions and also is an aid to deglutition. Although its pH level is slightly more acidic than blood—6.3 to 6.9—it is more basic than dental plaque and acts as a buffering agent within the oral cavity. Emotional disturbances affect the rate of salivary secretion either by stimulation of secretion or inhibition of activity, leading to xerostomia. A lowered rate of flow has been noted in patients suffering from depression, whereas a higher degree of salivary activity has been observed in patients with mania. However, most xerostomia is due to medications and is related to an increased caries risk.

saliva, lingual, *n* saliva secreted by von Ebner's glands and other serous glands of the tongue.

saliva, loss of CO_2 in, *n* a theory of calculus formation in which the loss of carbon dioxide (CO_2) from saliva reduces the salivary carbonic acid content and causes the calcium phosphate in solution in the saliva to become supersaturated; calcium phosphate then precipitates in areas of stasis of the saliva.

saliva, parotid, *n* saliva produced by the parotid gland. It is thinner and less viscous than are the other varieties and contains no mucin because the parotid gland is purely serous in its secretions.

saliva, supersaturated, n saliva overladen with mineral elements associated with calculus formation. With a loss of carbon dioxide (CO_2) and a rise in the pH level of saliva, precipitation of calcium, phosphates, and magnesium carbonate occur, thus providing the mineral components of salivary calculus.

saliva tests, n.pl See tests, colorimetric caries susceptibility.

saliva viscosity, n the relative thickness of saliva produced by the salivary glands. Saliva should be watery in order to aid in food digestion and to assist in the motor functions of chewing, swallowing, and speaking.

salivant (sal′ivənt), *adj* provoking a flow of saliva.

salivary duct openings, palatal (sal′əvar′ē), *n* minute, darkened areas distributed on the soft and hard palates.

salivary flow, *n* the amount of saliva naturally produced by the salivary glands. Saliva production is increased by the presence of food or irritating substances, such as vomit, in the oral cavity. A healthy individual produces approximately 700 mL of saliva each day.

salivary glands, *n.pl* three pairs of exocrine glands that produce saliva and empty it into the oral cavity. The parotid glands produce serous fluid, the sublingual glands produce mucous fluid, and the submandibular glands produce serous and mucous secretions. See also gland.

salivary glands, von Ebner's, n.pr the minor secretory glands located at the base of the circumvallate papillae on the posterior dorsal surface of the tongue. Also known as *Ebner's glands.*

salivary *Lactobacillus* count, *n* a determination of the number of *lactobacilli* per milliliter of saliva; an indicator of caries susceptibility. High lactobacillus counts generally correlate with high caries activity.

salivary percolation, *n* saliva bubbling from a dental implant's biologic seal, indicating that the implant is failing.

salivary stone, *n* a tiny, pebblelike mass of calcified saliva that forms in the major salivary ducts or glands. Mainly happens in the submandibular gland and its ducts. May cause a ranula or mucocele. Also called *sialolith.* See also ranula and mucus escape reaction.

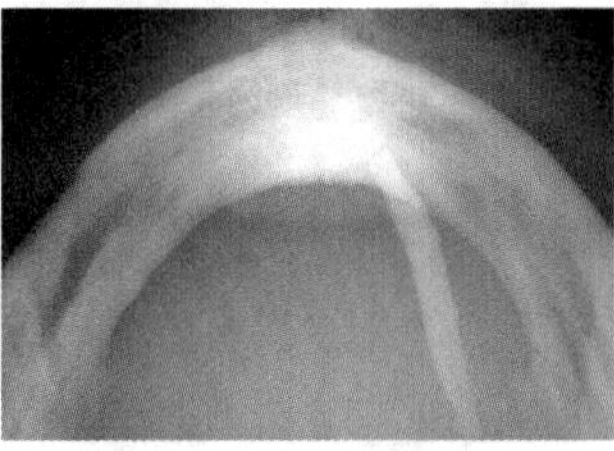

Salivary stone. (Courtesy Dr. Charles Babbush)

salivation (sal′ivā′shən), *n* the production of saliva.

salmeterol xinafoate (salmet′ərol′ zin′əfō′āt), *n brand name:* Serevent Inhalation Aerosol; *drug class:* long-acting selective β_2-agonist; *action:* relaxes bronchial smooth muscle by directly acting on β_2-adrenergic receptors; also inhibits release of mast cell mediators; *uses:* treatment of bronchospasm, maintenance treatment of asthma and exercise-induced bronchospasm.

Salmonella, *n* a genus of motile, gram-negative, rod-shaped bacteria that include species causing typhoid fever, paratyphoid fever, and other forms of gastroenteritis.

salmonellosis (sal′mənelō′sis), *n* an infection of the gastrointestinal tract caused by *Salmonella* bacteria, usually contracted by the ingestion of tainted food or drink. Symptoms include fever, bacteremia, and lesions.

salsalate (sal′səlāt), *n brand names:* Armigesic, Anaflex, Arthra-G, Mono-Gesic, Salflex, and Salsitab; *drug class:* salicylate, nonnarcotic analgesic; *action:* blocks formation of peripheral prostaglandins, which cause pain and inflammation; antipyretic action results from inhibition of hypothalamic heat-regulating center; does not inhibit platelet aggregation; *uses:* treatment of mild to moderate pain or fever, including arthritis and juvenile rheumatoid arthritis.

salt (sôlt), *n* a compound of a base and an acid; a compound of an acid, some of the replaceable hydrogen atoms of which have been substituted.

salt, basic, n a salt containing replaceable, or hydroxyl, groups.

salt depletion, n See depletion, salt.

salt solution, n a homemade mouthrinse consisting of one-half teaspoon salt and one-half cup of tepid water, used to decrease inflammation and promote healing.

sample, *n* a selected part of a population that is taken to be representative of the whole population.

sample, random, n a sample drawn by chance; a sample drawn in such a way that every item in the population has an equal and independent chance of being included in the sample.

sample, stratified, n a sample derived by dividing the population into a number of nonoverlapping classes or categories from which cases are selected at random, the number of cases selected from each category being proportional to the number therein.

sanguinaria (sang′gwiner′ēə) (bloodroot), *n Sanguinaria canadensis* contains an isoquinoline alkaloid thought to be useful in reducing plaque and gingivitis. Although it has been marketed, test results have been equivocal, and untoward side effects have been reported. It can be highly toxic if swallowed.

sanguine (sang′gwin), *adj* **1.** pertaining to an abundant and active blood circulation, ruddy complexion. *n* **2.** an attitude full of vitality and confidence.

sanitation, *n* the science of maintaining a healthful, disease- and hazard-free environment.

sanitization, *n* the process whereby pathogenic organisms are reduced to safe levels on inanimate objects, thereby reducing the likelihood of cross-infection.

saponification, *n* the production of soap.

saprophyte, *n* an organism that lives on dead organic matter.

saquinavir mesylate (səkwin′əvir mes′ilāt′), *n brand name:* Invirase; *drug class:* antiviral; *action:* inhibits human immunodeficiency virus (HIV) protease important for viral replication; *use:* used in combination with nucleoside analogues, zidovudine, or zalcitabine in the treatment of acquired immunodeficiency syndrome (AIDS).

SAR, *n* See relationship, structure-activity.

***Sarcina* (sär′sinə),** *n* bacterium belonging to the genus *Sarcina,* which encourages disease, dental caries, and periodontal inflammation.

sarcoadenoma (sar′kōad′ənō′mə), *n* a mixed tumor containing characteristics of both glandular and connective tissue.

sarcocarcinoma (sar′kōkär′sənō′mə), *n* a mixed tumor with characteristics of both sarcomas and carcinomas.

***Sarcodina* (sär′kōdī′nə, -dē′nə),** *n.pl* also called *amoebae,* a subphylum of sarcomastigophora of parasitic protozoa, which causes diseases such as dysentery and meningocephalitis by drinking, swimming, or bathing in water contaminated with feces.

sarcoidosis (sär′koidō′sis) (Besnier-Boeck-Schaumann disease, Boeck's sarcoid), *n* a chronic granulomatous disease of unknown etiology. Causes noncaseating granulomas in the skin, lymph nodes, salivary glands, eyes, lungs, and bones.

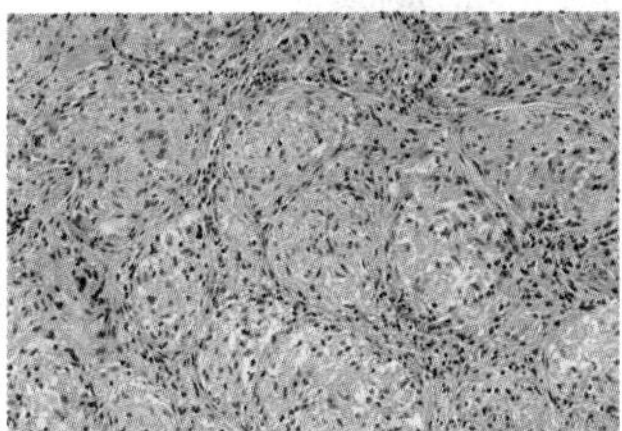

Sarcoidosis. (Regezi/Sciubba/Jordan, 2008)

sarcoma (särkō′mə), *n* **1.** a malignant neoplasm of connective tissue elements. **2.** a malignant neoplasm arising from mesenchyme or its derivatives.

sarcoma, ameloblastic, n a rare mixed tumor of odontogenic origin in which the mesenchymal component has undergone malignant transformation.

sarcoma, Ewing's, n.pr a rare, neuroectodermal malignancy of bone, caused by a translocation between chromosomes 11 and 22 [t(11, 22)].

It is characterized by pain, a radiographic appearance called *onion skinning,* and a histologic picture consisting of solid sheets of small round blue cells.

sarcoma, Kaposi's, n.pr a benign neoplasm of endothelial tissues. Skin lesions appear as multiple red-brown nodules ranging from a few mm to 1 cm in size. Histologically, endothelial proliferation in sheets or small vessels, hemosiderin deposits, fibroblastic proliferation, and an inflammatory infiltrate of lymphocytes are seen. Associated with HIV infection.

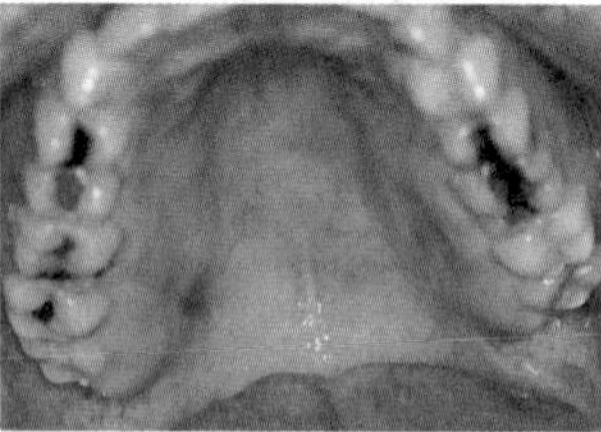

Kaposi's sarcoma. (Regezi/Sciubba/Jordan, 2008)

sarcoma, neurogenic (malignant schwannoma), n the malignant form of neurilemoma.

sarcoma, osteoblastic (osteogenic sarcoma), n an osteosarcoma in which atypical bone formation is the most evident histopathologic feature. See also osteosarcoma.

sarcoma, osteogenic, n a malignant connective tissue tumor that produces bone.

sarcoma, reticulum cell, n a malignant tumor of reticulum cells. It may occur as a primary neoplasm in soft tissue or bone.

***Sarcomastigophora* (sär'kōmas'tigof'ərə),** *n.pl* one of the four phyla of parasitic protozoa, to which the sarcodina and mastigophora subphyla belong. Capable of causing keratitis.

Sargenti technique, *n.pr* See N2.

satin finish, *n* See finish, satin.

satisfaction, *n* discharge of an obligation by actual payment of what is due or what is awarded by a court or other authority.

saturated (sach'ərā'tid), *adj* having all chemical affinities satisfied; unable to hold in solution any more of a given substance.

saturated fatty acid, *n* any of a number of glyceryl esters of certain organic acids in which all atoms are joined by single bonds. These fats are chiefly of animal origin but include cocoa butter, coconut oil, and palm oil.

saturation, *n* **1.** a condition in which a solution contains as much solute as can remain dissolved. **2.** a measure of the degree to which oxygen is bound to hemoglobin, expressed as a percentage of the possible limit. **3.** a chemical compound in which all the valency bonds have been filled.

saturation, color, n the quality of color that distinguishes the degree of vividness of hue.

saucerization (sôs'ərizā'shən), *n* an excavation of the tissue of a wound to form a shallow, saucerlike depression.

saucerization, pericervical, n the circular bone resorption that occurs about the necks of endosteal implants shortly after their insertion and continues slowly during the time of the implant's biologic presence.

saw, *n* a cutting blade with a toothed edge used to cut material too hard to slice with a knife.

saw, Gigli's wire, n.pr a flexible wire with teeth used for osteotomy procedures; often used in blind operations.

saw, gold, n an instrument with a thin sawlike blade used for removing surplus metal from the contact area of gold-foil restorations.

saw, Joseph, n.pr a nasal saw often used in ramusotomy of the mandible.

saw, Koeber's, n.pr a saw consisting of a thin, replaceable blade held in a frame; used to trim gross excess from the proximal portion of a Class II foil restoration in the preliminary stages of finishing and contouring.

saw, oscillating, n an oscillating blade in an electrical or compressed gas-driven unit; used to cut bone.

saw, rotary, n a rotary blade on a shaft in an electrical or compressed gas-driven unit; used to cut bone.

scabies (skā'bēz), *n* a contagious disease caused by *Sarcoptes scabiei,* the itch mite, characterized by intense itching of the skin.

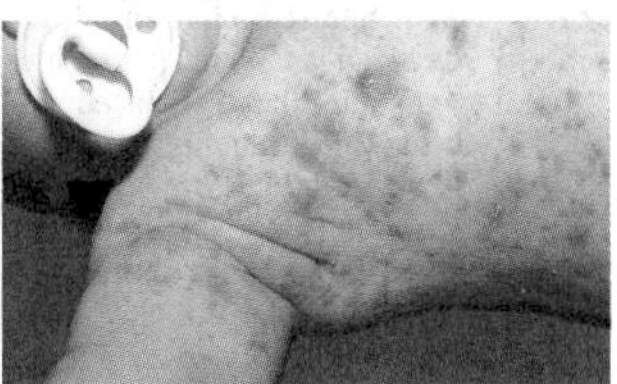

Scabies. (Zitelli/Davis, 2002)

scaffold, *n* a support, either natural or artificial, that maintains tissue contour.

scaler (skā'lur), *n* an instrument used to remove calculus from teeth.

scaler, hoe, *n* a double- or single-ended dental instrument used to remove heavy supragingival calculus; due to design limitations such as the shank angle; the straight, short, bulky blade; and the limited tactile sensitivity associated with this scaler, it is no longer used.

scaler, sickle, *n* a hand-activated, hook-shaped instrument available in various sizes and shapes; used for the removal of supragingival deposits; not suited for instrumentation apical to the gingival margin.

scaler, sickle, straight, *n* a sickle scaler that has an angled blade with a straight, flat face and two cutting edges that come to a point. Also called the *Jacquette scaler.*

scaler, sonic, *n.pl* an instrument that uses compressed air delivered from dental unit handpiece line to drive rotor system to move tip about 2500 to 7000 cycles per second in an elliptical pattern. Although sonic scalers do not get hot, they cause tissues to heat, requiring fluid for cooling tissues. This technology is generally not capable of removing heavy, hard deposits like the ultrasonic scaler is, but it removes softer, less tenacious deposits.

scaler, ultrasonic, *n* an electronic generator that transmits high-frequency vibrations from 25,000 to 40,000 or more cycles per second to a handpiece that is used to remove deposits from the surface of a tooth. Usually an insert is placed in the handle of the instrument to allow for specific instrumentation.

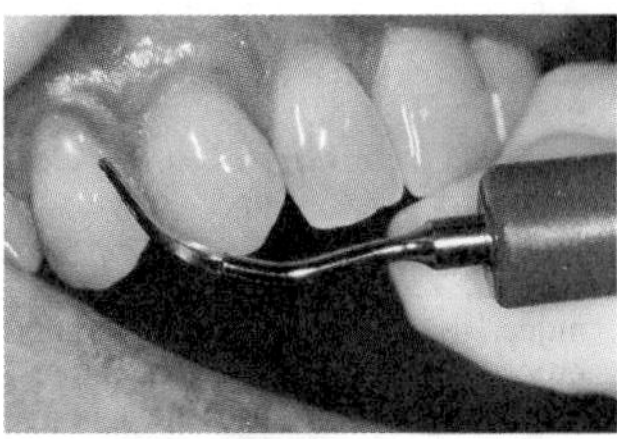

Ultrasonic scaler. (Bird/Robinson, 2005)

scaler, ultrasonic, chisel tip insert, *n* an instrument with a tip especially designed for removing deposits coronal to the gingival margin. It may also be used to remove overhanging restorations.

scaler, ultrasonic, contra-angled insert, *n* an instrument with a tip that is specially curved for removal of deposits on certain hard-to-reach tooth surfaces.

scaler, ultrasonic, magnetostrictive, *n* an instrument that uses a pulsing magnetic field applied to a metal "stack" that flexes to move tip in an elliptical pattern. It generates heat requiring fluid for cooling handpiece and tissues.

scaler, ultrasonic, piezoelectric, *n* an instrument that uses pulsing voltage applied to ceramic crystals that fly and move the tip in a reciprocating pattern. It causes the tissues to heat, requiring fluid for cooling them.

scaler, ultrasonic, plastic tip, *n* a plastic cover used on the working end of an ultrasonic scaler when removing deposits from the implant surface.

scaler, ultrasonic, probe tip insert, *n* an instrument with a thin, straight tip that is designed to provide access to subgingival deposits.

scaler, ultrasonic, straight insert, *n* an instrument with an arched tip that is designed for use in all parts of the oral cavity. Also called a *universal ultrasonic scaler insert.*

scaling, *n* the removal of deposits from the teeth.

scaling, channel, *n* a method of manual deposit removal in which the scaling instrument is applied in overlapping strokes across the surface of the tooth to ensure complete coverage and removal of all deposits.

S

scaling, coronal, *n* the removal of deposits from the clinical crowns of the teeth.

scaling, electrosurgical, *n* See electrosurgery and scalpel, electrosurgical.

scaling, reinforcement, *n* the technique used during instrumentation procedures in which the nondominant hand supports the instrument or the working hand, providing additional stability and control of the instrument.

scaling, root, *n* the removal of deposits from the accessible root surfaces of the teeth.

scaling, subgingival, *n* the removal of accretions and debris from the surfaces of the tooth apical to the gingival margin. This process accomplishes the removal of primary irritants to the gingival tissues and permits the reduction of inflammation in these tissues.

scaling, supragingival, *n* the removal of deposits from the surfaces of the teeth coronal to the gingival margin. This process accomplishes the removal of primary irritants to the gingival tissues and permits the reduction of inflammation in these tissues if there are no additional subgingival deposits.

scalpel (skal′pəl), *n* a delicate, razor-sharp, pointed knife, usually with a convex edge.

scalpel, electrosurgical, *n* a scalpel that severs tissue by means of an electrically heated wire.

scandium (Sc) (skan′dēəm), *n* a grayish metallic element. Its atomic number is 21 and its atomic weight is 44.956.

S

scanning, *n* a technique and protocol for carefully studying an area, organ, or system of the body by recording and displaying an image of the area using radioactive substances that have affinities for specific tissues.

scanning electron microscope (SEM), *n* See microscope, electron, scanning (SEM).

scar, *n* See cicatrix.

scar, apical, *n* the end product of wound repair. A radiolucent area characterized histologically by dense fibrous connective tissue. It is commonly noted in areas of tooth extraction.

scarify, *v* to make multiple superficial incisions into the skin.

scarlatina, *n* See scarlet fever.

scarlet fever, *n* an acute contagious disease of childhood caused by an erythrotoxin-producing strain of group A hemolytic *Streptococcus.* The infection is characterized by sore throat, fever, strawberry tongue, enlarged lymph nodes in the neck, prostration, and a diffuse bright red rash. See also strawberry tongue.

scattered radiation, *n* See radiation, scattered.

Schaumann's body, *n.pr* See body, Schaumann's.

Schaumann's disease, *n.pr* See sarcoidosis.

schedule, *n* **1.** the division of the working day into segments of time to enable the dental professional to provide treatment. **2.** a classification of drugs as determined by the Controlled Substances Act (CSA). **3.** a list of specifics.

Schedule I, *n* a category of drugs not considered legitimate for medical use. Included are heroin, lysergic acid diethylamide (LSD), and marijuana.

Schedule II, *n* a category of drugs considered to have a strong potential for abuse or addiction but that also have legitimate medical use. Included are opium, morphine, and cocaine.

Schedule III, *n* a category of drugs that have less potential for abuse or addiction than Schedule I or II drugs and have a useful medical purpose. Included are short-acting barbiturates and amphetamines.

Schedule IV, *n* a medically useful category of drugs that have less potential for abuse or addiction than those of Schedules I, II, and III. Included are diazepam and chloral hydrate.

Schedule V, *n* a medically useful catiegory of drugs that have less potential for abuse or addiction than those of Schedules I through IV. Included are antidiarrheals and antitussives with opioid derivatives.

schedule of allowances, *n* a list of specified amounts that will be paid toward the cost of dental services rendered; the patient pays the difference between the allowance and the actual cost of service. Also called *table of allowances.*

schedule of benefits, n a listing of the services for which payment will be made by a third party without specification of the amount to be paid.

schedule plan, n a plan that bases covered expenses on a schedule of allowances.

scheme, occlusal, *n* See system, occlusal.

Schick test (shik), *n.pr* a skin test used to determine immunity to diphtheria in which diphtheria toxin is injected intradermally. A positive reaction, indicating susceptibility, is marked by redness and swelling at the site of injection; a negative reaction, indicating immunity, is marked by absence of redness and swelling.

schistometer (shis′tom′ətur), *n* an instrument for measuring the aperture between the vocal cords.

schistosomiasis (shis′tōsōmī′əsis), *n* (bilharziasis), infestation with blood flukes of the genus *Schistosoma,* which causes cystitis, chronic dysentery, hepatosplenomegaly, and esophageal varices.

schizophrenia (skit′səfrē′nēə), *n* (dementia praecox), a functional psychosis (split personality) characterized by emotional distortion, withdrawal from reality, and disturbances of thought processes. It includes such disorders as hebephrenia, catatonia, and paranoia.

Schüller-Christian disease, *n.pr* See disease, Hand-Schüller-Christian.

Schüller's disease (shēl′ərz), *n.pr* See osteoporosis.

schwannoma (shwänō′mə), *n* See neurilemoma.

schwannoma, malignant, n See sarcoma, neurogenic.

sciatica (sīat′ikə), *n* an inflammation of the sciatic nerve, usually marked by pain and tenderness along the course of the nerve through the thigh and leg.

scientific method, *n* a formal style of study or research in which a problem is identified, pertinent information is assembled, a hypothesis is advanced and tested empirically, and the hypothesis is accepted or rejected.

scientific misconduct, *n* the fabrication, falsification, or plagiarism of research data, or other violations of ethical standards of the scientific community.

scissors, Fox, *n.pr* the delicate, fine-pointed scissors designed to gain access to interproximal areas and remove small tissue tabs or slight soft tissue deformities during gingivoplasty and gingivectomy. They also may be used to smooth the cut gingival surfaces.

sclera (skler′ə), *n* the opaque, fibrous, protective layer of the eye containing collagen and elastic fibers. It is commonly known as the white of the eye. Because the sclera is thinner in children, some of the underlying eye pigment is visible, making the eye appear slightly bluish. In older adults, fatty deposits on the sclera make it appear slightly yellowish.

scleroderma (skler′ōdur′mə), (dermatosclerosis, hidebound disease), *n* a collagen disease of unknown etiology; skin lesions are characterized by thickening, rigidity, and pigmentation in patches or diffuse areas. Dermal atrophy also may be seen. Periodontal lesions may simulate those of periodontosis, with widening of periodontal membrane space (verified by radiographic evidence), resulting from bone resorption, loss of architectural arrangement, and degeneration of periodontal fibers, with absence of inflammatory change in the gingivae and remaining periodontium. Thickening of the oral mucosa may also occur.

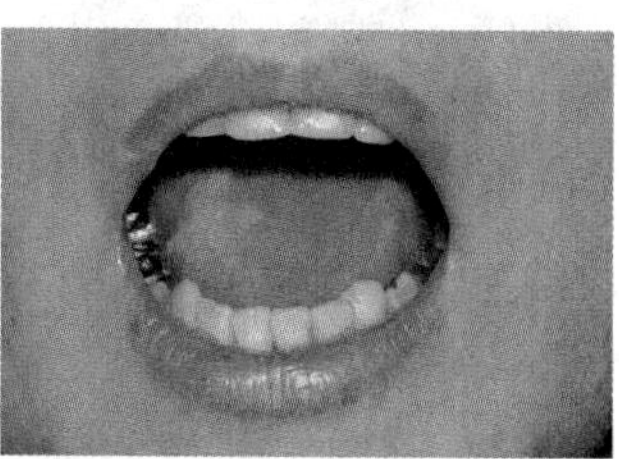

Scleroderma. (Regezi/Sciubba/Jordan, 2008)

sclerosing solution, *n* a liquid containing an irritant that causes inflammation and resulting fibrosis of tissues. It may be used in cauterizing ulcers, arresting hemorrhage, and treating hemangiomas.

sclerosis (sklerō'sis), *n* **1.** a hardening of a tissue. **2.** as applied to the jaws, sclerosis usually indicates an increased calcification centrally, with radiopacity. **3.** as applied to dentin, the tracts of increased density in the dentin are referred to as areas of *dentinal sclerosis.* It occurs beneath caries and with abfraction, abrasion, attrition, and erosion.

***sclerosis, dentinal* (den'tənəl),** *n* an occlusion of the dentinal tubules that inhibits outward fluid flow. It can occur naturally as root dentin ages but can also be caused by trauma, abrasion, or bacterial invasion. The sclerosing of the tubules produces translucent areas in the dentin.

sclerosis, multiple (MS), *n* a remitting and relapsing disease of the central nervous system affecting principally the white matter. Manifestations include sensory and motor incoordination and paresthesias; often dementia, blindness, paraplegia, and death result.

sclerotherapy, *n* the use of sclerosing chemicals to treat such varicosities as hemorrhoids and esophageal varices.

scoliosis (skō'lēō'sis), *n* a lateral curvature of the spine.

scopolamine (skōpol'əmēn), *n* an alkaloid found in the leaves and seeds of *Atropa belladonna* and other solanaceous plants having an action similar to atropine and used when spasmolytic or antisecretory effects are desired.

scopolamine, transdermal, *brand names:* Transderm-Scōp, Transderm-V; *drug class:* antiemetic, anticholinergic; *action:* competitive antagonism of acetylcholine at receptor sites in the eye, smooth muscle, cardiac muscle, glandular cells; inhibition of vestibular input to the central nervous system (CNS), resulting in inhibition of vomiting reflex; *use:* prevention of motion sickness.

scorbutic gingivitis (skôrbū'tik jin'jəvī'tis), *n* an abnormal condition, characterized by inflamed or bleeding gums; caused by vitamin C deficiency. See also scurvy.

scorbutus (skôrbyōō'təs), *n* See scurvy.

scratch test, *n* a skin test for identifying an allergen, performed by placing a small quantity of a solution containing a suspected allergen on a lightly scratched area of the skin. If a wheal forms within 15 minutes, allergy to the substance is indicated.

screen, intensifying, *n* a layer of fluorescent crystals (usually calcium tungstate) supported on a flat base. Used in intimate contact with light-sensitive radiographic film in a cassette. The crystals fluoresce when exposed to x-radiation and subsequently expose the film with light.

screen, oral, *n* a Plexiglas or acrylic resin appliance that fits into the vestibule of the oral cavity for the correction of oral cavity breathing.

screening, *n* **1.** an examination of individuals or their records to ascertain dental needs, assess treatment plans, or evaluate services rendered. Prescreening is the review by designated dental professionals of patients' examination records as a prerequisite to the authorization of some or all types of treatment. Postscreening is the examination by designated dental professionals, usually on a sample basis, of records to determine whether services have been rendered adequately and in accordance with prescribed administrative procedures. **2.** a sample survey to determine initial treatment needs of a group seeking coverage under a dental plan; used in setting the initial premium.

screw, expansion, *n* an orthodontic mechanism for achieving movement of teeth or arch segments, consisting of a threaded shaft and sleeve arrangement that permits controlled separation of elements of the appliance.

screw, implant, *n* a small screw 3 to 5 mm long that is used as a means for primary retention of the implant.

screw-retained, *n* the utilization of a screw in order to hold an abutment or prosthesis in place.

screwdriver, *n* See instrument, screwdriver.

scribe, *v* to write, trace, or mark by making a line or lines with a pointed instrument or carbon marker.

scrofula (skrof'ūlə), *n.* a primary tuberculosis complex occurring in the orocervical region and consisting of tuberculous cervical lymphadenopathy and tuberculosis of adjacent skin (lupus vulgaris), with chronic draining sinuses below the angle of the jaw and cervical region.

scurvy (skur′vē), *n* (scorbutus), a condition resulting from an ascorbic acid deficiency that is severe enough to desaturate the tissues. The development and manifestations depend on tissue storage of ascorbic acid and factors that influence the rate at which it is used in or released from the tissues. Manifestations of frank scurvy include weakness, poor wound healing, anemia, and hemorrhage under the skin and mucous membranes. Presence or severity of gingival changes is directly related to the presence of local irritants such as calculus. In a severe form and in infantile scurvy, painful subperiosteal hemorrhages occur.

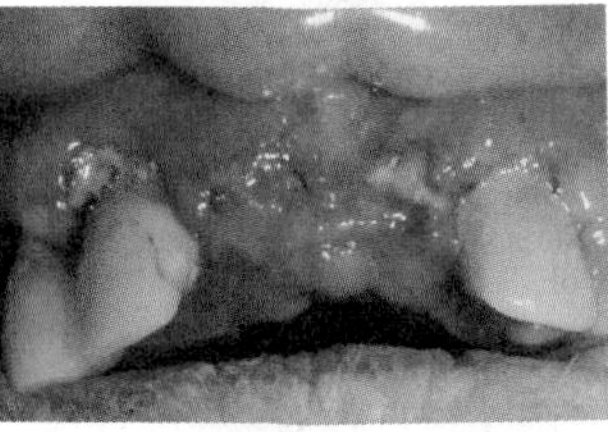

Scurvy. (Neville/Damm/Allen/Bouquot, 2002)

scurvy, infantile (Barlow's disease, Cheadle's disease, Moeller's disease), *n* a nutritional disease of infants caused by a deficiency of vitamin C in the diet. It has the same symptoms as scurvy does in adults.

scurvy, land, *n* See purpura, idiopathic thrombocytopenic.

seal, *n* **1.** something that firmly closes or secures. **2.** a tight and perfect closure. *v* **3.** to keep shut, enclosed, or confined.

seal, border, *n* See border seal.

seal, double, *n* a seal consisting of gutta-percha underneath another material such as temporary cement; used to close the coronal opening in a tooth during endodontic treatment.

seal, hermetic, *n* perfect and absolute obliteration of all space within a tooth.

seal, peripheral, *n* See border seal.

seal, posterior palatal, *n* the seal at the posterior border of a denture produced by displacing some of the soft tissue covering the palate by extra pressure developed in the impression or by scraping a groove along the posterior seal area in the cast on which the denture is to be processed.

seal, postpalatal, *n* See seal, posterior palatal.

sealant, enamel, *n* a resinous material designed for application to the occlusal surfaces of posterior teeth to seal the surface irregularities and prevent the carious process. Older term: *pit and fissure sealant.*

sealant, fluoride-releasing, *n* a type of sealant that contains fluoride for the purpose of resisting the development of caries in the tooth to which it is applied.

sealant, therapeutic, *n* See sealant, enamel.

sealant, unfilled, *n* a resin-based sealant that does not contain particles (as opposed to a filled sealant, which contains additional filler particles). It is less viscous and less resistant to water than a filled sealant and thus fills a fissure more effectively. Unfilled sealants typically do not require additional occlusional adjustments.

sealer, *n* a substance used to fill the space around silver or gutta-percha points in a pulp canal. Most contain some combination of zinc, barium, and bismuth salts and eugenol, Canadian balsam, and eucalyptol.

seasonal affective disorder (SAD), *n* a mood disorder associated with the shorter days and longer nights of autumn and winter. Symptoms include lethargy, depression, social withdrawal, and work difficulties.

seat, basal, *n* See basal seat.

seat, rest, *n* See area, rest.

sebaceous glands (sēbā′shəs), *n.pl* the exocrine glands of the skin, many of which open into the hair follicles and secrete an oily substance that coats the hair and surrounding epithelium, helping to prevent evaporation of sweat and retain body heat. In the oral cavity, these glands are known as *Fordyce's granules* or *Fordyce's spots* and can be seen with the unaided eye as yellowish-white in color and are more common in older adults on the buccal and labial mucosa. See also Fordyce granules.

seborrhea (seb′ərē′ə), *n* the skin conditions in which an overproduction of sebum results in excessive oiliness or dry scales.

seborrhea capitis, *n* seborrhea of the scalp often seen in infants. Also called *cradle cap.*

secobarbital/secobarbital sodium (sē′kōbär′bətal), *n brand names:* Novosecobarb, Seconal; *drug class:* sedative-hypnotic barbiturate, controlled substance Schedule II; *action:* nonselective depression of the central nervous system (CNS), ranging from sedation to hypnosis to anesthesia to coma depending on the dose; *uses:* treatment of insomnia, status epilepticus, and acute tetanus convulsions, sedation, preoperative medication.

second-opinion program, *n* an opinion about the appropriateness of a proposed treatment provided by a practitioner other than the one making the original recommendation; some benefit plans require such opinions for selected services.

secondary, *adj* **1.** not primary, immediately following the first position; supplemental. **2.** directly emerging or resulting from an original source or condition.

secondary bone, *n* a second layer of bone tissue that supersedes the original bone as part of the maturation process.

secondary cancer, *n* an opportunistic neoplasm imposed on a host with reduced health and resistance resulting from a preceding primary neoplasm or viral infection.

secondary deficiency, *n* an inadequacy of nutrients in the diet that is the result of the body's inability effectively to process and use the foods ingested, however healthy those foods might be; may be caused by disease, allergies, or interactions between drugs and nutrients or between two nutrients.

secondary dental caries, *n.pl* See caries, recurrent.

secondary dentition, *n* See dentition, permanent.

secondary hemorrhage, *n* bleeding that develops 24 hours or more after the original injury or surgery. It is often caused by an infection.

secondary infectious disease, *n* an opportunistic infection imposed on a host with reduced health and resistance resulting from a preceding infection by a more virulent organism.

secondary prevention, *n* an action performed to take care of early symptoms of a disease and preclude the development of possible irreparable medical conditions. See also primary health care and primary prevention.

secondary radiation, *n* See radiation, secondary.

secondary sex characteristic, *n* an external physical characteristic of sexual maturity that distinguishes one gender from the other, such as the distribution of hair and voice changes.

secretary-receptionist, *n* the auxiliary whose chief responsibilities are to receive patients into the office, handle the correspondence and bookkeeping, order supplies, supervise housekeeping, and answer the telephone.

secrete (sikrēt′), *v* to discharge or empty a substance into the bloodstream or a cavity or onto the surface of the body. The substance secreted is called a *secretion.* Glands that secrete internally are *endocrine* or *ductless glands*; glands that secrete into a cavity or onto the surface are *exocrine* or *duct glands.*

section, frontal, *n* the section of the body through any coronal (frontal) plane.

section, midsaggital, *n* the section of the body through the midsaggital (median) plane.

section, transverse, *n* the section of the body through any horizontal plane.

sectional arch wire, *n* an orthodontic wire that occupies less than a complete dental arch. It usually is attached to only a few teeth. Typically it spans one or both buccal segments of the dental arch or is limited to the anterior teeth. It facilitates the application of differential forces in effecting tooth movement.

sectional impression, *n* an impression made in two or more parts.

sectioning, surgical, *n* the action dividing a tooth to facilitate its removal. A variety of instruments, including osteotomes and power-driven burs, are used.

sedation (sedā′shən), *n* the production of a sedative effect; the act or process of calming.

sedation, conscious, n a condition induced by drugs or other means in which the patient retains a minimum level of consciousness while continuing to breathe on his or her own and to respond to verbal and physical prompts.

sedation, deep, n a condition induced by drugs or other means in which the patient enters a temporary state of semiconsciousness, causing partial loss of sensory perception and the inability to respond to verbal prompts.

sedative (sed′ətiv), *n* **1.** production of sedation. A drug that can produce sedation. **2.** a drug that produces cortical depression of varying degrees. **3.** a remedy that allays excitement and slows down the basal metabolic rate without impairing the cerebral cortex.

sedative-hypnotic, n a drug that reversibly depresses the activity of the central nervous system, used mainly to induce sleep and allay anxiety.

sediment, *n* a deposit of relatively insoluble material that settles to the bottom of a container of liquid.

sedimentation rate (SR), *n* the speed of settling of red blood cells in a vertical glass column of citrated plasma. It is used to monitor inflammatory or malignant disease.

seed, radon, *n* See radon seed.

segment, *n* a part into which a body naturally separates or is divided, either actually or by an imaginary line.

seizure, *n* See epilepsy.

seizure, absence, n a seizure characterized by sudden interruption of conscious physical and mental activities and a short period of unconsciousness. Formerly known as *petit mal,* sometimes simply called *absence.*

seizure, clonic phase, n a seizure's convulsion stage.

seizure, complex partial, n a seizure stemming from a localized part of the brain indicated by the presence of a state similar to a trance, varying degrees of awareness, and the manifestation of purposeless behaviors or motions. The seizure may be followed by an indeterminate period of confusion, garbled speech, poor mood, and an inability to recall the events of the episode.

seizure, generalized, n a nonfocalized, convulsive spell that has a simultaneous effect on the entire brain. Formerly known as *grand mal seizure.*

seizure, grand mal **(grand mäl, grän mäl),** *n* See seizure, generalized.

seizure, simple partial, n a type of seizure in which only one part of the brain is involved. Patients experiencing this type of seizure may feel intense emotions (joy, fear) or involuntary muscle spasms, depending on the region affected.

Seldane, *n.pr* a brand name for an oral antihistamine (terfenadine).

selection, *n* **1.** the act of choosing between or among a variety of options or alternatives. **2.** the process by which various factors or mechanisms determine and modify the reproductive ability of a genotype within a specific population. Also referred to as *natural selection.*

selection, shade (tooth color selection), n the determination of the color (hue, brilliance, saturation, translucency) of the artificial tooth or set of teeth for a given patient.

selection, tooth, n the selection of a tooth or teeth (shape, size, color) to harmonize with the individual characteristics of a patient.

selection, tooth color, n See selection, shade.

selective grinding, *n* See grinding, selective.

selectivity, sensory, *n* the property of the specialized receptor end-organ by which it responds to one type of stimulus rather than another.

selegiline HCl (silej′əlēn), *n brand names:* Eldepryl, SD-Deprenyl; *drug class:* antiparkinson agent; *action:* increased dopaminergic activity by inhibiting monoamine oxidase (MAO) type B activity; *uses:* adjunct management of Parkinson's disease in patients being treated with carbidopa-levodopa.

selenium (Se) (səlē′nēum), *n* a trace element used in the treatment of seborrhea and dandruff of the scalp. Selenium is toxic in large amounts.

***Selenomonas* (sel′enōmō′nas),** *n* a genus of gram-negative, anaerobic,

S

rod-shaped bacteria found in the oral cavity.

self-analysis, *n* an introspection on one's own behavior and actions in the total environment.

self-concept, *n* the composite of ideas, feelings, and attitudes that a person has about his or her own identity, worth, capabilities, and limitations.

self-curing resin, *n* See resin, autopolymerizing.

self-esteem, *n* the degree of worth and competence one attributes to oneself.

self-funding, *n* the method of providing employee benefits in which the sponsor does not purchase conventional insurance but rather elects to pay for the claims directly, generally through the services of a third-party administrator. Self-funded programs often have stop-loss insurance in place to cover abnormal risks.

self-history, *n* a patient's own accounting of his or her medical history, usually on a preprinted form.

self-injury, *n* the act of intentionally hurting oneself. One manifestation of this is known as *cutting.*

self-insurance, *n* the setting aside of funds by an individual or organization to meet anticipated dental care expenses or dental care claims, and accumulation of a fund to absorb fluctuations in the amount of expenses and claims. The funds set aside or accumulated are used to provide dental benefits directly instead of purchasing coverage from an insurance carrier.

self-limited disease, *n* a disease restricted in duration by its own pattern of characteristics and not by other influences or interventions.

self-mutilation, *n* the act of deliberately causing injury to oneself.

self-tapping implant, *n* an implant that cuts its own path into bone.

self-tapping screw, *n* a screw that cuts its own spiral threads into bone or tooth structure.

sella turcica (S) (sel'ə tur'sikə), *n* the pituitary fossa. The center is used as a cephalometric landmark.

sella turica, floor of, *n* the most inferior point on the internal contour of the sella turcica.

semantics (siman'tiks), *n* the study of language with special concern for the meanings of words and other symbols.

semicoma, *n* a mild coma from which the patient may be aroused.

semiconductor, *n* a solid crystalline substance the electrical conductivity of which is intermediate between that of a conductor and an insulator.

semipermeable (sem'ēpur'mēəbəl), *adj* permitting the passage of certain molecules and hindering that of others.

semisupine position (sem'ēsoopīn'), *n* an anatomic position in which a patient is face up with the body positioned at approximately a 45° angle, or midway between sitting and standing. Also called the *semi-Fowler's position.*

senescence (sənes'əns), *n* the process of growing old.

senescence, dental, *n* a condition of the teeth and associated structures in which deterioration results from aging or premature aging processes.

senile dental caries (sē'nīl), *n* See caries, root.

senile psychosis, *n* an organic mental disorder of aged people resulting from a generalized atrophy of the brain with no evidence of cerebrovascular disease.

senility (sənil'itē), *n* a term usually used to describe the cognitive and physiologic signs of advancing age.

sensation (sensā'shən), *n* an impression conveyed by an afferent nerve to the sensorium commune.

sensation, psychologic effects of, *n* an arousal, facilitation, and distortion of sensation by psychologic factors, the basis for which lies in the corticalization of the special senses.

sensation, referred, *n* a group of vaguely classified sensations that are a consequence of cortical experience. They are the sensory hallucinations, *paresthesias,* and the phenomenon called *phantom limb.* Nonspecific and poorly localized pain in the alveolar ridges, which have poor vascular supply, may be evidence of this phantom limb phenomenon associated with neurotic behavior.

sensation, specialized, *n* a sensation that is perceived by the specialized end organs associated with special senses such as vision, hearing, and smell.

sense (sens), *n* a faculty by which the conditions or properties of things are perceived. Hunger, thirst, malaise, and pain are varieties of sense.

sense, special, n one or all of the five senses: feeling, hearing, seeing, smell, and taste.

sensitive (sen′sitiv), *adj* able to receive or transmit a sensation; capable of feeling or responding to a sensation.

sensitivity, *n* **1.** the ability to feel or experience physical stimuli. **2.** compassion or thoughtfulness toward a person or situation.

sensitivity, tactile, n a capacity to sense the transference of vibrations from the parts of the instrument (e.g., handle, shank, and working end) to the fingers of the clinician.

sensitivity test, n a laboratory method for testing antibiotic effectiveness.

sensitivity, tooth, n the state of responsiveness of teeth to external influences such as heat, sugar, and trauma. May result from occlusal trauma, especially if the anatomic relation of the apical foramen to the traumatized tissue is such that the circulation of the pulp is disturbed.

sensitivity, tooth, hydrodynamic theory, n a theory that attributes tooth sensitivity to the expansion and contraction of fluids within the dentinal tubules, thus causing the nerve endings to trigger pain responses in the tooth pulp. See hypersensitivity, dentin.

sensitivity, tooth, neurophysiology theory of, n a theory that attributes tooth sensitivity to the stimulation of either A-type fibers, which cause short, sharp, localized pains, or C-type fibers, which produce dull, aching pains that may be spread across a wide area.

sensitivity training, n the use of group dynamics to experiment with and alter behavioral patterns and interpersonal reactions. Also called *T group.*

sensitization (sen′sitizā′shun), *n* the process of rendering a cell sensitive to the action of a complement by subjecting it to the action of a specific amboceptor; anaphylaxis.

sensorium (sensôr′ēum), *n* a sensory nerve center; more frequently, the whole sensory apparatus of the body.

sensory (sen′sərē), *n* that part of the nervous system that receives and perceives sensations such as sound, touch, smell, sight, pain, heat, cold, and vibration.

sensory innervation, n the distribution of nerves to an organ, muscle, or other body part conveying sensation to that area.

sensory threshold, n the point at which a stimulus triggers the start of an afferent nerve impulse. Absolute threshold is the lowest point at which response to a stimulus can be perceived.

separating medium, *n* See medium, separating.

separating spring, *n* a spring placed between adjacent teeth to obtain separation.

separating wire, *n* See wire, separating.

separator, *n* an instrument used to wedge teeth apart and out of normal contact by immediate separation; useful in the examination of proximal surfaces of teeth and in finishing proximal restorations. Must be used with care; it should be stabilized against the teeth with modeling compound to prevent tissue damage.

separator, Ferrier's, n.pr a set of balanced, double-bowed, adjustable separators designed by W.I. Ferrier.

separator, noninterfering, n See separator, True's.

separator, True's (noninterfering separator), n.pr a single-bowed separator designed to give greater access to the surface being operated on; designed by Harry A. True.

sepsis, oral (sep′sis), *n* an older term for a condition occurring within the oral cavity and adjacent areas characterized by the presence of pathogens.

septic sore throat, *n* a severe throat infection, usually caused by a *Streptococcus* strain, resulting in fever and marked exhaustion.

septicemia (sep′tisē′mēə), *n* a condition in which pathogenic bacteria and bacterial toxins circulate in the blood. Manifestations include high temperature, leukocytosis, malaise, rapid pulse, and subsequent diffuse systemic degenerative disturbances.

septum (pl. septa) (sep′təm, sep′tə), *n* a partition between two cavities or spaces.

septum, interdental (interdental alveolar septum), n the portion of the alveolar process extending between the roots of adjacent teeth.

septum, nasal, n the thin, vertical bony septum separating the right and left nasal cavities.

sequela (sikwel′ə), *n* an abnormal condition that follows and is the result of a disease, treatment, or injury, such as paralysis after poliomyelitis or scar formation after a laceration.

sequence, *n* the order of occurrence or performance.

sequence planning, n a method of identifying all the various dental treatments that a patient will need and putting those treatments in the most logical and effective order.

sequester, *v* **1.** to detach, separate, or isolate. A patient might be sequestered to prevent the spread of an infection. **2.** the isolation of a jury during the conduct of a trial.

sequestrum (sēkwes′trum), *n* a piece of dead bone that has become separated from vital bone. See also osteoradionecrosis.

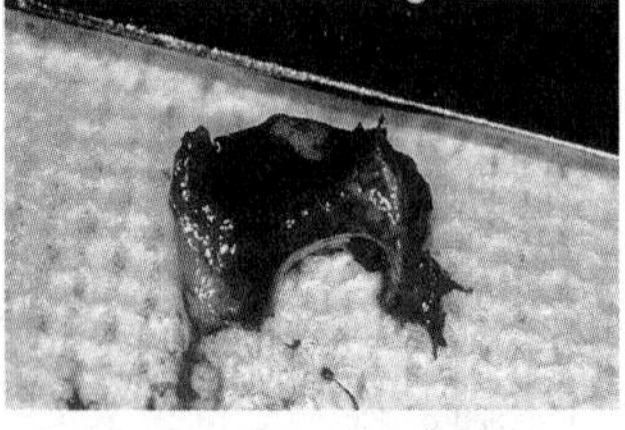

Sequestrum. (Newman/Takei/Klokkevold/Carranza, 2006)

serial extraction, *n* a program of selective extraction of primary and sometimes permanent teeth over time, with the objective of relieving crowding and facilitating the eruption of remaining teeth into improved positions. Close supervision of ensuing eruption is essential, because overclosure of the spaces and other sequelae may be expected in a significant number of cases. Comprehensive orthodontic treatment should almost always be initiated in the course of or after eruption for space management, control of the autonomous tipping usually induced by the procedure, and other malrelationships that commonly accompany these conditions.

serine (Ser) (serēn′), *n* a nonessential amino acid found in many proteins in the body. It is a precursor of the amino acids glycine and cysteine.

seroconversion (sir′ōkənvur′zhən), *n* a blood test in which the amount of time required for the blood to change from seronegative to seropositive is indicative of specific diseases.

serology tests (sērol′əjē), *n.pl* diagnostic tests of serum usually used to determine the immune or lytic properties of serum.

seronegative (sir′ōneg′ətiv), *n* serologic evidence of the lack of an antibody of a specific type in the serum; diagnostically useful in ruling out Lyme disease, syphilis, human immunodeficiency virus (HIV), serum hepatitis B, and many other viral diseases.

seropositive (sir′ōpoz′itiv), *n* serologic evidence of the presence of an antibody of a specific type in the serum; diagnostically useful in identifying many types of viral diseases.

seroprevalence rates (sir′ōprev′ələns), *n.pl* a statistical measure of the rate of occurrence of seropositive status in a population or sample; used as a criterion of comparison between populations or samples.

serotonergic drugs (ser′ətōnur′jik), *n.pl* the prescription drugs used for weight loss that contain serotonin, a vasoconstrictor that acts as an appetite suppressant; examples are fenfluramine and dexfenfluramine (the *fen* of Phen-fen), both of which have been removed from the U.S. market because of their links to heart valve disease, and fluoxetine, which has not been approved by the FDA for treatment of obesity.

serotonin (ser′ətō′nin), *n* (enteramine, thrombocytin), a local vasoconstrictor (5-hydroxytryptamine) and general hypotensive agent synthesized from tryptophan and found in tissues, rather than being transferred by blood to sites of action. Most serotonin is found in the gastrointestinal tract, although the kidney, liver, and brain also produce it. It is absorbed by platelets from the site of tissue damage, where it aids hemostasis locally by vasoconstriction and systemically by reducing blood pressure.

serotonin reuptake inhibitors, selective (SSRI), *n.pl.* a class of antidepressant drugs such as fluoxetine, sertraline, paroxetine, or voxamine.

serotonin serozyme **(sir'ōzīm),** *n* See factor VII.

serous (sēr'əs), *adj* relating to or resembling serum.

serous fluid, *n* a fluid that has the characteristics of serum in color and viscosity.

serous membrane, *n* a thin sheet of tissue that lines closed cavities of the body, such as the pleura lining the thoracic cavity and the pericardium lining the sac enclosing the heart.

serrated (ser'āted), *adj* having a jagged or notched edge; saw-toothed.

Serratia **(serā'shēə),** *n* a genus of motile, gram-negative bacilli capable of causing infection, including bacteremia, pneumonia, and urinary tract infections, in humans.

sertraline (ser'trəlēn'), *n brand name:* Zoloft; *drug class:* antidepressant; *action:* selectively inhibits the uptake of serotonin in the brain; *use:* treatment of major depression.

serum (sir'um), *n* the fluid component of the blood containing all stable constituents except fibrinogen. When blood is allowed to clot and stand, a clear yellowish fluid, the serum, separates.

serum accelerator globulin, *n* See accelerator, prothrombin conversion, I.

serum marker, *n* a specific indicator found in a blood test that identifies a disease.

serum protein determination, electrophoretic, *n* separation of serum protein fractions (albumin, α-globulin, β-globulin, and γ-globulin) based on their different isoelectric points and mobility in an electric field. Electrophoretic patterns and concentrations are of value in evaluating the hyperglobulinemias. Electrophoretic evaluation of serum protein abnormalities is usually related to moving-boundary or paper-strip separation patterns.

serum prothrombin conversion accelerator (SPCA) **(prōthrom'bin),** *n* See factor VII; thromboplastin, extrinsic.

serum sickness, *n* an anaphylactoid or allergic reaction after injection of foreign serum; marked by urticarial rashes, edema, adenitis, arthralgia, high fever, and prostration.

servant, *n* someone who is employed to perform personal services (other than those that would be rendered in an independent calling) for an employer and who, in that service, remains entirely under the control of the employer.

servant, loaned, *n* a person whose services have been granted by an employer to another person.

service, *n* the performance of labor for the benefit of another.

service, denture, *n* the diagnosis and treatment of edentulous and partially edentulous patients, including the diagnosis of existing and potential oral pathosis, planning of treatment for the preparation of the oral cavity for complete or partial dentures, fabrication and adjustment of the prostheses, and continuing observation of the changes in the oral conditions as the prostheses are in use.

service, gratuitous, *n* a service that does not involve a return, compensation, or consideration.

service of process, *n* the delivery of a writ, summons, or complaint to a defendant or witness. Service of process gives reasonable notice to allow the person to appear, testify, and be heard in court.

service, therapeutic, *n* treatment of a clinical nature deliberately performed to regulate or stop disease and sustain healthy oral tissues.

services, health, *n.pl* those services, including dentistry, that improve the general physical and mental well-being of the patient.

sessile lesion (ses'il), *n* a raised, wide-based lesion.

set, *n* term applied to the state of a plastic material after it has hardened or jelled by chemical action, cooling, or saponification. It is used in connection with impression materials, waxes, and gypsum materials.

set-square tooth numbering system, *n* See Palmer's tooth notation.

setoff, *n* See offset.

setting expansion, *n* See expansion, setting.

setting time, *n* See time, setting.

settlement, *n* an agreement made between parties to a suit before a judgment is rendered by a court.

setup, *n* **1.** the arrangement of teeth on a trial denture base. **2.** a laboratory procedure in which teeth are removed from a plaster cast and repositioned in wax. May be used as a diagnostic tool to evaluate alternatives, as when some teeth are missing; also used to produce the mold to make a positioner appliance. **3.** to prepare the armamentarium for a dental procedure.

sex, *n* a classification of an individual as male or female on the basis of anatomic, functional, hormonal, and chromosomal characteristics.

sex, anatomic, *n* (genotype), a classification of sex based on the sexual differentiation of the primary gonads.

sex, chromosomal, *n* the chromosomal characteristics involving normally 44 somatic and 2 sex chromosomes, the latter designated as XX for the normal female and XY for the normal male. The presence of the Y chromosome is associated with a male phenotype and its absence with a phenotypic female.

sex chromosomes, *n* the chromosomes responsible for sex classification—XX for female, XY for male.

sex, functional (phenotype), *n* the designation of sex based on the state of maturation and potential for use of the external genitalia.

sex, hormonal, *n* a contributory assignment of sex on the basis of adequate levels of estrogen and androgen for the development of typical phenotypic secondary sex characteristics.

sex hormones, *n.pl* See hormone(s), sex.

sex, legal, *n* the sex assigned at birth or legally by a court of law.

sex, nuclear, *n* the sex determination based on the presence or absence of the hyperchromatic nucleolar satellite in squamous cells from a buccal mucosa smear or of "drumsticks" in the polymorphonuclear neutrophil. Positives are normally seen in the female.

sex-linkage, *n* See linkage, sex.

sextant (seks′tənt), *n* one of the three sections into which each dental arch may be divided depending on its proximity to the midline of the arch.

sexual harassment, *n* the U.S. Supreme Court adopted the definition of sexual harassment formulated by the Equal Employment Opportunity Commission as follows: unwelcome sexual advances, requests for sexual favors, and other verbal or physical conduct of a sexual nature when (1) submission to such conduct is made either explicitly or implicitly a term or condition of an individual's employment, (2) submission to or rejection of such conduct by an individual is used as a basis for employment decisions affecting such individual (both quid pro quo harassment), or (3) such conduct has the purpose or effect of unreasonably interfering with an individual's work performance or creating an intimidating, hostile, or offensive working environment (condition of work harassment).

sexually transmitted diseases, *n.pl* contagious conditions acquired by sexual intercourse or genital contact. These include chancroid, gonorrhea, granuloma inguinale, herpes simplex type II, HIV, lymphogranuloma venereum, and syphilis. Older term: *venereal disease.*

shaken baby syndrome, *n* a condition of whiplash-type injuries ranging from bruises on the arms and trunk to retinal hemorrhages, coma, and convulsions, as observed in infants and children who have been violently shaken. Physicians are required by law to report cases of suspected child abuse and are granted immunity from liability for filing such reports. See also child abuse.

shallow breathing, *n* a respiration pattern marked by slow, shallow, and generally ineffective inspirations and expirations. It is usually caused by drugs and indicates depression of the medullary respiratory centers.

shank, *n* the part of the instrument that connects the working end to the handle.

shank flexibility, *n* the degree of rigidity that makes the shank of a hand-held instrument suited to a particular task. The thinner and more pliable the shank, the greater the tactile sensitivity of the instrument.

shank, lower, *n* the section of the working end of a dental instrument that is closest to the blade. Also called *terminal shank.*

shank, straight, *n* the linear, uncurved or unangled portion of an instrument that connects the working end to the handle. A straight shank is generally used in easily accessible areas while those with an angled shank are used in more confined areas.

shank, terminal, *n* See shank, lower.

shared services, *n.pl* the administrative, clinical, or other service functions that are common to two or more hospitals or their health care facilities and used jointly or cooperatively by them.

sharpening, instrument, *n* the act establishing or restoring a sharp edge on a cutting edge or blade of an instrument.

sharpening, instrument, automated technique, *n* a technique for sharpening using a device that secures both the instrument and stone during the process.

sharpening, instrument, moving stone technique, *n* a technique for sharpening with the stone moving against the cutting edge of an instrument placed at an angle on a secure surface.

sharpening, instrument, stationary flat stone technique, *n* a technique for sharpening with the stone flat on a secure surface and the finger resting on the edge or side of the stone; the cutting edge of the instrument is drawn over the face of the stone.

Sharpey's fiber, *n.pr* See fiber, Sharpey's.

sharpness, *n* the quality of a blade that has a thin, keen cutting edge; a cutting edge is suitably sharp when it functions efficiently and safely.

sharpness, visual test of, *n* an examination of the cutting edge of a blade (usually magnified) to determined its extent of sharpness. The cutting edge is sharp when the line of its edge is too fine to reflect light. Also called *glare test.*

sharps, *n.pl* any needles, scalpels, wires, endodontic files, or other articles that could cause wounds or punctures to personnel handing them.

sharps container, *n* a container in every clinic that is designed for the disposal of sharps; required and regulated by the Occupational Safety and Health Administration (OSHA).

shave biopsy, *n* the removal of a thin layer of tissue using a dermatome knife. See also biopsy, shave.

shear, *n* See strength, shear and strength, ultimate.

shearing cusps, *n.pl* the maxillary buccal cusps, mandibular lingual cusps, maxillary canines, and maxillary incisors. Each of these cusps helps form the fossae that receive the stamp cusps. In the post-canine teeth, the triangular ridges of the shearing cusps arm the fossae with cutting ridges.

sheath of Schwann, *n.pr* See neurilemma.

shedding, *n* See exfoliation.

sheep cell test, *n* a method that mixes human blood cells with the red blood cells of sheep to determine the absence or deficiency of human T-lymphocytes.

shelf, buccal, *n* the surface of the mandible from the residual alveolar ridge or alveolar ridge to the external oblique line in the region of the mandibular buccal vestibule. It is covered with cortical bone.

shelf life, *n* the length of time a material may be stored without deterioration; the length of time it remains usable.

shellac base, *n* See base, shellac.

shield, radiation, *n* a body of material used to prevent or reduce the passage of particles of radiation. A shield may be designated according to what it is intended to absorb (e.g., gamma ray, neutron shield) or according to the kind of protection it is intended to give (e.g., background, biologic, thermal shield). The shield of a nuclear reactor is a body of material surrounding the reactor to limit the escape of neutrons and radiation into the protected area. Shields may be required to protect personnel and reduce radiation sufficiently to allow use of counting instruments for research or for locating contamination or airborne radioactivity. See also apron, lead.

shift, axis, *n* See axis shift.

shift to right or left, *n* an arbitrary description of an increase in the number per unit volume of immature (shift to left) or mature (shift to right) forms of neutrophils, in the differential counting system of Schilling.

Shigella, *n* a genus of gram-negative pathogenic bacteria that causes gastroenteritis and bacterial dysentery.

shigellosis (shig′əlō′sis), *n* an infection of the gastrointestinal tract caused by *Shigella* bacteria, usually contracted by the ingestion of tainted food or drink. Symptoms include fever, abdominal pain, and diarrhea.

shingles, *n* See herpes zoster.

shock, *n* **1.** a state of collapse of the body after injury or trauma. Shock may be either primary or secondary. The principal effects of shock are slowing of the peripheral blood flow and reduction in cardiac output. **2.** a circulatory insufficiency caused by a disparity between circulating blood volume and vascular capacity.

shock, galvanic, *n* pain produced as a result of galvanic currents caused by similar or dissimilar metallic restorations.

shock, hemorrhagic, *n* an ineffectual circulating volume of blood resulting from loss of whole blood.

shock, insulin, *n* a coma resulting from too much insulin or an inadequate intake of food. Symptoms include wet or moist skin, hypersalivation or drooling, normal blood pressure, tremors, dilated pupils, normal or bounding pulse, and firm eyeballs. Sugar and acetoacetic acid may be present in bladder urine but are absent in the second specimen. The blood sugar is low (hypoglycemia). See also coma, diabetic.

shock, neurogenic, *n* shock caused by loss of nervous control of peripheral vessels, resulting in an increase in the vascular capacity. Onset is usually sudden but is quickly reversible if the cause is removed and treatment is instituted immediately.

shock, primary, *n* shock that has a neurogenic basis in which pain and psychic factors affect the vascular system. Occurs immediately after an injury.

shock, secondary, *n* shock that occurs some time after the injury (6 to 24 hours later). It is associated with changes in capillary permeability and subsequent loss of plasma into the tissue spaces. Changes in capillary permeability are probably related to histamine release associated with tissue injury.

shock, traumatic, *n* a shock produced by trauma, whether psychic or physical. In general usage, this term refers to shock following physical trauma, with hemorrhage, peripheral blood vessel dilation, and changes in capillary permeability.

shoeing cusps, *n.pl* See restoration of cusps.

short-bowel syndrome, *n* a loss of intestinal surface for absorption of nutrients caused by the surgical removal of a section of bowel.

short-cone technique, *n* See technique, short-cone.

shotgun therapy, *n* a treatment that has a wide range of effect and may be expected to correct the abnormal condition even though the particular cause is unknown.

shoulder, *n* **1.** the junction of the clavicle, scapula, and humerus where the arm attaches to the trunk of the body. **2.** in extracoronal cavity preparation of the ledge formed by the meeting of the gingival and axial walls at a right angle.

shoulder, linguogingival, *n* the portion of a prepared cavity in the proximal surface of an anterior tooth that is formed by the angular junction of the gingival and lingual walls. Developed to facilitate the dense compaction of gold in this area.

shrinkage, casting, *n* a volume change (contraction) that occurs when molten metal solidifies after being cast into a pattern mold. It is compensated for in three ways: by using the indicated water:powder ratio for the refractory investment to gain the maximal setting expansion of which that investment is capable; by exposing the investment to moisture as the refractory investment sets, causing some hydroscopic expansion; and by properly heating the mold to achieve thermal expansion. The total expansion must equal the contraction of the metal being cast.

shunt, *n* **1.** a hole or passageway that allows the movement of fluid, such as cerebrospinal fluid, from one body part to another. The term is used to describe congenital or acquired shunts, which may be either mechanical or biologic. **2.** a surgically implanted tube or catheter, such as those used to treat hydrocephalus, that allows the passage of fluid between body parts.

shunt, arteriovenous, *n* (arteriovenous aneurysm, arteriovenous fistula), an abnormal communication between an artery and a vein; usually caused by trauma.

shunt, ventriculoatrial **(ventrik'ūlōā'trēəl),** *n* a surgically manufactured passage made of plastic tubing between a cardiac atrium and cerebral ventricle for the treatment of hydrocephalus. See also ventriculoureterostomy.

shut, *n* the part of an anterior artificial tooth between the ridge lap and the shoulder. The pins for retaining the tooth in the base material are located in the shut.

sialadenitis (sī'əlad'ənī'tis), *n* inflammation of the salivary glands, especially the major glands, because of such trauma as surgery or infection. Noted in mumps due to viral infection.

sialagogue (sīal'əgog), *n* a substance that increases the flow of saliva.

sialoadenectomy (sī'əlōad'ənek'təmē), *n* an excision of a salivary gland.

sialoangiitis, *n* inflammation of salivary gland ducts.

sialodochoplasty (sī'əlōdō'kōplastē), *n* a surgical procedure for the repair of a defect or restoration of a portion of a salivary gland duct.

sialogram (sīal'əgram), a radiograph made to determine the presence or absence of calcareous deposits in a salivary gland or its ducts.

sialography (sīəlog'rəfē), *n* **1.** inspection of the salivary ducts and glands by radiographic examination after injection of a radiopaque medium. **2.** production of a sialogram.

sialolith (sīal'əlith), *n* See salivary stone.

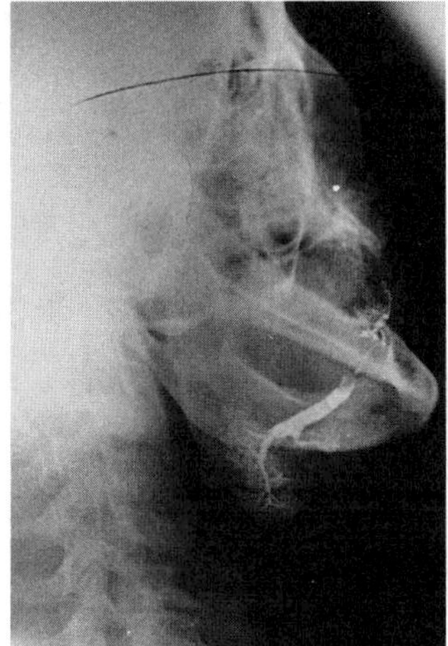

Sialogram. (Frommer/Stabulas-Savage, 2005)

sialolithiasis (sīal'əlithī'əsis), *n* the presence of one or more oval or round calcified structures (salivary stones) in a duct of a salivary gland.

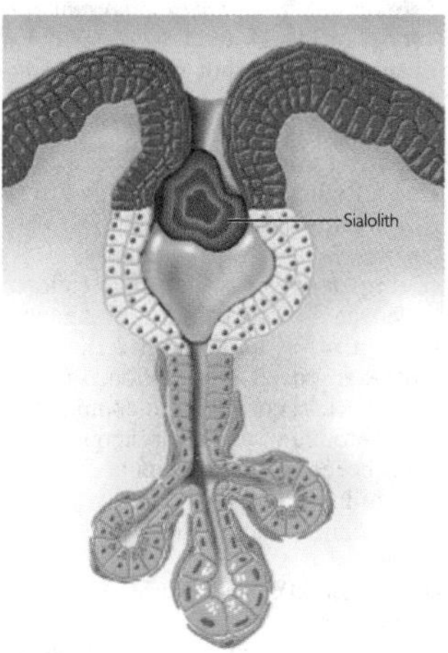

Sialolithiasis. (Sapp/Eversole/Wysocki, 2004)

sialolithotomy (sīaləlithôt'ōmē), *n* removal of calculus from a salivary gland or duct.

sialometaplasia, necrotizing (sī'əlōmet'əplā'zēə nek'rōtīzing), *n* an oral lesion due to a blood flow blockage to the region because of ischemia or trauma. The condition is indicated by localized tender swelling and pain and a well-defined ulcer, usually in the hard palate region.

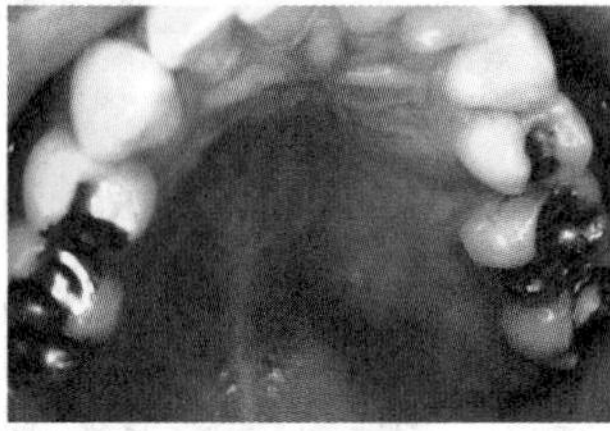

Necrotizing sialometaplasia. (Sams/Lynch, 1990)

sialorrhea (sīal′ərē′ə), *n* (hypersalivation, ptyalism), an excessive flow of saliva. It may be associated with acute inflammation of the oral cavity, mental retardation, neurologic disorders with lenticular involvement, mercurialism, pregnancy, ill-fitting dental appliances, dysautonomia, periodic diseases, cystic fibrosis of the pancreas, teething, alcoholism, and malnutrition.

sialorrhea, periodic, n recurrent episodes of hypersalivation; of unknown cause but probably related to recurrent parotitis and other so-called periodic diseases.

sibilant (sib′ilənt), *adj* accompanied by a hissing sound; especially a type of fricative speech sound. The phonemes /s/ and /z/ are sibilants.

sibling, *n* one of two or more children who have both parents in common.

sibutramine (sībū′trəmēn), *n* an FDA-approved prescription drug for weight loss containing a combination of serotonin and andronergics that has been shown to promote a feeling of fullness while apparently not influencing hunger; Meridia is an example.

sickle (sik′əl), *n* See scaler, sickle.

sickle cell anemia, *n* a severe, chronic, incurable, hemoglobinopathic, anemic condition that occurs in people homozygous for hemoglobin S (Hb S).

sickle cell crisis, *n* an acute, episodic condition that occurs in children with sickle cell anemia. The crisis may be vasoocclusive, resulting from the aggregation of misshapen erythrocytes, or anemic, resulting from bone marrow aplasia.

sickle cell trait, *n* the gene that carries sickle cell anemia. Only the presence of two genes in a person's genetic code leads to the manifestation of sickle cell anemia. See also sickle cell anemia.

sickle scaler, *n* a triangular-shaped dental instrument with two cutting edges and a pointed tip. They are designed primarily to remove deposits from teeth. Sickle scalers with straight shanks are used on the anterior teeth, and contraangled scalers (Jacquettes) are used on the posterior teeth.

sicklemia (siklē′mēə), *n* See sickle cell anemia.

side effect, *n* an effect not sought in the case under treatment that can complicate the prognosis.

side-shift, *n* an imprecise term for lateral thrust of the rotating condyle.

sidestream smoke, *n* the vaporous byproduct of burning tobacco that enters the air from the smoldering part of a tobacco product, such as the lit tip of a cigarette or cigar.

SIDS, *n* abbreviation for **s**udden **i**nfant **d**eath **s**yndrome.

sievert (Sv) (sē′vurt), *n* unit used for measuring the combined effects of various types of radiation, its quality and distribution, plus other relative factors.

sigh (sī), *n* an audible and prolonged inspiration followed by a shortened expiration.

sight, *n* the special sense that enables the shape, size, position, and color of objects to be perceived; the sense or faculty of vision.

sigmoid (sig′moid), *adj* of or pertaining to an S shape, as in the shape of the pelvic end of the colon prior to its joining the rectum.

sigmoid notch, n See notch, mandibular.

sign (sīn), *n* an indication of the existence of something; any objective evidence of a disease.

sign, Battle's, n.pr the ecchymosis that appears near the mastoid process of the temporal bone; indicative of a fracture of the base of the skull.

sign, Bell's, n.pr the turning up of the eyeball on the affected side when

S

a patient with Bell's palsy attempts to close the eyelid.

sign, Nikolsky's, n.pr a diagnostic feature wherein apparently normal epithelium may be rubbed off with finger pressure.

sign, Tinel's, n.pr a paresthesia in the area served by a sensory nerve when the site of a lesion or injury to the nerve is percussed. Indicative of partial injury of a nerve or regeneration of an injured nerve.

signa (sig′nə), *n* (signature), the portion of a prescription that contains a statement of the directions for use.

signature, *n* See signa.

signs and symptoms, diagnostic, *n.pl* the objective and subjective features of disease that are carefully evaluated to establish a diagnosis.

silex (sī′leks) (silicon dioxide), *n* a substance used in dental surface polishing due to its abrasive characteristics.

silica (sil′ikə) (quartz), *n* the purest of three major ingredients that make up dental porcelain. It imparts stiffness and hardness to the product and is the framework around which the kaolin and feldspar contract.

silicate cement (sil′ikāt), *n* See cement, silicate.

silicon (Si) (sil′ikon), *n* a nonmetallic element, second to oxygen as the most abundant of the elements. Its atomic number is 14, and its atomic weight is 28. It occurs in nature as silicon dioxide and in silicates. The silicates are used as detergents, corrosion inhibitors, adhesives, and sealants. Elemental silicon is used in metallurgy and in transistors and other electronic components. Protracted inhalation of silica dusts may cause silicosis, which increases susceptibility to other pulmonary diseases.

silicone (sil′ikōn), *n* a compound of organic structural character in which all or some of the positions that could be occupied by carbon atoms are occupied by silicon. A plastic containing silicons.

silicophosphate cement, *n* See cement, silicophosphate.

silicosis (sil′ikō′sis), *n* a lung disorder caused by continued, long-term inhalation of the dust of an inorganic compound silicon dioxide, which is found in sands, quartzes, flints, and many other stones.

silk suture, *n* a braided, fine black suture material, usually used to close incisions, wounds, and cuts in the skin. It is not absorbed by the body and is removed after approximately 7 days.

silver (Ag), *n* a whitish precious metal occurring mainly as a sulfide. Its atomic number is 47, and its atomic weight is 107.88. It is quite soft and is usually alloyed with small amounts of copper to increase its durability. It is used extensively in photography, radiography, and dentistry.

silver amalgam, n See amalgam, silver.

silver cones, n an endodontic filling material used in conjunction with gutta-percha points and sealing agents to effect a seal of the pulp chamber and canal. Also known as *master cones.*

silver halide crystals, n See crystal, silver halide.

silver nitrate, ammoniacal **(am′ōnī′əkəl),** *n* (ammoniated silver nitrate, Howe's silver nitrate), an ammonium compound of silver nitrate that is more readily reduced to silver and silver proteinates than is the usual silver nitrate; formerly used to disclose carious tooth structure and immunize incipient carious lesions of the enamel. It is highly irritating to the pulp and can permanently stain the oral mucosa.

silver nitrate, Howe's, n.pr See silver nitrate, ammoniacal.

silver points, n See silver cones.

simian crease (sim′ēən), *n* a single crease across the palm produced from the fusion of proximal and distal palmar creases, seen in such congenital disorders as Down syndrome.

Simmonds's disease, *n.pr* See disease, Simmonds's.

Simon's classification of malocclusion, *n* a classification of malocclusion in which tooth malpositions are related to three craniofacial planes: midsagittal, orbital, and Frankfort. Teeth too close to the midsagittal plane are in *contraction,* whereas those too far away are in *distraction.* Teeth too anterior to the orbital plane are in *protraction,* whereas those too posterior to the orbital plane are in *retraction.* Teeth too close to the Frankfort plane are in *attraction,* whereas those too distant are in *distraction.* See also malocclusion.

simple fracture, *n* an uncomplicated closed fracture in which the fractured ends of the bone do not break the skin.

simple reflex, *n* a reflex with a motor nerve component that involves only one muscle and level of the afferent and efferent nerve synapse.

simulation, *n* a mode of computer-assisted instruction in which a student receives basic information about a topic and then must interact with the computer to gain deeper understanding of the information and topic. It provides the student with the opportunity to gain experience at limited cost and with reduced risk.

simvastatin (sim′vəstat′ən), *n brand name:* Zocor; *drug class:* cholesterol-lowering agent; *action:* inhibits 3-hydroxy-3-methylglutaryl coenzyme A (HMG-CoA) reductase enzyme, which reduces cholesterol synthesis; *use:* as an adjunct in primary hypercholesterolemia types IIa and IIb.

single emulsion, *n* (film), See emulsion, single.

single-blind study, *n* an experiment in which the person collecting the data knows whether the subjects are in the control or experimental groups but the subjects do not.

single-crystal sapphire, *n* a single-crystal endosteal implant made of α-alumina oxide with a Knoop hardness number of 1.750. The implants are threaded and supplied in three sizes: 3, 4, and 5.

sinoatrial (SA) node (sī′nōā′trēəl), *n* a cluster of hundreds of cells located in the right atrial wall of the heart near the opening of the superior vena cava. It constitutes a knot of modified heart muscle that generates impulses, which travel swiftly throughout the muscle fibers of both atria, causing them to contract.

sinter (sin′tər), *v* to treat by applying heat below the boiling point to a powder in order to bond and fuse the particles together; this can be done with or without applying pressure.

sinus (sī′nus), *n* a cavity, recess, or hollow space.

sinus, alveolar, *n* a passage connecting a pathologic cavity in the alveolus with the oral or nasal cavity and penetrating the mucous membrane. See also fistula, alveolar.

sinus balloon, *n* See balloon, sinus.

sinus, carotid, *n* the swelling in the artery just before the common carotid artery bifurcates into the internal and external carotid arteries.

sinus, coronary, *n* the venous sinus in the groove between the left cardiac auricle and the left ventricle.

sinus(es), ethmoidal **(ethmoid′əl),** *n* an air space located within the ethmoid bone, which comprises the floor of the skull and the roof of the nose. There are four ethmoid sinuses: the anterior, middle, and two posterior sinuses. The anterior and middle sinuses drain directly into the middle meatus (opening) of the nose. The posterior sinuses drain into the superior meatus of the nose.

sinus(es), frontal, *n* an air space located within the frontal bone of the forehead.

sinus(es), maxillary (antrum of Highmore, maxillary antrum), *n* a large pyramidal cavity within the body of the maxilla. Its walls are thin and correspond to the orbital, nasal anterior, and infratemporal surfaces of the body of the maxilla. On dental radiographs the floor of the sinus is often observed approximating the root apices of the teeth and is seen to extend from the canine or premolar region posteriorly to the molar or tuberosity region.

sinus(es), paranasal, *n* the paired air cavities in various bones around the nose, including the maxillary sinus within the maxilla, the sphenoid sinus in the sphenoid bone, the ethmoid sinuses in the ethmoid bone, and the frontal sinus in the frontal bone.

sinus(es), sphenoid **(sfē′noid),** *n* an air space located within the wing-like sphenoid bone, located at the base of the skull. These sinuses are variable in shape and size, and are rarely symmetrical because of lateral displacement of the septum.

sinus tract, *n* See tract, sinus.

sinus pneumatization (nōō′məti-zā′shən), *n* an enlargement of the maxillary sinus, usually as part of the aging process and as a result of the loss of maxillary teeth.

sinusitis, *n* an inflammation of the sinus. Can be primary or secondary in origin.

site visit, *n* a visit to an institution by designated officials to evaluate or gather information about a program, department, or institution. A site visit is a step in the accreditation of an institution and in the funding of many major research and training projects. See accreditation.

Sjögren's syndrome (shœ′grenz), *n.pr* See syndrome, Sjögren's.

skeletal discrepancies, *n* an orthodontic term used to describe the nature of a malocclusion as being a malrelationship of the bony base rather than merely of the teeth.

skeletal relationships, *n.pl* the orientations of bony parts to one another; usually the mandible to the maxillae or to the bases with which they articulate.

skeletal system, *n* all bones and cartilage of the body that collectively provide the supporting framework for the muscles and organs.

skeleton, axial, *n* all bones that constitute the head and neck, including those that enclose the brain, face, and the neck bones. Some researchers include the entire midline vertebral column.

skill, *n* the practical knowledge of an art, science, profession, or trade and the ability to apply it properly in practice.

skill, reasonable, *n* the skill that is ordinarily possessed and exercised by persons of similar qualifications engaged in the same employment or profession.

skin, *n* the tough, supple cutaneous membrane that covers the entire surface of the body. It is the largest organ of the body and is composed of five layers of cells in the epidermis, which overlies the dermis. See also stratum.

slander, *n* an oral defamation; the saying of false and malicious words about another, resulting in injury to his or her reputation.

slant of occlusal plane, *n* the inclination measured by the angle the occlusal plane makes when extended to intersect with the axis-orbital plane.

sleep, *n* a period of rest for the body and mind, during which volition and consciousness are in partial or complete abeyance and the bodily functions partially suspended.

sleep apnea, *n* a sleep disorder characterized by periods of an absence of attempts to breathe. The person is momentarily unable to move respiratory muscles or maintain airflow through the nose and oral cavity.

sleep, twilight, *n* (seminarcosis), a state of amnesia and analgesia produced by an injection of scopolamine and morphine.

slice, *n* in cavity preparation a straight-line (plane) cut that removes a thin layer from an axial convexity.

slim disease, *n* a constitutional disease of acquired immunodeficiency syndrome (AIDS); also called *human immunodeficiency virus (HIV) wasting syndrome.* It is characterized by fever for more than 1 month, involuntary weight loss of greater than 10%, and diarrhea persisting for more than 1 month.

slope, lower ridge, *n* the slope of the mandibular residual ridge in the second and third molar region as seen from the buccal side.

slotted attachment, *n* See attachment, intracoronal.

slough (sluf), *n* **1.** the dead tissue that has been shed or discarded. *v* **2.** to remove dead tissue.

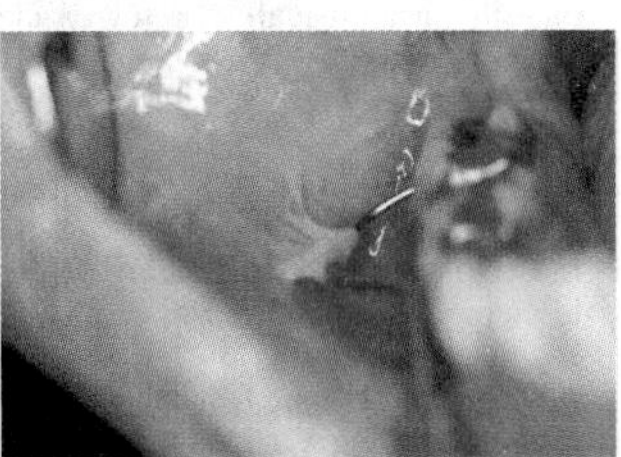

Slough. (Regezi/Sciubba/Jordan, 2008)

Sluder's neuralgia, *n.pr* See neuralgia, Sluder's.

slurry, *n* a thin mixture of insoluble material floating in liquid.

smallpox, *n* See variola.

smear, bacterial, *n* the act of taking bacteria taken from a lesion or area, spreading them on a slide, and staining them for microscopic examination.

smear layer, *n* a thin layer with small crystalline characteristics. It appears on the surface of teeth that have undergone dental instrumentation procedures, including root planing and cutting done with a dental bur. Not easily rinsed away, it must be removed by acid etching.

smell, *n* the special sense that enables odors to be perceived through the stimulation of the olfactory nerves.

smokeless tobacco, *n* chewing tobacco (leaves) or tobacco powder (snuff) that allows the nicotine to be absorbed through the mucous membrane of the oral cavity or digestive tract. It is related to a high risk of oral cancer. Can contain abrasives such as sand, pesticides, and sugar for taste. It is not a substitute for cigarettes. Impress upon the patient the social repugnance of the habit. The term *spit tobacco* is preferred.

smooth surface caries, *n* See caries, smooth surface.

sneeze, *n* an involuntary, sudden, violent expulsion of air through the oral cavity and nose; may be elicited during thiopental (Pentothal) anesthesia by corneal stimulation.

snuff, *n* See smokeless tobacco.

snuff dipper's lesion, *n* a white or discolored lesion of the oral mucosa occurring at the site at which the powdered tobacco is retained. Malignant transformations are not common but do occur, usually as low-grade verrucous carcinomas.

S

Snyder's test, *n.pr* See test, colorimetric caries susceptibility.

soap, *n* a salt or mixture of salts, of aliphatic acids, such as palmitic, stearic, or oleic acid, with sodium or potassium used for cleaning purposes.

soap, antimicrobial **(an′tīmīkrō′bēəl),** *n* hand cleanser infused with ingredients to reduce the number of microorganisms found on the skin.

sob, *n* a short, convulsive inspiration, attended by contraction of the diaphragm and spasmodic closure of the glottis.

social functioning, *n* the ability of the individual to interact in the normal or usual way in society; can be used as a measure of quality of care.

socialized medicine, *n* a system for the delivery of health care in which the expense of care is borne by a governmental agency supported by taxation rather than being paid directly by the client on a fee-for-service or contract basis.

socioeconomic status, *n* the position of an individual on a socioeconomic scale that measures such factors as education, income, type of occupation, place of residence, and in some populations, ethnicity and religion.

sociology, *n* the study of group behavior within a society.

socket, *n* **1.** the hollow part of a joint; the excavation in one bone of a joint that receives the articular end of another bone. **2.** a hollow or concavity into which another part fits, as the eyes. **3.** an alveolus; the cavity in the alveolar process of the jaw in which the root of a tooth is fixed.

socket, dry, *n* (alveolalgia, infected socket localized alveolar osteitis), an osteitis or periostitis associated with infection and disintegration of the clot after tooth extraction. Because of its painful nature, it also is called *alveolalgia.*

socket, infected, *n* See socket, dry.

socket preservation, *n* the protection of the contours of the ridge bone and soft tissue by implanting grafting material into the extraction socket as soon as a tooth is extracted; also known as ridge preservation, extraction socket graft, and socket graft.

soda, *n* a compound of sodium, particularly sodium bicarbonate, sodium carbonate, or sodium hydroxide.

sodium (Na) (sō′dēəm), *n* a soft, grayish metal of the alkaline metals group. Its atomic number is 11, and its atomic weight is 22.9898. Sodium is one of the most important elements in the body. Sodium ions are involved in acid-base balance, water balance, the transmission of nerve impulses, and the contraction of muscle. The recommended daily intake of sodium is 250 to 750 mg for infants, 900 to 2700 mg for children, and 1100 to 3300 mg for adults.

sodium aluminum fluoride **(flôr'īd, floor'īd),** *n* See cryolite.

sodium bicarbonate, *n* an antacid, electrolyte, and urinary alkalinizing agent.

sodium chloride, *n* common table salt.

sodium fluoride (NaF), *n* a white, odorless powder used in 2% aqueous solution and applied topically to teeth as a caries-preventing agent; used as 33% NaF in kaolin and glycerin as a desensitizing agent for hypersensitive dentin. In drinking water, one part per million of NaF is used as a caries-prophylactic substance.

sodium fluoride poisoning, *n* a chronic condition of fluorine poisoning that occurs in some communities where the fluorine concentration in the water supply exceeds one part per million. Signs of the condition include mottling of the tooth enamel and severe osteosclerosis.

sodium hypochlorite (NaOCl), *n* a popular chemical disinfectant made of a chlorine compound and usually combined with distilled water for enhanced stability. NaOCl is often used to clean dentures if they have no metal parts and to disinfect and decontaminate water lines. It is corrosive and toxic when applied directly to the skin. The chemical name for household bleach.

sodium iodide, *n* an iodine supplement to the diet, usually an additive to common table salt.

sodium lauryl sulfate (SLS) **(sō'-dēəm lor'əl sul'fāt),** *n* a surface-active substance used as an emulsifier, a detergent, or a wetting agent in most cosmetic products; toothpaste with sodium lauryl sulfate has a possible link to oral mucosal inflammation.

sodium monofluorophosphate **(mon'ōflŏŏr'ōfos'fāt),** *n* a form of fluoride added to oral care products at a strength of 1500 ppm, which is considered extra-strength.

sodium perborate **(purbôr'āt),** *n* an oxygen-liberating antiseptic that has been used in the treatment of necrotizing ulcerative gingivitis and other forms of gingival inflammation. Prolonged or indiscriminate use has produced burns of the oral mucosa and hyperplasia of the filiform papillae of the tongue (black hairy tongue). Also used to bleach pulpless teeth.

sodium pump, *n* a mechanism for transporting sodium ions across cell membranes against an opposing concentration gradient.

sodium thiosulfate **(thī'ōsul'fāt),** *n* a powdered chemical, commonly called *hypo,* that is an ingredient of the fixing solution used in film processing. It clears the film of undeveloped silver halide crystals.

soft deposits, *n* the nonmineralized material such as plaque biofilm, proteins, cellular material, and food debris that accumulates on the teeth, surrounding tissues, and dental restorations. The presence of bacteria can lead to gingival tissue infections and dental abscesses.

soft diet, *n* a diet that is soft in texture, low in fiber residue, easily digested, and well tolerated. It is commonly recommended for people who have gastrointestinal (GI) disturbances or after oral surgery.

soft palate, *n* the structure composed of mucous membranes, muscular fibers, and mucous glands, suspended from the posterior border of the hard palate forming the roof of the oral cavity. When the soft palate rises, as in swallowing, it separates the nasal cavity and nasopharynx from the posterior part of the oral cavity and oral portion of the pharynx. In sucking the soft palate and posterior superior surface of the tongue occlude the oral cavity from the orapharynx, creating a posterior seal. Thus it prevents the escape of fluid and food up through the nose and with the tongue allows fluid and food to collect in the oral cavity until swallowed.

soft radiation, *n* See radiation, soft.

soft tissue, *n* body tissue except bone, teeth, nails, hair, and cartilage.

soft tissue undercut, *n* See undercut, soft tissue.

soft water, *n* water that does not contain salts of calcium or magnesium, which precipitate soap solutions.

software, *n* the various programming aids supplied by manufacturers to facilitate the user's efficient operation of computer equipment. The collection of programs, routines, and documents associated with a computer (e.g., compilers, library routines).

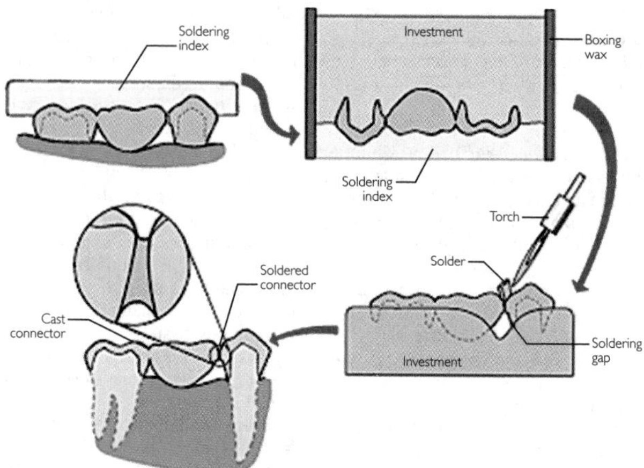

The soldering process. (Rosenstiel/Land/Fujimoto, 2006)

solar radiation, *n* the emission and diffusion of actinic rays from the sun. Overexposure may result in sunburn, keratosis, skin cancer, or lesions associated with photosensitivity.

solder (sod′ur), *n* a fusible alloy of metals used to unite the edges or surfaces of two pieces of metal.

soldering flux, *n* See flux, soldering.

soldering investment, *n* See investment, soldering and investment, refractory.

solubility (sol′ūbil′itē), *n* the quality or fact of being soluble; susceptible to being dissolved.

solute (sol′ūt), *n* the dissolved (usually the less abundant) constituent of a solution.

S

solution (səloo′shən), *n* the process of dissolving. In chemistry a homogeneous dispersion of two or more compounds. In pharmacy, usually a nonalcoholic solution. Solutions containing alcohol are variously called *elixirs, tinctures, spirits, essences,* or *hydroalcoholic solutions.*

solution, Carnoy's, *n.pr* a sclerosing solution; mild; does not cauterize normal oral mucosa if used judiciously. A mild hemostatic.

solution, cleansing, *n* a solution especially suited to the removal of adherent food particles by immersion of the denture to avoid damaging the denture by brushing.

solution, disclosing, *n* a topically applied dye used in aqueous solution to stain and reveal the extent of calcareous and mucinous deposition on the teeth.

solution, hardening, *n* an aqueous solution (often of 2% potassium sulfate) in which a hydrocolloid impression may be immersed to reduce or retard syneresis of the impression material.

solution, hypertonic, *n* a mixture containing a concentration of solute in excess of the concentration of the same solute in another mixture to which it is compared. When the two solutions are placed on opposite sides of a permeable membrane (either artificial or natural, as with cell membranes), the hypertonic solution attracts the solvent from the hypotonic solution, equalizing the concentration of the solute in both. See also solution, hypotonic; solution, isotonic; and osmosis.

solution, hypotonic, *n* a mixture containing a concentration of solute that is lower than the concentration of the same solute in another mixture to which it is compared. When two such solutions are separated by a permeable membrane, the solvent of the hypotonic solution flows through the membrane to the hypertonic solution, equalizing the concentration of the solute in both. See also solution, hypertonic; solution, isotonic; and osmosis.

solution, isotonic, n a mixture containing the same concentration of solute as another mixture to which it is compared. When separated by a permeable membrane, osmosis does not occur. See also solution, hypertonic; solution, hypotonic; and osmosis.

solution, parenteral, n a sterile solution or substance prepared for injection.

solution, physiologic saline, n a salt solution containing 0.9% sodium chloride in distilled water that exhibits the same molecular concentration as blood.

solution, pickling, n a solution of acid used for removing oxides and other impurities from dental castings (e.g., solutions of hydrochloric or sulfuric acid).

solution, sclerosing, n an agent that causes intense inflammation, resulting in fibrosis; used to treat subluxation of the temporomandibular joint, cauterize ulcers, arrest hemorrhage, and treat hemangiomas.

solution, Skinner's, n.pr an iodine preparation used as a disclosing agent, containing iodine crystals, potassium iodide, zinc iodide, water and glycerine. It is seldom used because of its bad taste.

solution, solid, n an alloy all of whose constituents are mutually soluble in the solid state.

solvent, *n* a substance capable of or used in dissolving or dispersing one or more other substances; a liquid component of a solution present in greater amount than the solute.

soma (sō′mə), *n* See somatic.

somatic (sōmat′ik), *n* derived from *soma,* meaning the body, as distinguished from the mind. Pertains to the framework of the body as distinguished from the viscera; hence the term *somatic nerves* describes the nerves associated with the musculoskeletal function of the muscles of the body.

somatotropin (sō′matōtrō′pin), *n* See hormone, growth.

somites (somīts), *n.pl* the paired cuboidal aggregates of cells differentiated from mesoderm that form along the neural tube of the embryo to create the vertebral column and other associated tissues.

somnambulism (somnam′būlizəm), *n* a habitual walking in the sleep; a hypnotic state in which the subject has full possession of senses but no subsequent recollection.

somnifacient (som′nifā′shənt), *adj* **1.** causing sleep; hypnotic. *n* **2.** a medicine that induces sleep.

somniferous (somnif′ərus), *adj* inducing or causing sleep.

somnolence (som′nəlens), *n* sleepiness; also unnatural drowsiness.

somnolism (som′nəlizəm), *n* a state of mesmeric or hypnotic trance.

sonant (son′ant), *n* a speech sound that has in it a component of tone generated by laryngeal vibrations (e.g., "a-a-a," "z-z-z").

sonic scaler, *n* See scaler, sonic and scaler, ultrasonic.

sonogram (son′ōgram), *n* the readily usable graph of the frequency bands (formants) produced by the sound spectrograph.

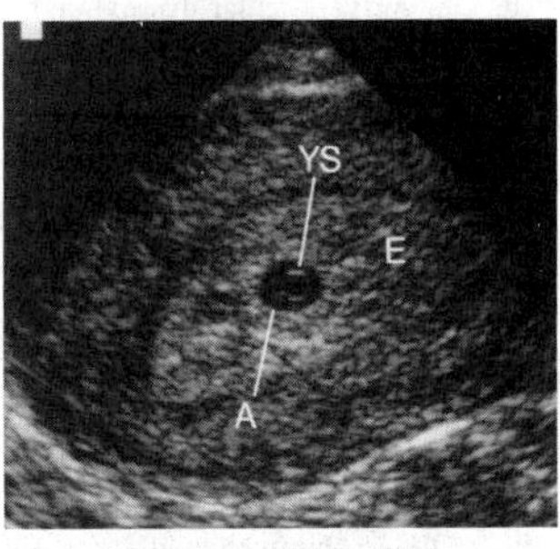

Sonogram. (Callen, 2000)

sonograph (son′ōgraf), *n* a wave analyzer that produces a permanent visual record showing the distribution of energy in both frequency and time.

soporific (sop′ərif′ik), *n* a sleep-producing drug.

sorbic acid, *n* a compound occurring naturally in berries of the mountain ash. Commercial sorbic acid is used in fungicides, food preservatives, lubricants, and plasticizers.

sordes (sôr′dēz), *n* an unclean material consisting of food particles, debris, skin, and microorganisms that forms a crust and gathers on the oral mucosa, lips, and teeth of a feverish or dehydrated individual with a chronic incapacitating condition.

sore, canker, *n* See ulcer, aphthous, recurrent.

sore, cold, *n* See herpes labialis.

sore, denture, *n* See ulcer, decubitus.

sort, *v* to arrange units of information according to rules dependent on a key or field contained in or with the information.

sort generator program, *n* a generalized program that can produce many different sorting programs in accordance with control information specified by the user.

sotalol HCl (sō′təlol′), *n brand name:* Betapace; *drug class:* nonselective β-adrenergic blocker; *action:* competitively blocks stimulation of β-adrenergic receptors in the heart and decreases renin activity, all of which may play a role in reducing systolic and diastolic blood pressure; inhibits β_2-receptors in the bronchial system; *use:* treatment of life-threatening ventricular dysrhythmias.

source file, *n* a file containing information used as input to a computer program.

source language, *n* a language that is an input to a given translation process.

source program, *n* a program coded in other than machine language that must be translated into machine language before being executed.

source-collimator distance (kol′əmā′tər), *n* distance from the focal spot to the diaphragm or collimator in a radiographic tube head.

S

source-film distance (SFD), *n* distance from the focal spot of a radiograph tube to the radiographic film. Also known as *target-film distance.*

source-object distance (SOD), *n* distance from focal spot to object of which a radiographic image is to be obtained. Also known as *target-object distance.*

Southern blot test, *n.pr* a gene analysis method used to identify specific deoxyribonucleic acid (DNA) fragments and diagnose cancers and hemoglobinopathies.

space, *n* a delimited, three-dimensional region.

space(s), fascial, *n* the spaces containing loose connective tissue that lie between the body's layers of fascia. The fascial spaces of the neck and head can be involved in the spread of dental infection.

space, freeway, *n* the interocclusal distance or separation between the occlusal surfaces of the teeth when the mandible is in its physiologic rest position. *Interocclusal distance* is the preferred term. See also distance, interocclusal; clearance, interocclusal.

space, interalveolar, *n* See distance, interarch.

space, interocclusal rest, *n* See distance, interocclusal.

space, interproximal, *n* the space between adjacent teeth in a dental arch. It is divided into the *embrasure* (occlusal to the contact point) and the *septal space* (gingival to the contact point).

space, interradicular, *n* the area between the roots of a multirooted tooth; it is normally occupied by bony septum and the periodontal membrane.

space, lattice, *n* See lattice space.

space maintainer, *n* a fixed or removable appliance designed to preserve the space created by the premature loss of a tooth.

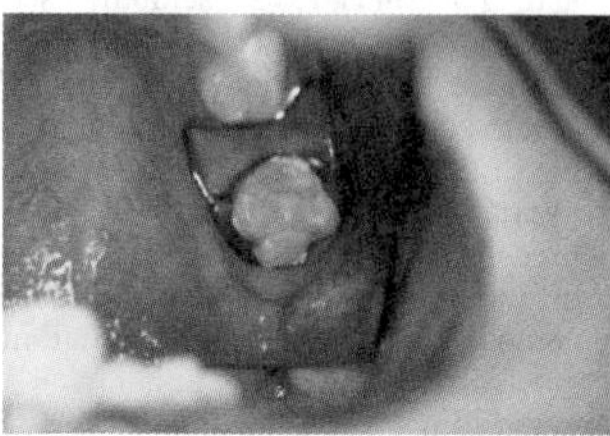

Space maintainer. (Cameron/Widmer, 2003)

space maintainer cast, *n* a type fabricated by a casting technique and cemented into place.

space maintainer, fixed, *n* a type not intended to be removable by the patient.

space maintainer, orthodontic, *n* a removable or fixed appliance fabricated to maintain space in the arch for erupting permanent teeth. The appliance may be designed to regain space needed to accommodate the erupting tooth or teeth.

space maintainer, removable, n a type designed for easy removal for cleaning and adjustment.

space, marrow, n spaces in the spongiosa of bone; in the mandible and maxilla the marrow spaces are occupied by fatty and hematogenic (blood-forming) marrow. When inflammation progresses into these spaces, the marrow becomes fibrous. The spaces enlarge in atrophy of disuse because of resorption of surrounding trabeculae, and the marrow remains fatty in nature.

space, masticator **(mas′tikā′tər),** *n* the area that contains the masticator muscles that attach to the ramus of the mandible. It is bounded by the superficial layer of deep cervical fascia.

space, mesiodistal **(mē′zēōdis′təl),** *n* the space between the mesial and distal surfaces of two teeth.

space obtainer, n an appliance used to increase the space between two teeth.

space, occupied, n the space that might be occupied by persons or radiation-sensitive materials and devices during the time that radiographic equipment is in operation or radiation is being emitted.

space, parapharyngeal **(par′əfərin′jēəl),** *n* an inverted-cone–shaped area that extends from the base of the skull to the hyoid bone and is bordered by the superior constrictor of the pharynx and the medial pterygoid muscle.

space, parotid, n the area that contains the facial nerve, the parotid lymph nodes, and the posterior facial vein. It is bounded by the superficial layer of the deep cervical fascia.

space, physiologic dead, n the air passages up to but not including the alveoli of the lungs; equal to about 150 ml.

space regainer, n a fixed or removable appliance capable of moving a displaced permanent tooth into its proper position in the dental arch.

space relief, n fabrication of a prosthesis so that certain predetermined, non–stress-bearing areas will not be contacted by the appliance.

space, retropharyngeal **(re′trōfərin′jēəl),** *n* the area behind the pharynx that contains the retropharyngeal lymph nodes. It is bounded by the prevertebral fascia and the buccopharyngeal fascia.

space, sublingual, n the superior part of the submandibular space, separated from the inferior part (the submaxillary space) by the mylohyoid muscle. It contains the sublingual gland and the tissue surrounding the tongue.

space, submandibular, n the area in the neck under the tongue that extends to the hyoid bone. It is bounded laterally and anteriorly by the mandible and is divided into two spaces: the sublingual and submaxillary.

space, submental, n the middle section of the submaxillary space. It contains the submental lymph nodes.

spasm (spaz′əm), *n* a sudden involuntary contraction of a muscle or muscle group. It may cause a twitch or close a canal or passage, depending on its location.

spasm, muscle, n the increased muscular tension and shortness that cannot be released voluntarily and prevents lengthening of the muscles involved. Caused by pain stimuli to the lower motor neurons.

spasmolysant (spazmol′izənt), *n* the relieving or relaxing spasms; an agent that relieves spasm.

spasmolytic (spaz′mōlit′ik), *adj* pertaining to a drug that reduces spasm in smooth or skeletal muscle.

spastic (spas′tik), *adj* characterized by a more or less constant state of hypertonic contraction of a muscle or group of muscles. The condition is regarded as abnormally heightened muscular tonus present even in states of inactivity.

spasticity (spastis′itē), *n* a form of muscular hypertonicity with increased resistance to stretch.

spatter, *n* droplets of airborne particulate matter larger than 50 µm that fall to the ground.

spatula (spach′ələ), *n* a flat-bladed instrument without sharp edges used for mixing certain dental materials (e.g., cement, plaster of paris, impression pastes).

spatulate (spach′oolāt), *v* to manipulate or mix with a spatala.

spatulation (spach′oolā′shən), *n* the manipulation of material with a

S

spatula to mix it into a homogeneous mass.

spatulator, *n* a mechanical device that mixes ingredients to form a homogeneous mass. Also called a *mechanical spatulator.*

SPCA, *n* an acronym for **s**erum **p**rothrombin **c**onversion **a**ccelerator. See also factor VIII; thromboplastin, extrinsic.

Spearman's rho, *n.pr* a statistical test for correlation between two rank-ordered scales. It yields a statement of the degree of interdependence of the scores of the two scales.

specialist, *n* a health care professional who is qualified to limit practice to a narrow spectrum of health care. A specialist usually has advanced clinical training and postgraduate education in the discipline or specialty.

specialization, *n* the limiting of professional services to one isolated and distinct phase of dental practice.

specialty, *n* a particular field of attention and endeavor to which a therapist's efforts are devoted.

specialty, dental, *n* the eight specialties recognized by organized dentistry: endodontics, public health dentistry, oral radiology, oral surgery, oral pathology, orthodontics, pediatric dentistry, periodontics, and prosthodontics.

specific dynamic energy (SDE), *n* the amount of energy an individual body must expend in order to process and use food; equal to approximately 10% of basal metabolism rate and activity energy components. Also called *nonshivering thermogenesis.*

specific gravity, *n* See gravity, specific.

spectrum, antibacterial, *n* the range of antimicrobial activity of a drug.

spectrum, electromagnetic, *n* a family of radiant energies that travel in wave form, have neither mass nor charge, and travel at the speed of light. Radiations within the spectrum vary only in wavelength. X-ray photons and light rays are examples of electromagnetic radiation.

Spee, curve of, *n.pr* See curve of Spee.

speech, *n* **1.** communication through conventional vocal and oral symbols. **2.** a basic biologic function of the maxillofacial structures. The essential characteristic of the speech function is the production and organization of sound into symbols.

speech aid, *n* See aid, speech.

speech, delayed, *n* failure of speech to develop at the expected age, usually resulting from slow maturation, hearing impairment, brain injury, mental retardation, or emotional disturbance.

speech device, *n* a prosthesis that assists in the management of speech disorders associated with congenital or acquired defects of the palate.

speech disorder, cerebrovascular, *n* a diminished capacity to speak due to the location of traumatic brain damage and the involvement of the throat, tongue, and oral cavity.

speech, infantile, *n* a speech defect characterized by substitution of speech sounds similar to those used by the child who speaks normally in the early stages of speech development.

speech pathology, *n* **1.** the study of abnormalities of speech or organs of speech. **2.** the diagnosis and treatment of abnormalities of speech as practiced by a speech pathologist or speech therapist.

speech phonation, *n* See phonation, speech.

speech reading, *n* See reading, lip.

speech resonance, *n* See resonance, speech.

speech, retarded, *n* slowness in speech development in which intelligibility is severely impaired; often preceded by late or delayed emergence of speech.

speech, slurred, *n* abnormal speech in which words are not enunciated clearly or completely but are run together or partially eliminated. The most common causes are alcohol toxicity and drug abuse. It may also be a sign of damage to a motor neuron or cerebellar disease.

speech therapy, *n* the application of treatments and counseling in the prevention or correction of speech and language disorders.

speech, visible, *n* audible speech patterns that have been transformed by electronic devices into visual patterns that may be read by people who are deaf.

speed, *n* the relative rapidity of action; rate of motion.

speed, film, *n* See film speed.

S

speed, high, *n* a relatively great rapidity of motion. In cavity preparations, rotary instruments are classified according to the number of revolutions per minute (rpm) made by the cutting tool. Designation of each speed range presently varies. In general, conventional speed is 10,000 to 60,000 rpm, high speed is 60,000 to 100,000 rpm, and ultrahigh speed is more than 100,000 rpm. May also be used to describe an evacuation system.

speed of light, *n* a speed of 186,300 miles/sec.

speed of radiation, *n* See radiation, speed of.

sperm, *n* the cells contained in the male's semen that fertilize the female's egg during the process of conception.

sphenoid bone (sfē′noid), *n* the single midline cranial bone with a body and several pairs of processes.

spherocytosis, hereditary (sfir′ōsī-tō′sis), *n* See jaundice, congenital hemolytic.

sphincter (sfingk′tər), *n* a circular band of muscle fibers that constricts a passage or closes a natural opening in the body.

sphygmomanometer (sfig′mōmə-nom′itər), *n* an instrument for indirect measurement of blood pressure. See also blood pressure cuff.

sphygmomanometer, aneroid manometer **(an′əroid mənom′itər),** *n* a portable, handheld blood pressure measurement unit consisting of a cuff that is easily applied with one hand, a built-in or attachable stethoscope, a valve that inflates and deflates the cuff automatically, and an easy-to-read data display screen.

sphygmomanometer, electronic manometer, *n* an instrument used to digitally measure blood pressure.

spicule (spik′ūl), *n* a small needle-shaped body.

spillway, *n* a channel or passageway through which food escapes from the occlusal surfaces of the teeth during mastication. The occlusal, developmental, and supplemental grooves, as well as the incisal, occlusal, labial, buccal, and lingual embrasures, become spillways during function.

spillway, axial, *n* a groove that first crosses a cusp ridge or marginal ridge and extends onto an axial (mesial or distal) surface of the tooth.

spillway, interdental, *n* a sluiceway formed by the interproximal contours of adjoining teeth and investing tissues.

spillway, occlusal, *n* a groove that crosses only a cusp ridge or marginal ridge of a tooth; numerous on marginal ridges, thus increasing masticatory function.

spina bifida, *n* a congenital neural tube defect characterized by a developmental anomaly in the posterior vertebral arch. It is relatively common.

spinal anesthesia, *n* a state of insensitivity to pain in the lower part of the body produced by injection of an analgesic or anesthetic drug into the subarachnoid space of the spinal cord. See anesthesia.

spinal cord, *n* See cord, spinal.

spinal cord injury, *n* the traumatic disruption of the spinal cord as a result of vertebral fractures and dislocations, usually associated with car accidents, sports injuries, and other violent impacts. The degree of paralysis is directly related to the level and severity of the injury. Injury below the first thoracic vertebra may produce paraplegia. Injuries above the first thoracic vertebra may cause quadriplegia.

spinal shock, *n* a reaction to a spinal cord injury in which the body's reflexes are lost, resulting in a limp paralysis below the point of injury. May last several hours.

spindle, *n* muscle, a fusiform body lying parallel to and between muscle fibers. It is composed of a conspicuously smaller modified muscle fiber that has its own motor end plate to cause it to contract and its own special sensory end organs (the flower spray ending and the anulospiral ending) that send information to the central nervous system regarding the state of contraction of the main muscle body.

spine, anterior nasal, *n* the small bony projection extending forward from the medial anterosuperior part of each maxilla. The tip of the anterior nasal spines may be seen on lateral radiographic head plates and cephalometric radiographs.

spine, posterior nasal, *n* the small, sharp, bony point projecting backward from the midline of the horizontal part of the palatine bone.

spirapril (spē′rəpril), *n brand name:* Renormax; *drug class:* angiotensin-converting enzyme (ACE) inhibitor; *action:* selectively suppresses the renin-angiotensin-aldosterone system; inhibits ACE, prevents conversion of angiotensin I to angiotensin II; results in dilation of arterial and venous vessels; *use:* treatment of hypertension.

Spirillum **(spīril′um),** *n* a genus of aerobic, gram-negative helix-shaped bacteria, found in fresh and salt waters.

spirit of ammonia, *n* a solution of 3% ammonium carbonate in alcohol with flavorings added. It is mixed with water for use as a stimulant and carminative.

spirochete (spī′rəkēt′), *n* a bacterium of the genus *Spirochaeta* that is motile and spiral shaped with flexible filaments. They include the organisms responsible for leprosy, relapsing fever, syphilis, and yaws.

spirograph (spī′rəgraf), *n* an instrument for registering respiratory movements.

spirography (spirog′rəfē), *n* the graphic measurement of breathing, including breathing movements and breathing capacity.

spirometry (spīrom′ətrē), *n* laboratory evaluation of the air capacity of the lungs by means of a spirometer.

spironolactone (spī′rənōlak′tōn), *n brand names:* Aldactone, Spirozide; *drug class:* potassium-sparing diuretic; *action:* competes with aldosterone at receptor sites in distal tubule, resulting in excretion of sodium chloride and water and retention of potassium and phosphate; *uses:* treatment for edema, hypertension, diuretic-induced hypokalemia, and cirrhosis of the liver with ascites.

S

spit tobacco, *n* See smokeless tobacco.

spleen, *n* a soft, highly vascular, roughly ovoid organ situated between the stomach and the diaphragm in the left hypochondriac region of the body. It is considered part of the lymphatic system.

splenomegaly (splē′nōmeg′əlē), *n* an abnormal enlargement of the spleen, usually associated with portal hypertension, hemolytic anemia, and malaria.

splint, *n* **1.** a rigid appliance for the fixation of displaced or movable parts. **2.** a support or brace used to fasten or confine. **3.** metal, acrylic resin, or modeling compound fashioned to retain in position teeth that may have been replanted or have fractured roots.

splint, abutment, *n* adjacent tooth restorations that have been rigidly united at their proximal contact areas to form a single abutment with multiple roots.

splint, acrylic resin bite-guard, *n* an appliance, usually fabricated of resin, designed to cover the occlusal and incisal surfaces of the teeth to immobilize and stabilize the teeth and thus prevent them from being subjected to the effects of trauma from occlusal forces.

splint, bridge, *n* See splint, fixed.

splint, buccal, *n* a material such as plaster that can be placed on the buccal surfaces of assembled fixed partial denture units and onto which these components can be assembled and held in accurate relation after hardening.

splint, cap, *n* a plastic or metallic fracture appliance designed to cover the crowns of the teeth; usually held in place by cementation.

splint, cast bar, *n* a provisional splint consisting of cast continuous clasps that follow the facial and lingual surfaces of the teeth at the height of contour. It is cemented onto the teeth to be splinted and simultaneously wired closed to bring the clasps into intimate contact with the teeth. May not be cemented in place to serve as a removable cast splint. Also called *Friedman splint.*

splint, continuous clasp, *n* a cast splint used for the provisional immobilization of teeth.

splint, copper band-acrylic, *n* a splint fabricated from copper bands and acrylic resin.

splint, crib, *n* an appliance used for temporary tooth stabilization; constructed of gold, acrylic resin, chrome-cobalt alloys, or combinations thereof. It consists of a continuous crib clasp covering the facial and lingual surfaces of the teeth to be splinted.

splint, cross arch bar, *n* a splint formed by a metal bar that unites one or more teeth of one side of the dental arch to one or more teeth of the opposite side. Used to stabilize weakened teeth against lateral tilting forces. See also connector, cross arch bar splint.

splint, cross arch bar, Bilson fixable-removable, *n.pr* a type of cross arch bar splint.

splint, dental, *n* an implement designed to hold teeth in place. It may be temporary or permanent.

splint, directive, *n* a splint used to hold condyles forward in order to correct condyle-disk alignment.

splint, fixed, *n* a fixed (nonremovable) restorative and replacement prosthesis used as a therapeutic aid in the treatment of periodontal disease. It serves to stabilize and immobilize the teeth and replace missing teeth.

splint, Friedman, *n.pr* See splint, cast bar.

splint, implant surgical, *n* See superstructure, temporary.

splint, inlay, *n* an inlay casting designed to give fixation or support to one or more approximating teeth. This may be accomplished by two inlays soldered together or a single casting made for prepared cavities.

splint, interdental, *n* an appliance made of plastic or metallic materials that is applied to the labial and lingual aspects of the teeth to provide points for applying mandibular and maxillofacial traction and fixation.

splint, labial, *n* an appliance of plastic, metal, or combinations of plastic and metal made to conform to the labial aspect of the dental arch. Used in the management of mandibular and maxillofacial injuries.

splint, lingual, *n* an appliance similar to a labial splint but conforming to the lingual aspect of the dental arch.

splint, provisional, *n* a splint placed for a relatively short period. It is used to stabilize the teeth either during the healing period after accidental or deliberate tooth evulsion and replantation or in conjunction with periodontal therapy. It also may be used during a period of observation to determine the prognosis of the involved teeth.

splint, Stader, *n.pr* See appliance, fracture.

splinting, *n* the ligating, tying, or joining of periodontally involved teeth to one another to stabilize and immobilize the teeth, thus preventing them from being adversely affected by occlusal forces. Splinting includes acrylic resin bite guards, orthodontic band splints, wire ligation, provisional splints, and fixed prostheses.

splinting, cross arch, *n* the stabilizing of weakened teeth against tilting movements caused by laterally directed occlusal stress loads. This is accomplished by the use of a rigid connector that projects to the opposite side of the dental arch where attachment is made to one or more teeth, thus producing effective counterleverage.

splinting of abutments, *n* the joining of two or more teeth into a rigid unit by means of fixed restorations.

split cast mounting, *n* See mounting, split cast.

split ring, *n* a casting ring made of three parts and designed to take advantage of the maximal expansion of the investment.

spondylitis (spon′dəlī′tis), *n* an inflammation of spinal vertebrae, usually characterized by stiffness and pain.

spongiosa (spun′jēō′sə), *n* bone, cancellous.

spoon, *n* an instrument with a round or ovoid working end; designed to be used for scraping or scooping.

spore, *n* **1.** a reproductive unit of some genera of fungi and protozoa. **2.** a form assumed by some bacteria that is resistant to heat, drying, and chemicals. Diseases caused by spore-forming bacteria include anthrax, botulism, gas gangrene, and tetanus.

spore testing, *n* a procedure in which test strips or receptacles containing microorganisms are checked for positive color changes or negative growth to verify that a sterilization technique is effective. See also *B. stearothermophilus.*

sporicide (spôr′əsīd), *n* a substance used to destroy spores.

S

sporotrichosis (spôr′ōtrikō′sis), *n* a fungal infection of the skin and nails caused by *Sporothrix schenckii.* Gardeners and farmers are most susceptible to the infection, which causes lesions in the tissue of the nails and extremities.

sports medicine, *n* a branch of medicine that specializes in the prevention and treatment of injuries from training and participation in athletic activities.

spot, *n* a small circular area.

spot, café-au-lait, n a group of brown-pigmented areas of the skin occurring particularly in neurofibromatosis.

spot, effective focal, n (prolonged focus), the apparent size and shape of the focal spot when viewed from a position in the useful beam. With the use of a suitably inclined anode face, the area from which the useful beam stems is sharply concentrated, if seen from the perspective of the useful beam. See also line, focus.

spot, focal, n the specific area of the face of the anode or target that is bombarded by the focused electron stream when a radiographic tube is in action. It is usually an insert of tungsten.

spot, Fordyce's, n.pr See Fordyce granules.

spot, Koplik's, n.pr an oral lesion of measles (rubeola); usually occurs on the buccal mucosa opposite the molar teeth as small white or bluish-white spots surrounded by red zones.

spot, pink, n See resorption, internal.

sprain, *n* an injury to a joint, with possible rupture of some of the ligaments or tendons but without dislocation or fracture. See also strain.

spray, *n* a liquid divided into smaller streams, as by a jet of air or steam.

spreader, *n* See condenser.

spring, *n* a piece of metal having the physical characteristic that when bent it returns to its original shape.

spring, auxiliary, n (finger spring), a short piece of wire, attached to an orthodontic appliance at one end, that serves as a lever to apply force to a tooth or teeth.

spring, coil, n a spiral winding of fine wire attached to an orthodontic appliance.

spring, finger, n See spring, auxiliary.

sprue (sproo), *n* in casting the ingate through which molten metal passes into the heated mold. The waste piece of metal cast in the ingate.

sprue base, n See sprue former and crucible former.

sprue former, n a cone-shaped base made of metal or plastic to which the sprue is attached. Forms a crucible in the investment material. Also called *crucible former.*

sprue pin, n See pin, sprue.

sputum (spū′təm), *n* a matter ejected from the oral cavity; saliva mixed with mucus and other substances from the respiratory tract.

squamous cell carcinoma (skwā′mus), *n* See carcinoma, squamous cell.

squeeze-releasing technique, *n* a procedure for releasing an orthodontic bracket from the adhesive resin. The squeeze-releasing technique uses a small pliers to bend the bracket wings together and cause the edges of the bracket to pull away from the surface of the tooth.

SRS-A, *n* an abbreviation for **s**low-**r**eacting **s**ubstance of **a**naphylaxis.

stabile (sta′bil), *adj* resistant to movement; fixed or stationary. See also stable.

stability, *n* the quality of being physically or emotionally predictable, orderly, not readily moved.

stability barriers, n.pl the specific conditions obstructing or interfering with the accessibility of services pertaining to oral health care, e.g., limited motion and assistive devices use, involuntary or abrupt movements, involuntary or violent actions potentially causing danger to the lives of the care provider and patient, and the inability of the patient to become comfortable with the space and procedures being performed.

stability, denture, n the characteristic of a removable denture that resists forces that tend to alter the relationship between the denture base and its supporting bony foundation.

stability, dimensional, n the property of a material that retains its size and form.

stability, emotional, n the state of an individual that enables him or her to

S

have appropriate feelings about common experiences and act in a rational manner.

stabilization, *n* **1.** the act or process of stabilizing; the state of being stabilized. **2.** the seating or fixation of a fixed or removable denture so that it does not tilt and is not displaced under pressure. **3.** the control of induced stress loads and development of measures to counteract these forces so effectively that the tilting of the teeth or the movement of a prosthesis is minimized to a point within tissue tolerance limits.

stabilized baseplate, *n* See baseplate, stabilized.

stabilizer (stā'bəlī'zər), *n* an instrument used in an radiograph unit to render the milliamperage output of the tube constant.

stabilizing, *n* the process of fixing movable parts; making firm and steady. The fixing of clamps, separators, or matrices to teeth by the application of tacky compound to the parts, then chilling the compound. In the case of clamps and separators, this distributes the force of operating over adjacent teeth and the one being operated on.

stabilizing circumferential clasp arm, *n* See clasp, circumferential, arm, stabilizing.

stable, *adj* the term applied to a substance that has no tendency to decompose spontaneously. As applied to chemical compounds, it denotes their ability to resist chemical alterations.

stable isotope, *n* See isotope.

stack, *n* a set of metal strips that is inserted into ultrasonic and sonic instruments. A stack converts magnetic fields into vibrations that move the tip of the instrument.

Stader splint (stā'dər), *n.pr* See appliance, fracture.

staff, *n* See personnel.

stage, surgical, *n* a period or distinct phase in the course of anesthesia.

staging, *n* a method for describing the growth and rate of metastasization of a tumor, as well as its prognosis. There are four stages, each evaluated according to size, amount of metastasis, and whether or not the lymph nodes are involved. See also TNM staging system.

stain, *v* **1.** to discolor with foreign matter. *n* **2.** a discoloration accumulating on the surface of teeth or dentures.

stain, alexidine **(əlek'sidēn),** *n* a brownish discoloration of the teeth and exposed roots that occurs as the result of using mouthrinses containing the antiplaque agent alexidine. Stains are more frequent on tooth surfaces that are difficult to reach during normal brushing.

stain, betel leaf **(bē'təl),** *n* the thick, hard, dark brown or black extrinsic stain left on the teeth after chewing the leaves of the betel palm; commonly seen in adults and children in the Eastern Hemisphere, where betel leaves and nuts are used as stimulants; must be removed by scaling.

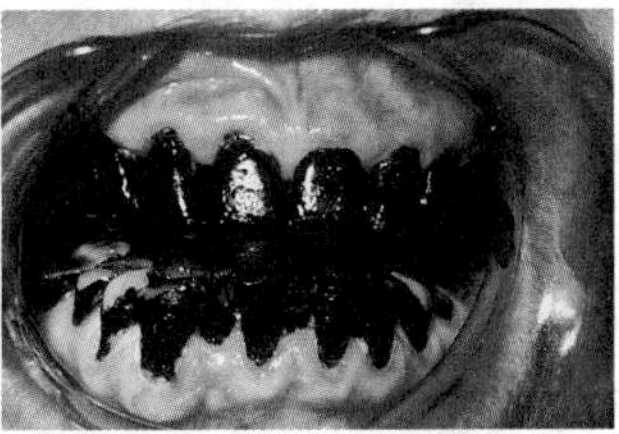

Betel leaf stain. (Daniel/Harfst/Wilder, 2008)

stain, black line dental, *n* a fine black or dark brown line composed of gram-positive microorganisms that appears along the gingival margin in adults and children who may be predisposed to this condition. The condition is not related to oral cleanliness or the presence of periodontal disease. Also called *black stain.* See also plaque, pigmented dental.

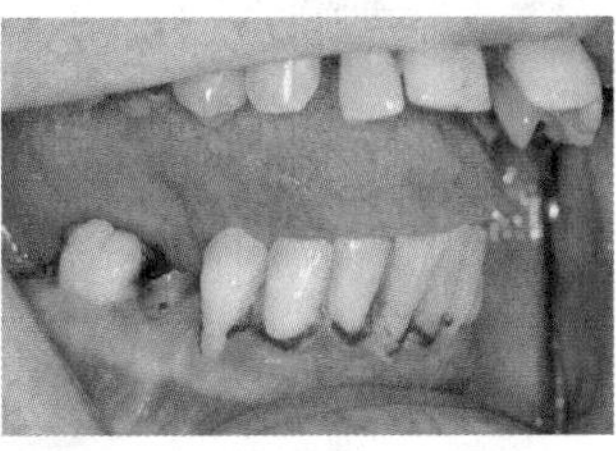

Black line stain. (Courtesy Dr. Charles Babbush)

stain, endogenous **(endoj′ənəs),** *n* a discolored area on a tooth that results from internal biologic conditions as opposed to outside or environmental factors. See also stain, intrinsic.

stain, exogenous **(eksoj′ənəs),** *n* a discolored area on a tooth caused by factors from outside the tooth. See also stain, extrinsic.

stain, extrinsic **(ekstrin′zik),** *n* a discolored area on the surface of a tooth that is caused by an external source such as cofee, tea, or tobacco, as opposed to an internal source, such as illness or genetic defects. These do respond to whitening, polishing, brushing, flossing, or scaling until they become more intrinsic over time.

stain, Gram's, *n.pr* a staining method for microorganisms that places them into two broad groups: *gram-positive,* which retains crystal violet stain, and *gram-negative,* which decolorizes but counterstains with a red dye.

stain, green dental, *n* a light to very dark green extrinsic stain appearing primarily on the labial surface of the teeth due to inadequate daily removal cleaning, chromogenic bacterial deposits, or decomposed hemoglobin. It may also represent stained enamel cuticle (Nasmyth's membrane). The condition is more common in children than adults.

stain, intrinsic, *n* a discolored area found on the inner layers of the dentin. They may be caused by certain medications, such as tetracycline or excessive fluoride exposure, or by illness or genetic defects. These do not respond to polishing, brushing, flossing, or scaling but can be lightened with dental whitening.

stain, metallic dental, *n* an uncommon, green, brown, yellow, or blue-green dental discoloration. Source is environmental, typically entering the individual's oral cavity through breathing air containing metals or metal salts.

stain, methyl violet, *n* a dye used to color bacteria for microscopic examination.

stain, orange dental, *n* an extrinsic stain of the cervical third caused by chromogenic bacteria.

stain, red dental, *n* an extrinsic stain caused by chromogenic bacteria; found at the cervical third.

stain, yellow dental, *n* a frequently occurring extrinsic stain of the teeth, generally caused by poor oral hygiene. If more orange in color, it may be due to topical use of stannous fluoride.

staining, *n* **1.** a modification of the color of the teeth or denture base to achieve a more lifelike appearance. **2.** amount of stain present on the teeth, either extrinsic or intrinsic in origin. See also stain.

stainless steel, *n* See steel, stainless.

stamp cusp, *n* a cusp made to work in a fossa. The maxillary lingual cusps are stamp cusps. In tooth-to-tooth occlusion all mandibular buccal cusps may stamp into fossae. In tooth-to-two-tooth occlusion the stamp cusps of the mandibular premolars may have their tips in embrasures and have only their shoulders in tiny fossae. See also cusp-fossa relations.

standard, *n* that which is established by authority, custom, or general acceptance as a model; criterion.

standard deviation (SD), *n* a computed measure of the dispersion or variability of a distribution of scores around a given point or line. It measures the way an individual score deviates from the most representative score (mean). A small SD indicates little individual deviation or a homogeneous group, and a large SD indicates much individual deviation or a heterogeneous group.

standard error, *n* a measure or estimate of the sampling errors affecting a statistic; a measure of the amount the statistic may be expected to differ by chance from the true value of the statistic.

standard error of estimate, *n* the standard deviation of the differences between the actual values of the dependent variables (results) and the predicted values. This statistic is associated with regression analysis.

standard error of the mean, *n* an estimate of the amount that an obtained mean may be expected to differ by chance from the true mean.

standard of care, *n* a written statement describing the rules, actions, and conditions that direct patient care. Standards of care guide practice and may be used to evaluate performance. Also referred to during the practice of dentistry when discussing quality of care.

standard operating procedure (SOP), *n* a method of functioning that has been established over time in order to execute a specific task or react to a specific set of circumstances.

standard orders, *n.pl* the rules, policies, procedures, regulations, and orders for the conduct of patient care in various stipulated clinical situations.

standard precautions, *n* a set of procedures designed by the Centers for Disease Control and Prevention (CDC) to prevent the spread of known and unknown sources of infections. It formerly was called *universal precautions* and applies to blood; body fluids, excretions, and secretions of the skin; and oral mucosa.

standard score, *n* a derived score indicating the degree of deviation of an individual score from the mean using the standard deviation as the unit of measure.

stanine (stā'nīn), *n* a unit consisting of one-ninth of the total range of the standard scores (SDs) of a normal distribution. The term is a condensation of "standard nine." The mean falls at 5, the SD at ±2. The stanine was developed by the U.S. Air Force and is used to report scores on the Dental Aptitude Test.

stannic oxide, *n* See tin oxide.

stannous fluoride (stan'us flôr'īd), *n* a fluoride salt of tin used in toothpaste and mouthrinses to reduce dental caries incidence can cause extrinsic stain when used topically. See also stain.

stanozolol (stan'əzō'lol), *n brand name:* Winstrol; *drug class:* androgenic anabolic steroid, controlled substance Schedule III; *action:* reverses catabolic tissue processes, promotes buildup of protein, increases erythropoietin production; *use:* hereditary angioedema prophylaxis.

Staphcillin, *n.pr* See methicillin.

S. albus* (staf'əlōkok'us al'bus) *(Staphylococcus pyogenes var. albus), *n* a species of bacteria of low pathogenicity, although occasional strains may be coagulase positive and produce hemolysis. Normally present as part of the oral flora and in mucosa-lined cavities such as the oral cavity and nasal cavity. May be isolated, along with *S. aureus,* streptococci, pneumococci, fusiform bacilli, *B. vincentii,* molds, and yeasts from the gingival crevices by cultural examination.

S. aureus* (ôr'ēus) *(Staphylococcus pyogenes var. aureus), *n* a pathogenic variety capable of producing suppurative lesions; cultured colonies are golden yellow. Produces hemolysis on blood agar, is coagulase positive, and may be resistant to commonly used antibiotics. Has been isolated with other microorganisms such as *S. albus* from the gingival crevice.

***S. epidermidis* (ep'idermī'dis),** *n* a bacterium normally present on the skin and in the oral cavity that causes oral infection when allowed to grow unchecked. Symptoms include inflammation of the mandible and parotid glands.

S. pyogenes var. albus, *n* See *S. albus.*

S. pyogenes var. aureus, *n* See *S. aureus.*

starch, *n* the principal molecule used for the storage of food in plants. Starch is a polysaccharide and is composed of long chains of glucose subunits.

***starch amylopectin* (am'ilōpek'tin),** *n* a component of starch that consists of glucose residues arranged in a branched chain.

***starch amylose* (am'ilōs),** *n* a component of starch that consists of glucose residues arranged in a straight chain.

starvation, *n* a condition resulting from the lack of essential nutrients over a long period and characterized by multiple physiologic and metabolic dysfunctions.

statement, *n* **1.** a printed form stating the balance of the account due the dental professional. **2.** in computer programming a meaningful expression or generalized instruction in a source language.

static electricity, *n* See film fault, static electricity.

stationary grid, *n* See grid, stationary.

stationary lingual arch, *n* an orthodontic arch wire designed to fit the lingual surface of the teeth and soldered to the associated anchor bands, which are then cemented to the molar teeth.

statistic, *n* a value or number that describes a series of quantitative observations or measures; a value calculated from a sample.

statistical significance, *n* a difference of such magnitude between two statistics, computed from separate samples, that the probability of the value obtained will not occur by chance alone with significant frequency and hence can be attributed to something other than chance. In modern investigation the generally accepted value for significance must have a probability of occurrence by chance factors equal to or less than five times in 100 ($p < 0.05$). Other significance levels commonly used are as follows: less than one chance in 100 ($p > 0.01$), less than five chances in 1000 ($p < 0.005$), and less than one chance in 1000 ($p < 0.001$).

statistically based utilization review, *n* a system that examines the distribution of treatment procedures based on claims information and, to be reasonably reliable, the application of such claims. Analyses of specific dental professionals should include data on type of practice, dental professional's experience, socioeconomic characteristics, and geographic location.

statistics, *n* the branch of mathematics that gathers, arranges, condenses, coordinates, and mathematically manipulates obtained facts so that the numerical relationships between those facts may be seen clearly and freed from anomalies resulting from chance factors.

statistics, descriptive, *n.pl* the statistics used to describe only the observed group or sample from which they were derived; summary statistics such as percent, averages, and measures of variability that are computed on a particular group of individuals.

statistics, inference, *n.pl* the inferences made regarding characteristics or general principles about an unseen population based on the characteristics of the observed sample. Statistical findings from a sample are generalized to pertain to the entire population. The process of drawing inferences, making predictions, and testing significance are examples of inferential statistics.

statistics, nonparametric, *n.pl* the statistical methods used when the statistician cannot assume that the variable being studied is normally distributed in a population. Also called *distribution-free statistics.*

status (stat′us), *n* state or condition.

status asthmaticus **(sta′tus azmat′ikus),** *n* a continual worsening of an asthmatic condition even with the use of medications for therapeutic purposes; may cause life-threatening situations; creates tremendous strain on the respiratory and circulatory systems.

status epilepticus **(sta′tus ep′ilep′tikus),** *n* a seizure lasting more than 30 minutes, or a series of seizures without pause between them. Patient often does not respond to medication.

status lymphaticus, *n* an enlargement of lymphoid tissue, particularly the thymus, in children. It may lead to sudden death under inhalation anesthesia.

status thymicolymphaticus, *n* a constitutional disturbance of controversial existence believed to be responsible in some way for sudden and unexplained deaths from trivial causes such as the extraction of teeth. Enlargement of the thymus and lymphoid tissue and underdevelopment of the adrenal glands, gonads, and cardiovascular system are evident.

statute (stach′ūt), *n* a law enacted and established by a legislative department of government.

statute of frauds, *n* a requirement that, for legal validity, contracts for conveying real property or contracts for the performance of personal services requiring a year or more to perform must be in writing.

statute of limitations, *n* a statute that sets a time limit within which legal action on certain causes of action must be brought.

statute, wrongful death, *n* a statute that provides for the recovery of damages by a party other than the party who received the fatal injuries.

statutory (in law) rape, *n* sexual intercourse with a child below the age of consent, which varies from state to state.

stavudine (stav′ūdēn′), *n brand name:* Zerit; *drug class:* antiviral; *action:* inhibits replication of human immunodeficiency virus (HIV); *uses:* treatment of adults with advanced HIV infection who are intolerant of other therapies or who have significant deterioration while receiving other therapies.

steady state, *n* a basic physiologic concept implying that the various forces and processes of life are in a state of homeostasis.

steam sterilization, *n* the destruction of all forms of microbial life on an object by exposing the object to moist heat (under pressure) for 15 minutes at 121° C.

steel crown, *n* See crown, stainless steel.

steel, stainless, *n* a steel that contains a minimum of 12% chromium and approximately 0.5% carbon to resist corrosion.

stellate reticulum (stel′āt ritik′-yələm), *n* one of the two layers between the outer and inner enamel epithelium of the enamel organ, which consists of star-shaped cells.

Stellite (stel′īt), *n.pr* **1.** a cobalt-chromium alloy. **2.** a very hard, noncorrosive alloy of cobalt, chromium, and sometimes tungsten used for special instruments, particularly surgical instruments.

stem, brain, *n* See brainstem.

stenosis (stenō′sis), *n* narrowing or stricture of a duct, canal, or vessel.

Stensen's duct, *n.pr* See duct, Stensen's.

stent (stent), *n* **1.** a device used to hold a skin graft placed to maintain a body orifice, cavity, or space. An acrylic resin appliance used as a positioning guide or support. **2.** an appliance that maintains tissue (e.g., to maintain a skin transplant in a predetermined position).

step, distal, *n* condition in which the mandibular second molar is in a distal position compared with the maxillary second molar, usually in reference to primary or mixed dentition. See also step, mesial.

step, mesial (mē′zēəl), *n* condition in which the mandibular second molar is in a mesial position compared with the maxillary second molar, usually in reference to primary or mixed dentition. See also step, distal.

step-up transformer, *n* See transformer, step-up.

stepwedge, *n* an aluminum device that, when exposed to roentgen rays, displays a range of exposure intensities on a radiograph. These "steps" are analyzed to determine the speed characteristics of the radiographic film. See also penetrometer.

stereognosis (ster′ēog′nōsis), *n* the ability to perceive and understand the form and nature of objects by the sense of touch.

stereoisomer, *n* See isomer.

stereoscope, *n* an optical instrument for viewing photographs or radiographs; it produces binocular vision, or a blending of images, so that new perspectives may be seen with an appearance of depth. It operates on the same principle as the eyes—that is, two views are registered on the retinas of the eyes, and the brain merges them into one.

stereoscopic microscope, *n* a microscope that produces three-dimensional images through the use of double eyepieces and double objectives, creating two independent light paths.

stereotype, *n* a generalization about a form of behavior, an individual, or a group.

sterile, *adj* free from viable microorganisms.

sterile field, *n* **1.** a specified area (such as within a tray or on a sterile towel) that is considered free of viable microorganisms. **2.** an area immediately around a patient that has been prepared for a surgical procedure.

sterilization, *n* the act or process of rendering sterile; the removal of viable microorganisms.

sterilization, chemical, *n* a method in which an object is immersed in a liquid containing sanitizing chemicals. Used for objects that cannot withstand high temperatures. Glutaraldehyde is one such sterilizer, which must be in contact with the instrument for at least 10 hours for proper sterilization. Other chemical sterilizers may require up to 24 hours of instrument contact. Colloquial term is *cold sterilization.*

sterilization, chemical vapor, *n* the process of destroying all living microorganisms through the use of chemicals heated under pressure to form a gaseous state. The various chemicals used include alcohol, formaldehyde, acetone, ketene, and water.

sterilization, steam, *n* application of moist heat at 121° F for 15 minutes to destroy all microorganisms on an object. It is typically conducted in an autoclave, which applies approximately 15 psi of pressure to achieve this temperature.

sterilizer for root canal instruments, *n* a special device for heat sterilization of root canal instruments and dressings; depends on molten metal, glass beads, salt, or fine sand for the conduction of the heat.

sternum, *n* the elongated, flattened bone forming the middle portion of the thorax. It supports the clavicles and articulates directly with the first seven pairs of ribs.

steroid (ster′oid), *n* a group name for compounds that resemble cholesterol chemically and also contain a hydrogenated cyclopentanoperhydrophenanthrene ring system. Included are cholesterol, ergosterol, bile acids, vitamin D, sex hormones, adrenocortical hormones, and cardiac glycosides.

steroid, 11-oxy, *n* the C-21 corticosteroids, all of which are oxygenated at carbon 11.

steroid, 17 α-hydroxycortico- (17-OHCS), *n* term used for cortisol and other 21-carbon steroids possessing a dihydroxyacetone group at carbon 17. Serum and urinary determinations give a direct measurement of adrenocortical activity.

steroid, 17-keto- (17-KS), *n* steroidal compounds with a ketone (carbonyl) group at carbon 17. Derived from cortisol and adrenal and testicular androgen. Urinary neutral 17-ketosteroids represent the catabolic end products of the endocrine glands. Produced by the adrenal cortex and testes. Increased values occur in adrenogenital syndromes, adrenocortical carcinoma, bilateral hyperplasia of the adrenal cortex, and Leydig cell tumors. Normal adult values for a 24-hour urine sample are 10 to 20 mg for men and 5 to 15 mg for women.

steroid, adrenocortical (adrenal corticosteroid), *n* **1.** a hormone extracted from the adrenal cortex or a synthetic substance similar in chemical structure and biologic activity to such a hormone. **2.** the biologically active steroid of the adrenal cortex, which include 11-dehydrocorticosterone (compound A), corticosterone (compound B), cortisone (compound E), 17 α-hydroxycorticosterone (compound F, hydroxycortisone, or cortisol), and aldosterone. The effects of the corticosteroids include increased resorption of sodium and chloride by the renal tubules and metabolic effects on protein, carbohydrate, and fat.

steroid, C-19 cortico- (anabolic protein, N hormone), *n* adrenocortical hormones similar in action to the male and female sex hormones. They cause nitrogen retention and, in excessive amounts, masculinization in the female.

steroid, C-21 cortico- (glycogenic steroid, sugar hormone), *n* 21-carbon adrenocortical hormones that are oxygenated at carbon 11 or at both carbon 11 and 17. They affect protein, carbohydrate, and fat metabolism; e.g., they elevate blood sugar, increase glyconeogenesis, decrease hepatic lipogenesis, mobilize depot fat, and increase protein metabolism.

steroid, glycogenic, *n* See steroid, C-21 cortico-.

sterols (ster′ôlz), *n.pl* steroids having one or more hydroxyl groups and no carbonyl or carboxyl groups (e.g., cholesterol).

stethoscope (steth′əskōp′), *n* an instrument used to assist the health care professional to listen to body sounds: heart, lungs, pulse, and gastrointestinal. It consists of two earpieces connected by means of flexible tubing to a diaphragm, which is placed against the skin of the patient at a location appropriate to pick up the sound.

Stevens-Johnson syndrome, *n.pr* See syndrome, Stevens-Johnson.

stillborn, *n* an infant who is born dead.

Stillman's cleft, *n.pr* See cleft, Stillman's.

stimulant (stim'ūlənt), *n* an agent that causes an increase in functional activity, usually of the central nervous system.

stimulant, abused, n the substances—such as amphetamines (e.g., methamphetamine or "ice"), cocaine (e.g., "crack" or "coke"), nicotine products (e.g., cigars, cigarettes, or chewing tobacco), and caffeine products (e.g., tea, soft drinks, and soda)—that are misused to increase the functioning of the central nervous system.

stimulant, psychomotor (steroid, psychomotor), n a drug that increases psychic activity.

stimulation, *n* **1.** an increased functioning of protoplasm induced by an extracellular substance or agent. **2.** the act of energizing or activating.

stimulator, interdental tip, *n* a rubber tip on the end of a plastic handle or toothbrush to remove plaque biofilm.

stimulus (stim'ūlus), *n* a chemical, thermal, electrical, or mechanical influence that changes the normal environment of irritable tissue and creates an impulse.

sting, *n* an injury caused by a sharp, painful penetration of the skin, often accompanied by exposure to an irritating chemical or the venom of an insect or other animal. Can also be considered a prick.

stippling (stip'ling), *n* **1.** an orange-peel appearance of the attached gingiva, believed to result from the bundles of collagen fibers that enter the connective tissue papillae. **2.** a roughening of the labial and buccal surfaces of denture bases to imitate the stippling of natural gingiva.

stippling, basophilic, n See basophilia.

stippling, gingival, n See gingiva, stippling.

stipulation, *n* an article in an agreement; an agreement in writing to do a certain thing.

stitch, *n* See suture.

stitch, blanket, n See suture, blanket.

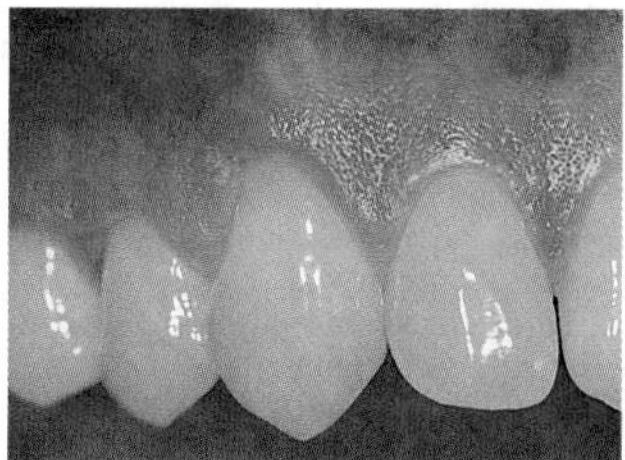

Stippling. (Daniel/Harfst/Wilder, 2008)

stock, *n* a security certificate that represents an equity ownership in a corporation.

stoma (sto'mə), *n* a tiny surface opening or pore. It may occur naturally or be the result of a surgical incision, as in a colostomy, or as the result of an abscess. *Stoma* is the Greek word for "oral cavity."

stomatitides (stō'mətit'idēz), *n.pl* an older term for the oral lesions associated with various forms of stomatitis.

stomatitis (stō'mətī'tis), *n* inflammation of the soft tissues of the oral cavity occurring as a result of mechanical, chemical, thermal, bacterial, viral, electrical, or radiation injury or reactions to allergens or as secondary manifestations of systemic disease.

stomatitis, acute herpetic, n (acute herpetic gingivostomatitis), the manifestations of clinically apparent primary herpes simplex characterized by regional lymphadenopathy, sore throat, and high temperature, followed by localized itching and burning, with the formation of small vesicles of an erythematous base that give way to plaques and then painful herpetic ulcers. The gingivae are swollen and erythematous, and they bleed easily. Manifestations subside in 7 to 10 days, and recovery usually occurs within 2 weeks.

stomatitis, aphthous (aphthae, canker sore), n refers to recurrent ulcers of the oral cavity that are limited to nonkeratinized mucosa and are thought to be immune related.

stomatitis, arsenical **(arsen'ikəl),** *n* oral manifestation of arsenic poisoning. The oral mucosa is dry, red, and painful. Ulceration, purpura, and mobility of teeth also may occur.

stomatitis, Atabrine **(at′əbrin),** *n.pr* a stomatitis considered by some to be associated with the use of the antimalarial and anthelmintic drug quinacrine hydrochloride (Atabrine) and characterized by oral changes simulating lichen planus.

stomatitis, bismuth, *n* a stomatitis resulting from systemic use of bismuth compounds over prolonged periods. Sulfides of bismuth are deposited in the gingival tissue, resulting in bluish-black pigmentation known as a bismuth line. Oral manifestations of bismuth poisoning include gingivostomatitis similar to that of Vincent's infection, a blue-black line on the inner aspect of the gingival sulcus or pigmentation of the buccal mucosa, a sore tongue, metallic taste, and a burning sensation of the oral cavity.

stomatitis, epidemic, *n* See disease, hand, foot, and oral cavity.

stomatitis, epizootic, *n* See disease, hand, foot, and oral cavity.

stomatitis, gangrenous (cancrum oris, noma), *n* See noma.

stomatitis, gonococcal, *n* an inflammation of the oral mucosa caused by gonococci.

stomatitis, herpetic, *n* **1.** the oral manifestation of primary herpes simplex infection. The term also is used by some for herpetiform ulcers considered to be oral manifestations of secondary or recurrent herpes simplex. See also ulcer, aphthous, recurrent. **2.** inflammation of the oral mucosa caused by herpesvirus. See also gingivostomatitis, herpetic.

stomatitis, iodine, *n* See iodism.

stomatitis, lead, *n* an oral manifestation of lead poisoning. Included are a bluish line along the free gingival margin, pigmentation of the mucosa in contact with the teeth, metallic taste, excessive salivation, and swelling of the salivary glands.

stomatitis medicamentosa **(med′ikəmentō′sə),** *n* an allergic response of the oral mucosa to a systemically administered drug. Possible manifestations include asthma, skin rashes, urticaria, pruritus, leukopenia, lymphadenopathy, thrombocytopenic purpura, and oral lesions (erythema, ulcerative lesions, vesicles, bullae, and angioneurotic edema).

stomatitis, membranous, *n* an inflammation of the oral cavity, accompanied by the formation of a pseudomembrane.

stomatitis, mercurial, *n* an oral manifestation of mercury poisoning, consisting of hypersalivation, metallic taste, ulceration and necrosis of the gingivae with a tendency to spread posteriorly and to the buccal mucosa and palate, glossodynia, and periodontitis with loosening of the teeth in severe cases of chronic intoxication.

stomatitis, mycotic, *n* an infection of the oral mucosa by a fungus, most commonly *C. albicans,* which produces moniliasis (thrush). See also moniliasis.

stomatitis, nicotinic, *n* an inflammation of the palatal minor salivary ducts caused by irritation by tobacco smoke or hot fluids and characterized by raised small palatal lesions with red centers and white borders. The palatal mucosa usually has a generalized keratosis accompanying the smaller lesions. Also called *stomatitis nicotina.*

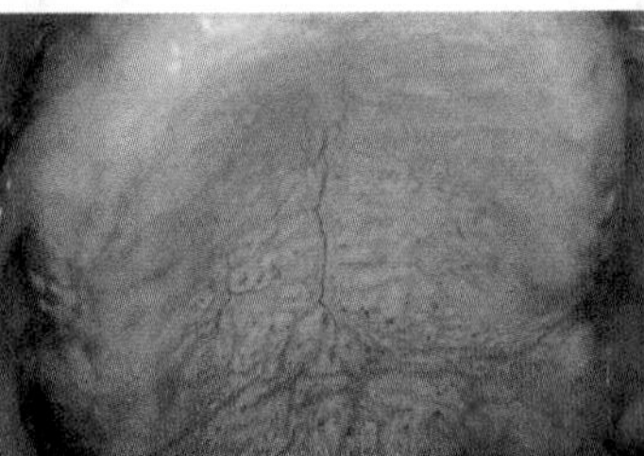

Nicotinic stomatitis. (Courtesy Dr. Charles Babbush)

stomatitis, recurrent, *n* recurrent manifestation of herpes simplex involving the lips and labial and buccal mucosa (fever blisters, cold sores). Episodes may result from fever, sunlight, menses, trauma, and gastrointestinal upset. Lesions begin as clear vesicles with an erythematous base that give way to ulcers and superficial crusts if the outer surfaces of the lips and skin are involved.

stomatitis, uremic, *n* an oral manifestation of uremia, consisting of varying degrees of erythema, exudation, ulceration, pseudomembrane formation, foul breath, and burning sensations. See also gingivitis, nephritic.

stomatitis venenata **(ven′ənat′ə),** *n* an inflammation of the oral mucosa as the result of contact allergy. The most common causative agents are volatile oils, iodides, dentifrices, mouthwashes, denture powders, and topical anesthetics. Possible manifestations include erythema, angioneurotic edema, burning sensations, ulcerations, and vesicles.

stomatodynia (stō′mətōdin′ēə), *n* an older term for a sore oral cavity.

stomatoglossitis (stō′mətōglôsī′tis), *n* an inflammation involving oral mucous membranes and the tongue. May be seen in nutritional disorders such as pellagra, beriberi, vitamin B complex deficiency, and infections.

stomatognathic system (stō′mətōnath′ik), *n* See system, stomatognathic.

stomatology (stō′mətol′əjē), *n* an older term for the study of the morphology, structure, function, and diseases of the contents and linings of the oral cavity.

stomion (stō′mēon), *n* the median point of the oral slit (opening) when the oral cavity is closed.

stomodeum (sto″mode′əm), *n* a superficial depression on the ectoderm of the developing embryo that later becomes the oral cavity; primitive mouth.

stone, *n* an abrading instrument or tool.

stone, Arkansas, *n.pr* a fine-grained stone, novaculite, used to make hones for the final sharpening of instruments.

stone, artificial, *n* (dental stone), a specially calcined gypsum derivative similar to plaster of paris. Because its grains are nonporous, the product is stronger than plaster of paris.

stone, Carborundum **(kärbərun′dəm),** *n.pr* **1.** a stone made of silicon carbide. **2.** an abrasive, handpiece-mounted rotary instrument of various sizes, shapes, and degrees of abrasiveness.

stone, dental, *n* (Hydrocal), **1.** α-hemihydrate of calcium sulfate. **2.** a gypsum product that, when combined with water in proper proportions, hardens in a plasterlike form. Used for making casts and dies.

stone, diamond, *n* rotary instruments containing diamond chips as the abrasive. Available in various sizes, shapes, and abrasive consistency. Used for tooth reduction in operative dentistry and crown and bridge prostheses, tooth contouring in the occlusal adjustment procedure, and osseous and gingival contouring in periodontal surgery.

stone die, *n* See die, stone.

stone, lathe, *n* (lathe wheel), a grindstone mounted on a chuck and used on a lathe.

stone, mounted point, *n* a small abrasive tooth of various shape and size bonded or cemented onto a shaft or mandrel.

stone, pulp, *n* See denticle.

stone, rotary, *n* the stone in a mandrel-mounted (power-driven) sharpening instrument.

stone, sharpening, *n* a hand stone, or a stone driven mechanically, that is used to sharpen instruments.

stones, sharpening cone, *n.pl* cylindrical or rounded rectangular stones used to sharpen curved blades.

stone, wheel, *n* a small grindstone of Carborundum or corundum of various grit, mounted on a mandrel; of various thickness, ranging in diameter from ½ to 1 inch (1.3 to 2.5 cm).

stop, *n* See rest.

stop, occlusal, *n* See rest, occlusal.

stop-loss, *n* a general term referring to that category of coverage that provides insurance protection (reinsurance) to an employer for a self-funded plan.

stopping, *n* temporary, gutta-percha mixed with zinc oxide, white wax, and coloring. Softens on heating and rehardens at room temperature. Used for temporary sealing of dressings in cavities. Lack of strength makes it ineffective in areas under occlusal stress. It has poor sealing properties.

storage, computer, *n* a device or portion of a device that is capable of receiving data, retaining them for an indefinite time, and supplying them on command. Also called *memory.*

strabismus (strəbiz′məs), *n* an abnormal ocular condition in which the eyes are crossed.

straight wire fixed orthodontic appliance, *n* See appliance, straight wire fixed.

straightening of teeth, *n* See orthodontics.

strain, *n* **1.** a deformation induced by an external force. **2.** deformation expressed as a pure number or ratio resulting from the application of a load. **3.** a traumatic stretching or compression of such tissues as the ligaments, capsule, or musculature associated with a joint. See also sprain.

strain hardening, *n* See hardening, strain.

strangulation, *n* a choking or throttling. The arrest of respiration resulting from occlusion of the air passage or arrest of the circulation in part because of compression.

stratum (strat′əm), *n.pl* (*pl* **strata**) a layer of the epidermis or the epithelium of the oral mucosa.

stratum basale, *n* the deepest of the five layers of the epidermis or epithelium of the oral mucosa, composed of a single layer of tall cylindrical cells or cubodial cells, respectively. This layer provides new cells by mitotic cell division. Also called the *basal layer* or *germative layer.*

stratum corneum, *n* the tough, outermost layer of the epidermis or epithelium of keratinized oral mucosa, composed of flat, closely packed, dead cells converted to keratin that continually flake away. Also called the *keratin layer* or *corneal layer.*

stratum granulosum, *n* one of the layers of the epidermis or the epithelium of the keratinized oral mucosa, situated just inferior to the stratum corneum in keratinized tissues except in the palms of the hands and the soles of the feet, where it lies just inferior to the stratum lucidum (transparent layer). Also called the *granular layer.*

stratum intermedium, *n* one of the two layers between the outer and inner enamel epithelium of the enamel organ that consists of a compressed layer of flat to cubodial cells.

stratum lucidum **(loo′sidəm),** *n* one of the layers of the epidermis situated just beneath the stratum corneum and present only in the thick skin of the palms of the hands and the soles of the feet. Also called the *transparent layer.*

stratum spinosum, *n* one of the layers of the epidermis or epithelium of oral mucosa, composed of several layers of polygonal cells. It lies on superior to the stratum basale. Also called the *prickle cell layer.*

stratum spongiosum, *n* one of the three layers of the endometrium of the uterus.

strawberry tongue, *n* a strawberry-like coloration of inflamed tongue papillae. It is a clinical sign of scarlet fever and also is seen in Kawasaki syndrome.

stray radiation, *n* See radiation leakage.

strength, *n* toughness; ability to withstand or apply force.

strength, biting, *n* **1.** the force available for application against food or other material placed between the teeth. See also force, masticatory. **2.** the amount of force the muscles of mastication are capable of exerting. See also force, masticatory.

strength, compressive (crushing strength), *n* the amount of resistance of a material to fracture under compression. See also strength, ultimate.

strength, crushing, *n* See strength, compressive.

strength, dry, *n* a term generally used in conjunction with materials whose strengths vary markedly in the wet and dry states. The strength of gypsum products is usually reported in both wet and dry states.

strength, edge, *n* a term indicative of the ability of fine margins to resist fracture or abrasion. No specific test is available to assess this property; it is a composite of ductility and shear, tensile, and other strength characteristics.

strength, gel, *n* usually, the ability of a material to withstand a load without rupture.

strength, impact, *n* the ability of a material to withstand a striking force.

S

strength, shear, *n* **1.** resistance to a tangential force. **2.** resistance to a twisting motion.

strength, tensile **(ten′səl),** *n* **1.** resistance to a pulling force. **2.** the amount of stress a material is able to withstand when being pulled lengthwise before permanent deformation results.

strength, ultimate, *n* the greatest stress that may be induced in a material or object before or during rupture; may be compressive, tensile, or shear strength. See also strength, tensile.

strength, wet, *n* compressive strength while water in excess of that required for hydration of the hemihydrate present in the specimen. Used in connection with gypsum products.

strength, yield, *n* a definite proportionality obtained by drawing a line parallel to the proportional limit line. Yield strength is reported in terms of the degree of strain.

strep throat, *n* an infection of the oral pharynx and tonsils caused by hemolytic species of *Streptococcus.* The infection is characterized by sore throat, chills, fever, swollen lymph nodes in the neck, and sometimes nausea and vomiting. See also fever, rheumatic.

***Streptococcus,* alpha-hemolytic (strep′tōkok′us al′fa-hē′mōlit′ik),** *n* a bacterium occurring in chains. Produces a zone of greenish discoloration around the colony in blood-agar medium. Part of an individual's normal oral flora; has been isolated from the gingival sulcus. Capable of producing bacterial endocarditis in patients at risk; thus antibiotic prophylactic therapy may be necessary.

***Streptococcus,* beta-hemolytic,** *n* a bacterium responsible for causing strep throat and scarlet fever, illnesses that are transmitted primarily through respiratory droplets spread from one person to another by direct contact. Also called *group A Streptococcus.*

***Streptococcus,* group A,** *n* See *Streptococcus,* beta-hemolytic.

***S. mitis* (mī′tis),** *n* a bacterium found on soft tissues of the oral cavity.

S. mutans, *n* a cariogenic bacteria found in plaque and one of two index organisms (*Lactobacillus* is the other) used to assess caries susceptibility. It is one of a few specialized organisms equipped with receptors for adhesion to the smooth surface of teeth. Sucrose is utilized by it to produce a sticky, extracellular dextran-based polysaccharide that allows them to cohere to each other, thus forming plaque. Conversely, many sugars (glucose, fructose, lactose, sucrose) can be digested by it to produce lactic acid as an end product. It is both aciduric and acidophilic. It is the combination of plaque and acid that leads to smooth surface caries.

***S. pneumoniae* (nəmō′nyē),** *n* the antigenic type of pneumococci that cause pneumonia and other diseases in humans.

***S. pyogenes* (pī′ōjēnz),** *n* a species of *Streptococcus* with many strains that are pathogenic to humans. It causes such suppurative disease as scarlet fever and strep throat.

***S. salivarius* (salivar′ēəs),** *n* a bacterium found in dental plaque that may cause endocarditis and dental caries.

S. sanguis, *n* a bacterium found in dental plaque that may cause endocarditis and dental caries.

***S. sobrinus* (sōbrī′nus),** *n* a mutans *Streptococcus* bacterium the role of which in dental decay is still being determined.

***S. viridans* (vir′idanz),** *n* See *Streptococcus,* alpha-hemolytic.

streptokinase (strep′tōkī′nās′), *n* a fibrinolytic activator that enhances the conversion of plasminogen to the fibrinolytic enzyme plasmin. It is used in the treatment of certain cases of pulmonary and coronary embolism.

streptokinase-streptodornase, *n.pl* two enzymes derived from a strain of *S. hemolyticus.* It is prescribed for debridement of purulent exudates, clotted blood, radiation necrosis, or fibrinous deposits resulting from trauma or infection.

***Streptomyces* (strep′tōmī′sēz),** *n* a genus of gram-positive, funguslike bacteria belonging to the order actinomycetales. Several antibiotics, such as tetracyclines and aminoglycosides, are produced from them.

streptomycin (strep′tōmī′sin), *n* an antimicrobial drug often used to treat infections caused by gram-negative bacteria (such as tuberculosis). Though no human studies have been conducted, streptomycin administered during pregnancy or breastfeeding may cause damage to the ear of the fetus or infant.

streptothricosis (strep′tōthrikō′sis), *n* See actinomycosis.

stress, *n* **1.** a force induced by or resisting an external force; measured in terms of force per unit area. **2.** the force of energy directed against a tissue structure or against the function of tissue as the result of injury and trauma associated with fracture, burn, infection, surgical procedure, pharmacologic action, or anxiety states. The response to stress involves local metabolic function, the hormonal activity of the endocrine system regulated by the pituitary gland, and the autonomic and central nervous systems. The stress phenomenon is often associated with the general adaptation syndrome. **3.** in prosthetic dentistry, forcibly exerted pressure (e.g., the pressure of the maxillary teeth against the mandibular teeth or the pressure contact of a distorted removable partial denture on the supporting teeth or ridge structures).

stress, axial, *n* excessive force applied vertically to the teeth and their periodontium.

stress, bone in, *n* the responses of bony structures to applied force. With application of excessive pressure stimuli to bone, adaptation may occur by the formation of thicker and more numerous trabeculae. If tissue components cannot compensate for excessive stress, bone resorption will occur.

stress, buccolingual, *n* an excessive pressure exerted against teeth and their attachment apparatus from a buccal or lingual aspect.

stress, compressive, *n* the internal induced force that opposes shortening of the material in a direction parallel to the direction of the stress.

stress control, *n* See control, stress.

stress, damage to restorations by, *n* a mechanical property that pertains to the capacity of substances used for restorative and preventive applications to loosen in response to continual pressure over time. See also strain.

stress response, *n* the physiologic changes that occur as a result of threatening situations, including rapid breathing, increased heart rate, and increased perspiration. Also known as the "fight or flight" response.

stress, shearing, *n* the internal induced force that opposes the sliding of one plane of the material on the adjacent plane in a direction parallel to the stress.

stress, tensile, *n* the internal induced force that opposes elongation of a material in a direction parallel to the direction of stress.

stress-bearing area, *n* See area, basal seat.

stressbreaker (stress equalizer, stress divider), *n* a device or system that is incorporated in a removable partial denture to relieve the abutment teeth of occlusal loads that may exceed their physiologic tolerance. See also connector, nonrigid.

stretch receptors, *n.pl* the specialized sensory nerve endings in muscle spindles and tendons that are stimulated by stretching movements. They are active in maintaining dynamic posture.

stretch reflex, *n* See reflex, stretch.

stretching, longitudinal, *n* the vertical elongations of gutta-percha that occur because of packing forces during the filling of large root canals. The material returns to the original form when force is released.

stretching pliers, *n* See pliers, stretching.

stridor (strī′dôr), *n* a peculiar, harsh, vibrating sound produced during respiration.

stridor, inspiratory, *n* the stridor heard in inspiration through a spasmodically closed glottis.

stridor, laryngeal, *n* a stridor resulting from laryngeal stenosis.

strip, *n* a thin, narrow, comparatively long piece of material.

strip, abrasive (linen strip), *n* a ribbonlike piece of linen of varying length and width, on one side of which are bonded abrasive particles of selected grit; used for contouring and polishing proximal surfaces of restorations.

strip, boxing, *n* a metal or wax strip used for making an enclosure to regulate the size and form of a cast.

strip, celluloid, *n* See strip, plastic.

strip, lightning, *n* (separating strip), a strip of steel with abrasive bonded on one side; used to open rough or improper contacts of proximal restorations or begin the reduction of proximal excess of a foil restoration.

strip, linen, *n* See strip, abrasive.

strip, plastic, *n* a clear plastic strip of celluloid or acrylic resin that is used as a matrix when silicate cement or acrylic resin cement is inserted into proximal prepared cavities in anterior teeth.

strip, polishing, *n* a strip with a very fine abrasive, such as crocus powder.

strip, separating, *n* See strip, lightning.

stripping, *n* **1.** the mechanical removal of a very small amount of enamel from the mesial or distal surfaces of teeth to alleviate crowding. **2.** (electrochemical) the process of subjecting the surface of a gold casting, attached to an anode from a rectifier and transformer unit, to the dissolving action of a heated cyanide solution, the metal container for which is the cathode of the unit. A microscopic amount of the surface of the alloy is removed by reverse electrolysis. The electrochemical stripping or milling is in contrast to electropolishing, wherein sharp edges are dissolved more rapidly than are broader areas.

stroke, *n* **1.** a single, unbroken movement made by an instrument or the mandible. **2.** a colloquial term for accident, cerebrovascular.

stroke, circular, *n* an unbroken spherical movement of approximately 1 to 2 mm in diameter, combined with pressure, that is used to apply paste in polishing.

stroke, circumferential **(serkum′-fəren′shəl),** *n* a movement used for root and gingival curettage; the blade of the periodontal curet is negotiated mesiodistally while it is in contact with either the root or the inner aspect of the soft tissue wall of the gingival or periodontal pocket.

stroke, exploratory, *n* a phase of subgingival root scaling in which the curet is held in a featherlike grasp to ascertain tactilely the amount and extent of the deposits on the root surface; the ingress stroke into the pocket area.

stroke, horizontal, *n* a short movement against a tooth that is made parallel to its occlusal surface.

stroke, oblique, *n* a single, continuous diagonal movement of an instrument over the external face of the object being worked on.

stroke, placement, *n* a single, continuous movement of an instrument over the surface of an object being worked on, which moves the instrument at the intended location.

stroke, power, *n* the phase of the working stroke that is designed to split or dislodge calculus from the root surface. It is prefaced by the exploratory stroke and followed by the shaving stroke.

stroke, probe walking, *n* the technique of assessing the progression and extent of disease within the oral cavity by inserting a periodontal probe into the sulcus or pocket of the tooth and moving the device up and down between 1 to 2 mm in height while simultaneously advancing forward in 1 mm increments.

stroke, pull, *n* a single, continuous movement of an instrument over the surface of an object being worked on. A pull stroke is enacted to remove calculus from the surface of a tooth.

stroke, push and pull, *n* the technique of using a subgingival explorer vertically or diagonally to assess a defect of the tooth's surface by inserting the lower shank of the instrument under the gingival margin and into the sulcus or pocket and moving the device up and down while simultaneously applying equal pressure and advancing forward.

stroke, shaving, *n* the phase of the working stroke of a periodontal curet that is designed to smooth or plane the root surface. It follows the power stroke, which is designed to dislodge calculus from the root surface.

stroke, vertical, *n* a single, continuous movement of an instrument over the external face being treated. The vertical stroke is in a direction that parallels the length of the tooth (from the root to the occlusal surface).

stroke volume, *n* the volume of blood put out by the heart per heartbeat. It is directly proportional to the volume of blood filling the heart during diastole.

stroke, working, *n* a single, continuous movement of an instrument that achieves a task or treatment.

strontium (Sr) (stron′chēəm), *n* a metallic element. Its atomic number is 38 and its atomic weight is 87.62. It is chemically similar to calcium and is found in bone tissue. Isotopes of strontium are used in radioisotope scanning procedures of bone.

structure, *n* the architectural arrangement of the component parts of a tissue, part, organ, or body. Also the individual components of the body.

structure, border, *n* See border structures.

structure, cored, *n* in metallurgy a grain structure with composition gradients resulting from the progressive freezing of the components in different proportions. Nonmetals used in dentistry (e.g., zinc phosphate, silicate cements) also are cored structures, in that they have a nucleus of undissolved powder particles surrounded by a matrix of reacted material.

structure, denture-supporting, *n* the tissues, including teeth and residual ridges, that serve as the foundation or basal seat for removable partial dentures.

structure, functional form of supporting, *n* the state of denture-supporting structures when they have been placed in such a position as to be able to begin resisting occlusal forces.

structure, histologic, *n* the microscopic structure of organic tissues.

structure, radiolucent, *n* the structures or substances that permit the penetration of x-radiation and are thus registered as relatively dark areas on the radiograph.

structure, radiopaque **(rā′dēōpāk′),** *n* structures of such density that roentgen rays cannot penetrate them, causing them to appear as light areas on the radiograph.

structure, supporting, *n* the tissues that maintain or assist in maintaining the teeth in position in the alveolus (e.g., gingivae, cementum of the tooth, periodontal ligament, alveolar and trabecular bone).

Stuart factor, *n.pr* See factor X.

study, *n* the pursuance of education; analysis.

study cast, *n* See cast, diagnostic.

study, graduate, *n* the baccalaureate educational efforts pursued for credit toward an advanced degree in institutions of higher learning.

study model, *n* See cast, diagnostic.

study, postgraduate, *n* postdoctoral educational endeavors that may or may not earn credits for advanced degrees.

study, time, *n* the technique of random sampling used for analysis of the time spent for rendering each phase of each of the various professional services performed by the dental professional.

stupor, *n* the condition of being only partly conscious or sensible; also, a condition of insensibility.

Sturge-Weber angiomatosis, *n.pr* See angiomatosis, Sturge-Weber.

Sturge-Weber-Dimitri disease, *n.pr* See disease, Sturge-Weber-Dimitri.

stuttering, *n* a speech dysfunction characterized by spasmodic enunciation of words, involving excessive hesitations, stumbling, repetition of the same syllables, and prolongation of sounds.

stylet, *n* a wire inserted into a soft catheter or cannula to secure rigidity; a fine wire inserted into a hollow needle to maintain patency.

stylohyoid ligament (stī′lōhī′oid), *n* the ligament attached to the tip of the styloid process of the temporal bone and the lesser cornu of the hyoid bone.

stylohyoid muscle (stī′lōhīoid′), *n* one of the four suprahyoid muscles. It is a slender muscle that arises from the styloid process and inserts into the hyoid bone. It serves to draw the hyoid bone up and back.

stylomandibular ligament, *n* one of a pair of specialized bands of cervical fascia, forming an accessory part of the temporomandibular joint. It extends from the styloid process of the temporal bone to the ramus of the mandible.

stylus, *n* an ancient writing instrument. It has assumed importance in gnathology because a well-pointed stylus can be slid on dust-covered glass with a minimum of friction, thereby making the jaw-writing data more accurate.

stylus, surgical indicator, n a small pointed instrument devised to mark the spot in the tissue where the intramucosal inserts will be placed. Styluses are seated in prepared depressions in the denture base and mark the mucosal tissue by puncturing it.

stylus tracer, n See tracer, needle point.

stylus tracing, n See tracing, needle point.

styptic, *n* a hemostatic astringent.

sub-, *pref* prefix signifying under, beneath, deficient, near, or almost.

subacute, *adj* less than acute.

subarachnoid hemorrhage (SAH), *n* an intracranial hemorrhage into the cerebrospinal fluid.

subclinical, *adj* pertaining to an illness or condition in its earliest stage; having no symptoms or readily discernible signs.

subconscious, *n* the state in which mental processes take place without the mind's being distinctly conscious of its own activity.

subculture, *n* an ethnic, regional, economic, or social group with characteristic patterns of behavior and ideals that distinguish it from the rest of the culture or society.

subdural, *adj* situated below the dura mater and above the arachnoid membrane.

subgingival (subjin′jivəl), *adj* at a level apical to the gingival margin.

subgingival calculus, n See calculus, subgingival.

subgingival curettage, n See curettage, subgingival.

subgingival irrigation, preanesthetic-antimicrobial, n a procedure for delivering a liquid antimicrobial agent to a subgingival area before; used to destroy or inhibit the growth of microorganisms and prevent contamination or infection. Not known if effects are long term.

subgingival scaling, n See scaling, subgingival.

subjective data collection, *n* the process in which information relating to the patient's problem is elicited from the patient.

subjects, *n.pl* the people, animals, or events selected for study to examine a particular variable or condition, such as the effects of a new medication or treatment.

subliminal, *adj* below the threshold of sensory perception or outside the range of conscious awareness.

sublingual (subling′gwəl), *adj* pertaining to the region of structures located beneath the tongue.

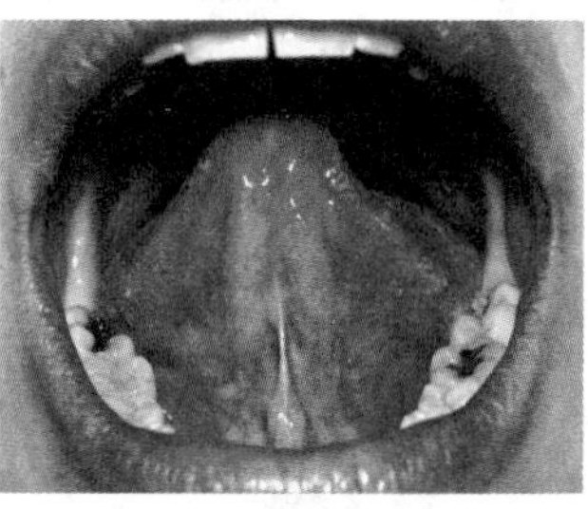

Sublingual. (Liebgott, 2001)

sublingual administration, n See administration, sublingual.

sublingual caruncle, n See caruncle, sublingual.

sublingual crescent, n See crescent, sublingual.

sublingual duct, n See duct, sublingual.

sublingual fold, n See fold, sublingual.

sublingual fossa, n See fossa, sublingual.

sublingual gland, n See salivary glands.

sublingual space, n See space, sublingual.

subluxation (sub′luksā′shən), *n* **1.** an incomplete dislocation of a joint. **2.** term applied to the temporomandibular joint, indicating relaxation of the capsular ligaments and improper relationship of the joint components, resulting in cracking and popping of the joint during movement.

submandibular (sub′mandib′yələr), *adj* inferior to the mandible.

submandibular caruncle, *n* See caruncle, submandibular.

submandibular duct, *n* See Wharton's duct.

submandibular fossa, *n* See fossa, submandibular.

submandibular fossa in image interpretation, *n* a radiolucent site within the region located in the body of the mandible that allows radiographs to gain a clear representation of the lingual depression of the salivary gland located within the submandibular area.

submandibular ganglion, *n* See ganglion, submaxillary.

submandibular lymph nodes, *n* the superficial cervical nodes located at the inferior border of the ramus of the mandible.

submandibular salivary gland, *n* See gland, submandibular salivary.

submandibular space, *n* See space, submandibular.

submandibular triangle, *n* See triangle, submandibular.

submarginal, *adj* pertaining to a deficiency of contour at the margin of a restoration or pattern.

submaxillary, *adj* situated deep to the maxilla.

submental, *adj* situated inferior to the chin.

submental lymph nodes, *n* the superficial cervical nodes located inferior to the chin.

submucosa (sub′mūkō′sə), *n* the tissue layer beneath the oral mucosa. It contains connective tissues, vessels, and accessory salivary glands.

submucous cleft, *n* a congenital anomaly in which the midportion of the soft or hard palate lacks proper mesodermal development. Nonunion of bone and muscle tissues of the soft and hard palates and concealment by the superficial intact mucoperiosteum. Also called *occult cleft.*

S

subnasion (sub′nā′zēon), *n* the point of the angle between the septum and the surface of the upper lip. It is sought at the point where a tangent applied to the septum meets the upper lip.

subocclusal connector (sub′əkloo′səl), *n* See connector, subocclusal.

subperiosteal (sub′perēos′tēəl), *adj* located or occurring beneath the periosteum.

subpoena (sub′pē′nə), *n* the process or writ issued by the court requiring the attendance of a witness at a certain time and place for testimony. It also may order him or her to bring books, records, or other relevant items as evidence.

subpoena duces tecum, *n* a subpoena commanding a person to bring books, papers, records, or other items to the court.

subroutine, *n* the set of instructions necessary to direct the computer to carry out a well-defined mathematical or logical operation; a subunit of a routine.

subscriber, *n* the person, usually the employee, who represents the family unit in relation to the prepayment plan. Other family members are *dependents.* Also called *certificate holders* or *enrollees.*

subsistence, *n* the state of being supported or remaining alive with a minimum of essentials.

subspecialty, *n* a limited portion of a narrowly defined professional discipline. E.g., surgery is a specialty of medicine and pediatric vascular surgery is a subspecialty.

subspinale (sub′spīnā′lē), *n* the deepest midline point on the premaxilla between the anterior nasal spine and the prosthion.

substance abuse, *n* See abuse, substance.

substance P, *n* an endogenous inflammatory substance thought to mediate or cause pain.

substandard, *adj* below an acceptable level of performance.

substantivity, *adj* pertaining to the capacity of an oral antimicrobial agent to continue its therapeutic activity for a prolonged period of time.

substitute, *n* one acting for or taking the place of another.

substitute, tinfoil, *n* alginate separating material painted on gypsum molds to serve as a liner in preventing both the penetration of monomers into the surrounding investing medium and the leakage of water into acrylic resin.

substitution, *n* a standard or nonstandard speech sound used for another consonant speech sound (e.g., *w* for *l* [*wady* for *lady*]).

substructure, *n* a structure built to serve as a base or foundation for another structure.

substructure, implant (implant denture substructure), *n* **1.** a skeletal frame of inert material that fits on the bone under the mucoperiosteum. **2.** the metal framework that is embedded beneath the soft tissues in contact with the bone for the purpose of supporting an implant superstructure.

substructure, implant, abutment, *n* the portion of the implant that extends from the surface of the mucosa into the oral cavity for the retention of crowns, bridges, or superstructure bearing the teeth of the denture.

substructure, implant, auxiliary rest, *n* a small metal protrusion through the mucosa connected to the labial or buccal and lingual (peripheral) frame to furnish additional support for the superstructure between the abutments.

substructure, implant, interspace, *n* a space between the primary and secondary struts that allows infiltration of tissue.

substructure, implant, neck (implant post, implant substructure, post), *n* the constriction that connects the implant frame with the implant abutment.

substructure, implant, part, *n* the root section shaped in the form of a wire loop. This part of the substructure sinks into the alveolar socket or sockets after the extraction of one or two remaining anterior teeth. Newly formed bone tissue grows through the loop and firmly affixes the implant.

substructure, implant, peripheral frame, *n* the labial, buccal, lingual, and distal outline of the frame.

substructure, implant, post, *n* See substructure, implant, neck.

substructure, implant, primary struts, *n* the main traverse struts that connect the implant necks or posts with the peripheral frame.

substructure, implant, secondary struts, *n* the additional smaller transverse, diagonal, and longitudinal struts that are added when necessary to give additional strength and rigidity to the implant, increase the area of bone support, and afford additional intermeshing of the mucoperiosteal tissue.

subtle, *adj* having a low intensity; not severe and having no serious sequelae.

succedaneous (suk′sidā′nēəs), *adj* replacing or substituting for something else; often used when referring to the permanent teeth that erupt to replace the milk teeth.

successional dental lamina (səksesh′ənəl lam′ənə), *n* an elongation of the primary tooth germ from which a permanent tooth will eventually take shape.

succinimides (suksin′imidz), *n* a class of drugs used in the treatment of epilepsy.

succinylcholine chloride (suk′sənilkō′lēn), *n* a skeletal muscle relaxant used as an adjunct to anesthesia, to reduce muscle contractions during surgery or mechanical ventilation and to facilitate endotracheal intubation.

sucralfate (sookral′fāt), *n brand name:* Carafate; *drug class:* protectant, aluminum salt of sulfated sucrose; *action:* forms an ulcer-adherent complex that covers and protects the ulcer site; *use:* treatment of duodenal ulcer.

sudden infant death syndrome (SIDS), *n* the unexpected and sudden death of an apparently normal and healthy infant that occurs during sleep and with no physical or autopsic evidence of disease. It is the most common cause of death of children in the United States between 2 weeks and 1 year of age.

sudorific (soo′dərif′ik), *n* an agent, substance, or condition, such as heat or emotional tension, that promotes sweating.

sufentanil citrate (soofen′tənil), *n* an intravenous analgesic and anesthetic used as an adjunct to general anesthesia and as a primary anesthetic with 100% oxygen.

suffocate, *v* asphyxiate; to prevent the exchange of air into the lungs, causing death.

suffocation, *n* interference with the entrance of air into the lungs.

sugar, *n* one of a number of water-soluble carbohydrates. Sugars are divided into two major categories, *monosaccharides* and *disaccharides.* Table sugar or sucrose is the principal disaccharide; glucose or blood sugar is the principal monosaccharide.

sugar alcohols, *n.pl* the nutritive sweeteners found in most grains, fruits, and vegetables that undergo natural fermentation as they are broken down by oral bacteria; not directly linked to the development of dental caries but may cause diarrhea if ingested in excessive amounts.

suggestion, *n* **1.** the process by which one thought or idea leads to another, as in the association of ideas. **2.** the use of persuasion to implant an idea, thought, attitude, or belief in the mind of another as a means of influencing or altering behavior or state of mind.

suicide, *n* the intentional taking of one's own life.

suit, *n* a proceeding in court in which the plaintiff pursues a remedy that the law gives for the redress of an injury or the enforcement of a right.

sulconazole nitrate (səlkon′əzōl), *n brand name:* Exelderm; *drug class:* topical antifungal; *action:* interferes with fungal cell membranes, increasing permeability and leaking of nutrients; *uses:* treatment of tinea pedis, tinea corporis, tinea cruris, and tinea versicolor.

sulcus (sul′kəs), *n* **1.** a furrow, trench, or groove, as on the surface of the brain or in the folds of mucous membranes. **2.** a groove or depression on the surface of a tooth. **3.** a groove in a portion of the oral cavity.

sulcus, alveololingual, *n* the space between the alveolar or residual alveolar ridge and the tongue. It extends from the lingual frenum to the retromylohyoid curtain and is a part of the floor of the oral cavity.

sulcus, gingival, *n* the shallow groove between the free gingiva and the surface of a tooth and extending around its circumference. Older term: *gingival crevice.* See also pocket.

sulcus, implant gingival, *n* a sulcus around the implant abutment post that resembles the sulcus around a healthy natural tooth.

sulcus, nasolabial (naz′ōlā′bēəl), *n* the groove that runs between the corner of the upper lip and the nose. Also known as *sulcus nasolabialis.*

sulcus, occlusal, *n* a groove or spillway on the occlusal surface of a tooth.

sulcus, terminalis, *n* a V-shaped shallow groove on the surface of the tongue that separates the distal third of the tongue from the proximal two-thirds.

sulfa (sul′fə), *adj/n* a colloquial term used to describe a group of antibacterial agents. See also sulfacetamide and sulfamethizole.

sulfacetamide sodium (ophthalmic), *n brand names:* Bleph-10, Cetamide, Isopto Cetamide; *drug class:* antibacterial sulfonamide; *action:* inhibits folic acid synthesis by preventing paraaminobenzoic acid (PABA) use, which is necessary for bacterial growth; *uses:* treatment of conjunctivitis, superficial eye infections, and corneal ulcers.

sulfamethizole (sul′fəmeth′izōl), *n brand name:* Thiosulfil Forte; *drug class:* sulfonamide, short acting; *action:* interferes with bacterial biosynthesis of proteins by competitive antagonism of paraaminobenzoic acid (PABA); *use:* treatment of urinary tract infections.

sulfamethoxazole (sul′fəmethok′səzōl), *n brand names:* Gamazole, Gantanol, Urabak; *drug class:* sulfonamide; *action:* interferes with bacterial biosynthesis of proteins by competitive antagonism of paraaminobenzoic acid (PABA); *uses:* treatment of urinary tract infections, lymphogranuloma venereum, and systemic infections.

sulfamethoxazole/trimethoprim, *n brand names:* Bactrim, Cotrim, Septra, Sulfatrim, Sulfamethoprim, Triazole, Uroplus SS; *drug class:* sulfonamide and folic acid antagonist; *action:* interferes with bacterial biosynthesis of proteins by competitive antagonism of paraaminobenzoic acid (PABA) when adequate levels are maintained; *uses:* treatment of urinary tract infections, otitis media.

sulfasalazine (sul′fəsal′əzēn), *n brand name:* Asulfi-dine-EN-Tabs, Azulfidine; *drug class:* sulfonamide derivative with antiinflammatory action; *action:* acts as a prodrug to deliver sulfapyridine and mesalamine (5-aminosalicylic acid) to the colon; *uses:* treatment of ulcerative colitis, Crohn's disease.

S

sulfhemoglobinemia (sulfēm′əglō′binē′mēə), *n* an abnormality of the heme moiety of the hemoglobin molecule resulting from inorganic sulfides (e.g., acetanilide).

sulfinpyrazone (sul′finpir′əzōn′), *n brand name:* Anturane; *drug class:* uricosuric; *action:* inhibits tubular reabsorption of urates, with increased excretion of uric acid; inhibits prostaglandin synthesis, which decreases platelet aggregation; *use:* treatment of chronic gouty arthritis.

sulfisoxazole (sul′fəsok′səzōl′), *n brand name:* Gantrisin; *drug class:* sulfonamide, short-acting; antiinfective; *action:* interferes with bacterial biosynthesis of proteins by competitive antagonism of paraaminobenzoic acid (PABA); *uses:* treatment of urinary tract, systemic infections; chancroid; trachoma; toxoplasmosis, acute otitis media; lymphogranuloma venereum; eye infections.

sulfonamide (sulfon′əmīd), *n* a derivative of sulfanilamide that is effective against microorganisms.

sulfonylureas (sul″fənilure′əs), *n* a class of medications used in the treatment of diabetes. They cause the pancreas to release more insulin. See also diabetes.

sulfur (S), *n* a nonmetallic, multivalent, tasteless, odorless chemical element that occurs abundantly in yellow crystalline form or in masses, especially in volcanic areas. Its atomic number is 16, and its atomic weight is 32.064. It has wide use in industry. Sulfur has been used in the treatment of gout, rheumatism, and bronchitis and as a mild laxative.

sulfur granules, *n* a yellow-white particle found in actinomycosis and diagnostic of actinomycosis infection. See also actinomycosis.

sulindac (səlin′dak), *n brand name:* Clinoril; *drug class:* nonsteroidal antiinflammatory; *action:* inhibits prostaglandin synthesis by interfering with cyclooxygenase, an enzyme needed for biosynthesis; possesses analgesic, antiinflammatory, and antipyretic properties; *uses:* osteoarthritis, rheumatoid, acute gouty arthrits, tendinitis, bursitis, ankylosing spondylitis.

sumatriptan succinate (soo′mətrip′tan suk′sənāt′), *n brand name:* Imitrex; *drug class:* serotonin agonist; *action:* selective agonist for the vascular 5-hydroxytryptamine (5-HT-1) (serotonin) receptor in cranial arteries, causing vasodilation with little or no effect on peripheral pressure; *use:* treatment of migraine headaches.

summary judgment, *n* a judgment requested by a party to a civil action to end the action when it is believed that no genuine issue or material fact is in dispute.

summary plan description, *n* See benefit plan summary.

summation, *n* the phenomenon in which similar actions of more than one drug result in a total action that may be expressed as the arithmetical sum of the effects of the individual drugs.

summons, *n* a writ requiring a proper officer to notify a defendant that an action has been begun against him or her in the court from which the writ was issued and that he or she is required to appear on a certain day to answer the complaint.

superficial, *adj* involving only the surface or to be minor in severity, not grave or dangerous.

superinfection, *n* an infection occurring during antimicrobial treatment for another infection.

superior, *adj* situated in a higher position on the body, closer to the head and farther from the feet.

supernumerary tooth, *n* a tooth in addition to the normal 32 teeth in the permanent dentition or the 20 teeth in the primary dentition. See also supplemental tooth.

superoxide, *n* a common form of oxygen that is created when molecular oxygen gains a single electron. Superoxide radicals may attack susceptible biologic targets, including lipids, proteins, and nucleic acids.

superoxol, *n* a 30% solution of hydrogen peroxide used to bleach endodontically treated teeth.

supersaturation, *n* the addition to or presence of an ingredient in a solution in greater quantity than the solvent can permanently take up.

superstructure, *n* a structure constructed on or over another structure.

superstructure casting, *n* in the subperiosteal implant, a surgical alloy bar designed with clasps to telescope over the four abutments. To this casting is processed the final denture superstructure.

superstructure, implant, *n* (implant denture superstructure), **1.** a removable denture that fits snugly onto the protruding implant abutments. Sometimes called the *implant denture.* **2.** the denture that is retained, supported, and stabilized by the implant denture substructure.

superstructure, implant, attaching material, *n* the denture resin by which the superstructure teeth are attached to the superstructure frame.

superstructure, implant, attachment, *n* a part of the superstructure that fits onto the implant abutments. May be a precision attachment coping, a conventional clasping, or a combination of a precision attachment with clasps.

superstructure, implant, connectors, *n* the rigid bars that unite the superstructure attachments into one strong element.

superstructure, implant, denture, *n* See superstructure, implant.

superstructure, implant, frame, *n* the metal skeleton of the superstructure, consisting of attachments and connectors.

superstructure, temporary (implant surgical splint), *n* an acrylic resin immediate appliance with six anterior teeth; has no metal clasps, precision coping, or frame; fitted closely over the implant abutments immediately after the surgical insertion of the substructure.

supervised neglect, *n* a case in which a patient is regularly examined and shows signs of a disease or other medical problems but is not informed of its presence or progress.

supervision, *n* the active administering and overseeing of all the functionings of the dental practice and the auxiliaries employed therein.

supine, *adj* lying horizontally on the back.

supplemental tooth, *n* a type of supernumerary tooth that is so well formed that it mimics a fully formed tooth. A supplemental tooth usually appears distal to a lateral incisor. Its detection requires the careful counting and identification of each tooth in the dental arch.

supplements, *n.pl* usually, dietary substances used to augment, enhance, or enrich the nutritional status of a patient.

support, *n* resistance to vertical components of masticatory force in a direction toward the basal seat.

support, ridge, *n* See area, supporting.

supporting area, *n* See area, supporting.

supporting bone, *n* See bone, cancellous.

supportive periodontal therapy, *n* See periodontal therapy.

suppressant (səpres′ənt), *n* an agent that retards or diminishes a physical or mental activity. Commonly used to describe a drug that inhibits coughing (cough suppressant).

suppuration (sup″ura′shən), *n* the formation and discharge of pus, a more commonly used term. See also pyogenic.

suprabulge (soo′prəbulj′), *n* the portion of the crown of a tooth that converges toward the occlusal surface from the height of contour of survey line.

supraclavicular lymph nodes (soo′prəklavik′ūlur), *n* the deep cervical nodes located along the clavicle.

supraclusion (soo′prəkloo′zhən), *n* a position occupied by a tooth that is too high in the line of occlusion.

supragingival calculus, *n* See calculus, supragingival.

supramentale (soo′prəməntā′lē), *n* the most posterior point in the concavity between infradentale and pogonion.

supraversion (soo′prəvur′zhən), *n* a condition in which teeth or other maxillary structures are situated above or below their normal vertical relationships.

suprofen (sooprō′fən), *n* an oral nonsteroidal antiinflammatory analgesic used in the treatment of mild to moderate pain and primary dysmenorrhea.

suramin sodium, *n* an antitrypanosomal and an antifilarial available from the Centers for Disease Control and Prevention. It is used primarily for treatment and prophylaxis of *Afri-*

can trypanosomiasis and *A. onchocerciasis.*

surcharge, *n* a stated dollar amount paid to the dental professional by the beneficiary in addition to other reimbursement received by third-party payers.

surface, *n* the outer portion of a mass or object.

surface, balancing occlusal, the surfaces of the teeth or denture bases that make contact to provide balancing contacts.

surface, basal, *n* See denture, basal surface of.

surface, buccal, *n* a surface adjacent to and facing the cheek.

surface, foundation, *n* See denture, basal surface of.

surface, implant-bearing, *n* the area of bone that has been selected from the surgical bone impression to be in direct contact with the implant frame.

surface, impression, *n* See denture, basal surface of.

surface markers, *n.pl* the identification labels applied to the external surfaces of dentures. They may be ink or engraved and may include name, initials, social security number, national registration number, date of birth, and so on.

surface, occlusal, *n* the anatomic superior surface of the mandibular posterior teeth and the inferior surface of the maxillary posterior teeth. These surfaces are limited mesially and distally by marginal ridges, and buccally and lingually by the buccal and lingual boundaries of the cusp eminences.

surface, proximal, *n* the surface of a tooth or the portion of a cavity that is nearest to the adjacent tooth; the mesial or distal surface of a tooth.

surface radiation exposure, *n* See exposure, entrance.

surface, smooth, *n* a surface of a tooth on which pits and fissures are not found normally.

surface, working occlusal, *n* the surface or surfaces of the teeth on which chewing can occur.

surfactant (surfak′tənt), *n* a surface-active agent.

surgeon, *n* a person whose profession is to cure diseases or injuries by manual operation or by medication.

surgery, *n* work performed by a surgeon.

surgery, access flap in osseous, *n* a full-thickness or split-thickness flap created for the purpose of gaining access to the alveolar bone when surgical remodeling is indicated.

surgery, apically repositioned flap in mucogingival, *n* a surgically created flap of gingival tissue that is repositioned apically to maintain or create a functionally adequate zone of attached gingiva. In the surgical procedure the existing attached and free gingiva is detached by employing a reverse bevel incision and apically repositioning the flap.

surgery, cosmetic, *n* surgery whose purpose is to improve external appearance rather than general health.

surgery, first-stage, *n* See surgery, stage-one.

surgery, full flap in mucogingival, *n* a flap in which all the soft tissue elements are raised and repositioned, as opposed to the split-thickness flap.

surgery, mucogingival, *n* surgical procedure designed to retain a functionally adequate zone of gingiva after surgical pocket elimination, create a functionally adequate zone of attached gingiva, alter the position of or eliminate a frenum, or deepen the vestibule.

surgery, oblique flap in mucogingival, *n* an increased band of attached gingiva created by preparing a narrow papillary flap (to avoid donor site radicular recession), which is then rotated 90° and sutured into the prepared recipient site.

surgery, osseous, *n* the therapeutic surgical measures used and designed to eliminate osseous deformities by means of ostectomy or osteoplasty or create a favorable environment by means of meticulous removal of the soft tissue contents of the infrabony osseous defect for the formation of new bone, periodontal membrane, and cementum to fill in the area of bone resorption.

surgery, pedicle flap in mucogingival, *n* an increased band of attached gingiva created to repair a cleft by using proximal gingiva situated mesial and distal to the cleft, because gingiva in either location alone is not wide enough to cover the cleft if repositioned. The pedicles are repositioned laterally and sutured. Also called a *double papilla procedure.*

surgery, second-stage, *n* See surgery, stage-two.

surgery, stage-one, *n* a surgical procedure in which an endosseous two-stage implant is placed in the bone and the soft tissue over the implant is sutured closed to allow osseointegration of the implant before the abutment and prosthesis are attached; also known as *first-stage surgery.*

surgery, stage-two, *n* a surgical procedure in which the soft tissue over a submerged implant is removed in order to place an abutment into the implant; also known as *second-stage surgery.*

surgical preparation, *n* See preparation, surgical.

surgical prosthesis (prosthē′sis), *n* See prosthesis, surgical.

surgical scrub, *n* a health care provider's first hand and arm wash of the day prior to entering a sterile surgical field. It involves a systematic routine in which a minimum of 10 minutes are spent lathering, soaking, and brushing one hand and arm and then the other.

surgical template, *n* See template, surgical.

surrogate (sur′əgit), *n* a substitute; a person or thing that replaces another.

survey, *n* the study and examination of an area of consideration, a diagnostic cast, or a radiograph.

survey, radiation, *n* evaluation of the radiation hazards incidental to the production, use, or existence of radioactive materials or other sources of radiation under a specific set of conditions.

survey, radiograph, *n* See survey, radiographic.

survey, radiographic, *n* the production of the minimal number of radiographic examinations necessary for a radiographic interpretation.

survey, roentgenographic, *n* See survey, radiographic.

survey, vertical bite-wing, *n* a series of oral radiographs in which the teeth are viewed and recorded from a series of positions: the *molar* position, where the film is positioned approximately over the center of the second molar on each side of the oral cavity; *premolar,* where the film is positioned over the mandibular premolar teeth on each side; *anterior,* where the film is centered between the canine and lateral teeth; and *central bite-wing,* where the film is placed at the midline.

survey line, *n* See line, survey.

surveying, *n* the procedure of studying the relative parallelism or lack of parallelism of the teeth and associated structures to select a path of placement for a restoration that will encounter the least tooth or tissue interference and provide adequate and balanced retention; locating guiding plane surfaces to direct placement and removal of the restoration and to achieve the best appearance possible.

surveyor (survā′ər), *n* an instrument used to determine the relative parallelism of two or more surfaces of teeth or other portions of a cast of the dental arch.

surveyor, Ney, *n.pr* the first commercially available dental cast surveyor designed to select a path of placement or insertion for a restoration.

survival rate, *n* See rate, survival.

susceptible, *adj* the opposite of immune; having little resistance to disease.

suspension (suspen′shən), *n* a mixture of two or more immiscible phases, such as a solid in a liquid or a liquid in a liquid. Suspensions differ from emulsions in that the former usually have to be shaken before each use.

sustenance, *n* the act or process of supporting or maintaining life and health.

Sutton's disease, *n.pr* See periadenitis mucosa necrotica recurrens.

suture (soo′chər), *n* **1.** a synarthrosis between two bones formed in a membrane, the uniting medium (which tends to disappear eventually) being a fibrous membrane continuous with the periosteum. **2.** a surgical stitch or seam. **3.** the material with which body structures are sewn, as after an operation or injury. *v* **4.** to sew up a wound.

suture, absorbable, *n* a suture that becomes dissolved in body fluids and disappears (e.g., catgut).

suture, approximation, *n* a suture

made to bring about apposition of the deeper tissues of an incision or laceration.

suture, blanket, *n* a suturing technique that loops each stitch over the previous one to create a succession of loops along one side and stitches across the incision. Also called *continuous lock stitch.*

suture, button, *n* a suture passed through buttonlike disks on the skin to prevent the suture cutting the soft tissue.

suture, chromic, *n* a chromatized sheepgut suture.

suture, circumferential, *n* a suture completely surrounding the tooth; generally used to suspend or retain a flap.

suture, continuous, *n* a suture in which an uninterrupted length of suture material is used to close an incision or laceration.

suture, craniofacial, *n* the line along which bones of the cranium or face articulate in an immovable articulation.

suture, frontomalar, *n* most lateral point of the suture between the frontal and zygoma (zygomatic bones).

suture, interdental, *n* a suture that joins two sides of the gingiva by passing between the teeth.

suture, interrupted, *n* individual stitches, each tied separately.

suture knot, *n* the tiny fastening used to hold a suture in place firmly but not too tightly. The specific type is dictated by procedure, incision location, and tension required to close the wound.

suture, mattress, *n* a continuous suture that is applied back and forth through the tissues in the same vertical plane but at a different depth, or in the same horizontal plane but at the same depth.

suture (median palatine suture), *n* the line of fusion of the two maxillae (two palatine processes), starting between the central incisors and extending posteriorly across the palate, separating the horizontal plates of the palatine bones into two nearly equal parts.

suture, monofilament, *n* refers to the single-strand composition of the material used to secure surgical stitches.

suture, multifilament, *n* refers to the multiple-strand composition of the material used to secure surgical stitches.

suture, natural, *n* a type of organic material used to secure surgical stitches that may react adversely with body tissue.

suture needle, conventional cut, *n* a suturing needle with three cutting edges, one on either side and a third located on the inside curve.

suture, nonabsorbable, *n* a suture that does not dissolve in body fluids (e.g., silk, tantalum, nylon).

suture, purse-string, *n* a horizontal mattress suture used generally about an implant cervix.

suture, shoelace, *n* a continuous surgical suture for depression of the tongue and retention and holding of the lingual flap out of the field of operation during the surgical impression.

suture, suspension (sling), *n* a type of surgical stitching used when the flap being repaired is open on the lingual or facial side; surrounds the tooth by passing between the surrounding teeth and gum tissue. The stitch is adjustable and allows for adjustment of the flap for proper healing.

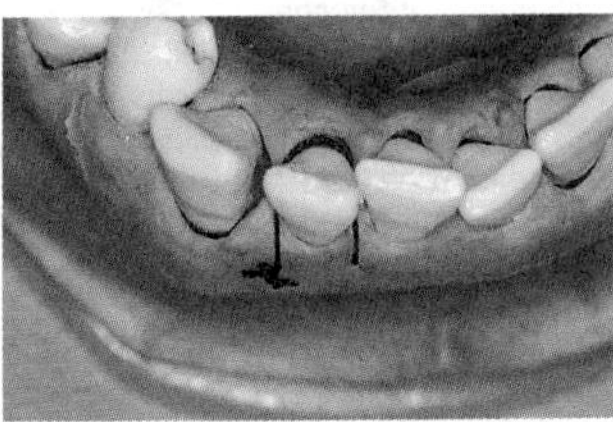

Suspension suture. (Daniel/Harfst/Wilder, 2008)

suture, synthetic, *n* new technology in surgical stitches developed to counteract the unreliable absorption rates and tissue sensitivity associated with natural stitches.

***suture, transverse palatine* (pal′ətīn),** *n* the line along which the bones of the palate and the superior maxilla articulate in an immovable articulation. Also known as *sutura palatina transversa.*

swage (swāj), *v* to shape metal by adapting or hammering it onto a die. Usually completed by forcing a counterdie into position on a die with the metal sheet interposed.

swager, *n* a laboratory instrument used for swaging.

swager, wax, *n* an instrument used to swage wax to a die.

swallowing, *n* See deglutition.

swallowing threshold, *n* See threshold, swallowing.

swear, *v* to take an oath; to become legally obligated by an oath properly administered.

sweat (swet), *n* perspiration. A clear liquid exuded or excreted from the sudoriferous glands. It possesses a characteristic odor and is slightly alkaline, salty to the taste, and, when mixed with sebaceous secretion, acidic. Sweating is under the control of the sympathetic nervous system, although it may be stimulated by parasympathetic drugs. Thermoregulatory sweating is influenced by the blood temperature's affecting the nervous centers and by reflexes associated with heat receptors in the skin.

sweating, gustatory, *n* See syndrome, auriculotemporal.

sweeteners, dietary, *n* the substances that provide the body with calories for energy; sources include sugars, other carbohydrates, sugar-alcohols, and nonnutritive sweeteners obtained from monosaccharides.

swelling, *n* one of the cardinal signs of acute inflammation; caused by the exudation of fluid from the capillary vessels into the tissue.

swelling, familial intraosseous, *n* See cherubism.

symbiotic relationship (sim′bīot′ik), *n* in implantology, that relationship assumed by an implant and the natural teeth to which it has been splinted. The continuing existence of their relationship is based on their independence.

symbolic coding, *n* instructions written in nonmachine language.

symmetric, *adj* evenly balanced or uniformly developed.

sympathectomy (sim′pəthek′təmē), *n* a surgical interruption of part of the sympathetic nerve pathways, performed for the relief of chronic pain or to promote vasodilation in vascular diseases.

sympathetic (sim′pəthet′ik), *adj* pertaining to the sympathetic nervous system.

sympathetic nervous system, *n* See autonomic nervous system.

sympatholytic (sim′pəthōlit′ik), *adj* pertaining to a drug that blocks the effects of stimulation of the sympathetic nervous system. See also adrenolytic.

sympathomimetic (sim′pəthōmimet′ik), *adj* resembling the effect produced by stimulation of the sympathetic nervous system. See also adrenergic.

sympathy, *n* the kind understanding of a patient.

symphysis (sim′fisis), *n* a line of union between two bony surfaces such as the symphysis of the mandible.

symptom, *n* any morbid phenomenon or departure from the normal in function, appearance, or sensation, experienced by the patient and indicative of disease. See also sign.

symptom, constitutional, *n* symptom related to the systemic effects of a disease (e.g., fever, malaise, anorexia, weight loss).

symptoms, diagnostic signs and, *n.pl* See signs and symptoms, diagnostic.

symptom, prodromal, *n* the first observable indicator of an illness; the initial manifestation of a disease.

synapse (sin′aps), *n* the region of contact between the processes of two adjacent neurons forming the place where a nervous impulse is transmitted from the axon of one neuron to the dendrites of another. It also is called the *synaptic junction.*

synarthrosis (sinärthrō′sis), *n* a joint formed by thin intervening layers of cartilage, connective tissue, or direct contact of bone to bone. It results in a rigid union, and little movement of the bones occurs except during growth. Suture lines may be obliterated in adults, with a synarthrodial joint when the bones joined together become fused.

synchondrosis (sing′kondrō′sis), *n* a cartilaginous joint between two immovable bones such as the union between the sphenoid and occipital bones at the base of the skull.

synchronous (sing′krənəs), *adj* having constant time intervals between events or occurrences.

synchronous device, *n* a term applied to a device in which the performance of a sequence of operations is controlled by equally spaced clock signals or pulses.

syncope (sing′kəpē), *n* fainting; temporary suspension of consciousness caused by cerebral anemia. See also shock.

syndactyly (sindak′təlē), *n* a congenital anomaly characterized by the fusion of fingers or toes, usually as a finding of a more complex congenital syndrome.

syndrome (sin′drōm), *n* a group of signs and symptoms that occur together and characterize a disease.

syndrome, adaptation, *n* See disease, adaptation; syndrome, general adaptation.

syndrome, adrenogenital, *n* disorder of sexual development or function associated with abnormal adrenocortical function resulting from bilateral adrenal hyperplasia, carcinoma, or adenoma. Pseudohermaphroditism occurs congenitally, and masculinization occurs later in females. Precocious sexual development and occasionally feminization occur in males.

syndrome, AHOP, *n.pr* **a**diposity, **h**yperthermia, **o**ligomenorrhea, and **p**arotitis appearing in females. Parotid gland enlargement begins at puberty and is followed by obesity, oligomenorrhea, and psychic disturbances.

syndrome, Apert, *n.pr* craniostenosis characterized by oxycephaly and syndactyly of the hands and feet. Facial manifestations include exophthalmos, high prominent forehead, small nose, and malformation of the mandible and oral cavity. Also called *acrocephalosyndactyly.*

syndrome, Ascher, *n.pr* syndrome consisting of double lip, a redundance of the skin of the eyelids (blepharochalasis), and nontoxic thyroid enlargement. The sagging eyelids are obvious when the eyes are open; the double lip is seen when the patient smiles.

syndrome, auriculotemporal, *n* See syndrome, Frey.

syndrome, autoimmune, *n* See disease, autoimmune.

syndrome, Behçet's **(bā′sets, bekh′chets)** ***(Behçet's disease),*** *n.pr* recurrent iritis and aphthous ulcers of the oral cavity and genitalia. Other manifestations include arthralgia, hydrarthrosis, swelling of the salivary glands, cutaneous eruptions, and central nervous system disorders.

syndrome, Bloch-Sulzberger (incontinentia pigmenti), *n.pr* syndrome in which pigmented skin lesions, defects of the eyes and central nervous system, skeletal anomalies, and hypoplasia of the teeth occur.

syndrome, Bogarad, *n.pr* See syndrome, auriculotemporal.

syndrome, Böök's **(bœks),** *n.pr* syndrome characterized by premature graying of the hair, hyperhidrosis, and premolar hypodontia.

syndrome, Bourneville-Pringle (epiloia), *n.pr* neurocutaneous complex consisting of adenoma sebaceum, mental deficiency, and epilepsy.

syndrome, burning mouth (BMS), *n* a condition characterized by a burning sensation in the oral cavity, despite the absence of any visible irritation to the mucous membranes.

syndrome, Caffey-Silverman, *n.pr* See hyperostosis, infantile cortical.

syndrome, Christ-Siemens-Touraine, *n.pr* See hypohidrotic ectodermal dysplasia.

syndrome, Costen's, *n.pr* discomfort, pain, and jaw pathosis claimed by Costen to be caused by lack of posterior occlusion, loss of vertical dimension, malocclusion, trismus, or muscle tremor.

syndrome, cracked tooth, *n* a condition caused by a cracked tooth, resulting in pain when chewing or applying other pressures or when in contact with cold substances. The crack may occur only on the enamel, or it may extend into the pulp.

syndrome, CREST, *n* a syndrome in which the initial letters of the clinical signs form the acronym CREST: **c**alcinosis, **R**aynaud's phenomenon, **e**sophageal dysfunction, **s**clerodactyly, and **t**elangiectasia; it is a slowly progressive disease in which calcium deposits usually form under the skin on the fingers and sometimes on other areas of the body; exposure to cold or stress causes pain in the fingers or toes; there is difficulty swallowing and acid reflux; there is tightening and thickening of the skin causing the fingers to bend; and small red spots form on the skin of the fingers, face, or inside of the oral cavity. It is a form of scleroderma that is diagnosed when at least two of these clinical signs are present.

syndrome, cri-du-chat **(krē-doo-shah′),** *n* clinical syndrome associated with the deletion of the short arm of a B chromosome. Manifestations include mental retardation, various congenital abnormalities, and an infant cry resembling the mewing of a cat.

syndrome, crocodile tears, *n* a syndrome in which a spontaneous lacrimation occurs with the normal salivation of eating. It follows facial paralysis and seems to result from straying of the regenerating nerve fibers, some of those destined for the salivary glands going to the lacrimal glands.

syndrome, Crouzon, *n.pr* a group of genetically inherited diseases characterized by midfacial hypoplasia, craniosynostosis, exophthalmos, and short head. Thought to be caused by a genetic mutation of the FGFRZ gene, located on chromosome 10.

syndrome, Cushing's (Cushing's disease), *n.pr* See hypercortisolism (Cushing syndrome).

syndrome, Down, *n.pr* See Down syndrome.

syndrome, Ehlers-Danlos, *n.pr* a congenital or familial disorder characterized by fragility of the skin and blood vessels, hyperlaxity of the joints, hyperelasticity of the skin, subcutaneous pseudotumors, and tendency to hemorrhage postoperatively.

syndrome, Ekman's, *n.pr* See osteogenesis imperfecta.

syndrome, Ellis-van Creveld, *n.pr* See chondroectodermal dysplasia.

syndrome, Feer's, *n.pr* See acrodynia.

syndrome, fetal hydantoin **(hīdan′-tōin),** *n* disorder developing in children who have been exposed to anticonvulsant therapy during the mother's pregnancy; indicated by mental deficiency, growth retardation, craniofacial abnormalities, cleft palate or lip, and congenital heart defects.

syndrome, Frey (auriculotemporal syndrome, gustatory sweating syndrome), *n.pr* sweating and flushing in the preauricular and temporal areas when certain foods are eaten. Thought to be related to parotid gland trauma or a complication of parotidectomy.

syndrome, Fröhlich's (adiposogenital dystrophy), *n.pr* adiposity and genital hypoplasia resulting from hypopituitarism or hypothalamohypophysdystrophy.

syndrome, Gardner's, *n.pr* the development of multiple osteomas, polyposis of the large bowel, epidermoid or sebaceous cysts, and cutaneous fibromas.

syndrome, general adaptation (adaptation syndrome, GAS), *n* a three-stage physiologic response to physical or psychologic stress. The first stage is the alarm reaction, consisting of bodily changes typical of emotion. A second stage is resistance to stress, wherein an attempt is made to adapt to the physiologic changes. Certain hormones of the anterior pituitary gland and the adrenal cortex hypersecrete to increase resistance. Such resistance leads to diseases of adaptation, such as hypertension. Continual stress results in the third stage, exhaustion.

syndrome, Goldscheider's, *n.pr* dystrophic form of epidermolysis bullosa, leading to scars. The disturbance is inherited on an autosomal dominant or recessive basis. This form of epidermolysis bullosa leads to retardation of mental and physical growth. See also syndrome, Weber-Cockayne.

syndrome, Gorlin (nevoid basal cell carcinoma syndrome), *n.pr* See syndrome, nevoid basal cell carcinoma.

syndrome, Greig's, *n.pr* a condition manifested by ocular hypertelorism, often mental retardation, ectodermal and mesodermal abnormalities, and dental and oral anomalies.

syndrome, Gunn's, *n.pr* See syndrome, jaw-winking.

syndrome, gustatory hyperhidrosis, *n* See syndrome, auriculotemporal.

syndrome, gustatory sweating, *n* See syndrome, auriculotemporal.

syndrome, Heerfordt's, *n.pr* See fever, uveoparotid.

syndrome, Horner's, *n.pr* a tetrad of symptoms resulting from paralysis of the cervical sympathetic trunk: pupillary constriction, ptosis of the upper eyelid, dilation of the orbital blood vessels (redness of conjunctiva), and blushing and anhidrosis of the side of the face.

syndrome, Hurler's (mucopolysaccharidosis I H, gargoylism, dysostosis multiplex), *n.pr* a heritable disorder of mucopolysaccharide metabolism in which excessive acid mucopolysaccharides—dermatan sulfate and heparitin sulfate—are made and stored in the tissues. Clinical manifestations include hypertelorism, open oral cavity with large-appearing tongue, thick eyelids and lips, anomalies of the teeth, and short, broad neck. The skeletal and facial deformities resemble the gargoyles of Gothic architecture. Mental retardation, corneal clouding, hepatosplenomegaly, deafness, and cardiac defects are present.

syndrome, Hutchinson-Gilford (progeria), *n.pr* syndrome of dwarfism, immaturity, and pseudosenility. Patient appears to be bald and elderly at an early age. Hypoplasia of the mandible occurs, and the face is small in relation to the neurocranium.

syndrome, jaw-winking (winking-jaw syndrome), *n* congenital unilateral ptosis and elevation of the lid on opening of the jaw or moving of the mandible to the contralateral side.

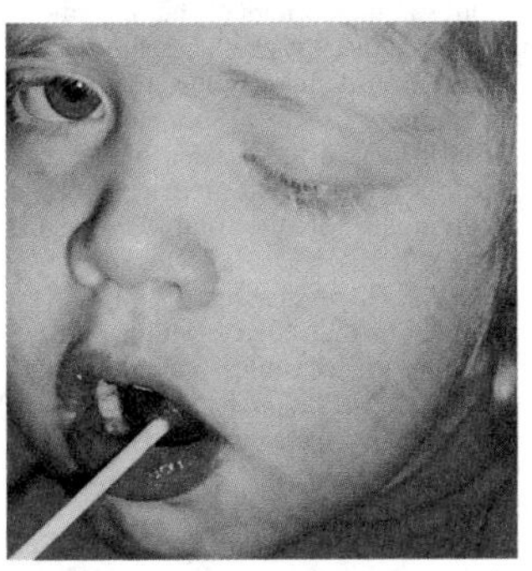

Jaw-winking syndrome. (Zitelli/Davis, 2002)

syndrome, Klinefelter's (XXY syndrome, chromatin-positive syndrome, medullary gonadal dysgenesis), *n.pr* presence in men of an abnormal sex-chromosome constitution. Persons with XXY constitution show the clinical signs of sterility, aspermatogenesis, variable gynecomastia, and often mental retardation. About 50% of subjects with XXXXY variant have cleft palate.

syndrome, Klippel-Feil, *n.pr* fusions of cervical vertebrae, short neck with limited head movement, and extension of the posterior hairline.

syndrome, Lobstein's, *n.pr* See osteogenesis imperfecta.

syndrome, Marfan, *n.pr* tall, thin stature, long, tapered fingers and toes (arachnodactyly), dislocation of the lens of the eye (ectopia lentis), and aneurysm leading to rupture of the aorta.

syndrome, McCune-Albright, *n.pr* a polyostotic form of fibrous dysplasia, usually associated with precocious puberty in females, endocrine disturbances influencing growth, and brown pigmentation of the skin.

syndrome, Melkersson-Rosenthal, *n.pr* transient facial edema, especially swelling of the upper lip, facial paralysis, and lingua plicata. Plicated swelling of the mucosa of the tongue, palate, and buccal mucosa may not be present, or the paralysis may be incomplete.

syndrome, Mikulicz's **(mē′koolich′əz),** *n.pr* a condition characterized by swelling of the parotid, submandibular, sublingual, and lacrimal glands; associated with lymphosarcoma, leukemia, tuberculosis, sarcoidosis, and syphilis.

syndrome, Möbius's, *n.pr* congenital facial diplegia consisting of facial paralysis as well as lingual and masticatory muscle paralysis, inability to abduct the eyes, and anomalies of the extremities.

syndrome, Munchausen **(moon′ chouzen),** *n.pr* a condition in which a patient repeatedly reports to a physician or hospital for treatment of an illness, the symptoms and history of which have been entirely fabricated.

syndrome, myeloproliferative **(mī′əlōprəlif′ərā′tiv),** *n* extramedullary myelopoiesis in adults. It may follow contact with benzol compounds or polycythemia, or it may precede leukemia.

syndrome, nephrotic **(nəfrot′ik),** *n* syndrome that includes proteinuria, hyperlipemia, hypoproteinemia, and edema. It occurs in a variety of conditions in which increased glomerular permeability and urinary loss of protein occur.

syndrome, nevoid basal cell carcinoma **(nē′void bā′zəl kar′si-nō′mə),** *n* a condition inherited as an autosomal dominant trait and characterized by a predisposition for keratocystic odontogenic tumors (odontogenic keratocysts) and skin cancers, especially basal cell carcinoma, as well as the presence of a number of abnormalities or tumors in the skeletal, nervous, endocrine, and other systems.

syndrome, nonarticular pain, *n* one of several painful disorders that limit joint motion and affect the periarticular structures: the tendons, tendon sheaths, bursae, connective tissue, and muscles. Patients commonly call this syndrome "muscular aches and pains." The pains are chronic and nagging and may occur in acute exacerbations. The neck, shoulder, back, thighs, hands, and legs are common sites of irritation. The nonarticular disorders are associated with fibrositis, tendinitis, tenosynovitis, and periarticular muscle spasm. The precipitating agents are often obscure and may be associated with postural or personality disorders. When the acute symptoms of pain, stiffness, and restricted motion are reduced, the tissues resume their normal function.

syndrome, Papillon-Lefèvre, **(päp′-ēyô′-ləfev′rə)** *n.pr* extensive periodontal disease in young patients (juvenile periodontosis) accompanied by keratotic lesions of the palmar and plantar surfaces. In some patients, changes similar to hereditary ectodermal dysplasia also are present.

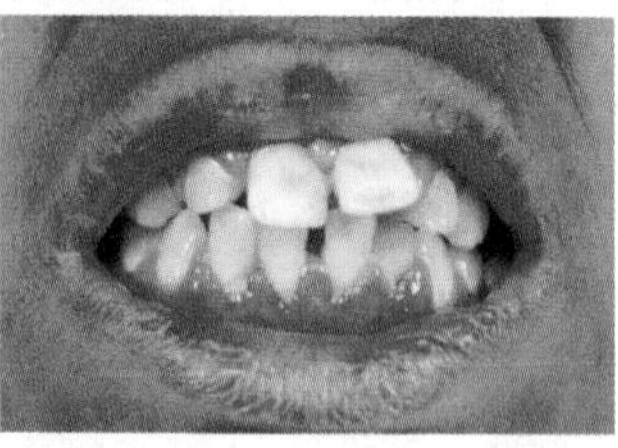

Papillon-Lefèvre syndrome. (Neville/Damm/Allen/Bouquot, 2002. Courtesy Dr. James L. Dickson)

syndrome, paratrigeminal **(par′ətrī′-jem′ənəl),** *n* trigeminal neuralgia, sensory loss, weakness and atrophy of the masticatory muscles, miosis, and ptosis of the upper eyelid on the affected side of the face resulting from a lesion of the semilunar ganglion and fibers of the carotid plexus.

syndrome, Patau's, *n.pr* See trisomy-D.

syndrome, Paterson-Kelly, *n.pr* See syndrome, Plummer-Vinson.

syndrome, Peutz-Jeghers, *n.pr* generalized multiple polyposis of the intestinal tract, consistently involving the jejunum, and associated with melanin spots of the lips, buccal mucosa, and fingers; autosomal dominant inheritance.

syndrome, PHC, *n* See syndrome, Böök's.

syndrome, Pierre Robin, *n.pr* micrognathia of the newborn. Congenital retrognathism associated with cleft palate, glossoptosis, difficulty in swallowing, respiratory obstruction, and cyanosis. This congenital micrognathia corrects itself during the growth of the child if proper care is provided.

syndrome, Plummer-Vinson, *n.pr* a symptom complex that includes fissures at the corners of the oral cavity, sore tongue, dysphagia, achlorhydria, and iron-deficiency anemia. Most commonly seen in females in the fourth and fifth decades of life and associated with a predisposition to carcinoma of the oral cavity and esophagus.

syndrome, premenstrual (PMS), *n* a condition that occurs within 10 days before menstruation and ends soon after menstruation begins. The most common physical and psychologic symptoms may include fatigue, heightened appetite, lack of coordination, headache, bloating or cramping of the abdomen, pain in the joints or back, pressure or pain in the breasts, depression, apprehension, and inappropriately aggressive behavior.

syndrome, radial tunnel, *n* a painful condition caused by the compression of the radial nerve that passes in various branches from the spine through the forearm, wrist, and hand.

syndrome, Ramsey-Hunt, *n.pr* herpetic inflammation of the geniculate ganglion, with herpes zoster of the soft palate, anterior faucial pillar, and auricular area.

syndrome, Reiter's, *n.pr* a syndrome that consists of arthritis (often of the rheumatoid type), conjunctivitis, nonspecific urethritis, and occasionally aphthous ulcers of the oral mucosa.

syndrome, Rieger's, *n.pr* a syndrome the characteristics of which include hypodontia, conical crowns, enamel hypoplasia, dysgenesis of the iris and cornea, and myotonic dystrophy.

syndrome, Riley-Day (familial dysautonomia), *n.pr* disturbances of the autonomic and central nervous systems consisting of hypersalivation, defective lacrimation, excessive sweating, erythematous blotching after emotional upset, relative indifference to pain, and hyporeflexia. Normal growth and motor development are retarded.

syndrome, Robin, *n.pr* See syndrome, Pierre Robin.

syndrome, Roger's, *n.pr* continuous excessive secretion of saliva as the result of cancer of the esophagus or other esophageal irritation.

syndrome, Rosenthal, *n.pr* See hemophilia C.

syndrome, rubella, *n* enamel defects of the primary teeth attributed to prolonged effect of the rubella virus on ameloblasts during fetal life and in the postnatal period.

syndrome, Scheuthauer-Marie-Sainton, *n.pr* See cleidocranial dysostosis.

syndrome, short face, *n* an abnormally short lower facial height relative to other face portions caused by increased levels of mandibular forward rotation during embryologic development.

syndrome, sicca, *n* See syndrome, Sjögren's.

syndrome, Sjögren's (sicca syndrome, xerodermostecisis) **(shur′-grenz),** *n.pr* condition related to deficient secretion of salivary, sweat, lacrimal, and mucous glands (xerostomia, keratoconjunctivitis, rhinitis, dysphagia), increased size of salivary glands, and polyarthritis.

syndrome, Smyth's, *n.pr* See hyperostosis, infantile cortical.

syndrome, Stevens-Johnson, *n.pr* an acute inflammatory disease characterized by oral, ocular, and genital lesions with severe generalized symptoms. The oral lesions are irregularly shaped, painful ulcers. See also erythema multiforme.

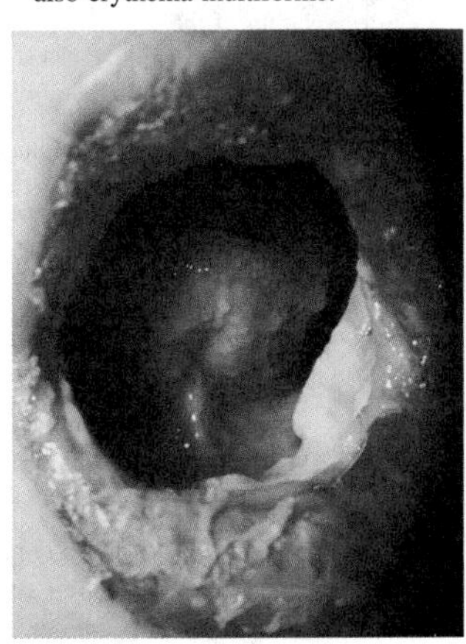

Stevens-Johnson syndrome. (Zitelli/Davis, 2002)

syndrome, Swift's, *n.pr* See acrodynia.

syndrome, temporomandibular joint, *n* an acute muscle spasm in the muscles associated with the protection and movement of the joint. It is believed to be caused by a postural (occlusal) imbalance associated with the muscular tension induced by psychologic stress. The principal symptoms are pain in the region of the joint, limitation of mobility of the mandible, crepitus, clicking sounds in the joint, and often tinnitus.

syndrome, thalassemia (Cooley's anemia, Mediterranean anemia, hereditary leptocytosis) **(thal′əsē′-mēə),** *n* a group of closely related and genetically determined disorders in which a specific decrease in one of the polypeptide chains constituting hemoglobin occurs. The defect results in hypochromic microcytic erythrocytes. Alpha, beta, and delta variants occur, as well as several subtypes based on biochemical techniques. See also thalassemia.

syndrome, Treacher Collins, *n.pr* See dysostosis, mandibulofacial.

syndrome, Turner's (XO syndrome, gonadal dysgenesis, genital dwarfism), *n.pr* a syndrome characterized by the absence of one of the X chromosomes, with affected females being sterile and short of stature and having various congenital anomalies, such as webbing of the neck, low-set ears, wide-set eyes, shieldlike chest, absence of breasts, and cubitus valgus. Common orofacial findings are hypoplastic mandible, high palatal vault, and dental anomalies.

syndrome, Ullrich-Feichtiger, *n.pr* a syndrome that has micrognathia, polydactyly, and genital malformations.

syndrome, Urbach-Wiethe, *n.pr* a syndrome characterized by hyalinosis of the skin and mucous membranes and hoarseness. The skin is infiltrated with yellowish, waxy nodules, and the oral tissues with similar plaques beginning before puberty and becoming increasingly severe. The teeth may be hypoplastic or may fail to develop.

syndrome, vestibular disorder, *n* one of several syndromes involving the vestibule of the ear. The two most common syndromes of vestibular disorders are seasickness, which results from the continuous movement of the endolymph in susceptible individuals (probably related to a disturbance in the reflex control of the eyeball movements), and Meniere's syndrome, of which paroxysmal vertigo is the principal sign but other associated vascular and metabolic disorders can occur.

syndrome, Waardenburg-Klein, *n.pr* a syndrome consisting of congenital deafness, white forelock, increased distance between the inner canthi, the iris of the same eye or of the two eyes having different color (heterochromic irides), and prognathism. Inherited as an autosomal dominant disorder.

syndrome, Weber-Cockayne, *n.pr* a simple nonscarring form of epidermolysis bullosa; transmitted as an autosomal dominant trait. See also syndrome, Goldscheider's.

syndrome, Weech's, *n.pr* See hypohidrotic ectodermal dysplasia.

syndrome, Witkop-von Sallman, *n.pr* a hereditary benign intraepithelial dyskeratosis with gelatinous plaques on hyperemic bulbar conjunctiva and white folds and plaques involving the oral mucosa.

syndrome, Zinsser-Engman-Cole, *n.pr* a syndrome consisting of reticular atrophy of the skin, with pigmentation, dystrophic fingernails and toenails, and oral leukoplakia. Hyperhidrosis of the palms and soles is present, as well as acrocyanosis of the hands and feet.

syneresis (siner′əsis), *n* a process by which a fluid exudate forms on the surface of a hydrocolloid gel, even when the gel is in water or in a humid atmosphere. It is accompanied by shrinkage of the gel.

synergism (sin′urjizəm), *n* a joint action of two drugs in such a manner that one supplements or enhances the action of the other to produce an effect greater than that which may be obtained with either one of the drugs in equivalent quantity or produce effects that could not be obtained with any safe quantity of either drug, or both. See also potentiation.

synergy, *n* the process in which two organs, substances, or agents work simultaneously to enhance the functions and effects of one another.

synostosis (sin′ōstō′sis), *n* the joining of two bones by the ossification of connecting tissues. It occurs normally in the fusion of cranial bones to form the adult skull.

synovial joint (sinō′vēəl), *n* a freely movable joint in which contiguous bony surfaces are covered by articular cartilage and connected by ligaments lined with synovial membrane. Also called *diarthrosis.* See also articulation, temporomandibular.

synovitis (sin′əvī′tis), *n* an inflammatory condition of the synovial membrane of a joint as the result of an aseptic wound or a traumatic injury, such as a sprain or severe strain.

syntax, *n* a property of language involving structural cues for the arrangement of words as elements in a phrase, clause, or sentence.

synthesis, *n* a putting together. The creation of a new entity or idea from elements not previously joined.

synthetic, *n* a substance that is produced by an artificial rather than a natural process or material.

synthetic porcelain, n See cement, silicate.

Synthodont, *n.pr* a brand name for a prefabricated ceramic implant.

syphilid (sif′ilid), *n* a cutaneous lesion of syphilis.

syphilis (sif′ilis) (lues), *n* a sexually transmitted disease caused by *T. pallidum* and usually transmitted by direct contact. Oral lesions include primary chancre, secondary mucous patches and split papule, and tertiary gumma.

syphilis, congenital, n a type that is transmitted prenatally by the mother to the fetus. Congenital syphilis may lead to Hutchinson's incisors, mulberry molars, or rhagades. See also chancre; gumma; incisors, Hutchinson's; molar, mulberry; patch, mucous; and *Treponema pallidum.*

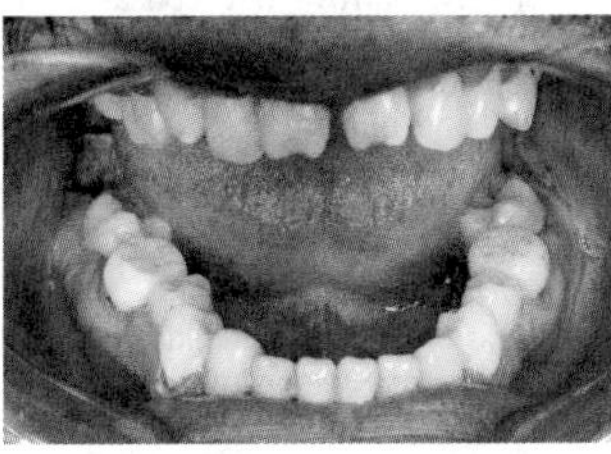

Congenital syphilis. (Regezi/Sciubba/Jordan, 2008)

syphilis, latent, n a stage in which no clinical signs or symptoms of the disease are present. It is usually discovered by serologic tests.

syphilis, primary, n a stage characterized by the appearance of a small painless pustule on the skin of a mucous membrane within 10 to 90 days after exposure. The lesion may appear anywhere on the body where contact with a lesion on an infected person has occurred, but it is most often seen in the anogenital region. It quickly erodes, forming a painless, bloodless ulcer, called a *chancre,* exuding a fluid that swarms with spirochetes. The disease is highly contagious during this stage.

syphilis, secondary, n a stage that occurs about 2 months after the primary stage. Secondary syphilis is characterized by general malaise, anorexia, nausea, fever, headache, alopecia, bone and joint pain, or the

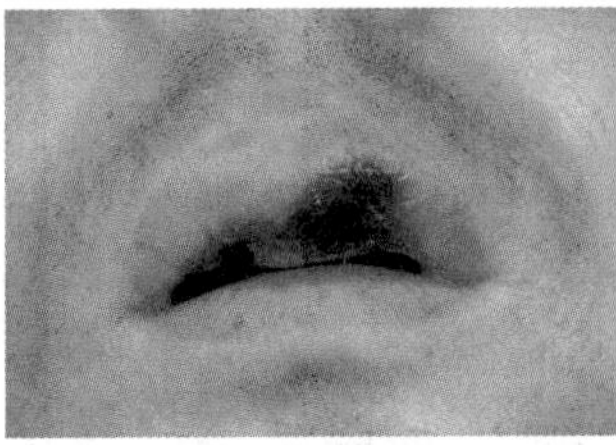

Primary syphilis. (Kerr/Ash/Millard, 1983)

appearance of a morbilliform rash that does not itch, flat white sores in the oral cavity and throat, and condylomata lata papules on the moist areas of the skin. The disease is highly contagious during this stage.

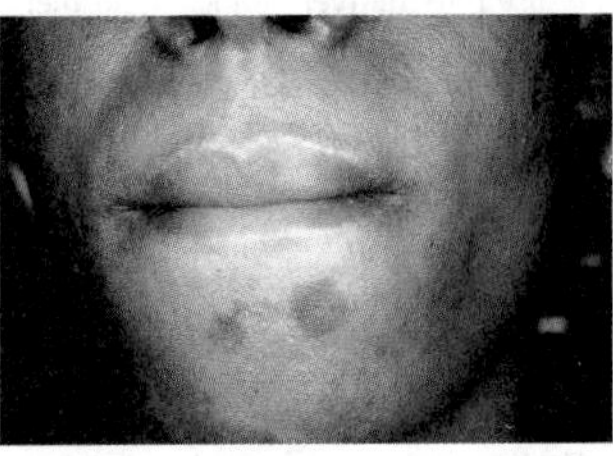

Secondary syphilis. (Regezi/Sciubba/Jordan, 2008)

syphilis, tertiary, n stage may not develop for 3 to 15 years after the initial infection. It is characterized by the appearance of soft, rubbery tumors, called *gummas;* the valves of the heart may be damaged, and late stages may lead to mental or physical disability and premature death.

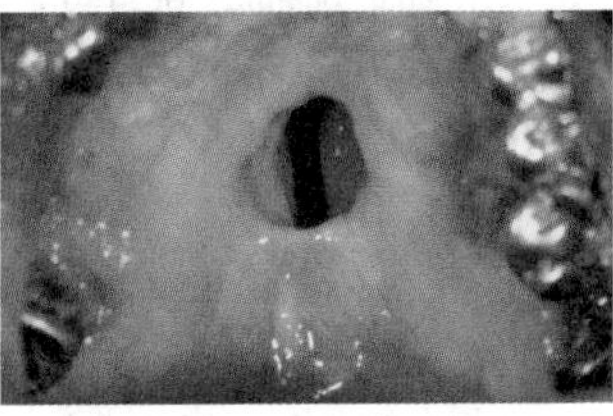

Tertiary syphilis. (Regezi/Sciubba/Jordan, 2008)

syringe (sirinj′), *n* an apparatus of metal, glass, or plastic material consisting of a nozzle, or needle, barrel, and plunger or rubber bulb; used to inject a liquid into a cavity or under the skin.

syringe, air, *n* a device by which air may be applied to a given area. An instrument supplied as part of the dental unit, consisting of a hand grip, nozzle, pressure-regulating valve, and hose connected to the compressed air supply.

syringe, air-water, *n* a device that delivers pressurized streams of water and air for use in dental procedures.

syringe, aspirating, *n* a type of hypodermic syringe used in local anesthesia that allows the user to confirm, in advance of delivering the anesthetic agent, that the needle has not entered a blood vessel.

syringe, aspirating, breech-loading, *n* an aspirating syringe, used to deliver a local anesthetic agent, that is assembled by inserting the rubber stopper end of the anesthetic cartridge first toward the thumb ring, then the diaphragm end toward the needle opening before setting the harpoon and attaching the needle.

syringe, combination, *n* a syringe that is usually part of the dental unit through which air, water, or a combination of the two may be delivered under pressure to the desired area.

syringe, hand air, *n* an air syringe consisting of a metal tube bent at one end, terminating in a reduced diameter, and enlarged at the other end to engage a rubber bulb. The bulb is compressed by hand to supply a controlled spurt of air to a given area.

syringe, jet injector, *n* a needle-free syringe that uses high pressure through small openings (jets) to administer a local anesthetic agent to oral mucosa.

S

syringe, nonaspirating **(nonas′pərā′ting),** *n* a syringe that does not aspirate before the local anesthetic agent is deposited because it does not contain a harpoon at the end of the piston; this type of syringe should never be used during dental procedures because it is not possible to be certain of the exact location of the needle tip.

syringe, warm air, *n* an air syringe equipped with an electric heating element to heat the air to any desired temperature.

syringe, water, *n* a device, usually part of the dental unit, permitting controlled application of water to a given area. It has a flow control, pressure regulator, and heating element.

system, *n* a set or series of organs or parts that unite in a common function.

system, acid-base buffer, *n* the system by which a virtually constant pH level of the blood and body fluids is maintained. The base and acid electrolytes associated with normal metabolism are continuously introduced into the bloodstream. Notwithstanding the marked amounts of base or acid or both introduced into the bloodstream during exercise, rest, hunger, or the ingestion of fluid and solid foods, the pH level of the blood remains rather constant between 7.3 and 7.5. Four means by which this relatively narrow but constant pH level is maintained are: the buffer system of the blood, tissue and cell fluids, and mineral salts of the bone matrix; excretion and retention of carbon dioxide by the lungs; excretion of an acid or alkaline urine; and the formation or excretion of ammonia and organic compounds.

system, apothecaries' **(əpoth′əkar′ēz),** *n* a nondecimal system of weights and measures traditionally used by druggists. See also system, avoirdupois.

system, autonomic nervous, *n* See autonomic nervous system (ANS).

system, avoirdupois **(av′ərdəpoiz′),** *n* a commercial nondecimal system of weights and measures. See also system, apothecaries'.

system, central nervous (CNS), *n* the brain and spinal cord, including their nerves and end organs; controls all voluntary acts.

system, circulatory, *n* the heart and blood vessels. Three major groups of blood vessels are defined: arteries, capillaries, and veins. The system transports metabolites to and from the tissue cells.

system, computer, *n* an assembly of procedures, processes, methods, routines, techniques, and equipment united by some form of regulated interaction to form an organized whole. It is an approach to a complex problem.

system, flowchart, *n* a pictorial diagram illustrating the flow of information into, through, and out of a system of programs.

system, hematopoietic **(hē′mətō′-poiet′ik),** *n* a term used to describe collectively the blood, bone marrow, lymph nodes, spleen, and reticuloendothelial cells.

system, masticatory, *n* the organs and structures primarily functioning in mastication: the jaws, teeth, and their supporting structures; temporomandibular articulation; mandibular musculature; tongue; lips; cheeks; and oral mucosa and their nerve supplies.

system, metric, *n* a decimal system of weights and measures almost universally used in scientific and professional work, including the writing of prescriptions. The individual units are based on an international set of standards, notably the meter, liter, and kilogram. In dentistry, measurement is done by the metric system.

system, musculoskeletal, *n* the system of body structures that provides the energy and movement necessary for the functions of life. The muscles, bones, and connective tissues of the body are grouped together into one system, and they are intimately connected in their individual and combined functions. E.g., for muscle to accomplish its ultimate purpose of movement by contraction, bone, leverage, and connective tissue are required to transmit the force that the contraction generates. In the oral cavity and its related structures the musculoskeletal tissues fulfill the mechanical and structural requirements for movement of the mandible and some related visceral functions, such as respiration and digestion.

system, neurohormonal, *n* the system by which the hormone secretions of the endocrine glands function in part as the regulators of both visceral and somatic function and have intimate anatomic and functional relationships with the nervous system by the union of the pituitary gland and the hypothalamus of the cerebrum. The pituitary gland has a pars nervosa, which is an extension of the anterior part of the hypothalamus, and a pars intermedia, which is an epithelial evagination of the secretory tissue from the stomodeum of the embryo. From its position in the cranial structures in the sella turcica, the pituitary gland regulates, by its union with the nervous system, the whole endocrine system, with its many glands; these glands in turn partially regulate the viscera and somatic muscle organs.

system, occlusal (occlusal scheme), *n* the form or design and arrangement of the occlusal and incisal units of a dentition or of the teeth on a denture. See also system, masticatory.

system, parasympathetic nervous, *n* one of the motor divisions of the autonomic nervous system. It is described as the *craniosacral division* and does not have the simplified structural apparatus of the strong sympathetic adrenal axis about which to function. It inhibits the heart, contracts the pupils, and, in emotional states, produces a vagus-insulin axis of activity. The several parts function rather independently. The ocular division relates to the midbrain, and the bulbar division relates to the hindbrain. The bulbar division supplies the facial, glossopharyngeal, and vagus nerves. It also supplies the secretory and vasodilator fibers of the salivary glands and mucous membranes of the oral cavity and pharynx. In conditions of very loud noise or unusual anxiety states, the parasympathetic system causes unaccounted-for spontaneous urination, excessive salivary and gastric juices, and either nausea or vomiting.

system, proaccelerin-accelerin, *n* See factor V.

system, proconvertin-convertin, *n* See factor VII.

system, stomatognathic, *n* the combination of all the structures involved in speech and the reception, mastication, and deglutition of food. The system is composed of the teeth, jaws, muscles of mastication, epithelium, and temporomandibular joints and nerves that control these structures.

system, sympathetic nervous, *n* one of the two opposing motor systems in the autonomic nervous system that mediate the activity of the viscera. (The other is the *parasympathetic* *system.*) It is composed of 21 or 22 ganglia in chains on each side of the spinal cord. The fibers connect with the spinal cord through these ganglia. The actions are closely allied to the action of the medulla of the adrenal gland; thus a sympathetic-adrenal axis that functions as a unit to protect and regulate the body environment may be conceived. The sympathetic control is modified by the volitional somatic control of the patient. The volitional control, superimposed on the autonomic control, gives rise to great variations in motor patterns, as seen in the face in the presence of emotional changes, such as in the blushing of shame and pallor of fear.

system, vascular, closed tube, *n* the type of vascular system, as in humans, in which the blood circulates through the vessels (or tubes) and is not dissipated into the tissues. The closed vascular tube system offers resistance to the pumping action of the heart because the pressures are cumulative with each pumping action. The elastic walls in the arterial vessels, particularly in the aorta, absorb the additional energy and release it slowly, thus creating the possibility of maintaining a fairly steady and safe pressure head throughout the vascular system. The high-pressure point at the height of cardiac contraction is the *systole,* and the low point before the ventricular contraction is the *diastole.*

system, vascular, open tube, *n* in some vertebrates a vascular system with an open end that causes the blood fluid to dissipate into the tissues. This system starts with a maximal head pressure that diminishes until inertia in the blood is overcome. The blood is returned to the heart by muscle function, gravity, and diffusion. The blood pressure in this system fluctuates from a maximum at the heart to a minimum at the tissue cell.

S

system, venous, *n* a system of interconnected blood vessels that returns blood to the heart from the tissue and capillary bed through progressively larger vessels. The following affect the return of blood to the heart: thoracic pressure, associated with respiration; gravity, associated with body posture; the valves, diameter of the lumen, and muscle structure of the veins; muscle contraction of the somatic structures; the pressures in the arteriole system and capillary bed; and the nervous and hormonal system controls that regulate cardiomuscular activity. The influences over the venous system circulation are collectively termed *venopressor mechanisms.*

systematic error (sis′təmat′ik), *n* a nonrandom statistical error that affects the mean of a population of data and defines the bias between the means of two populations.

systematically (sis′təmat′iklē), *adj* done in a well-organized, carefully followed pattern of procedure.

systemic lupus erythematosus (SLE) (sistem′ik loo′pus er′ə-them′ətō′sus), *n* an autoimmune disease that can be life threatening. Patients may have a distinctive pattern of facial redness and oral lesions. Endothelial damage to heart valves similar to that caused by rheumatic fever may occur.

systole (sis′təlē), *n* the period of contraction of the heart. The term specifically designates the contraction of the ventricles, as distinguished from auricular contraction. It occurs with the first heart sound. The pressure from the systolic contractions is taken up and stored as potential energy by the elastic properties of the aorta and other great vessels of the arterial system. This storage of energy protects the smaller, more fragile vessels from undue pressure. The even flow and steady pressure of the blood are sustained by the controlled release of the potential energy stored in the arterial walls into kinetic energy for movement of the blood during the diastolic phase of heart function. The pressure recorded at the height of the ventricular contraction is the systolic pressure. In the adult the normal blood pressure is 120/80 mm Hg (systolic/diastolic). It rises with advancing age to 135/89 at 60 years of age. See also diastole; pressure, blood, stage; and pressure, systolic blood.

T cell, *n* a small, circulating lymphocyte produced in the bone marrow that matures in the thymus. T cells primarily mediate cellular immune responses, such as graft rejection and delayed hypersensitivity.

T-4 cell, *n* a thymus-derived lymphocyte of the body's immune system with a role of destroying or neutralizing cells or substances identified as "nonself." The human immunodeficiency virus (HIV) commonly targets the T-4 cells, with the result that the body's immune defenses are severely damaged and opportunistic infections are allowed to flourish.

tabes, *n* a gradual, progressive wasting of the body in any chronic disease.

tabes dorsalis **(tā′bēz dôrsal′is)** ***(locomotor ataxia),*** *n* a form of neurosyphilis in which degeneration in the posterior roots of the spinal nerves and posterior column of the spinal cord exists. Manifestations include pain and paresthesia of the trunk, hands, and feet, abdominal pain crises, ataxia, Argyll Robertson pupil, atrophy of the optic nerve, and Charcot's joint.

table, occlusal, *n* the occlusal surfaces of the premolars and molars; the basic collective topography, including the form of the cusps, inclined planes, marginal ridges, and central fossae and grooves of the teeth.

table of allowances, *n* a list of covered services with an assigned dollar amount that represents the total obligation of the plan with respect to payment for such service but does not necessarily represent the dental professional's full fee for that service. Also called *schedule of allowances* and *indemnity schedule.*

tablet, *n* a small, solid dose form of a medication. It may be compressed or molded in its manufacture, and it may be of almost any size, shape, weight, and color. Most tablets are intended to be swallowed whole.

tachycardia (tak′ikär′dēə), *n* an excessively rapid action of the heart; the pulse rate is usually above 100 beats/min.

tachyphylaxis (tak′əfəlak′sis), *n* **1.** the rapid development of tolerance on administration of closely spaced successive doses of a drug or poison. **2.** a decreasing response that follows consecutive injections at short intervals.

tachypnea (tak′ipnē′ə), *n* an excessively rapid respiration. A respiratory neurosis marked by quick, shallow breathing.

tacrine HCl (tak′rēn), *n brand name:* Cognex; *drug class:* cholinesterase inhibitor; *action:* a centrally acting, reversible inhibitor of cholinesterase enzyme; *use:* treatment of mild to moderate cognitive defects associated with Alzheimer's disease.

tacrolimus (FK506), *n brand name:* Prograf; *drug class:* immunosuppressant; *action:* inhibits T-lymphocyte activation leading to immunosuppression; *use:* prophylaxis of organ rejection in patients receiving allogenic liver transplants.

tactile (tak′təl), *adj* pertaining to the sense of touch.

tailpiece, *n* See aid, speech, prosthetic, velar section.

Takahara's disease, *n.pr* See disease, Takahara's.

Talwin, *n.pr* the brand name for pentazocine lacatate, a potent analgesic, which is as effective as morphine. Talwin is a controlled substance.

tamoxifen citrate (təmok′səfen sit′rāt), *n brand name:* Nolvadex; *drug class:* antineoplastic, antiestrogen hormone; *action:* inhibits cell division by binding to cytoplasmic receptors, inhibits DNA synthesis; *use:* advanced breast cancer that has not responded to other therapy.

tang, *n* See connector, minor.

tank, processing, *n* a receptacle used in the photographic or radiographic darkroom for the chemical solutions used in the processing of films.

tannic acid, a vegetable tanning agent that attaches itself to collagen by hydrogen bonds. Tannic acid is used in dentistry as a cavity conditioner before placing a restoration.

tantalum (Ta) (tan′təlum), *n* a silvery metallic element, its atomic number is 73 and its atomic weight is 180.9479. Tantalum is a relatively inert, noncorrosive, malleable metal used in prosthetic devices, such as skull plates and wire sutures.

tantrum, *n* a sudden outburst or violent display of rage, frustration, and bad temper, usually occurring in a maladjusted child or immature or disturbed adult.

tape, dental, *n* a ribbon of waxed nylon or silk used to aid the prophylaxis of interproximal spaces and the proximal surfaces of the teeth. The flattened, wide form of dental floss. See also dental floss.

tapering, *n* a process of shaping a clasp arm the better to distribute flexure throughout its length, thus reducing fatigue, strain hardening, and resultant fracture.

tapering arch, *n* a dental arch that converges from the molars to the central incisors to such a degree that lines passing through the central grooves of the molars and premolars intersect within one inch anterior to the central incisors. See also arch, tapering.

tardive dyskinesia (tär′div dis′kinē′zēə, -zhə), *n* possible reaction to the extended use of antipsychotic medicines in which the muscles of the face, limbs, and trunk move uncontrollably.

target, *n* the small tungsten block, embedded in the face of the anode, that is bombarded by electrons from the cathode in a radiographic tube.

target cell, *n* **1.** also called *leptocyte,* an abnormal red blood cell characterized by a densely stained center surrounded by a pale, unstained ring that is encircled by a dark, irregular band. **2.** a cell having a specific receptor that reacts with a specific hormone, antigen, antibody, antibiotic, sensitized T cell, or other substance.

target group, *n* a set of persons who serve as the focal point for a particular program or service. This is a smaller sample than the target population.

target organ, *n* **1.** an organ intended to receive a therapeutic dose of irradiation. **2.** an organ intended to receive the greatest concentration of a diagnostic radioactive tracer.

target population, *n* all individuals belonging to a certain group who have a distinct set of qualities.

target symptoms, *n.pl* symptoms of an illness that are most likely to respond to a specific treatment.

target-film distance (TFD), *n* See distance, target-film; source-film distance.

target-object distance (TOD), *n* See source-object distance.

tarnish, *n* **1.** surface discoloration or loss of luster by metals. Under oral conditions, it often results from hard and soft deposits. **2.** a chemical process by which a metal surface is discolored or its luster destroyed.

tartar, *n* See calculus, dental.

taste, *n* the sense of perceiving different flavors in soluble substances that contact the tongue and trigger nerve impulses to special taste centers in the cortex and the thalamus of the brain. The four basic traditional tastes are sweet, salty, sour, and bitter.

taste bud, *n* any one of many peripheral taste organs distributed over the tongue and the roof of the oral cavity. See also lingual papillae.

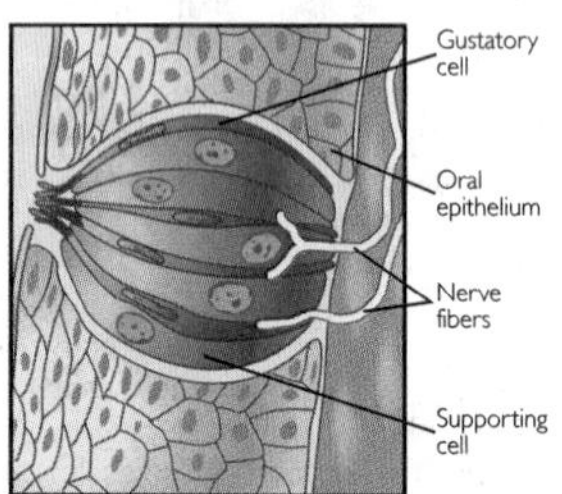

Taste bud. (Thibodeau/Patton, 2005)

taste enhancers, *n.pl* food additives that have little or no flavor of their own but when added to food bring out the taste of certain foods. Monosodium glutamate (MSG) is the most common flavor or taste enhancer.

tattoo, amalgam, *n* See amalgam tattoo.

taurodontism (tôr′ōdon′tizəm), *n* a tooth in which the pulp chamber is elongated and enlarged, and extends deeply into the region of the roots. A similar condition is seen in the teeth of cud-chewing animals.

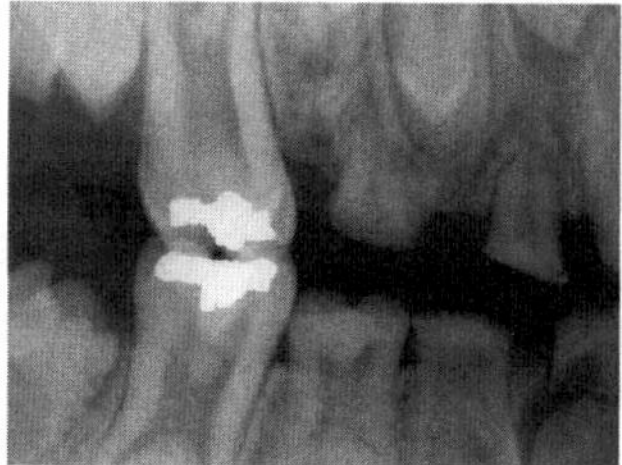

Taurodontism. (Regezi/Sciubba/Jordan, 2008)

tautomer (tôt′əmər), *n* structural isomers that differ only in the position of a hydrogen atom, or proton.

tax, *n* a ratable portion of the proceeds or value of the property and labor of the citizen; any contribution imposed by government for the use and service of the state.

tax brackets, n.pl the income intervals of the graduated income tax law that establish the rate of tax for each level of income.

Tax Equity and Fiscal Responsibility Act of 1982 (TEFRA), n.pr legislation (Public Law 97-248) affecting health maintenance organizations and the Medicare and Medicaid programs. Provides regulations for the development of HMO risk contracting with the Medicare program and, through an amendment, establishes new provisions for the foundation and operation of peer review organizations.

tax planning, n making business and investment decisions based on estimated income and current and projected tax laws.

tax shelter investments, n.pl investments that reduce, remove, or defer income from state and federal income tax liability.

taxes, *n.pl* the sum of monies collected by the various branches of a government.

taxonomy (takson′əmē), *n* a system for classifying organisms on the basis of natural relationships and assigning them appropriate names.

Tay-Sachs disease (tā-saks), *n.pr* an inherited, neurodegenerative disorder of lipid metabolism caused by a deficiency of the enzyme hexosaminidase A, which results in the accumulation of sphingolipids in the brain. The condition, which is transmitted as an autosomal recessive trait, occurs predominantly in families of Eastern European Jewish origin, specifically the Ashkenazic Jews.

teaching rounds, *n.pl* See rounds.

team practice, *n* professional practice by a group of complementary health care providers who collectively manage the care of a patient population.

tears, *n* the saline fluid excreted from the lacrimal glands that moistens, cleans, and protects the eyes.

technetium 99 (teknē′shēəm), *n* the radionuclide most commonly used to image the body in nuclear medicine scans. It is preferred because of its short half-life and because the emitted photon has an appropriate energy for imaging techniques.

technic (tek′nik), *n* See technique.

technical competence, *n* the ability of the practitioner, during the treatment phase of dental care and with respect to those procedures combining psychomotor and cognitive skills, consistently to provide services at a professionally acceptable level.

technical quality, *n* the degree to which the physically measurable attributes of procedures in dental care meet professionally acceptable standards.

technician, *n* a person skilled in the performance of technical procedures.

technician, dental, n See technician, dental laboratory.

technician, dental laboratory, n an individual skilled in the art of executing the dental professional's prescription for the mechanical fabrication of dental appliances.

technique (teknēk′), *n* **1.** a skillful and detailed method of executing procedures to accomplish a desired result. **2.** the method of performance of manipulation in any art; the terms *technique* and *technic* are used synonymously, but the word *technique* pertains more to the artistic skill involved.

technique, aseptic, n task performed in a sterile environment in order to avoid contact with harmful bacteria.

technique, bisection of the angle, n an intraoral radiographic technique whereby an angle formed by the mean plane of the tooth and the mean plane of the film is bisected, and the central ray is directed through the tooth perpendicular to the bisection. This is the application of Cieszynski's rule of isometry. See also rule of isometry, Cieszynski's.

technique, calibrated angle, *n* an intraoral radiographic technique using a specified degree in vertical angulation from the horizontal plane. It is a variation of the bisection of the angle technique and assumed to be the correct angulation for the majority of patients.

technique, chew-in, *n* See chew-in technique.

technique, double investing, *n* a method of investing wax patterns, whereby the pattern is covered with a primary layer of investment; this core is then invested, before or after the primary investment has set, in an outer, thinner mix of the same or a different type of investing material.

technique, dual impression, *n* a technique by which the anatomic form of the teeth and immediately adjacent structures is recorded and by which the free-end denture foundation areas are registered in their functional form.

technique, Eames's, *n.pr* in dental amalgam, a procedure using mercury and alloy in approximately a 1:1 ratio, thus not having residual mercury in the plastic mix.

technique, filling, *n* the method used to obliterate the space in the root of the tooth once occupied by the dental pulp.

technique, Fones's, *n.pr* See method, Fones's.

technique, Gow-Gates (GG) anesthetic, *n* the injection of a local anesthetic that anesthetizes the mandible, along with the floor of the oral cavity, the anterior two-thirds of the tongue, the skin covering the zygomatic bone, and corresponding facial, buccal, and lingual tissues.

technique, hydroflow, *n* See dentistry, washed-field.

technique, impression, *n* a method and manner used in making a negative likeness. The series of operations or procedures used for making an impression.

technique, long cone, *n* the use of an extended cone distance, generally 14 inches (35 cm) or more, in oral radiography. It is generally used with, but not confined to, parallel film placement.

technique metered spray, *n* refers to a topical anesthetic dispersal technique that controls the amount and rate at which a drug is administered.

technique, Miller's radiographic localization, *n* a method of identifying the buccolingual dimension of a tooth by taking a second radiographic image at an angle of 90° to the first. The technique is also useful for identifying the position of subgingival anomalies. Also called *right-angle technique; SLOB rule*, which stands for same **l**ingual, **o**pposite **b**uccal. See also localization, radiographic; technique, parallel.

technique, parallel (right-angle technique), *n* a technique in intraoral radiography in which the film is positioned parallel to the long axes of the teeth and the central ray is directed perpendicular to both the film and the teeth.

technique, periapical, *n* any of several methods for placing radiographic film to capture images of tooth root structure.

technique, punch, *n* a surgical incision of a circular area of soft tissue immediately above a submerged implant in order to expose the full diameter of the implant platform.

technique, scoop, *n* office jargon for a one-handed method of needle recap and disposal in which the needle is used in an upward sweep to lift a safety cap onto the needle. The needle is then removed and discarded into a sharps container.

technique, short cone, *n* the use of a short cone distance, usually 8 inches (20 cm) or less, that is supplied by the manufacturer as short cone. It is generally used with, but not confined to, the bisection of the angle technique.

technique, telephone, *n* the friendly but businesslike conveying of ideas over the telephone.

technique, thermal expansion, *n* a casting procedure whereby compensation is made for metal shrinkage by thermal expansion of the refractory investment mold.

technique, wax expansion, n a casting procedure whereby compensation is made for metal shrinkage by thermal expansion of the wax pattern before setting of the investment.

teeth, *n* See tooth.

teeth, hypermobile, n the propensity of teeth to abnormally move or shift positions within the alveolar bone. This condition can occur as a result of inflammation, metabolic abnormalities, or traumatic injury.

teeth, milk, n See teeth, primary.

teeth, opposing, n teeth that are opposite each other, one in the maxilla and one in the mandible, that ideally come into occlusal contact with each other.

teeth, short, n teeth that are severely worn from erosion or abrasion.

teeth, splayed anterior, n anterior teeth that have been forced to slope outward, usually as a result of pressure from the tongue.

teeth, tilted, n teeth that are at such an angle as to cause them to be out of centric contact with opposing teeth during occlusion.

teething (tēthing), *n* the eruption of primary teeth, which is preceded by increased salivation. Young children may become restless and irritable during this period. Inflammation of the gingival tissues before complete emergence of the crown may cause a temporary painful condition.

Teflon, *n.pr* brand name of a proprietary plastic material (polytetrafluoroethylene) used in reconstructive surgery of the jaw and chin.

Tegopen, *n.pr* the brand name for cloxacillin, an antistaphylococcal penicillin.

Tegretol, *n* See carbamazepine.

telangiectasia (təlan′jēektā′zhə), *n* **1.** the dilation of the capillaries and small arteries of a region. A hereditary form (hereditary hemorrhagic telangiectasia) may appear intraorally. **2.** a disorder characterized by cutaneous and mucosal vascular macules, nodules, and arterial spiders that tend to bleed sporadically.

telangiectasia, hereditary hemorrhagic (Rendu-Osler-Weber disease), n the dilation of small vessels and capillaries resulting from a genetic factor, with a tendency to bleed. Lesions may occur on the tongue as small, raised, red to bluish-red elevations.

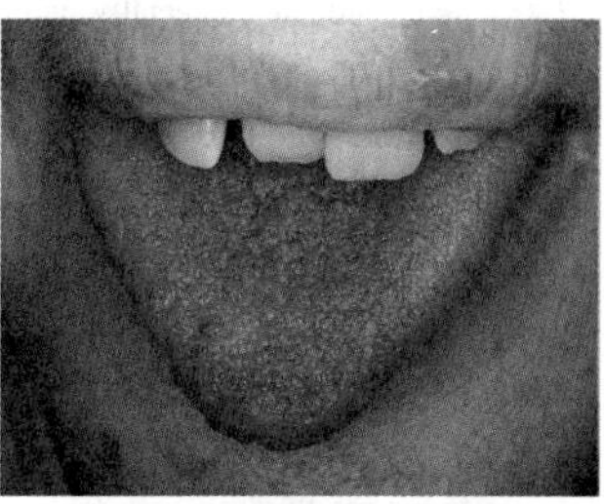

Hereditary hemorrhagic telangiectasia. (Regezi/Sciubba/Jordan, 2008)

Telecommunication Device for the Deaf (TDD), *n* a machine that converts written text to speech, enabling the deaf to use the telephone.

Telecommunication Relay Service (TRS), *n* a system that enables the deaf and hard of hearing to use the telephone. The caller talks to a third party, who types the information so the deaf party can read it on a TDD.

telemedicine, *n* the use of two-way television communication by which two or more physicians can consult on a patient. The consulting physicians have access to the diagnostic information as well as the ability to view and question the patient directly before making a diagnosis or offering a professional opinion.

telemetry (təlem′ətrē), *n* the electronic transmission of data between distant points.

teleradiography (tel′ərā′dēog′rəfē), *n* Radiography at a longer distance than is usually used (6 feet, or 1.8 m).

telic (tel′ik), *adj* (teleologic), assigning purpose to functions as if they were provided by a creative planner.

temazepam (təmaz′əpam′), *n brand name:* Restoril; *drug class:* benzodiazepine, sedative-hypnotic (Controlled Substance Schedule IV); *action:* produces central nervous system (CNS) depression at limbic, thalamic, hypothalamic levels of the CNS; *uses:* sedative and hypnotic for insomnia.

temperature, *n* the degree of sensible heat or cold.

temperature, body, n the measurable temperature of the body. Normal range of variations, 98°F to 99°F (35.5°C to 37°C) orally and 99°F to 100°F (37°C to 38°C) rectally, with much wider ranges for skin.

temperature, body, regulation, *n* homeostasis of body temperature. Results from a balance of heat production (external heat plus heat from muscle contraction and other chemical processes) and heat loss (through lungs, sweating, surface radiation, and excretions).

temperature, casting, *n* the required degree of heat necessary to bring a metal to proper fluidity for introduction into a refractory mold.

temperature, core, *n* the temperature of the internal tissues of the body, this temperature stays stable, unlike the temperature of the outer body surfaces, which are affected by the environment.

temperature, recrystallization, *n* the lowest temperature at which the distorted grain structure of a cold-worked metal is replaced by a new, strain-free grain structure during prolonged annealing. Time, purity of metal, and prior deformation are important factors.

tempering (hardening heat treatment), *n* the hardening or toughening of steels by heating. Treatment of an alloy in such a manner that solid-solid transformation occurs. Precipitation of intermetallic substances occurs, increasing the proportional limit and hardness of the alloy.

tempering, gold, *n* the hardening of gold alloys by cold working or by heating and then cooling slowly.

tempering, hydrocolloid, *n* storing of the material after liquefaction at a temperature that will increase the viscosity to the optimal manipulative degree of solidity.

tempering, steel, *n* counteracting of the hardening heat treatment to the extent needed for the particular tool or structure. It is heated to a predetermined temperature and then quenched in water or oil.

template (tem′plət), *n* a pattern or mold forming an accurate copy of an object or shape.

template, implant, *n* an early type of subperiosteal implant that was fabricated from a cast carved to simulate the host bone. Measurements made from radiographs taken with a template or wire mold resting on the soft tissues determined the carving of the cast.

template, occlusal, *n* a stone or metal (electroformed) occlusal table made from a wax occlusal path registration of jaw movements and against which the opposing supplied teeth are occluded.

template, orthodontics, *n* a cephalometric tracing of an age- and sex-normed facial and dental profile used in the analysis of facial and dentition variations in malocclusion.

template, prosthetic, *n* a curved or flat plate used as an aid in setting denture teeth.

template, surgical, *n* a thin transparent resin base shaped to duplicate the form of the impression surface of an immediate denture and used as a guide for surgically shaping the alveolar process and its soft tissue covering to fit an immediate denture.

template, viral, *n* the process of RNA/DNA replication associated with retrovirus activity.

template, wax, *n* a wax recording of the occlusion of the teeth.

temporal, *adj* pertaining to the sides of the skull behind the orbits.

temporal arteritis (tem′pərəl är′-tərī′tis), *n* a progressive inflammatory disorder of cranial blood vessels, principally the temporal artery, occurring most commonly in women over 70 years of age. The temporal artery is typically tender, swollen, and pulseless. Symptoms are intractable headache, difficulty in chewing, weakness, rheumatoid pain, and loss of vision if the central retinal artery becomes occluded.

temporal artery, *n* the arteries on each side of the head: the superficial temporal artery, the middle temporal artery, and the deep temporal artery.

temporal bone, *n* one of a pair of large bones forming part of the inferior portion of the cranium and containing various cavities and recesses associated with the ear. Each temporal bone consists of four portions: the mastoid, the squama, the petrous, and the tympanic.

temporal eminential angle, *n* the degree of slope between the axis-orbital plane and the discluding slope of the eminence.

temporal lobe, *n* the lateral region of the cerebrum, below the lateral fissure. It contains the center for smell, some association areas for memory and learning, and a region where choice is made of thoughts to express.

temporalis muscle (tempəral'is), *n* one of the four muscles of mastication. It arises in a fan-shaped pattern from the squama of the temporal bone and courses downward to insert along the anterior border of the ramus of the mandible. It is a major closing muscle of the jaw.

temporary, *adj* pertaining to the interim treatment used to protect a patient between appointments.

temporary base, *n* See baseplate.

temporary prosthesis, *n* See prosthesis, temporary.

temporary stopping, *n* See stopping, temporary.

temporary superstructure, *n* a prosthodontic appliance (removable or fixed) that is used, often immediately postoperatively, as a transitional appliance either for cosmetics or splinting, or both.

temporomandibular articulation (tem'pərōmandib'ūlur), *n* See articulation, temporomandibular.

temporomandibular disorder, *n* a disorder associated with one or both of the temporomandibular joints.

temporomandibular extraoral radiographic examination, *n* See examination, radiographic, extraoral, temporomandibular.

temporomandibular joint, *n* See articulation, temporomandibular.

temporomandibular joint (TMJ) arthrography, *n* a form of radiographic imaging using a compound of radioactive iodine that appears light-gray or whitish and contours soft tissues within the space between the joints.

temporomandibular ligament, *n* an oblique band of tissue that extends downward and backward from the zygomatic process to the neck of the mandible.

temporomandibular pain-dysfunction syndrome, *n* See temporomandibular disorder.

tender, legal, *n* coin or money that the law compels a creditor to accept in payment of a debt when offered by the debtor in the right amount.

tendon, *n* the white, glistening fibrous bands of tissue that attach muscle to bone.

tendonitis, *n* the inflammation of a tendon, usually stress or strain related.

tenosynovitis (ten'ōsī'nəvī'tis), *n* the inflammation of a tendon sheath caused by calcium deposits, repeated strain or trauma, high levels of blood cholesterol, rheumatoid arthritis, gout, or gonorrhea. Occasionally movement yields a crackling noise over the tendon.

tensile, *adj* having a degree of elasticity; having the ability to be extended or stretched.

tensile strength (ten'sil, -sīl), *n* See strength, tensile.

tension (ten'shən), *n* the state of being stretched, strained, or extended.

tension headache, *n* a pain that affects the head as the result of overwork or emotional strain, involving tension in the muscles of the neck, face, and shoulders.

tension, interfacial surface, *n* the tension or resistance to separation possessed by the film of liquid between two well-adapted surfaces (e.g., the thin film of saliva between the denture base and the tissues).

tentative, *adj* not final or definite, such as an experimental or clinical finding that has not been validated.

teratogenesis (ter'ətəjen'əsis), *n* the development of physical defects in the embryo.

teratogenic agents (ter'ətəjen'ik), *n.pl* See teratogens.

teratogenic effect, *n* the combined consequences of consuming a harmful substance, such as alcohol, on a developing fetus; may manifest itself as growth deficiency and/or mental retardation; fetal alcohol syndrome is an example.

teratogens (tərat'ōjens), *n.pl* agents that cause congenital malformations and developmental abnormalities if introduced during gestation.

teratology (ter'ətol'əjē), *n* the study of the causes and effects of congenital malformations and developmental abnormalities.

teratoma (ter′ətō′mə), *n* a tumor composed of cells capable of differentiating into any of the three primary germ layers. Teratomas in the ovary are usually benign dermoidal cysts; those in the testis are generally malignant.

terazosin HCl (terā′zəsin′), *n brand name:* Hytrin; *drug class:* antihypertensive, anti-adrenergic; *action:* decreases total vascular resistance, which is responsible for a decrease in blood pressure; *use:* hypertension as a single agent or in combination with diuretics or β-blockers.

terbinafine HCl (terbin′əfēn′), *n brand name:* Lamisil; *drug class:* antifungal; *action:* inhibits key enzyme, squalene epoxidase, involved with resultant fungal cell death; *uses:* tinea pedis, tinea cruris, tinea corporis.

terbutaline sulfate (terbū′təlēn′), *n brand names:* Brethaire, Brethine, Bricanyl; *drug class:* selective β_2-agonist; *action:* relaxes bronchial smooth muscle by direct action on β_2-adrenergic receptors; *uses:* bronchospasm, asthma prophylaxis, premature labor inhibitor.

terconazole (terkon′əzōl′), *n brand names:* Terazol 3, Terazol 7; *drug class:* local antifungal; *action:* interferes with fungal DNA replication; binds sterols in fungal cell membranes, which increases permeability, leaking of nutrients; *uses:* vaginal, vulvar, vulvovaginal candidiasis.

terfenadine (terfen′ədēn′), *n brand name:* Seldane; *drug class:* antihistamine; *action:* acts on blood vessels and gastrointestinal and respiratory systems by competing with histamine for peripheral H_1 receptor sites; decreases allergic response by blocking histamine; *uses:* rhinitis, allergy symptoms.

term infant, *n* a neonate, regardless of birth weight, born after the end of the thirty-seventh and before the beginning of the forty-third week of gestation.

terminal, *adj* **1.** near or approaching an end, such as a terminal bronchiole or a terminal illness. *n* **2.** an input/output device that has a two-way communication capability with a computer.

terminal, computer, n a device in a system or communications network at which data can either enter or leave.

terminal hinge position, n See position, hinge, terminal.

terminal illness, n an advanced stage of a disease with an unfavorable prognosis and no known cure.

terminal jaw relation record, n See record, terminal jaw relation.

terminal plane, n ideal molar relationship in the primary dentition when in centric occlusion.

termination date, *n* See expiration date.

terra alba (ter′ə al′bə), *n* gypsum added to plaster or stone to accelerate the setting reaction.

tertiary health care (ter′shēer′ē), *n* a specialized, highly technical level of health care that includes diagnosis and treatment of disease and disability in sophisticated large research and teaching hospitals. Specialized intensive care units, advanced diagnostic support services, and highly specialized personnel are characteristic of tertiary health care services.

tertiary syphilis (sif′əlis), *n* the most advanced stage of syphilis, resulting in infections of the cardiovascular and neurologic systems and marked by destructive lesions involving many tissues and organs.

test(s), *n* a clinical or laboratory procedure designed to evaluate constituents or functions of the body.

test, acetone, n See test, ketone bodies.

test, ACTH-stimulation (Thorn's test), n a test of adrenocortical reserve based on changes in the eosinophil count and urinary levels of 17-ketosteroids and 17-hydroxycorticoids as a result of intravenous infusion or intramuscular injection of ACTH.

test, allergy, intradermal, n a test for allergy performed by injecting a preparation containing the suspected allergen into the dermis.

test, amylase **(am′ilās),** *n* a determination of serum amylase, which is useful in the diagnosis of acute pancreatitis and after operations in which the pancreas might have been in-

T

jured. The Somogyi sarcogenic method is often used, and the results are given in *Somogyi* units, defined as the amount of amylase needed to digest 1.5 g of starch in 8 minutes at 37°C. The normal range is 60 to 200 units/100 ml. The serum amylase is also elevated in mumps and other diseases of the salivary glands.

test, amyloid **(am′iloid),** *n* See test, Congo red.

test, antiviral antibody, *n* antibody tests in viral diseases. Included are complement-fixation tests for poliomyelitis, psittacosis, and Coxsackie infections; hemagglutination-inhibition tests for mumps, influenza, and encephalitides; and neutralization tests.

test, Aschheim-Zondek **(ash′hīm-tson′dek),** *n.pr* See test, pregnancy.

test, ascorbic acid, intradermal, *n* a test for ascorbic acid deficiency based on the decoloration of an intradermal injection of a purple dye (2,6-dichlorphenol-indophenol). Normally with a wheal of 4 mm, using a dye concentration of N/300, decoloration occurs in 10 to 15 minutes.

test, basophilic aggregation **(bā′sō-fil′ik),** *n* a test for lead poisoning based on increased stippling of erythrocytes. More than 2% stippled cells are seen in lead poisoning. See also test, lead.

test, Bell's palsy, *n.pr* simple clinical tests, such as motor function tests, in which the patient is asked to whistle, pucker the lips, smile, or wrinkle the forehead; also sensory function tests in which the patient is asked to taste sweet with sugar, sour with citric acid, bitter with quinine, and salt with sodium chloride.

test, Benedict's, *n* a nonspecific copper reduction test for glucose in the urine. Cupric sulfate in the Benedict's reagent is reduced by glucose during the reaction to cuprous oxide, a reddish-orange precipitate.

test, bilirubin **(bil′iroo′bin),** *n* qualitative, presumptive, quantitative, or specific determinations for bilirubin in the urine and blood serum. Included are Gmelin's test and van den Bergh's test.

test, bleeding time, *n* techniques for determining the time interval required for hemostasis to occur after a standardized wound has been made in the capillary bed. See also test, Duke's and test, Ivy's.

test, Brinell hardness **(brinel′),** *n.pr* a means of determining surface hardness by measuring the amount of resistance to the indentation of a steel ball. Recorded as the Brinell hardness number (BHN); the higher the number, the harder the material. Generally indicative of abrasion resistance.

test, Bromsulphalein (BSP) **(brōm′-səlfal′ēən),** *n* a test of liver function based on the removal of a known quantity of Bromsulphalein from the blood in a measured period of time. Normal values are less than 5% retention at the end of 45 minutes with an intravenous dose of 5 mg/kg body weight. It is a useful test of hepatocellular disease and detoxifying ability but is not applicable in the presence of extrahepatic or intrahepatic obstructive jaundice.

test, Bunnell, *n.pr* See test, Paul-Bunnell.

test, capillary resistance (Rumpel-Leede-Hess test, Gothlin's test), *n* a test of capillary fragility based on the number of petechiae that develop when a standardized intraluminal positive pressure is applied to the capillaries either by a blood pressure cuff or a suction cup applied to the skin. See also test, tourniquet.

test, caries activity, *n* a test used to predict the probability of developing new or increased decay; may include assessments of saliva and plaque for the presence of certain designated microorganisms or studies of salivary secretion and sugar clearance.

test, CO_2 capacity (CO_2 combining power test), *n* a general measure of the alkalinity or acidity of the blood. Various normal adult ranges are given (e.g., 23 to 30 mEq/L of serum or 55 to 70 vol/100 ml of serum). A low value is found in diabetic acidosis, hyperventilation, certain kidney diseases, and severe diarrhea. A high value is found in excessive administration of ACTH or cortisone, intake of sodium bicarbonate, and persistent vomiting.

test, CO_2 combining power, *n* See test, CO_2 capacity.

test, cold bends, *n* a mechanical test used for assessing ductility.

test, colorimetric caries susceptibility (Snyder's test), *n* a method of determining the concentration of acid-producing bacteria in the saliva by use of bromcresol green in a culture medium. The reliability of this and other salivary bacterial tests for dental caries susceptibility is questionable.

test, Congo red, *n.pr* a test for amyloidosis based on the more rapid disappearance (excess of 60% injected dye in 1 hour) of Congo red from the serum of affected patients than from that of normal individuals. Gingival biopsy and positive staining with methyl violet or crystal violet also indicate amyloidosis.

test, creatinine clearance **(krēat′inin),** *n* a renal function test of exogenous creatinine clearance. It is a convenient clinical test of glomerular filtration rate. It is calculated as the quotient of the product of urine creatinine (mg/L) and urine volume (L/24 hr) divided by the serum creatinine concentration (mg/L). The normal value for young healthy adults of average size (1.73 M^2 body surface area) is 115 to 155 L/24 hr (±15%).

test, dermal, *n* See test, skin.

test, Dick's (scarlet fever test), *n* a skin test to determine susceptibility or immunity to scarlet fever. A positive test is indicated when an area of erythema and edema measuring more than 10 mm in diameter occurs 8 to 24 hours after an intradermal injection of a standardized erythrogenic toxin.

T

test, Duke's, *n.pr* a test of bleeding time as indicated by the time that elapses before a puncture wound of the earlobe ceases to bleed. Normal range is 2 to 4½ minutes.

test, electric, *n* a test to determine whether a pulp is vital.

test, erythrocyte sedimentation **(ərith′rōsīt′ sed′əməntā′shən),** *n* a macroscopic test of the blood used to detect certain pathologic conditions, particularly inflammation. The blood cells are allowed to settle in the presence of an anticoagulant and the time (sedimentation time) determined. The greater the time or rate, the more severe the condition. Pregnancy and menstruation affect the sedimentation.

test, flow, *n* used in the ADA specification for dental amalgam; measured as the percentage shortening of a cylinder of the material.

test, fluorescent treponemal antibody, absorbed (FTA-APS) **(trep′ənē′məl),** *n* a modification of the original FTA test for syphilis that employs a protein preparation from the Reiter treponeme.

test for trigeminal nerve function, *n.pl* three simple clinical tests for trigeminal nerve function: (1) *sensation:* apply gentle touch, pinpricks, or warm or cold objects to areas supplied by the nerve and note responses; (2) *reflex:* try the jaw jerk and eye and sneeze reflexes; (3) *motor function:* test the patient's ability to chew and work against resistance and observe contraction of the masseter and temporal muscles by visual examination and digital palpation.

test, Foshay's, *n.pr* a skin test for tularemia using the Foshay antigen.

test, Friedman's **(frēdmənz),** *n.pr* See test, pregnancy.

test, glare, *n* an examination of blade sharpness using a magnifying glass under light, which reveals dull edges as round, shiny, reflective surfaces.

test, glucose paper, *n* a test in which paper is impregnated with glucose oxidase and other reagents (TesTape, Clinistix). When the paper is moistened with fresh urine, the presence of glucose will cause a change in the color of the paper.

test, glucose tolerance (GTT), *n* a test for abnormalities of carbohydrate tolerance by glucose loading and subsequent serial measurements of the concentration of glucose in the blood. Graphic representation of the concentration and the elapsed time makes up the glucose tolerance curve. Abnormal curves occur in diabetes mellitus, thyrotoxicosis, Cushing syndrome, acromegaly, and pheochromocytoma.

test, Gothlin's, *n.pr* See test, capillary resistance.

test, hardness, *n* See hardness, Mohs; test, Brinell hardness; test,

Knoop hardness; and test, Vickers hardness.

test, Hess's, *n.pr* See test, capillary resistance.

test, histoplasmin **(his'tōplaz'min),** *n* a skin test to determine sensitization to *Histoplasma capsulatum.* A positive test indicates past or present infection (histoplasmosis).

test, infectious mononucleosis, *n* one of several tests for the diagnosis of infectious mononucleosis (e.g., Paul-Bunnell test).

test, intracutaneous, *n* See test, skin.

test, intradermal, *n* See test, skin.

test, Ivy's, *n.pr* a test of bleeding time performed by making a standard wound and touching the blood with filter paper every 30 seconds until no blood appears on the paper. Normal range is 3 to 7 minutes.

test, Janet's, *n.pr* a test to differentiate between functional and organic anesthesia. With the eyes closed, patients are instructed to say "yes" or "no" as they feel or do not feel the examiner's touch. In functional anesthesia, they will say "no," whereas in organic anesthesia, they will say nothing.

test, ketone bodies (acetone test, Rothera's test) **(kē'tōn),** *n* nitroprusside reaction tests for acetone and acetoacetic acid and the ferric chloride test for acetoacetic acid. Commercially prepared nitroprusside test tablets (Acetest) and powder (Acetone Test Denco) are available.

test, Kline's, *n.pr* a flocculation test for syphilis based on the combination of the cardiolipin antigen with reagin to form grossly visible aggregates.

test, Knoop hardness, *n.pr* a means of measuring surface hardness by resistance to the penetration of an indenting tool made of diamond. Produces an indentation that has a diamond or rhombic shape. Especially preferred for testing hardness of tooth structure.

test, laboratory, *n* investigative procedures performed in the laboratory that are useful in the diagnosis of disease, including biopsy examination of tissue specimens, determination of type and characteristics of associated microorganisms, serology, blood and urine chemistry, hemogram (red cell count, hemoglobin content, white cell count, differential white cell count), and metabolic studies (basal metabolic rate).

test, LE, *n* a test for lupus erythematosus based on the presence of a single (or multiple) homogenous basophilic inclusion(s) in polymorphonuclear leukocytes. Such LE cells have also been found in cases of rheumatoid arthritis, allergic reactions to penicillin, hydralazine toxicity, and "lupoid cirrhosis." Thus the test is not definitive for lupus only; it is one of the diagnostic tests for causation.

test, lead, *n* a test used to detect clinical lead poisoning or exposure to lead (e.g., coproporphyrinuria test, trace element analysis, urinary lead content test, and basophilic aggregation test).

test, Leede's, *n.pr* See test, capillary resistance.

test, Mann-Whitney U, *n.pr* a powerful nonparametric statistic test of significance between two means with unequal sample sizes.

test, Mantoux **(mäntoo'),** *n.pr* an intracutaneous tuberculin test using either old tuberculin (OT) or purified protein derivative (PPD). A positive reaction read 24 and 48 hours after injection shows erythema and edema greater than 5 mm in diameter and indicates past or present tuberculosis.

test, Mazzini's **(motsē'nēz),** *n.pr* a flocculation test for syphilis.

test, Mohs, *n.pr* See hardness, Mohs.

test, nontreponemal antigen, *n.pl* serologic tests for syphilis using nontreponemal antigens. Such tests are not absolutely specific or sensitive for syphilis. Included are the Kline, Kahn, and Kolmer tests, and the VDRL slide test.

test, one-stage, *n* See time, prothrombin.

test, oral glucose tolerance test (OGTT), *n* the application of glucose to the body, typically administered orally, in order to determine the rate at which glucose is metabolized. Can be used to diagnose diabetes mellitus.

test, patch, *n* (percutaneous test), a test for allergies that is performed by placing the suspected allergen in direct contact with the skin or mucosa. See also test, skin.

test, Paul-Bunnell, *n.pr* a test for infectious mononucleosis based on increased agglutination of sheep red blood cells resulting from heterophil antibodies in the serum. The test is considered positive if dilution of serum of 1:80 or higher agglutinates the sheep cells. Elevated agglutinin titers are more likely to be found during the second or third week of the disease, but the serum may not become positive until 7 weeks have elapsed.
test, percussion, *n* a method of examination executed by striking the tissues of the area being examined with the fingers or an instrument, listening for resulting sounds, and observing the response of the patient.
test, percutaneous **(pur'kūtā'nēus),** *n* See test, patch.
test, Phelan's **(fā'lənz),** *n.pr* a common test for diagnosing carpal tunnel syndrome. In a positive Phelan's test, tingling or numbness is felt within one minute when the subject's hands are held with the wrists flexed (usually at a 90° angle).
test, phenolsulfonphthalein (PSP) **(fē'nôlsul'fonthā'lēn),** *n* a renal test that roughly estimates glomerular function by measuring the rate of excretion of the dye after intravenous injection. Normally, after 15 minutes, 25% or more of the dye should be excreted in the urine.
test, plasma ketone *n* a test using nitroprusside for the detection of high levels of ketone bodies in the blood. The test is read 0 to 4 plus. A strongly positive reaction is seen in diabetic ketoacidosis.
test, prothrombin consumption (serum prothrombin time), *n* a convenient screening test of the first stage of blood coagulation as determined by the quantity of prothrombin remaining after coagulation. The test reflects the formation of plasma thromboplastin, provided the one-stage prothrombin time of plasma is normal. See also time, prothrombin.
test, pulp, *n* a diagnostic test to determine clinical pulp vitality and/or abnormality.
test, Reiter protein complement-fixation (RPCF) **(rī'tur),** *n.pr* treponemal antigen test for syphilis using extracts from the nonpathogenic Reiter treponeme.
test, reverse torque (RTT) (tork), *n* a test used to determine the degree of osseointegration of an implant by applying a rotational force in the opposite direction originally used to set the implant into the bone; in essence, it measures the shear strength at the point where the implant meets the bone.
test, Rockwell, *n* an indentation test for hardness of a material. A static load is placed on a steel ball or diamond point, and the depth of the indentation is measured on the instrument. The depth of the indentation is remeasured after the load is increased. The hardness number is related to the type of point used and to the depth of the indentation.
test, Rothera's, *n.pr* See test, ketone bodies.
test, routine, *n* a test or group of tests performed on most or all patients to detect relatively common disorders or to establish a base for further evaluation of a patient.
test, Rumpel-Leede-Hess, *n.pr* See test, capillary resistance.
test, scarlet fever, *n* See test, Dick's.
test, Schick, *n.pr* a skin test to demonstrate the presence or absence of an immunity to diphtheria.
test, scratch (skin test), *n* a test for allergies performed by placing a preparation containing the allergen on the skin and scratching the skin. A positive reaction is indicated by the formation of a wheal and flare.
test, serologic **(ser'əloj'ik),** *n* test of blood serum for the diagnosis of infectious diseases.
test, Snyder's, *n.pr* See test, colorimetric caries susceptibility.
test, sterilizer, *n* the periodic use of spore strip, color strip, or other microbial test to ensure that a sterilizer (autoclave, oven) is killing all microbes predictably.
test strip, *n* a blood test used to check blood sugar levels in diabetics. The patient places a drop of blood on the strip, and the strip changes color according to the level of blood sugar present.
test, subcutaneous, *n* See test, skin.
test, syphilis, *n* a serologic test for syphilis based on the presence

T

of a reagin, appearing during the second or third week of infection. Included are the Hinton, Kahn, Kline, Mazzini, Wassermann, and *Treponema pallidum* immobilization tests.

test, tension, *n* an evaluation used to determine the presence or absence of attached gingiva within the oral cavity. The tongue, cheek, and lip are retracted to apply pressure at the mucogingival junction and make the alveolar mucosa taut.

test, thermal, *n* the use of heat or cold as an aid in diagnosis (e.g., the use of heat or cold in testing the pulp).

test, Thorn's, *n.pr* See test, ACTH-stimulation.

test, thromboplastin generation **(throm′bōplas′tin),** *n* a test of the integrity of the first stage of blood coagulation and the nature of the defect. A patient's serum, plasma, or platelets are substituted in a system that is complete except for one of the factors to be tested for (antihemophilic factor, plasma thromboplastin antecedent, plasma thromboplastin component, or platelets), and the rate of thromboplastin generation is determined.

test, tourniquet **(tur′niket),** *n* a test for capillary fragility based on counting petechiae in a given area of the arm after application of the rubber cuff of a sphygmomanometer for 15 minutes.

test, transillumination, *n* a test for a pulpless tooth in which the use of transmitted light shows a shadow of the root when the pulp is necrotic or has been replaced by a filling (not always reliable).

test,* Treponema pallidum *immobilization (TPI) **(trep′ənē′mə pal-id′əm),** *n* a test to confirm syphilis by demonstrating the immobilization of *Treponema pallidum* by specific antibodies in the serum of an infected individual; not widely used.

test, tuberculin, *n* a test for past or present infection with tubercle bacilli. See also test, Mantoux.

test, tuberculin skin **(toobur′kūlin),** *n* an intradermal injection of old tuberculin (OT) or purified protein derivative (PPD) to determine a specific sensitivity or susceptibility to tuberculosis.

test, tularemia, *n* See test, Foshay's.

test, U, Mann-Whitney, *n.pr* See test, Mann-Whitney U.

test, urea clearance, *n* a clinical test of renal function determined by the clearance of urea from the plasma by the kidney each minute. Average normal value is 75 ml/min (75% to 125% of normal).

test, urine, routine, *n* the routine examination of the urine, including amount, appearance, pH level, specific gravity, qualitative tests for sugar and protein, and microscopic examination of sediment.

test, van den Bergh's, *n.pr* a test of hepatic function by measuring serum conjugated ("direct-reacting") 1-minute bilirubin, total serum bilirubin, and, by difference, unconjugated (indirect) bilirubin. Obstructive jaundice and hemolytic jaundice give abnormal values.

test, VDRL (Venereal Disease Research Laboratory), *n.pr* a serologic nontreponemal antigen test for the detection of syphilitic reagin by means of a reaction between the reagin and a standard antigen.

test, Vickers hardness, *n.pr* a penetration type of hardness test using a square-based pyramid made of diamond.

test, vitality, *n* the procedure using thermal, electrical, or mechanical stimuli to determine the response of the pulp in a tooth.

test, Wassermann, *n.pr* a complement-fixation test for syphilis.

test, Zondek's, *n.pr* See test, pregnancy.

tests, liver function, *n.pl* tests to measure the severity of liver disease, aid in the differential diagnosis of the various types of disease of the hepatobiliary system, and follow the course of liver disease. Screening tests include urine bile, urine urobilinogen, Bromsulphalein (BSP) excretion, serum transaminases, thymol turbidity, cephalin-cholesterol flocculation, and van den Bergh's reaction (1 minute direct and total).

tests, pancreatic function, *n.pl* tests of enzyme levels in blood and urine (amylase, lipase), fecal fat content, trypsin activity, nitrogen content, alteration of digestive capacity, and alteration of pancreatic secretion via duodenal intubation.

tests, pregnancy (Aschheim-Zondek test, Friedman's test), *n.pl* biologic or chemical tests that determine pregnancy. The tests are usually based on changes in the ovaries of an animal injected with the urine of a pregnant woman. Included are the Aschheim-Zondek test (using mice or rats) and the Friedman test (using virgin rabbits). Male frogs and female and male toads are also used. A saliva test has also been used.

tests, pulmonary function, *n.pl* tests used to evaluate respiratory function (e.g., tests of vital capacity, tidal volume, maximal breathing capacity, timed vital capacity, arterial blood gases).

tests, rapid reagin, *n.pl* serologic tests for syphilis that permit rapid and economic screening in the field. Included are the rapid plasma reagin (RPR) test and the unheated serum reagin (USR) test.

tests, renal function, *n.pl* quantitative tests including inulin or mannitol clearance for the glomerular filtration rate (GFR), paraaminohippurate (PAH) clearance for renal plasma flow, and the maximum rate of tubular excretion of paraaminohippurate and of reabsorption of glucose for the measurement of excretory and reabsorptive functions of the renal tubules. Clinical renal tests are used to assess the extent of renal impairment. They include blood urea nitrogen (BUN), nonprotein nitrogen (NPN), urea clearance, endogenous creatinine clearance, filtration fraction, phenolsulfonphthalein (PSP), and concentration tests.

tests, screening, *n.pl* a group of tests especially chosen to detect specific abnormalities.

tests, skin, *n.pl* tests to determine the sensitivity or susceptibility to infections by a specific agent, the presence of an allergy, or the presence of a nutritional deficiency. Included are the Mantoux, Schick, Dick, Frei, histoplasmin, and Foshay tests for infectious diseases (tests in which allergens are placed onto or into the skin) and the intradermal ascorbic acid, dermal, intradermal (intracutaneous), patch (percutaneous), scratch, and subcutaneous tests.

tests, thyroid function, *n.pl* tests for thyroid function (e.g., radioactive iodine uptake, protein-bound iodine, basal metabolic rate, serum cholesterol, triiodothyronine suppression, thyroid-stimulating hormone tests).

tests, transaminase **(transam′inās),** *n.pl* tests for serum glutamic oxaloacetic transaminase (SGOT) and serum glutamic pyruvic transaminase (SGPT). The normal value for serum glutamic oxaloacetic transaminase is 40 units or less; that for serum glutamic pyruvic transaminase is 35 units or less. The serum glutamic oxaloacetic transaminase value in myocardial infarction is 3 to 20 times the normal.

tests, treponemal antigen, *n.pl* tests for syphilis using *Treponema pallidum* or extracts from a treponeme as antigen. Included are *T. pallidum* immobilization (TPI), *T. pallidum* agglutination (TPA), fluorescent treponemal antibody (FTA), Reiter protein complement-fixation (RPCF), and *T. pallidum* complement-fixation (TPCF) tests.

testing stick, *n* in dentistry, a sterile plastic or acrylic rod that has a 3-inch length and a ¼-inch diameter and is used to determine the sharpness of an instrument.

testosterone/testosterone cypionate/testosterone enanthate/testosterone propionate (testôs′tərōn′ sip′ēōnāt′ inan′thāt prō′pēənāt′), *n brand names:* Andro-100, Histerone-50, Testamone-100, Testaqua, Testoject-50; *drug class:* androgen, anabolic steroid (Controlled Substance Schedule III); *action:* in many tissues, testosterone is converted to dihydrotestosterone, which interacts with cytoplasmic protein receptors to increase protein production; natural hormone that functions to regulate spermatogenesis and male secondary sex characteristics; also functions as an anabolic steroid; *uses:* treatment of androgen deficiency, delayed puberty, female breast cancer, certain anemias.

tetanic contraction (tetan′ik), *n* a condition of continuous contraction in a voluntary muscle caused by a steady stream of efferent nerve impulses.

tetanus (tet′ənəs), *n* an acute, potentially fatal infection of the central nervous system caused by tetanospasmin, which is an exotoxin, elaborated by an anaerobic bacillus, *C. tetani.*

tetanus and diphtheria toxoids (Td), n an active immunizing agent containing detoxified tetanus and diphtheria toxoids that slowly produce an antigenic response to the diseases. Typically administered as part of the immunization series of preschool children.

tetany, *n* a disorder characterized by hyperreflexia, muscle spasms and cramps, foot and ankle spasms, choreiform convulsions, and sometimes stridor. It is due to the malfunction of calcium metabolism. Possible causes are vitamin D deficiency, the ingestion of alkaline salts, hyperthyroidism, or alkalosis. There are many types of tetany.

tetany, hyperventilation **(hī′purven′tilā′shən tet′ənē),** *n* the neuromuscular irritability and tonic carpopedal muscle spasm resulting from the alkalosis that may be caused by forced respiration over an extended time.

tetracaine/tetracaine HCl (topical), *n brand name:* Pontocaine Cream; *drug class:* topical anesthetic (ester group); *action:* inhibits nerve impulses from sensory nerves, which produces anesthesia; *uses:* local anesthesia of mucous membranes, pruritus, sunburn, sore throat, cold sores, oral pain, rectal pain and irritation, control of gagging.

tetracycline (te′trəsī′klēn), *n* an antibiotic produced by certain strains of *Streptomyces.* Its administration during tooth formation may lead to intrinsic stain due to enamel discoloration that appears as brown to yellow horizontal lines.

tetracycline HCl, n brand names: Achromycin, Achromycin V, Tetracyn; *drug class:* tetracycline, broad-spectrum antibiotic; *action:* inhibits protein synthesis and phosphorylation in microorganisms, bacteriostatic; *uses:* syphilis, gonorrhea, lymphogranuloma venereum, rickettsial infections, acne, actinomycosis, anthrax, bronchitis, GU infections, sinusitis and many other infections.

tetracycline periodontal fiber, n brand name: Actisite; *drug class:* tetracycline, broad-spectrum antiinfective; *action:* antimicrobial effect related to inhibition of protein synthesis; decreases incidence of postsurgical inflammation and edema; suppresses bacteria and acts as a barrier to bacterial entry; acts on cementum or fibroblasts to enhance periodontal ligament regeneration; *use:* adjunctive treatment in adult periodontitis.

tetrology of Fallot (tetral′əjē falō), *n* a congenital heart problem in which four defects occur at the same time: a hole between the two ventricles, a narrowing below the pulmonary valve, a misaligned aorta, and an overdeveloped cardiac muscle tone.

Tg value, *n* the transition point of glass; in dentistry, the temperature at which resin becomes soft.

thalamus (thal′əmus), *n* an ovoid mass in the brain immediately lateral to the third ventricle that serves as the principal relay and integration station for the sensory systems in the body.

thalassemia (thal′əsē′mēə) (hereditary leptocytosis, hereditary microcytosis), *n* a hereditary, chronic, hemolytic anemia with erythroblastosis. A complex of hereditary disorders characterized by microcytosis and increased red blood cell destruction and often associated with abnormal hemoglobins and increased normal trace hemoglobins. These disorders are prevalent in people of Mediterranean, African, and Asian ancestry. Disorders include Cooley's anemia, Cooley's trait, hemoglobin H disease, Hb S-thalassemia, Hb C-thalassemia, and Hb E-thalassemia.

thalassemia major (Cooley's anemia, erythroblastic anemia, familial erythroblastic anemia, hereditary microcytosis, Mediterranean anemia, Mediterranean disease), n the severe homozygous form of thalassemia characterized by a marked microcytic hypochromic anemia, atypical nucleated red blood cells, marked increase in hemoglobin F, and skeletal changes (underdevelopment, mongoloid facies, anterior open bite).

thalassemia minor (Cooley's trait), *n* a heterozygous form of thalassemia that is a carried state with relatively mild manifestations; α_2 hemoglobin is elevated.

theophylline/theophylline sodium glycinate, *n brand names:* Aerolate Sr, Asmalix, Respbid, Slo-Bid, Theolair, Theovent, Uniphyl; others; *drug class:* xanthine; *action:* relaxes smooth muscle of respiratory system by blocking phosphodiesterase, which increases cAMP; *uses:* bronchial asthma, bronchospasm of chronic obstructive pulmonary disease, chronic bronchitis.

theorem (thē′ərəm), *n* **1.** a proposition to be proved by a chain of reasoning and analysis. **2.** a proven proposition used in the solution of a more advanced problem.

theory (thē′ərē), *n* an opinion or hypothesis not based on actual knowledge.

theory, Prothero "cone," *n.pr* See retention.

theory, quantum, *n* the theory that in emission or absorption of energy by atoms or molecules, the process is not continuous but takes place by steps, each step being the emission or absorption of an amount of energy called a *quantum.*

theory, somatotype, *n* the theory of W. H. Sheldon, suggesting that body structure is correlated with certain temperaments and predisposes to mental disorders.

therapeutic dose, *n* the amount of a medication required to produce the desired effect.

therapeutic endpoint, *n* the defining factors that denote the end of a therapeutic process, such as the return to gingival health, reduction of pocket depth, and a stable clinical attachment level.

therapeutic index (ther′əpū′tik), *n* See index, therapeutic.

therapeutic vehicle, *n* a device used to transport and retain some agent for therapeutic purposes (e.g., radium carrier).

therapeutics, *n* the art and science of treatment of disease.

therapist, *n* a person with special skills, obtained through education, training, and experience, in one or more areas of health care.

therapy (ther′əpē), *n* the treatment of disease, injury, or illness.

therapy, antibiotic, *n* the treatment of disease states by the local or systemic administration of antibodies.

therapy, antimicrobial, *n* a treatment modality that attacks the microorganisms responsible for a specific disease or condition.

therapy, chlorhexidine chip, *n* controlled delivery of the antimicrobial agent chlorhexidine in which a tiny, biodegradable dose of the drug is inserted into the periodontal pocket, where it continues to slowly release medication for approximately 7 to 10 days before disintegrating. This therapy is a means of attacking periodontal infection at its source without systemic involvement.

therapy, compromise periodontal maintenance, *n* a program of continuing periodontal treatment designed to slow disease progression in patients for whom surgery is not an option because of specific health concerns or economic restrictions.

therapy, doxycycline polymer, *n* delivery via syringe and cannula of a biodegradable liquid form of the antimicrobial agent doxycycline polymer directly into a periodontal pocket. The medication hardens upon contact with moisture, thus sealing the pocket and allowing the agent to destroy periodontal pathogens as it dissolves.

therapy, growth modification, *n* a treatment employed to modify the growth of the jaw or other bones as they are still developing, usually to treat cases of malocclusion.

therapy, hormonal replacement, *n* the administration of synthetic female hormones in order to ease the negative impacts of losing these hormones due to menopause, hysterectomy, or disease.

therapy, indirect pulpal, *n* the application of a drug that heals the pulpal cells beneath a layer of sound or carious dentin, as in a moderately deep preparation for a restoration.

therapy, megavoltage radiation, *n* a form of radiation therapy used in the treatment of oral cancer. It delivers a more precise point of contact than other forms.

therapy, myofunctional (myotherapeutic exercises), *n* the use of muscle exercises as an adjunct to mechanical correction of malocclusion.

therapy, oxygen, *n* the providing of additional oxygen for patients who need it.

therapy, periodontal, *n* the treatment of the periodontal lesion. Such therapy has two principal objectives: the eradication or arrest of the periodontal lesion with correction or cure of the deformity created by it, and the alteration in the oral cavity of the periodontal climate that was conducive or contributory to the periodontal breakdown.

therapy, periodontal, maintenance phase, *n* the part of periodontal therapy that is necessary for the preservation of the results obtained during active therapy and for the prevention of further periodontal disease; an extension of active periodontal therapy, requiring the combined efforts of both the periodontist and the patient.

therapy, pharmacotherapeutic nonsurgical pocket **(fär′məkōther′əpū′tik),** *n* the use of both systemic and topical antibiotic compounds to fight bacterial infections in periodontal pockets.

therapy, pocket, *n* the debridement or removal of deposits and endotoxins from the periodontal pocket in order to begin the healing process.

therapy, pulp canal, *n* See endodontology.

therapy putty, *n* a malleable, doughlike substance used in hand exercises to enhance the force and control of the hand muscles.

therapy, radiation (radiotherapy), *n* the treatment of disease with a type of radiation.

therapy, radiation, external beam, *n* a treatment for cancer in which a beam of high- or low-yield radiation is directed from outside the body at the site of the cancerous tumor or lesion; may cause unnecessary radiation to normal tissues.

therapy, radiation, internal, *n* a treatment for cancer in which the radiation source takes the form of an interstitial implant. It is placed in the body among the affected tissues to provide a directed dose of radiation that is not possible using external methods.

therapy, radiation, orthovoltage, *n* a form of cancer treatment in which a beam of low-yield radiation is directed from outside the body at a superficial lesion, such as those found in the oral cavity or on the lips.

therapy, radiation, supervoltage, *n* See therapy, radiation, megavoltage.

therapy, replacement, *n* the administration, as a therapeutic agent, of an essential constituent in which the body is deficient (e.g., insulin in diabetes mellitus).

therapy, root canal, *n* See endodontology.

therapy, speech, *n* the science that deals with the use of procedures, training, and remedies for the cure, alleviation, or prevention of speech disorders.

thermal conductivity, *n* See conductivity, thermal.

thermal expansion, *n* See expansion, thermal.

thermal sensitivity, *n* See sensitivity, tooth.

thermionic emission (thur′mīonik imish′ən), *n* the release of electrons when a material is heated (e.g., electron emission when the tungsten cathode filament of a radiographic tube is heated to incandescence by means of its low-voltage heating circuit).

thermistor (thur′mis′tər), *n* an electronic device, functioning as a thermometer, for measuring small changes in temperature. The resistance of a thermistor varies with the ambient temperature, thereby enabling accurate measurements of small temperature changes.

thermocoagulation, *n* the use of high-frequency electric currents to destroy tissue through heat coagulation. Also known as electrocautery.

thermocouple, *n* the joining of two dissimilar metals. The unequal thermal expansion of the two metals is used to indicate temperature changes.

thermography (thərmog′rəfē), *n* a technique for sensing and recording on film hot and cold areas of the body by means of an infrared detector that reacts to blood flow.

thermoluminescence (thur′mōloo′mines′əns), *n* the capability of certain crystalline compounds such as lithium fluoride to release stored energy as luminescent energy when heated.

thermoluminescent dosimetry (thur′mōloomines′ənt dōsim′ətrē), *n* the determination of the amount of radiation to which a thermoluminescent material has been exposed. This is accomplished by heating the material in a specially designed instrument that relates the amount of luminescence emitted from the material to the amount of radiation exposure.

thermometer, *n* instrument used for taking temperature readings. Varying designs of the thermometer allow the temperature to be taken in the oral cavity, rectum, or externally at the axillary or groin areas.

thermometer, external, *n* a reading from a thermometer taken at an external location (the armpit or groin) instead of by an internal method (the oral cavity or rectum).

thermometer, rectal, *n* a thermometer used to take temperature readings by insertion into the rectum of the patient.

thermoplastic (thur′mōplas′tik), *adj* the property of becoming soft with the application of heat, rigid at normal temperature, and again soft with the reapplication of heat. A reversible physical phenomenon.

thermosetting, *adj* having the property of becoming irreversibly rigid or hardened with the application of heat. In dentistry the term is used in connection with resins.

thiabendazole (thī′əben′dəzōl), *n* an anthelmintic agent most effective against infection with the roundworm *Strongyloides.* Its effectiveness in treating other roundworm infections is varied.

thiamine HCl (vitamin B_1) (thī′əmin), *n brand names:* Betalin S, Bewon, many others; *drug class:* vitamin B_1 water soluble; *action:* needed for carbohydrate metabolism; *uses:* treatment of vitamin B_1 deficiency or in prophylaxis, beriberi, and Wernicke-Korsakoff syndrome.

thiazides (thī′əzīdz), *n.pl* See diuretics.

thiazolidinediones (thī′əzō′lədē′dī-ōnēz′), *n.pl.* a class of medications used in the treatment of diabetes to make the tissues more reactive to insulin.

thickeners, *n.pl* See binder.

Thiersch's skin graft (tir′shəz), *n.pr* See graft, Thiersch's skin.

thiethylperazine maleate (thīeth′-ilperəzēn mā′lēāt), *n brand name:* Torecan; *drug class:* phenothiazine, antiemetic; *action:* acts centrally by blocking chemoreceptor trigger zone, which in turns acts on vomiting center; *uses:* treatment of nausea, vomiting.

thimble, *n* See coping.

thimble, ionization chamber, *n* See chamber, ionization, thimble.

thinking, *n* **1.** the cognitive process of forming mental images or concepts. **2.** the process of cognitive problem solving through the sorting, organizing, and classification of facts and relationships.

thiocyanate (thī′ōsī′ənāt), *n* compound present in tobacco smoke derived from hydrogen cyanide, used to confirm the use of tobacco by an individual.

Thiokol (thī′ōkôl), *n.pr* brand name for polysulfide polymer using a mercaptan bond. The basic ingredient of rubber-base impression materials. See also mercaptan.

thiopental sodium, *n* a potent ultrashort-acting barbiturate used as a general anesthetic for surgical procedures that are expected to require 15 minutes or less, as an induction agent for other general anesthetics, as a hypnotic component in balanced anesthesia, and as an adjunct to regional anesthesia.

thioridazine HCl (thī′ərid′əzēn′), *n brand names:* Mellaril, SK Thioridazine; *drug class:* phenothiazine antipsychotic; *action:* blocks neurotransmission at dopaminergic synapses in cerebral cortex, hypothalamus, and limbic system; exhibits strong peripheral α-adrenergic, anticholinergic blocking action; *uses:* treatment of psychotic disorders, schizophrenia, behavioral problems in children, alcohol withdrawal as adjunct, anxiety, major depressive disorders, organic brain syndrome.

thiothixene (thī′ōthik′sēn), *n brand name:* Navane; *drug class:* thioxanthene/antipsychotic; *action:* depresses the cerebral cortex, hypothalamus, and limbic system, which control activity and aggression; blocks neurotransmission produced by dopamine at the synapse; *uses:* treatment of psychotic disorders, schizophrenia, and acute agitation.

third party, *n* the party to a dental benefits contract that may collect premiums, assume financial risk, pay claims, and provide other administrative services. Also called *administrative agent carriers, insurers,* or *underwriters.*

third-party administrator (TPA), n claims payer who assumes responsibility for administering health benefit plans without assuming any financial risk. Some commercial insurance carriers and Blue Cross/Blue Shield plans also have TPA operations to accommodate self-funded employers seeking administrative services only (ASO) contracts.

third-party payer, n an organization other than the patient (first party) or health care provider (second party) involved in the financing of personal health services.

third-party payment, n payment for services by someone other than the beneficiary (e.g., when an employer or union makes such payment).

thixotrophic (thik′sōtrop′ik), *n* a type of gel with the ability to liquify when activated.

thoracic surgery, *n* the branch of surgery that deals with disease and injuries of the thoracic area, including the heart and major vessels and the lungs and respiratory tract.

thoracostomy (thôr′əkos′təmē), *n* an incision made into the chest wall to provide an opening for the purpose of drainage.

threat, *n* a menace; a statement of intention to harm or injure the person, property, or rights of another.

threonine (thrē′ōnīn), *n* one of the essential amino acids needed for proper growth in infants and maintenance of nitrogen balance in adults. See also amino acid.

threshold (thresh′ōld), *n* the lowest limit of stimulus capable of producing an impression on the consciousness or evoking a response in irritable tissue.

threshold dose, n See dose, threshhold.

threshold, high pain, n higher than average capacity to withstand pain; exceptional pain tolerance.

threshold, low pain, n lower than average capacity to withstand pain; minimal pain tolerance.

threshold, swallowing, n the minimal stimulation required to initiate the reflex action of deglutition.

thrill, *n* **1.** a vibration felt on the chest wall over the heart. It is caused by the eddy flow of the blood, which is produced by a structural defect in the heart. **2.** palpable high-frequency vibration that may accompany cardiac murmurs or vascular disease.

throat, *n* a portion of the neck located in front of the spinal column; contains the trachea, larynx, pharynx, and superior segment of the esophagus.

thrombasthenia (throm′basthē′nēə), *n* a hemorrhagic diathesis associated with qualitative abnormalities of the platelets.

thrombin (throm′bin), *n* a proteolytic enzyme formed from prothrombin by the action of thromboplastin, factor IV calcium (Ca^{++}), and other factors. Thrombin forms fibrin from fibrinogen, speeds up the disruption of platelets, and activates factor V.

thrombocatalysin (throm′bōkatal′isin), *n* See factor VIII.

thrombocytes (throm′bosīts), *n.pl* See platelets.

thrombocythemia (throm′bōsīthē′mēə), *n* an increase in the number of circulating blood platelets.

thrombocytin (throm′bōsī′tin), *n* See serotonin.

thrombocytopenia, *n* an abnormal hemotologic condition in which the number of platelets is reduced. Thrombocytopenia is the most common cause of bleeding disorders. See also purpura, thrombocytopenic.

thrombocytosis (throm′bōsītō′sis), *n* unusually large numbers of platelets in the circulating blood. It may occur after surgical procedures, parturition, and injury, or with thrombocythemia.

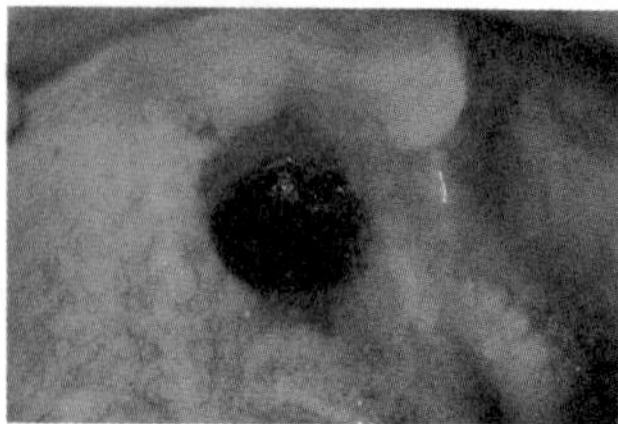

Thrombocytopenia. (Neville/Damm/Allen/Bouquot, 2002)

thromboembolism, *n* a condition in which a blood vessel is blocked by an embolus carried in the bloodstream from the site of formation of the clot. The obstruction of the pulmonary artery or one of its main branches may be fatal. Emboli are diagnosed by radiographs and other radiologic techniques.

thrombogen (throm′bōjen), *n* prothrombin. See also factor V.

thrombogene, *n* See factor V.

thrombokinase (throm′bōkin′ās), *n* See factor III.

thrombokinin (throm′bōkin′in), *n* See factor III.

thrombopenia, essential (throm′bōpē′nēə), *n* See purpura, thrombocytopenia.

thrombophlebitis (throm′bōfləbī′tis), *n* an inflammation of the vein in which the vein becomes closed or occluded resulting from the development of a clot or thrombus.

thromboplastic plasma component (TPC), *n* See factor VIII.

thromboplastin (throm′bōplas′tin), *n* a substance necessary to the coagulant activity of tissue extracts; also has been referred to as the direct activator of prothrombin and as a substance from plasma, platelets, and tissues that initiates thromboplastic activity in blood coagulation. See also thromboplastin, extrinsic.

thromboplastin, activated, *n* See thromboplastin, extrinsic.

thromboplastin, cofactor of, *n* See factor V.

thromboplastin, extrinsic, *n* a direct prothrombin activator formed by the interaction of brain extracts, factors V and VII, and factor IV calcium (Ca^{++}).

thromboplastin, incomplete, *n* tissue thromboplastin.

thromboplastin, intrinsic (plasma thromboplastin, intrinsic prothrombin activator), *n* a prothrombin activator formed from interaction of blood coagulation factors V, VIII, IX, and X and factor IV calcium (Ca^{++}) with a foreign surface.

thromboplastin, partial time (PTT), *n* a blood test used to determine von Willebrand disease, hemophilia, and to monitor anticoagulant medications. Normal coagulation time is 68 to 82 seconds. An updated form of the test, activated partial thromboplastin time (APTT), is replacing PTT.

thromboplastin, tissue, *n* a factor in tissue extract responsible for coagulation of blood.

thromboplastinogen (throm′bōplastin′ōjen), *n* See factor VIII.

thromboplastinogenase (throm′bōplastin′ōjənās), *n* See factor, platelet, 3.

thrombosis (thrombō′sis), *n* presence of a clot or deposit in a blood vessel, formed in situ and remaining in place. An abnormal vascular condition in which a thrombus (blood clot) develops within a blood vessel of the body.

thrombosis, cavernous sinus, *n* a blood clot in the cavernous sinus occasionally arising from maxillary periapical infection. The prognosis is poor but not so grave as before antibiotic therapy.

thrombosis, coronary, *n* thrombosis of the coronary artery; also called *heart attack* and *coronary occlusion.*

thrombotonin, *n* See serotonin.

thrombozyme (throm′bōzīm), *n* See factor II.

thrombus (throm′bus), *n* a blood clot in a vessel or in one of the chambers of the heart that remains at the point of its formation.

thrush, *n* (candidiasis, moniliasis), a disease caused by *Candida albicans* and characterized by white patches that scrape off with some difficulty, leaving bleeding bases. This term usually is used for the intraoral disease, whereas *moniliasis* is applied to the condition in other areas of infection by the yeast, as well as in the oral cavity. See also candidiasis; moniliasis.

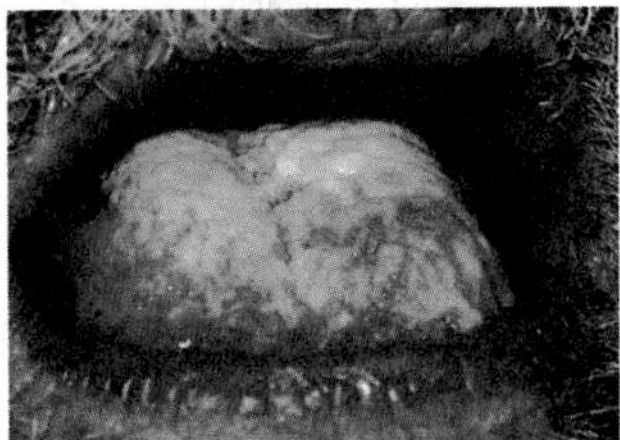

Thrush. (Sapp/Eversole/Wysocki, 2004)

thumb sucking, *n* See finger sucking.

thymol (thī′mol), *n* a synthetic or natural thyme oil, used as an antibacterial and antifungal. It is an ingredient in some over-the-counter preparations for the treatment of acne, hemorrhoids, and tinea pedis.

thymoma (thīmō′mə), *n* a usually benign tumor of the thymus gland that may be associated with myasthenia gravis or an immune deficiency disorder.

thymus (thī′məs), *n* a single unpaired gland located in the mediastinum that is the primary central gland of the lymphatic system. The T cells of the cell-mediated immune response develop in this gland before migrating to the lymph nodes and spleen.

thyroid cartilage, *n* the anterior midline prominence of the larnyx; also known as the *Adam's apple.*

thyroid collar, *n* a radiograph apron that covers the neck, especially the thyroid area, in order to reduce patient exposure during intraoral radiography.

thyroid crisis (thī′roid), *n* a sudden exacerbation of symptoms of thyrotoxicosis characterized by fever, sweating, tachycardia, extreme nervous excitability, and pulmonary edema. If untreated, the crisis often is fatal. Also called *thyroid storm.*

thyroid function test, *n* one of several tests to evaluate the function of the thyroid gland. These include protein-bound iodine, butanol-extractable iodine, radioactive iodine uptake, and radioactive iodine excretion.

thyroid gland, *n* a highly vascular organ at the front of the neck, consisting of bilateral lobes connected in the middle by a narrow isthmus. The thyroid gland secretes the hormone thyroxine directly into the blood. It is essential to normal body growth in infancy and childhood. It also regulates the metabolic rate in adults.

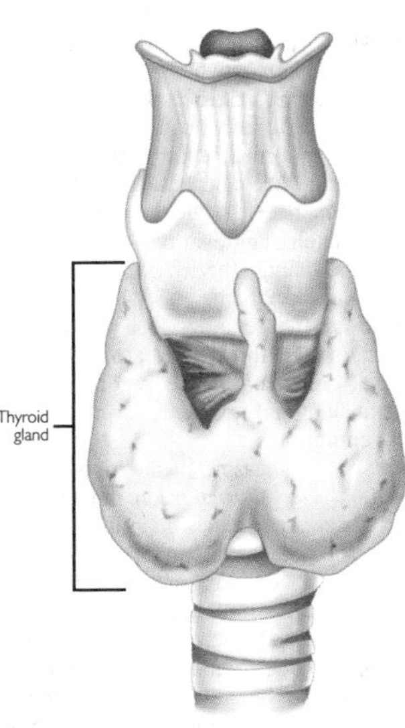

Thyroid gland. (Thibodeau/Patton, 2007)

thyroid, lingual, *n* presence of thyroid tissue in the tongue, which is related to abnormal embryonic activity of the thyroglossal duct.

thyroid USP (desiccated), *n brand names:* Armour Thyroid, Thyroid USP Enseals, Thryo-Teric, others; *drug class:* thyroid hormone; *action:* increases metabolic rate; increases cardiac output, oxygen consumption, body temperature, blood volume, and growth and development at cellular level; *uses:* treatment of hypothyroidism, cretinism, and myxedema.

thyroiditis, *n* inflammation of the thyroid gland.

thyrotoxicosis (thī′rōtok′sikō′sis), *n* See hyperthyroidism.

thyroxine (thīrok′sin), *n* the hormone secretion of the thyroid gland, L-3,5,3′,5′-tetraiodothyronine.

tic, *n* an involuntary, purposeless movement of muscle, usually occurring under emotional stress. It is a

T

survival in stereotyped form of a movement or muscle set once used voluntarily and purposefully.

tic douloureux, *n* spontaneous trigeminal neuralgia associated with a "trigger zone" and causing spasmodic contraction of the facial muscles. See also neuralgia, trigeminal.

ticarcillin (tik'ärsil'in), *n* an anti-*Pseudomonas* penicillin.

ticlopidine (tīklō'pədēn), *n brand name:* Ticlid; *drug class:* platelet aggregation inhibitor; *action:* inhibits first and second phases of adenosine diphosphate (ADP)-induced effects in platelet aggregation; *use:* effective in reducing the risk of stroke in high-risk patients.

t.i.d., *n* abbreviation for *ter in die,* Latin for "three times a day."

tidal volume, *n* the amount of air inhaled and exhaled during normal ventilation.

time, *n* a measure of duration.

time, clot retraction, *n* the time required for a given quantity of blood to separate in the tube in which it has been placed. For 3 ml of blood at room temperature, 1 hour is normal. It is very slow in thrombocytopenia.

time, coagulation, *n* the time required for blood clotting to begin in a capillary tube, normally 2 to 8 minutes. A coagulation time three times normal is a definite danger sign.

time, gel, *n* (gelation time), the interval of time required for a colloidal solution to become a solid or semisolid jelly or gel. Usually refers to the working time of a hydrocolloid or alginate impression material.

time, gelation, *n* See time, gel.

time limits, *n.pl* the periods within which a notice of claim must be filed.

time, median lethal, *n* (LD_{50} time, MLT), the time required for 50% of a large group of animals or organisms to die after administration of a specified dose of radiation.

time, prothrombin **(prōthrom'bin),** *n* (one-stage test), a gross but useful screening test of the completeness of the second and third stages of blood coagulation. Normal prothrombin time by the Quick method is 12 to 15 seconds. The time is affected by deficiencies of factor V or VII as well as of prothrombin. See also test, prothrombin consumption.

time, serum prothrombin, *n* See test, prothrombin consumption.

time, setting, *n* the length of time for a mixed preparation of materials to reach a state of hardness, measured from the start of the mixing. The end point for dental materials is usually determined by a penetration test.

timer, *n* radiographic timing device that functions as an automatic exposure timer and a switch to control the current to the high-tension transformer and filament transformer. The face of the timer is calibrated in seconds and fractions of seconds. The timer controls the total time that the current passes through the radiographic tube and thus the time during which the roentgen rays are emitted. The timer activates a switch or contractor that closes and opens the low-voltage circuit of the high voltage.

timer, electronic, *n* an electronic vacuum tube device, with no moving parts, that covers a time range of 1/20 to 10 seconds. It automatically sets itself, is more accurate than mechanical timers, and meets all the needs of modern high-speed dental techniques.

timer, foot, *n* a timer with an attachment that permits the timing device to be activated by foot pressure. This is the preferred type of timer.

timer, hand, *n* an attachment to or part of a timer that requires thumb or finger pressure to activate the timing device.

timer, mechanical, *n* a timer using a spring mechanism for determination of length of exposure. Accuracy of timing is not assumed in exposures of less than 1 second with a mechanical timer.

timolol maleate (tim'əlol), *n brand name:* Blocadren; *drug class:* nonselective β-adrenergic blocker; *action:* competitively blocks stimulation of β-adrenergic receptors in the heart and decreases renin activity, all of which may play a role in reducing systolic and diastolic blood pressure; inhibits β_2 receptors in the bronchial system; *uses:* treatment of mild to moderate hypertension, reduction of mortality after myocardial infarction (MI), and migraine prophylaxis.

timolol maleate (optic), *n brand names:* Betimol, Timoptic Solution, Timoptic-XE; *drug class:* β-adrenergic blocker; *action:* reduces production of aqueous humor by unknown mechanism; *uses:* treatment of ocular hypertension, chronic open-angle glaucoma, secondary glaucoma, and aphakic glaucoma.

tin octoate (ok′tōāt), *n* substance used to accomplish vulcanization of silicone rubber impression materials. It is not a true catalyst, because it becomes part of the final polymer.

tin oxide (SnO_2), *n* a polishing agent in the form of a purified white powder, prepared as a paste with glycerine or water.

tincture (tink′chur), *n* an alcoholic, hydroalcoholic, or ethereal solution of a drug.

tinea (tinē′ə), *n* a group of fungal skin diseases caused by dermatophytes of several kinds, characterized by itching, scaling, and sometimes painful lesions. *Tinea* is a general term that refers to infections of various causes, which are seen in several sites.

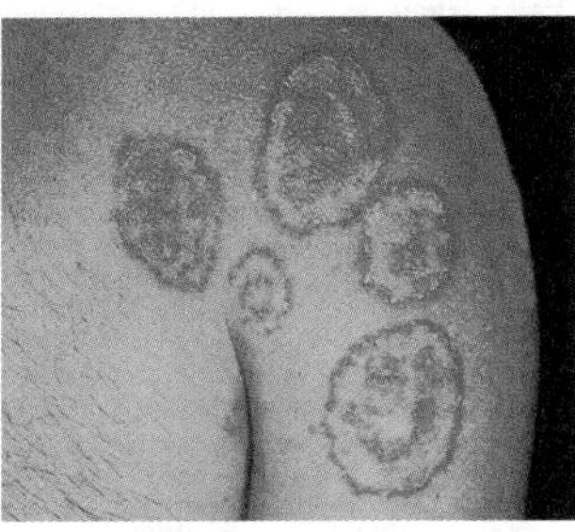

Tinea. (Habif, 2004)

tinea capitis, *n* a superficial fungal infection of the scalp seen most commonly in children.

tinea corporis, *n* a superficial fungal infection of the nonhairy skin of the body, most prevalent in hot, humid climates.

tinea cruris, *n* a superficial fungal infection of the groin.

tinea pedis, *n* a chronic superficial fungal infection of the foot, especially of the skin between the toes.

tinea unguium **(un′gwēəm),** *n* a superficial fungal infection of the nails.

tinea versicolor, *n* a fungal infection of the skin caused by *Malassezia furfur* and characterized by finely desquamating pale tan patches on the upper trunk and upper arms.

Tinel's sign (tinelz′), *n.pr* See sign, Tinel's.

tinfoil, *n* See foil, tin.

tinfoil substitute, *n* See substitute, tinfoil.

tinnitus (tin′itus), *n* noises or unpleasant sounds in the ears, such as ringing, buzzing, roaring, or clicking; usually high pitched. Heard by many persons with auditory impairment. Clicking tinnitus may be heard by others.

tinted denture base, *n* See base, denture, tinted.

tip frequency, *n* the measurement of the number of times the tip of an ultrasonic instrument moves back and forth to complete a cycle in one second.

tipping of cusps, *n* See restoration of cusps.

tissue (tish′oo), *n* an aggregation of similarly specialized cells united in the performance of a particular function.

tissue adhesives, *n* agents or materials that may be used to seal two cut tissue surfaces together or cover a surgically exposed surface such as butyl cyanoacrylate, which is used to cover palatal donor sites in periodontal surgery.

tissue, compression of, *n* See tissue displaceability.

tissue conditioning, *n* a disciplined program of patient-performed plaque control measures designed for gingiva that is soft, spongy, and bleeds easily from poor oral hygiene habits, in order to improve gingival health before subgingival scaling is performed.

tissue, connective, *n* the binding and supportive tissue of the body; derived from the mesoderm; depending on its location and function, it is composed of fibroblasts, primitive mesenchymal cells, collagen fibers, and elastic fibers, with associated blood and lymphatic vessels and nerve fibers.

tissue, critical, *n* tissue that reacts most unfavorably to radiation or by its nature attracts and absorbs specific radiochemicals.

tissue displaceability, *n* the quality of oral tissues that permits them to be placed in or assume other positions than their relaxed position.

tissue displacement, *n* change in the form or position of tissues as a result of pressure.

tissue, engineering, *n* the interdisciplinary field that uses life science and engineering principles in the development of biologic substitutes for tissue restoration or replacement.

tissue, flabby, *n* See tissue, hyperplastic.

tissue, hyperplastic, *n* in dentistry, excessively movable tissue about the mandible or maxillae resulting from increases in the number of normal cells.

tissue, interdental, *n* the gingivae, cementum of the teeth, free gingival and transseptal fibers of the periodontal membrane (ligament), and alveolar and supporting bone.

tissue molding, *n* See border molding.

tissue, peripheral, *n* See border structures.

tissue, redundant, *n* See epulis fissuratum.

tissue sloughing, *n* a surface layer of flesh peeling away. Possible causes are extensive exposure to topical anesthetic, overly abrasive toothpaste, smokeless tobacco, tissue burn, or mouthrinses. Also called *epithelial desquamation.*

tissue, subjacent, *n* the structures that underlie or are in border contact with a denture base; they may or may not have a supporting relationship to the overlying base.

tissue-borne partial denture, *n* See denture, partial, tissue-borne.

T

titanium, *n* a lightweight, strong, corrosion-resistant chemical element with a white-silver color and metallic luster. Commercially pure titanium and titanium alloys are used in the fabrication of dental implants. Titanium is also used in the manufacture of alloys, such as aluminum and iron, and in powdered form in materials such as graphite composites.

titanium mesh, *n* a woven net made of flexible titanium that is used during placement of bone grafts in order to ensure a predetermined volume of bone regeneration.

titanium plasma sprayed (TPS), *n* a process of applying a porous or dense coating of titanium onto a surface to be treated by using high temperature to melt titanium powders, which are then quickly resolidified.

titer (tī′tur), *n* the standard amount by volume of a material required to produce a desired reaction with another material.

titration (tītrā′shən), *n* incremental increase in drug dosage to a level that provides the optimal therapeutic effect.

TMJ facebow, *n* See facebow, kinematic.

TMJ pain-dysfunction syndrome, *n* See temporomandibular pain-dysfunction syndrome.

TMP-SMX, *n* acronym for trimethoprim-sulfamethoxazole.

TNF, *n* an abbreviation for **t**umor **n**ecrosis **f**actor, a genetic-triggered, tumor-killing agent produced by the body in small amounts to counteract neoplastic growth; an experimental agent used in the treatment of cancers.

TNM staging system, *n.pr* stands for **t**umor **n**ode **m**etastasis, a recognized method used to identify and predict the course of disease of a patient diagnosed with cancer.

tobacco pipe, *n* a small, handheld tobacco burning device that holds a burning, dried tobacco leaf in a small cup at one end, while user uses lips to draw smoke through a small cylinder attached to the side of the bowl.

tobacco use, *n* the practice of purposely using tobacco for its perceived physical and psychologic benefits—e.g., mental alertness, relaxation, weight control. Repeated use often leads to addiction. Product may be taken into the body by inhaling the smoke from burning tobacco or by chewing a variety of smokeless tobacco products. Tobacco use is linked to diseases occurring in nearly every system in the human body, including but not limited to cancer, emphysema, hypertension, sudden death syndrome (SIDS), and osteoporosis.

tobacco withdrawal syndrome, *n* a change in mood or performance associated with the cessation of or reduc-

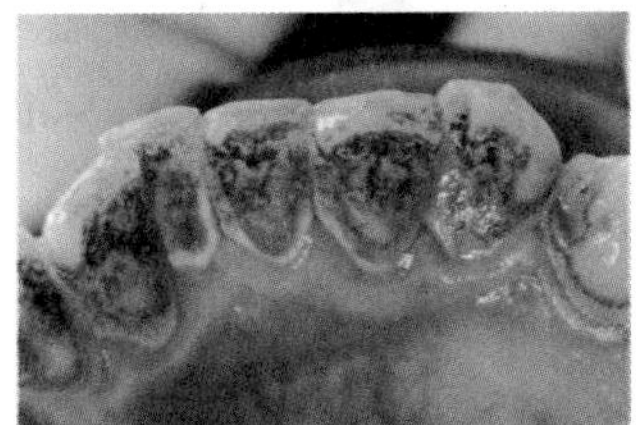

Tobacco use. (Neville/Damm/Allen/Bouquot, 2002)

tion in exposure to nicotine. Symptoms may range from lack of concentration to anxiety and temper outbursts.

tobramycin (ophthalmic), *n brand name:* Tobrax; *drug class:* antiinfective; *action:* inhibits bacterial protein synthesis; *use:* treatment of infection of the eye.

tocainide HCl (tōkā'nīd), *n brand name:* Tonocard; *drug class:* antidysrhythmic (Class IB), lidocaine analog; *action:* decreases sodium and potassium conductance, which decreases myocardial excitability; *use:* treatment of documented life-threatening ventricular dysrhythmias.

Togaviridae **(tō'gəvir'idā),** *n* a family of enveloped, linear, nonsegmented RNA viruses with icosahedral symmetry, which includes the rubella and yellow fever viruses.

toilet of cavity, *n* See cavity, toilet.

tolazamide (tōlaz'əmīd), *n brand name:* Tolinase; *drug class:* sulfonylurea (first generation) oral antidiabetic; *action:* causes functioning beta cells in pancreas to release insulin, leading to drop in blood glucose levels; *use:* treatment of type II diabetes mellitus.

tolbutamide (tolbū'təmīd'), *n brand name:* Orinase; *drug class:* sulfonylurea (first generation) oral antidiabetic; *action:* causes functioning beta cells in pancreas to release insulin, leading to drop in blood glucose levels; *use:* treatment of type II diabetes mellitus.

tolerance (tol'ərəns), *n* the ability to endure the influence of a drug or poison, particularly acquired by continued use of the substance. See also resistance.

tolerance, acquired, *n* tolerance that develops with successive doses of a drug. If it develops within a short span of time, such as 24 hours, it is called *tachyphylaxis.* Slowly acquired tolerance is sometimes called *mithridatism.*

tolerance, carbohydrate, *n* the ability of the body to use carbohydrates. A decrease in tolerance is seen in diabetes mellitus, liver damage, and some infections and in the presence of hyperactivity of the adrenal cortex or pituitary gland.

tolerance, cross, *n* tolerance to a number of drugs of similar mode of action or chemical structure.

tolerance, individual, *n* tolerance characteristic of an individual.

tolerance, pseudo-, *n* a state of apparent tolerance indicated due to failure of the drug to reach its usual receptor sites.

tolerance, species, *n* tolerance characteristic of a species of animal.

tolerance, tissue, *n* the ability of structures to endure environmental change without ill effect.

tolerance, upper intake level, *n* the specified limit of a given substance that an individual may consume and not suffer detrimental or toxic effects.

tolmetin sodium (tol'mətin), *n brand name:* Tolectin; *drug class:* nonsteroidal antiinflammatory; *action:* inhibits prostaglandin synthesis by interfering with cyclooxygenase needed for biosynthesis; *uses:* treatment of osteoarthritis, rheumatoid arthritis, juvenile rheumatoid arthritis.

tolnaftate (topical), *n brand name:* Aftate, Tinactin, Ting, others; *drug class:* antifungal, topical; *action:* interferes with fungal cell membrane, which increases permeability and leaking of cell nutrients; *uses:* treatment of tinea pedis, tinea cruris, tinea corporis, tinea capitis, tinea unguium, and tinea versicolor.

toluidine blue dye (tolū'idēn), *n* a chemical substance used to identify potentially malignant mucosal deviations; use as an oral cavity rinse or apply over the affected area with a cotton swab.

Tomes's granular layer (tōmz'əs), *n* a grainy appearing layer within dentin located in the root of the tooth beneath the dentinocemental junction. See also dentin.

tomogram, *n* See examination, radiographic, extraoral body section.

tomograph (tō′məgraf), *n* a radiograph produced while rotating the film and radiograph source in opposite directions around an axis located in the region of interest. This movement blurs outside structures while maintaining sharpness in the region of interest.

tomography (tōmog′rəfē), *n* a radiographic technique that produces a film representing a detailed cross section of tissue structures at a predetermined depth.

tongue (tung), *n* the muscular organ that is the main articulatory element in the production of speech and accounts for the clarity and fluidity of speech. Two groups of tongue muscles, the intrinsic and extrinsic, are united into one organ. Each group, however, has separate structural and functional characteristics.

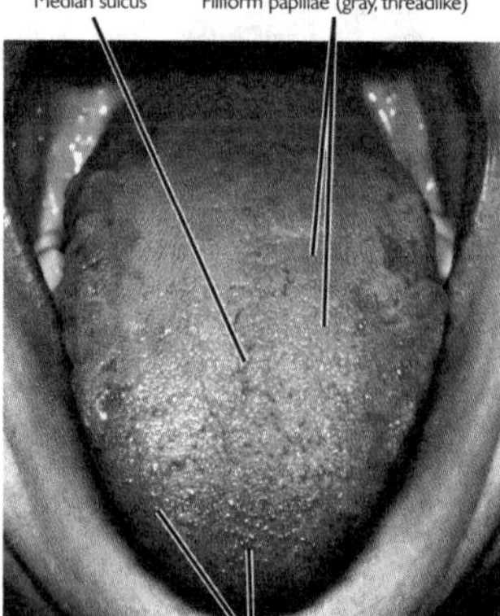

Tongue. (Liebgott, 2001)

tongue, amyloid (amyloid macroglossia), *n* enlargement of the tongue resulting from amyloidosis.

tongue, antibiotic, *n* a glossitis caused by sensitivity to an antibiotic, vitamin B complex deficiency associated with antibiotic therapy.

tongue, bald, *n* See glossitis, atrophic.

tongue, beefy, *n erythematous* or *atrophic glossitis.* See also glossitis, atrophic; glossitis, Moeller's.

tongue, bifid (cleft tongue), *n* a tongue divided by a midline cleft.

tongue, black hairy (lingua nigra), *n* a black appearance of the dorsal surface of the tongue; caused by elongated filiform papillae and an accumulation of dark pigments, microorganisms, and food debris.

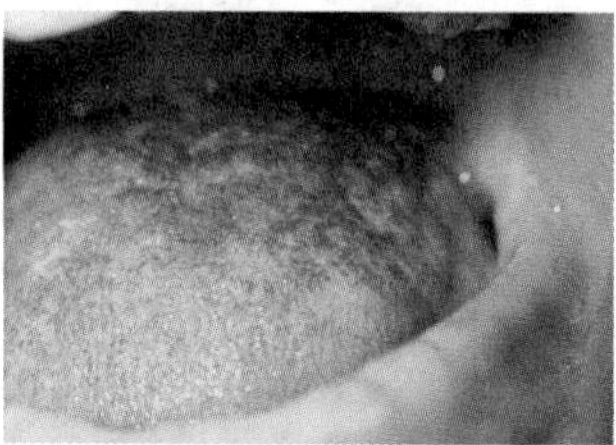

Black hairy tongue. (Courtesy Dr. Charles Babbush)

tongue blade, *n* a narrow, wooden instrument used by the patient to clean the tongue. Can also be used during an examination to aid in inspection of the teeth, gums, and oral cavity.

tongue, cleft, *n* See tongue, bifid.

tongue, coated, *n* nonspecific term used to describe the condition of the tongue resulting from whitish or otherwise discolored accumulations of food debris, bacterial plaques, and hyperplastic filiform papillae. Reduced function, as in general illness or laryngitis, is a primary cause.

tongue, cobblestone, *n* hyperplasia and hyperemia of fungiform and filiform papillae of the tongue in riboflavin deficiency. Formerly used to describe syphilitic glossitis with leukoplakia.

tongue crib, *n* an appliance used to limit undesirable tongue movements, usually constructed to prevent its protrusion between the anterior teeth.

tongue depressor, *n.pl* a flat wooden stick used to position the tongue so that the back of the throat may be seen. Several may be used together as oral cavity props.

tongue, fissured (furrowed tongue), *n* a tongue traversed by clefts that may be arranged like the veins of a leaf or give the tongue a "pavement block" appearance. It is seen in 5% of all dental patients but in 13% of those older than 50 years.

tongue, flat, *n* paralysis of the transverse lingual muscles such that the borders of the tongue cannot be rolled. The condition results from congenital syphilis.

tongue, furrowed, *n* See tongue, fissured.

tongue, geographic, *n* (benign migratory glossitis, glossitis areata exfoliativa, glossitis migrans, wandering rash), a condition characterized by a chronic, circumscribed, more or less circular desquamation of the superficial epithelium of the dorsum of the tongue. The spots of desquamation (redder areas) migrate continuously, usually passing from the region near the vallate papillae toward the tip of the tongue. This condition involves the filiform lingual papillae. The tongue can seem more sensitive than usual during times of exacerbation.

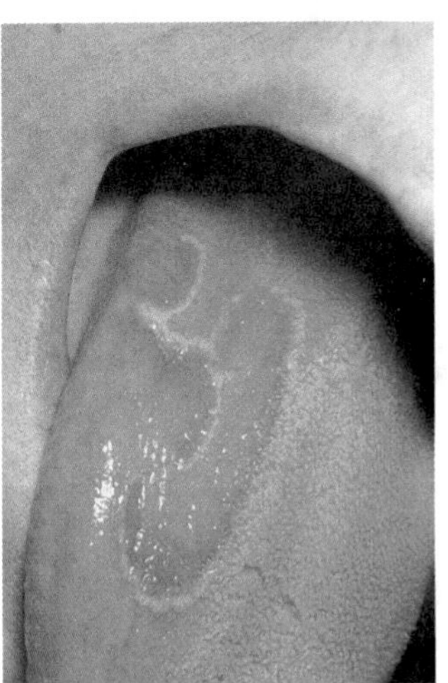

Geographic tongue. (Courtesy Dr. Charles Babbush)

tongue, hairy, *n* hyperplasia of the filiform lingual papillae, often associated with oral moniliasis and the use of antibiotics or tobacco.

***tongue, lobulated* (lob′yəlātid),** *n* a congenital defect, with a secondary lobe of the tongue arising from its surface.

tongue, magenta, *n* the reddish-purple tongue of riboflavin deficiency.

tongue margin, indentation, *n* See crenation of tongue.

tongue piercing, *n* a deliberate piercing of the tongue in order to wear tongue jewelry, which creates a high risk of life-threatening systemic effects, as well as dental abrasion, gingival recession, and fractured teeth, especially during athletic activities.

tongue room, *n* See tongue space.

tongue, Sandwith's bald, *n.pr* a condition in which the tongue is very smooth because of a loss of fusiform papillae and is fiery red and enlarged because of severe inflammation; seen in pellagra.

tongue scraper, *n* an oral hygiene implement drawn down the tongue from the back to the front in order to reduce oral cavity odors and plaque-producing bacteria.

tongue, smooth, *n* See glossitis, atrophic.

tongue space, *n* the space available for functioning of the tongue.

tongue, strawberry, *n* See strawberry tongue.

tongue thrust, *n* thrusting of the tongue between the anterior teeth, especially in the initial stage of swallowing. This action, often combined with a resting position also between the teeth, may inhibit normal eruption and produce an open bite.

tongue, white hairy (lingua alba, lingua villosa alba), *n* hairy tongue characterized by elongation of the filiform papillae but without the dark staining seen in lingua nigra (black hairy tongue). See also tongue, black hairy.

tonguetie, *n* See ankyloglossia.

tonguetie (tong′tī), *n* a condition in which a shorter-than-average lingual frenum connecting the tongue to the floor of the oral cavity limits tongue movement.

tonic convulsion, *n* a prolonged generalized contraction of the skeletal muscles.

tonofibril (ton′əfī′bril), *n* a fibril emanating from epithelial cells. Recent electron microscopy has shown such fibrils to be irregular formations of the cell membrane.

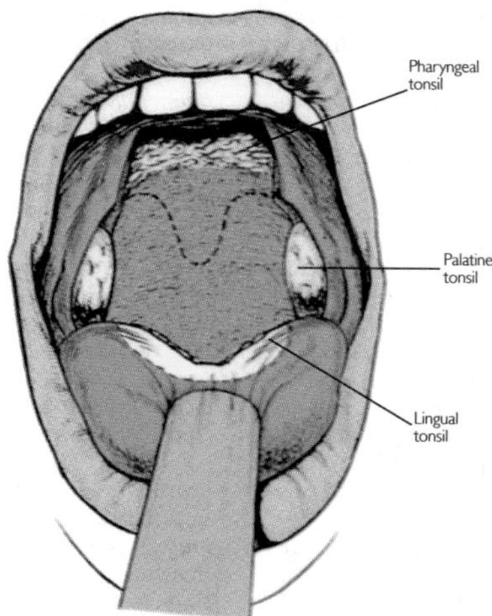

Tonsil. (Thibodeau/Patton, 2005)

tonsil (ton′sil), *n* a rounded mass of tissue, usually of a lymphoid nature.

tonsil, lingual, n a variable mass of lymphoid tissue at the base of the dorsal surface of the tongue.

tonsil, palatine, n one of two small tissue masses on opposite sides of the oropharynx, between the faucial pillars, which are believed to serve as the first line of defense against bacteria that enters the oral cavity via the oral cavity.

tonsil, pharyngeal **(fərin′jēəl),** *n* a mass of lymphoid tissue on the posterior wall of the nasopharynx; also known as the adenoids.

tonsillar (ton′sələr), *adj* of or relating to the tonsils.

tonsillar recess, n depressed region located between the posterior and anterior faucial pillars. This is the location of the paltine tonsils.

tonsillar region, n area surrounding the tonsils. See also fauces.

tonsillectomy (ton′səlek′təmē), *n* the surgical excision of the palatine tonsils, performed to prevent recurrent tonsillitis.

tonsillitis (ton′silī′tis), *n* an inflammation of the tonsils.

tonsillitis, lingual, n a form of tonsillitis at the posterior part of the base of the tongue in the lymphoid masses (lingual tonsils) located there.

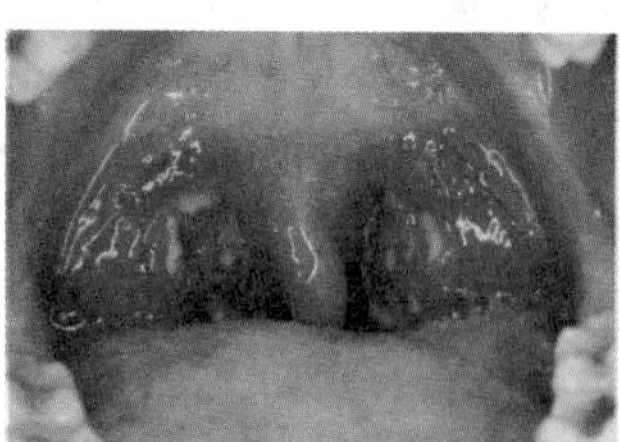
Tonsillitis. (Neville/Damm/Allen/Bouquot, 2002)

tooth (teeth), *n* one of the hard bodies or processes usually protruding from and attached to the alveolar process of the maxillae and the mandible; designed for the mastication of food.

teeth, anterior, n.pl the incisor or canine front teeth.

teeth, canine, n.pl the four canines; the third tooth located distal to the midline in any one of the four quadrants of the dentition.

teeth, deciduous, n See deciduous; tooth, primary.

teeth, drugs for sensitivity of, n.pl the medicaments used to treat hypersensitivity of the teeth. They should cause relatively little pain when applied; be easily applied, rapid in action, and permanently effective;

and not discolor the teeth or unduly irritate the pulp. Substances used include 33% sodium fluoride in kaolin and glycerin, a 25% aqueous solution of strontium chloride, hot medicinal olive oil, and 0.9% solution of sodium silicofluoride.

teeth, grinding of, *n* the selective modification of tooth form and contour in the occlusal adjustment operation to eliminate occlusal interferences and establish tooth contours conducive to the health of the periodontium. See also bruxism.

teeth, hereditary brown, *n.pl* See hypoplasia, enamel, hereditary.

teeth, neonatal, *n.pl* primary teeth that erupt into the oral cavity during the neonatal period (from birth to 30 days).

teeth, permanent, *n* See dentition, permanent.

teeth, polishing of, *n* See also polishing, coronal and polishing, selective.

teeth, posterior, *n.pl* the maxillary and mandibular premolars and molars of the permanent dentition or the premolars and molars of prostheses.

teeth, primary, *n.pl* **1.** term used by some in preference to deciduous teeth; however, it has not received the approval of preference by the American Dental Association. **2.** as a result of a survey of the terminology used to name the teeth of the first dentition, the College Committee Report of Dentistry for Children recommended in 1942 the use of *primary teeth* in place of deciduous, first, milk, temporary, baby, or foundation teeth. The term *primary* was suggested as a word "which may be acceptable to the dental profession, significant in its meaning, with no connotations of impermanence, and readily understood by nonprofessional people." See also deciduous.

teeth, sensitivity of, *n* a painful pulpal response to external stimuli such as heat, cold, and sweet substances. The most common clinical finding is a hyperesthetic state of the root surface resulting from loss of a portion of the cemental covering with exposure of the dentin. See also hypersensitivity, dentin.

teeth, separation of, *n* the action of moving a tooth mesially or distally out of contact with its neighboring tooth.

teeth, set of, *n* usually a full complement of maxillary and mandibular artificial teeth as they are carded by the manufacturer.

teeth, slow separation of, *n* drifting apart of teeth accomplished over a long period, usually by the wedging action of a material such as gutta-percha, orthodontic wire, thread, or fibers in orthodontic therapy.

teeth, supportive mechanisms of, *n.pl* the anatomic structures that function to maintain or aid in maintaining the teeth in position in their alveoli: the gingivae, cementum of the tooth, periodontal membrane, and alveolar and supporting bone. See also structures, supporting.

teeth, vital staining of, *n* the staining of enamel and dentin of primary and permanent teeth during development with vital stains (e.g., with bile pigment in Rh incompatibility or with tetracyclines).

tooth, abutment, *n* a tooth or teeth selected to support a prosthesis on the basis of the total surface areas of a healthy periodontium.

tooth, accessory **(akses′ərē),** *n* supernumerary teeth that do not resemble normal teeth in size, shape, or location. See also distomolar; mesiodens; paramolar; tooth,

tooth, acrylic resin **(əkril′ik),** *n* a tooth made of acrylic resin.

tooth, anatomic, *n* an artificial tooth that closely resembles the anatomic form of a natural unabraded tooth.

tooth, ankylosed **(ang′kəlōst′),** *n* abnormal calcification of the periodontal ligament resulting in abnormal fixation of a tooth.

tooth, artificial, *n* a tooth fabricated for use as a substitute for a natural tooth in a prosthesis; usually made of porcelain or plastic.

tooth-borne, *adj* term used to describe a prosthesis or a part of a prosthesis that depends entirely on the abutment teeth for support.

tooth-borne base, *n* the denture base restoring an edentulous area that has abutment teeth at each end for support. The tissue it covers is not used for support of the base.

tooth buds, *n.pl* embryonic teeth formed during the fifth and sixth weeks of embryo development. See also odontogenesis.

tooth, cap stage, *n* the second stage in the development of a tooth in which cells continue to proliferate to form the cap of a tooth.

tooth, conical (peg-shaped tooth), *n* failure of morphologic development of the tooth germ found in ectodermal dysplasia and other disorders and occasionally found in normal children.

tooth, cross-bite, *n.pl* the posterior teeth designed to permit the modified buccal cusps of the maxillary teeth to be positioned in the central fossae of the mandibular teeth.

tooth, cuspless, *n.pl* teeth designed without cuspal prominences on the masticatory surfaces.

tooth, devital, *n* See tooth, pulpless.

tooth, discoloration, *n* a stain or change in color of a tooth, which can be caused by bloodborne pigment or blood decomposition within the pulp, usage of certain drugs, and trauma. See also tooth, pigmentation.

tooth, drifting, *n* the migration of teeth from their normal positions in the dental arches as a result of such factors as loss of proximal support, loss of functional antagonists, occlusal traumatic tooth relationships, inflammatory and retrograde changes in the attachment apparatus, and oral habits.

tooth, embedded, *n* an unerupted tooth, usually one completely covered with bone; also spelled *imbedded.* See also tooth, impacted.

tooth eruption, *n* the process by which the tooth moves from its site of formation to its position of function. It can be active or passive.

tooth, evulsed (avulsed tooth), *n* a tooth that has been abnormally luxated from its alveolar support, commonly as a sequela to trauma.

tooth fairy, *n* a mythologic fairy said to leave small amounts of cash in exchange for a child's exfoliated primary tooth, which has been left under the pillow.

tooth form, *n* See form, tooth.

tooth fracture, *n* See fracture, tooth.

tooth, fulcrum, *n* the axis of movement of a tooth when lateral forces are applied to the tooth. The fulcrum is considered to be at the middle third of the portion of the root embedded in the alveolus and thus moves apically as the bone resorbs in periodontal disease.

tooth, fused, *n.pl* two teeth united during development by the union of their tooth germs. The teeth may be joined by the enamel of their crowns, root dentin, or both. Usually consists of a single large crown.

tooth germ, *n* the earliest evidence of a tooth. It includes the dental sac, dental papilla, and enamel organ.

tooth, geminated **(jem′inātəd),** *n* teeth with bifid crowns and confluent root canals resulting from the division of the enamel organ during the developmental period.

tooth, Hutchinson's, *n.pr* the defects of the permanent incisors associated with congenital syphilis. Dental hypoplasia affects primarily the incisors, canines, and first permanent molars. The incisors have a screwdriver or peg-shaped appearance. See also triad, Hutchinson.

tooth, hypersensitive, *n* a tooth that is painful when exposed to temperature changes, sweetness, or touch due to worn tooth enamel and, consequently, exposed dentin, usually near the cervix of the tooth.

tooth, hypoplasia of **(hī′pōplā′zhə),** *n* a reduction in the amount of enamel formed, resulting in irregular pits and grooves of the enamel.

tooth, immediate separation of, *n* separation of teeth accomplished by the rapid wedging action of an appliance during restorative procedures.

tooth, impacted, *n* a condition in which the unerupted or partially erupted tooth is positioned against another tooth, bone, or soft tissue so that complete eruption is unlikely. An impacted third molar tooth may be further described according to its position: buccoangular, distoangular, or vertical. An impacted maxillary canine tooth also may be further described according to its position: palatal (maxillary canine), lingual (mandibular canine), labial, or vertical.

tooth, inclination of, *n* the angle of slope of teeth from the vertical planes of reference. A tooth may be mesially, distally, lingually, buccally, or labially inclined.

tooth, loss of, *n* the separation of a tooth from its investing and supporting structures as a result of normal exfoliation attending loss of primary dentition, exfoliation as a sequela to excessive bone resorption and periapical migration of the epithelial attachment in periodontal disease, and instrumentation for extraction necessitated by pathologic involvement of the dental pulp, periodontium, or periapical tissues.

tooth, mesial movement of, *n* migration of teeth toward the midline, occurring as a phenomenon associated with the action of the anterior component of force. Mesial migration of teeth occurs with the wear of their proximal surfaces resulting from the buccolingual movements of the teeth.

tooth, metal insert, *n* an artificial tooth, usually of acrylic resin, containing an inserted ribbon of metal, or a cutting blade, in its occlusal surface, with one edge of the blade exposed; sometimes used in removable dentures.

tooth, migration of, *n* the movement of teeth into altered positions in relationship to the basal bone of the alveolar process and adjoining and opposing teeth as a result of loss of approximating or opposing teeth, occlusal interferences, habits, or inflammatory and dystrophic disease of the attaching and supporting structures of the teeth.

tooth, missing, *n* the absence of teeth from the dentition because of congenital factors, exfoliation, or extraction.

tooth mobility, *n* the movability of a tooth resulting from loss of all or a portion of its attachment and supportive apparatus. Seen in periodontitis, occlusal traumatism, and periodontosis.

tooth morphology, *n* the anatomic topography of the teeth.

tooth movement, *n* See movement, tooth.

tooth, natal, *n.pl* primary tooth found in the oral cavity at birth.

tooth, nonanatomic, *n* artificial teeth so designed that the occlusal surfaces are not copies from natural forms but are given forms that in the opinion of the designer seem more nearly to fulfill the requirements of mastication and tissue tolerance.

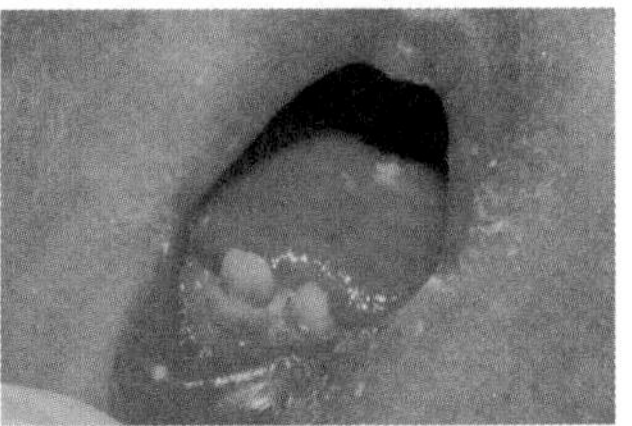

Natal tooth. (Neville/Damm/Allen/Bouquot, 2002)

tooth numbering systems, *n* the graphing techniques used to chart a patient's primary and permanent teeth, as well as record any clinical and radiographic findings; the American Dental Association used the Universal Numbering System (numbering teeth 1 to 32). Other tooth numbering systems include the International Numbering System (a two-digit system) and the Palmer Numbering System (teeth numbered 1 to 8 in different quadrants).

tooth, peg-shaped, *n* See tooth, conical.

tooth, pigmentation **(pig′məntā′shən),** *n* intrinsic discoloration of a tooth, which can be caused by bloodborne pigment or blood decomposition within the pulp, usage of certain drugs, and trauma.

tooth, pink, *n* See resorption, internal.

tooth, plastic, *n* artificial teeth constructed of synthetic resins.

tooth position, *n* See position, tooth.

tooth, pulpless, *n* a tooth from which the dental pulp has been removed or is necrotic.

tooth, replaced, *n* See tooth, supplied.

tooth, replanted, *n* a tooth that has been inserted back into the alveolus after accidentally being displaced.

tooth, rotated, *n* an altered position of the tooth in relation to the adjacent and opposing teeth and its basal alveolar process; in such an altered position the tooth has been turned on its long axis and is in a state of torsiversion. The result is an altered contact with adjacent teeth that produces a possible locus for food impaction between the teeth, with consequent gingival damage.

tooth selection, *n* See selection, tooth.

tooth, setting up of, *n* the arranging of teeth on a trial denture base; includes proper relation with occluding teeth.

tooth, shell, *n* a form of dentinal dysplasia characterized by large pulp chambers, meager coronal dentin, and usually no roots.

tooth size discrepancy, *n* lack of proportional harmony in the width of various teeth, causing relative spacing and crowding in different parts of the dentition.

tooth, submerged, *n* a tooth that has not erupted to the point of making contact with the opposing maxillary or mandibular tooth during mastication. Such a tooth may be immobile as a result of ankylosis to the mandible or maxilla.

tooth, succedaneous **(suk′sēdā′nēus),** *n* a permanent tooth with primary predecessors (i.e., premolars, canines, and incisors).

tooth, supernumerary, *n* extra erupted or unerupted teeth that resemble teeth of normal shape.

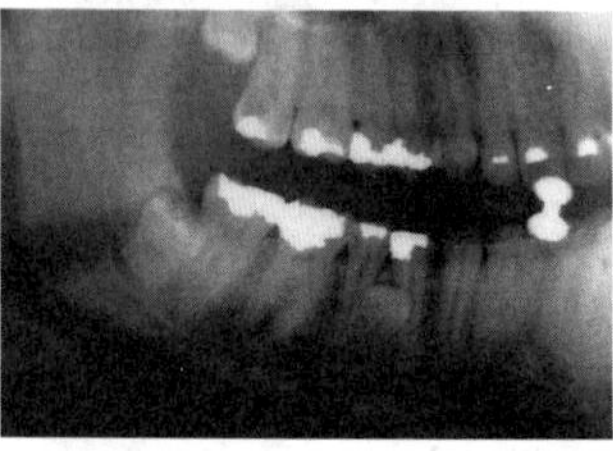

Supernumerary tooth. (Regezi/Sciubba/Jordan, 2008)

T

tooth, supplied (replaced teeth), *n.pl* an artificial replacement for natural teeth.

tooth surface pocket wall, *n* the portion of a narrow, infected sulcus that is adjacent to the surface of a tooth.

tooth, tube, *n.pl* artificial teeth constructed with a vertical, cylindric aperture extending from the center of the base into the body of the tooth into which a pin or cast post for the attachment of the tooth to a denture base may be placed.

tooth, Turner's, *n.pr* a permanent tooth showing hypoplasia resulting from injury or inflammation of the precedent primary tooth.

tooth wear, *n* the erosion of a tooth by chemical or mechanical processes.

tooth, zero degree, *n.pl* prosthetic teeth having no cusp angles in relation to the horizontal plane; cuspless teeth.

toothache, *n* pain located in the tooth or its surrounding supporting tissues. Dental pain may have a halo effect, making location of the precise source or location of the pain difficult. Determining the location may require several diagnostic tests.

toothache, nonodontogenic **(nonodon′tōjen′ik),** *n* pain that presents as a toothache but that is not of dental origin.

toothbrush, *n* a handheld device with an arrangement of bristles at one end, and a handle designed to reach effectively all exposed surfaces of the teeth and gingiva. A dentifrice is usually applied to the bristles for the purpose of cleaning the teeth and gingiva.

toothbrush, automatic, *n* an electric type. Also called *power-assisted toothbrush.*

toothbrush, bi-level orthodontic, *n* a type that is specifically designed to clean orthodontic appliances. The head of the tool features soft bristles that are shorter down the center, with hedges of taller bristles on either side, allowing the brush to pass over the appliance without causing abrasion to the teeth.

toothbrush, end-tuft, *n* a type that features a very small number of filaments. Handle may be angled to assist difficult-to-reach areas of both natural and replacement teeth. Also called *single-tuft* or *unituft.*

toothbrush head, *n* the section of the toothbrush that comes in direct contact with the teeth and gingiva, comprising various configurations of nylon bristles (filaments). The profile, or trim, of the head depends upon the number and height of bristle rows.

toothbrushing, *n* the use of a brush of varying design to brush the teeth and gingivae for cleanliness and to massage for oral hygiene. See also toothbrush.

toothbrushing, clock system, n a technique where a clock or timer is observed to ensure that brushing is sustained for a predetermined amount of time.

toothbrushing, faulty, n the improper performance of toothbrushing, resulting in defective cleansing, inadequate stimulation of the gingival tissues, and destructive effects on the teeth and marginal gingivae resulting from overzealous brushing.

toothbrushing, horizontal, n a method of teeth cleaning considered more harmful than beneficial. Characterized by long, parallel weight-bearing scrubbing movements that tend to damage teeth and gingiva while neglecting crucial areas between teeth.

toothbrushing, vertical, n See method, Leonard.

toothpaste, *n* See dentifrice.

toothpick, *n* a wood sliver used to cleanse the interdental space.

toothpick, balsa wood, n a triangular wedge of balsa wood used to clean the teeth interproximally and stimulate the interdental gingival tissues.

topical, *adj* **1.** of or pertaining to the surface of a part of the body. **2.** of or pertaining to a drug or treatment applied to the surface of a part of the body.

topical anesthesia, n See anesthesia, topical.

topographic anatomy, *n* the study of a specific region of a body structure, such as a lower leg, including all the systems in the part and their relationships to one another. Also referred to as *regional anatomy.*

topographic intraoral radiographic examination, *n* See examination, true occlusal topographic intraor.

topography (təpog′rəfē), *n* a detailed physical representation of anatomic features within a specific region.

torque (tôrk), *n* **1.** a force that produces or tends to produce rotation in a body. Such force applied to a tooth tends to cause rotation around its long axis. **2.** force applied to a tooth to produce rotation of a tooth on a mesiodistal or buccolingual (labiolingual) axis. **3.** a rotary force applied to a denture base.

torque driver (tork), *n* an electronic or manual instrument used to apply a rotational force.

torque wire, *n* an auxiliary wire used to torque the roots of the anterior teeth.

torque wrench, *n* See torque driver.

torsemide (tor′səmīd′), *n brand name:* Demadox; *drug class:* loop diuretic; *action:* acts on loop of Henle to decrease the reabsorption of chloride and sodium with resultant diuresis; *uses:* treatment of hypertension and edema associated with congestive heart failure (CHF), liver disease, and chronic renal failure.

torsion (tôr′shən), *n* in dentistry the twisting of a tooth on its long axis. Also, the loading of a wire by twisting it along its long axis.

torsion, clasp, n the twisting of the retentive clasp arm on its long axis. A retentive clasp may be formed so that it traverses a vertical distance before encircling the abutment to increase the torsion component of the clasp opening as compared with the flexure it experiences.

torsiversion (tôr′səvur′zhən), *n* an axially rotated tooth position.

tort, *n* a legal wrong perpetrated on a person or property, independent of contract.

torticollis (tôr′tikol′is), *n* an abnormal condition in which the head is inclined to one side as a result of the contraction of the muscles on that side of the neck.

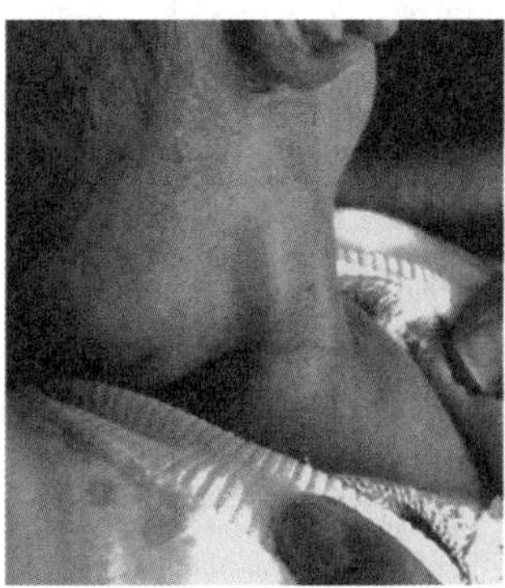

Torticollis. (Moore/Persaud, 2003)

torus (tôr′əs), *n* a bulging projection of bone.

torus mandibularis, *n* a bony enlargement (hyperostosis) appearing unilaterally or bilaterally on the lingual aspect of the mandible in the canine-premolar region of about 7% of the population.

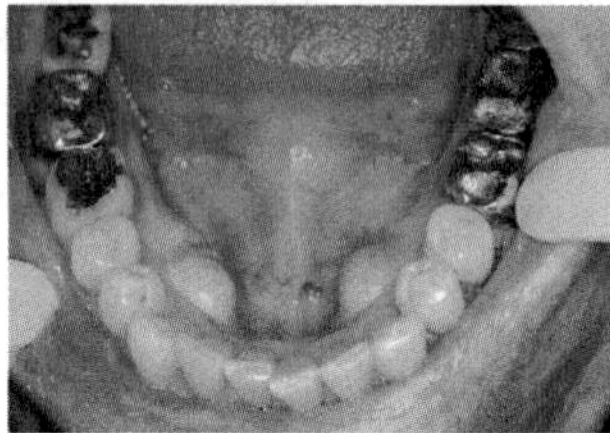

Torus mandibularis. (Regezi/Sciubba/Jordan, 2008)

torus palatinus, *n* a bony enlargement (hyperostosis) occurring in the midline of the hard palate in about 20% of the population.

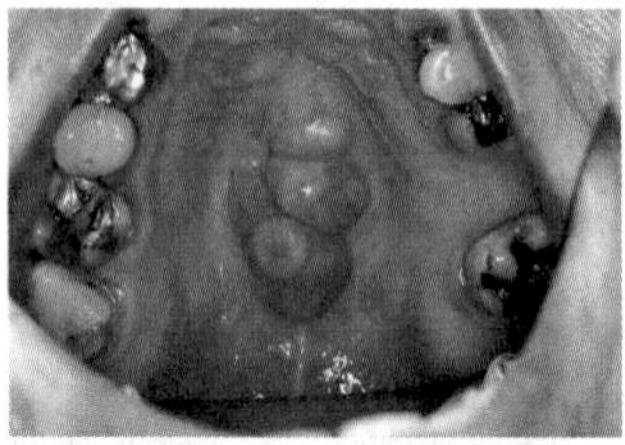

Torus palatinus. (Regezi/Sciubba/Jordan, 2008)

total filtration, *n* See filtration, total.

total hip arthroplasty, *n* total hip replacement; surgical reconstruction of the hip in which the ball-and-socket joint is replaced with a prosthesis.

total parenteral nutrition (TPN), *n* the administration of a nutritionally adequate hypertonic solution consisting of glucose, protein hydrolysates, minerals, and vitamins through an indwelling catheter into the superior vena cava.

total treatment plan, *n* a listing of all the necessary treatments and measures that dental staff must perform in order to restore full oral health to the patient.

touch, *n* the sense by which contact with an object provides evidence of its properties.

touch, light, *n* tactile sense. The principal organs of light touch are Meissner's corpuscles, which are large and oval. Each capsule receives several nerve fibers that shed their myelin sheaths and coil into a spiral complex network. Associated with Meissner's corpuscles in the perception of light touch are both Merkel's disks and a basketlike arrangement of nerve fibers around the hair follicles.

touch screen, *n* a type of screen on some video terminals that may be touched with the finger to specify the selection of an item from a displayed list.

Tourette's syndrome, *n* a condition in which the patient is unable to control numerous muscular and vocal tics, often resulting in twitching, grunting, or the making of inappropriate comments.

tourniquet (tur′nikit), *n* a device used in controlling hemorrhage, consisting of a wide constricting band applied to the limb proximal to the site of bleeding.

toxemia (toksē′mēə), *n* an abnormal condition in which there are toxic substances present in the blood.

toxic (tok′sik), *adj* poisonous; produced by a poison.

toxic delirium, *n* a symptom of disordered mental status as a result of poisoning.

toxic shock syndrome (TSS), *n* a severe, acute disease caused by infection with strains of *Staphylococcus aureus,* phage group I, that produce a unique toxin, enterotoxin F. It is most common in menstruating women using high-absorbency tampons but has occurred in infants, children, and men.

toxic waste, *n* refuse material that may be poisonous.

toxicity (toksis′itē), *n* the ability of a drug or poison to produce harm, especially to cause permanent injury or death. Usually distinguished from *allergenic properties.*

toxicity, acute, *n* a condition produced after short-term use of a toxic agent. See also dose, lethal, median; dose, lethal, minimum.

toxicity, chronic, *n* a condition produced after long-term use of a toxic agent.

toxicity, fluoride, *n* See fluoride toxicity.

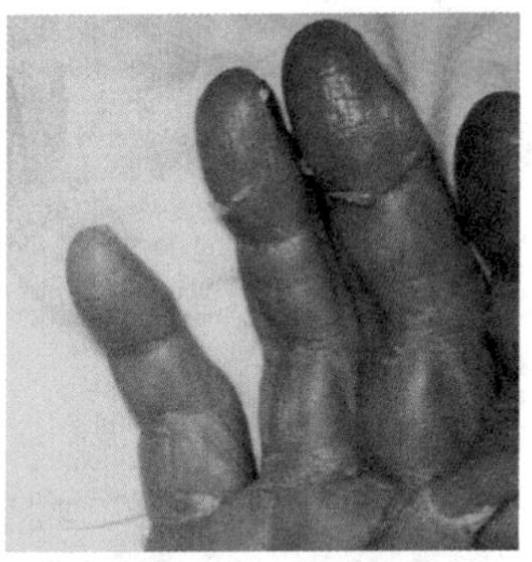

Toxic shock syndrome. (Zitelli/Davis, 2002. Courtesy Dr. George Pazin)

toxicologist (tok′sikol′əjist), *n* a person versed in toxicology.

toxicology (tok′sikol′əjē), *n* the scientific study of the nature and effects of poisons, their detection, and the treatment of their effects.

toxin (tok′sin), *n* a poisonous protein made by specific animals, higher levels of plants, and disease-causing bacteria.

toxoids (tok′soidz), *n.pl* toxins that have been treated to destroy their toxic properties but retain their ability to induce antibody production, thus creating an active immunity.

Toxoplasma gondii **(tok′sōplaz′mə gon′dēī),** *n* a protozoa commonly found in cat feces and undercooked meat. Pregnant women should avoid coming in contact with cat litter boxes, because the protozoa can cross the placenta and cause stillbirth or other serious physical or psychomotor defects in utero. See also toxoplasmosis.

toxoplasmosis (tok′sōplazmō′sis), *n* a disease caused by protozoa in the bloodstream and body tissues.

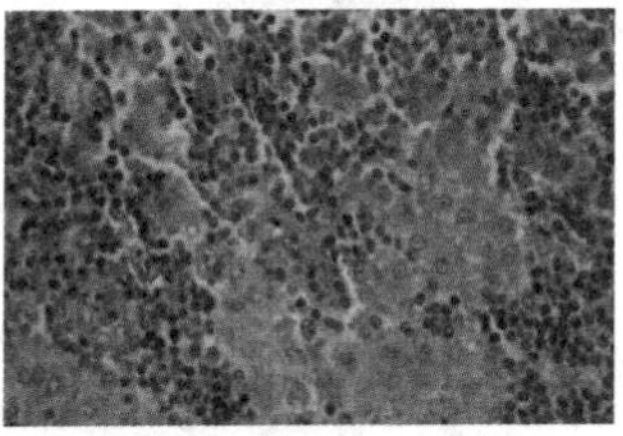

Toxoplasmosis. (Neville/Damm/Allen/Bouquot, 2002)

toxoplasmosis, neonatal, *n* an infection passed to the fetus during pregnancy via the placenta that can cause mental retardation, blindness, or an abnormally small head. See *Toxoplasma gondii.*

TPI, *n* See test, Treponema pallidum immobilization.

trabeculas (trəbek′yələs), *n* a thin, bar-shaped bony tissue in cancellous bone that intersects to form interconnected spaces filled with bone marrow.

trace element, *n* an element essential to nutrition or physiologic processes, found in such minute quantities that analysis yields a presence of virtually none.

tracer, *n* **1.** a mechanical device used to trace a pattern of mandibular movements. **2.** a foreign substance mixed with or attached to a given substance to enable the distribution or location of the latter to be determined subsequently. A radioactive tracer is a physical or chemical tracer having radioactivity as its distinctive property.

tracer, Gothic arch, *n* See tracer, needle point.

tracer, needle point, *n* a mechanical device consisting of a weighted or a spring-loaded needle that is attached to one jaw and a coated plate attached to the other jaw. Movement of the mandible causes a tracing to be formed on the horizontally placed plate. When the needle point is in the apex of the tracing, the mandible is said to be in the horizontal position of centric relation.

trachea (trā′kēə), *n* the windpipe; a cartilaginous and membranous tube extending from the lower end of the larynx to its division into two bronchi.

tracheo- (trā′kēō), *comb* combining form denoting connection with or relation to the trachea.

tracheobronchial (trā′kēōbrong′kēəl), *adj* pertaining to the trachea and a bronchus or bronchi.

tracheobronchoscopy (trā′kēōbrongkos′kəpē), *n* inspection of the interior of the trachea and bronchus.

tracheolaryngeal (trā′kēōlərin′jēəl), *adj* pertaining to the trachea and larynx.

tracheolaryngotomy (trā′kēōlərin-got′ōmē), *n* incision into the larynx and trachea; tracheotomy and laryngotomy.

tracheoscopy (trā′kēos′kəpē), *n* inspection of the interior of the trachea by means of a laryngoscopic mirror and reflected light or inspection through a bronchoscope.

tracheostenosis (trā′kēōstənō′sis), *n* abnormal constriction or narrowing of the trachea.

tracheostomy (trā′kēos′tōmē), *n* **1.** the formation of an opening into the trachea and the suturing of the edges of the opening to an opening in the skin of the neck. **2.** surgical formation of an opening into the trachea, usually through the tracheal rings below the cricoid cartilage, to give the patient an airway.

tracheotome (trā′kēōtōm), *n* **1.** a cutting instrument used in tracheotomy; a tracheotomy knife. **2.** an instrument for use in creating an airway through the skin into the trachea below the cricoid cartilage.

tracheotomy (trā′kēot′əmē), *n* the operation of cutting into the trachea to give the patient an airway.

tracing, *n* a line or lines or a pattern scribed by a pointed instrument or stylus on a tracing plate or tracing paper.

tracing, arrow point, *n* See tracing, needle point.

tracing, cephalometric **(sef′əlōmet′-rik),** *n* a line drawing of pertinent features of a cephalometric radiograph made on a piece of transparent paper placed over the radiograph.

tracing, extraoral, *n* a tracing of mandibular movements made outside the oral cavity.

tracing, Gothic arch, *n.pr* See tracing, needle point.

tracing, intraoral, *n* a tracing of mandibular movements made within the oral cavity. A tracing made by a mechanical device consisting of a weighted or spring-loaded stylus that is attached to one jaw and contacts a coated plate attached to the other jaw. Movement of the mandible causes a tracing to be formed on the horizontally placed coated plate. When the stylus point is in the apex of the tracing, the mandible is said to be in the horizontal position of centric relation. The shape of the tracing depends on the relative location of the marking point and tracing table. The various tracing shapes have been called *Gothic arch, arrow point,* and *sea gull tracings.* The apex of a properly made tracing indicates the most retruded unstrained relation of the mandible to the maxillae (i.e., the centric relation). The tracings are made by a stylus or needle point by the movement of the mandible. Unless otherwise designated, stylus tracings are made by lateral movements registered on a horizontal plate.

tracing, sea gull, *n* See tracing, needle point.

tracing, stylus, *n* See tracing, needle point.

tracings, pantographic, *n.pl* tracing of mandibular movements. A stylus is attached to the mandible traces line on vertical and horizontal plates attached to the maxilla, providing a graphic of the mandible's movements.

tract, sinus, *n* a communication between a pathologic space and an anatomic body cavity or between a pathologic space and the skin. A sinus tract may or may not be lined with epithelium.

traction, *n* the act of drawing (pulling).

traction, external, *n* a fracture reduction appliance principally used in the management of midfacial fractures. Points of fixation are located in the oral cavity and over the cranial area, and elastic or rigid connectors are placed between the cranial and oral points of fixation.

traction, intermaxillary, *n* See traction, maxillomandibular.

traction, internal, *n* a pulling force created by using one of the cranial bones above the point of fracture for anchorage.

traction, maxillomandibular (intermaxillary traction), *n* the technique for reducing fractures of the maxilla or mandible into functional relations with the opposing dental arch through the use of elastic or wire ligatures and interdental wiring or splints.

trade name, *n* **1.** the name under which a company conducts its business. **2.** the commercial name of a company's product.

trademark, *n* a word, symbol, or device assigned to a product by its manufacturer, possibly registered, as a part of its identity.

tragion (trā'jēon), *n* the notch just above the tragus of the ear. It lies 1 to 2 mm below the spina helicis, which may be easily palpated.

tragus (trā'gus), *n* a prominence in front of the opening of the external ear.

training grant, *n* an award of money or other resources to provide training in a particular field, usually in areas of public need or demand.

trait (trāt), *n* an inherited set of mental or bodily characteristics.

trait, Cooley's, *n.pr* See thalassemia minor.

trait, sickle cell, *n* a form of sickle cell disease in which patients are asymptomatic but their erythrocytes can be caused to assume a sickle shape under certain conditions. The trait is present when one parent has the gene (heterozygous condition) for sickle cell disease. See also disease, sickle cell.

tramadol HCl (tram'ədol), *n brand name:* Ultram; *drug class:* synthetic opioid analgesic; *action:* unknown, but it has been shown to bind to opioid receptors and inhibit the reuptake of norepinephrine and serotonin; *use:* treatment of moderate to severe pain.

tranquilizer (trang'kwilīzur), *n* one of a poorly defined group of drugs designed to control anxiety and reduce tension or stress. Tranquilizers tend to induce drowsiness and may cause physical and psychologic dependence. Most tranquilizers are controlled substances.

transaminase (transam'inās), *n* one of several enzymes involved in the reversible transfer of an amino (NH_2) group from an α-amino acid to an α-ketoacid, especially α-ketoglutaric acid. Characteristic high values are seen in myocardial infarction and viral hepatitis.

transamination (tranzam'inā'shən), *n* the reaction between an α-ketoacid and an amino acid in which the amino group moves to the α-ketoacid, creating a new amino acid and a new ketoacid.

transdermal delivery system, *n* a method of applying a drug to unbroken skin. The drug is absorbed through the skin and enters the body's systems. It is used particularly for the administration of nitroglycerin and in nicotine patches used to assist individuals to withdraw from the use of tobacco.

transducer (tranzdoo'sur), *n* a device that is activated by power from one system and then supplies a different form of power to a second system; used to convert electric energy into mechanical energy in ultrasonic and sonic scalers.

transfection (transfek'shən), *n* the process by which a bacterial cell is infected with purified deoxyribonucleic acid (DNA) or ribonucleic acid (RNA) isolated from a virus or a viral vector after a specific pretreatment.

transfer agreement, *n* a written contract between two health care institutions for the transfer of patients from one to the other and for the orderly exchange of pertinent clinical information on the patients transferred.

transfer belt, *n* a belt used to transfer a disabled person from one location to another by placing the belt around that person's waist and using it to hold on to while safely transferring the patient.

transfer coping, *n* See impression coping.

transferase (trans'fərās'), *n* a group of enzymes that catalyze the transfer of a chemical group or radical from one molecule to another.

transferrin (transfer'in), *n* a trace protein present in the blood that is essential in the transport of iron from the intestine into the bloodstream, making it available to the normoblasts in the bone marrow.

transformer, *n* an electrical device that increases or reduces the voltage of an alternating current by mutual induction between primary and secondary coils or windings.

transformer, auto-, *n* See autotransformer.

transformer, Coolidge filament, *n.pr* a step-down transformer that reduces line voltage of 110 volts to 12 volts, which in turn heats the tungsten filament of the Coolidge tube for the production of electrons.

transformer, step-down, n a transformer in which the secondary voltage is less than the primary voltage.

transformer, step-up, n a transformer in which the secondary voltage is greater than the primary voltage.

transforming growth factor (TGF), *n* a group of proteins produced by cells of a tumor that, when inoculated into a normal cell culture, causes a disorderly increase in the number of cells in the culture.

transforming growth factor beta (TGF-β), *n* a substance that is produced by bone cells and platelets to promote bone regeneration and wound healing.

transfusion (transfū′zhən), *n* the introduction into the bloodstream of whole blood or blood components such as plasma, platelets, or packed red cells. Infused donor blood must be matched to the recipient's blood type and antigen group.

transient (tran′zēənt), *adj* pertaining to a condition that is temporary or of short duration, usually not recurring.

transillumination (tran′siloo′minā′shən), *n* **1.** examination of an organ, cavity, or tissue (e.g., tooth or gingival tissue) by transmitted light. A valuable aid in detecting carious lesions, disclosing carious or demineralized dentin during cavity preparation, checking the finish or gingival margins of restorations, and revealing cement, debris, or calculus subgingivally. **2.** a test in which the use of transmitted light may disclose a discoloration of the coronal aspect, indicating dentinal tubular hemorrhage as a result of trauma, pulpal necrosis, or fracture. **3.** examination of tissues by means of a light placed so that the region under study is between the light source and the observer.

transition point, *n* See Tg value.

transitional dentition (mixed), *n* an older term for the final phase of the transition from primary to permanent teeth, in which most primary teeth have been lost or are in the process of shedding and the permanent successors are not yet in function.

translation, *n* movement of a rigid body in which all parts move in the same direction at the same speed.

translatory movement, *n* See movement, translatory.

translocation, *n* the rearrangement of genetic material within the same chromosome or the transfer of a segment of one chromosome to another nonhomologous one.

translucency (transloo′sənsē), *n* an object's ability to allow the passage of light through it.

transmission, *n* the transfer or conveyance of a thing or condition, such as an infectious or genetic disease or hereditary trait, from one person to another.

transmission, horizontal, n the transfer of an infection from person to person; direct transmission of a disease.

transmission, vertical, n the transmission of a disease from mother to child either during pregnancy, childbirth, or by breastfeeding.

transmission scanning electron microscope, *n* an instrument that transmits a highly magnified, well-resolved, three-dimensional image to a television screen, thus combining the advantages of the transmission electron and scanning electron microscopes.

transmission-based precautions, *n* a set of procedures whose goal is to prevent the communication of infectious diseases. They are to be used in addition to the standard precautions procedures.

transmucosal (tranz′mūkō′səl), *adj* administration of a substance, such as a drug, through the mucous membranes.

transosteal (transos′tēəl), *n* a type of dental implant whose metal posts pass through the mandible.

transosteal implant jig, *n* an instrument designed to guide a bone drill from the inferior border through the alveolar ridge to create a path for the seating of a transosteal implant.

transplant, *v* **1.** to remove and plant in another place, as from one body or part of a body to another. *n* **2.** implantation of living or nonliving tissue or bone into another part of the body; it then serves as a scaffold in the healing process and is progressively resorbed and replaced by newly formed bone. *v* **3.** to move a tooth or tissue from one site to another, often but not always autogenously.

transplantation, allogenic bone marrow (al′ōjen′ik), *n* the transfer of healthy bone marrow taken from a sibling in order to stimulate normal blood cell production.

transplantation, autogenous, *n* tooth, transplantation of a tooth from one position to another in the same individual.

transplantation, autologous bone marrow (ôtol′əgus), *n* the transfer of healthy bone marrow from one site to another in the same body in order to stimulate normal blood cell production.

transplantation, homogenous tooth, *n* transplantation of a tooth from one human to another.

transport, *n* the movement of biochemical substances from one site to another.

transport, active, *n* transport of substances through membranes or epithelium, requiring metabolic energy.

transport, passive, *n* transport along a gradient without the use of metabolic energy.

transseptal fiber, *n* See fiber, transseptal.

transudate (tran′soodāt), *n* any fluid substance that has passed through a membrane, possibly associated with inflammation. It is low in proteins and colloids and has a low specific gravity.

transverse (transvurs′), *adj* at right angles to the long axis of a common part.

transverse palatine suture, *n* See suture, transverse palatine.

transverse plane of space, *n* an imaginary plane that cuts the body in two, separating the superior half from the inferior half, and that lies at a right angle from the body's vertical axis.

transverse ridge, *n* ridge formed by the joining of two triangular ridges crossing the occlusal table transversely or from the labial to the lingual outline.

transversion, *n* eruption of a tooth in the wrong position

tranylcypromine sulfate (tran′əlsī′-prəmēn′), *n brand name:* Parnate; *drug class:* antidepressant, monoamine oxidase inhibitor (MAOI); *action:* increases concentrations of endogenous norepinephrine, serotonin, and dopamine in central nervous system (CNS) storage sites; *use:* treatment of depression (when uncontrolled by other means).

trauma (trou′mə, trô′mə), *n* a hurt; a wound; an injury; damage; impairment; external violence producing bodily injury or degeneration.

trauma, cumulative, *n* medical condition developing in the peripheral and autonomic nervous systems and musculoskeletal system due to forceful, awkward, and repetitive bodily motions as well as exposure to cold temperatures, mechanical stress, and vibrations.

trauma, injury in occlusal, *n* the damaging effects of occlusal trauma, which are of a dystrophic nature and affect the tooth and its periodontium. Lesions include wear facets on the tooth, root resorption, cemental tears, thrombosis of blood vessels of the periodontal membrane, necrosis and hyalinization of the periodontal membrane on the pressure side, and resorption of alveolar and supporting bone. Clinically, tooth mobility and migration may be evident; radiographically, evidence includes the widening of the periodontal membrane space and fraying or fuzziness of the lamina dura and formation of infrabony resorptive defects. Pocket formation is not a sequela to occlusal traumatism.

trauma, occlusal, *n* abnormal occlusal relationships of the teeth, causing injury to the periodontium.

traumatic (trômat′ik), *adj* of, pertaining to, or caused by an injury.

traumatic occlusion, *n* See occlusion, traumatic.

traumatic shock, *n* See shock, traumatic.

traumatism, *n* **1.** an injury. **2.** a wound produced by an injury; trauma.

traumatism by food, *n* impingement of the gingival margin by coarse foodstuff caused by improper contour of the tooth or faulty position of the tooth.

traumatism by food, occlusal, n lesions of the periodontium; caused by force placed on the tooth in excess of that which the supporting structures can withstand.

traumatism by food, periodontal, n the application of stress to the structures constituting the periodontium exceeding the adaptive capacities of the tissues, with resultant tissue destruction.

traumatism by food, primary occlusal, n force or forces caused by mandibular movement and resultant tooth percussion and capable of producing pathologic changes in the periodontium.

traumatism by food, secondary occlusal, n destruction of the periodontium by factors other than those of occlusion (e.g., periodontitis). In secondary occlusal traumatism, even the forces of mastication become pathologic in nature.

traumatogenic (trô′mətōjen′ik), *adj* capable of producing a wound or injury.

traumatogenic occlusion, n See occlusion, traumatic.

tray, *n* a receptacle or device that holds or carries.

tray, acrylic resin, n a tray made of acrylic resin.

tray, impression, n a receptacle or device that is used to carry impression material to the oral cavity, confine the material in apposition to the surfaces to be recorded, and control the impression material while it sets to form the impression.

tray, impression, maxillary, n a tray consisting of a body with a protruding edge and handle used to contain a material (e.g., rubber, hydrocolloid, or alginate) against the palatal tissues for making a mold of the maxillary arch structures.

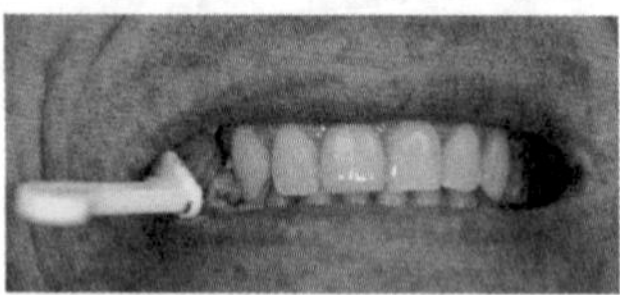

Triple tray. (Courtesy Dr. David Nunez)

tray, triple, n a tray used to make an impression of a prepared tooth as well as opposing teeth. Such impressions are then used to prepare fixed prostheses and to make a bite registration.

trazodone HCl (trā′zədōn′), *n brand names:* Desyrel, Trazon, Trialodine; *drug class:* antidepressant; *action:* selectively inhibits serotonin-specific reuptake in the brain; *use:* treatment of depression.

Treacher Collins syndrome, *n.pr* See syndrome, Treacher Collins.

treatment, *n* the mode or course pursued for remedial ends.

treatment, atraumatic restorative (ART), n a procedure for preventing and treating dental caries using hand instruments and adhesive filling material. Does not require electricity or anesthesia and may be performed in the field by trained health care workers or nondental personnel.

treatment, hardening heat, n See tempering.

treatment, heat, n **1.** subjecting a metal to a given controlled heat, followed by controlled sudden or gradual cooling to develop the desired qualities of the metal to the maximal degree. **2.** a process of giving a metal predetermined physical properties by controlled temperature changes.

treatment, homogenizing heat, n See anneal.

treatment, indirect pulp capping, n See capping, indirect pulp.

treatment, indirect, relationship, n an association between a health care provider and an individual in which the health care provided to the individual by the health care provider has been ordered by another provider.

treatment plan, n in dentistry a schedule of procedures and appointments designed to restore, step by step, the oral health of a patient.

treatment, prescription, n the formal outline of the projected treatment of a patient (e.g., the blueprint from which the dental professional projects treatment).

treatment, rest (sedative treatment), n use of a drug sealed into a root canal to relieve pain or discomfort; not used primarily for its antiseptic value.

treatment, root canal, n the techniques and pharmaceuticals used in removing pulp tissue, sterilizing the root canal, and preparing the root canal for filling.

treatment, sedative, n See treatment, rest.

treatment, softening heat, n See anneal.

trematodes (trem′ətōdz), *n* parasitic worms such as *Paragonimus westermani* that reside in contaminated water and can be transmitted to humans who are exposed to such water sources or who eat improperly cooked fish from the same.

tremolo (trem′əlō), *n* an irregular and exaggerated speech pattern that may be the symptom of an emotional disturbance or of various diseases affecting the nervous control of the organs of respiration and phonation.

tremor (trem′ər), *n* rhythmic, purposeless, quivering movements resulting from the involuntary alternating contraction and relaxation of opposing skeletal muscle groups.

trench mouth, *n* See gingivitis, acute necrotizing ulcerative.

Trendelenburg position (trendel′ənburg), *n.pr* See position, Trendelenburg.

trepanation (trephination), *n* the act of surgically cutting a round hole.

trephine (trefēn′), *n* a circle-cutting surgical instrument designed to remove a circumscribed portion of tissue. It permits the insertion of the heads of intramucosal inserts into the tissue.

***Treponema* (trep′ənē′mə),** *n* a genus of schizomycetes composed of parasitic and pathogenic spiral microorganisms.

Treponema microdentium, n a species found in the normal oral cavity.

Treponema mucosum, n a species found in periodontal infections in man.

Treponema pallidum, n the spirochete that causes syphilis in humans.

Treponema vincentii, n a spirochete associated with acute necrotizing ulcerative gingivitis.

tretinoin (vitamin A acid, retinoic acid), *n brand name:* Retin-A; *drug class:* vitamin A acid; *action:* decreases cohesiveness of follicular epithelium, decreases microcomedone formation; *use:* treatment of acne vulgaris.

triad, Hutchinson (trī′ad), *n.pr* a group of conditions that includes interstitial keratitis, deafness, and Hutchinson teeth resulting from congenital syphilis. Not current.

triage (trēäzh′), *n* **1.** (in military medicine) a classification of casualties of war and other disasters according to the gravity of injuries, urgency of treatment, and place for treatment. **2.** a process in which a group of patients is sorted according to need for care. The kind of illness or injury, severity of the problem, and facilities available govern the process, as in the emergency room of a hospital. **3.** (in disaster medicine) a process in which a large group of patients is sorted so that care may be concentrated on those who are likely to survive.

trial, *n* an examination before a competent tribunal of the facts or law in issue in a cause of action for the purpose of determining the issue.

trial base, *n* See baseplate.

triamcinolone (trī′amsin′əlōn′), *n* a synthetic adrenocorticosteroid that has a potent antiinflammatory effect and is used topically in the treatment of angular cheilosis.

triamcinolone acetonide (topical) (as′ətō′nīd), *n brand names:* Aristocort, Flutex, Kenalog, Kenalog in Orabase, Oracort, Triacet, Triderm, others; *drug class:* topical corticosteroid; *action:* interacts with steroid cytoplasmic receptors to induce antiinflammatory effects; possesses antipruritic and antiinflammatory actions; *uses:* treatment of psoriasis, eczema, contact dermatitis, pruritus; special dental paste used to treat nonviral inflammatory oral lesions, including aphthous stomatitis, lichen planus, and cicatrical pemphigoid.

triamcinolone/triamcinolone acetonide/triamcinolone diacetate/triamcinolone hexacetonide, *n brand names:* Triamcinolone (oral), Aristocort, Atolone, Kenacort, many others; *drug class:* glucocorticoid, intermediate-acting; *action:* decreases inflammation by suppressing macrophage and leukocyte migration, reduces capillary permeability and inhibits lysosomal enzymes and phagocytosis; *uses:* treatment of severe inflammation; immunosuppression; neoplasms; collagen, respiratory, and dermatologic disorders; and seasonal and perennial allergic rhinitis.

triamterene (trīam′tərēn′), *n brand name:* Dyrenium; *drug class:* potassium-sparing diuretic; *action:* acts on distal tubule to inhibit reabsorption of sodium, chlorine; increases potassium retention; *uses:* treatment of edema; hypertension.

triangle, *n* a three-cornered area.

triangle, anterior cervical, *n* one of two major triangles delineated by the sternocleidomastoid muscles, it extends approximately from the inferior part of the neck to the mandible.

triangle, Bolton, *n.pr* a triangle formed by drawing a line from the nasion to the sella turcica and from there to the Bolton point.

triangle, Bonwill, *n.pr* an equilateral triangle with 4-inch (10-cm) sides bounded by lines from the contact points of the mandibular central incisors (or the median line of the residual ridge of the mandible) to the condyle on either side and from one condyle to the other. It is the basis for Bonwill's theory of occlusion.

triangle, carotid, *n* also called the superior carotid triangle. The region of the neck bounded by the posterior belly of digastric muscle, the superior belly of the omohyoid muscle, and the anterior border of sternomastoid muscle. The carotid triangle contains numerous veins, arteries, and nerves.

triangle, cervical, posterior, *n* a region of the neck containing numerous vein, artery, and lymph node structures.

triangle, hyoid, *n* an area consisting of the hyoid bone and its ligaments, located in front of the throat above the Adam's apple. The presence of a raised, or positive, hyoid triangle is indicative of neck or jaw injury.

triangle, submandibular, *n* a region in the neck bounded by the mandible and the anterior and posterior bellies of the digastric muscle; contains the submandibular gland. Also known as the *digastric triangle* or the *submaxillary triangle.*

triangle, submental, *n* a region in the neck bounded by the anterior belly of the gastric muscle, the midline of the neck, and the hyoid bone. Its floor is the mylohyoid muscle, and it contains the submental lymph nodes, the anterior jugular vein, and the submental artery.

triangle, Tweed, *n.pr* a triangle formed by the mandibular plane, Frankfort plane, and long axis of the mandibular central incisor. Proposed as a diagnostic aid by C.H. Tweed.

triangular fossa, *n* fossa that has a triangular shape where the triangular grooves terminate.

triangular ridges, *n.pl* cusp ridges that descend from the cusp tips toward the central portion of the occlusal table.

triangulation (trīang′yəlā′shən), *n* a wedge-shaped area between the root surface and alveolar crest that permits the passage of radiographic rays.

triazolam (trī′az′əlam), *n brand name:* Halcion; *drug class:* benzodiazepine, sedative-hypnotic, controlled substance schedule IV; *action:* produces central nervous system (CNS) depression by interacting with a benzodiazepine receptor to facilitate the action of the inhibitory neurotransmitter gamma-aminobutyric acid (GABA); *use:* treatment of insomnia.

Trichinella spiralis **(trik′inel′ə spīral′is),** *n* a round worm found in raw or undercooked pork products. The worm resides in muscle tissue and is implicated in trichinosis food poisoning. Symptoms of infection, when they occur, are similar to those of food poisoning.

trichoepithelioma (trik′ōep′ithē′lēō′mə), *n* a benign skin tumor arising from the epithelium or hair follicles. See also epithelioma adenoides cysticum.

Trichuris **(trikyŏŏr′is),** *n* a genus of parasitic roundworms that infect the intestinal tract. Adult worms are 30 to 50 mm long and resemble whips with a threadlike anterior and a thicker posterior. Also called *whipworm.*

triclosan (trīklō′san), *n* an antibacterial agent, combined with a liquid, paste, or powder, used to clean the teeth by reducing gingivitis and plaque within the oral cavity. It can be used in combination with fluoride.

trident (trī′dənt), *n* a tooth with three cusps. Also called *tridentate* or *tricuspid.*

tridymite (trid′imīt), *n* a physical form of silica used in combination with cristobalite to limit thermal expansion.

trifluoperazine HCl (trī′floo′ōper′əzēn′), *n brand name:* Stelazine; *drug class:* phenothiazine antipsychotic; *action:* blocks neurotransmission at dopaminergic synapses in cerebral cortex, hypothalamus, and limbic system; *uses:* treatment of psychotic disorders, nonpsychotic anxiety, and schizophrenia.

triflupromazine HCl (trī′floo′prō′məzēn′), *n brand name:* Vesprin; *drug class:* phenothiazine, antipsychotic; *action:* blocks neurotransmission at dopaminergic synapses in the cerebral cortex, hypothalamus, and limbic system; *uses:* treatment of psychotic disorders, schizophrenia, acute agitation, nausea, and vomiting.

trifluridine (ophthalmic) (trī′floor′idēn′ ofthal′mik), *n brand name:* Viroptic ophthalmic solution; *drug class:* antiviral; *action:* inhibits viral deoxyribonucleic acid (DNA) synthesis and replication; *uses:* treatment of primary keratoconjunctivitis, recurring epithelial keratitis, and keratitis associated with herpes simplex virus types 1 and 2.

trifurcation, *n* division into three parts or branches, as the three roots of a maxillary first molar.

trigeminal nerve (trī′jem′ənəl), *n* See nerve, trigeminal.

trigeminal neuralgia, *n* a neurologic condition of the trigeminal nerve characterized by paroxysms of flashing, stablike, unilateral pain radiating along the course of a branch of the nerve. Any or all of the three branches may be affected. The attacks are initiated by stimuli, such as a light touch of the skin, chewing, washing the face, or brushing the teeth. In some individuals the attacks may be initiated by painless physical stimulation of specific areas that are located on the same side of the face as the pain. Also called *tic douloureux.*

trigger point, *n* See point, trigger.

trihexyphenidyl HCl, *n brand names:* Trihexane, Trihexy-5; *drug class:* antiparkinsonian, anticholinergic; *action:* blocks central muscarinic receptors, which decreases the severity of involuntary movements; *use:* treatment of Parkinson's disease symptoms.

triiodothyronine (trī′ī′ō′dōthī′rənēn′), *n* a hormone that helps regulate growth and development, control metabolism and body temperature, and by a negative-feedback system, inhibit the secretion of thyrotropin by the pituitary gland.

trilaminar embryonic disk (trī′lamənər), *n* a platelike area of ectoderm, mesoderm, and endoderm within a zygote that represents the first stage of embryonic development.

trilogy of Fallot, *n* a congenital cardiac anomaly consisting of a combination of pulmonic stenosis, interatrial septal defect, and right ventricular hypertrophy.

trimeprazine tartrate (trīmep′rəzēn′), *n brand name:* Temaril; *drug class:* antihistamine H_1 receptor antagonist; *action:* acts by competing with histamine for H_1 receptor sites; decreases allergic response by blocking histamine effects; *use:* treatment of pruritus.

trimester (trīmes′tər), *n* one of the three periods of approximately 3 months each into which pregnancy is divided.

trimethadione (trīmeth′ədī′ōn), *n brand name:* Tridione; *drug class:* anticonvulsant; *action:* increases the threshold for seizures initiated in the cortex, decreases central nervous system (CNS) synaptic stimulation to low-frequency impulses; *use:* treatment of refractory absence (petit mal) seizures.

trimethobenzamide (trīmeth′ōben′zəmīd′), *n brand name:* Arrestin, Bio-Gan, Stemetic, Ticon, Tigan, T-Gen, Triban, others; *drug class:* antiemetic; *action:* acts centrally by blocking the chemoreceptor trigger zone, which in turn acts on vomiting center; *uses:* treatment of nausea and vomiting and prevention of postoperative vomiting.

trimethoprim-sulfamethoxazole (trīmeth′əprim′ sul′fəmethok′səzōl), *n* a synthetic antibacterial combination effective in urinary tract infections; it is the drug of choice in the treatment of *Pneumocystis jiroveci* pneumonia, one of the opportunistic infections associated with acquired immunodeficiency syndrome (AIDS).

trimetrexate glucuronate (trī'mi-trek'sāt'), *n brand name:* Neutrexin; *drug class:* folate antogonist; *action:* inhibits the enzyme dihydrofolate reductase, which leads to interference with deoxyribonucleic acid (DNA), ribonucleic acid (RNA), and protein synthesis in the *Pneumocystis carinii* organism; *uses:* alternative therapy for *P. carinii* pneumonia in immunocompromised patients, including patients with acquired immunodeficiency syndrome (AIDS).

trimipramine maleate (trīmip'rə-mēn), *n brand name:* Surmontil; *drug class:* antidepressant-tricyclic; *action:* inhibits both norepinephrine and serotonin (5-HT) uptake in the brain; *uses:* treatment of depression and of enuresis in children.

trimmer, gingival margin, *n* (margin trimmer), a binangled, double-paired, chisel-shaped, single-beveled, double-planed lateral cutting instrument. The blade is curved left or right similar to a spoon excavator; the cutting edge is straight and not perpendicular to the axis of the blade. The pair with the end of the cutting edge farthest from the shaft forming an acute angle is termed *distal* and is used to bevel a distal gingival margin or accentuate a mesial axiogingival angle; the pair with the acute angle of the cutting edge closest to the shaft is called *mesial* and is used to bevel a mesial gingival margin or accentuate a distal axiogingival angle. When one of these trimmers is used, all four must be used.

T

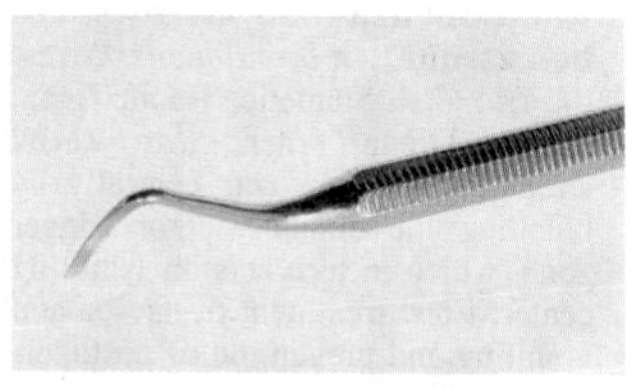

Gingival margin trimmer. (Bird/Robinson, 2005)

trimmer, margin, *n* See trimmer, gingival margin.

trimmer, model, *n* a device used to trim the edges of the full-scale stone or plaster reproduction of the teeth and nearby tissues. It may be a mechanical tool or plaster knife. See also cast, trimming diagnostic.

trimming, tissue, *n* See border molding.

tripelennamine HCl (trī'pelen'ə-mēn'), *n brand names:* PBZ, PBZ-SR, Pelamine; *drug class:* antihistamine, H_1 receptor antagonist; *action:* acts by competing with histamine for H_1 receptor sites; *uses:* treatment of rhinitis and allergy symptoms.

triplegia (trīplē'jēə), *n* a condition where three out of the four limbs are paralyzed.

tripoding (trī'pōding), *n* the marking of a cast at three points in the same plane as a means of repositioning the cast in that plane during subsequent procedures.

tripodism (trī'podiz'əm), *n* a widely used principle to gain instant stability on uneven terrains in all landings. It is referred to as a three-point landing. Stamp cusps in well-organized occlusion have only three-point contacts with their fossa brims (none with their tips).

triprolidine HCl (trīprō'lidēn), *n brand name:* Myidil; *drug class:* antihistamine, H_1 receptor antagonist; *action:* acts by competing with histamine for H_1 receptor sites; *uses:* treatment of rhinitis and allergy symptoms.

trismus (triz'məs), *n* spasms of the muscles of mastication resulting in the inability to open the oral cavity; often symptomatic of pericoronitis.

trisomy (trī'səmē), *n* an additional chromosome in the normal complement, so that in each nucleus a chromosome is represented three times rather than twice.

trisomy B, *n* (trisomy 13-15, Patau's syndrome) Clinical syndrome associated with an autosomal abnormality in which the extra chromosome occurs in the 13 to 15 group. Numerous anatomic defects are present, including hemangiomas, hernia, arrhinencephaly, eye anomalies, cleft lip and palate, and characteristic changes in the footprint and palm print.

trisomy syndrome, *n* a congenital condition caused by the addition of an extra member to a normal pair of homologous autosomes or to the sex chromosome or by the translocation of a portion of one chromosome to another. Trisomy 21 results in Down syndrome.

trituration (trich′oorā′shən), *n* the process of mixing together silver alloy fillings with mercury to produce amalgam.

trituration, hand, n the older method of mixing of constituents by hand in a mortar and pestle.

trituration, mechanical, n the newer method of mixing of constituents in a mechanical device or amalgamator.

troche (trō′kē), *n* See lozenge.

trophoblast layer (trof′oblast), *n* the layer of peripheral embryonic cells from which the placenta is formed.

true vocal cords, *n.pl* the vocal folds of the larynx as distinguished from the vestibular folds, called the *false vocal cords.*

True's separator, *n.pr* See separator, True's.

truss arm, *n* See connector, minor.

trust, *n* a relationship in which one person or entity holds fiduciary responsibility for another's property or enterprise.

try-in, *n* a preliminary placement of a trial denture (complete or removable partial), a partial denture casting, or a finished restoration to evaluate fit, appearance, and maxillomandibular relations.

try-in, mandibular tray, n the initial dry run to position a mandibular impression tray into the floor of the mouth to ensure the correct fit of a cast of the mandibular arch.

try-in, maxillary tray, n the initial dry run to position a maxillary impression tray into the palatal tissues to ensure the correct fit of a cast of the maxillary arch.

trypsin (trip′sin), *n* a proteolytic digestive enzyme produced by the exocrine pancreas that catalyzes in the small intestine the breakdown of dietary proteins to peptones, peptides, and amino acids.

tryptase (trip′tās), *n* See plasmin.

tryptophan, *n* one of the essential amino acids. See also amino acid.

TSH, *n* See hormone, thyrotropic.

t-test, *n* an inferential statistic used to test for differences between two means (groups) only. This statistic is used for small samples (e.g., $N < 30$). Also called *t-ratio, student's t.*

tub and tray system, *n* a system of instrument and supply management in which the instruments for a particular task are prearranged on a tray and the accompanying disposables are prearranged in an accompanying tub. The prepared trays and tubs are appropriately sterilized, stored, and delivered to the dental operatory at the proper time. May also use cartridges to facilitate the process. See also setup.

tube, *n* a hollow cylindrical structure.

tube, buccal, n a section of tubing attached to the buccal side of a molar band in a horizontal position, serving as an attachment for the labial arch wire, which slides into the tube.

tube, Coolidge, n.pr a radiographic tube in which the gas pressure is purposely made so low that it plays no role in the operation of the tube, the operation of which depends on the emission of electrons by the heated filament of the cathode. See also radiographic tube, Coolidge.

tube, discharge, n a vacuum tube in which a high-voltage electric current is discharged (e.g., a radiographic tube).

tube, endotracheal, n a plastic tube inserted into the trachea to permit the passage of air to and from the lungs. Tubes are available in varying diameters, depending on the size and age of the patient.

tube, horizontal, n a metal tube attachment that is placed in a horizontal position on the buccal surface of each anchor molar tooth to allow for the insertion of the labial arch wire.

tube, intubation, n a tube for insertion into the larynx through the oral cavity.

tube, line focus, n a radiographic tube in which the target face is about 20 inches (50 cm) from the cathode face. The focal spot is rectangular, with the length approximately three times the width. The acute angle provides an effective focal spot area approximately square and a fraction of the actual area in size.

tube, nasogastric **(naz′ōgas′trik),** *n* a plastic tube inserted through the nose, down the esophagus, and into the stomach. It is used to remove the stomach's contents or to pass food directly to the stomach. Also known as an *NG tube.*

tube, protective, housing, *n* a radiographic tube enclosure that provides radiation protection.

tube, protective, housing, diagnostic, *n* a tube housing that reduces the leakage of radiation to, at most, 0.10 r/hr at a distance of 1 mm from the tube target when the tube is operating at its maximal continuous rated voltage.

tube, protective, housing, therapeutic, *n* a tube housing that reduces the leakage of radiation to, at most, 1 r/hr at a distance of 1 m from the tube target when the tube is operating at its maximal continuous rated current for the maximal rated voltage.

tube, right-angle, *n* a radiographic tube in which the target is at right angles to the cathode.

tube tooth, *n* See tooth, tube.

tube, vertical, *n* an attachment that is usually placed on the lingual surface of the anchor band to allow for the insertion of the lingual wire.

tube, radiographic, *n* See radiographic tube.

tube feeding, *n* a method for supplying liquid nutrition through a tube that passes through the nasal passages and into the stomach. This method is utilized when ingesting food through the oral cavity is inadvisable or painful due to surgery or injury.

T

tubercle (too′burkəl), *n* **1.** a small rounded nodule or elevation on the surface of the skin, bone, or other tissue. **2.** the accessory cusps on the cingulum of certain anterior teeth or occlusal tables of permanent molars.

tubercle, genial **(jēnē′əl),** *n* (geniohyoid tubercle), a small rounded elevation on the lingual surface of the mandible on either side of the midline near the inferior border of the body of the mandible, serving as a point of insertion for the geniohyoid muscles.

tubercle, geniohyoid **(jē′nēōhī′oid),** *n* See tubercle, genial.

tubercle, superior genial, *n* the small spines on the lingual surface of the mandible that serve as the attachment for the genioglossus muscles. On resorbed mandibles, these tubercles may be at or above the crest of the residual ridge.

tubercle of the upper lip (superior labial), *n* midline thickening of the superior lip.

tuberculin skin test, *n* See test, tuberculin.

tuberculum impar, *n* a portion of the developing tongue located in the midline.

tuberculosis (toobur′kūlō′sis), *n* an infectious disease caused by *M. tuberculosis* and characterized by the formation of tubercles in the tissues.

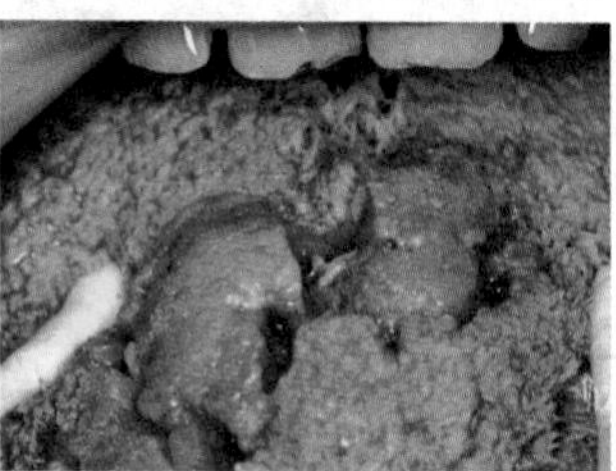

Tuberculosis of tongue. (Regezi/Sciubba/Pogrel, 2000)

tuberculous lymphadenitis **(tŏŏbur′kyələs),** *n* an inflammation of the lymph glands caused by the presence of *M. tuberculosis.*

tuberculosis, multidrug-resistant (MDR), *n* type that no longer responds to treatment due to incomplete or improper use of medication.

tuberculosis, reactivation, *n* a recurrence in a patient who has been symptom free for a period of years. Reactivation tuberculosis usually responds to treatment.

tuberosity (toobəros′itē), *n* a protuberance or elevation from the surface, usually of a bone.

tuberosity, maxillary, *n* the most distal aspect of the maxillary alveolar process, with its posterior border curving upward and distally.

tuberosity reduction, *n* a surgical excision of excessive fibrous or bony tissue in the area of the maxillary tuberosity before the construction of prosthetic appliances.

tubule (too′būl), *n* a small tube, such as one of the collecting tubules in the kidneys. The dentin of the tooth contains dentinal tubules that communicate from the pulp to the dentinoenamal interface.

tuft (toothbrush), *n* part of the toothbrush head, refers to the small, individual clusters of bristles that proceed from a single opening.

tumor, *n* a swelling. Through usage the term is now synonymous with *neoplasm.* See also neoplasm.

tumor, adenomatoid odontogenic (AOT) **(ad′ənō′mətoid′ ōdon′tō-jen′ik),** *n* a benign tumor that develops from odontogenic epithelium and usually surrounds the crown of an impacted tooth; histologically, it is composed of ducts lined by cuboidal or columnar cells. Also known as *adenoameloblastoma* and *ameloblastic adenomatoid tumor.*

tumor, basaloid mixed, *n* See carcinoma, adenocystic.

tumor, Brooke's, *n.pr* See epithelioma adenoides cysticum.

tumor, brown, *n* a central giant cell tumor of the bone; associated with parathyroidism.

tumor, carotid body, *n* a tumor formed about the carotid artery.

tumor, collision, *n* a rare condition in which two neoplasms, both growing in the same general area, collide with the tumor elements and become intermingled.

tumor, Ewing's (endothelioma, Ewing's sarcoma), *n.pr* See sarcoma, Ewing's.

tumor, giant cell, *n* a benign neoplasm of bone, producing resorption and characterized by giant cells.

tumor, granular cell, *n* a benign tumor of the oral soft tissue, most commonly the tongue. Usually of neural origin, these are characterized by the presence of large polygonal cells with a granular cytoplasm.

tumor, hormonal, *n* localized enlargements of the gingivae that have the appearance of neoplasms and are associated with hormonal imbalance during pregnancy. Not a true tumor.

tumor, inflammatory, *n.pl* a benign tissue growth made up of inflammatory cells; not a true tumor. The majority of oral growths fall into this category. See also granuloma, neoplasm.

tumor, keratocystic odontogenic, *n* See keratocystic odontogenic tumor.

tumor marker, *n* substances that are often found in elevated levels in the bloodstream, urine, or other bodily tissues when cancer is present in the body.

tumor, mixed, *n* **1.** one of a group of neoplasms of the salivary glands the histologic appearance of which suggests both epithelial and connective tissue origin, although they presently are considered of epithelial origin only. Benign and malignant types are possible. **2.** a tumor arising from cells derived from more than one germ layer.

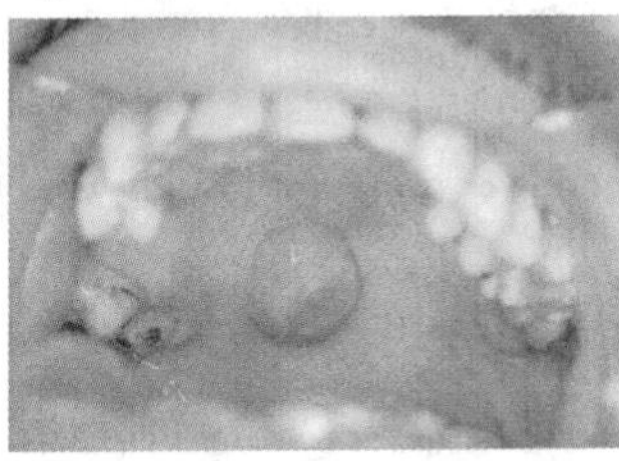

Mixed tumor. (Courtesy Dr. Charles Babbush)

tumor, mucoepidermoid, *n* See carcinoma, mucoepidermoid.

tumor, odontogenic **(ōdon′tōjen′ik),** *n* a neoplasm produced from tooth-forming tissues (e.g., odontogenic fibroma, odontogenic myxoma, ameloblastoma). See also calcifying epithelial odontogenic tumor.

tumor, turban, *n* See carcinoma, basal cell.

tumor, Warthin's, *n.pr* See cystadenoma, papillary, lymphomatosum.

tumor necrosis factor (TNF), *n* a natural body protein with anticancer effects. It is produced in the body in response to the presence of toxic substances, such as bacterial toxins. Adverse effects are toxic shock and cachexia.

tunica intima (too′nikə in′təmə), *n* the membrane lining an artery.

tunica media (too′nikə mē′dēə), *n* the muscular middle layer of an artery.

tunnel vision, *n* a defect in sight in which a great reduction occurs in the peripheral field of vision, as if one is looking through a hollow tube or tunnel.

turbidity (tur'biditē), *n* a condition of light scattering in a liquid resulting from the presence of suspended particles in the fluid.

turbulence, *n* casting term used to denote irregular flow of metal into a mold. May result in porosity.

turgor (tur'gər), *n* the normal resiliency of the skin caused by the outward pressure of the cells and interstitial fluid. Dehydration results in a decreased skin turgor, manifested by lax skin that, when grasped and raised between two fingers, slowly returns to a position level with the adjacent tissue.

Turner's tooth, *n.pr* See tooth, Turner's.

turnover time (of tissue), *n* the time required for all cells in a tissue to be lost and replaced.

Tweed triangle, *n.pr* See triangle, Tweed.

twilight sleep, *n* a light general anesthesia obtained by the parenteral administration of a mixture of morphine and scopolamine to reduce pain and obtund recall in childbirth.

twin-wire, *n* See appliance, twin-wire.

twins, *n.pl* the two siblings produced in the same pregnancy and developed from one egg (identical, monozygotic) or from two eggs fertilized at the same time (fraternal, dizygotic).

twist drill, *n* **1.** a drill having one or two deep helical grooves extending from the point to the smooth portion of the shank. **2.** a spiral bone bur.

twitch, *n* **1.** the contraction of small muscle units, manifested as a quick, simple, spasmodic contraction of a muscle. **2.** a short, sudden pull or jerk.

twitching, *n* an irregular spasm of a minor extent.

twitching, Trousseau's, n.pr a twitching of the face that the patient can exhibit at will and occurs obsessively to relieve tension.

Tylenol, *n.pr* See acetaminophen.

tympanic membrane, *n* a thin, semitransparent membrane in the middle ear that transmits sound vibrations to the internal ear by the means of the auditory ossicles. Also called the *eardrum.*

type A hepatitis, *n* See hepatitis, infectious.

type A personality, *n* a behavior pattern as associated with individuals who are highly competitive and work compulsively to meet deadlines. The condition is associated with a higher than usual incidence of coronary heart disease.

type B hepatitis, *n* See hepatitis, homologous serum.

type B personality, *n* a form of behavior associated with people who appear free of hostility and aggression and who lack a compulsion to meet deadlines, are not highly competitive at work or play, and have a lower risk of heart attack.

type E personality, *n* a form of behavior associated with people who fit neither type A nor type B personality categories but who have a marked sense of insecurity and strive to convince themselves that they are worthwhile.

typewriter ribbon as a marking medium, *n* typewriter ribbon is more desirable than carbon paper when setting teeth because the porcelain tooth that is being adjusted will not perforate the ribbon and abrade the surface of the stone template record of jaw movement.

typhoid carrier (tī'foid), *n* a person without signs or symptoms of typhoid fever who carries in the body the bacteria that cause the disease but sheds the pathogens in bodily excretions.

typhoid fever, *n* a bacterial infection usually caused by *Salmonella typhi;* transmitted by contaminated milk, water, or food and characterized by headache, delirium, cough, watery diarrhea, rash, and a high fever.

typhus (tī'fəs), *n* a group of acute infectious diseases caused by various species of *Rickettsia* and usually transmitted from infected rodents to humans by the bites of lice, fleas, mites, or ticks.

typical implant connective tissue, *n* the tendonlike condensed elongated avascular tissue formed in direct contact with implant infrastructure metal underlain by normal collagenous fibrous connective tissue.

typodont (tī'pōdont), *n* an artificial model containing artificial or natural teeth used for teaching technique exercises. Also called *dentoform.*

tyramine (tī'rəmēn'), *n* an amino acid synthesized in the body from the essential acid tyrosine. Tyramine stimulates the release of the catecholamines epinephrine and norepinephrine. It is important that people taking monoamine oxidase inhibitors avoid the ingestion of foods and beverages containing tyramine, particularly aged cheese, meats, bananas, yeast-containing products, and alcoholic beverages.

tyrosine (Tyr) (tī'rəsēn'), *n* an amino acid synthesized in the body from the essential amino acid phenylalanine. Tyrosine is found in most proteins and is a precursor of melanin and several hormones, including epinephrine and thyroxine.

tyrosinemia (tī'rōsinē'mēə), *n* a genetic disorder of amino acid metabolism in which tyrosine acid accumulates in the blood and urine at abnormally high levels; seen primarily in infants born prematurely; may respond to a low-protein diet and the administration of synthetic amino acids.

U

ugly duckling stage, *n* a stage of dental development preceding the eruption of the permanent canines, in which the lateral incisors may be tipped laterally because of crowding by the unerupted canine crowns. This tipping may cause spacing of the incisor crowns despite the crowding of the roots. The condition may be transitory in an otherwise normal dentition. It occurs during the mixed dentition stage of the dentition.

ulcer (ul'sur), *n* a loss of covering epithelium from the skin or mucous membranes, causing gradual disintegration and necrosis of the tissues.

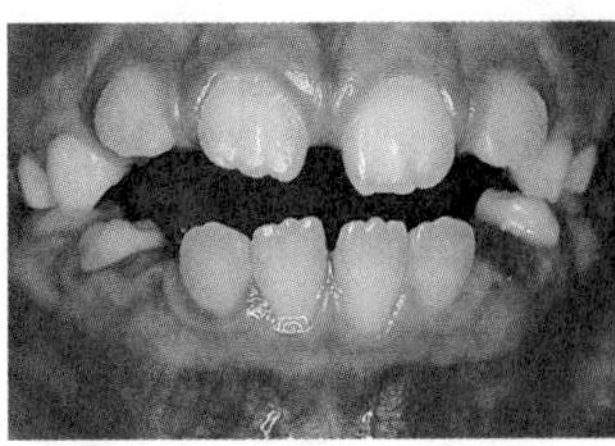

"Ugly duckling" stage of mixed dentition. (Daniel/Harfst/Wilder, 2008)

ulcer, aphthous **(af'thus),** *n* an open, shallow lesion in the oral cavity that causes pain; commonly known as a *canker sore.* The cause is unknown, and treatment is limited to alleviating the symptoms.

ulcer, aphthous, recurrent (RAU) **(af'thus),** *n* periodic episodes of aphthous lesions on nonkeratinized oral tissues lasting from 1 week to several months. Trauma and immunologic factors are involved in the etiology. The single or multiple discrete or confluent ulcers have a well-defined marginal erythema and a central area of necrosis with sloughing. Also called *canker sore* and *recurrent aphthae.*

ulcer, autochthonous **(ôtok'thənus),** *n* See chancre.

ulcer, decubitus **(dēkū'bitus),** *n* **1.** a bedsore. **2.** older term for a traumatic ulcer of the oral mucosa. More commonly called *traumatic ulcer.*

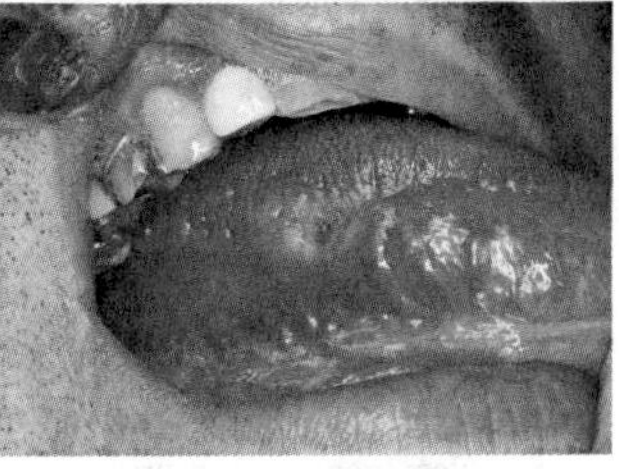

Decubitus ulcer. (Regezi/Sciubba/Jordan, 2008)

ulcer, diabetic **(dī'əbet'ik),** *n* an ulcer, usually of the lower extremities, associated with diabetes mellitus.

ulcer, herpetic **(hurpet'ik),** *n* an ulcer on keratinized orofacial tissues that is secondary to the vesicle of herpes simplex after the intact surface is broken by trauma to the lesion; a shallow ulcer with an irregular, erythematous border and a yellow-gray base. Contagious through all stages of lesion. Can be treated by topical acyclovir. Also called a *cold sore.*

ulcer, Mikulicz's **(mik′ūlichəz),** *n.pr* See periadenitis mucosa necrotica recurrens.

ulcer, pemphigoid aphthous, *n* a lesion located on the gingiva or mucous membranes due to a chronic disease of the autoimmune system. It is indicated by a wound with a thick wall that ruptures within 24 to 48 hours and leaves an eroded and painful surface area. It heals through the formation of a scar.

ulcer, peptic **(pep′tik),** *n* an ulcer of the stomach or duodenum. Most ulcers are associated with *H. pylori,* a spiral-shaped bacterium that lives in the acidic environment of the stomach. They can also be caused or worsened by drugs such as aspirin and other NSAIDs.

ulcer, pterygoid **(ter′igoid),** *n* See aphtha, Bednar's.

ulcer, rodent, *n* See carcinoma, basal cell.

ulcer, traumatic, *n* an ulcer that is caused by trauma. It can be due to faulty oral hygiene, rough foods, oral habits, poor-fitting dentures, or inadvertent mastication or biting of oral tissues. The offending cause may need to be removed by the patient or clinician. After this treatment, it must heal within a 2-week period to rule out any oral cancer concerns. The older term in dentistry is *decubitus ulcer.*

ulceration (ul′sərā′shən), the process of forming an ulcer or of becoming ulcerous.

ulcerative stomatitis, recurrent (ul′sərātiv, ul′sərətiv stō′mətī′tis), *n* See ulcer, aphthous, recurrent.

ulnar deviation (ul′nər), *n* a position of the hand in which the wrist bends toward the little finger. Continued ulnar deviation positioning may cause a repetitive strain injury.

ultimate strength, *n* See strength, ultimate.

ultra (ul′trə), *adj* beyond; in addition; in excess of.

ultra damages, *n* damages beyond those paid in court.

ultracentrifuge, *n* a high-speed centrifuge with a rotation rate fast enough to produce sedimentation of viruses, even in blood plasma. Many kinds of biochemical analyses use ultracentrifuge, including such analyses as the measurement and separation of some proteins and viruses.

ultrafiltrate (ul′trəfil′trāt), *n* a solution that has passed through a semipermeable membrane with very small pores. It usually contains only low-molecular-weight solutes.

ultrasonic (ul′trəson′ik), *adj* pertaining to sound frequencies so high (greater than 20 kHz) they cannot be perceived by the human ear.

ultrasonic cleaner, *n* an electronic generator that transmits high-energy and high-frequency vibrations to a fluid-filled container used to remove particulate matter from dental instruments and appliances.

ultrasonography, *n* the process of imaging deep structures of the body by measuring and recording the reflection of pulsed or continuous high-frequency sound waves. It is valuable in many medical situations, including the diagnosis of fetal abnormalities, gallstones, heart defects, and tumors. Also called *sonography.*

ultraviolet light, *n* light beyond the range of human vision, at the short end of the spectrum. It occurs naturally in sunlight; it burns and tans the skin and converts precursors in the skin to vitamin D. It is used in the treatment of psoriasis and other skin conditions. Prolonged or excessive exposure to ultraviolet light can damage the skin and increase the susceptibility of the skin to cancer.

unbundling of procedures, *n* the separating of a dental procedure into component parts with each part having a cost so that the cumulative cost of the components is greater than the total cost for the same procedure to patients who are not beneficiaries of a dental benefits plan.

uncompensated care, *n* health care services provided by a hospital, physician, dental professional, or other health care professional for which no charge is made and for which no payment is expected.

unconscious (unkon′shəs), *adj* insensible; not receiving any sensory impression and not having any subjective experiences.

undecylenic acid (topical) (un′desilen′ik), *n brand names:* Caldesene Medicated Powder, Cruex products, Desenex Aerosol Powder, others; *drug class:* local antifungal; *action:* interferes with fungal cell membrane permeability; *uses:* tinea cruris, tinea pedis, diaper rash, minor skin irritations.

underbite, *n* a nontechnical term for the vertical overlapping of mandibular teeth over upper teeth.

undercut, *n* **1.** the portion of a tooth that lies between its height of contour and the gingivae, only if that portion is of less circumference than the height of contour. **2.** the contour of a cross-section of a residual ridge of dental arch that would prevent the placement of a denture or other prosthesis. **3.** the contour of flasking stone that interlocks to prevent the separation of parts. **4.** the portion of a prepared cavity that creates a mechanical lock or area of retention; may be desirable in a cavity to be filled with gold foil or amalgam but is undesirable in a cavity prepared for a restoration to be cemented.

undercut gauge, *n* See gauge, undercut.

undercut, retentive, *n* an area of the abutment surface suitable for the location of a retentive clasp terminal, which in order to escape the undercut would be forced to flex and thus generate retention.

undercut, soft tissue, *n* an undercut in a residual ridge or soft-tissue covering of a dental arch that would prevent or influence the placement of a removable denture.

undercut, unusable, *n* the area of an abutment tooth or soft tissue across which a unit of the removable partial denture must pass without interference and hence must be blocked out (filled with wax or clay) before the master cast is duplicated. Use of a surveyor produces a surface that is parallel to the proposed path of a placement and removal.

underjet, *n* a malocclusion describing the positional relationship between the maxillary and mandibular incisors in which the maxillary incisors are measurably within the perimeter of the mandibular incisors.

undermine, *v* to separate surgically the skin or mucosa from its underlying stroma so that it can be stretched or moved to cover a defect or wound.

unemployment, *n* the state of being without a job or compensation for work, usually involuntarily.

unerupted, *adj* not having perforated the oral mucosa. In dentistry, used in reference to a normal developing tooth, an embedded tooth, or an impacted tooth.

unification, *n* the act of uniting or the condition of being united (e.g., the result of joining the components of a removable partial denture by connectors).

uniform dental recording, *v* completing a dental record whose contents are the same across dental practices. Uniform dental records facilitate the collection of data across dental practices.

unilateral, *adj* one-sided.

union-sponsored plan, *n* a program of dental benefits developed through a union's initiative. May be operated directly by the union or the union may contract for provision of the benefits. Funds to finance the benefits are usually paid out of a trust fund that receives its income from employer contributions, employer and union member contributions, or union members alone.

Unipen, *n.pr* See nafcillin.

unit, *n* one of the components of a whole.

unit, Ångstrom, (Å, a.u.) **(ang′strəm),** *n* the unit of measure of wavelengths; one one-hundred-millionth of a centimeter.

unit, dental, *n* **1.** basically, the tooth, periodontium, and gingival unit, all of which are necessary for proper masticatory activity. **2.** an article of equipment that contains an assembly of numerous items used in dental operations, such as a dental engine, operatory light, bracket, working table, saliva ejector, water supply, electric outlets, compressed air, or miscellaneous instruments. May or may not have a cuspidor.

unit, dentoperiodontal, *n* the tooth and periodontium together.

unit dosing, n a method for storing dental sealant materials and other products that lessens the risk of cross-contamination.

unit, gingival, n the tough collagenous and epithelial covering of the neck of the tooth and the underlying periodontium.

unit, partial denture, n the individual elements of the partial denture, each contributing some particular function.

unit, radiographic, n a device designed to produce radiographs.

unit, radiographic, calibration, n the determination of the kilovoltage peak (kVp) value of each autotransformer tap at various milliamperages, checking these values by means of a sphere gap or a prereading voltmeter.

United States Department of Agriculture (USDA), *n.pr* established in 1862, USDA is responsible for the safety of meat, poultry, and egg products. It conducts ongoing research in areas from human nutrition to new crop technologies and also helps ensure open markets for U.S. agricultural products.

United States Department of Health and Human Services (USDHHS), *n.pr* a cabinet-level government organization comprising 12 agencies, including the Food and Drug Administration and the Centers for Disease Control and Prevention.

United States dietary goals, *n.pr* the recommendation of a U.S. Senate committee in 1977 outlining the levels of consumption of complex carbohydrates, sugar, protein, fat, cholesterol, and salt for diets necessary to enhance the health status of Americans.

United States Food and Drug Administration (FDA), *n.pr* a unit of the Public Health Service created to protect the health of the nation against impure and unsafe foods, drugs, and cosmetics.

United States Health Resources and Services Administration (HRSA), *n.pr* a unit of the Public Health Service created to provide leadership and direction to programs and activities designed to improve the health services for all people of the United States and to develop health care and maintenance systems that are adequately financed, comprehensive, interrelated, and responsive to the needs of all members of American society.

United States Indian Health Service, *n.pr* a unit of the Department of Health and Human Services with 51 hospitals, 99 health centers, and several hundred field health stations established to improve the health status of the American Indian and Alaskan Native.

United States Occupational Safety and Health Administration (OSHA), *n.pr* a unit of the U.S. Department of Labor, created to develop and promulgate occupational safety and health standards, develop and issue regulations, conduct investigations and inspections to determine the status of compliance with safety and health standards and regulations, and issue citations and propose penalties for noncompliance with safety and health standards and regulations.

***United States Pharmacopeia* (USP) (far′məkəpē′ə),** *n.pr* a compendium officially recognized by the Federal Food, Drug, and Cosmetic Act that contains the descriptions, uses, strengths, and standards of purity for selected drugs.

United States Public Health Service (USPHS), *n.pr* a major division of the Department of Health and Human Services. The USPHS provides oversight of the following agencies: the Centers for Disease Control and Prevention (CDC); Food and Drug Administration (FDA); Health Resources and Services Administration (HRSA); Agency for Toxic Substances and Disease Registry; National Institutes of Health (NIH); Alcohol, Drug Abuse and Mental Health Administration; Health Care Financing Administration (HCFA); Social Security Administration; Office of Child Support Enforcement; and Office of Community Services.

universal donor, *n* a person with type O, Rh factor negative red blood cells. Packed red blood cells of this type may be used for emergency transfusion with minimal risk of incompatibility.

universal precautions, *n.pl* **1.** approaches to infection control designed to prevent transmission of bloodborne diseases, such as AIDS and hepatitis B in health care settings. Universal precautions were initially developed in 1987 by the Centers for Disease Control and Prevention (CDC) and in 1989 by the Bureau of Communicable Disease Epidemiology in Canada. The guidelines include specific recommendations for use of gloves and masks and protective eyewear when contact with blood or body secretions containing blood or blood elements is anticipated. In 1996 the CDC expanded the concept and changed the term to *standard precautions.* See also *standard precautions. n.pl* **2.** the protocols used to maintain an aseptic field and to prevent cross-contamination and cross-infection between health care providers, between health care providers and patients, and between patients. These include, but are not limited to, the sterilization of instruments and goods; the isolation and disinfection of the immediate clinical environment; the use of sterile disposables; scrubbing, masking, gowning, and gloving; and the proper disposal of contaminated waste.

universal recipient, *n* a person with blood type AB, who can receive a transfusion of blood of a group type without agglutination or precipitation effects.

universal strap, *n* a sling worn around the arm or wrist that provides stabilization for people who cannot hold devices by themselves.

universal tooth designation system, *n* a tooth numbering system in which each permanent tooth carries an Arabic numeral from 1 to 32, beginning with the maxillary right third molar and ending with the mandibular left third molar, and each primary tooth is identified by capital letters A through T.

unmedullated (unmed′ūlātəd), *adj* not possessing a medulla or medullary substance.

unpolarized, *adj* not polarized.

unsaturated fatty acid, *n* the glyceryl esters of certain organic acids in which some of the atoms are joined by double or triple valence bonds. These bonds are split easily in chemical reaction, and other substances are joined to them. Monounsaturated fatty acids have only one double or triple bond per molecule and are found in such foods as fowl, almonds, pecans, cashew nuts, peanuts, and olive oil. Polyunsaturated fatty acids have more than one double or triple bond per molecule and are found in fish, corn, walnuts, sunflower seeds, soybeans, and safflower oil.

unsaturated fatty acids, *n.pl* the double- or triple-bonded fatty acids contained primarily in vegetable oils and fish, which remain liquid at room temperature; linked to a reduction in the risk of developing heart disease.

unsharpness, geometric, *n* See geometric unsharpness.

unstable, *adj* **1.** not firm or fixed in one place; likely to move. **2.** capable of undergoing spontaneous change. A nuclide in an unstable state is called *radioactive.* An atom in an unstable state is called *excited.*

***unstable angina* (unstā′bəl anjī′nə),** *n* a form of pain that is prodromal to acute myocardial infarction. It typically has a sudden onset, sudden worsening, and stuttering recurrence over days and weeks. It carries a more severe short-term prognosis than stable chronic angina. Nearly one third of unstable angina patients experience myocardial infarction within 3 months of the first episode.

unstratified epithelium (unstrat′əfīd′ ep′əthē′lēəm), epithelium that consists of a single layer of cells.

upcode, *n* use of a procedure code that reflects a higher-intensity service than would normally be used for the services delivered.

upright arm, *n* See connector, minor.

uprighting spring, *n* an auxiliary wire used to torque roots mesially or distally.

uranium (U), *n* a heavy, radioactive metallic element. Its atomic number is 92 and its atomic weight is 238.0289. Uranium is the heaviest of the natural elements. Isotopes of uranium are used in nuclear power plants to provide neutrons for nuclear reactions that result in release of energy.

urban health, *n* the health of a population that lives and works closely together, usually in an incorporated area, such as a city or town, with a common water supply and with similar environmental conditions.

urban population, *n* the population of an incorporated area, such as a city or town.

urea (ūrē′ə), *n* a water-soluble compound that is the primary constituent of urine.

***Ureaplasma* (yoorē′əplaz′mə),** *n* gram-negative eubacteria from the family Mycoplasmataceae that serve as a hydrolitic for urea. The bacteria do not have cell walls.

urease, *n* an enzyme that divides urea into carbon dioxide and ammonia.

uremia (ūrē′mēə), *n* the presence of urinary components in the circulating blood and the resultant symptoms. Manifestations include weakness, headache, confusion, vomiting, and coma, and in terminal chronic renal disease, purpura and epistaxis may be present. Uremia is caused by insufficient urinary excretion for any reason. See also stomatitis, uremic.

ureteritis (yoorē′tərī′tis), *n* an inflammatory condition of a ureter caused by infection or by the mechanic irritation of a kidney stone as it passes through the ureter.

urethane (yoor′ithān′), *n* ethyl carbamate used as an anesthetic agent for laboratory animals, formerly used as a hypnotic in humans.

urethritis (yoor′ithrī′tis), *n* an inflammatory condition of the urethra that is characterized by dysuria, usually the result of an infection in the bladder or kidneys.

uric acid (yoor′ik), *n* a product of protein metabolism and present in the blood and urine. See also gout.

U

urinalysis (yoor′inal′isis), *n* a physical, microscopic, and chemical diagnostic examination of urine. Abnormal constituents indicate disease and can include ketone bodies, protein, bacteria, blood, glucose, suppuration, and certain types of crystals.

urinary tract, *n* all organs and ducts involved in the secretion and elimination of urine from the body, principally the kidney, ureter, bladder, and urethra.

urinary tract infection, *n* an infection of one or more structures in the urinary tract. Gram-negative bacteria cause most of these infections.

urine (yoor′in), *n* the fluid excreted by the kidneys. Normal urine is clear, straw-colored, and slightly acidic, and has the characteristic odor of urea.

Urised, *n.pr* a trademark for a urinary fixed-combination drug containing an antibacterial (methenamine), an analgesic (phenyl salicylate) anticholinergics (atropine sulfate and hyoscyamine), an antifungal (benzoic acid), and an antiseptic (methylene blue).

urobilin, *n* a brown pigment formed by the oxidation of urobilinogen, normally found in feces and, in small amounts, in urine.

urokinase (yoor′ōkī′nās), *n* an enzyme produced in the kidney and found in urine that is a potent plasminogen activator of the fibrinolytic system. A pharmaceutic preparation of urokinase is administered intravenously in the treatment of pulmonary embolism.

urology (yoorol′əjē), *n* the branch of medicine concerned with the study of the anatomy, physiology, and pathology of the urinary tract, with the care of the urinary tract of men and women; and with the care of the male genital tract.

ursodiol, *n brand names:* Actigall, Ursofalk; *drug class:* gallstone solubilizing agent; *action:* suppresses hepatic synthesis, secretion of cholesterol; inhibits intestinal absorption of cholesterol; *uses:* dissolution of radiolucent noncalcified gallstones of less than 20 mm in diameter, in which surgery is not indicated.

urticaria (ur′tiker′ēə), *n* a vascular reaction pattern of the skin marked by the transient appearance of smooth, slightly elevated patches that are more red or more pale than the surrounding skin and are accompanied by severe itching. Also called *hives.*

urticaria, bullosa, *n* a skin eruption in which the lesions are capped by blisters.

urticaria, giant, *n* See edema, angioneurotic.

USAN Council, *n.pr* the United States Adopted Names Council, re-

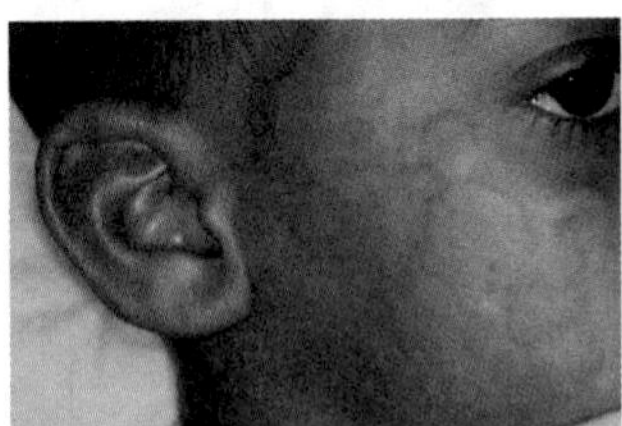

Urticaria. (Zitelli/Davis, 2002)

sponsible for the selection of appropriate nonproprietary names for drugs used in the United States.

USDA, *n.pr* See United States Department of Agriculture.

USDHHS, *n.pr* See United States Department of Health and Human Services.

useful beam, *n* See beam, useful.

USP, *n.pr* See *United States Pharmacopeia.*

usual, customary and reasonable (UCR) plan, *n* a dental benefits plan that determines benefits based on usual, customary, and reasonable fee criteria. See also usual fee, customary fee, and reasonable fee.

usual fee, *n* the fee that an individual dental professional most frequently charges for a given dental service. See also customary fee and reasonable fee.

ut dict., *n* abbreviation for *ut dictum,* Latin for "as directed."

utilization, *n* **1.** the extent to which a given group uses a particular service in a specified period. Although usually expressed as the number of services used per year per 100 or per 1000 persons eligible for the service, utilization rates may be expressed in other ratios. **2.** the extent to which the members of a covered group use a program over a stated time, specifically measured as a percentage determined by dividing the number of covered individuals who submitted one or more claims by the total number of covered individuals.

utilization management, *n* a set of techniques used by or on behalf of purchasers of health care benefits to manage the cost of health care before its provision by influencing patient-care decision making through case-by-case assessments of the appropriateness of care based on accepted dental practices.

utilization review (UR), *n* **1.** analysis of the necessity, appropriateness, and efficiency of medical and dental services, procedures, facilities, and practitioners. In a hospital, this includes review of the appropriateness of admissions, services ordered and provided, and length of stay and discharge practices, on concurrent and retrospective bases. **2.** a statistically based system that examines the distribution of treatment procedures based on claims information and, to be reasonably reliable, the application of such claims. Analyses of specific dental professionals should include data on type of practice, dental professionals' experience, socioeconomic characteristics, and geographic location.

uveitis (ū′vēī′tis), *n* inflammation of the uveal tract: the iris, ciliary body, and choroid of the eye.

uveoparotitis (ū′vēōper′ōtī′tis), *n* See fever, uveoparotid.

uvula (ū′vūlə), *n* a general term indicating a pendent fleshy mass.

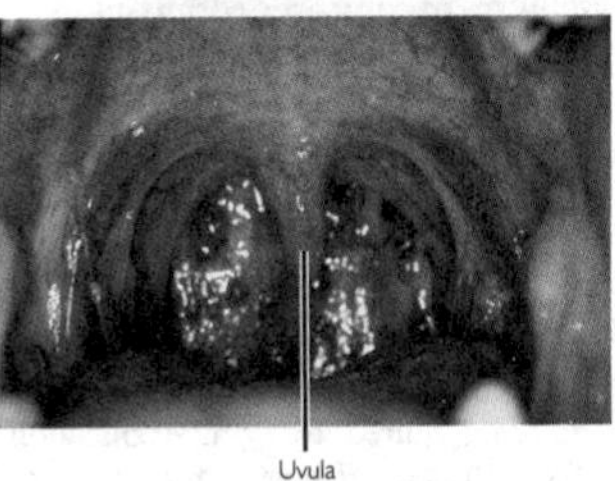

Uvula. (Liebgott, 2001)

uvula, bifid, *n* a congenital cleft resulting in a split uvula.

uvula, palatine, *n* a small, fleshy mass hanging from the posterior soft palate.

U

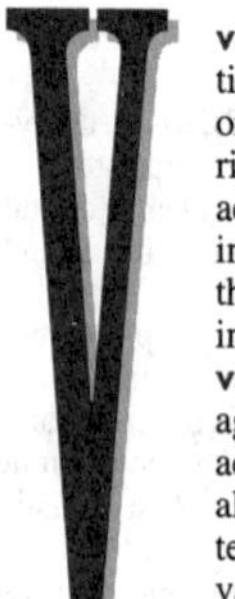

vaccination, *n* an injection of attenuated microorganisms, such as bacteria, viruses, or rickettsiae, administered to induce immunity or to reduce the effect of associated infectious diseases.

vaccine (vaksēn′), agent prepared to produce active immunity that usually kills microbes, attenuated live microbes, or variant strains of microbes and can induce antibody production without producing disease.

Vacudent (vak′ūdent), *n.pr* brand name for a high-volume suction device designed to remove strongly but gently any fluids and debris from an operating field.

vacuole (vak′ūōl′), *n* a clear space in the substance of a cell. It may stem from a degenerative process, or it may serve the cell as a temporary cell stomach for the digestion of a foreign body inclusion.

vacuum, *n* See oral evacuator.

vacuum mixing, *n* See mixing, vacuum.

vagomimetic (vā′gōməmet′ik), *adj* pertaining to a drug with actions similar to those produced by stimulation of the vagus nerve.

valacyclovir HCl (val′āsī′klōvir), *n brand names:* Valtrex, Zeilirex; *class:* antiviral; *action:* converted to acyclovir, which interferes with DNA synthesis required for viral replication; *uses:* herpes zoster in immunocompetent patients.

valence (vā′ləns), *n* **1.** in chemistry, a numeric expression of the capability of an element to combine chemically with atoms of hydrogen or their equivalent. *n* **2.** in immunology, an expression of the number of antigen-binding sites for one molecule of any given antibody or the number of antibody-binding sites for any given antigen.

validation, *n* an agreement of the listener with certain elements of the patient's communication.

validity, *n* the degree to which data or results of a study are correct or true.

valine (val′ēn), *n* one of the essential amino acids. See also amino acid.

Valium, *n.pr* See diazepam.

valproate sodium/valproate sodium-valproic acid/valproic acid (valprō′āt′ valprō′ik), *n brand names:* Depakene, Myproic Acid, Depakote; *class:* anticonvulsant; *action:* increased levels of λ-aminobutyric acid (GABA) in brain; *uses:* simple, complex (petit mal), absence, mixed seizures.

value system, *n* the accepted mode of conduct and the set of norms, goals, and values binding any social group that serves as a frame of reference for the individual in reaching decisions and achieving a meaningful life.

values, normal laboratory, *n.pl* generally, statistically and biologically significant qualitative and/or quantitative measurements of cellular and clinical components of the body. The values derived from such measurements are based on averages of a survey of presumably healthy persons. The concept of individual normal values is based on an acceptable response (comparable with known evidence of health or disease) of the individual to a known alteration of cellular and/or chemical components or systems.

values, phonetic (fənet′ik), *n.pl* the characteristics of vocal sounds.

valve, *n* a structure that controls flow of the contents of a canal or passage.

valve, exhalation, *n* a valve that permits escape of exhaled gases into the atmosphere and prevents them from being rebreathed.

valvular heart disease, *n* a potentially life-threatening cardiac valve disorder, characterized by the constriction or obstruction of blood vessels, in which a valve malfunctions so that blood is forced to flow backward rather than through the vessel. The condition may be present at birth or acquired as the result of an illness, such as rheumatic fever, syphilis, or bacterial endocarditis.

van den Bergh's test, *n.pr* See test, van den Bergh's.

vancomycin HCl, *n brand name:* Vancocin; *class:* glucopeptide-type antiinfective; *action:* inhibits bacterial cell wall synthesis; *uses:* resistant staphylococcal infections, pseudomembranous colitis, staphylococcal enterocolitis, endocarditis prophylaxis for dental procedures.

vapor, *n* **1.** the gaseous form assumed by a solid or liquid when sufficiently heated. *n* **2.** a visible emanation of fine particles of a liquid.

Vaquez' disease (vəkāz'), *n.pr* See erythremia.

variability, *n* the degree or range of divergence of an object from a given standard or average.

variable, *adj* **1.** changing; able to vary in quantity or magnitude. *n* **2.** a characteristic that may assume several values.

variable, continuous, *n* a variable for which it is possible to find an intermediate value between any two values. Continuous variables can be refined by more precise values. Length, weight, and time, and the points on a line are continuous variables.

variable costs, *n* costs, such as dental service claims, that generally increase or decrease as the size and composition of the enrollment fluctuates.

variable, dependent, *n* a variable whose value is consequent on change in the independent variable. The dependent variable is always the response or reaction to the independent variable. Also called *criterion variable.*

variable, discrete, *n* a variable that is expressed in whole units or mutually exclusive categories. Whole numbers and category designations such as sex and marital status are examples of discrete data.

variable, independent, *n* the variable being studied that is manipulated or controlled by an experimenter. In a drug study an investigator may give several doses of a drug (independent variable) to determine the most effective, symptom-reducing (dependent variable) level.

variables, control, *n.pl* those variables not being studied that are held constant so as not to influence the experimental outcome. Environmental conditions, intelligence quotients, and social and psychologic variables are examples of variables that must be controlled.

variation (genetic), *n* deviation from the genotype in structure, form, physiology, or behavior.

varicella (ver'isel'ə), *n* (chickenpox), an acute communicable disease with an incubation period of 2 or 3 weeks and caused by herpesvirus, usually found in children. Manifestations include coryza, fever, malaise, and headache, followed in 2 or 3 days by the eruption of macular vesicles.

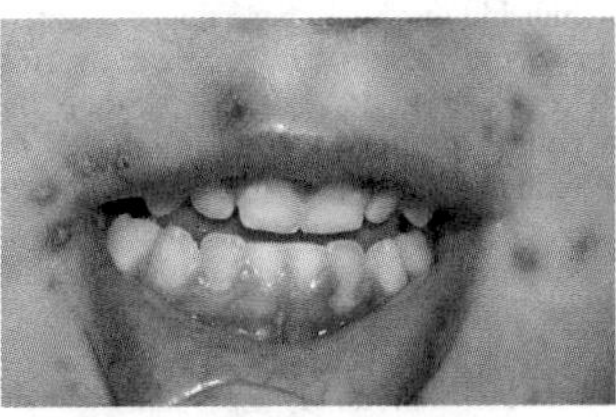

Varicella. (Regezi/Sciubba/Jordan, 2008)

varicosity (ver'ikos'itē), *n* an abnormal condition characterized by the presence of tortuous, abnormally dilated veins, usually in the legs or the lower trunk; may also appear in the esophagus.

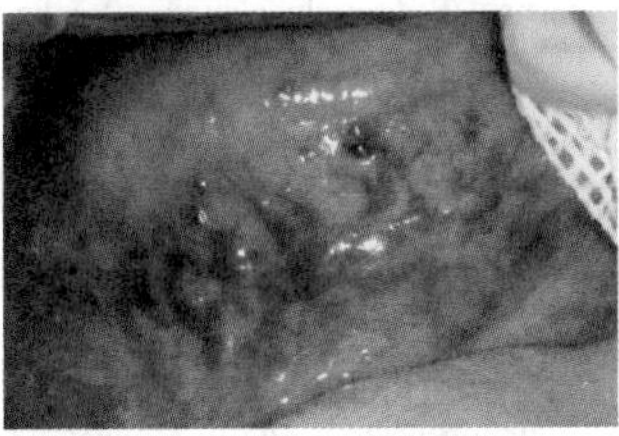

Varicosity. (Neville/Damm/Allen/Bouquot, 2002)

variola (ver'ēō'lə), *n* (smallpox), an acute, viral, contagious disease transmitted by the respiratory route and direct contact. The incubation period is 1 to 2 weeks. Manifestations include headache, chills, and temperature up to 106° F. On the third and fourth day, macules appear, which then become papules; then constitutional symptoms abate. On the sixth day the papules become vesicles. The vesicles then become pustules, with desquamation occurring in about 2 weeks. It has been eradicated in the United States due to vaccination.

varnish (vär'nish), *n* (cavity liner, cavity varnish), a clear solution of resinous material or natural gum, such as copal or rosin dissolved in acetone, ether, or chloroform, which is capable of hardening without losing its transparency. Varnish is used in cavity preparations to seal out dentinal tubules, reduce microleakage, and insulate the pulp against shock from thermal changes.

varnish, fluoride, *n* a sticky yellowish protective coating of 5% sodium fluoride in a resin base that is painted over the teeth to prevent dental caries in children and adults. It hardens on contact with saliva. It is also used to reduce root sensitivity. Its effects on enamel fluoride appear to provide a lower risk of accidental fluoride ingestion than most other topical fluoride treatments.

vascular diseases, *n.pl* diseases of the peripheral circulatory system.

vascular endothelial growth factors (VEGF) (en'dōthē'lēəl), *n* proteins that promote new blood vessel growth.

vascular reactions, *n.pl* the responses of the blood vessels to injury or introduction of chemical agents, particularly certain chemical mediators such as histamine and bradykinin.

vascular resistance, *n* the degree to which the blood vessels impede the flow of blood. High resistance causes an increase in blood pressure, which increases the workload of the heart.

vascular spasm, *n* a sudden constriction of the blood vessels causing reduction or stoppage in blood flow. A vascular spasm in vessels of the brain can result in a stroke; in the vessels of the heart it can result in a heart attack.

vasculitis (vas'kyəlī'tis), *n* an inflammatory condition of the blood vessels that is characteristic of certain systemic diseases or is caused by an allergic reaction.

vasoconstrictor (vā'zōkənstrik'tur), *n* (vasopressor), an agent that causes a rise in blood pressure by constricting the blood vessels. In local areas, it causes constriction of the arterioles and capillaries.

vasoconstrictor, adrenergic agents as, *n* adrenaline-mimicking drugs that increase the duration of local anesthesia by constricting the blood vessels, thereby safely concentrating the anesthetic agent for an extended duration and reducing hemorrhage. Excessive amounts can cause systemic toxicity, especially in certain medical conditions or when combined with certain medications. Also used in gingival retraction cord impregnated with epinephrine. In dentistry, this includes epinephrine and levonordefrin.

vasodepressor (vā'zōdēpres'ur), *n* an agent that depresses circulation and causes vasomotor depression.

vasodilator (vā'zōdī'lātur), *n* **1.** an agent that causes dilation of the blood vessels. *n* **2.** a drug that relaxes the smooth muscle walls of the blood vessels and increases their diameter.

vasomotor (vā'zōmōtur), *adj* pertaining to an agent or nerve that causes expansion or contraction of the walls of blood vessels.

vasopressin (vā'zōpres'in), *n* See hormone, antidiuretic.

vasopressor (vāz'ōpres'ur), *n* See vasoconstrictor.

vault, *n* **1.** an anatomic part resembling an arched roof or dome, such as the vault of a denture. *n* **2.** a cavity or specially prepared area within the jawbone for placement of an implant magnet.

V-bends, *n* V-shaped bends placed in an orthodontic arch wire, usually mesially to the canines. The V-bends create an adjustment site at which torquing bends may be placed.

VDRL test, *n.pr* abbreviation for Venereal Disease Research Laboratory test, a serologic flocculation test for syphilis or yaws.

vector (vek'tər), *n* a carrier that transmits a disease from one party to another.

vegan diet (vē'gən), *n* the strictest form of vegetarian diet, which prohibits the consumption of all animal products, including dairy, eggs, meat, poultry, fish, and animal fats. Care must be taken to avoid the risk of developing calcium, iron, zinc, or vitamin B_{12} deficiencies.

vehicle (vē'hikəl), *n* a pharmaceutic ingredient, usually a liquid, employed as a medium for dissolving or dispersing the active drug in a mass suitable for its administration.

Veillonella alcalescens **(vā′yənel′ə alkəles′enz),** *n* **1.** an organism of the genus *Veillonella.* *n* **2.** a schizomycete that has been found in the flora of the periodontal pocket and, by association, has been implicated in the origin and perpetuation of periodontitis in human beings.

vein (vān), *n* a blood vessel that conducts blood from the capillary bed to the heart. Size may range from the venules to small veins to large veins. See also each of the individual veins of the head and neck as they are listed.

vein, retromandibular **(ret′rōman-dib′ūlur),** *n* the vein formed posterior to the mandible by the joining of maxillary and superficial temporal veins. The posterior branch connects with the external jugular vein while the anterior branch enters the internal jugular vein.

velopharyngeal adequacy (vē′lōfərin′jēəl), *n* See closure, velopharyngeal.

velopharyngeal closure, *n* See closure, velopharyngeal.

velopharyngeal inadequacy, *n* See inadequacy, velopharyngeal.

velum (vē′lum), *n* a membranous cover that resembles a curtain or veil.

velum palatinum **(vē′lum pal′ətī′num),** *n* See soft palate.

velum platinum, *n* a membranous cover on the palate.

veneer (vənir′), *n* in the construction of crowns or pontics, a layer of tooth-colored material, usually porcelain or acrylic resin, attached to the surface by direct fusion, cementation, or mechanical retention.

venereal disease (vənir′ēəl), *n* See sexually transmitted disease.

venipuncture (ven′əpungkchur), *n* surgical or therapeutic puncture of a vein.

venlafaxine HCl (ven′ləfak′sēn), *n* *brand name:* Effexor; *class:* bicyclic antidepressant; *action:* inhibits both norepinephrine and serotonin (5-HT) uptake and, to a lesser extent, dopamine uptake; *use:* depression.

venous sinus (vē′nəs), *n* the space between two layers of tissue, which is filled with blood.

ventilate, *v* **1.** to provide with fresh air. *v* **2.** to provide the lungs with air from the atmosphere. *v* **3.** to open, to free, as in to openly express one's feelings.

ventilation (ven′tilā′shən), *n* the constant supplying of oxygen through the lungs.

ventilation, air, *n* the process of supplying alveoli with air or oxygen.

ventilation, mouth-to-mouth, *n* a method by which a rescuer uses the air in his or her own lungs to fill the lungs of another person who has stopped breathing in order to oxygenate that person's blood. See respiration, artificial.

ventilation, respiratory, *n* the process of getting air into and out of the lungs. The air enters the oral cavity and nose and must go through the conduction system (the pharynx, larynx, trachea, and bronchial tree) into the lungs. This ventilating process involves many other structures as well, including the abdomen, thorax, and maxillofacial tissues. The latter structures make two significant contributions to the respiratory process: they provide the portal of entry and egress for the air to and from the lungs, and they alter the physical properties of inspired air for protection of the very sensitive lung tissues.

venting, *n* an exit passage constructed in a casting mold to allow gases to escape during the casting process.

ventral, *adj* pertaining to the anterior part of a structure, or the part opposite the anatomic back.

ventricle (ven′trikəl), *n* a small cavity, such as one of the cavities filled with cerebrospinal fluid in the brain, or the right or left ventricle of the heart.

ventricular dysfunction, *n* an abnormality in contraction and wall motion within the ventricles.

ventricular fibrillation (VF), *n* a cardiac dysrhythmia marked by rapid, disorganized depolarizations of the ventricular myocardium. The condition is characterized by a complete lack of organized electric impulse, conduction, and ventricular contraction. Blood pressure falls to zero, resulting in unconsciousness. Death may occur within 4 minutes. Defibrillation and ventilation, i.e., cardiopulmonary resuscitation (CPR), must be initiated immediately.

ventricular function, *n* the cyclic contraction and relaxation of the ventricular myocardium.

ventricular septal defect (VSD), *n* an abnormal opening in the septum separating the ventricles of the heart. It is the most common congenital heart defect. Children with small defects are usually without symptoms. Large defects can prevent proper oxygenation of the blood and may initiate congestive heart failure, if not surgically corrected.

ventriculoureterostomy (ventrik′yəlō′yŏŏrē′təros′təmē), *n* a surgical procedure for directing cerebrospinal fluid into the general circulation; performed in the treatment of hydrocephalus, usually in the newborn.

venue (ven′ū), *n* the neighborhood, place, or county in which an injury is declared to have occurred or fact is declared to have happened; also designates the county in which an action or prosecution is presented for trial.

venule (ven′ūl), *n* the smallest of the venous blood vessels; consists of an endothelial tube enclosed in a variable amount of elastic and collagenous tissue. Smooth muscle is introduced in the media as the caliber of the vessel increases. The muscle fibers are distributed sparsely in the smaller vessels but coalesce into circumferential bands in the larger vessels.

veracity (vəras′itē), *n* legal principle that states that a health professional should be honest and give full disclosure to the patient, abstain from misrepresentation or deceit, and report known lapses of the standards of care to the proper agencies.

verapamil HCl (vərap′əmil′), *n brand names:* Calan, Isoptin, Calan SR, Isoptin SR, others; *class:* calcium-channel blocker; *action:* inhibits calcium ion influx across cell membranes during cardiac depolarization; produces relaxation of coronary vascular smooth muscle, dilates coronary arteries, decreases SA/AV node conduction, and dilates peripheral arteries; *uses:* chronic stable angina pectoris, vasospastic angina, dysrhythmias, hypertension.

verbal, *adj* by word of oral cavity; oral, as in a verbal agreement.

verdict, *n* the formal decision or finding of a jury on the matters or questions duly submitted to them at a trial.

vermilion border (vermil′yən), *n* the junction between the lip and the facial skin.

vermilion zone, *n* the external darkish area of the upper and lower lips, extending from the junction of the lips, with the surrounding facial skin on the exterior to the labial mucosa within the oral cavity.

vernier (vur′nēur), *n* See gauge, Boley.

verruca (vəroo′kə), *n* a benign, viral, warty skin lesion with a rough, papillomatous surface. It is caused by a common contagious papovavirus.

verruca senilis **(sənil′is),** *n* See keratosis, seborrheic.

verruca vulgaris, *n* (wart), a common wart of the skin or mucosa.

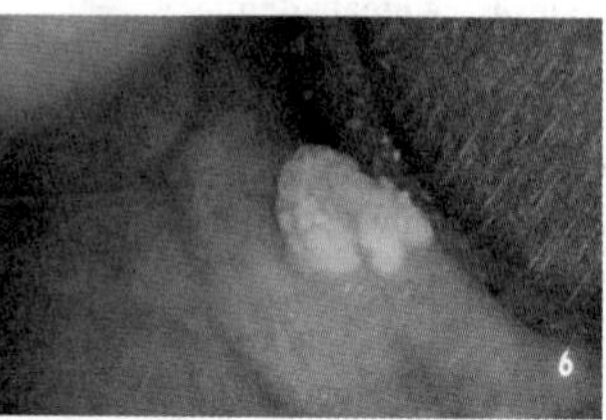

Verruca vulgaris. (Courtesy Dr. Charles Babbush)

verrucous (vəroo′kəs), *adj* **1.** covered with warty lesions. **2.** resembling a wart.

verrucous carcinoma (vəroo′kəs kär′sinō′mə), *n* See carcinoma, verrucous.

vertebra (vur′təbrə), *n* any one of the 33 bones of the spinal or vertebral column that comprises the 7 cervical, 12 thoracic, 5 lumbar, 5 sacral, and 4 coccygeal vertebrae.

vertical, *adj* perpendicular to the horizontal plane.

vertical angulation, *n* See angulation, vertical.

vertical bite-wing film, *n* a small, photosensitive piece of material that is used to take radiographs of the teeth at an angle that allows the viewing of any existing overhangs, root caries, crowns, furcation, and bone loss. The film is placed vertically rather than horizontally to get a more complete view of the root. See radiograph, bite-wing (BWX).

vertical bone loss, n an abnormal decrease in the alveolar crestal bone height indicated by a visible loss of bone on one tooth's proximal surface compared to the tooth on the adjacent side.

vertical dimension, n See dimension, vertical.

vertical lug, n See connector, minor.

vertical opening, n See dimension, vertical.

vertical overlap, n See overlap, vertical.

vertical plane of space, n the plane of space between the inferior and superior edges of the body when seen from the posterior, anterior, or lateral aspects.

vertical relation, See relation, vertical.

vertical-integrated health care, a health care delivery system in which the complete spectrum of care, including financial services, is provided within a single organization, such as a health maintenance organization (HMO).

vertigo (vur′təgō), *n* **1.** a sensation described as dizziness. *n* **2.** a sensation of the room revolving about the patient or the patient revolving in space. It is a form of dizziness, but the terms are not synonymous.

very low-density lipoproteins (VLDLs), *n.pl* lipoproteins containing approximately 9% protein that transport triglycerides from the liver to tissues throughout the body.

vesicant (ves′ikənt), *n* a chemically active substance that can produce blistering on direct contact with the skin or mucous membrane.

vesicle (ves′ikəl), *n* **1.** a small, blisterlike elevation of the skin or mucous membrane resulting from an intraepithelial collection of fluid. It is a primary type of lesion and may be seen in herpes simplex, recurrent herpes, recurrent aphthae, stomatitis medicamentosa, stomatitis venenata, erythema multiforme, Reiter's syndrome, Behçet's syndrome, Stevens-Johnson syndrome, herpangina, varicella, and many others. *n* **2.** a circumscribed, elevated lesion of the skin containing fluid and having a diameter of up to 5 mm.

vessel(s), *n* an avenue through which something can travel.

vessels, afferent, n.pl vessels that carry fluids such as lymph or blood toward a structure or a part.

vessels, blood, visualization of, n the methods by which the blood vessels are seen by the examiner. Direct visualization of blood vessels is possible only to a limited extent. The blood vessels in the retina can be directly visualized; the capillary loops in the fingernail can be seen by microscopy, and the blood vessels in the oral mucosa and gingivae can be visualized by infrared photography. More recently, radiography and cineradiography are used to visualize radiopaque substances. These methods can reveal the actual blood column, its width, variation in contour, and pathway. Arteriograms and venograms are useful in revealing spasms, obstructions, congenital defects, and collateral circulation of the deeper tissues.

vessels, efferent, n.pl vessels that carry fluids such as lymph or blood away from a body part.

vestibule, buccal, *n* the space between the alveolar ridge and teeth or between the residual ridge and the cheek distal to the buccal frenum.

vestibule, labial, *n* the space between the alveolar ridge and the teeth or the residual ridge and lips anterior to the buccal frenum.

vestibule, lower buccal, *n* the space between the mandibular alveolar ridge and teeth and the cheek; bounded anteriorly by the mandibular buccal frenum and posteriorly by the distobuccal end of the retromolar pad.

vestibule of the oral cavity, *n* the part of the oral cavity that lies between the teeth and gingivae and lips and cheeks or between the residual ridges and the lips and cheeks.

vestibule, upper buccal, *n* the space between the maxillary alveolar ridge and teeth or the residual ridge and the cheek; bounded anteriorly by the maxillary buccal frenum and posteriorly by the hamular notch.

vestibuloplasty (vestib′ūlōplastē), *n* any of a series of surgical procedures designed to restore alveolar ridge height by lowering the muscles attached to the buccal, labial, and lingual aspects of the jaws.

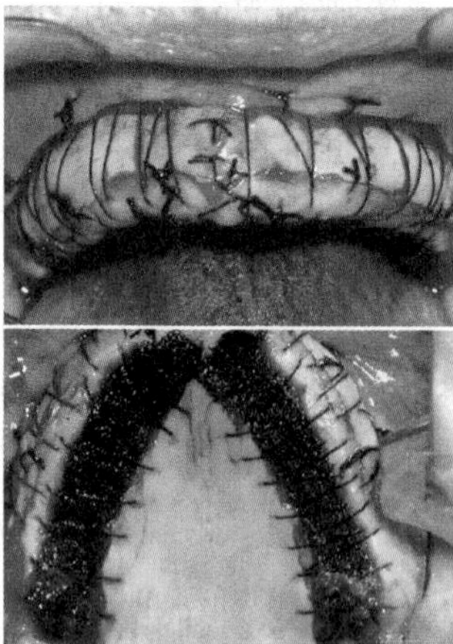

Vestibuloplasty. (Genco/Goldman/Cohen, 1990)

veteran, *n* **1.** a person who has a long period of service in an occupation or profession. *n* **2.** a person who has served in the armed forces, especially one who has fought for his or her country. *n* **3.** a long-serving member of a state legislature or the U.S. Congress.

veterinarian, *n* a Doctor of Veterinary Medicine (DVM), who is educated and trained to provide medical and surgical care for domestic and exotic animals.

viable (vī′əbəl), *adj* capable of life; able to live.

Viadent, *n.pr* brand name for an antiplaque mouthrinse containing sanguinarine, an alkaloid, as the active ingredient. See also sanguinarine.

vibrating line, *n* See line, vibrating.

vibrios (vib′rēōs′), *n.pl* bacteria belonging to the genus *Vibrio* found in plaque after 1 to 2 weeks of no flossing or brushing.

Vicat needle (vēkä), *n.pr* See needle, Vicat.

Vickers hardness number, *n.pr* See number, Vickers hardness.

Vickers hardness test, *n.pr* See test, Vickers hardness.

Vicodin, *n.pr* brand name for hydrocodone, a ketone derivative of codeine that is about six times more potent than codeine. Vicodin is a controlled substance.

vidarabine (vidar′əbēn′), *n* (ophthalmic), *brand name:* Vira-A Ophthalmic; *class:* antiviral; *action:* inhibits DNA synthesis by blocking DNA polymerase; *use:* keratoconjunctivitis due to herpes simplex virus.

viewbox, *n* used for viewing dental radiographs consisting of a tabletop box with a transparent surface through which light is transmitted. When radiographs are laid on the surface, visibility of important details is greatly increased, ensuring greater accuracy of interpretation.

Vincent's angina, *n.pr* See angina, Vincent's.

Vincent's bacillus, *n.pr* See *Fusobacterium fusiforme.*

Vincent's gingivitis, *n.pr* See gingivitis, necrotizing ulcerative.

Vincent's infection, *n.pr* See gingivitis, necrotizing ulcerative.

vinegar (as a solvent), *n* a warm, dilute solution of household vinegar; used as a substitute for acetic acid to dissolve accumulated dental calculus from a removable dental prosthesis.

Vinethene (vin′ethēn), *n.pr* brand name for vinyl ether.

vinyl resin (vī′nil), *n* See resin, vinyl.

violation, injury, *n* encroachment; breach of right, obligation, or law.

violence, *n* severe physical force; the forceful assault of a person.

violet, gentian (vīəlet, jen′shən), *n* a rosaniline dye, useful as a protective covering and an antiseptic in the treatment of minor lesions of the oral mucosa. It is an effective fungicide and is therefore of value in the treatment of moniliasis.

violet stain, *n* See stain, methyl violet.

viral hepatitis, *n* See hepatitis.

viral infection, *n* an infection by a pathogenic virus. A virus acts on the cell nucleus, taking over the genetic material within the nucleus and replicating itself.

viral shedding, *n* process that occurs when a virus is present in bodily fluids or open wounds and can thereby be transmitted to another person, as with herpetic lesions.

viremia (vīrē′mēə), *n* an elevation of virus levels occurring 2 to 4 weeks after infection with HIV.

virion (vir′ēon, vī′rē-), *n* the whole virus, including the inner nucleus and the outer shell.

virology (vīrol′əjē), *n* the scientific study of viruses and the diseases caused by viruses.

virulence (vir′yələns), *n* the power of a microorganism to produce disease.

virus (vī′rus), *n* one of a group of heterogeneous infective agents characterized by the lack of independent metabolism or the ability to replicate outside the host cell.

virus, herpes simplex, *n* See herpes simplex.

virus replication, *n* the ability of viruses to reproduce within a host cell.

viscera (vis′ərə), *n.pl* (*sg* **viscus**), the internal organs enclosed within a body cavity, primarily the abdominal organs.

viscerocranium (vis′ərōkrā′nēum), *n* the category of the 14 bones of the human skull that encircle the face. Also called the *facial bones.*

viscosity (viskos′itē), *n* the ability or inability of a fluid solution to flow easily. High viscosity indicates a slow-flowing fluid.

visible light, *n* the radiant energy in the electromagnetic spectrum that is visible to the human eye. The wavelengths cover a range of approximately 390 to 780 nm.

visible-light cure, *n* system designed to control the curing time of material that hardens over time; when light is withheld, the material is malleable for a longer duration; when light is applied, the material hardens rapidly.

vision (vizh′ən), *n* sight; the faculty of seeing.

vision, direct, *n* the category of sight in which an image is focused directly on the macula of the retina. Also called *central vision.*

vision, field of, *n* the portion of space that the fixed eye can see.

vision, indirect, *n* **1.** in dentistry, the capacity to see the treatment area by using a oral cavity mirror. *n* **2.** the category of sight in which an image is focused on an area of the retina other than the macula. Also called *peripheral vision.*

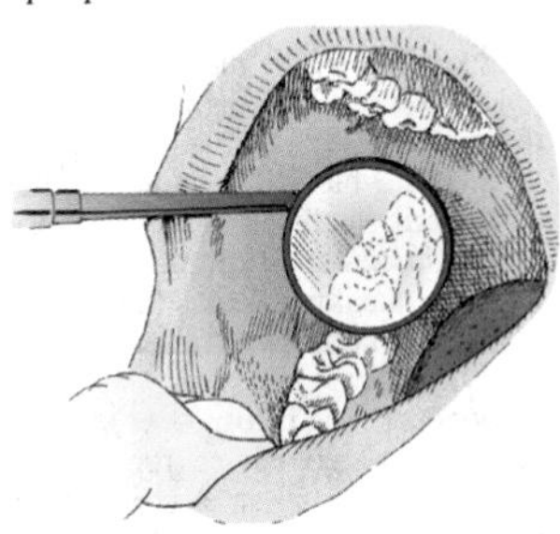

Indirect vision. (Bird/Robinson, 2005)

vision, stereoscopic, *n* vision in which the visual fields of the two eyes are unified. Sensations from a common object received by the two eyes are superimposed, and as a result of the slight differences in the fields and the superimposition of the fields, the effects of depth and shape of the object are attained.

visit, *n* a meeting between a health care professional and a patient for diagnostic, therapeutic, or consultative reasons, usually a scheduled appointment in a professional office. Also called *patient visit* or *patient encounter.*

visual acuity, *n* a measure of the resolving power of the eye, particularly its ability to distinguish letters and numbers at a given distance. See also acuity, visual.

visual analogue scale for pain (VAS), *n* a simple assessment tool consisting of a 10 cm line with 0 on one end, representing no pain, and 10 on the other, representing the worst pain ever experienced, which a patient indicates so the clinician knows the severity of his or her pain.

visual disorders, *n.pl* See disorders, visual.

visual treatment objective (VTO), *n* a diagnostic and communication aid, consisting of a cephalometric tracing, modified to show changes anticipated in the course of growth and treatment.

vital, *adj* necessary to or pertaining to life.

vital capacity, *n* a measurement of the amount of air that can be expelled at the normal rate of exhalation after a maximum inspiration, representing the greatest possible breathing capacity.

vital signs, *n.pl* the measurements of pulse rate, respiration rate, and body temperature. Although not strictly a vital sign, blood pressure is also customarily included in this category.

vital statistics, *n.pl* the data relating to births (natality), deaths (mortality), marriages, health, and disease (morbidity).

vitalometer (vī'təlom'əter), *n* an electric-powered device for delivering and measuring an electrical stimulus to a tooth. See also pulp tester.

vitalometry (vi'təlom'ətrē), *n* the use of high-frequency pulp-testing equipment to establish the vital condition of the pulp of a tooth.

vitamin (vi'təmin), *n* one of a number of unrelated organic substances that occur in small amounts in food and are required for normal metabolic activity. The vitamins may be water soluble or fat soluble.

vitamin A, *n* (retinal, retinol, retinoic acid), a fat-soluble substance, occurring in several chemical forms in food and function: retinal, an aldehyde; retinol, an alcohol; and retinoic acid, an acid. All three function in calcified and epithelial tissue growth. The aldehyde-alcohol (retinal-retinol) interconversion allows regeneration of rhodopsin (visual purple) in the rod cells of the retina. A deficiency results in hyperkeratinization of nonsecretory protective epithelium, deranged secretory function of the mucous membrane, dark dysadaptation (night blindness), and possibly, enamel hypoplasia. Dietary sources include liver, kidney, and lung as well as carotenes (provitamins A) from the plant kingdom.

vitamin, ascorbic acid **(əskôr'bik),** *n* (vitamin C, antiscorbutic factor), a water-soluble vitamin resembling glucose in structure; it is found in citrus fruits, tomatoes, cabbage, and other fresh fruits and vegetables. Necessary for hydroxylation of peptide-bound lysine and proline to hydroxylysine and hydroxyproline during collagen synthesis. A deficiency leads to scurvy, in which pathologic signs are confined mainly to the connective tissues with hemorrhages, loosening of teeth, gingivitis, and poor wound healing.

vitamin B_1, *n* See vitamin, thiamine.

vitamin B_2, *n* See vitamin, riboflavin.

vitamin B_6, *n* See vitamin, pyridoxine.

vitamin B_{12}, *n* See vitamin, cobalamin.

vitamin B complex, *n* collectively, the various B vitamins: thiamine, riboflavin, nicotinic acid, pyridoxine, biotin, paraaminobenzoic acid, folic acid, pantothenic acid, cyanocobalamin, pteroylglutamic acid, and others that are unknown.

vitamin, biotin **(bi'ətin),** *n* (vitamin H, anti-egg-white factor), one of the B complex vitamins found in organ meats (e.g., liver, heart, kidney), egg yolk, cauliflower, chocolate, and mushrooms. Its synthesis by intestinal bacteria makes human deficiency states rare, unless the diet contains significant raw egg white protein (avidin), which complexes the vitamin to prevent intestinal absorption. Dermatitis, retarded growth, and loss of hair and muscular control occur in experimental animals with deficiency. Biotin functions as a coenzyme for carboxylase enzymes that catalyze fixation of carbon dioxide (e.g., in fatty acid synthesis).

vitamin C, *n* See vitamin, ascorbic acid.

vitamin, calciferol, *n* See vitamin D.

vitamin, cholecalciferol, *n* See vitamin D.

vitamin, choline **(kō'lēn),** *n* not truly a vitamin, because it can be synthesized in the body if sufficient precursors are available. Prevents the accumulation of fat in the liver of certain animal species. Occurs as a constituent of lecithin, sphingomyelin, and acetylcholine.

vitamin, cobalamin **(kōbal'əmin),** *n* (antipernicious factor, vitamin B_{12}, cyanocobalamin, erythrocyte maturing factor [EMF], extrinsic factor) a vitamin that contains cobalt and is essential for the maturation of erythrocytes. Inability of the body to produce intrinsic factor, which is necessary for vitamin B_{12} absorption, results in pernicious anemia. Liver, kidney, muscle, and milk are good sources.

V

vitamin D (antirachitic factor, calciferol, cholecalciferol, ergosterol, ergocalciferol), *n* the group of lipid-soluble sterol compounds capable of preventing rickets. Of primary importance are D_2, or ergosterol, from plants and D_3, or cholecalciferol, from animal sources, especially fish liver oils. The latter is also formed in the skin from 7-dehydrocholesterol on exposure to ultraviolet light. Liver mitochondria further activate vitamin D to 25-(OH)-D, which in turn is metabolized to 1,25-$(OH)_2$-D by the kidney. The dihydroxy metabolites significantly increase dietary calcium absorption and bone resorption to maintain proper blood calcium and phosphorus levels. A primary vitamin D deficiency results from inadequate exposure to sunlight and low dietary intake. Secondary deficiencies occur from abnormalities of intestinal resorption and interference with vitamin D hydroxylation. The manifestations of rickets include enamel hypoplasia, poorly calcified bones, bowed legs, and a deformed rib cage with beadlike swellings of the ribs (rachitic rosary) in infants and children and osteomalacia in adults. Vitamin D intake in excess is toxic.

vitamin E, *n* (tocopherol, tocotrienol antisterility factor) the tocopherol and tocotrienols have varying degrees of vitamin E activity, but α-tocopherol is the most active. These fat-soluble compounds are found in eggs, muscle meats, liver, fish, chicken, oatmeal, and the oils of corn, soya, and cottonseed. In rats, the lack of vitamin E leads to fetus resorption in the female and atrophy of spermatogenic tissue with permanent sterility in the male. Vitamin E deficiency in humans is correlated with increased hemolysis of erythrocytes. The tocopherols prevent peroxidation of unsaturated fatty acids, and vitamin E requirements appear to be directly related to the dietary intake of unsaturated fatty acids. Although animals develop symptoms of muscular dystrophy on deficient diets, the vitamin has no effect on the human disease.

vitamin, ergocalciferol, *n* See vitamin D.

vitamin, folacin, *n* (adermine, folic acid, citrovorum factor, pteroylglutamic acid, vitamin M, vitamin B_c) occurs in many tissues as the free acid or is conjugated with one to seven glutamic acid molecules. Green, leafy vegetables; kidney; liver; and yeast are good sources, and bacterial synthesis in humans occurs readily. As a coenzyme, the vitamin serves as a carrier of one-carbon units (formyl, hydroxymethyl, formimino groups), especially in the synthesis of nucleoproteins. Inadequate folate levels produce a variety of species-dependent symptoms that include megaloblastic anemia in humans.

vitamin G, *n* See vitamin, riboflavin.

vitamin H, *n* See vitamin, biotin.

vitamin, inositol **(inō′sətôl),** *n* (*myo*-inositol, *meso*-inositol), a six-carbon alcohol closely related to the hexoses. Inositol is not truly a vitamin because the body can synthesize significant amounts from glucose. Its biologic role is not established, but it is essential to the growth of liver and bone marrow cells and helps alleviate fatty livers.

vitamin K, *n* (phytonadione, antihemorrhagic factor), one of the many fat-soluble naphthoquinone compounds with vitamin D activity. Vitamin K_1 is found primarily in leafy vegetables, K_2 is synthesized by human intestinal bacteria, and K_3 (menadione, N.F.) is a synthetic compound. Vitamin K is essential for the synthesis of prothrombin by the liver. A dietary deficiency of vitamin K is rare, however. The vitamin has been used in conjunction with extensive oral antibiotic therapy to treat hemorrhagic disease of the newborn, hemorrhage of obstructive jaundice, and sprue, and during anticoagulant therapy. Prothrombin, Stuart factor, Christmas factor, and serum prothrombin conversion accelerator require vitamin K for their synthesis.

vitamin, niacin **(nī′əsin),** *n* (nicotinic acid, nicotinamide, niacinamide, pellagra-preventive factor), a deficiency of niacin or its amide derivative, niacinamide, results in acute pellagra that is characterized by dermatitis, diarrhea, dementia, stomatitis, and glossitis. Dietary sources include liver, kidney, lean meats, wheat germ, yeast, soybeans, and peanuts. There is some intestinal synthesis by bacteria. Although the amino acid tryptophan contributes to the body supply of niacin, sufficient vitamin B_6 must be present for its metabolism. Niacin and niacinamide are interconvertible in the body, and the latter functions as a constituent of two coenzymes, NAD and NADP, which operate as hydrogen and electron transfer agents by virtue of their reversible oxidation and reduction in several enzyme systems.

vitamin, pantothenic acid **(pan′təthen′ik),** *n* (pantothen, panthenol), this vitamin is a component of coenzyme A and thereby functions in the metabolism of lipids, carbohydrates, and proteins. A deficiency is unusual because of its wide distribution, but a "burning feet syndrome" has been reported in people suffering from acute malnutrition.

vitamin, pyridoxine **(pir′ədok′sēn),** *n* (vitamin B_6, pyridoxal, pyridoxol, pyridoxamine) part of the B complex vitamins, the group includes three chemically related substances: pyridoxol, pyridoxal, and pyridoxamine, all of which serve as substrate in the formation of pyridoxal phosphate, the prosthetic group for several enzymes that decarboxylate, deaminate, transaminate, or desulfurate specific amino acids. It further functions in porphyrin, fatty acids, and cholesterol metabolism. Deficiency signs include an acrodynia-like syndrome, convulsive seizures, arteriosclerotic-like lesions, hypochromic microcytic anemia, and impaired antibody formation. Dietary sources include wheat; corn; liver; milk; eggs; and green, leafy vegetables.

vitamin, retinal, *n* See vitamin A.

vitamin, retinoic acid, *n* See vitamin A.

vitamin, retinol, *n* See vitamin A.

vitamin, riboflavin **(rī′bōflāvin),** *n* (vitamin B_2, vitamin G, lactoflavin) a heat-stable B complex vitamin that functions as a component of FAD and FMN for the reversible transfer of hydrogen and electrons in several enzyme systems. It is found in green, leafy vegetables; whole grains; eggs; liver; milk; and legumes; small amounts are synthesized in the intestinal tract by microorganisms. Signs of ariboflavinosis include angular stomatitis, seborrheic dermatitis of the face, and glossitis (magenta tongue).

vitamin, thiamine **(thī′əmin),** *n* (vitamin B_1, aneurine, antiberiberi factor, antineuritic factor) a B complex vitamin found primarily in plants, especially legumes; whole grains; and green, leafy vegetables; it is also synthesized by bacteria in the large intestine, which is not a reliable source. Thiamine pyrophosphate (TPP, cocarboxylase) is a coenzyme in the oxidative decarboxylation of pyruvate and α-ketoglutarate, in the transketolase reaction of glucose metabolism and in the metabolism of branched chained amino acids. A deficiency results in beriberi.

vitamin, tocopherol, *n* See vitamin E.

vitamin, tocotrienol, *n* See vitamin E.

vitiate (vish′ēāt), *v* to weaken; to make void or voidable.

vitiligo (vit′ilē′gō, vit′ilī′gō), *n* a skin condition characterized by spotty areas of depigmentation.

vitrification (vit′rifikā′shən), *n* the act, instance, art, or process of converting dental porcelain (frit) to a glassy substance; the process of becoming vitreous by heat and fusion.

VLDL, *n.pl* abbreviation for very-low-density lipids.

vocabulary, *n* **1.** the stock or range of words possessed by an individual or a culture used for self-expression or communication. *n* **2.** the sum of the distinct words related to a discipline or profession.

vocal cords, *n.pl* See cords, vocal.

voice, *n* sound produced primarily by the vibration of the vocal bands.

void, *n* **1.** empty or unfilled space. *n* **2.** space not filled with anything solid. *adj* **3.** ineffectual; having no legal, binding effect.

volatile (vol′ətil), *adj* having a tendency to evaporate rapidly.

volatile oil, *n* See oil, essential.

volatile sulfur compounds (VSCs), *n.pl* bad-smelling substances such as hydrogen sulfide, methyl mercaptan, dimethyl sulfide, and dimethyl disulfide that are produced by the metabolism of a microscopic organism.

Volkmann's canal, *n.pr* a passage distinct from a haversian canal that carries nutrients through bone.

volt (V), *n* the unit of electromotive force or electrical pressure; the force necessary to cause 1 ampere of current to flow against 1 ohm of resistance. A volt is the unit that is used to measure the tendency of a charge to move from one place to another.

volt, electron (eV), n the kinetic energy gained by an electron by falling through a potential difference of 1 volt. 1 eV is equivalent to 1.6×10^{-12} ergs; 1000 eV is referred to as 1 kilo electron volt, or keV, and 1,000,000 eV are referred to as 1 mega electron volt, or MeV.

voltage, *n* the potential of electromotive force of an electric charge, measured in volts.

volume, *n* measure of the quantity of space occupied by a substance, such as air.

volume, blood, n the total amount of blood in the body.

volume, expiratory reserve, n (reserve air, supplemental air, supplemental volume) the maximum volume that can be expired from the resting expiratory level.

volume, index of blood, n See blood, volume index of.

volume, inspiratory reserve, n (complemental air) the maximum volume that can be inspired from the end of tidal inspiration

volume, packed-cell, n See hematocrit.

volume, residual, n the volume of air in the lungs at the end of maximum expiration.

volume, stroke, n See stroke volume.

volume, supplemental, n See volume, expiratory reserve.

volume, tidal, n the volume of gas inspired or expired during each respiratory cycle.

vomer (vō′mər), *n* the single facial bone that forms the posterior portion of the nasal septum.

vomiting (vom′iting), *n* the forcible voluntary or involuntary emptying of the stomach contents through the oral cavity.

von Recklinghausen's disease of bone, *n.pr* See hyperparathyroidism and osteitis fibrosa cystica, generalized.

von Recklinghausen's disease of skin, *n.pr* See neurofibromatosis.

voucher, *n* a receipt or release that may serve as notice of payment of a debt or may prove the accuracy of accounts.

vowel, *n* a conventional vocal sound in the production of which the speech organs offer little obstruction to the airstream and form a series of resonators above the level of the larynx.

vs, *prep* an abbreviation for *versus* (against); commonly used in legal proceedings, particularly in designating the title of cases.

vulcanite (vul′kənīt), *n* a hard material with a form of rubber as the base; formerly used for denture bases.

vulcanization, *n* the process of treating crude rubber to improve such qualities as strength and hardness. This process usually involves heating the rubber with sulfur in the presence of moisture, the sulfur uniting with the rubber to produce saturated double bonds.

VZ virus, *n* varicella zoster virus, which causes chickenpox in humans. See varicella.

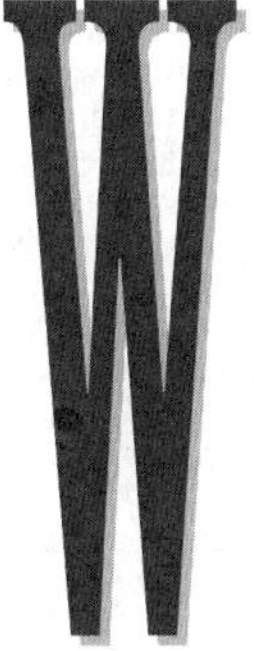

wages, *n* the compensation to an employee, agreed on by the employee and employer, for work completed by the employee.

waiting period, *n* the period between employment or enrollment in a dental program and the date when an insured person becomes eligible for benefits.

waiver (wā′vur), *n* **1.** repudiation, abandonment, or surrender of a claim, right, or privilege. *n* **2.** the intentional relinquishment of a known right.

walker, *n* an extremely light, movable device, about waist-high, made of metal tubing, used to assist a patient in walking. It has four widely placed, sturdy legs. The patient holds onto the walker, takes a step, then moves the walker forward, and takes another step.

wall, *n* the outside layer of material surrounding an object or space; a paries.

wall, cavity, n one of the enclosing sides of a prepared cavity. It takes the name of the surface of the tooth adjoining the surface involved and toward which it is placed. Parts of a surrounding or peripheral wall are the cavosurface angle, the enamel wall, the dentinoenamel junction, and the dentin wall.

wall, enamel, n the portion of the wall of a prepared cavity that consists of enamel.

wall, finish of enamel, n the planing of the enamel in finishing a cavity preparation; includes the treatment of the cavosurface angle.

wall, gingival cavity, n the peripheral wall that most closely approximates the apical end of the tooth.

wall, incisal, n the wall of a prepared cavity in an anterior tooth that is closest to or in direct relation to the incisal edge of the tooth.

wall, peripheral cavity, n See wall, surrounding cavity.

wall, surrounding cavity, n one of the external, bounding side walls of a cavity; one side forms a part of the cavosurface angle of the preparation. Also called *peripheral cavity wall.*

Walter Reed staging system, *n.pr* an alternative classification system used to describe various stages of HIV infection. See Centers for Disease Control and Prevention classification.

wandering rash, *n* See geographic tongue.

Wanscher's mask (vän′shuz), *n.pr* See mask, Wanscher's.

ward, *n* a person, especially a minor, placed by authority of law under the care of a guardian.

Ward's Wonderpack, *n.pr* brand name for a type of periodontal dressing used to cover and protect a surgical site; the basic components include tannic acid, zinc oxide, and powdered rosin.

warfarin sodium (wôr′fərin), *n brand names:* Coumadin, Panwarfin, Sofarin; *drug class:* oral anticoagulant; *action:* interferes with blood clotting by indirect means; depresses hepatic synthesis of vitamin K–dependent coagulation factors (II, VII, IX, and X); *uses:* pulmonary emboli, deep vein thrombosis, MI, atrial dysrhythmias.

warp, *n* uncontrolled torsional change of shape or outline, such as that which may occur in swaging sheet metal, in denture material, or in other materials exposed to varying temperatures.

wart, *n* See verruca vulgaris.

Warthin's tumor, *n.pr* See cystadenoma, papillary and lymphomatosum.

Wassermann test, *n.pr* See test, Wassermann.

waste disposal, *n* a removal of all potentially contaminated objects (e.g., objects soaked with saliva or blood) and placement in a secure site to prevent or decrease the risk of infection. See also sharps container.

waste, infectious, *n* waste that is contaminated with pathogenic microorganisms.

waste management, *n* protocol for the safe disposal of waste products, such as needles, tissue specimens, and instruments used in dental procedures.

waste products, *n.pl* the products of metabolic activity after oxygen and nutrients have been supplied to a cell. These include primarily carbon dioxide and water, along with sodium chloride and soluble nitrogenous salts, which are excreted in feces, urine, and exhaled air.

waste products, biohazard, n unusable biologic materials that can carry infection, which could then be transmitted to other organisms.

waste products, contaminated, n.pl **1.** instruments that have become nonsterile after coming into contact with blood, saliva, urine, or any other bodily fluids. *n.pl* **2.** the fluids or substances that contain the byproducts of metabolic activity. See also waste products.

waste products, infectious, n contaminated waste that may potentially cause infectious disease.

wasting, *n* a process of deterioration marked by weight loss and decreased physical vigor, appetite, and mental activity.

water, *n* a tasteless, odorless, colorless compound made of hydrogen and oxygen (H_2O), which freezes at 32°F (0°C) and boils at 212°F (100°C). The autonomic nervous system regulates water balance in the body.

water depletion, *n* cellular dehydration through decreased water intake, dysphagia, excessive sweating, and diuresis.

water, distilled, *n* a type of purified water that has undergone evaporation and recondensation prior to bottling.

water need, *n* the amount of water needed to maintain metabolism, approximately 1000 ml/day.

water, superoxidized **(soo′pərok′sədāzd),** *n* an electrolyzed saline solution used as a disinfectant.

water syringe, *n* See syringe, water.

water:powder ratio, *n* See ratio, water:powder.

Waters extraoral radiographic examination, *n.pr* See examination, Waters extraoral radiographic.

Waters view, *n.pr* See examination, Waters extraoral radiographic.

Watson-Crick helix, *n.pr* a model of the DNA molecule proposed by Watson and Crick as two right-handed polynucleotide chains coiled around the same axis as a double helix.

watt (W), *n* the unit of electric power or work; 1 watt of power is dissipated when a current of 1 ampere (A) flows across a difference in potential of 1 volt (V).

wave, electromagnetic, *n* energy manifested by movements in an advancing series of alternate elevations and depressions.

wavelength, *n* the distance between the peaks of waves in any wave form, such as light, roentgen rays, and other electromotive forms. In electromagnetic radiation, the wavelength is equal to the velocity of light divided by the frequency of the wave.

wavelength, effective, *n* the wavelength that would produce the same penetration as an average of the various wavelengths in a heterogeneous bundle of roentgen rays.

wax, *n* one of several esters of fatty acids with higher alcohols, usually monohydric alcohols. Dental waxes are combinations of various types of waxes compounded to provide the desired physical properties.

wax, baseplate, *n* a hard, pink wax used for making occlusion rims and baseplates for occlusion rims.

wax, bone, *n* a plastic mixture that may contain antiseptic and hemostatic drugs, designed for temporary application to freshly cut bone to prevent hemorrhage and infection.

wax, boxing, *n* a soft wax used for boxing impressions.

wax burnout, *n* See burnout, inlay and wax elimination.

wax, carnauba **(kärnô′bə, -nou′bə),** *n* a hard, high-melting wax used for control of the melting range of dental waxes.

wax, casting, *n* a composition containing various waxes with controlled properties of thermal expansion and contraction; used in making patterns to determine the shape of metal castings.

wax elimination, *n* the procedure of removing the wax from a wax pattern invested in a mold preparatory to the introduction of another material into the resulting cavity. This may be done by dry heat alone or by irrigation with boiling water followed by use of dry heat. Also called *wax burnout.*

wax expansion, *n* the enlargement of wax patterns to compensate for the shrinkage of gold during the casting process.

wax, fluid, *n* a series of waxes, each having different physical properties, used for making a correctable impression of the foundation structures that are to support a denture base. The term indicates that the wax is applied in fluid form as required.

wax inlay, *n* See wax casting.

wax out, *n* See blockout.

wax pattern, *n* See pattern, wax.

wax template, *n* See template, wax.

wax-bite, *n* See record, interocclusal.

waxing, *n* the contouring of a wax pattern or the wax base of a trial denture into the desired form. Also called *waxing up.*

WBC, *n* stands for **w**hite **b**lood **c**ell. See also leukocyte and white blood cell count.

wear, *n* a loss of substance or a diminishing through use, friction, or other destructive factors.

wear, abnormal occlusal, *n* wear that exceeds the physiologic wear patterns associated with the attritional effects of food substances; the excessive wear of the teeth occurring as a result of continued afunctional gyrations of the mandible.

wear, interproximal, *n* a loss of tooth substance in contact areas through functional wear and friction, resulting in broadening and flattening of the contacts and a decrease in the mesiodistal dimension of the teeth and the dentition as a whole.

wear, occlusal, *n* attritional loss of substance on opposing occlusal units or surfaces. See also abrasion and attrition.

wear pattern, *n* See pattern, wear.

wear, physiologic, *n* the attrition or abrasion of tooth substance occurring as a result of such conditions as the abrasive consistency of the normal diet or the slight buccolingual movement of the teeth possible in the masticatory process. It does not include the wear produced by such influences as habits or occlusal prematurities.

Weber's disease, *n.pr* See telangiectasia, hereditary hemorrhagic.

Weber-Dimitri disease, *n.pr* See disease, Sturge-Weber-Dimitri.

Wedelstaedt chisel (vēd'əlshtat), *n.pr* See chisel, Wedelstaedt.

wedge, *n* a small, pointed, triangular, contoured piece of wood used to seal the gingival margin of a cavity preparation before placement of an amalgam restoration.

wedge, step, *n* See penetrometer.

wedge stimulator, *n* an oral hygiene device made of plastic or wood used to stimulate and clean between teeth.

wedging, *n* packing or fixing tightly by driving in a wedge or wedges.

wedging effect, *n* See effect, wedging.

weekly permissible dose, *n* See dose, weekly permissible.

W

weight, *n* the product of the gravitational acceleration of one body and the mass of an attracted body; the measurement in pounds and ounces of how heavy an object is. In the metric system, weight (force) is measured in kg × m/sec^2.

weight, molecular **(məlek'ūlur),** *n* the sum of the atomic weights of all atoms in a molecule.

weight, rubber dam, *n* a piece of metal varying in shape and weight, attached to a clip that is hung on the bottom of a placed rubber dam to keep the field of operation clear.

Weil's disease (vīlz), *n.pr* See disease, Weil's.

welding, *n* a process used to join metals.

welding, arc and gas, *n* See welding, fusion.

welding, cold, *n* the property of welding at room temperature when clean surfaces are pressed into contact. This property is exhibited to the highest degree by gold in the form of foil or crystals.

welding, fusion, *n* a process in which parts are melted and fused together. Also called *arc and gas welding.*

welding, pressure, *n* a welding process in which the parts are not melted, although heat is usually required. Recrystallization across the interface occurs. Gold foil is welded by pressure without temperature elevation. Also called *resistance welding* and *spot welding.*

welding property, *n* the characteristic of certain materials, especially metals, to firmly unite together when subjected to heat or pressure in a suitable environment.

welding, resistance, *n* See welding, pressure.

welding, spot, *n* See welding, pressure.

Werlhof's disease (verl'hofs), *n.pr* See purpura, thrombocytopenic.

Wernicke-Korsakoff's syndrome (ver'nikē-kôr'səkôf), *n.pr* a disorder caused by a lack of thiamine due to long-term alcohol abuse in which the patient has difficulty in walking, seeing, or thinking clearly.

Western blot, *n.pr* a confirmatory test for HIV exposure that identifies antibodies to HIV proteins and glycoproteins.

wet strength, *n* See strength, wet.

wettability (wet'əbil'ətē), *n* the angle at which a droplet of liquid interfaces with a horizontal surface; the shape of the droplet varies depending on the type of liquid and surface, thereby influencing the contact angle and thus the wettability. The greater the angle past 90°, the greater the wettability.

wetting agent, *n* See agent, wetting.

Wharton's duct, *n* See duct, Wharton's.

wheal (w[h]ēl), *n* edematous elevation of the skin or mucosa. See also urticaria.

wheel, Burlew, *n.pr* See Burlew wheel.

wheel stone, *n* See stone, wheel.

wheelchair, *n* a mobile chair equipped with large wheels and brakes used to transport patients or to allow disabled persons to move themselves from one place to another. Federal law requires handicapped access to public buildings with ramps, doors, elevators, restrooms, and drinking fountains designed and constructed to allow patients in wheelchairs proper access.

wheelchair transfer, *n* the techniques for assisting a wheelchair-bound patient from the wheelchair to the dental chair.

wheeze, *n* a whistling sound made during breathing that is caused by a foreign substance in the trachea or bronchus.

white blood cell (WBC), *n* See leukocyte and white blood cell count.

white blood cell count, *n* a diagnostic clinical laboratory test to determine the number and types of leukocytes present in a measured sample of blood. Overall the normal number of leukocytes ranges from 5000 to $10{,}000/mm^3$. A differential white blood cell count identifies, counts, and determines the ratios of the various types of leukocytes present in a sample of blood. See also leukopenia and leukocytosis.

white lesions, *n.pl* lesions found on the mucosa that have a white coating. They require differential diagnosis because they may indicate trauma, infection, or a cancerous process.

white spot, *n* See enamel opacity.

whiting, *n* a grade of calcium carbonate used to polish dental surfaces.

whitlow (hwit'lō), *n* an inflammation of the end of a finger or toe that results in suppuration.

whitlow, herpetic, *n* an infection caused by the herpes simplex virus that enters the body through small breaks in the skin; usually appears as cracks in the skin around the fingernails; dental personnel are at risk of contracting the virus from an infected patient by direct contact with saliva or a lesion on the lip. See also herpes simplex.

whooping cough, *n* See pertussis.

Widman procedure (wid'mən), *n.pr* a surgical procedure in which a periodontal flap is made to gain better access to root surfaces for complete dèbridement and root planing.

will, *n* a legal document detailing one's wishes in the disposal of one's body and property and the care of one's minor children and dependents.

will, living, *n* a document that details one's wishes regarding the degree and amount of health care desired if one becomes mentally incapacitated.

willfully, *adv* intentionally; purposefully.

Wilson, curve of, *n.pr* a lateral curve of the occlusal table formed by the lingual inclination of the posterior teeth. Because the lingual cusps are lower than the buccal cusps, they form a curve with their antimeres. See also curve of Wilson theory.

window period, *n* the period between when a party is exposed to an infectious organism and when that organism becomes detectable via a serum marker. See incubation period.

winking, jaw, *n* See syndrome, jaw-winking.

wire, *n* slender and pliable rod or thread of metal.

wire, arch, *n* wire used in orthodontics as a source of force to direct teeth to move in desired directions. The wire may be described according to the shape of its cross-section, such as ribbon, rectangular, or round.

wire, diagnostic, *n* See wire, measuring.

wire edge, *n* a thin, rough ridge created by particles that have been rearranged during hand instrument sharpening and appear on the surface adjoining the cutting edge.

wire, internal suspension, *n* one of a network of wires placed inside the oral cavity connecting the zygoma and mandibular arch bar, which are used to immobilize the maxillary arch for healing after a LeFort I fracture. See also fracture, LeFort.

wire, Kirschner, *n.pr* a surgical steel wire of heavy gauge with pointed ends; used in the reduction and fixation of bone fragments by passing it through the cancellous portion of the bone and spanning the fracture site.

wire, ligature, *n* a soft, thin wire used to tie an arch wire to the band attachments.

wire, measuring, *n* a wire or other similar metal placed in a root canal to determine the length of the canal. A radiogram is used to make the determination.

wire, orthodontic, *n* stainless steel and wrought gold wire of various dimensions used in orthodontic treatment.

wire, Risdon **(riz′don),** *n.pr* a wire arch bar tied in the midline.

wire, separating, *n* wire threaded interproximally between two adjacent teeth and tightened by twisting the ends together to wedge the teeth slightly apart. Separating wire is used in preparation to adapt bands to teeth having tight contacts with adjacent teeth.

wire, transosseous **(tranzos′ēus),** *n* a thin, flexible thread of metal that is laced through a hole drilled into the bone to bridge a fracture line and stabilize bone fragments. See also wire, Kirschner and wiring, perialveolar.

wire, wrought, *n* **1.** a wire formed by drawing a cast structure through a die; used in dentistry for partial denture clasps and orthodontic appliances. *n* **2.** a form of metal resulting from the swaging, rolling, and drawing of a metal ingot into a desired shape and size.

wiring, *n* an arrangement of a wire or wires.

wiring, circumferential, *n* the placement of a wire around a bone contiguous to the oral cavity, with the ends exiting in the oral cavity to maintain mandibular and maxillofacial surgical appliances. Also known as *circumferential mandibular wiring* and *circumzygomatic wiring.*

wiring, continuous loop, *n* a technique of wiring the teeth for the reduction and fixation of fractures. Also called *multiple loop wire.*

wiring, craniofacial suspension, *n* a method of wiring using areas of bones not contiguous with the oral cavity for the support of fractured jaw segments (e.g., piriform aperture, zygomatic arch, zygomatic process of the frontal bone).

wiring, Ivy loop, *n.pr* a method using a wire around two adjacent teeth, providing a loop useful for fixation of a fracture.

wiring, multiple loop, *n* See wiring, continuous loop.

wiring, perialveolar **(per′ēalvē′əlur),** *n* a method of wiring a splint to the maxilla by passing a wire through the bone from the buccal plate to the palate.

wiring, piriform aperture **(pir′ifôrm),** *n* a method of wiring using that area of the nasal bones to stabilize fractures of the jaws.

wisdom tooth, *n* a colloquial term for the third molar tooth, the last tooth in each quadrant of each dental arch. It appears in the oral cavity at about 18 years of age.

witch hazel, *n* a shrub, *Hamamelis virginiana,* indigenous to North America, from which an astringent extract is derived.

withdrawal (abstinence) syndrome, *n* the somatic and psychosomatic symptoms recognizable after the abrupt termination of regular drug or other substance use. The types of symptoms are specific to the type of the withdrawn substance.

witness, *n* one who has knowledge of an event; a person whose declaration under oath is received as evidence for any purpose.

witness, expert, *n* a person whose education, training, and experience can provide the court with an assessment, opinion, or judgment within the area of his or her competence, which is not considered known or available to the general public.

witness, hostile, *n* witness who manifests so much hostility or prejudice under examination (in chief or direct) that the party who has called the witness is allowed to cross-examine the witness (i.e., to treat him or her as though he or she had been called by the opposite party).

witness, lay, *n* a witness who testifies only to firsthand knowledge of facts before judge and jury, different from an expert witness in that the witness is not allowed to testify to theories or hypothesize based on education or expertise.

witness marks, n.pl the small hemispheric depressions that may be prepared in the bone surface in lieu of abutment grooves as a guide for seating the abutment posts of the implant.

Wolff's law, *n.pr* See law, Wolff's.

Wolinella recta **(wō′linel′ə rek′tə),** *n* a microorganism associated with progressive periodontal destruction and refractory forms of periodontitis. A regimen combining antibiotic treatment, débridement, and home oral care seems to suppress or control periodontal infections. Also called *C. rectus.*

wooden interdental cleaner, *n* an implement made from birchwood and bass wood, used to clean between teeth, particularly when significant gum recession is indicated.

work hardening, *n* See hardening, work.

work sheet, *n* the office form used for a complete planning program for the completion of dental services.

work simplification, *n* the application of the principles of the scientific method to increase the ability to produce without sacrificing quality.

work stroke, *n* stroke used for removal of calculus or to reshape an overhanging margin.

working capital, *n* a firm's investment in short-term assets or cash, short-term securities, accounts receivable, and inventories. Gross working capital is defined as current assets minus current liabilities. If the term *working capital* is used without further qualification, it generally refers to gross working capital.

working contact, *n* See contact, working.

working end, *n* the section of an instrument that is used to accomplish the task for which the instrument is intended. A working end may be sharp (a blade) or dull (a nib).

working occlusal surface, *n* See surface, working occlusal.

working occlusion, *n* See occlusion, working.

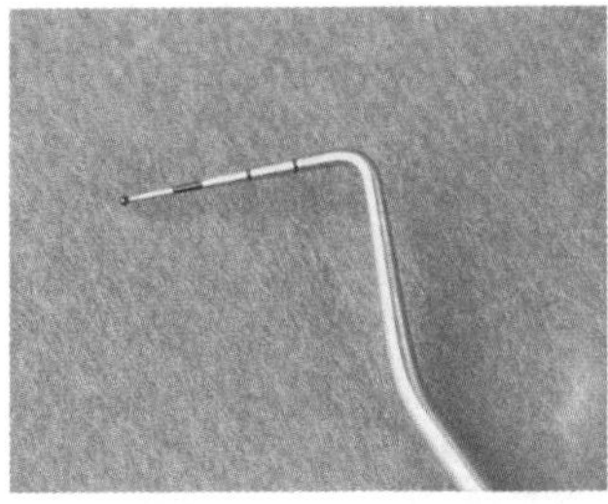

Working end of a periodontal probe. (Bird/Robinson, 2005)

working side, *n* the lateral segment of a denture or dentition toward which the mandible is moved.

Workmen's Compensation Board of Industrial Commission, *n.pr* an administrative body that receives claims for injuries and refers them to certain physicians or dental professionals for treatment, if indicated, with the express or implied assurance to the claimant that the expense will be defrayed by the employer under the Workmen's Compensation Law. The determination of the Industrial Commission is subject to an appeal to court. The federal agency overseeing these matters is the Bureau of Employees Compensation.

World Health Organization (WHO), *n.pr* an agency of the United Nations concerned with worldwide and regional health problems. Its functions include furnishing technical assistance, stimulating and advancing epidemiologic investigation of diseases, recommending health regulations, promoting cooperation among scientific and professional health groups, and providing information and counsel relating to health matters.

worms, *n* a family of parasites characterized by a long body, either flat (platyhelminthes) or round (nematodes). They primarily reside in the intestinal tract, but some types can also survive in other major organs and tissue, such as the brain or muscles, respectively.

wound, *n* an injury to the body of a person, especially one caused by violence.

wound, incised, *n* in medical jurisprudence, a cut or incision on a human body; a wound made by a cutting instrument.

wound repair, *n* restoration of the normal structure after an injury.

wrist drop, *n* a condition caused by paralysis of the extensor muscles of the hand and fingers or by injury of the radial nerve, resulting in flexion of the wrist.

writ of execution, *n* a mandatory precept in writing to implement the judgment or decree of a court.

writing, *n* a written or printed paper or document (e.g., contract, deed).

wrong, *n* an injury; a tort; a violation of right or of law; an injustice; a violation of right resulting in damage to another.

wrongful death status, *n* a statute existing in all states that provides that the death of a person can give rise to a cause of legal action brought by the person's beneficiaries in a civil suit against the person or persons whose willful or negligent acts caused the death.

wrought clasp (wrôt), *n* See clasp, wrought.

wrought wire, *n* See wire, wrought.

X

X chromosome, *n* a sex chromosome that in humans and many other species is present in both male and female. The male somatic cell consists of one X chromosome and one Y chromosome; the female somatic cell carries two X chromosomes. All female gametes carry the X chromosome, whereas half of the male gametes possess the X chromosome and the other half the Y chromosome.

X-bite, *n* See cross-bite.

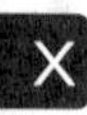

X-C-P film holder, *n.pr* See film holder, Rinn X-C-P.

xanthines (zan′thinz), *n.pl* a family of chemicals that includes caffeine, theophylline, and theobromine, which stimulate the central nervous system, act on the kidneys to produce diuresis, stimulate cardiac muscle, and relax smooth muscle.

xanthogranuloma (zan′thōgran′-ūlō′mə), *n* a benign lesion occurring in infancy, usually solitary and composed of lipid-laden histiocytes with varying numbers of Touton giant cells. In the oral cavity the lesion occurs most often on the tongue and regresses spontaneously.

xanthoma palpebrarum (pal′pə-brä′rəm), *n* a small, yellowish plaque on the eyelids resulting from an accumulation of lipids in reticuloendothelial cells. They often occur in persons with diabetes.

xanthomatosis (zan′thōmətō′sis), *n* a disease characterized by the accumulation of excess lipids. See also *histiocytosis X.*

xanthosis (zanthō′sis), *n* **1.** a yellowish discoloration sometimes seen in degenerating tissues of malignant diseases. *n* **2.** also called carotenosis, a reversible yellow discoloration of the skin most commonly caused by the ingestion of large amounts of yellow vegetables containing carotene pigment, usually in the form of carrot juice. It may be differentiated clinically from jaundice because the sclerae are colored yellow in jaundice but are not discolored in xanthosis.

xenograft (zen′əgraft′), *n* tissue from another species used as temporary graft in certain cases, as in treating a severely burned patient when sufficient tissue from the patient or from a tissue bank is not available. It is quickly rejected but provides a cover of the burn for the first few days, reducing the amount of fluid loss from the open wound. Also called *heterograft.*

xenophobia (zen′əfō′bēə), *n* an anxiety disorder characterized by a pervasive, irrational fear or uneasiness in the presence of strangers, especially foreigners, or in new surroundings.

xeroderma, *n* a chronic skin condition characterized by dryness and roughness.

xeroderma pigmentosum, *n* an eruption of exposed skin occurring in childhood and characterized by numerous pigmental spots resembling freckles, larger atrophic lesions eventually resulting in glossy white thinning of the skin surrounded by telangiectases, and multiple solar keratoses that undergo malignant changes at an early age. This results from a single-gene autosomal recessive disorder.

xerodermosteosis (zir′ōdurmos′-tēō′sis), *n* See syndrome, Sjögren's.

xerogenic (zir′ōjen′ik), *adj* indicates a substance that causes the oral cavity to be unusually dry.

xerography (zirog′rəfē), *n* a dry radiologic process in which an image is made on a metal plate coated with powdered selenium. The plate is electrically charged in a dark room. Exposure to light or roentgen rays causes the charge to be redistributed in a pattern proportional to the intensity of exposure in various areas of the plate. When "developed" in a cloud of charged particles, the particles are attracted to the areas discharged by radiation, producing the equivalent of a photographic negative.

xerophthalmia (zir′ofthal′mēə), *n* dryness of the conjunctiva caused by functional or organic disorders of the lacrimal apparatus. It may be found in vitamin A deficiency or Sjögren's syndrome and may follow chronic conjunctivitis.

xeroradiography, *n* the use of xerography to produce an image electrically rather than chemically, permitting lower exposure times and lower energy levels of roentgen rays.

xerostomia (zir′əstō′mēə), *n* dryness of the oral cavity resulting from functional or organic disturbances of the salivary glands and lack of the normal secretion, primarily caused by prescribed medications. Dryness, loss of basic environment, and resultant overgrowth of oral microorganisms frequently lead to rampant caries. See also hyposalivation.

xerotic keratitis (zirot′ik ker′ətī′-tis), *n* an inflammation of the cornea resulting from dryness of the conjunctiva. Underlying causes may be autoimmune diseases or a deficiency of vitamin A.

X-linkage, *n* See linkage, sex.

x-ray, *n* a type of electromagnetic radiation characterized by wavelengths between approximately 10^3 Å and 10^{-4} Å, corresponding to photon energies of about 20 eV to 125 MeV.

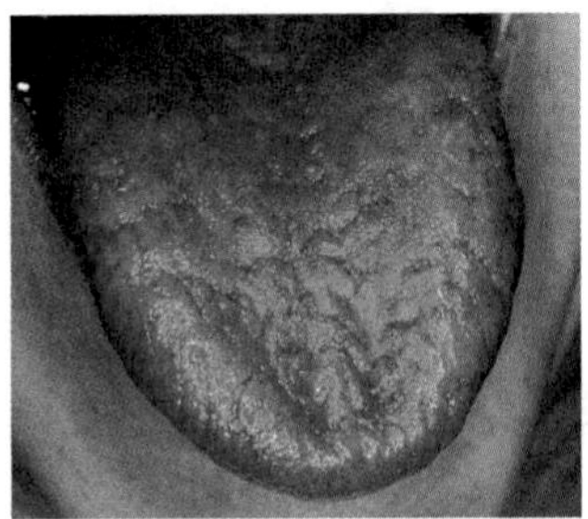

Xerostomia. (Ibsen/Phelan, 2004)

X-rays are invisible; penetrative, especially at higher photon energies; and travel with the same speed as visible light. Typical production involves bombarding a target of high atomic number with fast electrons in a high vacuum; they are also emitted as a product of some radioactive disintegrations (specifically originating from the extranuclear part of the atom). X-rays were first discovered by Wilhelm C. Roentgen in 1895; hence the term *roentgen rays,* often applied to mechanically generated radiographs. Roentgen called them *x-rays* after the mathematic symbol *x* for an unknown. Also the colloquial term for radiograph. See also radiograph.

radiograph, low-voltage filament circuit, *n* the lower-energy circuit in a radiography machine that uses a step-down transformer to lower the line voltage to around 3 volts, just enough to heat the filament and produce an electron cloud.

radiograph, monochromatic, *n* a radiograph that has a single wavelength or an extremely narrow band of wavelengths.

x-ray beam, *n* the spatial distribution of radiation emerging from a radiograph generator or source. The colloquial term for radiographic beam. See radiographic beam.

radiographic beam, central, *n* the straight line passing through the center of the source and the center of the final beam-limiting diaphragm.

radiographic beam, edges, *n* the lines joining the center of the anterior face of the source to the diaphragm edges farthest from the source.

radiographic beam, field size, n the geometric projection, on a plane perpendicular to the central ray, of the distal end of the limiting diaphragm as seen from the center of the front surface of the source. The field is thus the same shape as the aperture of the collimator, and it can be defined at any distance from the source.

radiographic beam, principal plane, n a plane that contains the central ray and, in the case of rectangular section beams, is parallel to one side of the rectangle.

x-ray film, full-mouth, *n* See survey, radiographic.

x-ray mount, *n* See mount, radiographic.

x-ray tube, *n* an electronic tube in which roentgen rays can be generated. See radiographic tube.

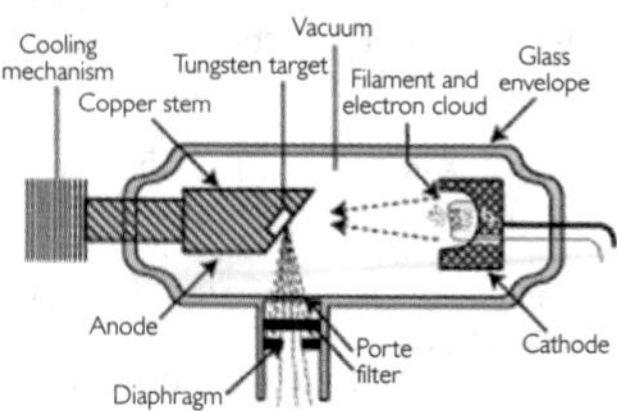

X-ray (radiographic) tube. (Frommer/Stabulas-Savage, 2005)

radiographic tube, Coolidge, n.pr a vacuum tube in which roentgen rays are generated when the target (integral with the anode) is bombarded by electrons that are emitted from a heated filament (on the cathode) and accelerated toward the anode across a high-potential difference. Modern radiograph tubes are of this type. See also tube, Coolidge.

radiographic tube, Crookes', n.pr a vacuum discharge tube used by Sir William Crookes in early experimental work with cathode rays. Wilhelm C. Roentgen first discovered that in addition to the production of cathode rays, radiographs were emitted during the operation of these tubes.

radiographic tube, gas, n an early type of radiographic tube in which electrons were derived from residual gases within the tube.

x-ray unit, *n* See unit, radiographic.

xylene (zīʹlēn), *n* a colorless, flammable fluid used as a solvent and clarifying agent in the preparation of tissue sections for microscopic study. Also called *xylol;* $C_6H_4[CH_3]_2$ *dimethylbenzene.*

xylitol, *n* a low-calorie sweetener that reduces caries activity and the growth and transmission of *S. mutans.*

Xylocaine, *n.pr* See lidocaine.

xylol (zīʹlôl), *n* See xylene.

xylose (zīʹlōsʹ), *n* wood or beechwood sugar; an aldopentose, isomeric with ribose, obtained by fermentation or hydrolysis of naturally occurring carbohydrate substances such as wood fiber.

xylulose (zilʹyəlōs), *n* a substance that appears in the urine of patients with essential pentosuria; its presence is diagnostic.

Y

Y axis, *n* See axis, Y.

Y chromosome, *n* a sex chromosome that in humans and many other species is present only in the male, appearing singly in the normal male. It is carried as a sex determinant by one half of the male gametes. None of the female gametes contain a Y chromosome.

yawn, *n* an involuntary act of opening the oral cavity wide and taking a deep breath. It tends to occur when a person is bored, drowsy, or depressed and may be accompanied by upper body movements to aid chest expansion.

yaws (yôz), *n* a disease caused by *T. pertenue.* It occurs in hot regions; raspberry-like excrescences occur on the hands, face, feet, and external genitalia.

yeast, *n* a general term denoting true fungi of the family *Saccharomycetaceae.* Because of their ability to ferment carbohydrates, some yeasts are important to the brewing and baking industries.

***Yersinia enterocolitica* (yərsinʹēə enʹtərōkōlitʹikə),** *n.pl* bacteria that causes *Yersinia enterocolitis,* contracted from contaminated food or water. Symptoms of infection often mimic acute appendicitis and are most common in children younger than age 7. A sister bacteria, *Y. pestis,* was the cause of the historic bubonic plague. From the genus *Yersinia,* these motile and nonmotile, non–spore-forming bacteria contain gram-negative, unencapsulated, ovoid- to rod-shaped cells. These organisms are parasitic on humans and other animals.

yield point, *n* See point, yield.

yield strength, *n* See strength, yield.

yogurt, *n* a slightly acid, semisolid curdled milk preparation made from either whole or skimmed cow's milk and milk solids by fermentation with organisms from the genus *Lactobacillus.* It is rich in B-complex vitamins and is a good source of protein. It provides a medium in the gastrointestinal tract that retards the growth of harmful bacteria and aids in the absorption of minerals. Also spelled *yoghurt.*

yohimbine (yōhim′bēn′), *n* an alkaloid, the active principle comes from the bark of *Corynanthe johimbe.* It produces a competitive blockage of limited duration of α-adrenergic receptors. It has also been used for its alleged aphrodisiac properties.

yoke, *n* **1.** something that connects or binds. *n* **2.** an assembly of metal clamps with adjustable screws that secure the cylinders to the device or reducing valves. They are equipped with nipples that fit snugly into the inlet socket or part of the cylinder valve. In dentistry, used with the nitrous oxide cylinders.

Young's modulus, *n* See elasticity, modulus of.

Young's rule, *n* See rule, Young's.

Y-plasty, *n* a method of surgical revision of a scar, using a Y-shaped incision to reduce scar contractures. See also Z-plasty.

ytterbium (Yb) (itur′bēəm), *n* a metallic element of the lanthamide group with an atomic number of 70 and an atomic weight of 173.04.

yttrium (Y) (it′rēəm), *n* a scaly, grayish metallic element with an atomic number of 39 and an atomic weight of 88.9059. Radioactive isotopes of yttrium have been used in cancer therapy.

Z

Z, *n* a symbol for atomic number.

zalcitabine (zal′sitəbēn′), *n brand name:* Hivid; *drug class:* synthetic pyrimidine antiviral; *action:* converted by cellular enzymes to active drug; functions as antimetabolite to inhibit replication of HIV in vitro; *uses:* used in combination with zidovudine in advanced HIV infection, second-line monotherapy if AZT tolerant.

zero, *n* **1.** a symbol for nothing or for the starting point. **2.** the point on most scales from which measurements begin. **3.** absolute zero, the temperature at which there is no molecular movement, corresponding to –273.15 on the Kelvin scale.

zidovudine (zidō′voodēn′), *n brand names:* AZT, Retrovir; *drug class:* antiviral thymidine analog; *action:* inhibits replication of viral DNA; *uses:* symptomatic HIV infections (AIDS, ARC), confirmed *P. jiroveci* pneumonia, or absolute CD4 lymphocytes of less than 200 ml; prevention of HIV transmission from an infected mother to her baby.

zinc (Zn) (zingk), *n* a bluish-white chemical element used in medicine in the form of various salts and as a component in some silver amalgams.

zinc oxide, *n* a zinc compound used as a topical protectant; prescribed for a wide range of minor skin irritations.

zinc oxide and eugenol **(zingk ok′sīd ū′jənol),** *n* two substances that react chemically to form a relatively hard mass. When modified by certain additives, the material is used for impression pastes, root canal fillings, surgical dressings, temporary filling materials, and cementing media.

zinc oxide-eugenol cement, See cement, dental, zinc oxide-eugenol.

zinc oxyphosphate **(zingk ok′sēfos′fāt),** *n* See cements.

zinc phosphate cement **(zingk fos′fāt),** *n* See cement, zinc phosphate.

zinc polycarbonate cement **(zingk pol′ēkär′bənāt),** *n* See cements.

Zinsser-Cole-Engman syndrome, *n.pr* See syndrome, Zinsser-Cole-Engman.

zirconium (Zr), *n* a metallic element with an atomic number of 40 and an atomic weight of 91.22. It is widely distributed in nature, although no concentrations are found in any one place.

ZOE, *n* See zinc oxide and eugenol.

Zollinger-Ellison syndrome, *n.pr* a condition characterized by severe peptic ulceration, gastric hypersecretion, elevated serum gastrin, and gastrinoma of the pancreas or the duodenum. It may occur in early childhood but is seen more commonly in people between 20 and 50 years of age. Two thirds of the tumors are malignant. Total gastrectomy may be necessary, but the administration of cimetidine in large doses may control gastric hypersecretion and allow the ulcers to heal.

zolpidem, *n brand name:* Ambien; *drug class:* nonbarbiturate, nonbenzodiazepine sedative/hypnotic; *action:* presumed to interact with subunit of GABA-benzodiazepine receptor; *use:* insomnia.

zone (zōn), *n* a region or area with specific characteristics or boundary.

zone, incubation, *n* an area that provides a favorable environment for growth of microorganisms and is thus conducive to initiation or perpetuation of a pathologic process (e.g., gingival flap over a partly erupted third molar).

zone, neutral, *n* the potential space between the lips and cheeks on one side and the tongue on the other. Natural or artificial teeth in this zone are subject to equal and opposite forces from the surrounding musculature.

zone of reference, *n* the area of perceived pain referred by a trigger point. See also trigger point.

zone, subsurface, *n* the area of the tooth lying immediately below the outer covering of enamel; usually an area affected initially by caries.

zonography (zōnog′rəfē), *n* a radiographic-imaging technique used to produce films of body sections similar to those made by tomography.

zoster, See herpes zoster.

zoster (shingles) (zos′tur), See herpes zoster.

Z-plasty, *n* a surgical procedure using the transposition of tissue flaps to ensure the release of contractures, as in the repair of a cleft lip or in ankyloglossia.

z-score, *n* a standard score based on the normal distribution; the difference between the obtained score and the mean, divided by the standard deviation. Standard scores computed for different variables are comparable; used to determine statistical significance in large samples.

zygoma (zīgō′mə), *n* **1.** a long, slender process of the temporal bone, arising from the lower part of the squamous portion of the temporal bone and passing forward horizontally to join with the malar or zygomatic bone. **2.** the zygomatic or malar bone that forms the prominence of the cheek.

zygomatic arch, *n* the arch formed by articulation of the temporal process of the zygomatic bone with the zygomatic process of the temporal bone. The colloquial term is *cheekbone.*

zygomaxillare (zī′gōmaksəler′ē), *n* See ridge, key.

APPENDIX A

Symbols and Abbreviations*

Table A-1 Symbols

Symbol	*Meaning*
@	At
ʒ	Dram
fʒ	Fluid dram
℥	Ounce
f℥	Fluid ounce
0	Pint
lb	Pound
℞	Recipe; take
M	Misce; mix
A, Å	Angstrom unit
E_0	Electroaffinity
F_1	First filial generation
F_2	Second filial generation
mμ	Millimicron, micromillimeter
μg	Microgram
mEq	Milliequivalent
mg	Milligram
m%	Milligrams percent; milligrams per 100 ml
$Q\ O_2$	Oxygen consumption
m-	Meta-
o-	Ortho-
p-	Para-
Po_2	Partial pressure of oxygen
Pco_2	Partial pressure of carbon dioxide
μm	Micrometer
μ	Micron
μμ	Micromicron
+	Plus; excess; acid reaction, positive
−	Minus; deficiency; alkaline reaction; negative
±	Plus or minus; either positive or negative; indefinite
↑	Increased
↓	Decreased
→	Yields; leads to
←	Resulting from; secondary to
Δ	Change
#	Number; following a number, pounds
÷	Divided by
×	Multiplied by; magnification
=	Equals
≅	Approximately equals
≠	Not equal to
>	Greater than; from which is derived
<	Less than; derived from
≮	Not less than
≯	Not greater than
≦, ≤	Equal to or less than

**Continued*

**Mosby's Dictionary of Medicine, Nursing & Health Professions,* ed 7, St Louis, 2006, Mosby.

Table A-1 Symbols—cont'd

Symbol	*Meaning*
≧, ≥	Equal to or greater than
/	Divided by; per
$\sqrt{}$	Root; square root; radical
$\sqrt[2]{}$	Square root
$\sqrt[3]{}$	Cube root
∞	Infinity
:	Ratio; "is to"
∴	Therefore
°	Degree
%	Percent
π	3.1416—ratio of circumference of a circle to its diameter; pi
□, ♂	Male
O, ♀	Female
⇌	A reversible reaction

Table A-2 Abbreviations

Note: Abbreviations in common use can vary widely from place to place. Each institution's list of acceptable abbreviations is the best authority for its records.

Abbreviation	*Meaning*
A	Accommodation; acetum; Ångström unit; anode; anterior
a	Accommodation; ampere; anterior; area
ā	Before
A_2	Aortic second sound
abd	Abdominal/abdomen
ABG	Arterial blood gases
ABO	Three basic blood groups
AC	Alternating current; air conduction; axiocervical; adrenal cortex
acc.	Accommodation
ACE	Adrenocortical extract; angiotensin-converting enzyme
ACh	Acetylcholine
ACH	Adrenocortical hormone
ACLS	Advanced cardiac life support
ACTH	Adrenocorticotropic hormone
AD	Right ear *(auris dextra)*
ADD	Attention deficit disorder
add	Add to *(adde)*
ADDH	Attention deficit disorder, hyperactivity
ADH	Antidiuretic hormone
ADHD	Attention deficit hyperactivity disorder
ADL	Activities of daily living
ADS	Antidiuretic substance
AF	Atrial fibrillation
AFB	Acid-fast bacillus
AFP	Alpha-fetoprotein
A/G; A-G ratio	Albumin/globulin ratio
Ag	Silver, antigen
$AgNO_3$	Silver nitrate
ah	Hypermetropic astigmatism
AHF	Antihemophilic factor
AICD	Automatic implantable cardiac defibrillator
AIDS	Acquired immunodeficiency syndrome
aj	Ankle jerk
AK	Above the knee
Al	Aluminum
Alb	Albumin
ALH	Combined sex hormone of the anterior lobe of the hypophysis
ALS	Advanced life support, amyotrophic lateral sclerosis
ALT	Alamine aminotransferase (formerly SGPT)
alt. dieb.	Every other day *(alternis diebus)*
alt. hor.	Alternate hours *(alternis horis)*
alt. noct.	Alternate nights *(alternis noctes)*
Am	Mixed astigmatism
AM	Morning
ama	Against medical advice
AMI	Acute myocardial infarction
amp	Ampule; amputation
amp.	Ampere
amt	Amount
ANA	Antinuclear antibody
ana	So much of each, or āā
anat	Anatomy or anatomic
ant.	Anterior
AO	Anodal opening; atrioventricular valve openings
AOP	Anodal opening picture
AOS	Anodal opening sound
A-P; AP; A/P	Anterior-posterior
A.P.	Anterior pituitary gland
APA	Antipernicious anemia factor
AQ	Achievement quotient
AR	Alarm reaction
ARC	Anomalous retinal correspondence, AIDS-related complex
ARD	Acute respiratory disease
arg	Silver
As	Arsenic

Continued

Table A-2 Abbreviations—cont'd

Abbreviation	*Meaning*
As.	Astigmatism
AS	Left ear *(auris sinistra)*
ASCVD	Arteriosclerotic cardiovascular disease
ASD	Atrial septal defect
AsH	Hypermetropic astigmatism
ASHD	Arteriosclerotic heart disease
AsM	Myopic astigmatism
ASS	Anterior superior spine
AST	Aspartate aminotransferase (formerly SGOT)
Ast	Astigmatism
ATS	Anxiety tension state; antitetanic serum
Au	Gold
A-V; AV; A/V	Arteriovenous; atrioventricular
Av	Average or avoirdupois
ax	Axis
B	Boron; bacillus
Ba	Barium
BAC	Buccoaxiocervical
Bact	Bacterium
BBB	Blood-brain barrier
BBT	Basal body temperature
BCLS	Basic cardiac life support
BE	Barium enema
Be	Beryllium

Abbreviation	*Meaning*
BFP	Biologically false positivity (in syphilis tests)
Bi	Bismuth
Bib	Drink
bid; b.i.d.	Twice a day *(bis in die)*
BK	Below the knee
BM	Bowel movement
BMR	Basal metabolic rate
BP	Blood pressure; buccopulpal
bp	Boiling point
BPH	Benign prostatic hypertrophy
bpm	Beats per minute
BRP	Bathroom privileges
BSA	Body surface area
BSE	Breast self-examination
BSP	Bromsulphalein
BUN	Blood urea nitrogen
BW	Birthweight
Bx	Biopsy
C	Carbon; centigrade; Celsius
$\bar{c}$	With
C_{alb}	Albumin clearance
C_{cr}	Creatinine clearance
C_{in}	Inulin clearance
CA	Chronologic age; cervicoaxial
Ca	Calcium; cancer; carcinoma
CABG	Coronary artery bypass graft
CABS	Coronary artery bypass surgery

Abbreviation	*Meaning*
$CaCO_3$	Calcium carbonate
CAD	Coronary artery disease
CAH	Chronic active hepatitis
Cal	Large calorie
cal	Small calorie
C&S	Culture and sensitivity
CAT	Computed (axial) tomography
cath.	Catheter
CBC or cbc	Complete blood cell count
CC	Chief complaint
CCI_4	Carbon tetrachloride
CCU	Coronary care unit; critical care unit
CF	Cystic fibrosis
cf	Compare or bring together
CFT	Complement-fixation test
Cg; Cgm	Centigram
CH	Crown-heel (length of fetus)
$CHCL_3$	Chloroform
CH_3COOH	Acetic acid
CHD	Congenital heart disease; coronary heart disease
ChE	Cholinesterase
CHF	Congestive heart failure
$C_5H_4N_4O_3$	Uric acid
CHO	Carbohydrate
C_2H_6O	Ethyl alcohol
CH_2O	Formaldehyde

Abbreviation	Meaning
CH_4O	Methyl alcohol
CI	Cardiac index; cardiac insufficiency; cerebral infarction
CK	Creatinine kinase
Cl	Chlorine
cm	Centimeter
CMR	Cerebral metabolic rate
CMV	Cytomegalovirus
CNS	Central nervous system
c/o	Complaints of
CO	Carbon monoxide; cardiac output
CO_2	Carbon dioxide
Co	Cobalt
COLD	Chronic obstructive lung disease
COPD	Chronic obstructive pulmonary disease
CP	Cerebral palsy; cleft palate
CPAP	Continuous positive airway pressure
CPC	Clinicopathologic conference
CPD	Cephalopelvic disproportion
CPK	Creatinine phosphokinase
CPR	Cardiopulmonary resuscitation
CR	Crown-rump length (length of fetus)
CS	Cesarean section
CSF	Cerebrospinal fluid
CSM	Cerebrospinal meningitis
CT	Computed tomography
Cu	Copper
$CuSO_4$	Copper sulfate
CV	Cardiovascular; closing volume
CVA	Cerebrovascular accident; costovertebral angle
CVP	Central venous pressure
CVS	Chorionic villi sampling; clean voided specimen
CXR	Chest x-ray
cyl	Cylinder
D	Dose; vitamin D; right *(dexter)*
d	Day; diem
DAH	Disordered action of the heart
D & C	Dilation (dilatation) and curettage
db, dB	Decibel
DC	Direct current
dc, DC, D/C	Discontinue
DCA	Deoxycorticosterone acetate
Dcg	Degeneration; degree
dg	Decigram
DIC	Desseminated intravascular coagulation
diff	Differential blood count
dil	Dilute or dissolve
dim	One half
DJD	Degenerative joint disease
DKA	Diabetic ketoacidosis
dL	Deciliter
DM	Diabetes mellitus, diastolic murmur
DNA	Deoxyribonucleic acid
DNR	Do not resuscitate
DOA	Dead on arrival
DOB	Date of birth
DOE	Dyspnea on exertion
DPT	Diphtheria-pertussis-tetanus
dr	Dram
DRG	Diagnosis-related groups
DSD	Discharge summary dictated, dry sterile dressing
DT	Delirium tremens
DTR	Deep tendon reflex
D5W	Dextrose 5% in water
Dx	Diagnosis
E	Eye
EAHF	Eczema, asthma, and hayfever
EBV	Epstein-Barr virus
EC	Electroconvulsive therapy
ECF	Extended care facility; extracellular fluid
ECG	Electrocardiogram, electrocardiograph
ECHO	Echocardiography
ECMO	Extracorporeal membrane oxygenation
ECT	Electroconvulsive therapy
ED	Emergency department; erythema dose; effective dose
ED_{50}	Median effective dose
EDD	Estimated date of delivery (formerly EDC, estimated date of confinement)

Continued

Table A-2 Abbreviations—cont'd

Abbreviation	*Meaning*
EEG	Electroencephalogram, electroencephalograph
EENT	Eye, ear, nose, and throat
EKG	Electrocardiogram, electrocardiograph
ELISA	Enzyme-linked immunosorbent assay
Em	Emmetropia
EMB	Eosin-methylene blue
EMC	Encephalomyocarditis
EMF	Erythrocyte maturation factor
EMG	Electromyogram
EMS	Emergency medical service
ENT	Ear, nose, and throat
EOM	Extraocular movement
EPR	Electrophrenic respiration
ER/ED	Emergency room/department (hospital); external resistance
ERG	Electroretinogram
ERPF	Effective renal plasma flow
ERV	Expiratory reserve volume
ESR	Erythrocyte sedimentation rate
ESRD	End-stage renal disease
EST	Electroshock therapy
Et	Ethyl
ext	Extract
F	Fahrenheit; field of vision; formula

Abbreviation	*Meaning*
FA	Fatty acid
FANA	Fluorescent antinuclear antibody test
F & R	Force and rhythm (pulse)
FAS	Fetal alcohol syndrome
FBS	Fasting blood sugar
FD	Fatal dose; focal distance
Fe	Iron
$FeCl_3$	Ferric chloride
ferv.	Boiling
FEV	Forced expiratory volume
FH, Fhx	Family history
FHR	Fetal heart rate
Fl, fld	Fluid
fl dr	Fluid dram
fl oz	Fluid ounce
FR	Flocculation reaction
FSH	Follicle-stimulating hormone
ft	Foot
FTT	Failure to thrive
FUO	Fever of unknown origin
fx	Fracture
Gm; g; gm	Gram
GA	Gingivoaxial
Galv	Galvanic
GB	Gallbladder
GBS	Gallbladder series
GC	Gonococcus or gonorrheal

Abbreviation	*Meaning*
GDM	Gestational diabetes mellitus
GFR	Glomerular filtration rate
GH	Growth hormone
GI	Gastrointestinal
GL	Greatest length (small flexed embryo)
GLA	Gingivolinguoaxial
GP	General practitioner; general paresis
G6PD	Glucose-6-phosphate dehydrogenase
gr	Grain
Grad	By degrees *(gradatim)*
GRAS	Generally recognized as safe
Grav I, II, III, etc.	Pregnancy one, two, three, etc. *(Gravida)*
GSW	Gunshot wound
gt	Drop *(gutta)*
GTT	Glucose tolerance test
gtt	Drops *(guttae)*
GU	Genitourinary
Gyn	Gynecology
H	Hydrogen
H^+	Hydrogen ion
H & E	Hematoxylin and eosin stain
H & P	History and physical
HAV	Hepatitis A virus
Hb; Hgb	Hemoglobin

H_3BO_3	Boric acid
HBV	Hepatitis B virus
HC	Hospital corps
HCG	Human chorionic gonadotropin
HCHO	Formaldehyde
HCl	Hydrochloric acid
HCN	Hydrocyanic acid
H_2CO_3	Carbonic acid
HCT	Hematocrit
HD	Hearing distance
HDL	High-density lipoprotein
HDLW	Distance at which a watch is heard by the left ear
HDRW	Distance at which a watch is heard by the right ear
He	Helium
HEENT	Head, eye, ear, nose, and throat
Hg	Mercury
Hgb	Hemoglobin
HHC	Home health care
Hib	*Haemophilus influenzae* type B
HIV	Human immunodeficiency virus
HME	Home medical equipment
HNO_3	Nitric acid
h/o	History of
H_2O	Water
H_2O_2	Hydrogen peroxide
HOP	High oxygen pressure
HPI	History of present illness
HR	Heart rate
H_2SO_4	Sulfuric acid
HSV	Herpes simplex virus
Ht	Total hyperopia
HT, HTN	Hypertension
HTLV-III	Human T-lymphotropic virus type III
hx, Hx	History
Hy	Hyperopia
I	Iodine
^{131}I	Radioactive isotope of iodine (atomic weight 131)
^{132}I	Radioactive isotope of iodine (atomic weight 132)
I & O	Intake and output
IB	Inclusion body
IBW	Ideal body weight
IC	Inspiratory capacity; intracutaneous
ICP	Intracranial pressure
ICS	Intercostal space
ICSH	Interstitial cell-stimulating hormone
ICT	Inflammation of connective tissue
ICU	Intensive care unit
Id.	The same *(idem)*
IDDM	Insulin-dependent diabetes mellitus
Ig	Immunoglobulin
IH	Infectious hepatitis
IM	Intramuscular; infectious mononucleosis
IOP	Intraocular pressure
IPPB	Intermittent positive pressure breathing
IQ	Intelligence quotient
IRV	Inspiratory reserve volume
IS	Intercostal space
IUD	Intrauterine device
IV	Intravenous
IVP	Intravenous pyelogram, intravenous push
IVT	Intravenous transfusion
IVU	Intravenous urogram/urography
JRA	Juvenile rheumatoid arthritis
K	Potassium
k	Constant
Ka	Cathode or kathode
KBr	Potassium bromide
kc	Kilocycle
KCl	Potassium chloride
kev	Kilo electron volts
kg	Kilogram
KI	Potassium iodide
kj	Knee jerk
km	Kilometer
KOH	Potassium hydroxide
KUB	Kidney, ureter, and bladder
kV	Kilovolt
KVO	Keep vein open
kw	Kilowatt
L	Left; liter; length; lumbar; lethal; pound
lab	Laboratory

Continued

Table A-2 Abbreviations—cont'd

Abbreviation	Meaning
L & A	Light and accommodation
L & D	Labor and delivery
lat.	Lateral
lb	Pound *(libra)*
LB	Large bowel (x-ray film)
LBW	Low birth weight
LCM	Left costal margin
LD	Lethal dose; perception of light difference
LDL	Low-density lipoprotein
LE	Lower extremity; lupus erythematosus
le	Left extremity
l.e.s.	Local excitatory state
LFD	Least fatal dose of a toxin
LGA	Large for gestational age
LH	Luteinizing hormone
Li	Lithium
LIF	Left iliac fossa
lig	Ligament
Liq	Liquor
LLE	Left lower extremity
LLL	Left lower lobe
LLQ	Left lower quadrant
LMP	Last menstrual period
LNMP	Last normal menstrual period
LOC	Level/loss of consciousness

Abbreviation	Meaning
LP	Lumbar puncture
LPF	Leukocytosis-promoting factor
LR	Lactated Ringer's
LTD	Lowest tolerated dose
LTH	Luteotrophic hormone
LUE	Left upper extremity
LUL	Left upper lobe
LUQ	Left upper quadrant
LV	Left ventricle
LVH	Left ventricular hypertrophy
L & W	Living and well
M	Myopia; meter; muscle; thousand
m	Meter
MA	Mental age
Mag	Large *(magnus)*
MAP	Mean arterial pressure
MBD	Minimal brain dysfunction
mc; mCi	Millicurie
μc	Microcurie
mcg	Microgram
MCH	Mean corpuscular hemoglobin
MCHC	Mean corpuscular hemoglobin concentration
MCV	Mean corpuscular volume
MD	Muscular dystrophy
MDI	Medium-dose inhalants; metered-dose inhaler

Abbreviation	Meaning
Me	Methyl
MED	Minimal erythema dose; minimal effective dose
mEq	Milliequivalent
μEq	Microequivalent
mEq/L	Milliequivalent per liter
ME ratio	Myeloid/erythroid ratio
Mg	Magnesium
mg	Milligram
mcg	Microgram
MHD	Minimal hemolytic dose
MI	Myocardial infarction
MID	Minimum infective dose
ML	Midline
mL	Milliliter
MLD	Median or minimum lethal dose
MM	Mucous membrane
mm	Millimeter, muscles
mm Hg	Millimeters of mercury
mmm	Millimicron
MMR	Maternal mortality rate; measles-mumps-rubella
mμ	Millimicron
μm	Micrometer
μμ	Micromicron
Mn	Manganese
mN	Millinormal

MRI	Magnetic resonance imaging
MS	Multiple sclerosis
MSL	Midsternal line
MT	Medical technologist; membrane tympani
mu	Mouse unit
MVA	Motor vehicle accident
MW	Molecular weight
My	Myopia
N	Nitrogen
n	Normal
N/A	Not applicable
Na	Sodium
NaBr	Sodium bromide
NaCl	Sodium chloride
Na_2CO_3	Sodium carbonate
$Na_2C_2O_4$	Sodium oxalate
NAD	No appreciable disease
NaF	Sodium fluoride
$NaHCO_3$	Sodium bicarbonate
Na_2HPO_4	Sodium phosphate
NAI	Sodium iodide
N & V, N/V	Nausea and vomiting
$NaNO_3$	Sodium nitrate
Na_2O_2	Sodium peroxide
NaOH	Sodium hydroxide
Na_2SO_4	Sodium sulfate
n.b.	Note well
NCA	Neurocirculatory asthenia
Ne	Neon
NG, ng	Nasogastric
NH_3	Ammonia
Ni	Nickel
NICU	Neonatal intensive care unit
NIDDM	Non–insulin-dependent diabetes mellitus
NIH	National Institutes of Health
NKA	No known allergies
nm	Nanometer
NMR	Nuclear magnetic resonance
N.O.	Nursing order
NPN	Nonprotein nitrogen
NPO; n.p.o.	Nothing by mouth *(non per os)*
NRC	Normal retinal correspondence
NS	Normal saline
NSAID	Nonsteroidal antiinflammatory drug
NSR	Normal sinus rhythm
NTP	Normal temperature and pressure
NYD	Not yet diagnosed
O	Oxygen; oculus; pint
O_2	Oxygen; both eyes
O_3	Ozone
OB	Obstetrics
OBS	Organic brain syndrome
OD	Optical density; overdose; right eye *(Oculus dexter)*
OOB	Out of bed
OPD	Outpatient department
OR	Operating room
ORIF	Open reduction and internal fixation
OS	Left eye *(oculus sinister)*
Os	Osmium
OT	Occupational therapy
OTC	Over-the-counter
OTD	Organ tolerance dose
OU	Each eye *(oculus uterque)*
oz; ℥	Ounce
P	Phosphorus; pulse; pupil
p	After
P_2	Pulmonic second sound
P-A; P/A; PA	Posterior-anterior
PAB; PABA	Para-aminobenzoic acid
PALS	Pediatric Advanced Life Support
P & A	Percussion and auscultation
Pap test	Papanicolaou smear
Para I, II, III, etc.	Unipara, bipara, tripara, etc.
PAS; PASA	Para-aminosalicylic acid
PAT	Paroxysmal atrial tachycardia
Pb	Lead
PBI	Protein-bound iodine
PCA	Patient-controlled analgesia
PCP	Phencyclidine, *Pneumocystis carinii (jiroveci)* pneumonia, primary care physician, pulmonary capillary pressure
PCV	Packed cell volume

Continued

Table A-2 Abbreviations—cont'd

Abbreviation	Meaning
PCWP	Pulmonary capillary wedge pressure
PD	Interpupillary distance
pd	Prism diopter; pupillary distance
PDA	Patent ductus arteriosus
PDR	*Physician's Desk Reference*
PE	Physical examination
PEEP	Positive end expiratory pressure
PEFR	Peak expiratory flow rate
PEG	Pneumoencephalography
PERRLA	Pupils equal, regular, react to light and accommodation
PET	Positron emission tomography
PFF	Protein-free filtrate
PGA	Pteroylglutamic acid (folic acid)
PH	Past history
pH	Hydrogen ion concentration (alkalinity and acidity in urine and blood analysis)
Pharm; Phar.	Pharmacy
PI	Previous illness; protamine insulin
PICC	Percutaneously inserted central catheter
PID	Pelvic inflammatory disease
PK	Psychokinesis
PKU	Phenylketonuria
PL	Light perception
PM	Postmortem; evening
PMB	Polymorphonuclear basophil leukocytes
PME	Polymorphonuclear eosinophil leukocytes
PMH	Past medical history
PMI	Point of maximal impulse
PMN	Polymorphonuclear neutrophil leukocytes (polys)
PMS	Premenstrual syndrome
PN	Percussion note
PND	Paroxysmal nocturnal dyspnea
PNH	Paroxysmal nocturnal hemoglobinuria
PO; p.o.	Orally *(per os)*
PPD	Purified protein derivative (TB test)
ppm	Parts per million
Pr	Presbyopia; prism
PRN, p.r.n.	As required *(pro re nata)*
pro time	Prothrombin time
PSA	Prostate-specific antigen
PSP	Phenolsulfonphthalein
pt	Pint
Pt	Platinum; patient
PT	Prothrombin time; physical therapy
PTA	Plasma thromboplastin antecedent
PTC	Plasma thromboplastin component
PTT	Partial thromboplastin time
Pu	Plutonium
PUO	Pyrexia of unknown origin
PVC	Premature ventricular contraction
Px	Pneumothorax
PZI	Protamine zinc insulin
Q	Electric quantity
q	Every
qns	Quantity not sufficient
q.o.d.	Every other day
qt	Quart
Quat	Four *(quattuor)*
R	Respiration; right; *Rickettsia;* roentgen
℞	Take
RA	Rheumatoid arthritis
Ra	Radium
rad	Unit of measurement of the absorbed dose of ionizing radiation; root
RAI	Radioactive iodine
RAIU	Radioactive iodine uptake
RBC; rbc	Red blood cell; red blood count
RCD	Relative cardiac dullness
RCM	Right costal margin

Abbreviation	Meaning
RDA	Recommended daily/dietary allowance
RDS	Respiratory distress syndrome
RE	Right eye; reticuloendothelial tissue or cell
Re	Rhenium
re	Right extremity
Rect	Rectified
Reg umb	Umbilical region
RES	Reticuloendothelial system
Rh	Symbol of rhesus factor; symbol for rhodium
RhA	Rheumatoid arthritis
RHD	Relative hepatic dullness; rheumatic heart disease
RLE	Right lower extremity
RLL	Right lower lobe
RLQ	Right lower quadrant
RM	Respiratory movement
RML	Right middle lobe of lung
Rn	Radon
RNA	Ribonucleic acid
R/O	Rule out
ROM	Range of motion
ROS	Review of systems
RPF	Renal plasma flow
RPM; rpm	Revolutions per minute
RPR	Rapid plasma reagin
RPS	Renal pressor substance
RQ	Respiratory quotient
RR	Recovery room; respiratory rate
RT	Radiation therapy; reading test; respiratory therapy
R/T	Related to
RU	Rat unit
RUE	Right upper extremity
RUL	Right upper lobe
RUQ	Right upper quadrant
S	Sulfur
S.	Sacral
$\bar{s}$	Without
S-A; S/A; SA	Sinoatrial
SAS	Sodium acetate solution
SB	Small bowel (x-ray film); sternal border
Sb	Antimony
SD	Skin dose
Se	Selenium
Sed rate	Sedimentation rate
SGA	Small for gestational age
SGOT	Serum glutamic oxaloacetic transaminase
SGPT	Serum glutamic pyruvic transaminase
SH	Serum hepatitis
SI	International system of units (stroke index)
S.I.	Soluble insulin
Si	Silicon
SIDS	Sudden infant death syndrome
SLE	Systemic lupus erythematosus
SLP	Speech-language pathology
Sn	Tin
SNF	Skilled nursing facility
SOB	Shortness of breath
sol	Solution, dissolved
SP	Spirit
sp. gr., SG, s.g.	Specific gravity
sph	Spherical
SPI	Serum precipitable iodine
spir	Spirit
SR	Sedimentation rate
Sr	Strontium
s/s	Signs and symptoms
SSS	Specific soluble substance, sick sinus syndrome
sss	Layer upon layer *(stratum super stratum)*
St	Let it stand *(stet; stent)*
Staph	*Staphylococcus*
stat	Immediately *(statim)*
STD	Sexually transmitted disease; skin test dose
STH	Somatotrophic hormone
Strep	*Streptococcus*
STS	Serologic test for syphilis
STU	Skin test unit
SV	Stroke volume; supraventricular

Continued

Table A-2 Abbreviations—cont'd

Abbreviation	*Meaning*
sv	Alcoholic spirit (*spiritus vini)*
Sx	Symptoms
Sym	Symmetrical
T	Temperature; thoracic
t	Temporal
T_3	Triiodothyronine
T_4	Thyroxine
TA	Toxin-antitoxin
Ta	Tantalum
TAB	Vaccine against typhoid, paratyphoid A and B
Tab	Tablet
TAH	Total abdominal hysterectomy
TAM	Toxoid-antitoxoid mixture
T & A	Tonsillectomy and adenoidectomy
TAT	Toxin-antitoxin, tetanus antitoxin
TB	Tuberculin; tuberculosis; tubercle bacillus
Tb	Terbium
TCA	Tetrachloracetic acid
Te	Tellurium; tetanus
TEM	Triethylene melamine
TENS	Transcutaneous electrical nerve stimulation
Th	Thorium
TIA	Transient ischemic attack
TIBC	Total iron-binding capacity
Tl	Thallium
TM	Tympanic membrane
Tm	Thulium; symbol for maximal tubular excretory capacity (kidneys)
TMJ	Temporomandibular joint
TNT	Trinitrotoluene
TNTM	Too numerous to mention
TP	Tuberculin precipitation
TPI	*Treponema pallidum* immobilization test for syphilis
TPN	Total parenteral nutrition
TPR	Temperature, pulse, and respiration
tr	Tincture
Trans D	Transverse diameter
TRU	Turbidity reducing unit
TS	Test solution
TSE	Testicular self-examination
TSH	Thyroid-stimulating hormone
TSP	Trisodium phosphate
TST	Triple sugar iron test
TUR; TURP	Transurethral resection
Tx	Treatment
U	Uranium
UA	Urinalysis
UBI	Ultraviolet blood irradiation
UE	Upper extremity
UIBC	Unsaturated iron-binding capacity

Umb; umb	Umbilicus
URI	Upper respiratory infection
US	Ultrasonic
USP	*U.S. Pharmacopeia*
UTI	Urinary tract infection
UV	Ultraviolet
V	Vanadium; vision; visual acuity
v	Volt
VA	Visual acuity
V & T	Volume and tension
VC	Vital capacity
VD	Venereal disease
VDA	Visual discriminatory acuity
VDG	Venereal disease—gonorrhea
VDM	Vasodepressor material
VDRL	Venereal Disease Research Laboratories (sometimes used loosely to mean venereal disease report)
VDS	Venereal disease—syphilis
VEM	Vasoexciter material
Vf	Field of vision
VHD	Valvular heart disease
VIA	Virus inactivating agent
VLBW	Very low birth weight
VLDL	Very-low-density lipoprotein
VMA	Vanillylmandelic acid
vol	Volume
VR	Vocal resonance
VS	Volumetric solution
VS, v.s.	Vital signs
Vs	Venisection
VsB	Bleeding in arm *(venaesectio brachii)*
VSD	Ventricular septal defect
VW	Vessel wall
VZIG	Varicella zoster immune globulin
W	Tungsten
w	Watt
WBC; wbc	White blood cell; white blood cell count
WD	Well developed
WL	Wavelength
WN	Well nourished
WNL	Within normal limits
WR	Wassermann reaction
wt	Weight
X-ray	Roentgen ray
y, yr	Year
yo	Years old
Z	Symbol for atomic number
Zn	Zinc
Zz	Ginger

APPENDIX B

American Dental Association (ADA) Dental Codes

Table B-1 Coding system

CDT-2007/2008 is organized by a numbered system with 12 categories. The categories are as follows:

	Category of Service	*Code Series*
I.	Diagnostic	D0100–D0999
II.	Preventive	D1000–D1999
III.	Restorative	D2000–D2999
IV.	Endodontics	D3000–D3999
V.	Periodontics	D4000–D4999
VI.	Prosthodontics, Removable	D5000–D5899
VII.	Maxillofacial Prosthetics	D5900–D5999
VIII.	Implant Services	D6000–D6199
IX.	Prosthodontics, Fixed	D6200–D6999
X.	Oral and Maxillofacial Surgery	D7000–D7999
XI.	Orthodontics	D8000–D8999
XII.	Adjunctive General Services	D9000–D9999

Note how the coding system is arranged so that each procedure is identified by five numbers. Each number begins with D, which tells the payer that the service is a dental procedure. The dental category—such as orthodontics or periodontics—of the service is indicated by the second numeral of each code; unclassifiable services are coded with the number 9 as the second digit. CDT-2007/2008 is functional for all services that can be performed by a licensed dentist.

From *CDT-2007/2008: Current dental terminology,* 2006, American Dental Association.

APPENDIX C

Anxiety and Pain Management*

Table C-1 Mandibular injections

Injection	*Needle*	*Structures anesthetized*	*Penetration site*	*Terminal deposition site*	*Amount deposited*
Inferior alveolar (**IA**) and Lingual (**L**)	**Long**	1. Mandibular teeth 2. Facial gingiva of mandibular anterior teeth and first premolar 3. Skin of chin 4. Lower lip 5. Lingual gingiva of mandibular teeth 6. Floor of mouth 7. Anterior ⅔ of tongue	Pterygotemporal depression; place thumb in coronoid notch and roll medially to temporal crest	Approach from opposite canine/premolar area; needle path is parallel to occlusal plane of mandibular teeth and 6-10 mm superior; site is directly above mandibular foramen between sphenomandibular ligament and ramus of mandible; approximately ¾ of long needle is inserted	⅞ cartridge (1.5 mL) Wait 1-5 minutes
Buccal (**B**)	**Long**	1. Facial gingiva of mandibular molars 2. Skin of cheek	Mucobuccal fold, 2-3 mm posterior to distobuccal root of last molar adjacent to retromolar pad	2-3 mm penetration; needle is held parallel and inferior to horizontal plane of occlusal surfaces when directed toward penetration site	⅛ cartridge (0.3 mL) Wait 1-5 minutes
Incisive (**I**)	**Short**	1. Mandibular anterior teeth and premolars 2. Facial gingiva of mandibular anterior teeth and first premolar 3. Skin of chin 4. Lower lip	From the horizontal approach, mucobuccal fold at apex of first premolar	Directly over mental foramen	⅓ cartridge (0.6 mL) Wait 1-5 minutes

*From Darby ML: *Mosby's comprehensive review of dental hygiene,* ed 6, St Louis, 2006, Mosby.

Table C-2 Maxillary injections

Injection	*Needle*	*Structures anesthetized*	*Penetration site*	*Terminal deposition site*	*Amount deposited*
Anterior superior alveolar (**ASA**)	**Short**	1. Facial gingiva of maxillary anterior teeth 2. Maxillary anterior teeth	Mucolabial fold anterior and parallel to canine eminence	Apex of the canine tooth	½-⅔ cartridge (0.9-1.2 mL) Wait 1-5 min
Middle superior alveolar (**MSA**)	**Short**	1. Facial gingiva of maxillary premolars and mucobuccal root of first molar 2. Maxillary premolars and mucobuccal root of first molar	Mucobuccal fold parallel to apex of second premolar	3-5 mm superior to apex of the second premolar	½-⅔ cartridge (0.9-1.2 mL) Wait 1-5 min
Infraorbital (**IO**)	**Long**	1. Facial gingiva of maxillary anteriors, premolars, and mucobuccal root of first molar 2. Maxillary anteriors, premolars, and mucobuccal root of first molar 3. Side of nose 4. Upper lip 5. Lower eyelid	Mucobuccal fold parallel to apex of first premolar	Infraorbital foramen; keep needle parallel with tooth; approximately ½ of long needle	½-⅔ cartridge (0.9-1.2 mL) Wait 1-5 min
Posterior superior alveolar (**PSA**)	**Short**	1. Facial gingiva of maxillary molars, *except* for mucobuccal root of first molar 2. Maxillary molars, *except* for the mucobuccal root of first molar	Within the soft tissue depression just distal to the maxillary second molar	Insert needle 45° to midsagittal plane and 45° to horizontal plane of maxillary occlusal surfaces Approximately ½ of short needle	½-1 cartridge (0.9-1.8 mL) Wait 1-5 min
Greater palatine (**GP**)	**Short**	1. Lingual gingiva of maxillary posterior teeth 2. Palatal mucosa to the midline	Pressure anesthesia (1 min); 2-3 mm anterior to the greater palatine foramen	Approximately 2 mm (until bevel is covered)	¼-⅓ cartridge (0.45-0.6 mL) Wait 1-5 min
Nasopalatine (**NP**)	**Short**	1. Lingual gingiva of maxillary anterior teeth 2. Palatal mucosa in the premaxillary area	Pressure anesthesia (1 min); incisive papilla at base and into fattest portion	Approximately 2 mm (until bevel is covered)	½ cartridge (0.45 mL) Wait 1-5 min

Table C-3 Color-coding of local anesthetic cartridges, as per American Dental Association Council on Scientific Affairs

Local Anesthetic Solution	Color of Cartridge Band
Articaine HCl 4% with epinephrine 1:100,000	Gold
Bupivacaine 0.5% with epinephrine 1:200,000	Blue
Lidocaine HCl 2%	Light blue
Lidocaine HCl 2% with epinephrine 1:50,000	Green
Lidocaine HCl 2% with epinephrine 1:100,000	Red
Mepivacaine HCl 3%	Tan
Mepivacaine HCl 2% with levonordefrin 1:20,000	Brown
Prilocaine HCl 4%	Black
Prilocaine HCl 4% with epinephrine 1:200,000	Yellow

From Malamed SF: Handbook of local anesthesia, ed 5, St Louis, 2004, Mosby.

Table C-4 Comparison of frequently used local anesthetic agents in dentistry

Generic name	*Color code*	*Concentrations (ml)*	*Chemical classification*	*Vasoconstrictor*	*Concentrations of vasoconstrictor*	*Onset of action*
Articaine	Gold	4	Amide	Epinephrine	1:100,000	1-3 min
Lidocaine	Green	2	Amide	Epinephrine	1:50,000	2 min
	Red				1:100,000	
Mepivacaine	Brown	2	Amide	Levonordefrin	1:20,000	1½-2 min
	Tan	3	Amide	—	—	
Prilocaine	Yellow	4	Amide	Epinephrine	1:200,000	2-4 min
	Black	4	Amide	—	—	

Approximate duration					*Maximum safe dose for normal adult patient*	
Without vasoconstrictor	*With vasoconstrictor*	*Toxicity*	*Method of metabolism*	*Cartridge vol. (mg)*	*mg; ml*	*No. cartridges*
Pulpal = 5-10 min	Pulpal = 60 min	2.0	Liver	36	300 mg; 15 mL	8.3
Soft tissue = 60-120 min	Soft tissue = 3-5 hr					
Pulpal = 20-40 min	Pulpal = 60-90 min	1.5-2.0	Liver	36	300 mg; 15 mL	8.3
Soft tissue = 2-3 hr	Soft tissue = 3-5 hr	1.5-2.0	Liver	54	360 mg; 12 mL	6.6
Pulpal = 40-60 min	Pulpal = 60-90 min	1.0	Liver and lung	72	400 mg; 10 mL	5.5
Soft tissue = 2-4 hr	Soft tissue = 3-8 hr	1.0	Liver and lung		400 mg; 10 mL	5.5

APPENDIX D

Clinical Oral Structures*

Table D-1 Oral structures

Structure	*Clinical description*	*Clinical consideration*
	Lips, Cheeks, and Oral Mucosa	
Philtrum	Midline vertical depression of the skin between the nose and upper lip	A cleft lip can occur to the left or the right of the philtrum
Vermilion zone	Transition area between skin of the face and oral mucosa of the lips; medium pink in light-skinned individuals and pigmented with melanin in darker-skinned individuals	The junction between the vermilion zone and the skin of the face is a frequent site of herpetic lesions; the lower lip is a frequent site of oral cancer Fordyce's granules or spots (small white spots of ectopic sebaceous material) may be present
Labial commissure	Junction of the upper and lower lips at the corner of the mouth	Frequent site of chafing, herpetic lesions, and cracking (angular cheilitis); avoid pulling with instrument handle
Vestibule	Space bounded by the cheeks, lips, and facial surfaces of the teeth and gingiva	Frequent site of aphthous ulcers
Labial mucosa	Mucosal lining of the inner lip; vascular; small elevations are external manifestation of numerous labial salivary glands	Frequent site of mucoceles, mucus-retention cysts, aphthous ulcers, and scars
Labial frenum (maxillary and mandibular)	Fold of tissue at the midline (maxillary and mandibular) between the inner surface of the lip and the alveolar mucosa	Maxillary fold is sometimes overdeveloped, which results in a space between the central incisors called a *diastema;* frequently has an extra flap of tissue If overextended onto the attached gingiva mandibular fold may cause recession
Buccal mucosa	Mucus membrance lining of the inner cheek	Frequent site of linea alba, cheek bites, and Fordyce's granules

*From Darby ML: *Mosby's comprehensive review of dental hygiene,* ed 6, St Louis, 2006, Mosby.

Continued

Table D-1 Oral structures—cont'd

Structure	*Clinical description*	*Clinical consideration*
Parotid papilla	Flap of tissue on the cheek opposite the maxillary first molars; contains the opening of Stenson's duct, which carries saliva from the parotid gland	Large amounts of mainly serous saliva come from this duct The opening often can be seen as a dark spot
Buccal frena (muscle attachments)	Folds of epithelium between the cheek and attached gingiva (maxillary and mandibular) in the first premolar area	Overextension may cause gingival recession
Mucobuccal fold	Fold or "gutter" area between the alveolar and buccal or labial mucosa	The height of the mucobuccal fold above a maxillary tooth area to be anesthetized is the needle insertion area The mental foramen of the mandible can be palpated in the mucobuccal fold area, facial to the mandibular premolars; this is the needle insertion site for a mental nerve block
Alveolar mucosa	Thin movable mucosal lining covering the alveolar bone; between the attached gingiva and mucobuccal fold on the facial of the maxillary and mandibular arches; and between the attached gingiva and floor of the mouth on the lingual aspect of the mandibular arch	Very thin and fragile epithelium Frequent site of aphthous ulcers Mandibular lingual lining is the site of tori (bony projections), which may interfere with exposing radiographs or taking impressions
Gingiva	Keratinized mucosa that surrounds the teeth and alveolar bone	Ideally, except for a narrow band around the necks of the teeth, it is firmly attached to tooth and bone
Mucogingival line or junction	A visible line where the pink keratinized gingiva meets the more vascular alveolar mucosa	Found on the maxillary facial and the mandibular facial and lingual areas
Gingival margin or crest	The most crownward (coronal) edge of the keratinized gingivae	Mandibular lingual lining is the site of tori (bony projections), which may interfere with exposing radiographs or taking impressions
	Tongue	
The tongue is a flat, muscular organ of speech and taste; the lateral border and undersurface are frequent sites of oral cancer		
Median sulcus	Midline depression on the dorsum of the tongue	Presence and depth vary Additional deep depressions are called *fissures;* a fissured tongue
Fungiform papillae	Mushroom-shaped, red to dark-brown elevations scattered over the anterior third of the dorsum of the tongue	In darker-skinned individuals they may contain melanin pigmentation Function in taste sensations of sweet, sour, and salt

Filiform papillae	Fringelike keratinized projections concentrated in the middle third of the dorsum of the tongue	Readily collect plaque and stain Moving patches devoid of these papillae is called a *geographic tongue*
Circumvallate papillae	8-10 large papillae arranged in an inverted V-shaped row posterior to the filiform papillae	Function in taste sensation of bitter Ducts of von Ebner's salivary glands open around them and secrete serous saliva
Foliate papillae	Vertical ridges on the lateral borders of the tongue	Function in taste sensation of sour May be a site of precancerous or cancerous findings (white or red areas, ulcers, masses, pigmentations)
Lingual tonsils	Mass of lymphoid tissue on the base of the tongue, posterior to the circumvallate papillae	Difficult to observe; extend and move the tongue to the right and left to examine
Lingual frenum	Thin fold of epithelium attaching the undersurface of the tongue to the floor of the mouth	A short frenum limits movement (*ankyloglossia,* tongue-tied) and makes exposing of radiographs and taking impressions difficult
Sublingual folds	Two ridges of tissue on the floor of the mouth arranged in a V-shaped direction, from the lingual frenum to the base of the tongue	Contains submandibular duct from the submandibular salivary gland and the ducts and openings of the sublingual salivary glands Limited amounts of mixed saliva secreted here
Sublingual caruncle	Round elevation of the floor of the mouth on either side of the lingual frena Contains the opening for Wharton's ducts	Submandibular duct carries large amounts of saliva from the submandibular salivary gland
Lingual veins	Blue line on the undersurface of the tongue on either side of the lingual frenum	With age this vein becomes more prominent in size and color; varicosities may be present
Plica fimbriatae	Fringelike projections on the undersurface of the tongue, lateral to the lingual vein	May be dark-colored, with more melanin pigmentation
Palate		
Anterior two thirds of the roof of the mouth is hard palate; posterior third is soft palate; a frequent site of oral cancer		
Incisive papillae	Midline pad of tissue lingual to the maxillary central incisors	Often burned or traumatized when eating Protect the nasopalatine nerve, which enters through the underlying *incisive foramen;* the palatal mucosa immediately lateral to the papilla is the needle insertion site for nasopalatine nerve-block anesthesia

Continued

Table D-1 Oral structures—cont'd

Structure	*Clinical description*	*Clinical consideration*
Rugae	Firm irregular ridges of masticatory mucosa on the anterior half of the hard palate	If prominent, rugae may be burned or traumatized more easily
Palatine fovea	Small dimple on either side of the midline at the junction of the hard and soft palates	Touching the posterior area of this may initiate the gag reflex
Palatal salivary duct openings	Small dark spots scattered on the hard and soft palates	Represent the duct openings of the minor palatal salivary glands
Palatine raphe	Hard linear elevation along the midline of the hard palate; external manifestation of the palatine suture, which joins the right and left maxillary and palatine bones	Excess bone *(tori)* or a deep depression may be present here Site of hyperkeratinization or associated nicotinic stomatitis
Maxillary tuberosity	Protuberance of the alveolar bone distal to the last maxillary molar	Erupting third molar may be present here
Tonsillar Region		
Retromolar area	Triangular area of bone and pad of tissue distal to the last mandibular molar	Erupting third molar may be present, and a flap of tissue *(operculum)* often is associated with an infection in this area
Pterygomandibular raphe	Fold of tissue from the retromolar area to an area near the maxillary tuberosity; separates the soft palate from the cheek; lies medial to the posterior border of the ramus of the mandible	Covers a ligament from the mandible to the sphenoid bone Used as a guide to identify the posterior border of the ramus of the mandible when targeting the area for needle insertion for inferior alveolar-nerve anesthesia

Anterior or glossopalatine arch	Thin fold of epithelium extending laterally and inferiorly from both sides of the soft palate to the base of the tongue	Marks the entry into the pharynx; the anterior boundary of the tonsillar recess
Posterior or pharyngopalatine arch	Thin fold of epithelium that is more posterior and narrower than the anterior arch	Marks the posterior boundary of the palatine tonsillar recess
Tonsillar recess	Recessed area between the anterior and posterior arches	May or may not contain palatine tonsils
Palatine tonsils	Globules of lymphoid tissue in the tonsillar recess	Vary greatly in size Not visible if removed or atrophied, or may be so large the fauces is very narrow
Uvula	Fleshy tissue suspended from the midline of the posterior border of the soft palate	Closes the opening to the nasopharynx when swallowing Varies in size and shape
Pharyngeal tonsils	Globules of lymphoid tissue on the oropharyngeal wall	Lay term is *adenoids* Appear as globules of reddish-orange tissue Mucosal secretions from the sinuses may be seen here
Fauces or faucial isthmus	Isthmus (narrowing) of the space from the oral cavity into the pharynx	

APPENDIX E

Dental Professional Organizations

Table E-1 Dental professional organizations

Abbreviation	*Organization*	*Website*
AADS	American Association for Dental Schools	http://www.aads.jhu.edu
AAE	American Association of Endodontists	http://www.aae.org
AAO	American Association of Orthodontists	http://www.braces.org
AAOMP	American Association of Oral and Maxillofacial Pathology	http://www.aaomp.org
AAOMR	American Association of Oral and Maxillofacial Radiology	http://www.aaomr.org
AAOMS	American Association of Oral and Maxillofacial Surgeons	http://www.aaoms.org
AAP	American Academy of Periodontology	http://www.perio.org
AAPD	American Academy of Pediatric Dentistry	http://www.aapd.org
AAPHD	American Association of Public Health Dentistry	http://www.aaphd.org
ABPD	American Board of Pediatric Dentistry	http://www.abpd.org
ACP	American College of Prosthodontics	http://www.prosthodontics.org
ADA	American Dental Association	http://www.ada.org
ADAA	American Dental Assistants' Association	http://www.dentalassistant.org
ADEA	American Dental Education Association	http://www.adea.org
ADHA	American Dental Hygienists' Association	http://www.adha.org
AGD	Academy of General Dentistry	http://www.agd.org
ASDA	American Student Dental Association	http://www.asdanet.org
ASDA	American Society of Dentist Anesthesiologists	http://www.asdahq.org
IADR	International Association of Dental Research	http://www.iadr.com
IAO	International Association for Orthodontics	http://www.iaortho.com
ICOI	International Congress of Oral Implantologists	http://www.icoi.org
WFO	World Federation of Orthodontists	http://www.wfo.org

Table E-2 Federal and international organizations

Abbreviation	*Organization*	*Website*
CDC	Centers for Disease Control and Prevention	http://www.cdc.gov
FDA	Food and Drug Administration	http://www.fda.gov
Library of Congress	THOMAS	http://thomas.loc.gov
NHIC	National Health Information Center	http://www.health.gov/nhic
NIDRC	National Institute of Dental Research and Craniofacial	http://www.nidcr.nih.gov
NIH	National Institutes of Health	http://www.nih.gov
NLM	National Library of Medicine	http://www.nlm.nih.gov
NOHIC	National Oral Health Information Clearinghouse	http://www.nohic.nidcr.nih.gov
OSHA	Occupational Safety and Health Administration	http://www.osha.gov
WHO	World Health Organization	http://www.who.int/en

APPENDIX F

Health Insurance Portability and Accountability Act of 1996

The Health Insurance Portability and Accountability Act (HIPAA) of 1996 was signed into law by President Bill Clinton on August 21, 1996. Conclusive regulations were issued on August 17, 2000, to be instated by October 16, 2002. HIPAA requires that the transactions of all patient health care information be formatted in a standardized electronic style. In addition to protecting the privacy and security of patient information, HIPAA includes legislation on the formation of medical savings accounts, the authorization of a fraud and abuse control program, the easy transport of health insurance coverage, and the simplification of administrative terms and conditions.

HIPAA encompasses three primary areas, and its privacy requirements can be broken down into three types: privacy standards, patients' rights, and administrative requirements.

1. Privacy Standards. A central concern of HIPAA is the careful use and disclosure of protected health information (PHI), which generally is electronically controlled health information that is able to be distinguished individually. PHI also refers to verbal communication, although the HIPAA Privacy Rule is not intended to hinder necessary verbal communication. The U.S. Department of Health and Human Services (USDHHS) does not require restructuring, such as soundproofing, architectural changes, and so forth, but some caution is necessary when exchanging health information by conversation.

An Acknowledgement of Receipt Notice of Privacy Practices, which allows patient information to be used or divulged for treatment, payment, or health care operations (TPO), should be procured from each patient. A detailed and time-sensitive authorization can also be issued, which allows the dentist to release information in special circumstances other than TPOs. A *written consent* is also an option. Dentists can disclose PHI *without* acknowledgement, consent, or authorization in very special situations—for example, perceived child abuse, public health supervision, fraud investigation, or law enforcement with valid permission (i.e., a warrant). When divulging PHI, a dentist must try to disclose only the *minimum necessary* information, to help safeguard the patient's information as much as possible.

It is important that dental professionals adhere to HIPAA standards because health care providers (as well as health care clearinghouses and health care plans) who convey *electronically* formatted health information via an outside billing service or merchant are considered *covered entities.* Covered entities may be dealt serious civil and criminal penalties for violation of HIPAA legislation. Failure to comply with HIPAA privacy requirements may result in civil penalties of up to $100 per offense with an annual maximum of $25,000 for repeated failure to comply with the same requirement. Criminal penalties resulting from the illegal mishandling of private health information can range from $50,000 and/or 1 year in prison to $250,000 and/or 10 years in prison.

2. Patients' Rights. HIPAA allows patients, authorized representatives, and parents of minors, as well as minors, to become more aware of the health information privacy to which they are entitled. These rights include, but are not limited to, the right to view and copy their health information, the right to dispute alleged breaches of policies and regulations, and the right to request alternative forms of communicating with their dentist. If any health information is released for any reason other than TPO, the patient is entitled to an account of the transaction. Therefore it is important for dentists to keep accurate records of such information and to provide them when necessary.

The HIPAA Privacy Rule determines that the parents of a minor have access to their child's health information. This privilege may be overruled, for example, in cases where there is suspected child abuse or the parent consents to a term of confidentiality between the dentist and the minor. The parents' rights to access their child's PHI also may be restricted in situations when a legal entity, such as a court, intervenes and when a law does not require a parent's consent. For a full list of patient rights provided by HIPAA, be sure to acquire a copy of the law and to understand it well.

3. Administrative Requirements. Complying with HIPAA legislation may seem like a chore, but it does not need to be so. It is recommended that you become appropriately familiar with the law, organize the requirements into simpler tasks, begin compliance early, and document your progress in compliance. An important first step is to evaluate the current information and practices of your office.

Dentists will need to write a *privacy policy* for their office, a document for their patients detailing the office's practices concerning PHI. The American Dental Association's (ADA) *HIPAA Privacy Kit* includes forms that you (the dentist) can use to customize your privacy policy. It is useful to try to understand the role of health care information for your patients and the ways in which they deal with the information while they are visiting your office. Train your staff; make sure they are familiar with the terms of HIPAA and your office's privacy policy and related forms. HIPAA requires that you designate a *privacy officer,* a person in your office who will be responsible for applying the new policies in your office, fielding complaints, and making choices involving the minimum necessary requirements. Another person with the role of *contact person* will process complaints.

A *Notice of Privacy Practices*—a document detailing the patient's rights and the dental office's obligations concerning PHI—also must be drawn up. Further, any role of a third party with access to PHI must be clearly documented. This third party is known as a *business associate* (BA) and is defined as any entity who, on behalf of the dentist, takes part in any activity that involves exposure of PHI. The *HIPAA Privacy Kit* provides a copy of the USDHHS "Business Associate Contract Terms," which provides a concrete format for detailing BA interactions.

The main HIPAA privacy compliance date, including all staff training, was April 14, 2003, although many covered entities who submitted a request and a compliance plan by October 15, 2002, were granted 1-year extensions. Contact your local branch of the ADA for details. It is recommended that dentists prepare their offices ahead of time for all deadlines, which include preparing privacy policies and forms, business associate contracts, and employee training sessions.

For a comprehensive discussion of all these terms and requirements, a complete list of HIPAA policies and procedures, and a full collection of HIPAA privacy forms, contact the ADA for a *HIPAA Privacy Kit*. The relevant ADA website is www.ada.org/prof/resources/topics/hipaa/index.asp. Other websites that may contain useful information about HIPAA are the following:

- USDHHS Office of Civil Rights, www.hhs.gov/ocr/hipaa
- Work Group on Electronic Data Interchange, www.wedi.org/snip/public/articles/index.shtml
- Phoenix Health, www.hipaadvisory.com
- USDHHS Office of the Assistant Secretary for Planning and Evaluation, http://aspe.hhs.gov/_ /index.cfm

Sources used:

1. *HIPAA Privacy Kit*
2. http://www.ada.org/prof/resources/topics/hipaa/index.asp

APPENDIX G

Infection Control

One of the most important areas in dentistry today is infection control, maintaining a healthy, disease-free work zone that protects both patients and dental workers. The process encompasses not only common communicable infections, such as influenza and strep throat, and long-term life-threatening illnesses, such as human immunodeficiency virus (HIV) and hepatitis, but also the handling of biohazard and hazardous materials. Two national organizations, the Occupational Safety and Health Administration (OSHA) and the Centers for Disease Control and Prevention (CDC), are committed to protecting dental hygienists and technicians from these daily risks and produce a number of publications that focus on making dentistry a healthy and safe environment in which to work. Here are links to these governing bodies and the informational materials with which every dental professional should be familiar.

Table G-1 Infection control resources

Organization	*Website*	*Description*
OSHA	http://www.osha.gov	This is the link to the main OSHA website. There is a search function available to quickly locate whatever information you need.
OSHA on dentistry	http://www.osha.gov/SLTC/dentistry/index.html	Covering all the risks in and requirements for dental offices, OSHA provides dentistry with its own articles that educate a dental professional about topics including potential hazards, workplace violence, and noise control.
OSHA standards for bloodborne pathogens	http://www.osha.gov/pls/oshaweb/owadisp.show_document?p_table=STANDARDS&p_id=10051	This explains OSHA's requirements for businesses that work with potential infectious agents, such as blood and needles, to have a plan to protect their employees.

Continued

Table G-1 Infection control resources—cont'd

Organization	*Website*	*Description*
OSHA plan for safe health care facilities	http://www.osha.gov/SLTC/healthcarefacilities/index.html	This link covers how to establish a safe health care facility. The page covers identifying potential hazards, developing plans to address those hazards, and providing training for employees about the risks in their work environment.
OSHA guidelines for workplace exposure to anesthetic gases	http://www.osha.gov/dts/osta/anestheticgases/index.html	Focusing on educating employees about the damaging materials around them, this page describes and teaches dental professionals about the risks and realities of contact with the inhaled anesthetics in their dental office.
OSHA and bloodborne pathogens and needlestick prevention	http://www.osha.gov/SLTC/bloodbornepathogens/recognition.html	This page provides an overview of the risks associated with bloodborne pathogens as well as a number of links to electronic pamphlets and other sites containing guidelines for preventing needlestick injuries.
CDC	http://www.cdc.gov	The link to the main CDC website has the latest information in the health care world as well as a wealth of information and resource materials on training and employment.
CDC's recommended infection control practices for dentistry	http://www.cdc.gov/oralhealth/infectioncontrol/guidelines/index.htm	These are the CDC's updated recommendations for dental practices' guidelines for infection control.
CDC on exposure to blood	http://www.cdc.gov/ncidod/dhqp/pdf/bbp/Exp_to_Blood.pdf	This electronic pamphlet covers all of the bases that a health care worker needs to know about blood exposure. It gives detailed answers to questions about HIV and hepatitis.

Table G-2 OSAP Surface disinfectant reference chart—2006

PRODUCT CLASSIFICATION	*PRODUCT BRAND INFORMATION*				
Category	*Brand (packaged as)*	*EPA #*	*Dilution*	*TB Claim*	*Manufacturer or Distributor*
Accelerated Hydrogen Peroxide	**Optim 33 TB**	74559-1-83259	RTU	5 min	SciCan
Citric Acid Citric acid, hydroxyacetic acid, diprooylene glycol n-butyl ether	**Lysol IC Ready to Use Disinfectant Cleaner**	675-55	RTU	10 min	Sultan Healthcare
Iodophors Alpha- (p-nonylphenyl)-omega-hydroxypoly (oxethylene) iodine	**IodoFive Surface Disinfectant/Cleaner**	4959-16-50611	1:213	10 min	Certol International
Phenolics (Dual) Water-Based Phenylphenol and benzylchlorophenol or tertiary amylphenol	**Birex SE Concentrate**	1043-92-51003	1:256	10 min	Biotrol International
	DisCide Germicidal Foaming Cleaner	33176-6	RTU	10 min	Palmero Health Care
	ProSpray C-60 Conc. Surface Disinfectant	46851-1-50611	1:32	10 min	Certol International
	ProSpray Surface Disinfectant Spray	46851-5-50611	RTU	10 min	Certol International
	ProSpray Wipes	46851-10	RTU	10 min	Certol International
Phenolics (Dual) Alcohol-Based Tertiary amylphenol and/or phenylphenol + ethyl alcohol or isopropyl alcohol	**Coe Spray II (Pump)**	11694-98-10214	RTU	6 min	GC America
	DisCide Disinfectant Spray	706-69-10492	RTU	10 min	Palmero Health Care
Quaternaries Dual or Synergized Plus Alcohol Diisobutylphenoxyethoxyethyl dimethylbenzyl ammonium chloride; isopropanol or ethanol; alkyldimethyl benzyl ammonium chloride	**CaviCide Spray**	46781-6	RTU	5 min	TotalCare/Pinnacle/Metrex
	CaviWipes	46781-8	RTU	5 min	TotalCare/Pinnacle/Metrex
	Cetylcide II Broad Spectrum Disinfectant	61178-1-3150	2 oz/gal	NOL	Cetylite Industries
	Clorox Disinfecting Spray	67619-3	RTU	10 min	Harry J. Bosworth Company
	DisCide ULTRA Spray	10492-5	RTU	1 min	Palmero Health Care
	DisCide ULTRA Wipes	10492-4	RTU	1 min	Palmero Health Care
	DisCide V Detergent Disinfectant	1839-83-10492	RTU	5 min	Palmero Health Care
	GC Spray-Cide	1130-15-10214	RTU	6 min	GC America

Continued

Table G-2 OSAP Surface disinfectant reference chart—2006—cont'd

PRODUCT CLASSIFICATION	*PRODUCT BRAND INFORMATION*				
Category	*Brand (packaged as)*	*EPA #*	*Dilution*	*TB Claim*	*Manufacturer or Distributor*
Quaternaries Dual or Synergized Plus Alcohol—cont'd Diisobutylphenoxyethoxyethyl dimethylbenzyl ammonium chloride; isopropanol or ethanol; alkyldimethyl benzyl ammonium chloride	**Lysol IC Disinfectant Spray**	777-72-675	RTU	10 min	Sultan Healthcare
	Maxispray Plus	46781-6-10597	RTU	5 min	Sullivan-Schein Dental
	Maxiwipe Germicidal Cloth	9480-4-10597	RTU	5 min	Sullivan-Schein Dental
	Opti-Cide-3 Spray	70144-1	RTU	3 min	Micro Scientific Industries
	PDCare Surface Disinfectant Spray	46781-6-43100	RTU	5 min	Patterson Dental
	PDCare Wipes	46781-8-43100	RTU	5 min	Patterson Dental
	Sanitex Plus Spray	1130-150-64285	RTU	6 min	Crosstex International
	Sanitex Plus Wipes	9480-4-64285	RTU	5 min	Crosstex International
	Sani-Cloth HB Wipes	61178-4-9480	RTU	NOL	PDI International
	Sani-Cloth Plus Wipes	9480-6	RTU	5 min	PDI International
	Super Sani-Cloth Wipes	9480-4	RTU	2 min	PDI International
Sodium Hypochlorite	**Clorox Germicidal Spray**	67619-13	RTU	30 sec	Harry J. Bosworth Company
	Clorox Germicidal Wipes	67619-12	RTU	2 min	Harry J. Bosworth Company
Sodium Bromide & Chlorine	**Microstat 2 Tablets**	70369-1	2 tabs/ qt water	5 min	Septodont

IMPORTANT INFORMATION: Listing does not imply endorsement, recommendation or warranty. Other products are available. Only OSAP member *Hospital Disinfectants* are represented in this chart. Purchasers are legally required to consult label and package insert for changes in formulation and recommended use. Check compatibility of material before use on dental/medical equipment.

KEY: RTU = Ready to Use; NOL = Not on label, e.g., one or both of the HIV/HBV claims is not provided on the label. OSAP is using the CDC guidelines. Be sure to use a disinfectant with a TB claim if there is any blood or OPIM present.

This chart is a publication of the Organization for Safety & Asepsis Procedures (OSAP). OSAP assumes no liability for actions taken based on the information herein.

APPENDIX H

Legal and Ethical Issues

Table H-1 Differentiating between ethics and law*

	Ethics	*Law*
Definition	Individual interpretation of the nature of right and wrong and rules of conduct	Rules and regulations by which society is governed, set forth in a formal and legally binding manner
Source	Internalized; individual nature and beliefs	Externalized rules and regulations of society
Emphasis	Individual moral behavior for the good of the individual within society	Social behaviors that are good for society as a whole
Conduct	Motives and reasons why the individual behaves the way he or she does	Overt conduct of the individual; what a person actually did or failed to do
Sanctions	Professional organization—expulsion from the organization	Judicial and administrative bodies—criminal sanctions such as fines and imprisonment imposed by the courts; civil sanctions such as monetary damages imposed by the courts; disciplinary sanctions such as fines, license suspension, or license revocation by a board of dentistry

*From Darby ML: *Mosby's comprehensive review of dental hygiene,* ed 6, St Louis, 2006, Mosby.

Table H-2 Historical court cases

Category of law	*Court case*	*Issue*	*Decision in favor of*	*Precedent established*
Civil/affirmative action/age discrimination	*M. Bennett v Hardy* (1990)	Unlawful discharge	Defendant	Burden of proof was lacking.
Civil/contract/disability	*Hansen v Gordon* (1992)	Work-related impairment	Plaintiff	Disease impairment covered under worker's compensation.
Civil/contract/employment rights	*Murphy v Birdtree Dental* (1997)	Breach of contract	Plaintiff	Contractual right confirmed by policy handbook.
Civil/contract/insurance coverage	*Hawkins v Berkshire Life Ins. Co.* (1999)	Full disclosure	Defendant	Contract void if full disclosure is not given.
Civil/contract/insurance coverage	*Freidin v Pan-Am Ins.* (1992)	Full disclosure	Plaintiff	Facts did not support claims of the defendant.
Civil/contract/unemployment benefits	*Stagner v Highfill* (1990)	Work rules	Defendant	Reasonable work rules are contractually valid.
Civil/malpractice/breach of practice act*	*Edwards v Pennsylvania Dental Examining Board* (1983)	Unlawful action	Pennsylvania Dental Examining Board	Police power of the state upheld.
Civil/malpractice/breach of practice act*	*Bach v Florida State Board of Dentistry* (1979)	Unlawful action	Florida State Board of Dentistry	Police power of the state upheld.
Civil/malpractice/breach of practice act*	*Barletta v State of LA/School of Dentistry* (1988)	Unlawful action	Defendant	Due process affirmed.
Civil/malpractice/breach of practice act*	*Oppenheim, Sloan v Pennsylvania Dental Examining Board* (1983)	Unlawful action	Pennsylvania Dental Examining Board	Police power of the state upheld.
Civil/malpractice/negligence/personal injury	*Myers v Dunscombe* (1983)	Unlawful action	Defendant	Police power of the state upheld.

Civil/restraint of trade	*CDA v CDHA* (1990)	Freedom of association	Defendant	Collective bargaining right in professional organizations affirmed.
Civil/state practice act	*Fosket v State Board of Dentistry* (1977)	Independent practice	Defendant	Police power of the state upheld.
Civil/tort/negligence/ personal injury	*Campbell v Pommier* (1985)	Reasonable care	Defendant	Burden of proof lies with plaintiff.
Civil/tort/negligence/ personal injury	*Sirkin and Levine v Timmons* (1994)	Work environment risk	Plaintiff	Reasonable precautions required of employers.
Civil/tort/negligence/ personal injury	*Flor v Holguin* (2000)	Work environment risk	Plaintiff	Reasonable precautions required of employers.
Civil/tort/negligence/ personal injury	*Kilburn v U.S.* (1991)	Full disclosure	Defendant	Plaintiff did not show probable cause.
Civil/tort/negligence/ personal injury	*Ryan v Hiller* (1994)	Dual capacity doctrine	Defendant	Transporting an employee to another office is work related.
Civil/tort/negligence/ personal injury	*Parker v Frelich* (2002)	Respondent superior	Plaintiff	Liability is assumed if not explicitly informed of independence.
Civil/tort/negligence/ personal injury	*Austin v AANS* (2001)	Expert testimony	Plaintiff	Misrepresentation is actionable.
Civil/tort/work-related injury	*Colwell v Trotman* (1980)	Working conditions	Plaintiff	Two employers may be jointly liable.
Civil/vendor-proximate cause/injury	*Falcone v Baxter Healthcare Corp. et al.* (1996)	Defective product	Remanded to State Court	

*Although these cases were adjudicated in civil court, criminal charges of fraud and/or assault could have been levied. The reason for adjudication in civil court was the possibility of restitution or remuneration rather than only retribution.

Furthermore, the burden of proof is higher in a criminal proceeding (beyond a reasonable doubt) than in a civil proceeding (by the preponderance of evidence).

APPENDIX I

How Dental Terms Are Made and Read

Dental terminology is a hybrid speech. Most of the words also are common to medical terminology and as such are largely made up of Greek and Latin stems, prefixes, and suffixes. However, many words have been borrowed from other languages as well. Dental terminology also is dynamic in the sense that many new words are coined as necessity demands. Generally, technical words can be analyzed for their meanings by dividing them into their component parts and determining the meaning of each part.

To build or analyze any vocabulary, the five elements that can be used to form words must be understood: the word root, combining vowel, combining form, prefix, and suffix.

WORD ROOT

The word root is the basic core of any word and gives it its primary meaning. (Some compound words may be made up of more than one root.) For instance, in the words *stomatitis, adenitis,* and *pulpitis* the word roots are *stomat* (meaning "mouth"), *aden* (meaning "gland"), and *pulp* (meaning "the soft tissue within a tooth").

COMBINING VOWEL

Certain combinations of word roots are difficult to pronounce, especially when the first word root ends in a consonant and the second begins with a consonant. This awkwardness of pronunciation necessitates the insertion of a vowel called a combining vowel. Usually the combining vowel is an *o,* although *a, e, i, u,* and *y* may be encountered occasionally. Combining vowels are encountered in everyday words. Instead of joining the two word roots *speed* and *meter* directly, the combining vowel *o* is inserted to create *speedometer.* Another example is *megal* and *glossia,* which become *megaloglossia.*

COMBINING FORM

The combination of word root plus combining vowel is known as the combining form.

Word root	+	*Combining vowel*	=	*Combining form*
-gnath-		O		-gnatho-
-micr-		O		-micro-
-dent-		O		-dento-
-arthr-		O		-arthro-

SUFFIX

A suffix is a syllable or syllables added at the end of a word root or combining form to change the meaning of the root, give it grammatical function, or form a new word. *Play, read,* and *speak* are word roots; by adding the suffix *-er* (meaning "one who") the words are changed to "one who plays," "one who reads," and "one who speaks." If the suffix *-able* (meaning "capable of being") were added, the words mean "capable of being played," "capable of being read," and "capable of being spoken." In the words *microtome, dermatome,* and *arthrotome,* -tome is a suffix meaning "instrument for cutting." Notice that the suffix is added to the combining form rather than the word root:

Word root	+	*Combining vowel*	+	*Suffix*	=	*Meaning*
micr-		O		-tome		instrument to cut very fine sections
derm-		O		-tome		instrument to cut skin
arthr-		O		-tome		instrument to cut joints

PREFIX

A prefix is a syllable or syllables placed before a word or word root to alter its meaning or create a new word. If the prefixes *over-, re-,* and *out-* are added before the words *play, read,* and *speak,* three new words are created—*overplay, reread,* and *outspeak.* Any number of these five elements can be combined to form new words.

Auto-bi-o-graph-ic-al		*Sub-strat-o-spher-e*		*Electr-o-cardi-o-gram*	
auto-	prefix	sub-	prefix	electr-	word root
-bi-	word root	-strat-	word root	-o-	combining vowel
-o-	combining vowel	-o-	combining vowel	-cardi-	word root
-graph-	word root	-spher-	word root	-o-	combining vowel
-ic	suffix	-e	suffix	-gram	suffix
-al	suffix				

WORD AND ROOT ORDER

The order in which the various elements of compound words are placed is of great importance. Observe the consequences if the order of the elements in the following words were reversed:

leg iron	became	iron leg
motorboat	became	boat motor
snake poison	became	poison snake
pig iron	became	iron pig
zoo animal	became	animal zoo
eyeglass	became	glass eye
house dog	became	dog house

In all of these instances the order of the elements may be reversed and still arrive at a sensible word, although the subject in each example has changed. Other compound words such as the following may become nonsensical if the order of their elements is changed:

shoulder blade	cannot become	blade shoulder
nerve tonic	cannot become	tonic nerve
chickenpox	cannot become	pox chicken
headache	cannot become	achehead

The following is a list of combining forms for anatomic structures and body fluids, prefixes, suffixes, verbs, and adjectives. Although the combining form generally appears at the beginning of a term, it may appear within a term or at the end of it.*

---

*From Young CG, Austin MG: *Learning medical terminology step by step,* ed 4, St Louis, 1979, Mosby.

adeno- gland
adreno- adrenal gland
angio- vessel
ano- anus
arterio- artery
arthro- joint
balano- glans penis
blepharo- eyelid
broncho- bronchus (windpipe)
cantho- canthus (angle at either end of slit between eyelids)
capit- head
cardi-, cardio- heart
carpo- wrist
cephalo- head
cerebello- cerebellum (part of brain)
cerebro- cerebrum (part of brain)
cheilo- lip (mouth)
chole- bile (NOTE: *chole-* + *cyst* meaning "bladder," = gallbladder; *chole-* + *doch,* meaning "duct," = choledocho, or common bile duct.)
chondro- cartilage
chordo- cord or string (generally used in connection with the vocal cord or spermatic cord)
cilia- hair (Latin)
cleido- collarbone
coccygo- coccyx (end bone of the spinal column)
colpo- vagina
cordo- cord (usually vocal cord)
coxa- hip (Latin)
cranio- head
cysto- sac, cyst, or bladder (most often used in connection with the urinary bladder)
cyto- cell
dacryo- tear (used commonly in relation to tear duct or sac)
dento-, donto- tooth
derma- skin
duodeno- duodenum (part of small intestine)
emia- blood
encephalo- brain
entero- intestines
fascia- sheet or band of fibrous tissue (Latin)
fibro- fibers
gastro- stomach
genu- knee (Latin)
gingivo- gums
glomerulo- glomerulus (often a structure of the kidney)
glosso- tongue
gnatho- jaw
hem-, hema-, hemo-, hemato- blood
hepato- liver
hilus- pit or depression in an organ where vessels and nerves enter (Latin)
histio- tissue
hystero- uterus (NOTE: This term may also pertain to hysteria.)
ileo- ileum (part of small intestine)
ilio- flank or ilium (bone of pelvis)
jejuno- jejunum (part of small intestine)
kerato- cornea or horny layer of the skin
labio- lips (either of mouth or vulva)
lacrimo- tears (used also in connection with tear ducts or sacs)
laparo- loin or flank (also refers to abdomen)
laryngo- larynx
linguo- tongue
lympho- lymph
masto- breast
meningo- meninges (coverings of the brain and spinal cord)
metra-, metro- uterus
morpho- form
myelo- bone marrow and spinal cord (NOTE: Use of this term will determine which tissue is meant.)
myo- muscle (NOTE: The Latin word for muscle is *mus.*)
myringo- eardrum
naso- nose
nephro- kidney
neuro- nerve
oculo- eye
odonto- tooth
omphalo- navel or umbilicus
onycho- nails
oophoro- ovary
ophthalmo- eye
ora-, oro- mouth

orthio-, orchido- testis
os- bone or mouth
osteo- bone
oto- ear
ovario- ovary
palato- palate of mouth
palpebro- eyelid
pectus- breast, chest, or thorax (Latin)
pharyngo- pharynx
phlebo- vein
pilo- hair
pleuro- pleura of lung (relates also to side or rib)
pneumo-, pneumono- lungs (also used in referring to air or breath)
procto- rectum
pyelo- pelvis of kidney
pyloro- pylorus (part of stomach just before duodenum)
rhino- nose
sacro- sacrum
salpingo- fallopian tube or oviduct
sialo- saliva (used in connection with a salivary duct or gland)
splanchno- viscera
spleno- spleen
sterno- sternum
stoma- mouth
tarso- instep of foot; ankle (also edge of eyelid)
teno-, tenonto- tendon
thoraco- thorax or chest
thyro- thyroid
trachelo- neck, particularly the neck of the uterus or bladder
tracheo- trachea
unguis- nail
uretero- ureter
urethro- urethra
uro- urine, urinary
utero- uterus
vaso- vessel
veno- vein
ventriculo- ventricle of heart or brain
viscero- viscera

PREFIXES

Prefixes, the most frequently used elements in the formation of medical-dental words, are one or more syllables (prepositions or adverbs) placed before words or roots to show various kinds of relationships. They are never used independently, but when added before verbs, adjectives, or nouns, they modify the meaning. Most prefixes are a part of words in ordinary speech and do not refer specifically to medical-dental or scientific terminology, but many also occur frequently in medical terminology. Studying them is an important step in learning medical terms and building a medical-dental vocabulary.

Prefix	*Translation*	*Examples*
a- (an- before vowel)	Without, lack of	Apathy (lack of feeling), apnea (without breath), aphasia (without speech), anemia (lack of blood)
ab-	Away from	Abductor (leading away from), aboral (away from mouth)
ad-	To, toward, near to	Adductor (leading toward), adhesion (sticking to), adnexa (structures joined to), adrenal (near the kidney)
ambi-	Both	Ambidextrous (ability to use hands equally), ambilaterally (both sides)
amphi-	About, on both sides, both	Amphibious (living on both land and water)
ampho-	Both	Amphogenic (producing offspring of both sexes)
ana-	Up, back, again, excessive	Anatomy (a cutting up), anagenesis (reproduction of tissue), anasarca (excessive serum in cellular tissues of body)
ante-	Before, forward	Antecubital (before elbow), anteflexion (forward bending)
anti-	Against, opposed to, reversed	Antiperistalsis (reversed peristalsis), antisepsis (against infection)

apo-	From, away from	Aponeurosis (away from tendon), apochromatic (abnormal color)
bi-	Twice, double	Biarticulate (double joint), bifocal (two foci), bifurcation (two branches)
cata-	Down, according to, complete	Catabolism (breaking down), catalepsia (complete seizure), catarrh (flowing down)
circum-	Around, about	Circumflex (winding about), circumference (surrounding), circumarticular (around joint)
com-	With, together	Commissure (sending or coming together)
con-	With, together	Conductor (leading together), concrescence (growing together), concentric (having a common center)
contra-	Against, opposite	Contralateral (opposite side), contraception (prevention of conception), contraindicated (not indicated)
de-	Away from	Dehydrate (remove water from), decompensation (failure of compensation)
di-	Twice, double	Diplopia (double vision), dichromatic (two colors), digastric (double stomach)
dia-	Through, apart, across, completely	Diaphragm (wall across), diapedesis (ooze through), diagnosis (complete knowledge)
dis-	Reversal, apart from, separation	Disinfection (apart from infection), disparity (apart from equality), dissect (cut apart)
dys-	Bad, difficult, disordered	Dyspepsia (bad digestion), dyspnea (difficult breathing), dystopia (disordered position)
e-, ex-	Out, away from	Enucleate (remove from), eviscerate (take out viscera or bowels), exostosis (outgrowth of bone)
ec-	Out from	Ectopic (out of place), eccentric (away from center), ectasia (stretching out or dilation)
ecto-	On outside, situated on	Ectoderm (outer skin), ectoretina (outer layer of retina)
em-, en-	In	Empyema (pus in), encephalon (in the head)
endo-	Within	Endocardium (within heart), endometrium (within uterus), endodont (within tooth)
epi-	Upon, on	Epidural (upon dura), epidermis (on skin)
exo-	Outside, on outer side, outer layer	Exogenous (produced outside), exocolitis (inflammation of outer coat of colon)
extra-	Outside	Extracellular (outside cell), extrapleural (outside pleura)
hemi-	Half	Hemiplegia (partial paralysis), hemianesthesia (loss of feeling on one side of body)
hyper-	Over, above, excessive	Hyperemia (excessive blood), hypertrophy (overgrowth), hyperplasia (excessive formation)
hypo-	Under, below, deficient	Hypotension (low blood pressure), hypothyroidism (deficiency or underfunction of thyroid)
im-, in-	In, into	Immersion (act of dipping in), infiltration (act of filtering in), injection (act of forcing liquid into)
im-, in-	Not	Immature (not mature), involuntary (not voluntary), inability (not able)
infra-	Below	Infraorbital (below eye), infraclavicular (below clavicle or collarbone)
inter-	Between	Intercostal (between ribs), intervene (come between)
intra-	Within	Intracerebral (within cerebrum), intraocular (within eyes), intraventricular (within ventricles)
intro-	Into, within	Introversion (turning inward), introduce (lead into)
meta-	Beyond, after, change	Metamorphosis (change of form), metastasis (beyond original position), metacarpal (beyond wrist)

opistho-	Behind, backward	Opisthotic (behind ears), opisthognathous (behind jaws)
para-	Beside, by side	Paraplegia (paralysis of both sides), paracentesis (puncture along side of), parathyroid (beside thyroid)
per-	Through, excessive	Permeate (pass through), perforate (bore through), peracute (excessively acute)
peri-	Around	Periosteum (around bone), periatrial (around atrium), peribronchial (around bronchus)
post-	After, behind	Postoperative (after operation), postpartum (after childbirth), postocular (behind eye)
pre-	Before, in front of	Premaxillary (in front of maxilla), preoral (in front of mouth)
pro-	Before, in front of	Prognosis (foreknowledge), prophase (appear before)
re-	Back, again, contrary	Reflex (bend back), revert (turn again to), regurgitation (backward flowing, contrary to normal)
retro-	Backward, located behind	Retrocervical (located behind cervix), retrograde (going backward), retrolingual (behind tongue)
semi-	Half	Semicartilaginous (half cartilage), semilunar (half moon), semiconscious (half conscious)
sub-	Under	Subcutaneous (under skin), subarachnoid (under arachnoid), subungual (under nail)
super-	Above, upper, excessive	Supercilia (upper brows), supernumerary (excessive number), supermedial (above middle)
supra-	Above, upon	Suprarenal (above kidney), suprasternal (above sternum), suprascapular (on upper part of scapula)
sym-, syn-	Together, with	Symphysis (growing together), synapsis (joining together), synarthrosis (articulation of joints together)
trans-	Across, through	Transection (cut across), transduodenal (through duodenum), transmit (send beyond)
ultra-	Beyond, in	Ultraviolet (beyond violet end of spectrum), ultraligation (ligation of vessel beyond point of origin), ultrasonic (sound waves beyond the upper frequency of hearing by human ear)

SUFFIXES

Suffixes are the one or more syllables or elements added to the root, or stem, of a word (the part that indicates the essential meaning) to alter the meaning or indicate the intended part of speech.

To make it pronounceable the last letter or letters of the root to which the suffix is attached may be changed. The last vowel may be changed to an *o,* or *o* may be inserted if it is not already present before a suffix beginning with a consonant, as in *cardiology.* The final vowel in the root may be dropped before a suffix beginning with a vowel, as in *neuritis.*

Most suffixes are in common use in English, but some are peculiar to medical science. The suffixes most commonly used to indicate disease are *-itis,* meaning "inflammation," *-oma,* meaning "tumor," and *-osis,* meaning "a condition," usually morbid. The following suffixes occur often in medical-dental terminology, but they are also in use in ordinary language:

Suffix	*Use*	*Examples*
-ise, -ate	Added to nouns or adjectives to make verbs expressing to use and to act like; to subject to; make into	Visualize (able to see), impersonate (act like), hypnotize (put into state of hypnosis)

-ist, -or, -er	Added to verbs to make nouns expressing agent or person concerned or instrument	Anesthetist (one who practices the science of anesthesia), dissector (instrument that dissects or person who dissects), donor (giver)
-ent	Added to verbs to make adjectives or nouns of agency	Recipient (one who receives), concurrent (happening at the same time)
-sia, -y	Added to verbs to make nouns expressing action, process, or condition	Therapy (treatment), anesthesia (process or condition of feeling)
-ia, -ity	Added to adjectives or nouns to make nouns expressing quality or condition	Septicemia (poisoning of blood), disparity (inequality), acidity (condition of excess acid), neuralgia (pain in nerves)
-ma, mata, -men, -mina, -ment, -ure	Added to verbs to make nouns expressing result of action or object of action	Trauma (injury), foramina (openings), ligament (tough fibrous band holding bone or viscera together), fissure (groove)
-ium, -olus, -olum, -culus, -culum, -cule, -cle	Added to nouns to make diminutive nouns	Bacterium, alveolus (air sac), follicle (little bag), cerebellum (little brain), molecule (little mass), ossicle (little bone)
-ible, -ile	Added to verbs to make adjectives expressing ability or capacity	Contractile (ability to contract), edible (capable of being eaten), flexible (capable of being bent)
-al, -c, -ious, -tic	Added to nouns to make adjectives expressing relationship, concern, or pertaining to	Neural (referring to nerve), neoplastic (referring to neoplasm), cardiac (referring to heart), delirious (suffering from delirium)
-id	Added to verbs or nouns to make adjectives expressing state or condition	Flaccid (state of being weak or lax), fluid (state of being fluid or liquid)
-tic	Added to verbs to make adjectives showing relationships	Caustic (referring to burn), acoustic (referring to sound or hearing)
-oid, -form	Added to nouns to make adjectives expressing resemblance	Polypoid (resembling polyp), plexiform (resembling a plexus), fusiform (resembling a fusion), epidermoid (resembling epidermis)
-ous	Added to nouns to make adjectives expressing material	Ferrous (composed of iron), serous (composed of serum), mucinous (composed of mucin)

The following verbs or combining forms of verbs are derived from Greek or Latin. They may be attached to other roots to form words, or suffixes and prefixes may be added to them to form words. In the following examples, the part or root of the word to which the verb is attached is italicized and the meaning, if not clear, is given in parentheses:

Root	*Translation*	*Examples*
-algia-	Pain	*Cardi*algia (heart), *gastr*algia (stomach), *neur*algia (nerve)
-dynia-	Pain	*Masto*dynia (breast), *pleuro*dynia (chest), *esophago*dynia (esophagus), *coccygo*dynia (coccyx)
-audi-, -audio-	Hear, hearing	Audio*meter* (measure), audio*phone* (voice instrument for deaf)
-bio-	Live	*Bio*logy (study of living), *bio*statistics (vital statistics), *bio*genesis (origin)
cau-, -caus-	Burn	Caus*tic* (suffix added to make adjective), caut*erization;* caus*algia* (burning pain), *electro*cautery

-centesis-	Puncture, perforate	Thoracentesis (chest), pneumocentesis (lung), arthrocentesis (joint), enterocentesis (intestine)
-clas-, -claz-	Smash, break	Osteoclasis (bone), odontoclasis (tooth)
-duct-	Lead	Ductal (suffix added to make adjective), oviduct (egg uterine tube or fallopian tube), periductal (peri means "around"), abduct (prefix meaning lead away from)
-ecta-, -ectas-	Dilate	Venectasia (dilation of vein), cardiectasis (heart), ectatic (suffix added for adjective)
-edem-	Swell	Myoedema (muscle), lymphedema (lymph) (a is a suffix added to make a noun)
-esthes-	Feel	Esthesia (suffix added to make noun), anesthesia (an is a prefix)
-fiss-	Split	Fissure, fission (suffixes added to make nouns)
-flex-, -flec-	Bend	Flexion (suffix added to make noun), flexor (suffix added), anteflect (prefix added meaning "before" bending forward)
-flu-, -flux-	Flow	Fluctuate, fluxion, affluent (abundant flowing)
-geno-, -genesis-	Produce, origin	Genotype, homogenesis (same origin), pathogenesis (disease, origin of disease), heterogenesis (prefix added meaning "other," alteration of generation)
-iatro-, -iatr-	Treat, cure	Geriatrics (old age), pediatrics (children)
-kine-, -kino-, -kineto-, -kinesio	Move	Kinetogenic (producing movement), kinetic (suffix added to make adjective), kinesiology (study)
-liga-	Bind	Ligament (suffix added to make noun) ligate, ligature
-logy-	Study	Parasitology (parasites), bacteriology (bacteria), histology (tissues)
-lysis-	Breaking up, dissolving	Hemolysis (blood), glycolysis (sugar), autolysis (self-destruction of cells)
-morph-, -morpho-	Form	Morphology, amorphous (not definite form), pleomorphic (more, occurring in various forms), polymorphic (many)
-olfact-	Smell	Olfactophobia (fear), olfactory (suffix added to make adjective)
-op-, -opto-	See	Amblyopia (dull, dimness of vision), presbyopia (old, impairment of vision in old age), optic, myopia (myo, to wink, half close the eyes)
-palpit-	Flutter	Palpitation
-par-, -partus-	Labor	Postpartum (after birth), parturition (act of giving birth) (NOTE: para I, II, III, IV, etc., are symbols for number of births.)
-pep-	Digest	Dyspepsia (bad, difficult), peptic (suffix added to make adjective)
-pexy-	Fix	Mastopexy (fixation of breast), nephrosplenopexy (surgical fixation of kidney and spleen)
-phag-, -phago-	Eat	Phagocytosis (eating of cells), phagomania (madness, mad craving for food or to eat), dysphagia (difficult eating or swallowing)
-phan-	Appear, visible	Phanerosis (act of becoming visible), phantasia, phantasy
-phas-	Speak, utter	Aphasia (unable to speak), dysphasia (difficulty in speaking)
-phil-	Like, love	Hemophilia (blood, a hereditary disease characterized by delayed clotting of blood), acidophilia (acid stain, liking or straining with acid stains), philanthropy (love of mankind)
-phobia-	Fear	Hydrophobia (fear of water), photophobia (fear of light), claustrophobia (closeness, fear of close places)
-phrax-, -phrag-	Fence off, wall off	Diaphragm (across, partition separating thorax from abdomen), phragmoplast (formed)
-plas-	Form, grow	Neoplasm (new growth), rhinoplasty (nose operation for formation of nose), otoplasty (ear), choledochoplasty (common bile duct)
-plegia-	Paralyze	Paraplegia (paralysis of lower limbs), ophthalmoplegia (eye), hemiplegia (partial paralysis)

-pne-, -pneo-	Breathe	*Dyspnea* (difficult breathing), *apnea* (lack of breathing), *hyperpnea* (overbreathing)
-poie-	Make	*Hemato*poiesis (blood), *erythro*poiesis (red blood cells), *leuko*poiesis (making white cells)
-ptosis-	Fall	*Procto*ptosis (anus, prolapse of anus), *splanchno*ptosis (viscera)
-rrhagia-	Burst forth, pour	Meno*rrhagia* (abnormal bleeding during menstruation), *menometro*rrhagia (abnormal uterine bleeding), *hemo*rrhage (blood)
-rrhaphy-	Suture	*Hernio*rrhaphy (suturing or repair of hernia), *hepato*rrhaphy (liver), *nephro*rrhaphy (kidney)
-rrhea-	Flow, discharge	*Leuko*rrhea (white discharge from vagina), *galacto*rrhea (milk discharge), *rhino*rrhea (nasal discharge)
-rrhexis-	Rupture	*Entero*rrhexis (intestines), *metro*rrhexis (uterus)
-schiz-	Split, divide	Schizo*phrenia* (mind, split personality), schiz*onychia* (nails), schizo*trichia* (hair)
-scope-	Examine	*Micro*scopic, *cardio*scope, *endo*scope (*endo* means "within," an instrument for examining the interior of a hollow internal organ)
-stasis-	Stop, stand still	*Hemato*static (pertaining to stagnation of blood), *epi*stasis (checking or stopping of any discharge)
-stazien-	Drop	*Epi*staxis (nosebleed)
-teg-, -tect-	Cover	Teg*men*, tect*um* (rooflike structure), *in*tegu*ment* (skin covering)
-therap-	Treat, cure	Therapy, *neuro*therapy (nerves), *chemo*therapy (chemicals), *physio*therapy
-tomy-	Cut, incise	*Phlebo*tomy (incision of vein), *arthro*tomy (joint), *appendec*tomy (*ectomy*, meaning "cutout," excision of appendix), *oophorec*tomy (excision of ovary), *ileoceco*stomy (*ostomy*, meaning "creation of an artifical opening," *os*, meaning "opening or mouth"; ileocecostomy is an anatomosis of ileum and cecum)
-topo-	Place	Topo*graphy*, topo*narcosis* (numbing, hence numbing of a part or localized anesthesia)
-tropho-	Nourish	*Hyper*trophy (enlargement or overnourishment), *a*trophy (undernourishment), *dys*trophy (difficult or bad)
-volv-	Turn	*In*volution, volv*ulus* (twisting of an organ, as in intestinal obstruction with twisting of the bowel or twisting of the esophagus)

The following roots and combining forms are derived from Greek or Latin adjectives. Adjectives appear most often in compounds and are joined to nouns or verbs. Suffixes may be added to make them into nouns.

In the following examples, the part or root of the word that the adjective modifies is italicized, and the meaning, if not clear, is given in parentheses:

Root	*Translation*	*Examples*
-auto-	Self	Auto*infection*, auto*lysis*, auto*pathy* (disease), auto*psy* (view, postmortem examination)
-brachy-	Short	Brachy*cephalia* (head), brachy*dactylia* (fingers), brachy*chelia* (lip), brachy*gnathous* (jaw)
-brady-	Slow	Brady*pnea* (breath), brady*pragia* (action), brady*uria* (urine), brady*pepsia* (digestion)
-brevis-	Short	Brevi*ty*, brevi*flexor* (short flexor muscle)
-cavus-	Hollow	Cavi*ty*, cave*rnous*, *vena* cava (vein)
-coel-	Hollow	Coel*arium* (lining membrane of body cavity), coel*om* (body cavity of embryo)
-cryo-	Cold	Cryo*therapy*, cryo*tolerant*, cryo*meter*

-crypto-	Hidden, concealed	Crypt*orchid* (testis), crypto*genic* (origin obscure or doubtful), crypto*phthalmos* (eye)
-dextro-	Right	*Ambi*dextrous (using both hands with equal ease), dextro*phobia* (fear of objects on right side), dextro*cardia* (heart)
-dys-	Difficult, bad, disordered, painful	Dys*arthria* (speech), dys*hidrosis* (sweat), dys*kinesia* (motion), dys*tocia* (birth), dys*phasia* (speech), dys*pepsia* (digestion)
-eu-	Well, good	Eu*phoria* (well-being), eu*phagia,* eu*pnea* (breath), eu*thyroid* (normal thyroid), eu*tocia* (normal birth)
-eury-	Broad, wide	Eury*cephalic* (head), eury*opia* (vision), eury*somatic* (body, squat thickset body)
-glyco-	Sugar, sweet	Glyco*hemia* (sugar in blood), glyco*penia* (poverty of sugar, low blood sugar level)
-gravis-	Heavy	Gravid*a* (pregnant woman), gravid*ism* (pregnancy)
-haplo-	Single, simple	Haplo*id* (having a single set of chromosomes), haplo*dont* (teeth without simple crowns), haplo*pathy* (simple, uncomplicated disease)
-hetero-	Other, different	Hetero*geneous* (kind, dissimilar elements), hetero*inoculation,* hetero*logy* (abnormality of structure), hetero*intoxication*
-homo-	Same	Homo*geneous* (same kind or quality throughout), homo*zygous* (possessing identical pair of genes), homo*logous* (corresponding in structure)
-hydro-	Wet, water	Hydro*nephrosis* (kidney, collection of urine in kidney pelvis), hydro*pneumothorax* (fluid in chest), hydro*phobia* (fear of water, water causes painful reaction in this disease)
-iso-	Equal	Iso*cellular* (similar cells), iso*dontic* (all teeth alike), iso*cytosis* (equality of size of cells), iso*chromatic* (having same color throughout)
-latus-	Broad	Lati*tude,* latiss*imus* dorsi (muscle adducting humerus)
-leio-	Smooth	Leio*myosarcoma* (smooth muscle, fleshy malignant tumor), leio*myofibroma* (tumor of muscle and fiber elements), leio*myoma* (tumor of unstriped muscle)
-lepto-	Slender	Lepto*somatic* (body), lepto*dactylous* (fingers)
-levo-	Left	Levo*cardia* (heart), levo*rotation* (turning to left)
-longus-	Long	*Adductor* longus (muscle of thigh), longi*tude*
-macro-	Large, abnormal size	Maco*cephalic* (head), macro*cheiria* (hands), macro*mastia* (breast), macro*nychia* (nails)
-magna-	Large, great	Magni*tude, adductor* magnus (thigh muscle)
-malaco-	Soft	Malac*ia* (softening), *osteo*malac*ia* (bones)
-malus-	Bad	Mal*ady,* mal*aise,* mal*ignant,* mal*formation*
-medius-	Middle	Median, medium, *gluteus* medius (femur muscle)
-mega-	Great	Mega*colon* (large colon), mega*cephaly* (head)
-megalo-	Huge	Megalo*mania* (delusion of grandeur), *hepato*megaly (enlarged liver), *spleno*megaly (enlarged spleen)
-meso-	Middle, mid	Meso*carpal* (wrist), meso*derm* (skin), meso*thelium* (a lining membrane of cavities)
-micro-	Small	Micro*glossia* (tongue), micro*blepharia* (eyelids), micro*organism,* micro*phonia* (voice)
-minimus-	Smallest	*Gluteus* minimus (smallest muscle of hip), *adductor* minimus (muscle of thigh)
-mio-	Less	Mio*lecithal* (egg with little yolk), mio*pragia* (perform, decreased activity)
-mono-	One, single, limited to one part	Mono*chromatic* (color), mono*brachia* (arm)
-multi-	Many, much	Multi*para* (bear, woman who has borne many children), multi*lobar* (numerous lobes), multi*centric* (many centers)
-necro-	Dead	Necro*sed,* necro*sis,* necro*psy* (postmortem examination), necro*phobia* (fear of death)
-neo-	New	Neo*formation,* neo*morphism* (form), neo*natal* (first 4 weeks of life), neo*pathy* (disease)

-oligo-	Few, scanty, little	Oligo*phrenia* (mind), oligo*pnea* (breath), oli*guria* (urine), oligo*dipsia* (thirst)
-ortho-	Straight, normal, correct	Ortho*dontic* (teeth, normal), ortho*genesis* (progressive evolution in a given direction), ortho*grade* (walk, carrying body upright), ortho*pnea* (breath, unable to breathe unless in an upright position)
-oxy-	Sharp, quick	Oxy*esthesia* (feel), oxy*opia* (vision), oxy*osmia* (smell)
-pachy-	Thick	Pachy*derm* (skin), pachy*sulemia* (blood), pachy*pleuritis* (inflammation of pleura), pachy*cholia* (bile), pachy*otia* (ears)
-paleo-	Old	Paleo*genetic* (origin in the past), paleo*pathology* (study of diseases in mummies)
-platy-	Flat	Platy*basia* (skull base), platy*coria* (pupil), platy*crania* (skull)
-pleo-	More	Pleo*morphism* (forms), pleo*chromocytoma* (tumor composed of different colored cells)
-poikilo-	Varied	Poikilo*derma* (skin mottling), poikilo*thermal* (heat, variable body temperature)
-poly-	Many, much	Poly*hedral* (many bases or faces), poly*mastia* (more than two breasts), poly*melia* (supernumerary limbs), poly*myalgia* (pain in many muscles)
-pronus-	Face down	Prone, pron*ation*
-pseudo-	False, spurious	Pseudo*stratified* (layered), pseudo*cirrhosis* (apparent cirrhosis of liver), pseudo*hypertrophy*
-sclero-	Hard	Scler*osis* (hardening), *arterio*sclerosis (artery), sclero*nychia* (nails), sclero*derma* (skin)
-scolio-	Twisted, crooked	Scolio*dontic* (teeth), scoli*osis*, scolio*kyphosis* (curvature of spine)
-sinistro-	Left	Sinistro*cardia*, sinistro*manual* (left handed), sinistr*aural* (hearing better in left ear)
-steno-	Narrow	Sten*osis*, steno*stomia* (mouth), mitral sten*osis* (mitral valve in heart)
-stereo-	Solid, three dimensions	Stereo*scope*, stereo*meter*
-supinus-	Face up	Supine, supin*ation*, supin*ator* longus (muscle in arm)
-tachy-	Fast, swift	Tachy*cardia* (heart), tachy*phrasia* (speech)
-tele-	End, far away	Tele*pathy*, tele*cardiogram*
-telo-	Complete	Telo*phase*
-thermo-	Heat, warm	Therm*al*, thermo*meter*, thermo*biosis* (ability to live in high temperature)
-trachy-	Rough	Trachy*phonia* (voice), trachy*chromatic* (deeply staining)
-xero-	Dry	Xero*phagia* (eating of dry foods) xero*stomia* (mouth), xero*derma* (skin)

PRONUNCIATION OF MEDICAL-DENTAL TERMS

Medical terms are hard to pronounce, especially if a person has read them but never heard them spoken. Following are some helpful shortcuts:

ch is sometimes pronounced like *k*. Examples: chromatin, chronic.
ps is pronounced like *s*. Examples: psychiatry, psychology.
pn is pronounced with only the *n* sound. Example: pneumonia.
c and *g* are given the soft sound of *s* and *j*, respectively, before *e*, *i*, and *y* in words of both Greek and Latin origin. Examples: cycle, cytoplasm, giant, generic.
c and *g* have a harsh sound before other letters. Examples: gastric, gonad, cast, cardiac.
ae and *oe* are pronounced *ee*. Examples: coelom, fasciae.
i at the end of a word (to form a plural) is pronounced *eye*. Examples: alveoli, glomeruli, fasciculi.
e and *es*, when forming the final letters or letter of a word, are often pronounced as separate syllables. Examples: rete (reetee), nares (nayreez).

PLURALS

In most English words the plurals are formed by merely adding an *s* or *es,* but in Greek and Latin the plural may be designated by changing the ending.

- *-ae,* as in fasciae (singular form, fascia). *-ia,* as in crania (singular form, cranium).
- *-i,* as in glomeruli (singular form, glomerulus). When the singular form ends in *us,* the plural form is made by adding *i* and dropping the *us.*
- *-ata,* as in adenomata (singular form, adenoma).

SPELLING

The aforementioned rules for pronunciation and the formation of plurals are essential for spelling, but the professional should consult a medical dictionary if unsure. Phonetic spelling has no place in medicine, because a misspelled word may give the wrong meaning to a diagnosis. Furthermore, some terms are pronounced alike but spelled differently; for example, ileum is a part of the intestinal tract, but ilium is a pelvic bone.

APPENDIX J

Nutrition and Nutritional Counseling

Table J-1 Body Mass Index classification chart

	Obesity class	*Body Mass Index (BMI) (1 kg/m^2)*
Underweight	—	<18.5
Normal	—	18.5-24.9
Overweight	—	25.0-25.9
Obesity	I	30.3-34.9
	II	35.0-39.9
Extreme obesity	III	>40

Adapted from National Institutes of Health: *Clinical guidelines on the identification, evaluation, and treatment of overweight and obesity in adults: Obesity Initiative.* Washington, DC, 1998, NIH.

Table J-2 Effects of nutrients on oral tissues and their role in tooth formation

Nutrients	*Effects on oral soft and hard tissue*	*Role in tooth formation*
Vitamin A	• Synthesis and function of epithelial cells • Maintenance of the integrity of the sulcus • Normal growth and function of salivary glands • Essential for activity of epiphyseal cartilage cells and normal endochondral bone growth	• Normal growth of dentin and enamel • Normal growth of periodontal tissues and maintenance of epithelium
Vitamin D	• No effects noted	• Controls calcification of dentin and enamel by regulating calcium absorption at the intestines
Vitamin C	• Synthesis of connective tissue • Essential for integrity of capillaries and oral mucosa • Needed for normal bone matrix formation • Needed for normal phagocytic function and antibody synthesis in host defense system	• Integrity of blood vessels in gingival and pulpal tissues • Hydroxylation of proline and lysine in collagen synthesis • Normal formation of dentin
B-complex vitamins		
Niacin	• Integrity of oral tissues	• No effects noted
Folacin	• Normal synthesis of protein compounds in oral tissues (e.g., hemoglobin and enzymes)	• No effects noted
Thiamin	• Normal energy metabolism during development and maintenance of oral tissue	• No effects noted
Riboflavin	• Energy metabolism of oral tissues	• No effects noted
Pyridoxine	• Normal carbohydrate metabolism and hemoglobin synthesis in oral tissues	• No effects noted
Cobalamin	• Integrity of nerve tissue and normal red blood cell formation in oral tissues	• No effects noted
Calcium: phosphorus ratio	• No effects noted	• Normal tooth and bone mineralization
Fluoride	• No effects noted	• Forms dentin and enamel
Iron	• Normal hemoglobin formation and carbon dioxide transport to tissue	• No effects noted
Fiber	• Stimulates salivary flow and maintains integrity of periodontal tissues	• No effects noted
Protein	• Synthesis of antibodies and leukocytes • Synthesis of epithelial and connective tissues in the healing process • Maintains integrity of periodontal tissues	• Formation of matrix of dentin and enamel • Collagen formation

Data from DePaola DP, Faine MP, Palmer CA: Nutrition in relation to dental medicine. *In* Shils ME, et al (eds): *Modern nutrition in health and disease,* ed 9, Baltimore, 1998, Williams & Wilkins, p 1114; *and from* Lee M, Stanmeyer W, Weght A: *Nutrition and dental health.* Chapel Hill, 1982, Health Sciences Consortium.

Table J-3 Dietary Reference intake, adequate intake, and tolerable upper limits of nutrients specific to bone health

Nutrient	*Dietary Reference Intake (DRI)/Recommended Dietary Allowance (RDA)§*	*Therapeutic range‡ (adequate intake)*	*Tolerable upper limit*
Calcium (g/d)	—	*210-1300	2.5 for children and adults
Phosphorous (g/d)	460-1250 for most healthy children and adults	*100-275	†3-4 for healthy individuals
Magnesium (mg/d)	80-420 for most healthy children and adults	*30-75	†65-350 for healthy individuals
Vitamin D (μg/d)	—	*5-15	†25-50 for healthy individuals
Fluoride (mg/d)	—	*0.01-4	†0.7-10 for healthy individuals

From Darby ML: *Mosby's comprehensive review of dental hygiene,* ed 5, St Louis, 2002, Mosby.

*Lower number represents the adequate intake for infants and children, and the higher range of numbers will vary depending on life stage and gender group. Refer to the National Academy Press website (http://www.nap/edu/info/browse.htm) for more in-depth information. The therapeutic range, also referred to as adequate intake, is the dose at which there may be physiologic benefits for healthy individuals and decreased risk for toxicity.

†Lower number represents upper limit for infants and children, and higher number represents upper limit for males and females (pregnant and lactating). The tolerable upper limit is the highest level of daily nutrient intake that is likely to pose no risk of adverse health effects.

‡Adequate intake (AI), also known as a therapeutic range, is the mean intake for healthy individuals that is used when an RDA cannot be determined.

§Recommended dietary allowance values meet the needs of 97% of individuals in a group. Daily reference intake values are groups of values that provide quantitative estimates of nutrient intake for planning and assessing diets for all healthy individuals.

APPENDIX K

Pharmacology

Box K-1 Formulas for drug calculations

Surface area rule:

$$\text{Child dose} = \frac{\text{Surface area (m}^2\text{)}}{1.73\ \text{m}^2} \times \text{Adult dose}$$

Calculating strength of a solution:

Solution Strength: *Desired Solution:*

$$\frac{x}{100} = \frac{\text{Amount of drug desired}}{\text{Amount of finished solution}}$$

Calculating flow rate for IV:

$$\text{Rate of flow} = \frac{\text{Amount of fluid} \times \text{Administration set calibration}}{\text{Running time}}$$

$$\frac{x}{1} = \frac{\text{(ml) (gtt/min)}}{\text{min}}$$

Calculation of medication dosages:
Formula method:

$$\frac{\text{Amount ordered}}{\text{Amount on hand}} \times \text{Vehicle} = \text{Number of tablets, capsules, or amount of liquid}$$

Vehicle is the drug form or amount of liquid containing the dosage. Amounts used in calculation by formula must be in same system.

Ratio-proportion method:
1 tablet:tablet in mg on hand::x tablet order in mg
Know or have::Want to know or order

Multiply means and extremes, divide both sides by known amount to get x. Amounts used in equation must be in same system.

Dimensional analysis method:

$$\text{Order in mg} \times \frac{\text{1 tablet or capsule}}{\text{What 1 tablet or capsule is in mg}} = \text{Tablets or capsules to be given}$$

If amounts are in different systems:

$$\text{Order in mg} \times \frac{\text{1 tablet or capsule}}{\text{What 1 tablet or capsule is in g}} \times \frac{1}{\text{1000 mg}} = \text{Tablets or capsules to be given}$$

From Skidmore-Roth L: *Mosby's 2006 nursing drug reference,* St Louis, 2006, Mosby.

Table K-1 Common abbreviations used in writing prescriptions

Abbreviation	*Derivation*	*Meaning*	*Abbreviation*	*Derivation*	*Meaning*
āā	ana	of each	o.m.	omni mane	every morning
a.	ante	before	o.n.	omni nocte	every night
a.c.	ante cibum	before meals	o.s.	oculus sinister	left eye
ad	ad	to, up to	os	os	mouth
A.D.	auris dextra	right ear	o.u.	oculus uterque	each eye
ad lib.	ad libitum	freely as desired	oz	uncia	ounce
agit. ante sum.	agitare ante	shake before taking	p.c.	post cibum	after meals
A.L.	auris laeva	left ear	per	per	through or by
alt. dieb.	alternis diebus	every other day	pil.	pilula	pill
alt. hor.	alternis horis	alternate hours	p.o.	per os	orally
alt. noct.	alternis noctibus	alternate nights	p.r.		by rectum
aq.	aqua	water	p.r.n.	pro re nata	when required
aq. dest.	aqua destillata	distilled water	q	quaque	every
b.i.d.	bis in die	two times a day	q.d.	quaque die	every day
b.i.n.	bis in nocte	two times a night	q.h.	quaque hora	every hour
c., c̄	cum	with	q. 2 h.		every 2 hours
Cap.	capiat	let him take	q. 3 h.		every 3 hours
caps.	capsula	capsule	q. 4 h.		every 4 hours
c.m.s.	cras mane sumendus	to be taken tomorrow morning	q. 6 h.		every 6 hours
c.n.	cras nocte	tomorrow night	q.i.d.	quater in die	four times a day
c.n.s.	cras nocte sumendus	to be taken tomorrow night	q.o.d.		every other day
comp.	compositus	compound	q.l.	quantum libet	as much as desired
Det.	detur	let it be given	q.n.	quaque nocte	every night

Dieb. tert.	diebus tertiis	every third day
dil.	dilutus	dilute
elix.	elixir	elixir
ext.	extractum	extract
fld.	fluidus	fluid
Ft.	fiat	make
g	gramme	gram
gr	granum	grain
gt	gutta	a drop
gtt	guttae	drops
h.	hora	hour
h.d.	hora decubitus	at bedtime
h.s.	hora somni	hour of sleep (bedtime)
M.	misce	mix
m.	minimum	a minim
mist.	mistura	mixture
non rep.	non repetatur	not to be repeated
noct.	nocte	in the night
O	octarius	pint
o.d.	oculus dexter	right eye
ol.	oleum	oil
o.d.	omni die	every day
o.h.	omni hora	every hour
q.p.	quantum placeat	as much as desired
q.v.	quantum vis	as much as you please
q.s.	quantum sufficit	as much as is required
℞	recipe	take
Rep.	repetatur	let it be repeated
s, s̄	sine	without
seq. luce.	sequenti luce	the following day
Sig. or S.	signa	write on label
sl.		sublingual
s.o.s.	si opus sit	if necessary
sp.	spiritus	spirits
supp.		suppository
ss	semis	a half
stat.	statim	immediately
syr.	syrupus	syrup
t.d.s.	ter die sumendum	to be taken three times daily
t.i.d.	ter in die	three times a day
t.i.n.	ter in nocte	three times a night
tr. or tinct.	tinctura	tincture
ung.	unguentum	ointment
ut. dict. or u.d.	ut dictum	as directed
vin.	vini	of wine

Adapted from *Mosby's dictionary of medicine, nursing, and health professions,* ed 7, St Louis, 2006, Mosby. Daniel SJ, Harfst SA: *Mosby's dental hygiene: Concepts, cases, and competencies,* St Louis, 2002, Mosby.

Table K-2 Use of drugs in pediatric dentistry

Drug	*Route*	*Dose*	*Frequency*	*Notes*
Antibiotics				
Amoxycillin	PO	25-50 mg/kg/day	tds	Syrup or chewable tablets for young children
	IV	100-400 mg/kg/day	tds	
	PO, IV	50 mg/kg up to adult dose 2 g	1 hour before	Endocarditis prophylaxis, parenteral use in susceptible patients
Amoxycillin plus clavulanic acid	PO	20-40 mg/kg/day	tds	For beta-lactam-resistant organisms only
Ampicillin	IV	50-100 mg/kg/day	qid	
	IV	50 mg/kg up to adult dose 2 g	stat	Endocarditis prophylaxis
Benzylpenicillin	IV	15-350 mg/kg/day 20,000-500,000 U/kg/day	qid	First IV drug of choice for odontogenic infections
Penicillin VK	PO	<5 years 500 mg/day >5 years 1-2 g/day	qid	Give 1 hour before meals
Cephalexin	PO	25-50 mg/kg/day	qid	
Cephalothin IV	IV	40-80 mg/kg/day	qid	Not for use in pregnancy
Erythromycin	PO	25-40 mg/kg/day	qid	Ethylsuccinate is readily absorbed
Metronidazole	IV	22.5 mg/kg/day	tds	Not for use in pregnancy
	PO	10-15 mg/kg/day	tds	
Gentamicin	IV	1.5 mg/kg (children) up to 120 mg maximum	stat	Endocarditis prophylaxis in highly susceptible patients in conjunction with ampicillin. Follow-up dose of ampicillin or amoxycillin required 6 hours later

Clindamycin	PO, IV	15-40 mg/kg/day	qid	Risk of pseudomembranous colitis
	PO, IV	10 mg/kg up to adult dose 600 mg	oral 1 hour before IV stat	Endocarditis prophylaxis in susceptible patients
Vancomycin	IV	20 mg/kg up to adult dose 1 g	infused over 1 hour	Endocarditis prophylaxis, susceptible patients allergic to penicillin
Antifungals				
Nystatin	Tablets	500,000 U	tds	Nilstat, Mycostatin
	Mixture	100,000 U/mL	6-hrly	Apply to affected area
Amphotericin B	Lozenges	10 mg	6-hrly	Apply to affected area Fungilin
	Suspension	100 mg/mL	6-hrly	Apply to affected area
	Ointment	3%	6-hrly	Apply to affected area
Analgesics and sedatives				
Aspirin				Should not be used in children under 12 years of age because of the risk of Reye's syndrome
Paracetamol	PO, PR	15 mg/kg	4-hrly	Hepatotoxic if overdose
Codeine phosphate	PO	1-1.5 mg/kg single dose 1-3 mg/kg/day	4-6 divided doses	Similar side effects to narcotics, including nausea and constipation
Pethidine	IV, IM	1 mg/kg	3-4 hrly	Maximum 100 mg
Morphine	IV, IM	0.1-0.2 mg/kg	6-hrly	Should only be used in hospitalized patients
Naloxone	IM, IV	1-10 μg/kg	stat	May be repeated at 2-3-minute intervals if necessary
Midazolam	PO	0.3 mg/kg	single dose	Sedation, may be given intranasally
	PN	0.2 mg/kg		
	IV, IM	0.1-0.2 mg/kg		
Chloral hydrate	PO	30-50 mg/kg/day, 15-20 mg/kg single dose	4-6 hrly	Sedation

Continued

Table K-2 Use of drugs in pediatric dentistry—cont'd

Drug	*Route*	*Dose*	*Frequency*	*Notes*
Analgesics and sedatives				
Trimeprazine	PO	3-4 mg/kg	single dose	Vallergan, sedation
Metoclopramide	PO, IM	3-5 years 2 mg 5-9 years 2.5 mg 9-14 years 5 mg 15-19 years 10 mg	single dose	Single dose after narcotic if vomiting or nausea. Dystonic reactions may occur
Other medications				
Kenalog in Orabase	Ointment	Triamcinolone 0.1%	4-6 hrly	Recurrent severe oral ulceration in children, apply to ulcer but do not rub ointment in
ε aminocaproic acid	IV	30 mg/kg		Antifibrinolytic, loading dose of 100 mg/kg
Tranexamic acid	PO	15-20 mg/kg	qid	Antifibrinolytic
DDAVP	IV	0.3 μg/kg		Infused over 1 hour before surgery
Heparin	IV	50-100 U/kg	4-6 hrly	Anticoagulant
Tetanus toxoid	IM	0.5 mL	single dose	If immunization protocol not complete, course should be given. Otherwise, a booster may be required for tetanus-prone wounds if >2 years since last booster

Adapted from Cameron AC, Widmer RP: *Handbook of pediatric dentistry,* ed 2, London, 2003, Mosby.

The table that forms Table K-2 is a guide to the administration of commonly used drugs in pediatric dentistry. Medications for children should always be prescribed in relation to weight. It is of utmost importance that clinicians understand the contraindications and precautions relevant to the drugs they are prescribing and should consult prescribing information supplied by the pharmaceutical manufacturers and relevant pharmacopeia. In the table, PO = oral, IV = intravenous, IM = intramuscular, tds = ×3 daily, qid = ×4 daily, and stat = immediately.

APPENDIX L

Radiology and Radiography

Box L-1 Criteria for intraoral radiographs*

1. The radiograph should show proper definition and detail and a degree of density and contrast so that all structures can be delineated easily.
2. The structures should not be distorted either by elongation or by foreshortening.
3. The radiograph should show the teeth from the occlusal or incisal edges to 2 to 3 mm beyond their apices.
4. In a full-mouth survey, the entire alveolar processes of the mandible and maxilla must be seen—as far distal as the tuberosity in the maxilla and the beginning of the ascending ramus in the mandible.
5. All interproximal surfaces of the teeth should be seen without overlapping, providing the teeth are not overlapped in the mouth.
6. The x-ray beam should be centered on the film so that there are no unexposed parts of the film ("cone cuts" or "collimator cutoff").
7. The radiograph should not be cracked or bent or have any other artifacts.
8. The radiograph should be processed properly.

Box L-2 Time and temperature chart*

Temperature of Developer	Time in Developer
80° F	2½ minutes
75° F	3 minutes
70° F	4 minutes (optimum)
68° F	4½ minutes
60° F	6 minutes

*From Frommer HH, Stabulas-Savage II: *Radiology for the dental professional,* ed 8, St Louis, 2005, Mosby.

Table L-1 Guidelines for prescribing dental radiographs

The recommendations in this chart are subject to clinical judgment and may not apply to every patient. They are to be used by dentists only after reviewing the patient's health history and completing a clinical examination. Because every precaution should be taken to minimize radiation exposure, protective thyroid collars and aprons should be used whenever possible. This practice is strongly recommended for children, women of childbearing age, and pregnant women.

	Patient age and dental developmental stage				
Type of encounter	***Child with primary dentition*** *(prior to eruption of first permanent tooth)*	***Child with transitional dentition*** *(after eruption of first permanent tooth)*	***Adolescent with permanent dentition*** *(prior to eruption of third molars)*	***Adult, dentate or partially edentulous***	***Adult, edentulous***
New patient* being evaluated for dental diseases and dental development	Individualized radiographic exam consisting of selected periapical/occlusal views and/or posterior bitewings if proximal surfaces cannot be visualized or probed. Patients without evidence of disease and with open proximal contacts may not require a radiographic exam at this time.	Individualized radiographic exam consisting of posterior bitewings with panoramic exam or posterior bitewings and selected periapical images.	Individualized radiographic exam consisting of posterior bitewings with panoramic exam or posterior bitewings and selected periapical images. A full-mouth intraoral radiographic exam is preferred when the patient has clinical evidence of generalized dental disease or a history of extensive dental treatment.		Individualized radiographic exam, based on clinical signs and symptoms.
Recall patient* with clinical caries or at increased risk for caries[†]	Posterior bitewing exam at 6-12 month intervals if proximal surfaces cannot be examined visually or with a probe.			Posterior bitewing exam at 6-18 month intervals.	Not applicable.

Recall patient* with no clinical caries and not at increased risk for caries[†]	Posterior bitewing exam at 12-24 month intervals if proximal surfaces cannot be examined visually or with a probe.	Posterior bitewing exam at 18-36 month intervals.	Posterior bitewing exam at 24-36 month intervals.	Not applicable.
Recall patient* with periodontal disease	Clinical judgment as to the need for and type of radiographic images for the evaluation of periodontal disease. Imaging may consist of, but is not limited to, selected bitewing and/or periapical images of areas where periodontal disease (other than nonspecific gingivitis) can be identified clinically.			Not applicable.
Patient requiring monitoring of growth and development	Clinical judgment regarding need for and type of radiographic images for evaluation and/or monitoring of dentofacial growth and development.	Clinical judgment regarding need for and type of radiographic images for evaluation and/or monitoring of dentofacial growth and development. Panoramic or periapical exam to assess developing third molars.	Usually not indicated.	

Continued

Table L-1 Guidelines for prescribing dental radiographs—cont'd

	Patient age and dental developmental stage				
Type of encounter	***Child with primary dentition*** *(prior to eruption of first permanent tooth)*	***Child with transitional dentition*** *(after eruption of first permanent tooth)*	***Adolescent with permanent dentition*** *(prior to eruption of third molars)*	***Adult, dentate or partially edentulous***	***Adult, edentulous***
Patient with other circumstances, including but not limited to proposed or existing implants, pathology, restorative/endodontic needs, treated periodontal disease, and caries remineralization	Clinical judgment regarding need for and type of radiographic images for evaluation and/or monitoring in these circumstances.				

From American Dental Association, U.S. Food & Drug Administration: *The selection of patients for dental radiograph examinations.* Available on www.ada.org.

***Clinical situations for which radiographs may be indicated include but are not limited to:**

A. Positive Historical Findings

1. Previous periodontal or endodontic treatment
2. History of pain or trauma
3. Familial history of dental anomalies
4. Postoperative evaluation of healing
5. Remineralization monitoring
6. Presence of implants or evaluation for implant placement

B. Positive Clinical Signs/Symptoms

1. Clinical evidence of periodontal disease
2. Large or deep restorations
3. Deep carious lesions
4. Malposed or clinically impacted teeth
5. Swelling
6. Evidence of dental/facial trauma
7. Mobility of teeth
8. Sinus tract ("fistula")
9. Clinically suspected sinus pathology
10. Growth abnormalities
11. Oral involvement in known or suspected systemic disease
12. Positive neurologic findings in the head and neck
13. Evidence of foreign objects
14. Pain and/or dysfunction of the temporomandibular joint
15. Facial asymmetry
16. Abutment teeth for fixed or removable partial prosthesis
17. Unexplained bleeding
18. Unexplained sensitivity of teeth
19. Unusual eruption, spacing, or migration of teeth
20. Unusual tooth morphology, calcification or color
21. Unexplained absence of teeth
22. Clinical erosion

†Factors increasing risk for caries may include but are not limited to:

1. High level of caries experience or demineralization
2. History of recurrent caries
3. High titers of cariogenic bacteria
4. Existing restoration(s) of poor quality
5. Poor oral hygiene
6. Inadequate fluoride exposure
7. Prolonged nursing (bottle or breast)
8. Frequent high sucrose content in diet
9. Poor family dental health
10. Developmental or acquired enamel defects
11. Developmental or acquired disability
12. Xerostomia
13. Genetic abnormality of teeth
14. Many multisurface restorations
15. Chemotherapy or radiation therapy
16. Eating disorders
17. Drug/alcohol abuse
18. Irregular dental care

APPENDIX M

Tooth Numbering Systems and Explanation for Mounting Radiographs

TOOTH NUMBERING

According to a resolution passed by the 1968 American Dental Association (ADA) House of Delegates, teeth should be numbered as follows:

Permanent Dentition

Permanent teeth should be numbered from 1 to 32, starting with the patient's upper right third molar (1), following around the upper arch to the patient's upper left third molar (16), descending to the patient's lower left third molar (17), and following around the lower arch to the patient's lower right third molar (32).

Primary Dentition

In the same manner as described for permanent dentition, primary teeth should be lettered with uppercase letters A through T, with A being the patient's upper right second primary molar and T being the patient's lower right second primary molar.

MOUNTING RADIOGRAPHS

According to the same resolution from the 1968 ADA House of Delegates, radiographs should be mounted as follows:

Looking at the teeth from outside the mouth, radiographs should be viewed in the same manner, and so mounted.

NOTE: The raised dot in the film should be toward you when mounting radiographs.

PERMANENT DENTITION

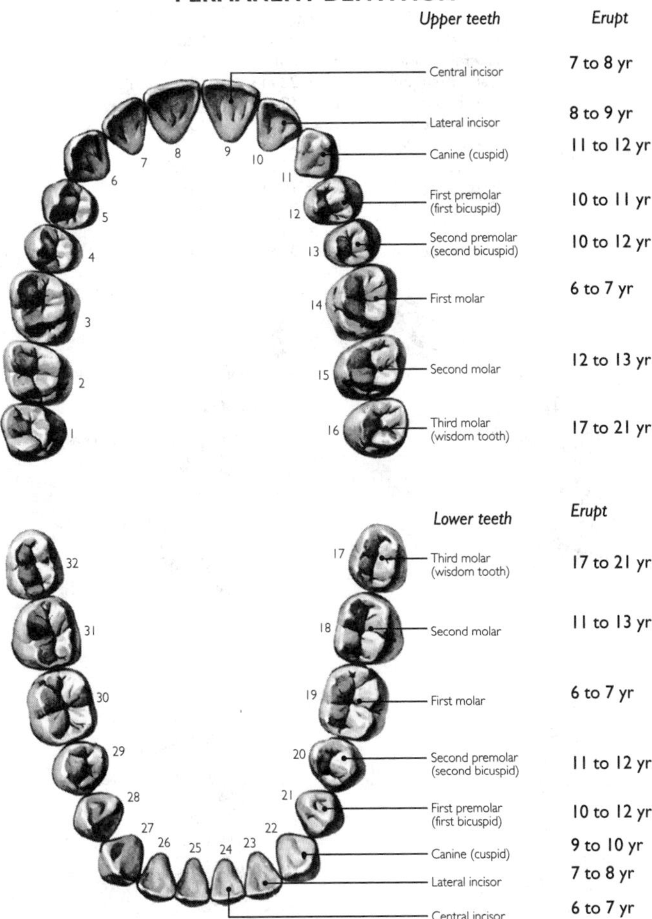

Universal Numbering System.

PRIMARY DENTITION

Upper teeth	*Erupt*	*Shed*
Central incisor	8 to 12 mo	6 to 7 yr
Lateral incisor	9 to 13 mo	7 to 8 yr
Canine (cuspid)	16 to 22 mo	10 to 12 yr
First molar	13 to 19 mo	9 to 11 yr
Second molar	25 to 33 mo	10 to 12 yr
Lower teeth	*Erupt*	*Shed*
Second molar	23 to 31 mo	10 to 12 yr
First molar	14 to 18 mo	9 to 11 yr
Canine (cuspid)	17 to 23 mo	9 to 12 yr
Lateral incisor	10 to 16 mo	7 to 8 yr
Central incisor	6 to 10 mo	6 to 7 yr

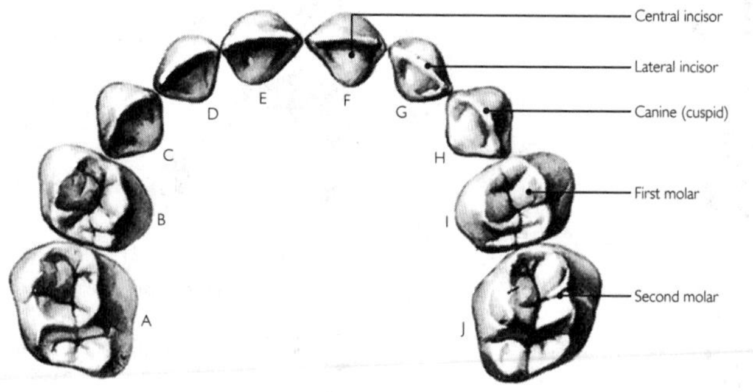

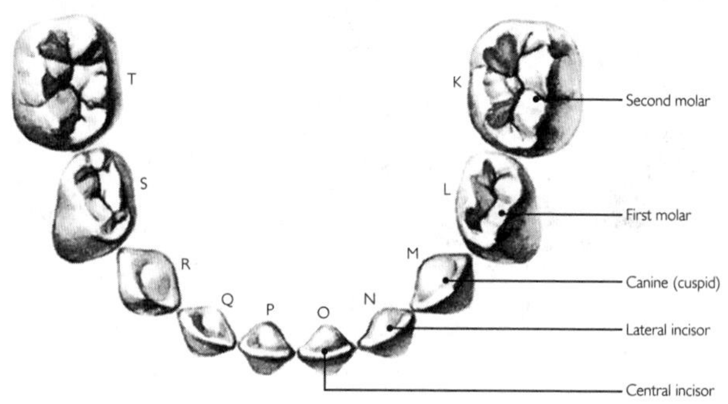

Universal Numbering System.

APPENDIX N

Implant Prosthetics

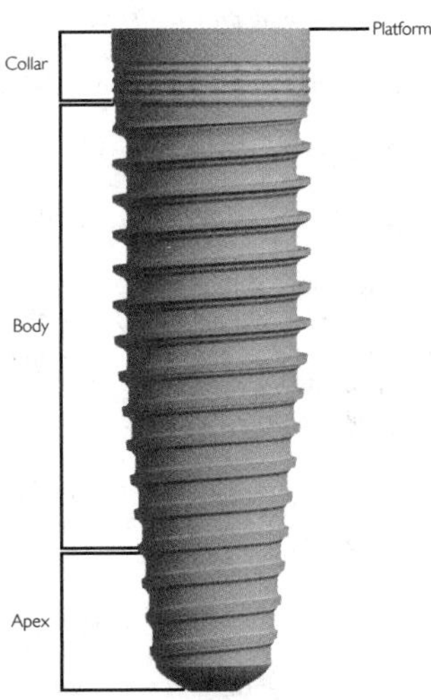

Fig. N-1. Implant body. The portion of the dental implant designed to be placed into the bone to anchor prosthetic components. The implant body has a platform, collar, body, and apex.

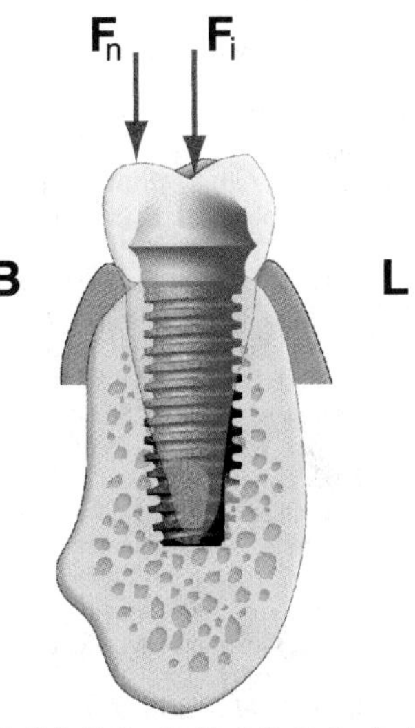

Fig. N-2. Ideal occlusal load. The ideal occlusal load on an implant prosthesis is direct over the implant body and is accomplished with a cemented prosthesis (F_i). When a screw hole is placed to retain the restoration, the primary occlusal contact is often located on the buccal cusp in the mandible (F_n), which is an offset load that magnifies the force applied to the implant component interfaces (and fixation screw). *B,* Buccal; *L,* lingual.

Table N-1 Terminology for implant failure

	Time	*Cause*
Surgical failure	Stage I surgery	Surgical complication
Osseous healing failure	Healing phase to Stage II	Trauma (heat-surgery) healing micromotion, infection
Early loading failure	First year prosthetic loading (transitional prosthesis)	Overload/bacteria
Intermediate failure	Year 1 until year 5 in function	Overload/bacteria
Late failure	Year 5 until year 10 in function	—
Long-term failure	>10 years in function	—

From Misch CE: *Dental implant prosthetics*, St. Louis, 2005, Mosby.

Illustration Credits

Applegate EJ: *The anatomy and physiology learning system,* ed 3, Philadelphia, 2006, Saunders.

Bath-Balogh M, Fehrenbach MJ: *Illustrated dental embryology, histology, and anatomy,* ed 2, St. Louis, 2006, Saunders.

Bird DL, Robinson DS: *Torres & Ehrlich modern dental assisting,* ed 8, St Louis, 2005 Saunders.

Boyd LB: *Dental instruments: a pocket guide,* ed 2, St. Louis, 2005, Saunders.

Callen PW (ed): *Ultrasonography in obstetrics and gynecology,* ed 4, Philadelphia, 2000, Saunders.

Cameron AC, Widmer RP: *Handbook of pediatric dentistry,* ed 2, London, 2003, Mosby International Ltd.

Chester GA: *Modern medical assisting,* Philadelphia, 1998, Saunders.

Christensen GJ: *A consumer's guide to dentistry,* ed 2, St Louis, 2002, Mosby.

Daniel SJ, Harfst SA, Wilder R: *Mosby's dental hygiene: concepts, cases and competencies,* ed 2, St Louis, 2008, Mosby.

Darby ML, Walsh MM: *Dental hygiene: theory and practice,* ed 2, St. Louis, 2003, Sanders.

Fehrenbach MJ, Herring SW: *Illustrated anatomy of the head and neck,* ed 3, St. Louis, 2007, Saunders.

Frommer HH, Stabulas-Savage JJ: *Radiology for the dental professional,* ed 8, St Louis, 2005, Mosby.

Genco RJ, Goldman HM, Cohen DW: *Contemporary periodontics,* St Louis, 1990, Mosby.

Habif TP: *Clinical dermatology: a color guide to diagnosis and therapy,* ed 4, St Louis, 2004, Mosby.

Iannucci J, Jansen Howerton L: *Dental radiography: principles and techniques,* ed 3, St. Louis, 2006, Saunders.

Ibsen OAC, Phelan JA: *Oral pathology for the dental hygienist,* ed 4, Philadelphia, 2004, Saunders.

Kerr DA, Ash MM, Millard HD: *Oral diagnosis,* ed 3, St Louis, 1983, Mosby.

Liebgott B: *The anatomical basis of dentistry,* ed 2, St Louis, 2001, Mosby.

Malamed SF: *Handbook of local anesthesia,* ed 5, St. Louis, 2004, Mosby.

Moore KL, Persaud TVN: *Before we are born: essentials of embryology and birth defects,* ed 6, Philadelphia, 2003, Saunders.

Neville BW, Damm DD, Allen CM, et al: *Oral & maxillofacial pathology,* ed 2, Philadelphia, 2002, Saunders.

Newman MG, Takei H, Klokkevold PR, Carranza FA: *Carranza's clinical periodontology,* ed 10, St. Louis, 2006, Saunders.

Perry DA, Beemsterboer PL: *Periodontology for the dental hygienist,* ed 3, St. Louis, 2007, Saunders.

Proffit WR, Fields HW, Sarver DM: *Contemporary orthodontics,* ed 4, St Louis, 2007, Mosby.

Proffit WR, White RP, Sarver DM: *Contemporary treatment of dentofacial deformity,* St Louis, 2003, Mosby.

Regezi JA, Sciubba JJ, Jordan RCK: *Oral pathology-clinical pathologic correlations,* ed 5, St Louis, 2008, Saunders.

Regezi JA, Sciubba JJ, Pogrel MA: *Atlas of oral and maxillofacial pathology,* Philadelphia, 2000, Saunders.

Roberson TM, Heymann HO, Swift EJ: *Sturdevant's art and science of operative dentistry,* ed 5, St Louis, 2006, Mosby.

Rosenstiel SF, Land MF, Fujimoto J: *Contemporary fixed prosthodontics,* ed 4, St Louis, 2006, Mosby.

Sapp JP, Wysocki GP, Eversole LR: *Contemporary oral and maxillofacial pathology,* ed 2, St Louis, 2003, Mosby.

Sams WM, Lynch P (eds): *Principles of dermatology,* New York, 1990, Churchill Livingstone.

Sanders MJ: *Mosby's paramedic textbook,* ed 3 (revised reprint), St. Louis, 2007, Mosby.

Seidel HM, Ball JW, Dains JE, et al: *Mosby's guide to physical examination,* ed 6, St Louis, 2006, Mosby.

Stepp CA, Woods M: *Laboratory procedures for medical office personnel,* Philadelphia, 1998, Saunders.

Thibodeau GA, Patton KT: *Anatomy and physiology,* ed 6, St Louis, 2007, Mosby.

Thibodeau GA, Patton KT: *The human body in health and disease,* ed 4, St Louis, 2005, Mosby.

Tyldesley WR: *Colour atlas of orofacial diseases,* ed 2, St Louis, 1991, Mosby [Wolfe].

Young AP: *Kinn's the administrative medical assistant: an applied learning approach,* ed 10, St. Louis, 2007, Saunders.

Zitelli BJ, Davis HW: *Atlas of pediatric physical diagnosis,* ed 45, St Louis, 2002, Mosby.

	Molars		Canine	Incisors				Canine	Molars	
	Maxillary Arch									
I	A	B	C	D	E	F	G	H	I	J
II	55	54	53	52	51	61	62	63	64	65
III	E┘	D┘	C┘	B┘	A┘	└A	└B	└C	└D	└E

III	E┐	D┐	C┐	B┐	A┐	┌A	┌B	┌C	┌D	┌E
II	85	84	83	82	81	71	72	73	74	75
I	T	S	R	Q	P	O	N	M	L	K
	Mandibular Arch									
	Right					Left				

A

I Universal tooth designation system

II International Standards Organization designation system

III Palmer Method

The Universal Tooth Designation System, International Standards Organization Designation System, and Palmer Method for the primary (A) and permanent (B) teeth. (From Bath-Balogh M, Fehrenbach MJ: Illustrated Dental Embryology, Histology, and Anatomy, ed 2, Elsevier Saunders, St. Louis, 2006.)